W9-BYC-745

Assistive Technologies:

Principles and Practice

Assistive Technologies:

Principles and Practice

Fourth Edition

Albert M. Cook, PhD, PE
Professor, Communication Sciences and Disorders
University of Alberta
Edmonton, Alberta
Canada

Janice M. Polgar, PhD, OT Reg. (Ont.), FCAOT
Professor, School of Occupational Therapy
Faculty of Health Sciences
Western University
London, Ontario
Canada

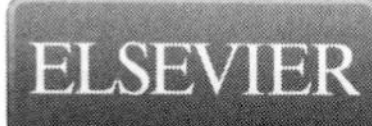

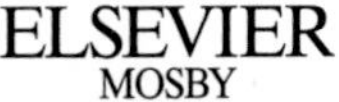

ELSEVIER
MOSBY

3251 Riverport Lane
St. Louis, Missouri 63043

ASSISTIVE TECHNOLOGIES: PRINCIPLES AND PRACTICE, FOURTH EDITION ISBN: 978-0-323-09631-7

Notices

Knowledge and best practice in this field are constantly changing. As new research and experience broaden our understanding, changes in research methods, professional practices, or medical treatment may become necessary.

Practitioners and researchers must always rely on their own experience and knowledge in evaluating and using any information, methods, compounds, or experiments described herein. In using such information or methods they should be mindful of their own safety and the safety of others, including parties for whom they have a professional responsibility.

With respect to any drug or pharmaceutical products identified, readers are advised to check the most current information provided (i) on procedures featured or (ii) by the manufacturer of each product to be administered, to verify the recommended dose or formula, the method and duration of administration, and contraindications. It is the responsibility of practitioners, relying on their own experience and knowledge of their patients, to make diagnoses, to determine dosages and the best treatment for each individual patient, and to take all appropriate safety precautions.

To the fullest extent of the law, neither the Publisher nor the authors, contributors, or editors, assume any liability for any injury and/or damage to persons or property as a matter of products liability, negligence or otherwise, or from any use or operation of any methods, products, instructions, or ideas contained in the material herein.

Library of Congress Cataloging-in-Publication Data

Cook, Albert M., 1943- , author.
[Cook & Hussey's assistive technologies]
Assistive technologies : principles and practice / Albert M. Cook, Janice M. Polgar. -- Fourth edition.
p. ; cm.
Preceded by: Cook & Hussey's assistive technologies : principles and practice / Albert M. Cook and Jan Miller Polgar ; author emerita, Susan M. Hussey. 3rd ed. c2008.
Includes bibliographical references and index.
ISBN 978-0-323-09631-7 (hardcover : alk. paper)
I. Polgar, Jan Miller, author. II. Title.
[DNLM: 1. Self-Help Devices. 2. Disabled Persons--rehabilitation. WB 320]
RM698
617'.033--dc23

2014039969

Content Strategist: Penny Rudolph
Content Development Manager: Jolynn Gower
Publishing Services Manager: Hemamalini Rajendrababu
Project Manager: Kiruthiga Kasthuriswamy
Designer: Margaret Reid

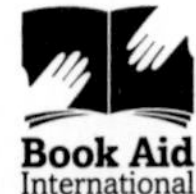

Printed in the United States of America

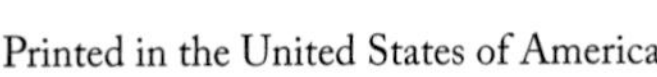

Last digit is the print number: 9 8 7 6 5 4 3 2

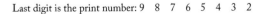

For giving us the reason and the direction for this work,
we dedicate this book to all of our students and to consumers of assistive technologies,
especially Elizabeth Cook, Brian Cook, Charles and Evelyn Miller.

Preface

Writing is no trouble: you just jot down ideas as they occur to you. The jotting is simplicity itself—it is the occurring which is difficult.

Stephen Leacock

Technology use is pervasive in almost everything we do. Technology development occurs at a rapid pace, making it difficult to keep current with the latest devices and software. The field of assistive technology (AT), commonly considered to be technology designed for individuals with some form of impairment, is expanding at a similarly rapid pace. The revisions in this latest edition of *Assistive Technologies: Principles and Practice* reflect the constant and rapid pace of change as well as the changing perspective of what constitutes AT. The book is written to support students in rehabilitation, engineering, and other relevant programs and service providers in the acquisition and application of knowledge that supports the provision of AT services.

Both of us are from North America and primarily understand AT issues from that perspective. However, in the years since the first edition of this textbook was published, we know that it has been used outside of this context and has been translated into multiple languages. Similarly, events such as the signing and ratification of the United Nations Convention on the Rights of Persons with Disabilities by many nations and the publication of the World Health Organization's *Report on Disability* position AT provision and use as global concerns. Consequently, we have attempted to provide a more global perspective to this edition through descriptions of processes that can be applied in different contexts and discussions of issues of appropriate and sustainable AT service delivery. The rapid development of AT applications for mainstream technologies has also made AT more accessible in underresourced countries. These topics are evident throughout the first few chapters discussing the Human Activity Assistive Technology (HAAT) components, ethical issues in AT and AT service delivery, as well as in the discussion of different categories of AT.

Assistive technology service delivery is founded on five principles that are clearly articulated in this book. Earlier editions contained three basic principles describing a person-centered approach, focused on functional outcomes supported by evidence, to which we have added two more reflecting ethical and sustainable service delivery practices. We have attempted to make the application of these principles more explicit throughout this edition in the description of the elements of the HAAT model and the service delivery process and in the discussion of categories of AT. Chapter 1 presents foundational ideas for the subsequent chapters in this edition. In addition to the principles and the HAAT model, definitions of AT, complementary models of health and functioning, legislative aspects, and a summary of some of the research applying the HAAT model are covered in this introductory chapter.

The HAAT model guides assessment and evaluation of AT use by clients. It provides a framework for assessing the usability of technology and guides product research and development. The basic structure of the HAAT model remains unchanged from earlier editions. However, in this edition, we have provided considerably more depth to the discussion of each of the individual elements. Furthermore, we discuss how the elements interact with and influence each other to support a human doing an activity in context using AT. Chapters 2 to 4 expand significantly on the concepts and application of the HAAT model.

Chapter 2 introduces AT, discussing the blurring of technology that is designed specifically for persons with impairments and mainstream technology. Everyone knows about the "explosion" of mainstream technologies. When our previous edition was written, tablet computers did not exist, cell phones were not all that smart, and the Internet and connectivity were just beginning their global expansion. Today these things are old news, but they have dramatically impacted the technology options for people with various disabilities. There are both positive and negative consequences for people with disabilities. Particular attention is paid to the international impact that these developments might have for people with disabilities in underresourced countries.

Chapter 3 discusses the activity, human, and context components of the HAAT model, including how they influence and interact with each other. Here we apply ideas of social and occupational justice to the access to and use of AT, understanding the ability to access affordable, appropriate AT to be a right for all individuals for whom the technology will support engagement in daily activities and participation in their communities. The social and cultural components of the context element of the HAAT model were enhanced to reflect issues of sustainability that affect AT provision and use. AT provision has to make sense for the context in which it will be used: technology that works well in an urban area may be quite useless in remote areas such as the outback of Australia, remote areas of South American or African countries, or the far north of Canada. We sought to bring issues of AT service provision in underresourced areas to the forefront in Chapter 3 and in other relevant sections of this book, recognizing that all we can do is scratch the surface of this topic in a book of this complexity.

As technologies become more and more pervasive and consequently have a greater and greater impact on the ways people with disabilities live and interact with the world around them, ethical considerations become important. Some of these are the direct result of the application of AT in particular ways, for example, monitoring or tracking of individuals with dementia. Other ethical concerns are related to secondary effects of AT application such as the dependence on technology for storage and retrieval of private information. Still other ethical issues arise as a result of particular disabilities such as cognitive limitations. We have added Chapter 4 to explore these ethical issues in some depth.

The application of the HAAT model is made explicit in each of the chapters discussing different types of AT. A consistent format is followed in these chapters to (1) discuss the activities supported by the technology that is the chapter focus; (2) describe the individuals who benefit from use of the technology, as well as impairments that affect the ability to engage in the activity supported by the technology; (3) discuss contextual factors that influence use and service provision; (4) discuss assessment to identify the need for and most appropriate AT; (5) discuss specific technologies; (6) describe outcome evaluation; and finally (7) summarize the research to support the use of the specific technology. In some chapters, the format is followed in the order in which it was just stated; however, in others, the order of these within chapter topics varies to fit the specific topic area.

In Chapter 6, we discuss the various ways in which individuals who have upper extremity motor limitations can access controls for electronic ATs. Chapter 7 describes the major approaches to the design of control interfaces that are used with ATs for computer access, power mobility, communication, and environmental control. In Chapter 8, we focus on the general principles underlying the utilization of mainstream technologies as ATs as well as computer access for individuals with motor disabilities.

Chapter 9 discusses seating and positioning technology, including both the different types of seating and positioning systems and hardware as well as the features of materials and construction techniques. Chapter 10 describes the structure of and means to control manual and powered wheelchairs. It identifies principles to guide recommendation of these technologies and introduces advances in these areas. Chapter 11 has two main components: (1) technology for safe transportation when traveling in a vehicle, either while seated in the vehicle seat or in a wheelchair, and (2) technology for driving.

In Chapter 12, we discuss the use of ATs to replace or augment manipulative ability. This area has seen a huge expansion of available technologies and applications since the previous edition. We include both low- and high-technology devices, but here greater attention is given to the devices that are used to manipulate the environment, such as smart technology as their availability and use become more prevalent. We also discuss advances in robotics that will be available to individuals in their homes, and study and work locations.

Chapter 13 provides an overview of technologies to support individuals with low vision or blindness. The increasing use of mainstream technologies has created a need for visually accessible design in tablets and smartphones for those with low vision and for alternatives to visual access for those who are blind. In Chapter 14, we discuss technologies that aid individuals who are hard of hearing or deaf. Developments in hearing technologies have expanded the options for treatment for both partial and total hearing loss. The area of deaf-blind communication has been significantly impacted by the utilization of mainstream technologies.

Chapter 15 addresses the area of AT applications for individuals who have cognitive disabilities. Again, the use of mainstream technologies with appropriate apps has dramatically expanded the options in this area. The use of monitoring technologies for individuals with dementia has also grown. The area of augmentative communication has perhaps had the greatest impact of mainstream technologies with many new communication applications appearing almost daily. However, in this area, the very practice of assessment and implementation of communication alternatives for those with speech and language difficulties has been impacted by the changing technology landscape. This topic is analyzed in Chapter 16.

It is our hope that individuals familiar with ATs will find something *new* in this text and that readers who are new to this subject will develop *familiarity* with ATs and appreciate their potential.

Acknowledgments

We received tremendous support from two of our doctoral students, both of whom successfully completed and defended their own work during the completion of this edition, Dr. Liliana Alvarez and Dr. Laura Titus. Lili has experience in both clinical practice of occupational therapy in Colombia and as a professor at Rossairo University in Bogota, where she taught assistive technologies (ATs) using the previous edition of this text. The breadth of her background was valuable in helping us understand the global perspective of AT application, and her assistance in finding and reviewing the current research literature in AT enriched the content of the text. Laura is an experienced clinician whose own research explores why and how individuals use power tilt on wheelchairs in their daily lives. She was always ready for a discussion about seating and mobility technologies, pointing out what should and should not be included, identifying key resources, and providing feedback on drafts of the seating and mobility chapters. When pictures were needed, she arranged to have devices available so these pictures could be taken. Laura's support, knowledge, and friendship made the writing of seating and mobility chapters easier and their content stronger.

The contributions of others who supported the writing of this edition are also acknowledged and appreciated. Linda Norton, from Shopper's Home Health and a doctoral student at Western University, was a valuable resource on the topic of wound prevention and pressure redistribution technologies. Dave Farr of Motion Specialties and Andrew Smith of Thames Valley Children's Centre in London Ontario opened up their stock room and clinic to provide access to seating and mobility technologies for pictures. Drs. Alex Mihailidis, University of Toronto; Ian Mitchell, University of British Columbia; and Pooja Viswanathan, University of Toronto provided current information on smart wheelchair technologies.

Work of this magnitude does not happen in isolation. We were privileged to work with Jolynn Gower, our editor from Elsevier, who guided us through the publication process. Jolynn's support was invaluable as she offered guidance on various resources, helped us make decisions, and was always understanding when life circumstances intervened and deadlines had to be changed.

Albert M. Cook
Janice M. Polgar

Jan Polgar and I have collaborated on both the third and fourth editions of this book and *Essentials of Assistive Technology*. The fact that we have continued to find ways to work together speaks to the value I have for Jan as a collaborator. Collaboration is always challenging and often produces unexpected outcomes, especially when it occurs by phone and email rather than face to face. Jan has made that collaboration easy and productive. She is thoughtful, critical, and highly productive, all qualities that contribute to quality outcomes. An added bonus—that got us through those impossible deadlines—is her sense of humor and her consistently positive attitude. Working with Jan has been a delight from start to finish. Always thoughtful, always critical, and most important always kind, she has made many major improvements to the parts that I wrote and shown her typical insight and care in the parts she led. Thank you, Jan, for all of the effort and for the quality product that resulted.

I cannot adequately express the appreciation I have for the continuing support, love, and understanding of my wife, Nancy, and the support of my daughters, Barbara and Jennifer. Finally, my son, Brian, continues to inspire me to understand the ways in which technology can ameliorate the problems faced by individuals who have disabilities.

Albert M. Cook

Again, it has been an absolute pleasure to write a book with Al Cook. This book is the third collaboration between Al and me. As we begin each revision, we spend considerable time discussing changes to the content and the organization of the book. Our conversations with this revision were particularly energizing as we discussed and debated the changes in theory, practice, and technology that influenced how we modified the content and organization of this book. Issues of global provision of AT, blurring of mainstream and AT, and ethics are more prominent in this edition. The ideas discussed are the results of much lively discussion and debate.

Anyone who has engaged in and completed a project that spans a significant length of time knows the ebb and flow of enthusiasm for the work involved. Al's presence as my coauthor was most welcome during those times in the past couple of years when my energy for writing flagged. Al is a generous man. Most appreciated are his generosity of time and his unending support. When work and personal issues competed for my time for writing, Al stepped in, taking on additional responsibilities. He is generous with his knowledge and experience; as the senior author of this book, he frequently guided me through the pragmatic aspects of writing a book. He was always generous with his feedback—constructive comments, of course. I continue to feel fortunate that Al asked me to come on board as a coauthor several years ago and value the friendship that has coalesced over those years.

My family continues to make my life meaningful and full. As my parents, Charles and Evelyn Miller, age and become users of AT themselves, the importance of focusing on the person using the technology is reinforced. I value the ongoing love and support of my husband Roger and my children Andrea and Alex, both of whom completed secondary school and moved on to university during this project. Our lively dinner debates, adventures, and many occasions of laughter are the great joys of my life.

Janice M. Polgar

Contents

CHAPTER 1

Principles of Assistive Technology: Introducing the Human Activity Assistive Technology Model

CHAPTER OUTLINE

LEARNING OBJECTIVES

On completing this chapter, you will be able to do the following:

1. Define assistive technology (AT).
2. Describe key principles of AT service delivery.
3. Describe contributions of existing ecological models of health to the conceptualization of the Human Activity Assistive Technology (HAAT) model.
4. Describe the purpose of the HAAT model.
5. Describe the activity, human, context, and AT components of the HAAT model.
6. Describe four applications of the HAAT model for AT research and clinical applications.

KEY TERMS

Activity
Activity Output
Assessment
Assistive Technology
Assistive Technology Service
Beneficence
Context
Enabler
Ecological Models
Environmental Interface
Evidence Informed
Ethics
High Technology
Human
Human Rights
Human Technology Interface
Low Technology
Mainstream Technology
Nonmaleficence
Outcome Evaluation
Processor
Social Justice
Usability

INTRODUCTION

Contextual Background of the Book

Disability is seen as a socially constructed phenomenon that results from barriers that are present in the environment. This view of disability locates it within the environment rather than within the person. The World Health Organization's (WHO's) International Classification of Functioning, Disability and Impairment (ICF) views disability as the result of an interaction between the person and his environment. Viewed this way, disability is possible in everyone's experience (Bickenbach et al., 1999).

The worldwide prevalence of disability is difficult to estimate because of challenges of definition of cohesive definitions of disability and technical aspects of data collection. However, the WHO *Report on Disability* (2011) estimates that approximately 720 million people worldwide experience some form of disability (WHO, 2011, p. 27). Furthermore, approximately 190 million (or 3.8% of the world's population) experience "severe disability" that limits their ability to participate in daily activities.

People with disabilities are much more likely to live in countries that are considered to be of low or middle income. Estimates suggest that 89% of people with vision impairment, 76% with hearing impairment, and 92% of those with a disability resulting from an intentional or unintentional injury live in a low- or middle-income country (Samant, Matter, & Harris, 2012, p. 1). Similarly, women, older adults, and people living in poverty have a greater prevalence of disability (WHO, 2011).

Disability has significant consequences on an individual's life. Persons with a disability have a greater likelihood of being under- or unemployed; they and their families are more likely to have a lower socioeconomic status; they experience poorer health; they are less likely to receive an education; and they experience more social isolation, less community participation, and less safety and security (they are more likely to experience physical, mental, or financial abuse).

Assistive technology (AT) is one of many opportunities that are necessary to reduce the disabling influence of many environments. Technology is a ubiquitous part of our everyday lives, which for the most part, makes our daily tasks simpler to do. This book focuses on the different aspects of using technology to meet the needs of individuals with a variety of disabilities. We will present a model that guides service delivery, **outcome evaluation**, and research and development of AT.

CONSTRUCTS OF DISABILITY IN KEY DOCUMENTS

The United Nations (UN) Convention on the Rights of Persons with Disabilities (CRPD) opens with a statement that recognizes the "inherent dignity and worth and the equal and inalienable **rights** of all members of the human family as the foundation of freedom, justice, and peace in the world" (UN, 2007, p. 1). It recognizes that disability occurs at the intersection of the person and the **context** in which they live and consequently, that the extent of disability is different for individuals living in different contexts. This document describes rights of persons with disabilities, with the explicit expectation that member states who are signatories to the document will enact legislation, regulations, and other measures to ensure these rights for their citizens.

The CRPD enshrines the rights of persons with disabilities to be treated as equals before the law and to be "entitled without any discrimination to the equal protection and equal benefit of the law." Persons with disabilities have the right to be recognized as "persons before the law" (UN CRPD, p. 8). In other words, the presence of a disability does not nullify the state's recognition that the individual is entitled to the full benefits and responsibilities of citizenship. This convention prevents a member state from declaring a person with a disability to be a nonperson, which means he or she is not entitled to vote, own property, participate in civic governance, or enter into a legal contract. If you recall the limitations on the rights of women before the suffragette movements of the early 1900s, you will better understand the intent of this particular article of the CRPD.

Women and children with disabilities are given particular attention given their vulnerability to discrimination and abuse because of gender or age.

Beyond rights and protections afforded to all global citizens, the CPRD identifies several that are specific to persons with disabilities (Table 1-1) and describes the articles that are relevant to AT use, service delivery, and research and development.

Assistive technology is mentioned specifically in many of the sections of this convention, calling for research and development of all types of AT, requiring many other forms of technology (information and communication technology in particular) to be accessible in terms of use, availability, and information; promotion of AT accessibility; and provision of information about AT in accessible formats. It further calls for education of professionals to support all aspects of AT service delivery (UN, 2007).

DEFINITIONS OF ASSISTIVE TECHNOLOGY

Formal Definitions

Definitions allow us to frame the construct of interest and convey to others what we include and exclude in the use of a term. In a legislative or policy context, definitions delimit the scope of the law or policy, influencing how each is interpreted and applied. For example, in jurisdictions where AT funding is supported through government, a definition is used to determine what constitutes an assistive device that is eligible for funding versus one that is not. Definitions outside of this context can also help to conceptualize the term and understand the perspective of the individual or collective that conceived the definition.

Two formal definitions of AT, which are commonly used, come from the United States legislation The Assistive Technology Act of 1998, as amended (2004) and from the WHO. The US legislation defines AT as: "Any item, piece of equipment or product system whether acquired commercially off the shelf, modified, or customized that is used to increase, maintain or improve functional capabilities of individuals with disabilities."

Similarly, the WHO (2001) defines AT as "any product, instrument, equipment, or technology adapted or specially designed for improving functioning of a disabled person." These two definitions both focus exclusively on the technology and limit it to a tangible object that is usable by a person with a disability. The US definition is more inclusive of mainstream technologies than the WHO version.

TABLE 1-1 Articles of the United Nations Convention on the Rights of Persons with Disabilities Relevant to Assistive Technology

Article Number	Article Title	Relevance to Assistive Technology
4	General Obligations	Articulates agreement to undertake research and development of assistive technologies, with emphasis on affordable devices Agreement to provide information about AT and related services and supports in an accessible format
9	Accessibility	In support of full participation by all, member countries agree to provide equitable access to transportation, information (and information communication technology), public buildings, and services.
19	Living independently and being included in the community	Persons with disabilities have the right to choose where they live in the community and to participate fully in necessary and chosen life activities.
20	Personal mobility	Requires provision of personal mobility choices, including mode of mobility and time, with an affordable cost Quality mobility aids will be accessible and affordable. Persons with disabilities will receive training in the use of mobility aids. Requires production of mobility aids to consider the full range of mobility requirements of persons with disabilities
21	Freedom of expression and opinion and access to information	Persons with disabilities have the same rights to express their ideas and opinions as others, in a manner of their choice. Information will be provided in accessible formats. Use of alternate forms of communication (e.g., Braille, sign language, alternative and augmentative communication) is required for all official interactions. Private enterprise will be encouraged to similarly use these alternate forms of communication; mass media, including the Internet, is encouraged to use and accept alternate access and forms of communication. Sign language is used and promoted.
24	Education	Persons with disabilities have equal access to an education. Reasonable accommodation to educational needs of persons with disabilities is made, including individualized programs as required.
25	Health	Persons with disabilities have the right to the "highest attainable standard of health" (p. 14).
26	Habilitation and rehabilitation	Member states will support habilitation and rehabilitation with the desired outcome of achievement and maintenance of maximal functional independence. Availability, knowledge, and use of AT will be supported.
27	Work and employment	Persons with disabilities have the right to equal access to gainful employment of their own choice. Reasonable accommodation of needs of the person with disability is required in the workplace.
29	Participation in political and public life	Ensures accessibility of location and means to enable persons with disabilities to exercise their right to participate in political activities, including their right to vote Active promotion of an environment that enables full participation in community activities of choice
30	Participation in cultural life, recreation, leisure, and sports	Accessible formats, materials, and environments are required to support the participation of persons with disabilities in all aspects of cultural life, recreation, leisure, and sports.

AT, Assistive technology.
From United Nations: *Convention on the rights of persons with disabilities (CRPD)*, Resolution 61/106, New York: United Nations, 2007. Available from: www.un.org/disabilities/convention/conventionfull.shtml.

Informal Definitions

Hersh and Johnson (2008a) argue that these formal definitions link AT too tightly to a medical model, which highlights the use of AT to overcome limitations and improve function for the individual. The definitions cited above, although useful in some contexts, also limit our concept of AT to simply the technology. Hersh and Johnson propose a definition of AT that is inclusive of products, environmental modifications, services, and processes that enable access to and use of these products, specifically by persons with disabilities and older adults (2008a). They further describe the use of AT to assist users to overcome infrastructure barriers to enable full societal participation and to accomplish activities safely and easily.

This broader understanding of AT is congruent with the position we take of AT. We understand AT as inclusive of mainstream technologies and those developed specifically for persons with some form of impairment. The importance of services and infrastructure is highlighted in this book; it is not simply the provision of a device; the opportunity to use it for desired occupations, across multiple environments, and without prejudice is critical. Throughout this book, we focus on activities broadly categorized as communication, cognitive, mobility, and manipulation and the technologies that enable them. However, we do so by incorporating mainstream and specialized technologies and by presenting the evidence that supports their effectiveness in enabling users to engage in the political, social, and economic occupations of their communities.

Differentiating Assistive Technology from Other Technologies

Discussions and writings about participation and function of individuals with disabilities include a vast array of terms that include constructs of technology. Some of these include rehabilitation technologies, educational technologies, accessible and universal design. The latter two will be discussed in more detail in Chapter 2 where we engage in a more detailed discussion of the AT component of the Human Activity Assistive Technology model (see later in this chapter for an overview of this model). Sanford (2012) adds a dimension to the conceptualization of AT that helps differentiate it within the concepts of accessible and universal designs. He describes AT as "individualized and usually follows the person" (Sanford, 2012, p. 55) in contrast to designs that make environments more accessible to individuals with a variety of abilities such as automatic door openers and ramps that stay fixed in a location and are used by many users who come to that particular location.

We do not include rehabilitation or educational technologies in this book, although some of the devices that we discuss do have application in a rehabilitation or educational setting. We understand rehabilitation technologies to be devices that have a primary use in a clinical setting, such as parallel bars, overhead slings, and tilt tables, and that are primarily used for habilitation or rehabilitation purposes. Educational technologies are those that make educational materials more accessible, such as software programs that provide educational curricula in some alternative, accessible format. Many of the devices that promote communication, positioning, and computer access; support cognitive activities; and augment hearing and vision assist the learner to engage with these educational technologies with the difference being the emphasis on enabling participation versus achieving specific education goals.

Summary

Formal definitions of AT are used by different groups to delimit what constitutes AT for the purposes of funding and regulation of requirements to make environments and services accessible to individuals with a broad range of disabilities. Their focus is on the promotion of function of an individual with a disability. Informal definitions add context to the formal definitions and are inclusive of social and other environmental dimensions that affect AT design, use, and implementation. Although both formal and informal definitions are inclusive of **mainstream technology**, it is more apparent in the informal definition presented. This book discusses both mainstream technology and that designed specifically for persons with disabilities, describing different types of technology, and a service delivery process, with a focus on how technology use enables full participation in desired activities.

PRINCIPLES OF ASSISTIVE TECHNOLOGY SERVICE DELIVERY

Assistive technology is presented in this book primarily from the perspective of the application of a clinical process to identify the need for AT, determining the most appropriate device(s), obtaining the device and then providing follow-up and outcome evaluation to ensure the user is able to use the device. Service delivery is formally defined as "any service that directly assists an individual with a disability in the selection, acquisition, or use of an assistive technology (AT) device" (118 STAT. 1170).

We propose several principles that foreground **AT service delivery**: (1) the process is **person centered,** not AT centered, (2) the outcome is enablement of participation in desired activities, (3) an **evidence-informed** process is used for service delivery, (4) AT service delivery is provided in an ethical manner, and (5) AT services are provided in a sustainable manner. These principles are introduced here, explored in greater detail in chapters 4 and 5, and applied in subsequent chapters that discuss specific categories of AT. They should be interpreted from the context within which AT services are provided.

Person Centered, Not Assistive Technology Centered

The provision and development of AT are not about fitting the person to the technology. Rather, they are about using a process with the outcome of meeting the needs of the user when engaging in relevant activities across necessary contexts.

On the product development side, technology that is developed without the input of consumers throughout the design process or without knowledge of how the technology will be used is less likely to be adopted for its intended purpose. The resulting technology may be designed to meet a need that does not exist for the intended user.

On the service delivery side, AT that is recommended or prescribed without input from the user and relevant others ends up abandoned or not used to its full potential. One participant in a project that collected stories of individuals with spinal cord injuries and their use of AT illustrated this point well. He described his abandonment of complex technology that did not provide him with any perceived advantage over simpler devices. Furthermore, the necessary devices were not recommended before returning to live at home; some devices were not needed, and others that were useful had not been acquired (SCIPILOT, nd). More will be said about device discontinuance in a later chapter. There are many reasons stated for device discontinuance; a large proportion of them are the result of a process that does not adequately involve users of AT.

Focus Is on the Functional Outcome and Participation

Similar to the ideas expressed in the first principle, this second principle indicates that what a person does with a device is important rather than simply providing access to the device. Our conceptualization of AT includes the activities in which the user engages. It is important to understand what a person wants and needs and is expected to do throughout the AT service delivery process. More important, though, is the recognition that simply noting whether a person is able to use a device for a particular function is insufficient.

It is more important to understand how the person is using the device and whether it is used in a manner of her choosing. For example, an alternative and augmentative communication device can support the user's ability to engage in a conversation (i.e., the function of conversation is supported by the device). However, it is equally important to understand whether the device supports the user's vocabulary, inflection, and pace of speech. The idea here is that the device becomes an extension of the person for some users (i.e., it conveys part of their image). When its use contributes to an undesired self-image, it is not used to the full advantage. It is not sufficient for the device to enable function; it must do so in a manner that supports how the user wants to engage in that function. This concept is discussed in more detail in Chapter 3.

Evidence-Informed Process

Use of an **evidence-informed** process benefits the user of AT through ensuring that elements of AT service comprehensively include steps to identify technology that is most appropriate for the user; to provide necessary training and support for initial and ongoing use of the technology; and to evaluate adequately the outcome of the technology, not only for the individual user but for aggregate groups as well. Evidence may come from data collected systematically through the service delivery process and through research studies investigating a wide range of questions surrounding AT. The different types of evidence and research that support them are discussed in Chapter 5.

Amassing aggregate data concerning different aspects of the AT service delivery process is key to building the evidence base. Evidence is present to support the AT assessment and recommendation processes, training, ongoing evaluation, and functional outcomes. This evidence is presented throughout this book for different AT applications. As will be seen and as professionals experienced in AT are aware, more research is necessary to support this area. Funders frequently require evidence that supports specific outcomes of AT use before they will support the purchase of AT.

Ethical Process

An ethical process includes multiple perspectives: professional or clinical code of ethics along with embodying constructs of beneficience and nonmaleficence and broader philosophical and ethical worldviews that speak to means of creating an inclusive society that enables meaningful engagement in community participation for all. Key ideas that form the background for ethical AT service delivery are introduced briefly here. We expand on these ideas in Chapter 4.

Professional and Clinical Code of Ethics

Many reading this book are engineering or health care professionals or students whose practice is guided by a formal code of **ethics**. A review of several different codes of ethics (e.g., from Rehabilitation Engineering and Assistive Technology Society of North America [RESNA], Canadian Association of Occupational Therapists, American Physical Therapy Association, World Confederation of Physical Therapy, and Swedish Association of Occupational Therapists) uncovered many commonalities across the various codes. Box 1-1 shows the RESNA Code of Ethics.

The principles of **beneficence** (do only good) and **nonmaleficence** (do no harm) are prominent in these professional codes. These principles are translated into practice through actions that embody professional integrity, accountability, and maintenance of continuing competence and professional standards.

They explicitly describe the client/patient–clinician/provider relationship. Simply stated, this relationship is guided by respect for the welfare, rights, and self-determination of the client. In practice, the clinician recognizes the client's autonomy and right to be fully engaged in the clinical or service delivery process. The clinician or service provider acts in a trustworthy and truthful manner, maintaining client confidentiality. These codes assert the balance between client–service provider roles while concurrently declaring the responsibilities for providing competent, honest, and respectful service.

BOX 1-1 RESNA Code of Ethics

RESNA is an interdisciplinary association for the advancement of rehabilitation and assistive technology. It adheres to and promotes the highest standards of ethical conduct. Its members:

- Hold paramount the welfare of persons served professionally.
- Practice only in their area(s) of competence and maintain high standards.
- Maintain the confidentiality of privileged information.
- Engage in no conduct that constitutes as a conflict of interest or that adversely reflects on the profession.
- Seek deserved and reasonable remuneration for services.
- Inform and educate the public on rehabilitation and assistive technology and its applications.
- Issue public statements in an objective and truthful manner.
- Comply with the laws and policies that guide the profession.

Modified from Summary of RESNA Code of Ethics. Available from: http://resna.org/certification/RESNA_Code_of_Ethics.pdf

RESNA, Rehabilitation Engineering and Assistive Technology Society of North America.

Some codes *suggest* that practice be based on principles of **social justice**, which is described in more detail in the following sections. Social justice in this context refers to accessibility of AT services for all who require it. The code of ethics of the American Occupational Therapy Association (AOTA, 2010) specifically mentions that practice is guided by principles of distributive justice (see later discussion); the Philippine Physical Therapy Association states that physical therapy services will be accessible to all (PPTA, 2009).

Social Justice

John Rawls expressed foundational principles of social justice that inform our discussion. Social justice concepts were initially framed from an economic perspective, referring to equitable access to rights and resources (e.g., income and material goods) within society (Rawls, 1999). Capability theory advances Rawls' ideas to further suggest that all individuals have equal access to basic rights and freedom of choice (Nussbaum, 2011; Sen, 2009).

Applying these ideas to persons with disabilities (i.e., persons who use AT in their daily lives) recognizes the economic disadvantage they experience through fewer opportunities to participate in income-generating activities and the concomitant reductions in their incomes because of the greater expenses incurred because of the disability. Lack of access to AT keeps some people with disabilities in poverty (Samant et al., 2012). Specifically, the lack of availability of or access to AT services and technology limits the ability of a person with a disability to engage in community occupations, in particular, it limits his or her ability to participate in economic activities that in turn afford sufficient resources to support themselves or their families (Samant et al., 2012; WHO, 2011). For example, a person who has difficulty communicating with unfamiliar others, but who could do so with the use of an augmentative and alternative communication (AAC) device is barred from employment and other civic activities (among other things) when access to such a device is not available. In this situation, societal elements are the limiting factor, restricting the individual's full participation in his community and beyond.

A second source of inequity is seen in a situation in which two people with the same level of income, one with a disability (or who supports a family member with a disability) and one without, will have very different incomes when the costs associated with the disability are taken into account (Samant et al., 2012; WHO, 2011). Persons with disabilities have many expenses that those without disabilities do not encounter, such as personal assistant costs; higher transportation costs; home modification costs; and, of course, the cost of AT, which is significant. Globally, the purchase of these devices is inconsistently supported, with the result that a person or family that must obtain AT will have less disposable income than someone without a disability with the same level of income who does not need to purchase AT.

A formal approach to social justice is seen in legislation such as the Americans with Disabilities Act of 1990 that attempts to legislate formal mechanisms to remove barriers to full participation in society for individuals with disabilities (Danermark & Gellerstedt, 2004). Similarly, the UN CRPD identifies basic rights that all member countries must support for their citizens and explicitly states that AT must be accessible regardless of gender, age, or impairment. Throughout this book, we identify and apply formal social justice mechanisms as they relate to AT service delivery. In Chapter 3, we identify key pieces of legislation that aim to legislate accessibility for persons with disabilities and discuss the aspects of the legislation (e.g., the definition of disability and who is eligible for consideration under the legislation) that need to be identified and applied in clinical practice. When relevant, we discuss these issues as they relate to individual categories of AT.

Distributive Justice

Distributive justice is a second theory of social justice. This theory is premised on the idea that inequities occur at the intersection of the person with a disability and the context in which he or she lives. One way of reducing the influence of these inequities is more equitable distribution of resources, which include financial resources as well as opportunities for education, employment, and health and access to infrastructure that supports full social participation. Distributive justice advocates for a redistribution of resources to account for this inequity. It is based on principles "designed to guide the allocation of the benefits and burdens of economic activity" (Cook, 2009, p. 10).

Assistive Technology Services Are Provided in a Sustainable Manner

In general, **sustainability** means providing AT products and services in a manner that ensures that people who need them have access in a timely and continuing manner. This basic idea is enacted somewhat differently in well-resourced and underresourced economies. Many well-resourced countries face a population shift that is well known; their populations are aging, with the largest proportional increase seen in the "old-old" (i.e., persons older than age 75 years). These individuals experience a greater incidence of disability, including multiple disabilities, and account for the largest proportion of health care spending. The cost of health care is significant in developing countries to the point that current systems are not sustainable.

Some of the health care dollars in these countries are used to support the cost of selected AT products and services associated with **assessment** of and training in the use of AT. Clinicians contribute to sustainability by balancing the rights and needs of clients with the reality of limited health care dollars. This statement does not mean not advocating for the needs of clients; rather, it means use of an evidence-informed process to identify AT that will meet the client's needs, including the client in this process, to ensure that devices obtained are used (i.e., do not end up in a closet, drawer, or the garage) and are used to their maximal potential.

In underresourced economies, sustainability often means development and establishment of AT services. Products and services that are readily available in developed countries may not be present in these emerging economies, generally because of cost, legislation, lack of infrastructure, and other resource limitations (Samant et al., 2012). Establishment of AT services and an AT industry means working with local manufacturers, using local materials, and designing products that are functional in the local context (Borg, Lindstrom, & Larson, 2011, Owen & Simonds, 2010; Samant et al., 2012). It also means providing technology that can be maintained and repaired using local knowledge, technology, and materials (Owen & Simonds, 2010). Furthermore, it means provision of products and services that are affordable by persons with disabilities (WHO, 2011).

THE HUMAN ACTIVITY ASSISTIVE TECHNOLOGY MODEL

Cook and Hussey (1995) introduced the Human Activity Assistive Technology (HAAT) model in the first edition of *Assistive Technology: Principles and Practices* (1995). The model describes someone (**human**) doing something (**activity**) in a context using AT. This simplistic explanation of the HAAT model is deliberately worded to demonstrate where AT fits in the model. The emphasis of the model is on the person engaged in an activity within chosen environments. Consequently, any application of the model starts with someone doing something in context and then introduces the AT.

This order prevents the AT from assuming prime importance with the result that the person adapts to the technology rather than the technology meeting the needs of the person. The model has been used to development of AT, research, and assessment involving the initial selection of AT and ongoing evaluation of the outcome of its use. Figure 1-1 illustrates this model.

The HAAT model is introduced briefly in this chapter. Chapter 2 provides foundational ideas related to AT. Chapter 3 discusses the activity, human, and context elements in greater detail as well as the interactions among all of these elements. The model is applied to specific categories of AT in the middle section of the book.

Foundational Concepts

The HAAT model shares many features of other models that integrate activity (occupation), the person, and the environment. It has evolved in parallel with influential models such as the WHO's ICF (WHO, 2001), Canadian Model of Occupational Performance and Enablement (CMOP-E) (Townsend & Polatajko, 2002, 2013), and Person-Environment-Occupational Performance (PEOP) model (Baum & Christiansen, 2005). These related models inform the different elements that comprise the HAAT model, which differs from these other models through its explicit consideration of AT.

International Classification of Functioning, Disability, and Health

The WHO's ICF (WHO, 2001) is a well-recognized and frequently applied model that classifies components of body structures and functions, activities and participation, and the environment in terms of their influence on health. Four aims are stated for the ICF, two of which have relevance to our discussion: to provide a basis for research on health and its determinants and to establish a common language that will foster effective communication across different users (WHO). Relevant components of the ICF are described in greater detail in subsequent chapters that discuss the components of the HAAT model.

The WHO definition of AT was described earlier in this chapter. AT is located in the environment component of the ICF, which can pose a challenge when thinking about and providing AT. Specifically, AT is primarily located in Chapter 1 of the ICF, "Products and Technology of the Environmental Factor." AT for certain participation contexts, such as education, is also identified. The ICF describes environmental factors as external to the person. The challenging aspect of this concept when considering AT is that although AT is certainly external to the user, it is much more personal than other elements of the environment, such as an elevator that is adapted to meet the needs of individuals with mobility or vision impairments. AT is commonly recommended for a specific person who brings the technology with him or her to different situations. Similar to other environmental elements, AT is designed and modified to suit the needs of the person. However, the personal nature of most devices requires the consideration of the person using a certain device when thinking about activities and participation within and across environments.

Ecological Models in Occupational Therapy

Models that describe the relationships among the person, the environment, and occupation inform the practice of occupational therapy. Two particularly influential models are the CMOP-E (Townsend & Polatajko, 2002, 2013) and the Person-Environment-Occupation-Performance (PEOP) model (Baum & Christiansen, 2005). The CMOP-E does not explicitly identify AT; however, the PEOP, which is based on the ICF, locates AT within the environmental component.

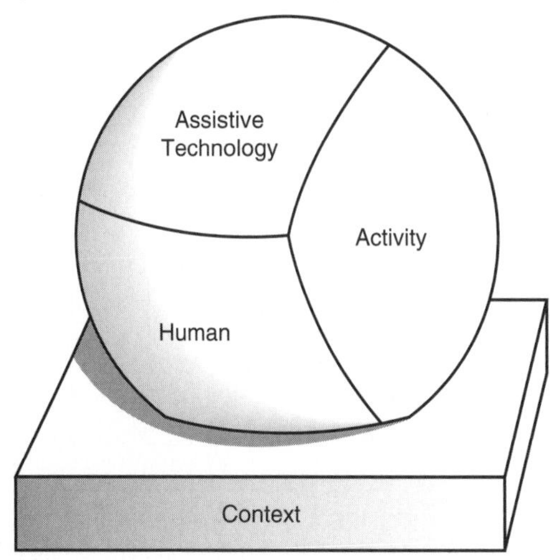

FIGURE 1-1 The Human Activity Assistive Technology model.

Similar to the HAAT model, the CMOP-E and PEOP are **ecological models**; specifically, they consider the influence of the interaction of a number of elements on occupational performance, participation, health, quality of life, and well-being. It is the transactional nature of the person, environment, and occupation that results in the occupational performance outcome. Figure 1-2 demonstrates a comparison of the main components and subcomponents of each of these models.

In addition to the central constructs of person, environment, and occupation, these models share other ideas. Both articulate notions of environmental enablers and barriers, which are features of the environment that facilitate occupation or limit it. Occupation, or activity, is seen as the bridge between the person and environment, the means by which the person is part of the world. They help guide clinical practice by articulating a practice process. The CMOP-E articulates different roles the clinician plays in the client–therapist relationship (Townsend & Polatajko, 2002, 2013). The PEOP articulates a top-down approach that guides the intervention process of enabling occupational performance and participation (Baum & Christiansen, 2005). Although both are linked to the ICF, the link is stronger for the PEOP.

Models such as the PEOP and the CMOP-E influence our recent articulations of the HAAT model by informing the notion of activity to move beyond the classification to incorporate the complexity of the phenomenon of occupation, which helps us understand the place of AT in the performance of occupation and the enablement of participation. They require us to think not just about how the AT supplements the performance of an activity (e.g., how a calendar application can supplement memory by reminding the user of upcoming events) but to also consider how the user views the occupation and the influence of the different aspects of the environment (or context using HAAT terminology). Similar to the ICF, these models move the emphasis away from the technology and back to the person doing something in a context, which is the essence of the HAAT model.

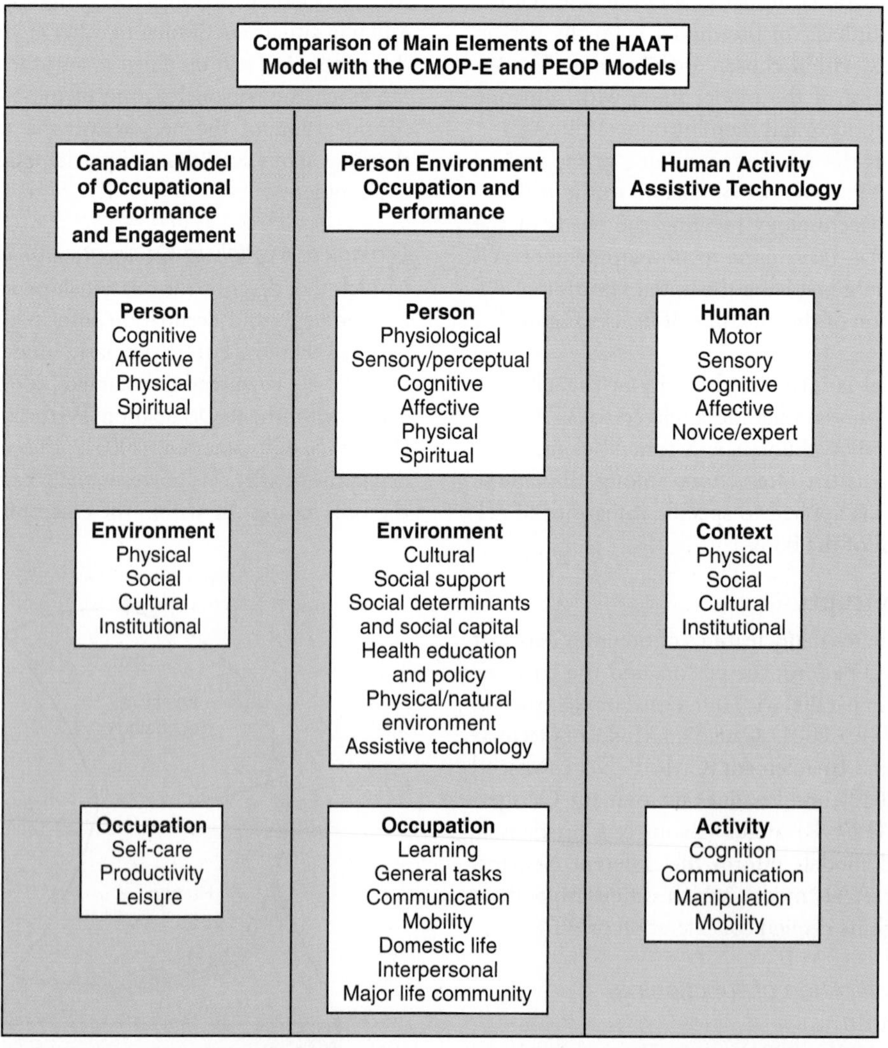

FIGURE 1-2 Comparison of the Canadian Model of Occupational Performance and Enablement (CMOP-E), Person-Environment-Occupational Performance (PEOP), and Human Activity Assistive Technology (HAAT) models.

The HAAT model is built on four components: the activity, the human, the AT, and the context. The model is conceptualized as transactional in nature to capture the experience of the individual as he or she engages in activities. This transactional nature broadens our understanding of a person's participation as enabled by AT through the recognition of the dynamic nature of the person's experience in a situation as he or she interacts with other people and nonhuman aspects of the context. The current situation is influenced by past experiences and the individual's understanding of the experience in the present, a concept labeled "situated knowledge" by Cutchin (2008).

Activity

Activities are described in the ICF as the execution of tasks, which along with the ICF notion of participation (*involvement in a life situation*) is congruent with the construct of occupation. The ICF and occupational therapy models such as the CMOP-E and the PEOP model are useful guides here to identify the activities in which a person who uses AT wants or needs to complete. Commonly, activities of daily living are separated into self-care, productivity (work, volunteer activities, or education), and leisure, although this categorization scheme has been recently challenged as being too limiting. It also suggests that activities are separate in time, space, and place. Many of us experience the need to perform multiple tasks concurrently (as I write this section, I am also providing assistance to my son as he prepares to leave for university), suggesting that this notion of separation is artificial, something that allows us to discuss activity conveniently. Although we will discuss different categories of activities to aid understanding of the concepts and the application to AT, it is understood that the person may engage in multiple activities concurrently; that engagement in activity is dynamic, with participation flowing among different activities.

It is important to understand the activity to be supported, the activity in which the person wants or needs to engage. The activity component of the HAAT model assists the understanding of the tasks in which the user of AT participates. It guides product research and development, selection of AT, identification of functional outcomes to evaluate AT use, and definition of the research question. It helps us think about what the user does with the AT, bearing in mind that sometimes the doing is not observable.

The activity component also includes temporal aspects of length and frequency of participation in activity (e.g., multiple times a day, weekly, monthly, seasonally). Consideration is given to whether engagement in this activity involves other people. Knowledge of where the activity occurs is necessary to determine the contextual influences on activity performance and the effect on use of AT across these contexts, as well as issues affecting transportation of the device as required.

Human

The human component includes the user's abilities in motor, sensory, cognitive, and affective areas. Analysis of performance in sensory, motor, cognitive, and affective areas is part of initial and ongoing assessment and outcome evaluation. Chapter 3 describes these areas in more detail. Understanding of the human's function in these foundational areas is necessary to guide the recommendation of effective AT and to develop training programs. Assessment here also includes acknowledgement of whether change in ability is expected to occur (i.e., improvement through developmental changes or recovery or decline through age-related changes or due to the nature of a progressive condition). Function of these basis elements is interpreted in terms of their ability to support performance of desired and necessary occupations, enabled through the use of AT.

Beyond knowledge of body function, an understanding of the person's roles in life and her experience with technology, motivation, and use of a lifespan perspective are important aspects of the human component of the HAAT model. Roles involve the combination of many activities across different contexts and contribute to a person's identity. Common roles include parent, worker, student, and consumer. Motivation is an important aspect of the human and is understood from two perspectives, motivation to return to performance of specific activities and motivation to use AT.

A lifespan perspective directs the clinician to consider the developmental aspects of the human. A young child's skills and abilities are developing, necessitating his reliance on his parents to support activity performance and AT use. An older adult with age-related functional losses will have different needs for AT design and support. In addition, the use of AT may be perceived as a visible sign of loss related to aging.

The concepts of novice and expert technology user influence the balance between clinician and user input into the assessment and training processes. A novice user relies more on the clinician for information because of her lack of knowledge and experience. In contrast, an experienced user knows what she wants the technology to do and is more active in driving the AT acquisition process.

Context

The HAAT model uses the term **context** in contrast to many other models that use the term *environment*. When the model was first developed, the term *environment* was perceived to be too limiting, with the potential to be interpreted as meaning the physical environment. The notion of context was considered to be more inclusive, including social and cultural contexts, and dynamic, thus a better fit with a model used to guide AT applications.

Understanding of mechanisms of disability has shifted in the past decades, although not fully. The medical model of disability locates the "problem" in the individual, as some impairment that needs to be fixed. Intervention that focuses solely on making changes to the individual follows a medical model. Although these interventions are certainly useful and often necessary, use of the medical model exclusively limits recognition of other causes of impairment that lie outside of the individual's body structures and function (Whalley Hammel 2006; McColl & Jongbloed, 2006).

A social model of disability moves the location of the disability out of the person and into social structures. It recognizes that social perceptions, attitudes, institutions, and policies all contribute to the creation of disability. Furthermore, disability creation results from a dynamic combination of personal characteristics, physical settings, and cultural norms that is "situational and interactive" (Fougeyrollas & Gray, 1998). These situations lead to exclusionary practices that limit the activity and community participation of individuals on the basis of their impairments. The context presents physical, attitudinal, cultural, infrastructure, and institutional barriers that exclude persons with disabilities from full participation in society.

The HAAT model reflects the social model of disability by making the contextual aspects of AT design, service delivery, and use explicit and prominent. Four contextual components are included: (1) physical context, including natural and built surroundings and physical parameters; (2) social context (with peers, with strangers); (3) cultural context; and (4) the institutional context, including formal legal, legislative acts, and regulations; policies, practice, and procedures at other institutional levels such as educational, work, organizational, and community settings; and sociocultural institutions such as religious institutions.

The **physical context** includes elements of the natural and built environments that support or hinder participation. These elements include inclusive design features such as Braille signage or ramped building entrances but also include physical aspects such as different natural terrains (e.g., snow, ice, sand) that affect mobility. Physical parameters of noise, light, and temperature also form the physical context.

The **social context** includes individuals in the environment who affect activity participation and AT use. Direct and indirect interactions are distinguished here, with recognition that interaction with others face to face, remotely, or indirectly all have an influence. Individuals who exert an influence indirectly are those responsible for the development and enactment of policies and procedures that affect the participation of persons with disabilities. The social context also includes consideration of the society in which the individual lives and the social values and attitudes that affect his full social inclusion.

The **cultural context** involves systems of shared meanings (Bruner, 1990; Jonsson & Josephsson, 2005) that include beliefs, rituals, and values that are broadly held and that do not change as quickly as socially held attitudes and practices. Although similarities exist among social and cultural contexts, cultural beliefs transcend social settings, formed as part of membership in a group, such as a religious or ethnic group, rather than living in a particular social context. Actions and attitudes are influenced by perception of time and space, rights and responsibilities of different members of a group, independence and autonomy, and beliefs about the causality of life situations such as disability (Jonsson & Josephsson, 2005).

The final element of the context is the **institutional context,** which involves two key areas, (1) legislation and related regulations and (2) policies and funding. Relevant legislation affects individuals with disabilities by requiring access to key rights such as education, health care, and employment. It also details requirements for inclusion of individuals with disabilities in most aspects of community and social life. On the funding side, legislation, regulation, and policy define who and what are eligible for funding and the process whereby funding is obtained.

Assistive Technology

Assistive technology in the HAAT model is viewed as an **enabler** for a human doing an activity in context. This component has four aspects: the human/technology interface (HTI), the **processor**, the **environmental interface,** and the activity output. Interaction with the human is by the HTI, which forms the boundary between the human and the AT. A two-way interaction occurs at this boundary (i.e., information and forces are directed from the human to the technology and vice versa).

The technology supports activity performance through an **activity output,** which is cognition, communication, manipulation, or mobility. The HTI and the activity output are linked by the processor, which translates information and forces received from the human into signals that are used to control the activity output. Some assistive technologies (e.g., sensory aids) must also be capable of detecting external environmental data. The environmental interface accomplishes this function. After the external data are detected, the processor interprets and formats them so they can be provided to the user through the HTI. Not all assistive technologies have all of these components. However, all of them have at least one of these components, and most have two or three.

Assistive technologies can also be considered on a continuum that identifies technology produced for the mass market, or mainstream technology, to technology that is created for a single individual. As will be seen in Chapter 2, increasingly, individuals with disabilities can use technology that is mass produced, intended for a wide consumer audience. In particular, information and communication technologies and computer technologies are useful for individuals with a wide range of abilities. These devices are typically easier to obtain and less expensive than devices that are produced specifically for individuals with disabilities. On the midrange of this continuum are products that are produced for individuals with disabilities that are usually used "off the shelf" with minimal or no modifications necessary. At the other end of this continuum are devices that are created for a single individual (or a very small number) that meet very specific needs of that person. These devices tend to be more expensive and more difficult to obtain because they are custom made and produced in very low numbers. Figure 1-3 illustrates this continuum.

The complexity of the technology is another consideration of this component of the HAAT model. A continuum of complexity ranges from simple to complex in terms of ease of use and the configuration of the AT hardware. Devices

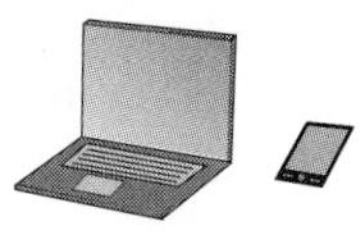
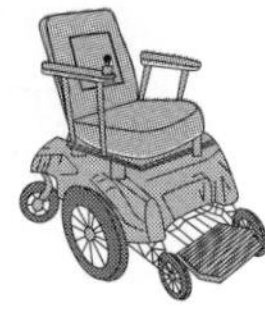
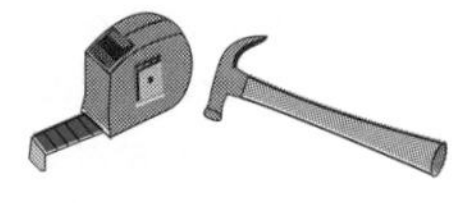

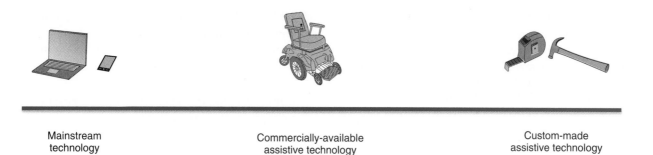

FIGURE 1-3 Continuum illustrating the progression from mainstream to custom-made technology.

that are simple to use tend to be more acceptable to the user and less likely to be used incorrectly.

Another way of considering complexity is by describing technology as low tech or high tech. Low-tech devices are simple to operate and construct, often are manually driven, are easy to acquire, and are low cost. Examples of low-tech devices are mouthsticks, adapted utensils, and computer keyguards. In contrast, high-tech devices are more complex to use; frequently are electrically powered or feature electronics; have multiple functions, including functions that are defined by the user; are more difficult to acquire; and are more expensive. AAC devices, powered wheelchairs, electronic aids to daily living, and robotic devices are all examples of high-tech devices.

A final distinction is made between hard and soft technologies. **Hard technology** refers to the actual, tangible device, such as computer hardware, an AAC device, a hearing aid, or a mobility device. Most of the formal definitions of AT refer to these hard technologies. In contrast, **soft technology** refers to less tangible aspects that support the use of a device, including other people, written or auditory materials, and computer software. These technologies involve decision making, strategies, training, concept formation, and service delivery that are used in the research and development of new products, decision making when making a product recommendation or purchase, and then the activities involved when learning how to use the new device. Initially, a new user or clinician may depend heavily on external resources, such as this textbook, to learn about device use. With greater confidence and knowledge, additional strategies and flexibility are applied to device use and to the service delivery process.

Reassembling the Human Activity Assistive Technology Model

The HAAT model describes a complex and dynamic framework for understanding the place of AT in the lives of persons with disabilities, guiding both clinical applications and research. It includes several different elements that affect use of AT. The dynamic nature of the model reminds us that these elements interact and influence each other and that the degree of influence changes. For example, in the summer, the weather, which is part of the physical environment, may have little influence on the outdoor mobility of a person who uses a device that supports mobility for either vision or movement reasons. However, in the winter when snow, ice, and cold are present, the physical context has a much greater influence on outdoor mobility. The institutional context supports activity participation via AT use when public funding is provided for device acquisition but becomes a hindrance when devices are not funded at a sufficient level.

Collectively, the elements of the human, activity, and context affect the selection and success of the AT as an enabler of human activity. A consistent process for product design and recommendation is described that recognizes the importance of understanding the activity the person wants and needs to perform, the capabilities of the individual, and the influence of the different aspects of the context on device acquisition and use. Understanding the activity ensures that the device will support the performance of something useful. Understanding the person results in knowledge not only about her abilities, skills, and knowledge but also about her stage in life; experience with technology; the roles she enacts; and the meaning she holds for the activity, her disability, and use of AT. Understanding the context results in knowledge of how the physical, social, cultural, and institutional contexts individually and collectively support or limit activity participation of an individual with a disability as well as the acquisition and use of AT.

Client- or user-centered approaches are primary themes in the application of the HAAT model. It is important to understand the client's goals and her perception of her own needs as a starting point in the service delivery and research process. Technology that does not meet the client's needs or expectations will not be useful to support the client's full potential. Most of us probably have devices that we thought would be useful when purchased but that did not meet our expectations and were put aside. In the case of AT, particularly for devices that are acquired with public funds, such device abandonment has greater implications if the user's activity performance is compromised or scarce health care funds are wasted.

In the next two chapters, the different elements of the model are presented individually, and then their mutual interactions are described. Although we do separate the components in order to discuss the key ideas of each, it is important to understand that the model is intended to be considered as a unit, with each element contributing to the desired outcome of activity performance and community participation of the technology user.

Ecological Models of Assistive Technology

Two other models were developed specifically to address AT assessment and service delivery, the Matching Person and Technology (MPT) model (Scherer & Glueckauf, 2005) and the Comprehensive Assistive Technology (CAT) model (Hersh and Johnson, 2008a, 2008b). Both of these models incorporate elements of the person, the environment, and the technology. CAT also incorporates the activity component.

The MPT was developed to support an AT assessment process that is goal directed, client centered, and designed to facilitate the identification of AT that is most likely to be used by the individual. The model incorporates three key elements: person (preferences and needs), milieu (elements of the environment that affect AT use and function), and AT (features and function) (Scherer & Glueckauf, 2005).

Several assessments are available that are based on the model. Commonly, these assessments require input from both the potential user or client and the professional assisting with the identification of appropriate AT. The assessments include evaluation of current use of technology and a series of tools that evaluate the attitude and experience with general, educational, and workplace technologies. These assessments are discussed in greater detail in Chapter 5 on service delivery. Matching Technology and Child (MATCH) assessments are a recent development from this group.

The MPT approach is consistent with HAAT in that it considers a complex situation (use of technology), identifies critical elements that affect the situation, and understands that making changes in one element will effect change (positive and negative) in other elements. The MPT does not specifically discuss activities, which are explicit in the HAAT model; however, links to the WHO Activities and Participation categories have been made with different MPT measures (Scherer & Glueckauf, 2005).

The CAT model was developed by two electronics and electrical engineers. It is primarily designed to categorize and describe different features that influence the use of AT. Design specification, initial assessment, and outcome evaluation are identified as the prime applications of CAT (Hersh & Johnson, 2008a). CAT is modeled closely on the WHO ICF. It is organized in a tree and branch structure, with different options of display (e.g., chart, table, and engineering flow diagram), depending on the user's needs and preferences. The model's main categories are activities, human, context, and AT. There are three levels of categories—the main areas listed above and then sublevels under each.

Hersh and Johnson (2008b) demonstrate the different applications of the model, with benefits of identifying key elements to consider when designing, selecting, or evaluating AT. They show how the model can be used to describe relevant features for a specific purpose.

Conceptually, the CAT model is very similar to the HAAT model because it contains very similar main categories. Both models can be used for similar applications of device design and development, guidance of the service delivery process, and outcome evaluation. The main difference between these models is in the supporting description—whereas the HAAT model posits a more dynamic interaction among the different components, CAT seems to provide more description of the individual categories in a situation rather than describing an interaction among these categories.

APPLICATION OF THE HUMAN ACTIVITY ASSISTIVE TECHNOLOGY MODEL

The HAAT model has four primary applications: (1) product research and development; (2) product **usability** studies; (3) client assessment; and (4) outcome evaluation, which can include individual and collective outcomes of AT use. The general process for each of these is similar—identification of the desired activity, consideration of the individual or collective user characteristics, and determination of the contextual factors that influence the device acquisition and use all precede consideration of the AT.

Product Research and Development

Products that are developed without consideration of the activity, human, or contextual needs, and influences are less likely to meet the needs of the user. For this reason, we advocate conducting preparatory studies that investigate these needs before a produce is designed. Two of the foundational principles of this book—AT design and service delivery processes that are person centered and function based—are influential here. The lived experiences of individuals with disabilities are critical parts of the AT research and development process to support identification of the need for a product and to evaluate the success of each design iteration to meet that need.

Although not explicitly based on the HAAT model, the process used to develop a toileting system for children with seating needs illustrates a user-centered and function-based approach (Lee et al., 2002). The process started with parents of young children providing their opinion on toileting needs, including how they needed to be able to use a toileting product (e.g., it needed to be easily removed from a toilet so others in the household could use the toilet). These opinions were then translated into design features that led to the development of an initial prototype and an evaluation instrument that could be used to critique the prototype. The prototype, along with other currently available products, was then evaluated by parents using the criteria that had been developed in the initial phase. Concurrently, the children who might benefit from the device were seated in it so that an experienced physiotherapist could evaluate the positioning and the children could indicate their opinion of the device. The final stage of the development of the product, before the technology was transferred, involved use of the device in the home over an extended timeframe so the parents and children could provide feedback on the utility and usability of the device (Lee et al., 2002). The extensive feedback obtained at each stage and the identification of key aspects of the activity, human user, and the contexts in which the device was used resulted in a product that ultimately met its intended outcome.

Usability

Fisk et al. (2009) distinguish between device utility and usability. Whereas utility describes how well the device meets its intended function, usability describes how well the user is able to access the device's functionality (Fisk et al., 2009). They identify five key features of usability:

1. *Learnabilty*: All functions of the device are easily learned. We would add consideration of the effectiveness of soft technologies to support learning here.
2. *Efficiency*: The user meets the intended goals of device use in a reasonable amount of time with minimal frustration, effort, and frustration.
3. *Memorability*: How the device is used can be easily remembered, particularly when a function has not been used over a long period of time. An example of memorability involves programming a particular function on a smart phone. When the programming process is easily retained or retrieved from memory, this aspect of usability is satisfied.
4. *Errors*: This aspect refers to incorrect actions the user makes or actions that are omitted that limit or prevent a device from functioning as intended. It is important that errors can be recognized, that the effect of an error is minimal, that feedback is given to signal an error is made, and that the user can repair an error made.
5. *Satisfaction:* The user has a positive experience when using the device, which we interpret as satisfaction with how the device functions as well as the image that the device use conveys to the user (Miller Polgar, 2010).
6. *Ease of use*: In addition to the five criteria listed above, identified by Fisk et al. (2009), we add ease of use. This last criterion involves many of the ideas above, but it also makes explicit the idea that a device must be simple to use on a regular basis, which we interpret as minimizing the number of steps required to generate the desired output.

Two major perspectives of usability analysis are described. In the first instance, the goal is to identify and rectify problems that a person encounters when using the device. The second involves performing a number of tasks with the device and measuring the user's performance. Although both will provide useful information on problems with device use, the second type of analysis provides details on steps necessary to use the device as well as cognitive, communicative, sensory, and physical demands of device use (Fisk et al., 2009).

Clinical Assessment

The assessment process is described in greater detail in Chapter 5. The basic process involves identification of the need to be addressed by AT use, assessment of key aspects, synthesis of the assessment results, and device recommendation. Assessment is user centered, which means that the user of AT—and others as appropriate such as a parent, child, or spouse—are equal partners on the assessment team and that their goals for device use are paramount in driving the assessment process.

Assessment can include both formal and informal instruments, with formal instruments interpreted as tests that have been developed using rigorous procedures with established measurement properties and that are administered and interpreted in a standardized manner. Informal assessment involves observation and interview to gather input and information.

The clinical team includes the AT users (and relevant others), audiologists, occupational and physical therapists, speech language pathologists, nurses, physicians, teachers, rehabilitation engineers, and rehabilitation and educational assistants. Institutional policies and practices determine who is present during an assessment and what their responsibilities are regarding different aspects of the assessment.

Assessment culminates in device recommendation and acquisition. When possible, the assessment process also results in procurement of funding. This component requires knowledge of who is responsible to request funding and what is required to make that request.

Outcome Evaluation

Outcome evaluation involves two aspects, evaluation of the outcome of device use by an individual client and outcome of device use for a group of individuals. In the latter case, this evaluation forms part of the evidence base that is increasingly necessary to justify requests for funding of AT.

Outcome evaluation of an individual client ideally occurs at several points after acquisition of the device: immediately after acquisition and short- and long-term follow-up. In reality, the possibility of conducting these evaluations depends on funding, institutional policies, and clinician workload. Unfortunately, often the only time a clinician is able to follow up with the client is at the time the device is delivered, which limits the ability to evaluate how well the device has been integrated into the client's life.

Outcome evaluation is based on the goals identified by the client regarding the acquisition of the device. This evaluation determines how well these goals have been met. In addition, other outcomes, such as satisfaction with the device and the psychosocial impact of the device use, which are discussed in greater detail in Chapter 5, can also be incorporated into the individual client evaluation. Carpe et al. (2010) used the HAAT model to interpret their data in a study of children's perceptions of their use of writing and communication aids. The HAAT model was useful to identify barriers and enablers to the use of these devices.

On a larger scale, evaluation of the outcomes of device use with a sample of clients provides information on device use, the ability of the device to meet the intended need, and feedback on device design for future development. Commonly, this type of evaluation is conducted as part of a formal research study with the purpose of building an evidence base related to the AT use. This evidence base supports clinical decisions, influences policy, and justifies new and continued public funding of assistive devices and services.

Lenker et al. (2012) reviewed the service delivery process associated with the HAAT model along with other models relevant to AT service delivery. They concluded that it provides useful information to support a client-focused approach. The model and associated process will benefit from continued development of more specific processes and methods to support outcome evaluation research (Lenker et al.).

SUMMARY

Technology is ubiquitous in the performance of our daily activities. Very few activities are performed without the support of technology. AT is defined formally as technology designed specifically for individuals with disabilities to augment or replace function. This definition commonly is used to identify devices that are required by different pieces of legislation or regulations that support accessibility and inclusivity of individuals with disabilities. However, increasingly, devices that are developed for mainstream use (i.e., that are not developed specifically for individuals with disabilities) are useful by persons with a wide range of abilities. In particular, information communication and computing technologies have features included that make them accessible to individuals with varying abilities.

Several key principles guide the design, assessment, and evaluation of assistive technologies. These principles include (1) person-centered processes, (2) function as the outcome, (3) use of an evidence-informed process, (4) use of an ethical process, and (5) provision of AT in a sustainable manner. These key principles can be used by professionals involved in device design and development, clinical applications, and policy makers to ensure that devices meet their intended functional goals, are accepted by the intended users, and are congruent with the context in which they are used.

The HAAT model is the framework applied in this book. It describes a human doing an activity in a context using AT. It has four main components: (1) activity, (2) human, (3) context, and (4) AT. The model is based on ecological and transactional constructs, emphasizing the dynamic and integrative nature of its components. The model is applied in the research and development, device usability, clinical assessment, and outcome evaluation processes.

The next several chapters of this book describe the HAAT model in detail and discuss ethical and service delivery issues relevant to AT. These chapters make the application process of the HAAT model explicit. The remainder of the book focuses on specific categories of AT. Each chapter is organized to reflect the HAAT model, starting with the activities that are supported by the AT discussed, attributes of the human user of that particular category of technology, contextual considerations, and assessment and outcome evaluation. The bulk of each chapter is devoted to description of the technology that is currently available as well as emerging technology. This organization is deliberate to illustrate the process inherent in the HAAT model and to provide sufficient detail about the different technologies to support their clinical application.

STUDY QUESTIONS

1. Contrast the concept of disability as understood from a medical versus a social model. Describe how each influences AT use and service delivery.
2. Discuss how the presence of a disability influences the life circumstances of a person with a disability.
3. Identify the elements of formal definitions of AT. Contrast these with information definitions of AT.
4. Identify and describe the key components of the ICF, CMOP-E, and PEOP. Discuss their influence on the HAAT model.
5. Describe each of the four principles that guide AT service delivery. Give an example of each.
6. Describe each component of the HAAT model and give an example of each. Describe each of the four contextual components. Give an example of each.
7. Identify and describe each of the four applications of the HAAT model.

REFERENCES

American Occupational Therapy Association: Occupational therapy code of ethics, *Am J Occup Ther* 64:S17–S26, 2010.

Americans with Disabilities Act of 1990, 42 U.S.C. §§ 12101 et seq.

Assistive Technology Act of 1998, as amended, PL 108-364, §3, 118 stat 1707, 2004.

Baum C, Christiansen C: Person-Environment-Occupation-Performance: An occupation-based framework for practice. In Christiansen CH, Baum CM, Bass-Haugen J, editors: *Occupational therapy: Performance, participation, and well-being*, Thorofare, NJ, 2005, SLACK, pp 242–267.

Bickenbach J, Chatterji S, Badley EM, et al.: Models of disablement, universalism and the international classification of impairment, disabilities and handicaps, *Soc Sci Med* 48:1173, 1999.

Borg J, Lindstrom A, Larsson S: Assistive technology in developing countries: A review from the perspective of the Convention on the Rights of Persons with Disabilities, *Prosthet Orthot Int* 35:20–29, 2011.

Bruner J: *Acts of meaning*, Cambridge, MA, 1990, Harvard University Press.

Carpe A, Harder K, Tam C, Reid D: Perceptions of writing and communication aid use among children with a physical disability, *Assist Technol* 22:87–98, 2010.

Cook AM: Ethical issues related to the use/non-use of assistive technologies, *Dev Disabil Bull* 37:127–152, 2009.

Cook AM, Hussey S: Assistive Technologies: Principles and Practice, St. Louis MO, 1995, Mosby.

Cutchin M: John Dewey's metaphysical ground-map and its implications for geographical inquiry, *Geoforum* 39:1555–1569, 2008.

Danermark B, Gellerstedt LC: Social justice: Redistribution and recognition—a non-reductionist perspective on disability, *Disabil Soc* 19:339–353, 2004.

Fisk AD, Rogers WA, Charness N, et al.: *Designing for older adults: Principles and creative human factors approaches*, ed 2, Boca Raton, FL, 2009, CRC Press.

Lee DF, Ryan S, Polgar JM, Leibel G: Consumer-based approaches used in the development of an adaptive toileting system for children with positioning problems, *Phys Occup Ther Pediatr* 22:5–24, 2002.

Fougeyrollas P, Gray DB: Classification systems, environmental factors and social change. In Gray DB, Quantrano LA, Lieberman ML, editors: *Designing and using assistive technology: The human perspective*, Baltimore, 1998, Paul H. Brookes, pp 13–28.

Hersh MA, Johnson MA: On modelling assistive technology systems—Part 1: Modelling framework, *Technol Disabil* 20:193–215, 2008a.

Hersh MA, Johnson MA: On modelling assistive technology systems—Part 2: Applications of the comprehensive assistive technology model, *Technol Disabil* 20:251–270, 2008b.

Jonsson H, Josephsson S: Occupation and meaning. In Christiansen CH, Baum CM, Bass-Haugen J, editors: *Occupational therapy: Performance, participation, and well-being*, Thorofare, NJ, 2005, SLACK, pp 116–133.

Lenker J, Shoemaker LL, Fuher MJ, et al.: Classification of Assistive Technology services, *Technol Disabil* 24:59–70, 2012.

McColl MA, Jongbloed L: *Disability and social policy in Canada*, Concord, ON, 2006, Captus University Publishers. 2.

Miller Polgar J: The myth of neutral technology. In Oishi MMK, Mitchell IM, Van der Loos HFM, editors: *Design and use of assistive technology: Social, technical, ethical, and economic challenges*, Boca Raton, FL, 2010, Springer, pp 17–24.

Nussbaum M: *Creating capabilities: The human development approach*, Cambridge MA, 2011, The Belknap Press of Harvard University Press.

Owen J, Simonds C: Beyond the wheelchair: Development of motorised transport for people with severe mobility impairments in developing countries, *Disabil Rehabil Assist Technol* 5:254–257, 2010.

Phillipine Physical Therapy Association: *Code of ethics*, 2009. Available from www.philpta.org/?page_id=62. Accessed November 5, 2012.

Rawls J: *A theory of justice*, Cambridge MA, 1999, Belknap Press of the Harvard University Press.

RESNA: Code of ethics, nd. Available from: http://resna.org/certification/RESNA_Code_of_Ethics.pdf. Accessed December 27, 2013.

Samant D, Matter R, Harniss M: Realizing the potential of accessible ICTs in developing countries, *Disabil Rehabil Assist Technol* 1–10, 2012.

Sanford J: *Universal design as a rehabilitation strategy: Design for the ages*, New York, 2012, Springer.

Scherer MJ, Glueckauf R: Assessing the benefits of assistive technologies for activities and participation, *Rehabil Psychol* 50:132–141, 2005.

SCIPILOT: *Luther: Navigating the system*. Available from www.scipilot.com/_g/cons-g/036.php, 2013. Accessed December 27.

Sen A: The idea of justice, Cambridge, MA: The Belknap Press of Harvard University Press, 2009.

Townsend E, Polatajko HJ: *Enabling occupation II: Advancing occupational therapy vision for health, well-being and justice through occupation*, Ottawa, ON, 2002, CAOT Publications ACE.

Townsend E, Polatajko HJ: *Enabling occupation II: Advancing occupational therapy vision for health, well-being and justice through occupation,* ed 2, Ottawa, ON, 2013, CAOT Publications ACE.

United Nations: *Convention on the Rights of Persons with Disabilities (CRPD),* Resolution 61/106, New York, 2007, United Nations. Available from www.un.org/disabilities/convention/conventionfull.shtml.

Whalley Hammel K: *Perspectives on disability and rehabilitation: Contesting assumptions, challenging practice*, London, UK, 2006, Churchill Livingstone.

WHO, 2011.

World Health Organization: *International classification of Functioning, disability and health*, Geneva, 2001, World Health Organization.

World Health Organization: *World Report on Disability*, Geneva, 2011, WHO Press.

CHAPTER 2

Technologies That Assist People Who Have Disabilities

CHAPTER OUTLINE

LEARNING OBJECTIVES

On completing this chapter, you will be able to do the following:

1. Describe the various technology options that are available for meeting the needs of people with disabilities.
2. Define assistive technology (AT).
3. Understand the principles of universal design and their application to meeting the needs of people with disabilities.
4. Describe the changing demographics that affect the development of AT applications globally.
5. Distinguish between hard and soft AT and describe each.
6. Identify and describe the major functional parts of AT devices.
7. Describe the major categories of soft technologies.
8. Understand the technology options for meeting the needs of individuals with disabilities through technology.

KEY TERMS

Assistive technologies (ATs)
Activity output
Control interface
Environmental sensor
Function allocation
Human/technology interface (HTI)
Information and communication technologies (ICTs)
Mainstream technologies
Mainstream smart phones
Mechanisms
Mobile technologies
Processor
Smart wheelchairs
Soft technologies
Universal design
User display

In the 21st century, the world is moving from a machine-based or manufacturing economy to a knowledge-based economy (Ungson and Trudel, 1999). The focus of the development of the knowledge economy is to overcome traditional societal barriers, including spatial distribution of citizens, language or knowledge barriers, handicaps resulting from disabilities or environmental conditions, social status, and economic power (Weber, 2006).

There is also a trend from a regional or national scope to a global scope. This may mean that the "digital divide" between developed and emerging countries is narrowed. If the information age brings significant growth and improvement in living conditions in underresourced countries, will people with disabilities be included? The answer will only be "yes" if sufficient attention is paid to accessibility.

Information and communication technologies (ICTs), including computers (desktop and notebook), standard and smart cell phones, and tablets, are the gateway to the knowledge-based economy. Access to the Internet is more critical for people with disabilities than for the general population because they lack alternatives for information retrieval or participation in general (Weber, 2006). In Chapter 8, we discuss ways in which ICTs are being made accessible and are being used as **assistive technologies (ATs).**

Another important factor is that technologies are changing rapidly. These technologies are tools. Tools that dramatically affect the way we learn, work, and play. The ability to make tools is what distinguishes us as human, but our tools ultimately control us by making us dependent on them (Wright, 2004). If you do not believe it, give up your computer and mobile phone for 24 hours or more and see if you can survive without them. This dependence on technology may be optional for most of us, but it is much less so for people with disabilities because they often depend on technologies to access work, perform tasks of daily living, and participate fully in the community.

It is not only ICTs that are changing the technology options for people with disabilities. New materials are also making it possible to provide greater comfort and avoid skin breakdown in seating systems. Lighter materials are making wheelchairs and other mobility products easier to use and transport in vehicles. Changes in mainstream products for home use (e.g., food preparation and consumption, self-care) are being designed to accommodate for older individuals with arthritis or loss of visual or hearing ability. Most significantly, many more products from automobiles to home appliances are being designed with features that increase their accessibility and usability for individuals who have disabilities. The end result of these factors is that there are many more technology options available to meet the needs of individuals who have disabilities. Some of these are mainstream products, and some are specially designed for people with disabilities.

The constellation of functions in ICTs such as a smart phone is typical of those required for many ATs whether based on mainstream technology or specially designed devices. We already know how to make many devices accessible; we just need to make sure it happens with new technologies. In this chapter, we consider the broad scope of technological capability that is emerging and the specific implications that those technologies have for people with disabilities. Pullin (2009) observed that "despite a proliferation of technology and consumption that is so worrying in other ways, many people remain excluded and disabled by design that does not acknowledge their abilities" (p. 69). Addressing this challenge by accessing mainstream as well as specialized technologies can enable people who have disabilities to participate more fully in all aspects of society.

THE CHANGING WORLD OF ASSISTIVE TECHNOLOGIES AND ITS IMPACT ON PERSONS WITH DISABILITIES

An often used definition of *assistive technology* (AT) comes from US Public Law (PL) 100-407, the Technical Assistance to the States Act in the United States:

> *Any item, piece of equipment or product system whether acquired commercially off the shelf, modified or customized that is used to increase, maintain or improve functional capabilities of individuals with disabilities.*

When this definition was developed in the 1990s there were few adaptations built into mainstream products, and most of the ATs were specially designed to meet the unique needs of people with disabilities (Cook & Hussey, 1995). Over time many of the special adaptations developed for people with disabilities have become standard features incorporated into mainstream products. A partial listing of these features and both their AT and mainstream uses are shown in Table 2-1. Table 2.2 lists some mainstream derivatives of accommodations originally made in public buildings for people with disabilities.

This bidirectional exchange of functionality is longstanding (Newell, 2011). Cassette tapes and long-playing records were developed to support talking books for the blind. The typewriter was developed for a blind Italian countess, the ballpoint pen for people who could not use a pen with a point because of poor manual skills, and a carpenter's miter blocks for those who could not use two hands for sawing were all developed first for people with disabilities. The introduction of the telephone was originally intended to help individuals who were hard of hearing, but its impact was felt mainly in the mainstream population, actually marginalizing those who had difficulty hearing (Emiliani, 2006). However, the same technology that made the telephone possible was also useful in sensing sound and making it available for amplification in hearing aids. Furthermore, the problems of profoundly deaf people were ameliorated by the discovery that telephone lines could be used to transmit digital data via modems. This made the TTY (see Chapter 14) possible as a visual substitute for auditory information communicated over telephone lines. It also made possible the use of SMS (texting) on cell phones. The contribution to the mainstream of design concepts, materials, and approaches that were originally intended for people with disabilities includes material and manufacturing techniques as well. Pullin (2009) describes how plywood manufacturing techniques developed for splints during World War II led to the design and mass manufacture of unique furniture in the 1940s and 1950s. This "migration" of features from ATs to the mainstream technology world and back has contributed to a larger trend that is based on **universal design.**

UNIVERSAL DESIGN

Over the past 20 years, mainstream off-the-shelf technologies have become increasingly more accessible to people with disabilities. To lead full and productive lives, persons with disabilities need to have the same access to **mainstream technologies** as the rest of the population. Of particular importance are mobile devices (smart phones, tablets) and computer and information technologies because of the impact they are having on worldwide development and international commerce. We discuss the implications for this access in Chapter 8.

Commercial products may be designed according to the principles of universal design: "The design of products and environments to be usable by all people, to the greatest extent possible, without the need for adaptation or specialized design" (Sanford, 2012, p. 66).

In this approach, features that make a product more useful to persons who have disabilities (e.g., larger knobs; a variety of display options such as visual, tactile, or auditory; alternatives to reading text such as icons or pictures) are built into the product.

In some countries (e.g., those in Europe), universal design is known as "design for all." The North Carolina State University Center for Universal Design, in conjunction with advocates of universal design, has compiled a set of

TABLE 2-1 Mainstream Derivatives of Assistive Technology

Technology Name	Assistive Use	Mainstream Use
Closed captioning	Textual translation of voice and sounds on TV for people who are deaf or hard of hearing	Television screens in lounges and gyms (more used here than by people who are deaf)
Voice recognition	Text entry for those who are unable to use their hands to type on a keyboard	Anyone wanting to enter text faster than they can type; widely used by lawyers; telephone prompt systems
On-screen keyboards	Text entry for those who are unable to use their hands to type on a keyboard	Tablets and personal digital assistants (PDAs); many emerging computing platforms do not have a keyboard attached and require the use of an onscreen keyboard for text entry
Speech synthesis	Computer-generated speech used to communicate for those unable to speak using their own voices	Voice prompt telephone systems; many software applications where verbal feedback is provided
Digitized speech	Computer-generated speech used to communicate for those unable to speak using their own voices	Voice prompt telephone systems; many software applications in which verbal feedback is provided
Computer keyboard equivalents	Keyboard access and control of menu items for people who are unable to use a mouse or see the screen	Shortcuts to save time by anyone (e.g., Control-S to save)
Mouse keys	Control of the cursor via the numeric keypad for people who are unable to use the mouse	Graphic designers who wish to move the cursor a single pixel at a time and have difficulty doing so with a mouse
Sticky keys	Assist one-handed typists in accomplishing key combinations, such as Shift-A	Anyone who is a two-finger typist can use this feature (and there are many)
T9 disambiguation	A quick way to enter text using scanning by someone who is unable to use a keyboard (fewer keys means less time scanning)	The majority of cell phone companies in the world have now licensed this technology to speed text entry using the numbers on the telephone keypad.
Word prediction	Speed text entry for people who are unable to use their hands to type on a keyboard	Used everywhere from spreadsheets to language learning software. Word completion and word prediction help speed text entry for everyone.
Abbreviation expansion	Speed text entry for people who are unable to use their hands to type on a keyboard	Now a standard feature in most mainstream word processing applications; type common terms, such as your name and address, with a single abbreviation
Single latches on laptops	Allow people with only one arm to open the lid on a laptop	Ever had one arm full of papers and tried to open your laptop lid? You will immediately appreciate this feature when you do.
On/off push button toggle switches	Ability for people with limited motor control to turn on/off computers (instead of the traditional rocker switches in the rear)	Now almost every computer made uses this type of switch because it is simply easier for everyone
Call-out control descriptions	Allow people who are blind to have the description of a control icon read to them via speech synthesis	Anyone wondering what a certain toolbar icon is supposed to mean can now dwell over it and get the text description
Screen enlargement	Allows people with low vision problems to more easily see the screen of the computer	Often used during presentations or in kiosks to make certain parts of the computer screen more viewable by the public
System color schemes	Allow people who are color blind or have low vision to see the computer screen easier	Who do you know who has not played with the system colors and customized them to their own tastes? High-contrast modes are often used in presentations to large audiences when the screen must be seen from large distances.
Wearable computers	Allow someone with a disability who is using a computer for communication to have it with them at all times (e.g., glasses-mounted displays)	This is just emerging. There are specialized uses for it now, such as the military, but it will become more common for everyone in the future.
Head tracking devices	Allow someone without the use of their hands to control the cursor	Gamers who are using their hands for other things such as firing buttons can still control the cursor. Also used by database entry clerks and other computer operators who must have their hands on the keyboard at all times. Used in hazardous environments where the computer is behind a window yet can still be controlled.

Continued

TABLE 2-1 Mainstream Derivatives of Assistive Technology—cont'd

Technology Name	Assistive Use	Mainstream Use
Brainwave recognition units	Allow someone without the use of their hands to control a computer through thought	This is just emerging as well. One can only imagine the possibilities.
Single-switch hardware interfaces	Allow people with physical disabilities who are unable to use a pointing device or keyboard to control the computer using a single switch	Used as a simple data acquisition solution for anyone needing to plug a switch into a computer. One known example: a TV weatherman who changes slides on the weather map he is standing in front of using a small switch in his hand.
Swype text input for touch screens	People who have difficulty using a standard keyboard (e.g., people with spinal cord injury, learning disabilities, amyotrophic lateral sclerosis) can enter text using head tracking or touch much faster than traditional uses of on-screen keyboards	Smart phones and the proliferation of touch-screen devices (e.g., iPads) do not have keyboards. Swype is used for all people using these devices to enter text much faster than alternative methods.

Compiled by Randy Marsden, Edmonton, AB, Canada.

TABLE 2-2 Mainstream Derivatives of Public Building Accommodations

Technology Name	Assistive Use	Mainstream Use
Pay telephone volume adjustments	Allow people who are hard of hearing to use the public telephone	Most public phones are in noisy environments (e.g., traffic noise), so turning up the earpiece volume is used by anyone talking on the phone
Sidewalk curb cuts	Allow people in wheelchairs to cross the street	Skateboarders, parents with baby strollers, people pushing shopping carts, bicyclers, and rollerbladders all thought they were put there for them
Automatic doors	Allow people in wheelchairs to enter a building	A study showed that people without apparent physical disabilities preferred to use an automatic door over an adjacent revolving door 97% of the time
Low buttons on elevators	Allow people in wheelchairs to select floors on the elevator keypad	Children who insist on pressing the desired floor in an elevator can now reach the buttons without a parent having to pick them up
Music played in conjunction with crosswalk signals	Allows people who are blind to know when it is okay to cross the street	Anyone not paying attention now has an audible cue when the walk signal changes
Elevators in two-story buildings	Allow people in wheelchairs to access the second floor	Even though most people can manage a flight of stairs (in 95% of homes), most still use the elevator in public buildings
Enlarged bathroom stalls	Allow people in wheelchairs to transfer from the chair to the toilet	Ever been going through an airport with a bunch of carry-on luggage and tried to fit in a normal sized stall? Enough said.

principles of universal design, shown in Box 2-1. This center also maintains a website on universal design (http://www.design.ncsu.edu/cud).

Universal design can be less expensive than modifying a product after production to meet the needs of a person with a disability. However, the increased emphasis on economic sustainability and profit worldwide has caused a level of skepticism in industry regarding the cost–benefit ratio of universal design (Emiliani, Stephanidis, & Vanderheiden, 2011). Companies faced with limited profits and very competitive markets have adopted the concept that "people with limitations should be a duty of the welfare system in the different countries and should not be an obstacle to the main aim of industry, i.e., to the generation of profit" (Emiliani et al., 2011, p. 108). In some areas (e.g., telecommunications equipment), companies may be mandated by legislation to make products accessible to a wide range of users "without much difficulty or expense." To

BOX 2-1 Principles of Universal Design

1. Equitable use: The design is useful and marketable to people with diverse abilities.
2. Flexibility in use: The design accommodates a wide range of individual preferences and abilities.
3. Simple and intuitive use: Use of the design is easy to understand regardless of the user's experience, knowledge, language skills, or current concentration level.
4. Perceptible information: The design communicates necessary information effectively to the user regardless of ambient conditions or the user's sensory abilities.
5. Tolerance for error: The design minimizes hazards and the adverse consequences of accidental or unintended actions.
6. Low physical effort: The design can be used efficiently and comfortably and with a minimum of fatigue.
7. Size and space for approach and use: Appropriate size and space is provided for approach, reach, manipulation, and use regardless of user's body size, posture, or mobility.

accomplish this goal, companies must look at the costs and the resources available to address accessibility (Schaefer, 2006). Large companies with more resources will be expected to do more than small companies with limited budgets because large mainstream companies "being forced (e.g., by legislation) to take into account all users is considered by them an undue interference in their goal (serving the mainstream customer and maximizing profits)" (Emiliani et al., 2011, p. 107).

According to Pullin (2009), universal design mixes two concepts: (1) different people have different skills and abilities, and some designs may exclude some individuals, and (2) different people have different needs and desires that may or may not be related to their abilities (i.e., they may just want different things from a product or service). These two concepts are addressed by different approaches. The first can be addressed by flexible interfaces that use different sensory, cognitive, and physical modalities. This type of personalization can be found on websites such as Amazon related to content (e.g., "You might also like these similar items") (Emiliani et al., 2011). By expanding this concept, personalized interfaces may be developed for websites and for other downloadable applications for mainstream technologies ". . . provide alternative and personal user interfaces in an economically feasible fashion" (Emiliani et al., 2011, p. 106). This approach takes advantage of technology advances in mainstream products while also allowing users with a wide range of abilities to access the product through specialized interfaces. One example cited by Emilani et al. is the Universal Remote Console (URC) framework (see Chapter 12).

The second need cited by Pullin (2009) (i.e., different people have different needs and desires that may or may not be related to their abilities) is addressed through multimodal platforms that have many features and flexible configurations. Inexpensive AT devices will have to be based on mainstream devices such as smart phones equipped with a variety of sensors; a GPS antenna built in; and features such as voice recognition, word prediction, and speech output that make them ideal platforms (Emiliani et al., 2011). Customization of the platform to meet AT goals will be provided through software apps. Examples of applications to meet specific needs are discussed in later chapters.

Product development time and cost can also be affected by the inclusion of universal design principles. Björk (2009) evaluated the design of two supportive seating products. One used a universal design approach, and the other was developed as a modular solution that could be adjusted to fit a variety of users. The development of the universally designed system took four times as long as the design and development of the modular system.

When telecommunication product developers do not focus on the needs and preferences of users who have disabilities, design flaws occur (Lee, Jhangiani, Smith-Jackson, Nussbaum, & Tomioka, 2006). One example that could be resolved by simple changes in design is the inability to change font types on most mobile phones. From a universal design point of view, this feature would help individuals with low vision from a variety of causes (including not having their reading glasses handy when the phone rings).

A major distinguishing feature between ATs and universal design is the focus. ATs are developed and applied to maximize societal participation by individuals with disabilities in carrying out the functional tasks of daily living. Universal design has a focus on the functionality of design for as wide a segment of the population as possible without concern for individual needs (Sanford, 2012). Much of universal design addresses the built environment. That aspect is beyond the scope of this book.

Universal design also applies to products and services such as ICT. Because of the increasing universality of many mainstream products, largely because of the application of concepts originally developed for ATs, many needs of individuals who have disabilities can be addressed by mainstream commercially available products. In this book, we will deal with the continuum of technologies from mainstream to highly specialized ***with a focus on meeting the needs of individuals who have disabilities.***

General Design Concepts and Usability of Everyday Things

The concept of design of everyday things was originated by Donald Norman in the 1990s (Norman, 2002). Concerned with the difficulty he and others experienced in using common objects that were poorly designed, he set out to improve the design of the things that we all encounter daily. Norman observed that the operation of many products was neither obvious nor easy to figure out. He used the concept of "affordances" to describe this mismatch between observed properties and functional operation. Affordances are "perceived and actual properties of the thing" (Norman, 2002, p. 9). If a designer follows Norman's principles, then the operation of the device will be conveyed to the user by the design itself.

Norman used the term *constraints* to identify the limits on the possible number of uses for an object. Classes of constraints used by Norman include physical (rely on the properties of the physical world), semantic (based on meaning), cultural (rely on accepted conventions), and logical (Norman, 2002). The latter category describes the relationship between the spatial and functional layout of components and the functions that they control or affect. If these constraints are viewed in terms of the wide range of skills and abilities of persons with disabilities, then they can contribute to the universality of products. Norman also considered the role of design in system errors. He defined two types of errors, slips and mistakes. Slips result when the user has the correct goal but the wrong execution. Mistakes result from the wrong goal. He discusses these types of errors in terms of the device affordances, operator patterns of action, and user device features.

To improve design, Norman proposed that a mapping of the relationships between affordances and constraints be used to yield possible operations of any object. He also described the concept of perceptual models that allow us to predict the effect of our actions on an object. Associated with the perception of the object is the sensory feedback that the object provides to the user. This feedback can be tactile (e.g., the click of a switch or the force encountered in turning a knob), visual (e.g., movement when activated, lights or other indicators), or auditory (e.g., a click when a knob is turned, auditory alarms or signals). The principles of universal design in Box 2-1 are supported by the ideas of affordances, constraints, and the classification of errors developed by Norman. His concepts of design of everyday things and the principles of universal design in Box 2-1 have made a significant contribution to functionality in tasks of daily living for persons with disabilities.

Disability Demographics and Assistive Technologies

The characteristics of the population served by ATs are changing in several important ways. The demographics of the world population are changing with a significant shift to an older population. Because many individuals in this age range require some sort of assistance, this growth is presenting particular challenges for AT providers. With the possibility of mainstream technologies enabled by specialized applications taking the role of ATs, the opportunity to reach a larger percentage of the world's disabled population is significantly increased. Over the past 5 to 10 years, the needs of individuals with cognitive disabilities have begun to be addressed. This segment of the AT market is also increasing, and there is potential for mainstream technologies to be used in meeting these needs. The impacts of these three demographic changes are discussed in this section.

Increasing Older Global Population

The emerging group of elderly individuals (i.e., "baby boomers") is generally more experienced with computers and other technologies than earlier generations, and they will insist on greater performance and adaptability from both ATs and mainstream technologies such as **mobile technologies** (e.g., cell phones, smart phones, tablets, and embedded technologies). This age-driven increase in the size of the "disabled community" has been characterized as the "new old" (Cravit, 2008). These individuals will have greater technological competence and experience, higher expectations for technology performance, more active [lifestyles], and a longer life span than previous "older populations". The latter will lead to more dependence on technologies related to aging. Older adults also have an increase in holistic judgment, a lifetime of experience, and a release of creative abilities and energies because of reduced work and family responsibilities (Newell, 2011). Meeting the needs of this population will require innovative approaches to both universal design and ATs. Mainstream technologies should not frighten seniors who need to use them (Newell, 2011). Future requirements depend on personality as well as disability of users, and they must be accommodated as the demographics change and more users are older than 65 years of age and eventually older than 80 years of age. The varying responses of seniors to technology advances are illustrated in Figure 2-1.

Despite the changing attitudes of tomorrow's seniors, there are major needs that this group will have that might be addressed by technology, particularly ICTs (Newell, 2011). Remaining connected to family and community through communication networks can help reduce feelings of isolation. Access to shopping and services from home via Internet connectivity is an advantage for those with restricted mobility. The possibility of working from home can contribute to greater financial security. All of these advantages depend on ICTs that are available, accessible, and affordable for a senior population.

Vicente and López (2010) investigated the differences between Internet users with and without disabilities and elderly adults in Spain. In contrast to the "new old" concept of Cravit (2008), this study included elderly individuals with limited technology experience. Affordability is an issue because people with disabilities have lower incomes, and they may also lack training and support. People with disabilities and elderly individuals have attitudes toward the Internet that can limit its usefulness to them. In general, they have a lack of interest, low motivation, and anxiety about technology use. Specific problems in computer use include difficulties in reading text on the screen, selecting targets and perceiving icons and toolbars, hearing auditory prompts, clicking and dragging using a mouse, and finding relevant information in confusing and complex programs (Newell, 2011). All of these factors also depend on socioeconomic background because it influences computer experience. The functional limitations of this group are not the same as those of younger individuals who have disabilities. Disabilities associated with aging include visual (acuity, color sensitivity, and ocular motor control), visual search and identification of targets, manual dexterity, hearing (high frequencies blocking out noise), cognitive functioning, and requirements for mobility and stability (use of a walker, avoiding long periods of standing) (Newell, 2011).

Once online, factors of Internet use come into play. Digital skills decline with age and differ by gender. Vicente and López found that online patterns of use compared with users without disabilities showed no difference. Previous studies had indicated lower e-commerce, educational use, information retrieval, and email use for people with disabilities and elderly adults. This study indicates that the situation is changing, and more people with disabilities and older individuals are increasingly finding use of the Internet to be useful and accessible.

A 2004 study of use of cell phones by elders with disabilities revealed that 60% valued their cell phones, one third used their phones daily, and a large percentage (87%) used their phones for emergencies (Mann et al., 2004). Participants were also asked for suggestions for improving phone design. The size of the buttons was a concern for 50% of the participants. Fewer (20%–30%) suggested that the size of the display and overall size of the phone be increased and that the complexity be decreased.

Because some markets (e.g., mobile phones) are very volatile with competition driving almost constant innovation and change, devices with accessible futures built in tend to become obsolete quickly and disappear (Pedlow, Kasnitz, & Shuttleworth, 2010). Although many of the features required by seniors (including those with disabilities) are available in mainstream cell phones, they are not often all available in the same phone but rather are spread across several different manufacturers and may be difficult to access on mobile handset

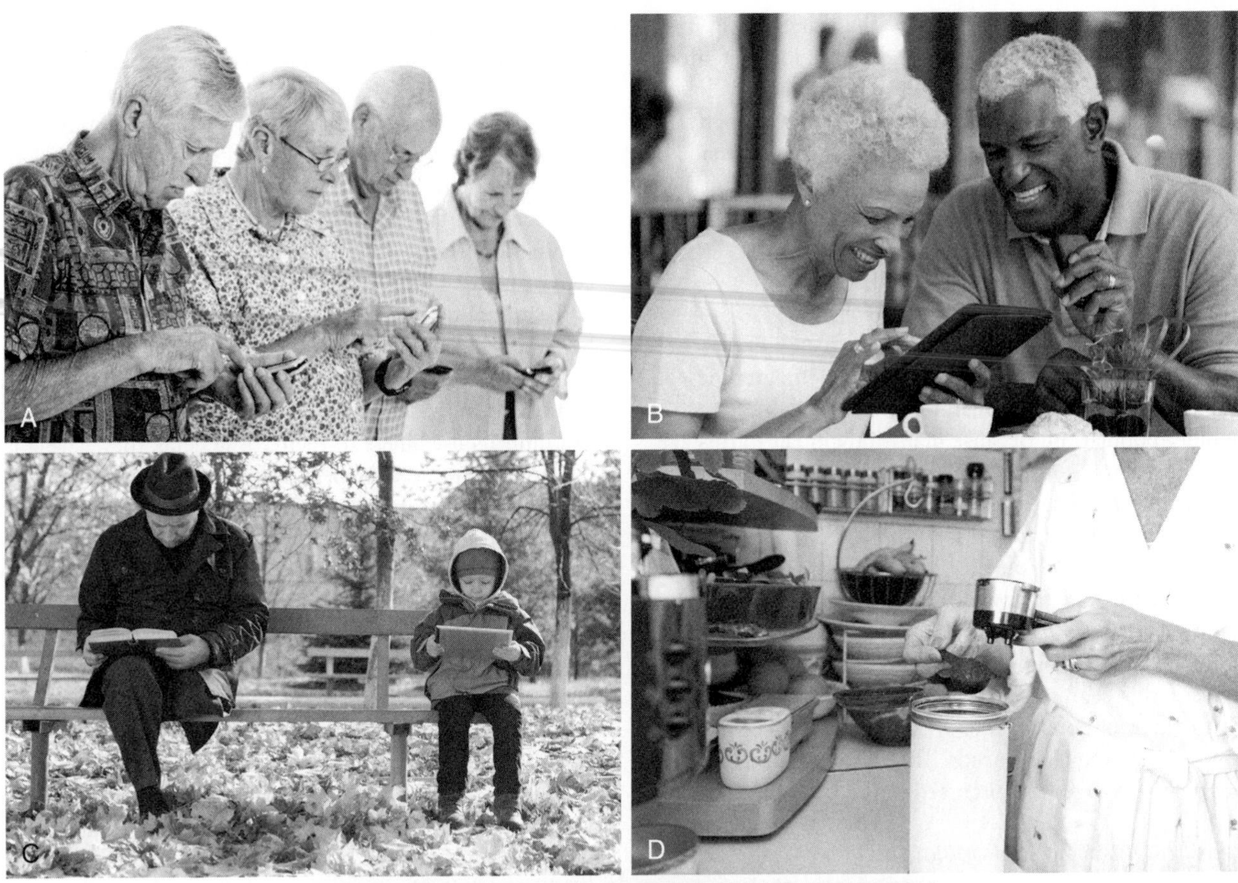

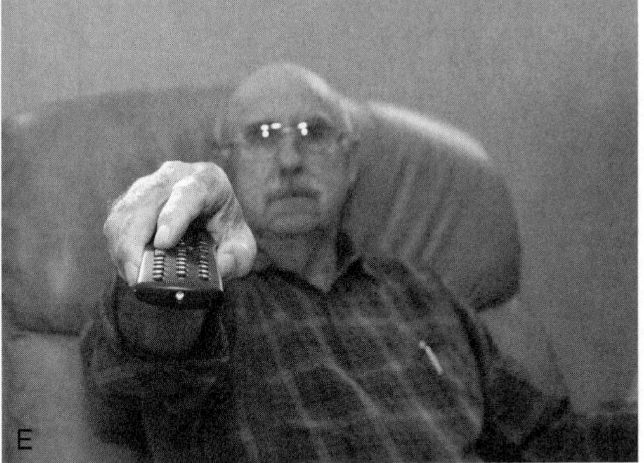

FIGURE 2-1 Seniors have varying responses to mainstream technology from total acceptance and success of use to confusion and distrust. **A:** Some seniors embrace mobile phones enthusiastically. **B:** Technologies like tablets can keep grandparents in touch with grandchildren. **C:** Technologies also differ by generation -a book for grandpa, a tablet for grandson. **D:** Even kitchen appliances are becoming smarter providing a challenge for some seniors to keep up, **E:** Entertainment is no longer just a clicker and a TV, with hundreds of channels streaming movies, new formats for music and video things are changing constantly and seniors long for the simpler times.

menus. It can also be difficult to find information about accessible features in descriptions of technical specifications.

Meeting the Needs of Individuals with Intellectual Disabilities

With the proliferation of mainstream applications, there is increased interest in meeting the needs of people with intellectual or cognitive disabilities using these devices. Cognitive ATs, some based on mainstream applications, have become more widespread (see Chapter 15). However, for many individuals with intellectual disabilities, access to mainstream mobile technologies is limited because of deficits in literacy or numerical comprehension and inherent features of the technology such as shrinking size and escalating complexity in features (Stock, Davies, Wehmeyer, & Palmer, 2008).

Stock et al. (2008) developed a multimedia cell phone with accessibility and universal design features specifically for people with intellectual disabilities. A comparison of this specially designed phone with a standard cell phone was carried out by 22 individuals with intellectual disabilities. Participants required significantly less assistance and made significantly fewer errors using the specially designed multimedia phone compared with the mainstream cell phone. Stock et al. (2008) concluded that a usability focus and the potential to use universal design principles could increase the benefits of mobile technology use for individuals with intellectual disabilities.

Because some smart phone technology operating systems are more open to application developers (e.g., Android-based devices), it is possible to develop personalized ATs based on individualized user profiles (Lewis, Sullivan, & Hoehl, 2009). Personalized profiles, possibly with features downloaded from the cloud as needed and integrated with sensors such as cameras and GPS receivers and internal features such as phone and calendar, can support a range of activities for individuals with intellectual disabilities. These features could support reminders of activities on specific days or specific times or provide navigation assistance via GPS location and a second key feature, spoken presentation of information. Lewis et al. (2009) also describe the need for applications to be useable on different manufacturers' phones, referred to as cross-platform software support. Specific benefits of cloud-based information include user preferences stored in the cloud and downloaded to any device being used, the availability of audio presentation of data across applications, and providing access to definitions of unfamiliar words (Lewis & Ward, 2011). Applications such as these are discussed further in Chapter 15.

Addressing a Global Need

"An estimated 80 per cent of all people with disabilities in the world live in rural areas of developing countries and have limited or no access to services they need" (International Labor Office, 2007, p. 1). ATs are available to meet the needs of people with disabilities, especially in the developed world. However, because these devices are very expensive, much of the world cannot acquire AT. Because it is less expensive, there is a need to use mainstream technology to meet the needs of people with disabilities through apps that function like AT devices.

Mainstream technology is globally pervasive, and its capability, especially for ICTs, is constantly increasing. (see Figure 2-2) However, much of this technology is not accessible to individuals with disabilities. Advances in technologies that are not accessible to those with disabilities can increase the gap in available resources for work, school, and community living between people who have disabilities and those who do not. As advances occur more quickly, the gap widens faster, and the people who are poor or disabled lose out even more completely and quickly. This is a characteristic of cultural and societal "progress" over centuries—technology drives change and creates both positive and negative outcomes in the process (Wright, 2004).

Primarily because of cost and the availability of suppliers, much of the world has not had access to ATs. There have been some efforts to produce products, primarily wheelchairs, using local materials and local craftspeople (Armstrong et al., 2008). Although these efforts have been locally successful in some regions, there are many types of ATs, primarily those based on computer technology, that have not been available to much of the world's population. Computer-based AT includes computer access, environmental control, cognitive ATs, and augmentative communication.

Similar to smart phones and tablets, ICTs have the capability of running AT applications previously requiring laptop or desktop computers (International Telecommunication Union [ITU], 2011). Among the thousands of applications ("apps") developed for these devices, many are directly related to addressing the needs of people with disabilities. Many more can be of benefit to people with disabilities even though they were developed for the general population. There is also recognition that ICTs can be a critical enabler to developing countries that are moving toward an information-based society. They can also provide access to society (work, family, leisure) for persons with disabilities.

Achieving widespread global availability of AT applications at an affordable local price will have to be based on mainstream devices (Emiliani et al., 2011). The largest area of growth internationally is mobile broadband Internet access, and some countries advanced between 2008 and 2010 (ITU, 2011). "Wireless-broadband access, including prepaid mobile broadband, is mushrooming in developing countries and Internet users are shifting more and more from fixed to wireless connections and devices" (p. 1). This is good news for the global application of ATs based on smart phones and tablets. However, the cost of these technologies is still too high in many developing countries, and there is a need to develop more affordable devices (ITU, 2011).

The ITU, the United Nations' specialized agency for information and communication technologies, provides an annual overview of the world's use of ICTs (ITU, 2012). The ITU has developed the ICT Development Index (IDI) that compiles 11 indicators of development in communication and technology within a country, divided into access (40%), use (40%; percentage of use of the Internet, broadband, and fixed or wired ICT), and skills (20%; based on literacy and enrollment in secondary and postsecondary education). The IDI allows a more detailed look at ICT development than measures based strictly on the number of cell phones or computers.

All of the subindices for developing countries increased between 2008 and 2011. The ITU (2012) report presents the IDI score and rank for 152 countries broken into four levels based on IDI levels. The two top levels of ICT use, penetration and skills based on the IDI, have 26% of the world's population, and the lower two levels have 74%. There is still a long way to go before the "digital divide" is narrowed substantially.

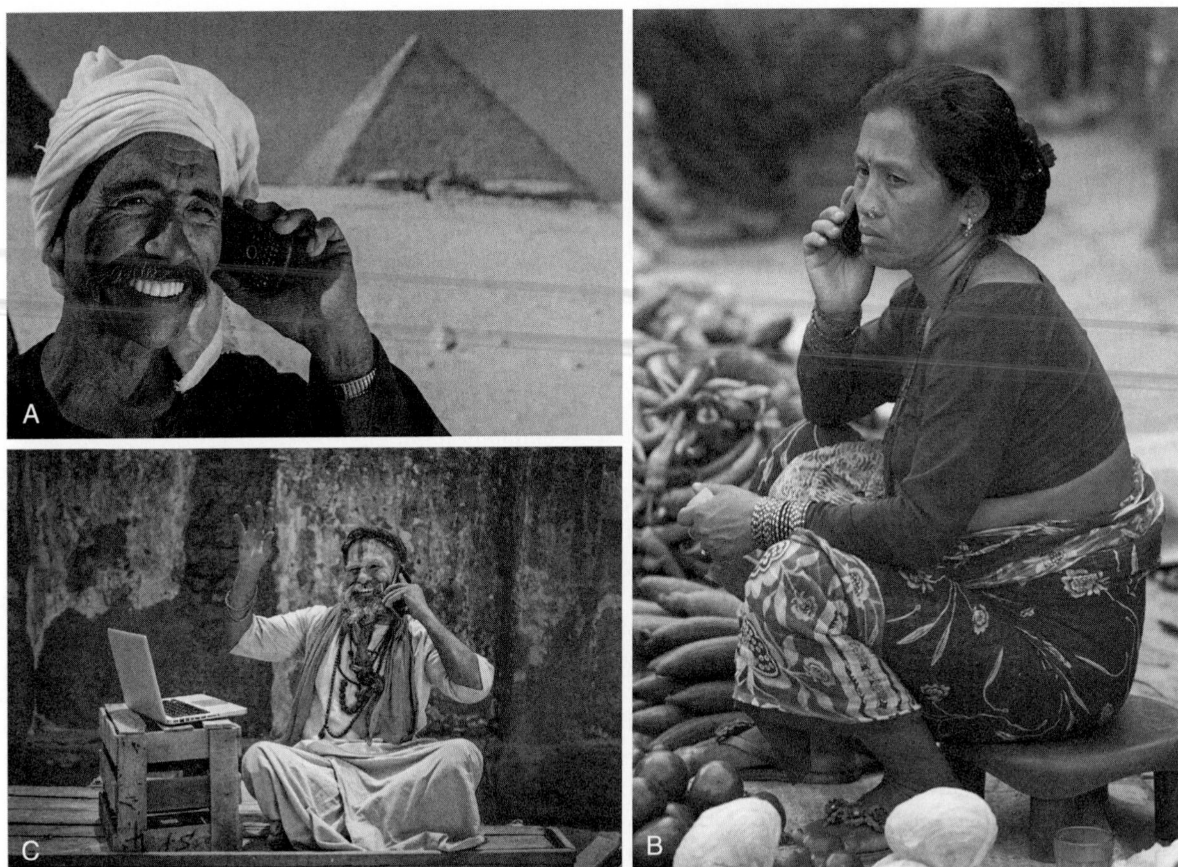

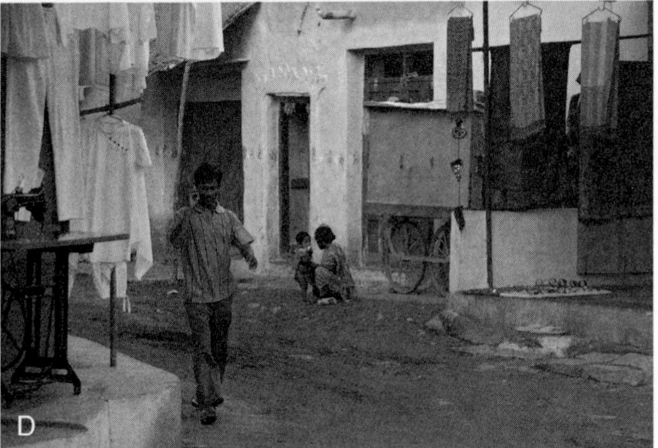

FIGURE 2-2 Use of mainstream technologies in underresourced countries has provided a platform for the development of ATs based on smart phone and tablet applications. **A:** Cell phone coverage now includes remote areas, **B:** A farmer's market is connected via mobile phone, **C:** Multiple mobile technologies are seen on the streets of under resourced countries, **D:** It is as likely to see someone walking down the street with phone to their ear in under-resourced countries as it used to be only in the developed world.

Individuals with Complex Needs

Some individuals have multiple disabilities that make design and use of technology more challenging. Medical advances have made it possible to save the lives of infants with significant pre-, peri-, and neonatal problems and of people who sustain significant trauma or insult such as traumatic brain injury or stroke. These individual are often left with impairments in multiple systems—sensory, motor, and cognitive. These multiple impairments compound limitations of activity and participation and make identification and use of AT more complex. The increased complexity of AT may be structural, resulting in additional requirements for positioning, or functionally requiring accommodation for other components such as a ventilator. Increased AT complexity might also be seen in the electronic and control components if multiple AT devices are required such as a combination of power mobility, augmentative communication, and environmental control. For example, a person with a severe disability may use a powered wheelchair controlled by a hand-operated joystick, a communication device controlled by an optical head pointer, and a remote control for TV and other appliances activated by a switch located next to the head. This array of controls and procedures for accessing them can be difficult if there is cognitive limitation as part of the disability.

Because of the increased needs and challenges presented by individuals with complex needs, the cognitive demands of operating the AT might also need to be addressed. An example is a person with a cognitive or visual impairment who may not be able to use a wheelchair independently because of the challenge of accounting for the cognitive or visual impairment when making the recommendation and use of the chair. Likewise, the recommendation of an augmentative communication device for someone with a communication impairment will be complicated by the presence of a vision impairment.

A FUNCTIONAL FRAMEWORK FOR ASSISTIVE TECHNOLOGIES

The range of technology options that provide functional assistance to individuals with disabilities is growing. Mainstream commercial devices are being used to provide functional assistance that traditionally required specially designed assistive devices. However, specialized ATs are still required in many situations. As we describe below, this combination of technologies is able to meet a continuum of needs. At one extreme are devices that provide some limited assistance or augment the individual's ability to perform a task. For example, an individual with cerebral palsy may be able to speak, but occasionally his speech may be difficult to understand. In these instances, he may clarify his speech using a letter board to spell out words not understood. Or a person with respiratory problems may be able to ambulate inside her house but, because of low endurance, may require a powered wheelchair to be able to do her grocery shopping independently. Many grocery stores now provide powered carts for individuals who need this type of augmented mobility. At the other extreme are ATs that replace significant amounts of ability to generate functional outcomes. For example, some individuals have no verbal communication ability and may require a device to be able to communicate. Likewise, some individuals are totally dependent on a manual or powered wheelchair for their personal mobility.

Hard and Soft Technologies

Odor (1984) has distinguished between *hard technologies* and *soft technologies.* Hard technologies are readily available components that can be purchased and assembled into AT systems. This includes everything from simple mouth sticks to computers and software. The PL 100-407 definition of an AT device applies primarily to hard technologies as we have defined them. The main distinguishing feature of hard technologies is that they are tangible. On the other hand, soft technologies are the human areas of decision making, strategies, training, concept formation, and service delivery as described earlier in this chapter. Soft technologies are generally captured in one of three forms: (1) people, (2) written, and (3) computer (Bailey, 1996). AT services as defined in PL 100-407 are basically soft technologies. These aspects of technology, without which the hard technology cannot be successful, are much harder to obtain because they are highly dependent on human knowledge rather than tangible objects. This knowledge is obtained slowly through formal training, experience, and textbooks such as this one. The development of effective strategies of use also has a major effect on AT system success. Initially, the formulation of these strategies may rely heavily on the knowledge, experience, and ingenuity of the AT practitioner. With growing experience, the AT user originates strategies that facilitate successful device use. The roles of both hard and soft technologies as integral portions of AT systems are discussed in later chapters.

Allocation of Functions

In any human/device system, we can allocate some functions to the human, some to the device, and some to a personal assistant. Bailey (1996) defines several approaches to **function allocation** that are used in general human factors design. Several of these are applicable to the design of AT systems and are useful when determining how and what type of AT will be beneficial to an individual. The simplest approach is *comparison allocation.* Here each task to be carried out is assigned completely to the human or the device. The user's skills define the task that can be assigned to her, and the characteristics of the technology determine which capabilities are assigned to it. For example, a telephone is designed with the assumption that the user can hold the phone, press the buttons to dial, hear the other person, and speak into the telephone. These are all functions assigned to the user. However, if the user cannot perform any of these tasks, the AT must provide an alternative set of tasks. For example, assume that a particular consumer is able to carry out all the functions except holding the phone and dialing. A Bluetooth speaker would avoid the need to hold the handset, and automatic speech recognition (see Chapter 8) could be used for entering numbers and controlling the menus. These constitute the AT component of this system. We often use comparison allocation when matching characteristics of technology to a consumer's skills.

A second allocation approach is *leftover allocation,* in which as many functions as possible are assigned to the human, and the device carries out the remainder. In AT system design, this approach is often followed to give the consumer as much natural control over his activities as possible but to provide assistance when needed. For example, some manual wheelchairs are equipped with power assist wheels that amplify the user's propulsion strokes. Thus, a person who has limited strength and endurance can propel the wheelchair manually, but the power assist wheels augment the person's abilities.

A third approach is *economic allocation,* in which the basic consideration is whether it is cheaper to select, train, and pay a personal assistant to do the activity or to design an AT system for this purpose. Often the economic analysis initially

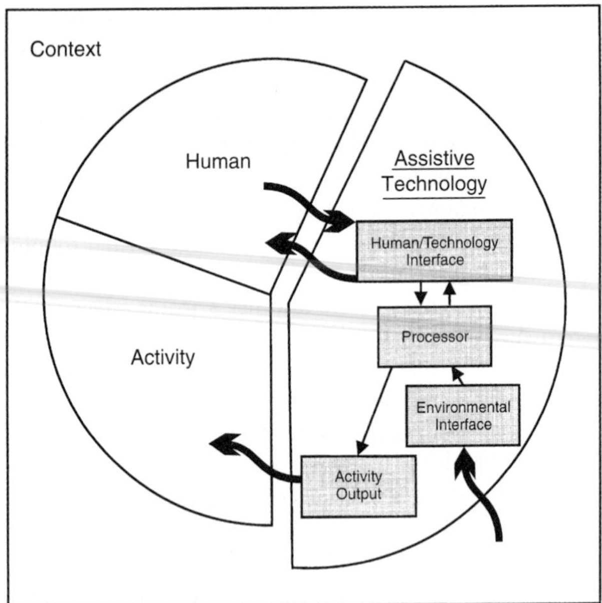

FIGURE 2-3 HAAT model with assistive technology components: identified.

favors the personal assistant because the purchase cost of the technology is relatively high. However, if the technology cost is amortized over its useful life, the technological approach may be significantly less expensive because the personal assistant cost (salary) rises over time.

The final approach is *flexible allocation.* In this approach, the user can vary his or her degree of participation in the activity based on skills and needs. Whenever possible, we use this approach in AT systems, and we couple the use of the AT system with personal assistant services (PAS). The human and technology components are not fixed in scope; rather, they change based on the specific activities and tasks to be carried out. Initially, the novice user of a cell phone may rely on intuitive skills and only use the most basic features such as dialing each number. As knowledge of the device operation increases and strategies are developed, more advanced features such as contact lists, texting, and others can be used. In this way, more tasks such as remembering numbers are assigned to the device, and the user is free to do other things.

Hard Assistive Technologies

In Chapter 1, we describe the basic structure of an AT system in terms of the four components of the HAAT model: someone (*human*) doing something (*activity*) in a specific *context* using *technology* as an enabler. Regardless of whether the technology is based on a mainstream device or is specially designed for people with disabilities and whether it is a tangible device (phone, computer, wheelchair) or a software program, we can conceptualize the AT functionality in a systematic way. Figure 2-3 illustrates the elements of the AT component.

The Human/Technology Interface

The boundary between the human user and the AT is called the **human/technology interface (HTI).** The HTI can play any of several roles in a specific AT system. It can include the means through which the user can control the AT system, the support provided to the user by the system, mounting of components for easy access by the user, and feedback provided to the user of the system regarding the environment (e.g., speech output of a scanned book for a user who is blind) or the operation of the device (e.g., a visual display of the current mode of operation in a power wheelchair, auditory feedback for alarms like low battery). When considering an assistive device for a specific individual, consideration must be made as to whether the user can see information displayed on an HTI, hear auditory output, exert sufficient force and control when manipulation is required, is properly positioned to be able to access the HTI, and has sufficient cognitive abilities to control and interpret information from the HTI.

For electronically controlled ATs (e.g., powered wheelchairs, communication devices), this element (e.g., joystick, keyboard) is the **control interface** (see Chapter 7). For electronic systems, the HTI may also include other elements. As discussed earlier in this chapter, the typical smart phone HTI has many features common to electronic ATs and requires skills consistent with those needed for those technologies.

As in a smart phone, an HTI provides input via a **user display** that portrays information to the user. For individuals with low vision (see Chapter 13) and those with hearing loss (see Chapter 14), a visual user display is usually adequate if the size is large enough. For those who are blind, the user display must be converted to either synthesized speech or a Braille display (see Chapter 13).

Reducing the complexity of the HTI can increase access for those with cognitive disabilities and for individuals who are learning to use the device. This suggestion goes against the trend to have more and more features on devices. "More thought should go into simplifying an interface, not always augmenting it" (Pullin, 2009, p. 80). To illustrate this point, Pullin uses the example of a single station radio with the physical appearance of a radio from the 1940s. This radio is usable by individuals who have dementia but intact longer term memory sufficient to remember how to turn it on and off. It is simple to use, just on/off with no tuning to find the station, and it can be used without thought. Unfortunately, "Pressure by consumer markets to compete on the basis of 'so-called' features" (Pullin, 2009, p. 69) in both ATs and mainstream products leads to more and more features that are used by fewer and fewer people.

With increasing complexity of mobile technologies, especially in the number of features and functions available, even the "average" user may become confused by the complexity (Hellman, 2007). Older individuals may have less experience with technology and have some limitations in cognitive functioning that make the use of mobile technologies even more challenging. Devices that are too complex are frequently abandoned or not used to their full potential. They take too long to learn, their use is difficult to remember if an individual hast not used them in a while, and many people do not bother to learn how to use all the functions in the first place (Hellman, 2007).

For a mechanical system such as a manual wheelchair, the HTI is the push rims used to drive the chair (see Chapter 10). Mechanical HTIs can also accommodate for differing needs. The diameter of the push rim and its location can change the mechanical advantage for the wheelchair rider. Wheelchair athletes make use of this concept in the design of their chairs. A wheelchair for sprinting will have a mechanism (hand rim diameter, wheel location and size, seat height) that differs from a wheelchair designed for marathons. A wheelchair for basketball will also differ because of the need for quick moves over shorter distances. The diameter of the hand rim tubing also affects use (Medola, Paschoarelli, Silva, Elui, & Fortulan, 2011). A larger diameter hand rim is ergonomically more effective because it distributes pressure across the hand more effectively. Experienced wheelchair users found the ergonomically designed hand rim made propulsion easier and more comfortable. For individuals with partial paralysis, a one-armed drive with a linkage between wheels can be used. Each of these mechanical mechanisms must be related to the needs of the individual user.

Another mechanical interface is hand controls for driving (see Chapter 11). These devices substitute hand function for foot function. Because the upper extremity is not as strong as the lower and the brake and accelerator of the car are designed for the lower extremity, the hand controls must provide a mechanical advantage. They are also designed to fit the hand and to allow use while also steering. This is another HTI but with a very different function than electronic controls.

Another function of the AT HTI is provision of structural support for the user (see Chapter 9). Two important factors are the amount of support required (depends on the individual) and the materials used—for longevity of the HTI and for the comfort and support to the individual. The HTI for seating also includes the interface between the person and the seat and the back of the sitting surface. The design of this interface can play a major role in minimizing acute pressure areas and redistributing overall seated pressure. The choice of materials to meet these criteria is discussed in Chapter 9.

The HTI also needs to position the control interface where it can be easily accessed (see Chapter 7). For mounting of technology (devices, controls, and displays), issues that impact access by the user are important such as flexibility, capability of moving the mounting for transfers in or out of a wheelchair, and stability for continued use (see Chapter 10).

Environmental Sensor

An **environmental sensor** is a device that can detect energy of various forms. The most common examples in mobile technologies are light sensors (cameras), sound sensors (microphones), motion sensors (accelerometers), and location sensors (GPS receivers). A major use of environmental sensing is in sensory aids for individuals with vision or hearing limitations (see Chapters 13 and 14). In the case of vision loss, the required sensor is a camera that provides an image of text on a page or objects in the environment. The environmental sensor for hearing loss is a microphone that can detect speech and other sounds.

Assistive technology applications make use of individual sensors or combinations of several sensors. An example is the iWalk smart phone app that is a navigation system for low-vision users (Stent, Azenkot, & Stern, 2010). This application combines the built-in GPS capability of the phone with automatic speech recognition and voice output to provide assistance finding and navigating to a destination for users with low vision. The user speaks information about a business destination into the microphone on the phone and the device recognizes the speech and accesses a cloud-based database and determines the user's current location via GPS. The top 10 possible business locations accessed from the cloud are presented to the user via speech output, and she can select the one to which she wishes to travel. The iWalk program then determines a routing and provides verbal directions to navigate to the desired destination.

Individuals who have cognitive disabilities also need navigation assistance that can be provided by a smart phone with GPS and speech output capability (Boulos, Anastasiou, Bekiaris, & Panou, 2011). The system also includes assistance with emergency calling for people with cognitive disabilities, including elderly adults. In some applications, environmental sensors are used to provide automatic or semiautomatic control of ATs.

Smart wheelchairs are another example of the use of environmental sensors. Defined as "either a standard power wheelchair to which a computer and a collection of [environmental sensors] have been added or a mobile robot base to which a seat has been attached" (Simpson, 2005, p. 424), these devices are useful for wheelchair users who have low vision or a severely restricted visual field, have motor impairments such as excessive tone or tremor, or who have cognitive impairments that limit their ability to navigate a wheelchair safely. Sensors on these wheelchairs are used to guide navigation in a known environment and to avoid collisions. For example, a problem often faced by individuals who have cognitive limitations (e.g., caused by dementia) and need to use a powered wheelchair is the avoidance of obstacles, including other residents. One approach to this problem is to use a "sensor skirt" added to a powered wheelchair to detect obstacles and avoid collisions (Wang, Gorski, Holliday, & Fernie, 2011).

Environmental sensing is also used in monitoring systems designed to aid a user in performing common tasks of daily living by assessing the person's current physiological state and the state of various utilities throughout the home and providing the user with feedback if he becomes disoriented or confused on a given task (Haigh, Kiff, & Ho, 2006). Sensors can also be used to detect whether an individual has taken medication and inform the caregiver. There are also significant ethics concerns about this type of invasive monitoring that we discuss in Chapter 4.

The Processor or Mechanism

In many AT systems, the input from the HTI must be altered in some way to generate an activity output. For electronic AT applications, we refer to this component as the **processor**. The processor may be relatively straightforward such as the

TABLE 2-3 Typical Processor Functions for Electronic AT

Function Name	Description	Examples
Transformation	Conversion from one type of energy (e.g., electrical) to another (e.g., mechanical) or visual to auditory or tactile or vice versa	Braille reader that converts visual information from a camera to tactile information on a Braille display (see Chapter 13)
Amplification	Increases the strength of the required mechanical or electrical energy	Hearing aid (see Chapter 14), screen magnifier (see Chapter 13), power assist wheelchair rims (see Chapter 10)
Managing information	Storage and retrieval of data from internal or cloud-based sources	Vocabulary for augmentative communication (see Chapter 16), configurations for individual users of smart phones (see Chapter 8), stored functions in controller for power wheelchair (see Chapter 10) or for electronic aids for daily living (see Chapter 12), maps or routing information for navigation (see Chapters 13 and 15)
Configuration	Loads user profiles that include ideal parameters for a particular user	Setup for computer access or controller for power wheelchair
Output	Generates control signals for activity outputs	Motor control signals sent to powered wheelchair motors based on an internal controller
Manipulate data	Software programs that perform functions necessary to process sensory information and generate appropriate outputs	Optical character recognition software for screen readers, automatic speech recognition software, and digital processing of speech in a hearing aid to separate speech from noise; powered wheelchair motor speed control based on joystick input

TABLE 2-4 Typical Mechanism Functions for Mechanical Assistive Technologies

Function Name	Description	Examples
Transformation	Converts one type of mechanical energy (e.g., translation) to another (rotation) to accommodate for motor abilities	Lever arms used for manual wheelchair propulsion
Augmentation	Increases mechanical advantage	Relative size of push rim diameter to wheel diameter determines "gearing" like a bicycle hub
Linkage	Connects the user action to the desired output	The internal linkage in a mechanical reacher that converts user grip to reacher end effector grasp

amplification of sound from a microphone in a hearing aid (see Chapter 14) or very complex such as the control required for the smart wheelchair (see Chapter 10). In all cases, the input signal is received from the user, it is modified in some way by the processor, and then an activity output is generated.

With advances in electronics, much more sophisticated processing can be accomplished. For example, hearing aids can be designed to separate speech from background noise (see Chapter 14). Navigation systems such as iWalk (Stent et al., 2010) use sophisticated processing embedded in software programs. Typical processor functions are listed in Table 2-3. Various combinations of these functions may be found in computers, mobile technologies such as smart phones and tablets, and purpose-built ATs. Increasingly, processor functions receive input information from embedded intelligence (e.g., the cloud) as well as data stored in the device.

Some mechanical AT systems have no need for any processing (e.g., simple aids to daily living). For other mechanical AT systems, there are processor-like functions that we refer to as **mechanisms.** One definition of a mechanism is "the arrangement of connected parts in a machine" (http://www.thefreedictionary.com/mechanism). The linkages that connect the hand rims on a manual wheelchair to the wheels are an example of an AT mechanism. Another example is the linkage between the gripper and the claw end on a mechanical reacher. Just as for the processor, the mechanism has functions that can aid the user of the AT. Some typical mechanism functions are shown in Table 2-4.

Activity Outputs

As a result of the input by the user through the HTI and the internal processing of relevant information, the AT generates an output that is relevant to the chosen activity. We call this the **activity output.** Types of activity outputs from the user to the environment are communication (see Chapter 16), mobility (see Chapters 10 and 11), manipulation (see Chapter 12), and cognitive processing (see Chapter 15). The output may be in the form of mechanical energy causing movement (e.g., powered wheelchair motors, motor to lift a spoon in feeding device, motors for a robotic arm) or mechanical pins used to render text in Braille. Alternatively, the output may be in electronic form (e.g., synthetic speech for communication devices or screen readers for the blind, visual images on a screen) or printed (e.g., a map for orientation and mobility assistance in cognitive disability or prompting commands for cognitive assist in task completion). The purpose of these output components is to link human interactions (e.g., pressing a switch) to activity (e.g., moving or speaking) in an assistive or augmentative way.

Soft Assistive Technologies

Assistive technology services are defined in the United States AT law, PL 100-407 as "Any service that directly assists an individual with a disability in the selection, acquisition or use of an AT device."

The law also includes several specific examples that further clarify this definition. These include (1) evaluating needs and skills for AT; (2) acquiring ATs; (3) selecting, designing, repairing, and fabricating AT systems; (4) coordinating services with other therapies; and (5) training both individuals with disabilities and those working with them to use the technologies effectively. The United Nations Convention on the Rights of Persons with Disabilities (UNCRPD) also specifies access to training in the use of AT as well as access to service delivery and training of professionals to prescribe and support the use of AT.

To account for these aspects of AT services, Odor (1984) called these areas of service delivery **soft technologies.** Hard technologies are those that we have discussed in the majority of this chapter; they are readily available components that can be purchased and assembled into AT systems. This includes everything from simple mouth sticks to computers and software. The definition of an AT device applies primarily to hard technologies as we have defined them. The main distinguishing feature of hard technologies is that they are tangible. On the other hand, soft technologies are the human areas of decision making, strategies, and concept formation applied to service delivery in proper assessment, system or device selection, and fitting or setup. Training, mentoring, and technical support are ongoing forms of soft technologies. Soft technologies can be provided in a number of forms such as (1) directly through people (e.g., professional providers, family, informal care providers); (2) written manuals, tip sheets, and other documents; or (3) electronic (e.g.. built-in help screens, online help, websites). By labeling these aspects as another technology, they become more tangible. Without these aspects of technology, the full potential benefit of the use of hard technology is limited. Many people do not receive education or training in the use of their devices, so they do not realize the full potential benefit of the AT.

Soft technologies are difficult to acquire because they are highly dependent on human knowledge rather than tangible objects. This knowledge is obtained slowly through formal training, experience, and textbooks such as this one. The development of effective strategies of use also has a major effect on AT system success. Initially, the formulation of these strategies may rely heavily on the knowledge, experience, and ingenuity of the AT practitioner. With growing experience, the AT user originates strategies that facilitate successful device use. For example, Norman (2002) found that people tend to blame themselves for errors in a system and fail to report a system failure because they think it is their fault. In AT applications, this is the direct result of inadequate soft technologies.

A major area of soft technology application is the fitting of assistive devices to meet the needs of individual users. For example, current wheelchairs (see Chapter 10) are often multifunctional, with a number of components on the wheelchair being adjustable. Some adjustments and settings are made in the factory before shipping, but typically the provider of the wheelchair will need to make modifications to fit the chair to the user after it arrives from the factory. Adjustments to the wheelchair that can make a difference in user comfort, safety, and performance include axle position, wheel chamber, and wheel alignment.

Another major form of soft technology is training of the user to successfully use the hard technology. Effective use of a wheelchair requires a systematic training program (see Chapter 10). In some cases, this soft technology is available as a program. One well-researched training program is the Wheelchair Skills Program (Kirby, 2005), which is available from http://www.wheelchairskillsprogram.ca. The program teaches wheelchair users basic use of a wheelchair, such as applying and releasing the brakes, removing footrests, and folding the chair. It teaches basic propulsion such as rolling forward and backward and turning and maneuvering through doorways. More advanced skills include propulsion on an incline, level changes, performance of a wheelie, and various wheelie skills.

To overcome the challenges of lack of access to mobile phones and use of features by individuals with disabilities and seniors, thoughtfully developed and implemented training programs are required. In one study of individuals age 14 to 80 years learning cell phone functions, the importance of soft technologies was underlined. The training began with a matching of the user's motor, sensory, and cognitive skills to a cell phone type. The basic features were taught until they were understood. Advanced features (e.g., speed dialing, SMS texting, storage and retrieval of numbers) were taught in subsequent sessions. An ABA pre-post evaluation was conducted. "The successful outcomes obtained required knowledge of all of the features on the available phones, a careful assessment of the participant's needs and comprehensive user training, both initially and when requested" (Nguyen, Garrett, Downing, Walker, & Hobbs, 2007, p. 90).

Pedlow et al. (2010) provided a cell phone, airtime, and individual support to seniors from 66 to 90 years of age who had a variety of impairments. The 1-month trial identified barriers that included a realization that this group is "deterred from cell phone use as much by the confusing structure of the industry as by the lack of certain handset features" (p. 147). Pedlow et al. concluded that availability of what we are calling soft technology supports can make a difference, but the specific kinds of support needed and how best to deliver it has not been determined.

One of the major types of soft technologies is assessment to determine the specific needs of an individual and to match ATs to those needs. We discuss general characteristics of this process in Chapter 5 and factors related to specific types of ATs in subsequent chapters. Ineffective or inappropriate assessment can have significant impacts for disabled consumers. For example, the choice of a seating system to ensure tissue integrity requires expertise in seated pressure management, biomechanical principles, and clinical insight (see Chapter 9). No matter how good the hard technology (e.g., a pressure redistribution cushion) is, errors in the soft technology areas of assessment, fitting, and training (e.g., pressure redistribution strategies) can result in skin breakdown with loss of work, possible hospitalization, and other significant impacts.

Assistive technologies for vision may serve either reading or mobility (see Chapter 13). Errors in assessment and training for a reading application may result in loss of information for the user. Although this is a significant factor, it is not the same as the possible impact of errors in mobility that could result in failure to detect a drop off or a street crossing resulting in injury or death. That is why there is an entire soft technology discipline devoted to orientation and mobility training for individuals with significant visual limitations.

Technology Options for Meeting the Needs of Individuals Who Have Disabilities

Technologies that assist individuals who have disabilities can come from two main sources, mainstream or products designed specifically for individuals with disabilities. Mainstream off-the-shelf products, including those with universal design principles incorporated, can often meet the needs of individuals who have a wide range of disabilities. The greater the diversity of the people who are to have access to technologies, the more complex the technology is likely to become. Figure 2-4 illustrates some of the design features that can impact usability of technologies by persons with disabilities. All of the technology options can be considered functionally within the AT framework presented in the previous section.

The Virtue of Simplicity

Sometimes clinicians focus on the AT and prescribe devices with the laudable aim of enabling function. What is often forgotten is that people have different tolerances for complexity of devices and varying beliefs regarding the utility of technology. These aspects need to be factored in when making AT recommendations. There is a term that originated in prosthetics called *gadget tolerance*. What this means is the degree to which an individual can tolerate complexity in technology. For AT, it also means the amount of "stuff" that can be in and around a person's personal space and still be comfortable. For example, a person faced with multiple controls for several devices, including a powered wheelchair (hand-operated joystick), a communication device (optical head pointer), and an entertainment remote control (activated by a switch located next to the head) may be overwhelmed, but other individuals actually enjoy the complexity of control.

We value simplicity because of the complexity of the world in general. "Fitness for purpose not only implies that something does what it needs to do well, but also that it is not compromised by doing more than it has to" (Pullin, 2009, p. 67). For example, seniors often do not use phone features that would help them because they find them difficult to understand (Nguyen et al., 2007). One approach to decreasing complexity is to limit operation to only basic functions initially and then add additional features as needed (Leung, Findlater, McGranere, Graf, & Yang, 2010). Another option is to build "senior-friendly" phones that have larger buttons; fewer, more intuitive functions; and larger screens (Pedlow et al., 2010). A number of these are available in Europe, North America, and Japanese markets. The downside of these applications is that they can stigmatize seniors as being less functional because they require "special" technologies.

Complementary Approaches

Mainstream design is increasing the ways it can meet the needs of a range of people by broadening the concept of user-centered design from physical ergonomics to include cultural diversity and individual identity (Pullin, 2009). But ATs that are designed for narrow populations are generally more expensive and have fewer capabilities than mainstream technologies. The dilemma of a specialized design that meets the needs of a few versus a more general design that meets the needs of many but not all and often increases complexity in doing so has been approached from a different point of view by Pullin (2009, p. 92).

> *I would like to propose the term resonant design for a design intended to address the needs of some people with a particular disability and other people without that disability but perhaps finding themselves in particular circumstances. So this is neither design just for able-bodied people nor design for the whole population; nor even does it assume that everyone with a particular disability will have the same needs. It is something between these extremes, not as a compromise, but as a fundamental aspiration.*

Pullin is saying that specialized features may be of interest to individuals who are not disabled as well as those who are. This approach recognizes that disability is not a constant state of being but is dynamic and changing under environmental, physiological, or social conditions for each of us. Within any context, our abilities change depending on our state of mind, the activity, and all of the other environmental and human characteristics. Pullin (2009) cites the example of an "urban mobility cape," a garment that could be used by wheelchair riders, cyclists, and scooter riders to protect them from rain. The design of such an item would be driven by the need for protection from the weather, not by whether the person had a disability or not or for that matter whether the person used a wheelchair, bicycle, or scooter. "Ergonomically designed" food preparation utensils such as can openers, slicers, peelers, and large-button microwave oven panels make cooking easier for all of us, but they are of particular value to individuals with limited hand strength or fine motor control because of disability or aging. Resonant design addresses needs and functional abilities, not compensation for disability as in ATs or meeting everyone's needs as in universal design.

For electronic ATs (e.g., augmentative communication, computer access, appliance control, sensory aids, cognitive ATs), inclusion of the principles of universal design together with the incorporation of accessibility features in mainstream products has opened new opportunities for people with disabilities. However, universal design

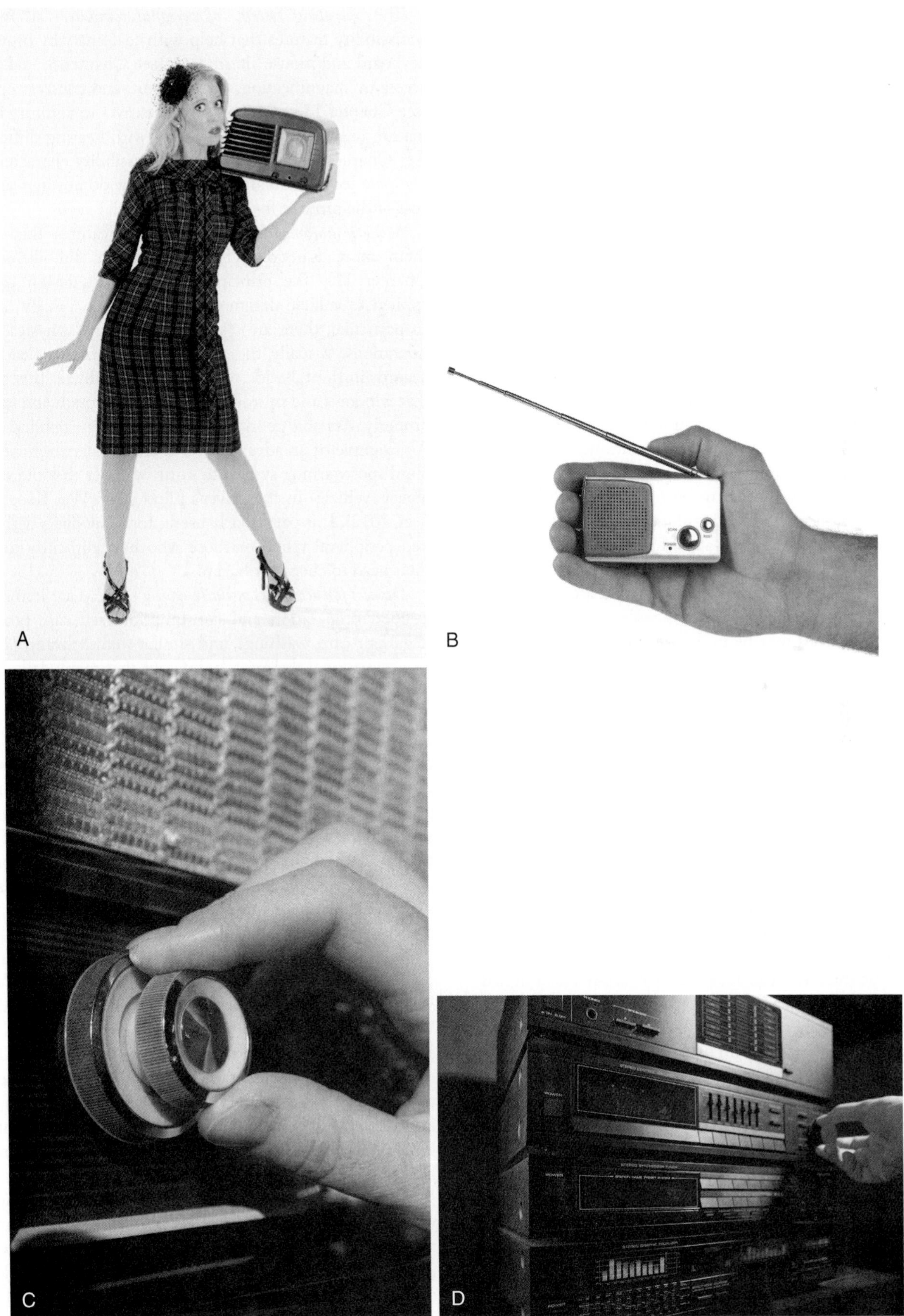

FIGURE 2-4 The variety of design approaches that can help or hinder applications for individuals with disabilities include overall size (**A** and **B**) and the degree of complexity of controls (**C** and **D**).

does not completely eliminate the need for ATs because the variety and complexity of individual needs are too great for inclusion in a single product (Emiliani, 2006). For these AT application areas, two complementary approaches—universal design and specialized ATs—are required (Emiliani et al., 2011). Both approaches require the use of mainstream technologies because low-cost AT depends on the use of mainstream products that have useful AT application features. Mainstream products are likely to be more accessible to people with disabilities even if they are not specifically designed with those individuals in mind, that is, using universal design principles (Emiliani et al., 2011).

The result of the combination of mainstream and specialized technologies is a much broader range of available options. Figure 2-5 illustrates this concept. Each row represents a level of adaptation in technology to more closely meet individual needs. Each column represents the degree to which the technology focuses specifically on disability applications. The first column, mainstream commercial products, has no specific focus on disability but may have universal design features. This column also includes mainstream application software (apps) for mobile technologies such as smart phones and tablet computers. The middle column describes software applications that are specifically developed to meet the needs of people with disabilities. These applications may be in the form of a computer program that runs on notebook computers, apps for tablet or smart phone technologies, or applications that are embedded in the environment (i.e., cloud applications) (Emiliani et al., 2011).

Commercially Available Mainstream Products

Using technologies to meet the needs of persons with disabilities can be seen from two different perspectives, the AT perspective and universal design. The first row of Figure 2-5 describes commercially available mainstream products that can be purchased for use directly by an individual with a disability without any additional modifications. *Commercially available* refers to devices that are mass produced and available off the shelf. These include commercial devices designed for the general population (standard commercially available devices) and commercially available AT devices that are mass produced for individuals with disabilities. The entries shown in Figure 2-5 illustrate the diversity of mainstream products that have features that make them usable by a range of people with disabilities.

Features That Make Off-the-Shelf Products Useful for Persons with Disabilities

The AT portion of the HAAT models that we described earlier in this chapter provides a framework for looking at useful features of mainstream products. The degree to which mainstream products meet the characteristics described for the ATs, the more likely they will be useful for people with disabilities. Figure 2-6 shows examples of mainstream technology advances that benefit people who have disabilities.

The *operating systems of personal computers* all include accessibility features that help with text entry by providing keyboard and mouse alternatives (see Chapter 8); aid visual access by magnification, voice output, and contrast options (see Chapter 13); and provide alternatives to auditory information (e.g., alerts) for individuals with hearing difficulties (see Chapter 14). Because these accessibility characteristics are included as premarket features, they do not increase the cost of the product for people with special needs.

Modern automobiles have standard features that make them more functional for people with disabilities (see Chapter 11). The principles of universal design can be applied to vehicle design (Polgar, Shaw, & Vrkljan, 2005). In particular, there are visual, cognitive, and physical considerations. Visually, the driver must be able to clearly see hazards in front, beside, and behind the vehicle. This means that windows and mirrors must be large enough and located properly to enable good sightlines and minimize blind spots. An example of an advanced feature in modern vehicles is a blind spot warning system to notify a driver that there is an object (vehicle) in the driver's blind spot (Wu, Kao, Li, & Tsai, 2012). It is particularly useful for individuals with limited peripheral vision or those who have difficulty turning their head to check for hazards.

Devices for activities of daily living (ADLs) are items used in food preparation and consumption, self-care products (e.g., hair care, washing), and similar items. Swann (2007), an occupational therapist, points out that many daily living products such as suction nail brushes, nonslip matting, water temperature detectors, swivel-bladed vegetable peelers, and long-handled dustpans and brushes were once thought of as assistive devices but are now available in supermarkets and pharmacies. Often these items have enlarged handles for grasping, designs that require less force to operate, or nonslip grips. While making use easier for everyone, they are of particular benefit to individuals with limited fine motor control or hand strength or reach (e.g., a long-handled hair brush or shoe horn). Most people have items at home that began as assistive devices.

User-friendly websites are accessible to everyone, including those with motor, sensory, or cognitive disabilities. The World Wide Web Consortium Web Accessibility Initiative (W3C WAI; http://www.w3.org/WAI) develops guidelines that serve as the international standard for web accessibility. Their support materials include special considerations for specific disabilities and for aging individuals. The WAI also provides information for evaluating websites for accessibility, guidelines for developing accessible websites, and many documents aimed at making the web as accessible to everyone as possible.

The characteristics of **mainstream smart phones** equipped with a variety of sensors and a GPS antenna provide opportunities to create capabilities equivalent to special purpose AT (Doughty, 2011). Features of smart phones and capabilities of operating systems vary by manufacturer. Limitations of this approach include flexibility of the user interface (see Chapter 8), uniform mobile coverage across rural and urban regions and countries, and increasing power demands because apps use

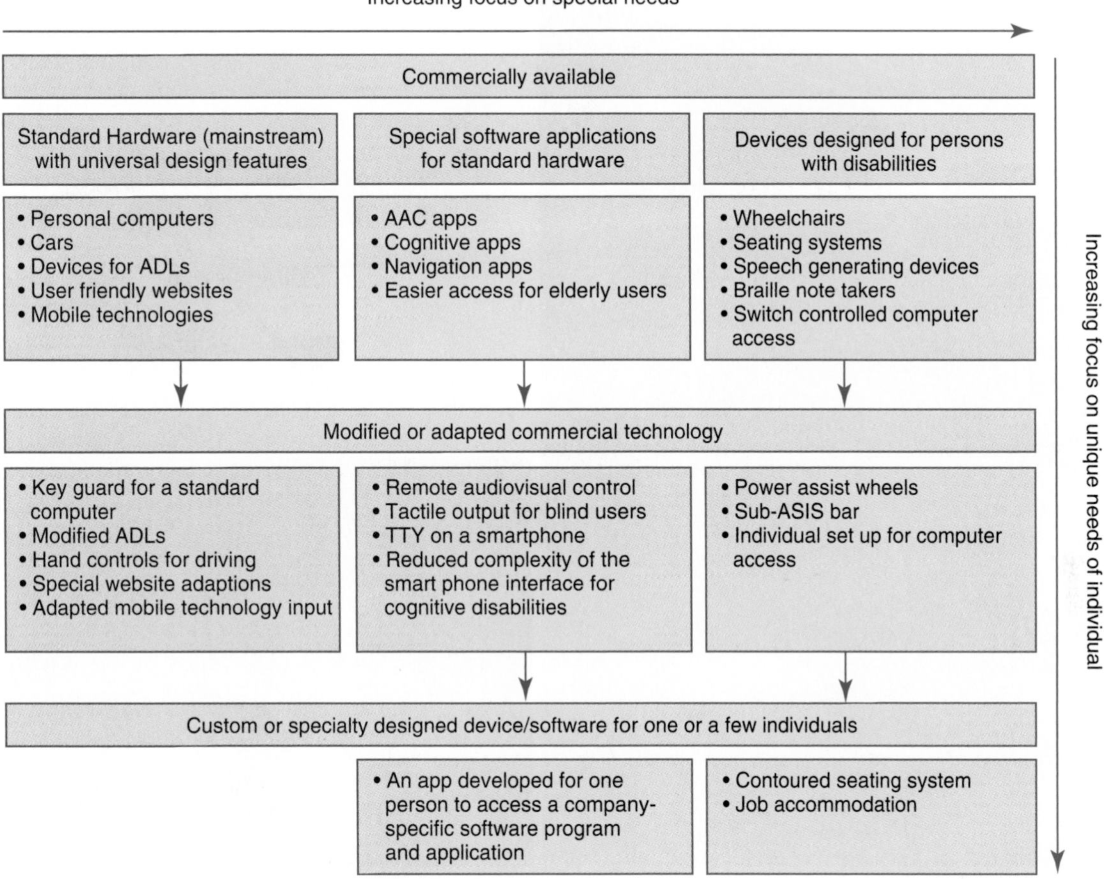

FIGURE 2-5 The range of technology options available to meet the need of individuals who have disabilities. See text. Entries are examples in each of the major categories.

more phone resources and sensors and are used for longer periods of time in AT applications than standard shorter interactions typical of voice or text messaging (Doughty, 2011).

Modified or Adapted Mainstream Commercial Technology

The middle row of Figure 2-5 describes specific modifications to the items in the first row to allow them to meet the needs of people with disabilities whose abilities do not match the functional requirements of the basic commercial products in the first row. Sanford (2012) argues that whereas specialized design increases the function of design for individuals or groups of individuals by allowing the person to adapt to everyday design, universal design (embodied in the first row in Figure 2-5) aims to increase functionality of everyday design for everyone. The reason that specialized designs exists is that universal design is not completely universal. There will always be individuals who fall outside of the broad design parameters of universal design. Fortunately, the scope of universally designed products continues to broaden, and more and more individuals are able to take advantage of more usable products. For the foreseeable future, the middle row of Figure 2-5 will be required, and as we have pointed out, more and more advances in ATs will find their way into the mainstream, contributing to the achievement of the principles of universal design in mainstream products. The device modifications in the middle row of Figure 2-5 are sometimes called *specialized design*.

Some persons may be able to select individual keys directly, but they may occasionally miss the desired key and enter the wrong key. An example of an adaptation to a standard keyboard is for individuals who have difficulty in accurately targeting and activating keys is a *key guard* placed over the keyboard that helps by isolating each key and guiding the person's movement. A key guard is also useful for individuals who produce a lot of extraneous movement each time they bring their hands off the keyboard in their attempt to target a new key. Key guards are commercially available for common computer keyboards (see Chapter 7).

Modified ADLs for food preparations include one-handed holders for can and jar opening, brushes with suction cups for one-handed scrubbing of vegetables, bowls with suction cup bottoms for stability while stirring with one hand, bowl and pan holders (some of which tilt for pouring), and cutting boards that stabilize food during cutting. Modified handles are available for knives and serving spoons, as well as for other utensils. Modifications to plates include suction cups for stability, enlarged rims that make it easier to scoop food onto a utensil, and removable rims that attach to any plate. Drinking aids include cups with caps and "snorkel" lids through which

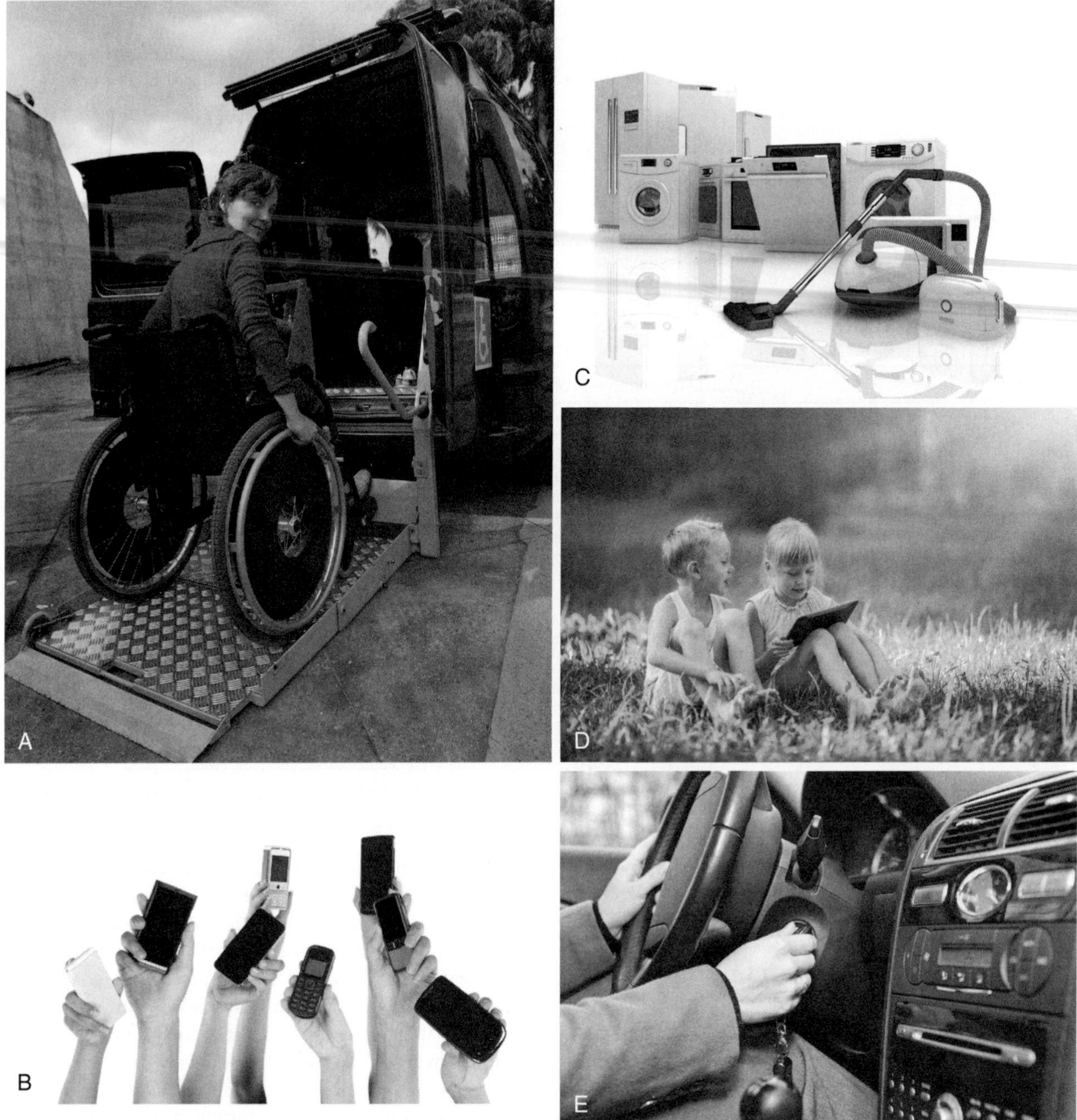

FIGURE 2-6 Advances in mainstream technologies that make them more useable by individuals with disabilities of all ages include information and communication technologies, appliances, and automobiles. **A:** Automobile are adapted to accommodate wheelchairs, **B:** There are many more options for all types of mobile technologies like cell phones, **C:** Home appliances are "smarter" and require less physical ability to use, **D:** Mobile devices like tablets are becoming more and more user friendly to accommodative a range of cognitive abilities, **E:** Mainstream automobiles are also smarter with more options that help individuals with dishabilles.

fluid can be sucked, nose cutouts that allow drinking to occur without tipping the head back, double-handled cups for two-handed use, and cups modified at the bottom with a quad grasp to allow lifting and tipping with limited hand function (see Chapter 12).

Adaptations to the standard automobile may be necessary for individuals who have lower extremity weakness or paralysis. *Hand controls* for accelerators and brakes consist of a mechanical linkage connected to each pedal, a control handle, and associated connecting hardware (see Chapter 11). The driver activates the brakes by pushing on a lever in a direction directly away from him parallel to the steering column. Acceleration is accomplished by pulling back on the control, rotating it, or pulling downward at a right angle to the steering column. The weight of the user's hand is sufficient to maintain a constant velocity.

Despite the continuing developments in mainstream computer and mobile technologies, there are still challenges for use by individuals who have motor disabilities. One approach, called Tecla (http://komodoopenlab.com/tecla), provides *adapted mobility technology input* by creating an alternative access interface for mobile technologies that also links to all the available apps. The Tecla shield allows an individual to use her standard AT interface (e.g., wheelchair joystick or single switches) to control either an iOS (iPhone, iPod Touch, or iPad) or Android device. This and similar devices are discussed further in Chapter 8.

Commercially Available Software Applications ("Apps") That Assist People with Disabilities

Assistive Technology Software Applications for Standard Hardware

The middle column of Figure 2-5 describes software applications that enable AT applications for mainstream technologies. Included in this category are applications for desktop and laptop computers, smart phones, and tablets. This area is expanding quickly with tablets, smart phones, and other platforms in addition to laptop computers. Commercial versions of these programs have traditionally been available thorough specific manufacturers. Programs written to convert standard computers into *augmentative communication systems* have been in existence for more than 25 years. More recently, the availability of more sophisticated mobile technologies (smart phones and tablets) has resulted in an explosion of "apps," which are application programs that perform some augmentative communication functions (see Chapter 16) (Gosnell, Costello, & Shane, 2011). For the past 10 years or so, there have been applications on personal digital assistants (PDAs) for individuals who have cognitive limitations. Many of these are now available as *cognitive assist* apps (Stock et al., 2008). Because most mobile technologies now include GPS capability, embedded systems can also support *navigation assistance* for individuals who are blind (Angin & Bhargava, 2011) or those with cognitive limitations such as dementia (Boulos et al., 2011). Smart phone apps can also provide easier *access for elderly users* (Olwal, Lachanas, & Zacharouli, 2011). Applications designed to meet the needs of specific populations are discussed in subsequent chapters.

The model for delivery of these programs has shifted from independent companies—as in the case of the augmentative communication applications—to "app stores" that provide access to a large number of downloadable programs (iTunes for the iPhone, iPod, and iPad, http://store.apple.com/ca; https://play.google.com/store for Android-based smart phones). Many apps developed for the general population can be useful to individuals with disabilities. These include productivity, educational, and recreational apps. Some AT manufacturers also supply apps for specific applications. These are described in subsequent chapters. A note of caution to readers: it can be difficult to determine easily if an app will work or not until it is bought and downloaded.

The primary motor and sensory access challenges in this area are those described earlier in relation to access to mainstream technologies by individuals with various disabilities. The cognitive demands of various apps are extremely variable and must be considered before recommending a specific app for an individual with a cognitive disability (see Chapter 16).

The major attraction of these apps and the associated mainstream technology is that they are typically much less expensive than purpose-built ATs, and they can easily be purchased by individuals. This can lead to families buying an app hoping that it will meet their child's need and then taking it to a clinician to implement it. This process bypasses the typical assessment process based on needs and skills (see Chapter 5). The clinician is faced with the dilemma of either conducting a proper assessment, the outcome of which might a recommendation of the mobile technology and app that the parents have purchased, but assessment might also lead to another choice of AT judged to more appropriately meet the needs of the child. It is not simply a matter of making an app work for a child; rather, it is a case of choosing an app that will most appropriately meet the needs of the child. "Some service providers for people with disabilities have also been reluctant in exploiting the full potential of [mobile technology apps], as their role and incentives is based on having clients come to them for evaluation and fitting of special assistive technologies" (Emiliani et al., 2011, p. 108).

The proliferation of apps also has resulted in a widely variable level of quality. Apps vary in how robust they are, how reliable they are, and how much support is available. Training in the use of an application is not available if the app is downloaded by a family directly. For complex applications such as augmentative communication, training and ongoing support are essential for success (see Chapter 16). Often the need for training and ongoing support is not recognized. Public funding sources (e.g., Medicare in the United States) will often support the purchase of commercially available AT products. The same sources of funding will often refuse to purchase mainstream technologies with equivalent functionality despite a significantly lower cost. They also do not routinely cover the cost of training in the use of the technology. Despite these limitations, there is value in many of the apps if they are truly matched to the needs of the person with a disability. A number of clinicians have worked to develop databases about apps with user information and evaluations. Many of these are discussed in subsequent chapters.

Modified or Adapted Software Application Programs

The vast majority of apps for mobile phones and tablets do not require any additional hardware or adaptation. There are some cases, however, in which the built-in mobile technology capabilities do not meet the individual's need. One of those is *remote controls for audiovisual equipment*. These controls are essential elements in electronic aids to daily living (EADLs) (see Chapter 12) because they can be used by individuals with limited mobility or fine motor skills to control appliances. Many home entertainment centers (DVD players, Blu-ray disc players, CD players) use infrared control signals, a feature not found in mobile technologies. There are apps that replace the standard remote, but they all require an additional infrared transmitter to allow sending infrared commands (Kumin, 2010).

Individuals who are blind often make use of electromechanical devices that present Braille characters based on text output for computers (see Chapter 13). These devices are not portable in general and can be very expensive. An alternative is to develop tactile output methods for use with mobile technologies (Rantala et al., 2009). Various approaches to this problem are discussed in Chapter 13.

Individuals who are deaf often use text messaging, but there is also a special format for texting used by these individuals called TTY (see Chapter 14). TTY phones can be cumbersome and not very portable. They also lack many of the features of current smart phones. Zafrulla, Etherton, and Starner (2008) developed an app that emulates *TTY on a smart phone.* An important feature of this app is that it links to TTY technology installed in all emergency call centers in the United States and elsewhere.

Apps can also *reduce the complexity of the smart phone interface* for people with cognitive disabilities (Verstockt, Decoo, Van Nieuwenhuyse, De Pauw, & Van De Wall, 2009). The physical interface is made more usable and additional features, such as photo-based GPS and other content management features useful to people with cognitive disabilities and seniors, are added.

Custom- or Specially Designed Software for One or a Few Individuals

In some works settings, it may be necessary to develop a *specialized software application* to allow a user's device to interface to the company computer. This is most likely in computer-controlled manufacture ring operations.

Technology Specifically Designed for Persons with Disabilities

When an individual's needs for technology assistance cannot be met with a mainstream commercial device, we attempt to meet their needs with special devices that are mass produced and specifically designed for persons with disabilities. Examples are shown in the right column of Figure 2-5. Small AT device manufacturers must often develop technically sophisticated products for small disability markets of individuals with complex needs (Bauer & Lane, 2006). They are very familiar with the segment of the disabled population they serve, including reimbursement and distribution issues. However, they often lack the financial and technical resources of mainstream manufacturers. The changing demographics related to aging and disability are making AT markets more attractive to mainstream manufacturers. Collaborative relationships combining the resources of large corporations with the specialized expertise of niche-focused AT companies are developing. This will create the opportunity for new AT products to be developed in shorter timeframes, with broader distribution (Bauer & Lane, 2006).

Commercially Available Assistive Technology Products

When an off-the-shelf mainstream product, including an assistive application program is not available, there are many devices specifically designed to meet the needs of individuals who have disabilities. Examples of these devices are shown in the first row of the right-hand column of Figure 2-5. The major categories of ATs covered in this text are seating and positioning systems (see Chapter 9); adapted human user interface for computer and mobile mainstream technologies (see Chapters 6 to 8); devices that assist upper extremity function for manipulative tasks, including EADLs (see Chapter 11), assisted mobility (personal using walkers, manual and powered wheelchairs) (see Chapter 10) and adaptations for vehicle transportation (see Chapter 11); sensory aids for vision (see Chapter 13) and hearing (see Chapter 14); cognitive ATs (see Chapter 15); and alternative and augmentative communication (see Chapter 16).

Modified or Adapted Assistive Technology

Although ATs meet the needs of a wide range of individuals, some require additional adaptations to make the AT effective for them. Several examples are listed in Figure 2-5.

Individuals who use a manual wheelchair can develop shoulder pain. One option for individuals with shoulder pain that limits their ability to propel a manual wheelchair but for whom an electrically powered wheelchair is not desirable is push rim-activated power-assist wheels (see Chapter 10). These wheels are interchanged with those of a manual wheelchair. A motor is located in the hub of the rear wheels that is linked to the hand rims (Algood, Cooper, Fitzgerald, Cooper, & Boninger, 2005). The *power-assist wheels* supply power to the manual wheelchair as needed by the user. When the user applies force above a preset level to the hand rims, such as when going up an incline, the motors engage and help to propel the wheelchair.

In some cases, a simple lap belt or other similar accessory does not provide sufficient stability in a seating system. A rigid pelvic positioning device, also called *a sub-ASIS bar,* is typically a close-fitting, padded metal bar that is attached to the wheelchair frame or seat insert to position the pelvis below the individual's ASIS (see Chapter 9). It is designed to be used in conjunction with a complete seat and back system for individuals who require greater control to maintain the neutral position of the pelvis and to prevent pelvic rotation.

Some individuals require an *individualized setup for computer access.* This may be a typing stick or splint or mouth stick for typing (de Jonge, Sheerer, & Rodger, 2007) (see Chapter 7). Other possible adaptations are adjustment of the height of the workstation to accommodate a wheelchair, positioning of the keyboard or mouse for access, and use of alternatives to the mouse or keyboard. These are discussed in Chapters 7 and 8.

Another important difference between modified or custom devices and commercial devices is the level of technical support that is available with each. A commercially produced device generally has written documentation and online operating manuals and help screens available. Although the quality of these written materials varies widely, some documentation is better than none, and modified or custom devices often have none. The manufacturer or supplier of commercial equipment provides technical support and repair. Because modified or custom devices are one of a kind, technical support may be hard to obtain, especially if the original designer and builder is no longer available (e.g., if the user moves to a new area).

Custom- or Specially Designed Devices for One or a Few Individuals

There are also cases in which neither commercial mainstream or AT products nor specialized designs will meet the needs of an individual person with a disability. This approach results in a custom device. The bottom row of Figure 2-5 lists examples of custom AT software or hardware devices that might be developed for one individual.

When an individual has significant seating needs (e.g., fixed deformities, contractures, or other musculoskeletal problems), it may not be possible to position him using a standard contoured seating system (see Chapter 9). In these cases, a *custom contoured seating system* may be used. This system provides the greatest amount of body contact and therefore the most support because it is custom contoured to the individual's body. These cushions are much more costly to make, and they take longer to obtain. The need for these cushions is diminishing with the development of back components of seating systems that can be adjusted to meet the posture needs of the user.

The use of ATs for *job accommodation* is typically individualized because it is dependent on the functional level of the individual's impairment and the specific nature of the job task(s) (Zolna, Sanford, Sabata, & Goldthwaite, 2007). For mild to moderate impairments, common mainstream technologies (e.g., letter-folding machines, electric staplers, adaptive keyboards, telephone, headsets, material lifts, ergonomically designed tools and chairs, and anti-fatigue mats) are readily available. For workers who have cognitive disabilities, weighing and counting tasks in manufacturing and assembly can be difficult. One approach is to use a talking scale connected to a controller that provides prompting and feedback as necessary (Erlandson & Stant, 1998). For counting tasks, a bin that holds just the right number of items is weighed. If the bin is properly filled, the weight is correct, and the user is prompted to proceed with the next step. If the weight is too low, the user is told to add to the bin, and if it is too high, the user is prompted to be sure it is not overfilled. Erlandson and Stant (1998) describe the successful use of this system in a nail counting task for a construction supply company by a woman with a mild intellectual disability.

SUMMARY

The technology options available to clinicians to use in meeting the needs of persons with disabilities have dramatically expanded in recent years. The increase in functionality of mainstream mobile technologies (e.g., smart phones, tablets) has opened up possibilities for meeting the needs of a greater portion of the global disability community through the development of application software. The continued development of universal design is resulting in more and more mainstream products usable by persons with disabilities. Together with the continued availability and improvement in specialized ATs, the opportunities for meeting the needs of persons with disabilities through technology are greater than ever before.

STUDY QUESTIONS

1. As we describe, technologies are changing rapidly. Explain both the advantages and the risks this has for people with disabilities.
2. Look at Table 2-1. Pick three of these AT applications to mainstream technologies that you use every day and tell someone that they came from assistive technologies. What reaction did you get?
3. Universal design (design for all) has many advantages, especially for the built environment. However, there are also costs of universal design that limit its effectiveness in some situations. Describe both the advantages and limitations of universal design.
4. What is the most fundamental difference between universal design and the design of specialized assistive technologies?
5. What do we mean by the terms "affordances" and "constraints" when describing the use of everyday objects?
6. List three reasons that older people might require assistive technologies.
7. How do the needs of older individuals affect the design, delivery, and support of assistive technologies?
8. What is meant by the term "the digital divide?"
9. What factors are important in reducing the "digital divide" between developed and underresourced countries? How can people who have disabilities be included as this divide is narrowed?
10. Distinguish between hard and soft technologies.
11. What is meant by the term "function allocation," and how is it applied to AT systems?
12. What are the major approaches to function allocation? What are the strengths and weaknesses of each approach when used in AT system design?
13. What are the four components of the AT portion of the HAAT model?
14. Describe the key elements of the human technology interface for:
    a. Electronic assistive technologies
    b. Assistive technologies that provide support
    c. Mechanical assistive technologies
15. List three types of environmental sensors used for different AT applications.
16. What is the function of the processor or mechanical mechanism in an assistive device?
17. List three types of soft technologies.

18. What is meant by resonant design, and how does it differ from universal design?
19. Refer to Figure 2-5. Distinguish between specific purpose and general purpose technologies.
20. What are the two main sources of technologies that can assist individuals with disabilities?
21. What is meant by the term "the virtue of simplicity?"
22. Refer to Figure 2-5. Why does the cost of technology increase from left to right in the figure when the actual number of functions is often less going from left to right in the figure?
23. Can you think of technologies that you use regularly that have features that might make them useful to people with disabilities? What are the features, and who might they help?
24. Pick a particular disability and a need that a person with that disability might have and find two or three phone or tablet apps that would be useful.
25. What is a "jig," and how is it useful to people who have intellectual disabilities?

REFERENCES

Algood SD, Cooper RA, Fitzgerald SA, et al.: Effect of a pushrim-activated power-assist wheelchair on the functional capabilities of persons with tetraplegia, *Arch Phys Med Rehabil* 86:380–386, 2005.

Angin P, Bhargava BK: Real-time mobile-cloud computing for context-aware blind. *Proceedings of the Federated Conference on Computer Science and Information Systems*, Szczecin, Poland 985–989, 2011.

Armstrong W, Borg J, Krizack M, et al.: *Guidelines on the provision of manual wheelchairs in less resourced settings*, Geneva, 2008, WHO.

Bailey RW: *Human performance engineering*, ed 3, Englewood Cliffs, NJ, 1996, Prentice Hall.

Bauer S, Lane J: Convergence of assistive devices and mainstream products: keys to university participation in research, development and commercialization, *Technol Disabil* 18(2):67–77, 2006.

Björk E: Why did it take four times longer to create the Universal Design solution? *Technol Disabil* 21(4):159–170, 2009.

Boulos MNK, Anastasiou A, Bekiaris E: Panou, M: Geo-enabled technologies for independent living: Examples from four European projects, *Technol Disabil* 23(1):7–17, 2011.

Cook AM, Hussey SM: *Assistive technologies: Principles and practice*, St. Louis, 1995, Mosby.

Cravit D: *The new old: How the boomers are changing everything... again*, Toronto, 2008, ECW Press.

de Jonge D, Scherer MJ, Rodger S: *Assistive technology in the workplace*, St Louis, 2007, Elsevier.

Doughty K: SPAs (smart phone applications)—a new form of assistive technology, *J Assist Technol* 5(2):88–94, 2011.

Emiliani P: Assistive technology (AT) versus mainstream technology (MST): The research perspective, *Technol Disabil* 18(1):19–29, 2006.

Emiliani P, Stephanidis C, Vanderheiden G: Technology and inclusion—Past, present and foreseeable future, *Technol Disabil* 23(3):101–114, 2011.

Erlandson RF, Stant D: Polka-yoke process controller: Designed for individuals with cognitive impairments, *Assist Technol* 10:102–112, 1998.

Gosnell J, Costello J, Shane H: Using a clinical approach to answer "what communication apps should we use?" *Perspect Augment Altern Commun* 20:87–96, 2011.

Haigh KZ, Kiff LM, Ho G: The independent lifestyle assistant: Lessons learned, *Assist Technol* 18:87–106, 2006.

Hellman R: Universal design and mobile devices, *Lecture Notes in Computer Science* (including subseries Lecture Notes in Artificial Intelligence and Lecture Notes in Bioinformatics), 4554 LNCS, part 1:147–156, 2007.

International Labor Office: *Facts on disability in the world of work*, Geneva, 2007, http://www.ilo.org/wcmsp5/groups/public/---dgreports---/dcomm/documents/publication/wcms_087707.pdf. Accessed September 7, 2012.

International Telecommunication Union: *Measuring the information society*, Geneva, 2012, International Telecommunication Union.

International Telecommunication Union: *Percentage of individuals using the Internet report. Per country report and comparative data over the past 10 years*, Geneva, 2011, International Telecommunication Union.

Kirby RL: *Wheelchair skills program,*, version 3.2, 2005. http://www.wheelchairskillsprogram.ca.

Kumin D: *Review: The best iPhone universal remote apps*, http://www.soundandvisionmag.com/article/review-best-iphone-universal-remote-apps?page=0,0 Accessed September 24, 2012.

Lee YS, Jhangiani I, Smith-Jackson TL, et al: Design considerations for accessible mobile phones, *Proceedings of the Human Factors and Ergonomics Society*, 2178–2182, 2006.

Leung R, Findlater L, McGranere J, et al: Multi-layered interfaces to improve older adult's initial learnability of mobile applications, *ACM Transactions on Accessible Computing*, 3(1):1–30, 2010

Lewis C, Sullivan J, Hoehl J: Mobile technology for people with cognitive disabilities and their caregivers, *HCI issues, Lecture Notes in Computer Science* (including subseries *Lecture Notes in Artificial Intelligence and Lecture Notes in Bioinformatics),* 5614 LNCS, part 1, 385–394, 2009.

Lewis C, Ward N: Opportunities in cloud computing for people with cognitive disabilities: Designer and user perspective. part II, HCII 2011. In Stephanidis C, editor: *Universal access in HCI*, LNCS, 6766, pp 326–331, 2011.

Mann WC, Helal S, Davenport RD, et al.: Use of cell phones by elders with impairments: Overall appraisal, satisfaction, and suggestions, *Technol Disabil* 16(1):49–57, 2004.

Medola FO, Paschoarelli LC, Silva DC, et al: Pressure on hands during manual wheelchair propulsion: a comparative study with two types of handrim, *European Seating Symposium*, 63–65, 2011.

Newell AF: *Design and the digital divide: Insights from 40 years in computer support for older and disabled people*, Morgan & Claypool Publishers, San Rafael, California, 2011.

Norman D: *Design of everyday things*, New York, 2002, Basic Books.

Nguyen T, Garrett R, Downing AD, et al.: Research into telecommunications options for people with physical disabilities, *Asst Technol* 19:78–93, 2007.

Odor P: Hard and soft technology for education and communication for disabled people. *Proceedings of the International Computer Conference*, Perth, Australia, 1984.

Olwal A, Lachanas D, Zacharouli E. OldGen: Mobile phone personalization for older adults, *Proceedings Conference on Human Factors in Computing Systems*, 3393–3396, 2011.

Pedlow R, Kasnitz D, Shuttleworth R: Barriers to the adoption of cell phones for older people with impairments in the USA: Results from an expert review and field study, *Technol Disabil* 22(3):147–158, 2010.

Polgar JM, Shaw L, Vrkljan B: Implications of universal design principles to vehicle design, *OT Now*, September-October: 31–32, 2005.

Pullin G: *Design meets disability*, Cambridge, MA, 2009, MIT Press.

Rantala J, Raisamo R, Lylykangas J, et al: Methods for presenting braille characters on a mobile device with a touchscreen and tactile feedback, IEEE TRANSACTIONS ON HAPTICS, 2:128–139, 2009.

Sanford JA: *Universal design as a rehabilitation strategy*, New York, 2012, Springer.

Schaefer K: Market-based solutions for improving telecommunications access and choice for consumers with disabilities, *J Disabil Policy Studies* 17(2):116–126, 2006.

Simpson R: Smart wheelchairs: A literature review, *J Rehab Res Dev* 42(4):423–435, 2005.

Stent A, Azenkot S, Stern B: iWalk: A lightweight navigation system for low-vision users. I, ASSETS 10, *Proceedings of the 12th International ACM SIGACCESS Conference on Computers and Accessibility*, 269–270, 2010.

Stock SE, Davies DK, Wehmeyer ML, Palmer SB: Evaluation of cognitively accessible software to increase independent access to cellphone technology for people with intellectual disability, *J Intellect Disabil Res* 52(12):1155–1164, 2008.

Swann J: Inclusive design of tools for daily living, *Int J Ther Rehabil* 14(60):285–289, 2007.

Ungson GR, Trudel JD: The emerging knowledge-based economy, *IEEE Spectrum* 36(5):60–65, 1999.

Verstockt S, Decoo D, Van Nieuwenhuyse D, et al: Assistive smartphone for people with special needs: The personal social assistant, *Proceedings of 2nd Conference on Human System Interactions, HSI '09*, 331–337, 2009.

Vicente MR, López AJ: A multidimensional analysis of the disability digital divide: Some evidence for Internet use, *Information Society* 26(1):48–64, 2010.

Wang RH, Gorski SM, Holliday PJ, Fernie GR: Evaluation of a contact sensor skirt for an anti-collision power wheelchair for older adult nursing home residents with dementia: Safety and mobility, *Assist Technol* 23:117–134, 2011.

Weber H: Providing access to the internet for people with disabilities: short and medium term research demands, *Theoret Issues Ergonom Sci* 7(5):491–498, 2006.

Wright RA: *Short history of progress*, Anansi Pub, Toronto, ON, Canada, 2004.

Wu B, Kao C, Li Y, Tsai MY: A real-time embedded blind spot safety assistance system, International Journal of Vehicular Technology, Volume 2012 (2012), http://dx.doi.org/10.1155/2012/506235. Article ID 506235, 15 pages 2012.

Zafrulla Z, Etherton J, Starner T: TTY phone—direct, equal emergency access for the deaf, *ASSETS'08: 10th International ACM SIGACCESS Conference on Computers and Accessibility*, 277–278, 2008.

Zolna J, Sanford J, Sabata D, Goldthwaite J: Review of accommodation strategies in the workplace for persons with mobility and dexterity impairments: Application to criteria for universal design, *Technol Disabil* 19(4):189–198, 2007.

CHAPTER 3

Activity, Human, and Context: The Human Doing an Activity in Context

CHAPTER OUTLINE

LEARNING OBJECTIVES

On completing this chapter, you will be able to do the following:

1. Identify and describe the components of the HAAT model.
2. Discuss how each individual component of the HAAT model affects assistive technology (AT) design, use, and service delivery.
3. Discuss how the individual components interact to affect AT design, use, and service delivery.
4. Identify major performance areas for which AT is used.
5. Describe the contexts in which AT is used.

KEY TERMS

Activity
Activity Analysis
Body Structures and Functions
Capability Theory
Capacity
Contexts
Co-occupation
Cultural Context
Expert
Free and Appropriate Public Education (FAPE)
Habits
Human Activity Assistive Technology (HAAT) Model
Individualized Education Plan (IEP)
Individualized Plans for Employment
Institutional Context
International Classification of Functioning, Disability and Impairment (ICF)
Least Restrictive Environment
Leisure
Lifespan
Linguistic Competence
Marginalization
Meaning
Novice
Occupation
Occupational Alienation
Occupational Apartheid
Occupational Balance
Occupational Deprivation
Occupational Engagement
Occupational Imbalance
Occupational Injustice
Occupational Justice
Occupational Performance
Occupational Satisfaction
Operational Competence
Participation
Performance
Physical Context
Productivity
Reasonable Accommodation
Roles
Self-care
Self-efficacy
Social Context
Social Competence
Stigma
Strategic Competence

INTRODUCTION

This chapter describes the activity, human, and context elements of the **Human Activity Assistive Technology (HAAT) model**. The previous chapter introduced key concepts related to assistive technology (AT). As stated in Chapter 1, the HAAT model describes a human doing something in a context using AT. In this chapter, we deconstruct the elements of the human, the **activity**, and the context to understand their individual influence on the design, assessment and evaluation, and use of AT. However, as you can see from Figure 3-1, the HAAT model is depicted as an integration of the human, activity, and AT, nested in the context. Consequently, the chapter concludes with a reconstruction of the model elements to describe and understand the transactional nature of their mutual influence on doing and their collective influence on AT. Although it is possible to discuss each element in isolation, it is only in uncovering their connections that the complexity of the place of AT in a person's life is revealed.

The order in which the HAAT elements are presented is deliberate. Whether applying the HAAT to device design, assessment resulting in AT recommendation, or outcome evaluation, the order of consideration and integration of the HAAT elements is consistent. The activity or need is identified first followed by the aspects of the human that affect the ability to perform and engage in the activity. The contextual influences that affect the human's performance of that activity are then considered. The AT design and recommendation come last, signifying technology's place to enable activity participation and engagement.

ACTIVITY

Classifications of Activity

International Classification of Functioning, Disability and Impairment

The **International Classification of Functioning, Disability and Impairment (ICF)** (World Health Organization [WHO], 2001) is a well-known system for coding and classifying elements of the person, activity, and environment that influence health. The activities and **participation** components are useful for identification and organization of activities that a person needs or wants to do. Furthermore, the ICF provides a common language for communication around these activities.

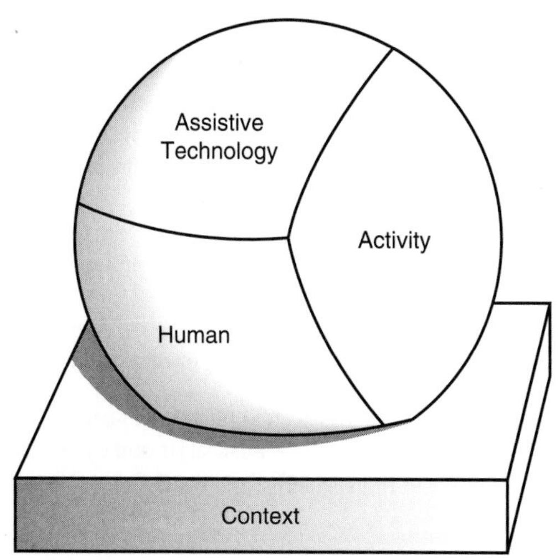

FIGURE 3-1 The Human Activity Assistive Technology (HAAT) model.

The ICF defines *activities* as: "the execution of a task or action by an individual" (WHO, 2001, p. 10) and *participation* as "involvement in a life situation" (WHO, 2001, p. 10). In addition to the identification of different domains of activities and participation, the ICF includes two types of qualifiers that assist the characterization of the person's involvement in the activity and participation domains: **performance** describes what the person actual does, and **capacity** describes the person's potential optimal performance given favorable and supportive circumstances.

The major ICF activity and performance domains include:
- Learning and applying knowledge
- General tasks and demands
- Communication
- Mobility
- Self-care
- Domestic life
- Interpersonal interactions and relationships
- Major life areas
- Community, social, and civic life

Each of the domains and subdomains is defined to provide a consistent understanding, which is intended to make the ICF transferable across professions, organizations, and cultures. Table 3-1 provides examples of subdomains in each of these areas.

Occupational Therapy Classifications

Occupational therapists also classify activity or **occupation** into areas of self-care, productivity, and leisure. Other professional groups have also adapted the use of these categories. Typically, **self-care** occupations include activities of daily living (ADLs) and instrumental ADLs; **productivity** includes occupations at work, school, or in nonpaid activities that contribute to society; and **leisure** are activities done for recreation (American Occupational Therapy Association [AOTA], 2002; Townsend & Polatajko, 2002, 2013).

The HAAT model includes four activity output areas to organize our discussion of AT in this book: communication, cognitive abilities, manipulation, and mobility. Table 3-2 compares the HAAT classification of activities with selected domains and subdomains of the ICF. Figure 3-2 shows the HAAT model with the elements of the activity component identified.

Activity Analysis

Activity analysis has been a foundational skill of occupational therapists for decades. It is complementary to methods used by human factors engineers in analysis of tasks, hierarchical task analysis being one example (Fisk et al., 2009; Stanton, 2006). These methods of analysis begin with a deconstruction of the activity to understand the different steps necessary to complete it. A hierarchical task analysis may produce a flow chart that depicts the process of doing an activity, showing different paths resulting from different choices made. An occupational therapy activity analysis provides a narrative of these steps.

Additional background information includes listing the materials and equipment that are used to do the activity, describing the context in which it is completed and who is doing the activity. The occupational therapy analysis proceeds into describing the different performance components (e.g., cognitive, physical, sensory, perceptual, communicative, and affective) that are used to perform each step of the activity. These analyses are useful for two main purposes: (1) understanding the performance of an activity generally (i.e., detailing the performance process) and (2) understanding how a specific individual or group of individuals completes an activity.

An analysis is useful in the process of determining appropriate AT as it assists the clinician to determine the skills and abilities possessed by the client to complete the task and those that require supplementation or replacement by AT for successful performance. This process is time consuming, so it is recognized that activity analysis as presented here is rarely completed for a single activity in practice. However, possessing a framework for such an analysis of a single activity supports the clinician during the assessment and evaluation processes to understand the activities in which the client needs and wishes to engage and the skills and abilities that are required for successful performance of those activities. Several schemes for conducting an occupational or activity

TABLE 3-1 International Classification of Functioning, Disability and Impairment (ICF) Activities and Participation Domains with Examples

ICF Domain	Examples Relevant to Assistive Technology
Learning and applying knowledge	• *Basic learning skills*, such as learning how to read, write, and do arithmetic operations; skill acquisition • *Applying knowledge*, such as reading, attending to a learning situation, thinking, writing, problem solving, doing arithmetic operations, and decision making
General tasks and demands	• *Performing a single task*, which involves steps required to do one thing; including acquisition and organization of materials; initiating, maintaining, and completing task; sequencing the task; and the place, space, and pacing • *Performing multiple tasks*, including skills and knowledge required to perform many tasks either concurrently or consecutively • *Performing a daily routine*, involving performance of all the activities that make up one's day • *Handling stress or other psychological demands*; involves the ability to deal effectively with stress, demands, and distractions of daily tasks
Communication	• *Reception of communicative messages*, including spoken, written, signed language, or other means • *Expression of communicative messages*, including oral, written, signed, or other means • *Conversation and use of communication devices and techniques*; classification includes use of telephones and writing implements but not devices that would necessarily be considered assistive technology
Mobility	• Ability to move from one position to another (e.g., sit to stand) or maintain one position • Transfers from one surface to another • Lift, hold, handle, and carry objects, including use of both upper and lower extremities for this purpose; upper extremity classification includes manipulation • Activities of the hands and arms, including motions such as reaching, grasping, pinching, and rotating • *Walking and moving*, including walking or moving by other means such as crawling or running in different environments and using equipment such as skates as well as a wheelchair or walker • *Use of transportation for mobility*, including transportation use as a passenger or driver as well as use of an animal for transport
Self-care	• Includes basic activities of daily living, such as bathing, eating, dressing, toileting, and personal health promotion activities
Domestic life	• *Acquiring necessities*, including securing a place to live; necessary goods to support daily life; and home management activities as well as providing assistance to others, such as child care
Major life areas	• *Education*, including formal and informal educational opportunities • *Work and employment*, including work training, job acquisition, and remunerative and nonremunerative work • Management of personal finances
Community, social, and civic life	• *Community life*, including participation in formal and informal organizations such as service clubs • *Recreation and leisure*, including participation in organized or informal play, leisure, or recreational activities • *Religion and spirituality*, including both formal and informal activities • *Human rights*, including participation in rights as identified in declarations such as the United Nations Convention on the Rights of Persons with Disabilities; excludes rights related to political life and citizenship • *Political life and citizenship*, includes participation in all forms of political activity and rights accorded to persons with citizenship status in a particular country

United Nations Declaration on the RIghts of Persons with Disabilities, 2006.

From: International Classification of Functioning, Disability and Health, WHO, 2001. More information on the ICF is available on the World Health Organization's website at www.who.int/classifications/icf.

analysis are found in the literature (e.g., Hersch, Lamport, & Coffey, 2005).

Understanding Activity Beyond Its Classification

Use of the ICF or other systems that classify activity or occupation helps name and organize what a person does. However, a simple classification does not provide the full picture. When the consideration of activity stops at classification, other factors that influence doing activity are lost. The personal **meaning** attributed to doing activity, its complexity and flow, and the situated nature of doing within a context are not evident within a classification system. A number of questions help further define the activity. These questions guide the gathering of information about performance of the activity as well as how its performance relates to engagement in other activities.

TABLE 3-2 Comparison of International Classification of Functioning, Disability and Impairment (ICF) and the Human Activity Assistive Technology (HAAT) Model

ICF	HAAT Model
Learning and applying knowledge	Cognition Communication
General tasks and demands	Cognition
Communication	Communication
Mobility	Manipulation Mobility
Self-care	Cognition Communication Manipulation
Domestic life	Cognition Communication Manipulation Mobility
Interpersonal interactions and relationships	Cognition Communication Manipulation Mobility
Major life areas	Cognition Communication Manipulation Mobility
Community, social, and civic life	Cognition Communication Manipulation Mobility

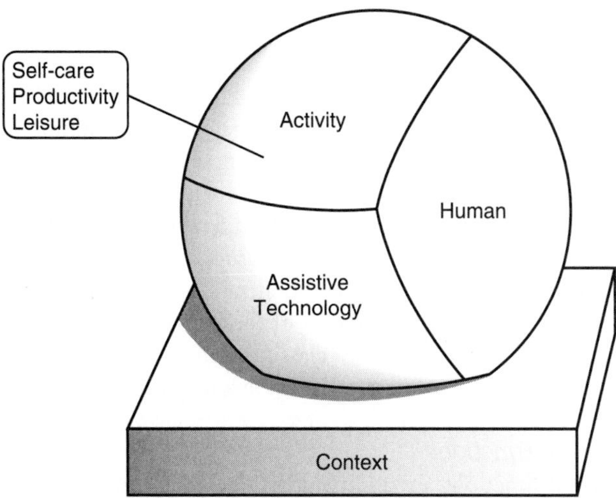

FIGURE 3-2 The Human Activity Assistive Technology (HAAT) model with elements of the activity component identified.

Why is this activity performed? Here a distinction is made between a person *wanting to do an activity* versus *needing to do an activity*. Because the individual herself has some influence on required versus chosen activities, we will return to this idea when we discuss the meaning of the activity. The individual has more choice in whether to perform certain activities than others. Getting up and going to work is a required activity for many adults.

At work, specific activities are expected as part of the requirements of the job. Engaging in training to complete a marathon is an activity that some individuals choose (Figure 3-3). Even within activities, there is an element of choice. For example, for most children younger than a certain age, as defined by local legislation, attending school is a required occupation. There is no choice. However, choice is exerted (at least by older children) around how much or to what extent required school activities are completed.

How is the activity performed? Is it important for the client to perform the activity independently, or will he accept assistance from others or technology? When he does accept assistance from others, it is important to determine whether this assistance is provided by family, friends, or a personal care attendant. If the activity is a sensitive one, such as toileting, the person may be very particular about the person from whom he will accept this assistance. Another aspect of this question is whether the activity is performed alone or with others. For example, reading is something that can be done alone, but having a conversation requires a minimum of two people. The concept of a co-occupation (Pierce, 2009) is a relatively new idea from occupational science that explores performance of an occupation by two or more people.

Temporal aspects. Timing issues related to activity performance give guidance about how frequently the person engages in that activity. Frequency is one indicator of the importance of an activity to the individual. One that is completed regularly and frequently is usually of higher priority than something that is only done infrequently. It is also useful to ask how long it takes the person to complete the task and whether she is willing to invest that amount of time required to do it without assistance. Similarly, does the time to complete the task take away from time available for other activities? For example, a client may be able to dress herself by adapting to the activity but only with much effort over an extended period of time. This amount of time can be problematic when she is getting ready for school or work—if dressing takes a long time, doing it herself either means getting up very early to dress or risk being late for some commitment. Similarly, this length of time means she is not able to do other activities.

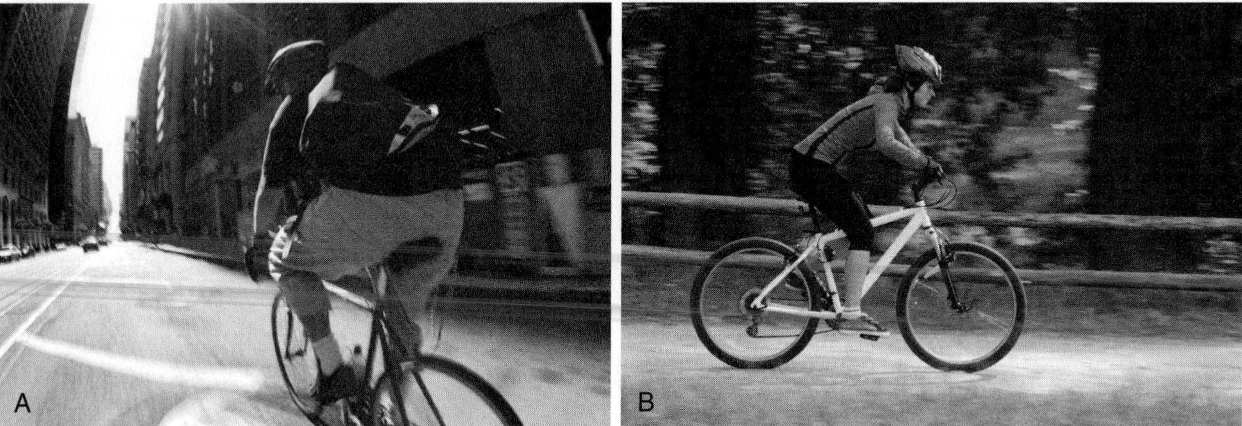

FIGURE 3-3 Doing an activity involves different levels of choice. **A,** Less choice in the work environment. **B,** Greater choice in leisure pursuits.

A final consideration relates to the preference the client has to how frequently an activity is performed. Individual preference often determines how frequently an activity, such as exercising or bathing, is performed. A change in abilities that affects cognitive, communicative, manipulative, or mobility skills can alter the ability of a person to exercise choice regarding the frequency with which certain activities are performed. For example, when a person lives in a skilled nursing facility, the institutional routines dictate the frequency of many activities, including personal care activities. The resident has limited opportunity to exercise choice over this temporal component.

Where does the occupation take place? We will explore the implications of place on activity when we discuss context. Here we identify the considerations required when considering place. An activity may be performed differently in a public versus a private place.

The presence of others in the place where the activity occurs can mean that there are individuals available to provide assistance. The opinion and knowledge of others about AT may hinder or enable its use. Place may also limit the choice of AT because some technologies that use voice input or activation may be obtrusive in a quiet place, and their use may restrict the privacy of the user. The physical aspects of place may also enable or hinder the performance of the activity.

What other activities are supported by the performance of a given activity? The performance of complex activities depends on the ability to perform more basic ones. For example, the ability to sit supports many other activities a person does to look after herself, socialize with others, volunteer, or engage in work or educational activities. Similarly, the ability to speak and manipulate materials are basic skills used in more complex activities.

Seeking the answers to these questions moves beyond simply knowing what activities a person needs or wants to do. They also assist the clinician to understand other elements of the performance of an activity and how they will enable or hinder the use of any AT.

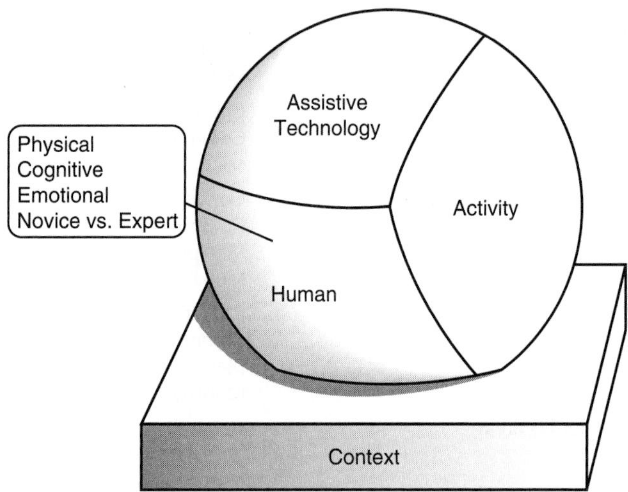

FIGURE 3-4 The Human Activity Assistive Technology (HAAT) model with elements of the human component identified.

THE HUMAN USER

ICF Body Structures and Functions

The ICF (WHO, 2001) is a good starting place to understand the human user. The classification provides a useful way to organize the functions of the human body that affect the ability to perform an activity, engage in the community, and use AT. The ICF defines body functions as "the physiological functions of body systems (including psychological functions)" (WHO, 2001, p. 10). In this chapter, we cover the classifications of body functions that support AT applications as described by the human component of the HAAT model. Figure 3-4 shows the elements of the human component of the HAAT model. Relevant classifications of body functions are discussed in greater detail in individual chapters.

Mental Functions

Mental functions are abilities that enable the individual to be alert and focus on his environment, perceive and interpret sensory phenomena, feel and regulate emotions, and perform higher level functions that enable him to organize and control his behavior and action and to learn, reason, and synthesize information (WHO, 2001).

At a very basic level, mental functions involve a level of consciousness (being able to attend to one's surroundings); orientation to place, person, and time; and general intellectual functions that enable an individual to process, remember, and understand information. The ability to perceive and interpret sensory stimulation, including auditory, visual, tactile, and visual-spatial, are basic functions that help a person organize and respond to her world (AOTA, 2002; WHO, 2001).

Higher level cognitive functions enable the individual to synthesize and integrate information, to reason and learn. These executive functions enable a person to regulate and organize his behavior and to exercise judgment. Mental functions as they relate to written and spoken language, mathematical functions, and the ability to organize and sequence movement (praxis) form part of this category. The ICF also includes classifications of personality and temperament here (AOTA, 2002; WHO, 2001).

Seeing Functions

Seeing classifications involve functions related to vision. Acuity is the ability to see clearly, including monocular and binocular near distant vision (AOTA, 2002; WHO, 2001). This visual function is probably the one with which most people are familiar. Individuals who are "near sighted" can see objects up close but perceive distant objects as blurry. "Far-sighted" vision is the opposite. As individuals age, the ability to focus on objects up close declines. You might hear a middle-aged person saying her "arms are too short," referring to the fact that she must hold materials at a distance to be able to read them.

Visual field describes the span an individual is able to see when the eyes are fixed in a certain direction, including visual information that is directly in front and in the peripheral field (WHO, 2001). The quality of vision relates to the ability to detect color, sensitivity to light, and visual contrast. Light sensitivity refers to the amount of light that is required to be able to see clearly; with age, individuals often require a greater amount of light to see clearly. It also refers to the reaction to light—some individuals with light sensitivity problems have difficulty seeing clearly in high light conditions, for example, on a sunny day in the snow or on the beach. Light contrast refers to the amount of contrast required between a figure in the foreground and the background to enable a person to distinguish the figure from the background. Light contrast is particularly important for AT with an interface with a visual display.

Hearing Functions

The functions of hearing include both auditory (hearing) functions and those related to vestibular function in the inner ear that have implications for balance, movement, and position in space (WHO, 2001). At the most basic level, these classifications involve detecting that a sound has occurred and discriminating among sounds that are in the environment (e.g., the ability to focus on a conversation in a noisy restaurant).

Localization of sound is the ability to determine where a sound is coming from, and lateralization of sound is the ability to determine if it is coming from the right or left side. Hearing includes the ability to discriminate between sounds that are language and those that are not (e.g., laughing, crying) (WHO, 2001).

The structures of the inner ear detect movement and position relative to gravity to assist a person to move through space and to maintain balance. They enable her to detect whether she is upright or not and assist her to retain body alignment in terms of keeping her head in an upright position, regardless of the body position, to maintain a useful line of sight. The ability to detect the body's movement through space and whether the body is supported on a flat or tilted surface assists with balance and movement. Think about the difficulty a child has retaining an upright position after spinning; in this situation, the vestibular apparatus and visual information are not providing consistent information to enable the child to maintain balance. Another example of vestibular function (or dysfunction) is the phenomenon of motion sickness. When the vestibular input and the visual input conflict, a person might feel nauseous. For example, sitting in a moving vehicle or on an amusement park ride, where the body is not moving relative to the car but the visual information conveys movement, can result in motion sickness because of the disconnect between vestibular and visual stimuli.

Additional Sensory Functions

The ICF identifies several other sensory functions, although we are only including the sensations here that are pertinent to the scope of this book. Tactile functions involve the ability to detect various physical stimuli, including temperature, vibration, pressure, and noxious stimuli. Proprioception is the ability to sense the position of body parts in relation to each other. For example, if you close your eyes and your friend flexes your elbow to 90 degrees, proprioception is what tells you that your arm is bent and not straight. The ability to detect movement of the parts of the body is called kinesthesia. Sensations associated with pain are a separate classification in the ICF (WHO, 2001).

Voice Functions

Voice functions refer to the production of different sounds in order to speak or vocalize. It involves enunciation of various sounds and articulation of phonemes. The rhythm of speech, fluency, speed, and intonation are included here. In addition to vocalizations that produce speech, this classification group includes alternative forms of vocalizations such as babbling, crying, screaming, producing musical notes, and humming (WHO, 2001).

Neuromusculoskeletal Functions

The final body function classification that we will present describes neuromusculoskeletal and movement-related functions. Several of these classifications involve functions that are necessary for the production of movement, such as bone and joint functions (mobility and stability around a joint and bone mobility, which refers to the mobility of specific joints in the body, including the scapular, pelvic, carpal, and tarsal joints) (WHO, 2001).

Muscle functions include muscle tone, power, and endurance (AOTA, 2002; WHO, 2001). Movement-related functions include reflex and other involuntary motor reactions, involuntary movement such as tremors, tics, and simple to complex voluntary movements, including gait (WHO, 2001).

The ICF classification system is useful in terms of categorizing the many different body functions that influence the ability to engage in activity in one's community and to use AT. But it does not tell the whole story. It is important to understand the implications of cognitive, physical, and sensory performance when conducting an assessment that results in the recommendation of an assistive device, evaluating the outcome of AT use, or designing AT. Other aspects of a person also affect the person's ability and willingness to use AT.

Lifespan Perspective

The ability and desire to use technology is not the same across the **lifespan.** Although it is important to remember that chronological age does not necessarily have the strongest influence on activity performance or AT use, it certainly has an effect and deserves consideration.

Children are acquiring skills that affect their ability to perform activities and use AT. Young children and infants have limited abilities to express themselves, control their movement for mobility and manipulation, and perform cognitive functions. AT that is aimed at children must take into account their ability to interact and control it.

Technology that is complex to use, involving multiple steps to operate, may be beyond the ability of a young child. The experience a child has with performing different actions or activities can also affect her ability to use AT. Along with skill acquisition, it is important to consider the opportunities a child has had to engage in activities. Age should not be a restriction to the use of AT. Rather, AT should support a child to engage in activities in which her peers are also participating. For example, as children start to explore production of language, simple language boards can help very young children begin to express themselves. Similarly, a powered wheelchair can give a young child mobility, although perhaps not at the same time as her peers (Rosen et al., 2009).

Parents enable activities in children, and the meaning of AT use for the child may not be the same as for the parent. Children do not carry the same viewpoint that activities are performed in only one way or that there is stigma in how they engage in activity when they use some form of device. Parents, on the other hand, may view AT as a visible sign that their child has a disability. It may be interpreted as a sign that their dreams of the future for their child may not be realized. AT might be fun and interesting to a child, but the stigma of its use may make it difficult for a parent to accept it for her child.

Adolescence is an interesting age for most young people; it is a time when they seek independence from their family, at least to some degree, and think about their future as a worker, a partner, and a contributor to the community. It is also a time when they explore their identity, often striving for a sense of belonging with a certain group. Adolescence can be a time when a child with a disability becomes aware that he is different from his peers, although often this awareness comes at a younger age (King, Brown, & Smith, 2003). Although adolescents often have the body function to control their AT, if it becomes a symbol for them that they are different, then it might not be used. On the other hand, if AT enables them to do the activities they want to do, such as communicate with friends with an augmentative and alternative communication (AAC) device or with computer access technology or go out with friends with the use of a wheelchair, device use is more likely.

At the other end of the age spectrum, older adults have changing needs that affect their ability to use AT (Fisk et al., 2009). Surveys such as the Canadian Physical Activity and Limitations Survey (PALS) (Statistics Canada, 2007) and US National Health Interview Survey (Ervin, 2006; Shoenborn & Heyman, 2009) reveal that older adults account for the highest proportion of individuals who have a disability, and as they get older, they are likely to experience more than one impairment. Vision and mobility are the most common physical limitations experienced by older adults (Statistics Canada, 2007). Pain, cognitive impairment, and hearing impairment also affect the ability of older adults to perform activities and use AT. These age-related impairments are introduced here and discussed in greater detail in later chapters.

The most common causes of low vision in older adults are age-related macular degeneration, glaucoma, cataracts, and diabetic retinopathy. Low vision is defined as corrected vision (i.e., wearing corrective lenses) of 20/200 or worse. Age-related macular degeneration occurs when the macula of the eye deteriorates, resulting in loss of vision in the central visual field.

Cataract occurs when the lens of the eye hardens and becomes opaque. The changes to the lens block light from getting to the retina, resulting in a visual field that seems to be seen through a dirty lens, like through glasses that are smudged or a windshield that is dirty. Glaucoma results from increased pressure on the optic nerve caused by a buildup of the fluid in the eye, the vitreous gel. The resulting visual impairment is loss of vision in the peripheral fields, which over time limits sight to the central field, what is commonly called "tunnel vision."

Diabetic retinopathy is not only associated with older adults, but the incidence does increase with age. In this disease, increased glucose levels cause the blood vessels of the eye to swell and leak. New blood vessels may also form. These changes result in random loss of vision, dark patches in the visual field, blurred vision, or blindness.

The most common causes of mobility impairment in older adults are musculoskeletal conditions, such as osteoarthritis and other forms of arthritis. Mobility can also be impaired by neurological conditions such as stroke, Parkinson's disease, and multiple sclerosis. Mobility is impaired through loss of coordination, balance or stability, and decreased strength and range of motion. Pain is also a contributing factor for limited mobility.

Cognitive impairment is frequently the result of some form of dementia, most commonly Alzheimer's dementia. An individual may be diagnosed with a mild cognitive impairment (MCI) when others notice problems with memory, behavior, and executive functions. When MCI progresses to a dementia, these problems become more evident and restrict the ability to engage in activity to a greater degree. At the onset, devices that assist memory can be useful; however, as the disease progresses, even simple activities are a challenge to perform, and other devices, such as mobility devices, can become necessary.

Hearing impairment associated with aging is sensorineuronal hearing loss. In this situation, damage occurs to the cochlea or the auditory nerve, which limits the ability of the person to hear sounds. Sounds that are perceptible may seem muffled. This situation is not treatable and requires the use of hearing aids as the condition progresses.

How an older adult performs in each of these areas is a consideration in the assessment process as well as in the AT design process. The ability of an older adult to see the screen on a controller, to generate the force required to propel a manual wheelchair, or to see or hear instructions or feedback provided by the device are essential considerations for both assessment and design.

The presence of a disability can magnify the effects of age-related impairments. Individuals who are aging with a disability experience secondary impairments that affect their ability to function and to use AT. These secondary impairments make it appear that age-related changes occur earlier in individuals with a congenital disability or one acquired as a child or young adult. Common related impairments are osteoporosis, joint immobility, and contractures as a result of limited movement and weight bearing. Increased pain is commonly reported. Furthermore, individuals aging with a disability are at greater risk of obesity because of fewer opportunities to exercise (Klingbeil, Baer, & Wilson 2004).

Older adults with Down syndrome have a higher incidence of Alzheimer's disease (AD) than other older adults. The compound influence of the original cognitive impairment and the acquired AD affects new and continued use of devices.

The meaning of technology use for older adults may reflect loss, diminishing of abilities, and perhaps generate a feeling of being less capable or valued. Not only does AT device use signal a person is no longer able to perform activities in the manner to which she is familiar, but it may also limit the ability to engage in desired activities when the use of the device is not supported in a particular environment. For example, an older woman who enjoys attending musical theater may find herself unable to continue to engage in this activity if she requires the use of a wheelchair for mobility and the theater is not accessible. Similarly, another adult may choose not to engage in activities if it means he must use AT. A common example here is the use of a hearing aid; some older adults may choose not to go into a social situation because of the stigma of using a hearing aid.

A final consideration with older adults is prior experience with technology use. It is not appropriate to assume that an older person will not wish to use technology or is unable to learn to use new technology. Many older adults thrive with the use of a computer, using it to keep in touch with family and to explore information and ideas on the Internet. Stereotyping older adults as non-users of technology limits their potential for continued engagement in and new possibilities for activity.

Novice versus Expert

Another human characteristic important in the selection or evaluation of AT is whether a person is a **novice** or **expert** user of the specific technology. The term *novice* describes a user of an AT system who has little or no experience with that particular system or the task for which it is used. A novice user may have no idea of the possibilities for performing activities that have become difficult or impossible because of injury, illness, or some other condition. Although devices such as wheelchairs and hearing aids are common in most areas, AT such as alternative communication systems, computer access systems, and devices that help control the environment is not as familiar. If a person has a newly developed impairment, the lack of knowledge of different types of AT can be a limiting factor in regaining function.

Another aspect of a novice user is the tendency to use the device in a limited manner because of the lack of familiarity and experience with its use. The full range of functionality may not be available to the individual because of his knowledge of how to use the device or lack of training. A new user of a smart phone may restrict himself to the functions of the phone that are familiar, easy to learn to use, and most useful. A novice is more likely to use the system in prescribed ways, relying on soft technologies (instructions or others with expertise) to use it effectively. He is less likely to generalize use of the system from one task to another and must use more conscious effort to control it.

As a user practices and gains more experience, she may become an *expert* user, that is, she demonstrates a high degree of skill in the use of the system. An expert takes more risks with the equipment in terms of stretching the way it is used and trying new activities with the system (Figure 3-5). For example, a skilled manual wheelchair user will take her chair up or down an escalator rather than use an elevator. A skilled communication aid operator will develop strategies to increase her rate of communication.

An expert technology user also knows how he wants a device to perform and what he wants it to do. An expert has an opinion on how the technology should look; how fast it performs; and, with devices like seating and mobility

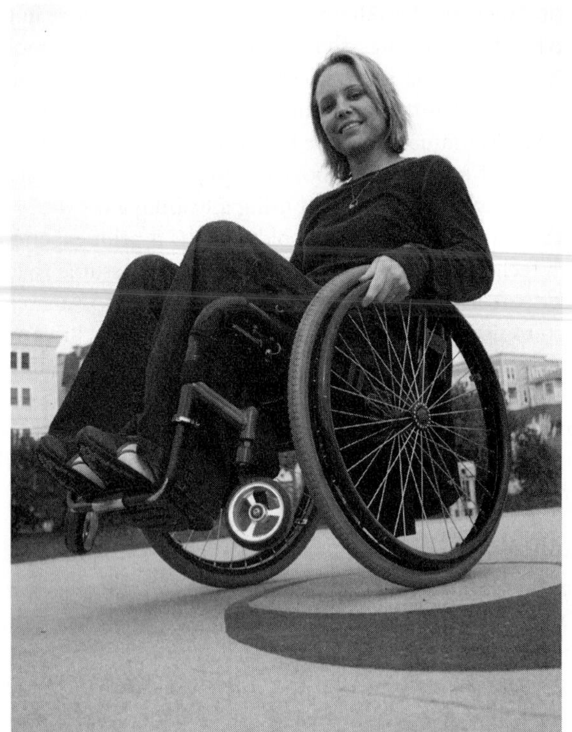

FIGURE 3-5 A skilled AT user will use technology in complex and challenging ways.

technology, how it should fit. An expert also feels comfortable to modify the technology and often has ideas about how to improve the technology, building on his familiarity and experience with using a device in many different situations.

Understanding the differences between a novice and expert user has important implications for teaching people how to use a system and the development of strategies (soft technologies). An expert user exerts less conscious effort in the operation of the system—because she does not need to do so. Analysis of the strategies of an expert user and translation of these into teaching programs can be an effective means of assisting a novice to become an expert user of a system. The pervasive nature of technology in our lives provides an opportunity when recommending a technology and teaching an individual to use it. Previous experience with technology and a willingness to try new technology are important considerations during the assessment process and can be used to support the development of new skills.

Roles

The concept of **roles** has been defined as "a set of socially agreed upon [expectations], functions, or obligations that involve patterns, scripts, or codes of behavior, routines, **habits**, and occupation that a person assumes and which become part of that person's social identity" (Reed, 2005, p. 596). Roles can express a vocational position (e.g., apprentice, worker, retiree), an educational position, a position in society (e.g., someone who lives in poverty, person of influence), a familial position (e.g., mother, brother, aunt), or a position in a social context (e.g., leader, follower, donor, recipient).

If we look at the definition of role above, we note several key words that influence the human doing something and then implications of doing activity with AT. *Socially agreed* conveys the importance of the social, contextual understanding of a given role. Social expectations define how the role is enacted. For example, a student is expected to attend school on a regular basis, interact with teachers and peers in a particular manner, engage in the learning process in school, perhaps engage in extracurricular activities, and complete homework as set out by the teacher. The intersection of the roles of teacher and student are also socially defined, and although education in some areas is moving into a student-centered direction, the expectation that the teacher directs the educational experience and the student is the recipient remains a dominant model of education. The advent of online methods of delivering educational materials challenges the social conventions of teaching and learning, changing the understanding of these roles. This example illustrates the power of the social construction of a particular role and the social expectations that define how a role is enacted. Yet it also illustrates the opportunity for flexibility of how roles are enacted, leaving room for alternate ways of doing.

The definition indicates that roles "involve patterns, scripts, or codes of behavior, routines, habits, and occupation." These words suggest that there is a particular way of doing an activity or performing a role, that is, we can articulate how a role is performed. With the exception of the word *occupation*, all of the other words suggest a prescribed manner of doing something. This certainty of how a role is performed is useful in one sense; it helps understand or anticipate what is expected of someone in a given situation.

For example, someone in the role of worker is expected to show up to work on time, to dress in a particular style, to interact with others in an acceptable way, and to perform work tasks within a range of acceptable competency. On the other hand, this scripting of how a role is performed is limiting; it may make it difficult for someone to perform a role in a different way based on his abilities. Think about how a person most commonly inputs information on a computer—he makes desired keystrokes on the keyboard and uses the mouse to navigate and select different areas on the screen. An individual who does not have the fine motor coordination to access a keyboard may have limited opportunities to enact the worker role if that role requires him to use a computer and necessary alternative access methods are unavailable.

The last part of this definition is the notion of "social identity." Often, one of the first things a person asks when meeting someone for the first time is: "What do you do?" The response commonly indicates a profession or, if the person is a student, where and what she studies. Individuals obtain their identity and status through their roles. When an older adult retires, her social identity shifts with the cessation of employment. She may believe she no longer has a role in society. The notion of social identity here conveys both how the individual perceives herself within her society and how others perceive her.

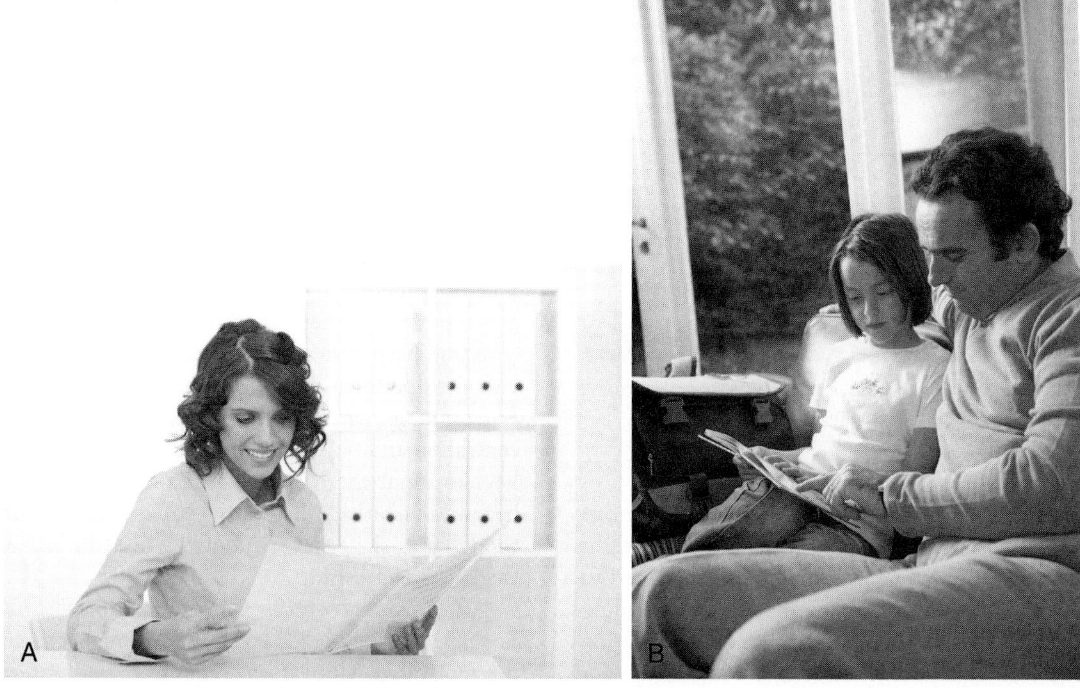

FIGURE 3-6 Activities have different meanings when performed as part of different roles. **A,** Reading in the worker role. **B,** Reading in the parent role.

We all have multiple roles, for example, we can be student, parent, child, sibling, employee, friend, and homemaker. Within each exists a set of performance expectations. Although the same activity may be present in the enactment of multiple roles, how it is enacted may change. Performance of an activity may differ depending on the nature of the role in which it is performed. For example, a parent reading to her child reads in a different way than when she reads as part of the role of worker or student (Figure 3-6).

Integration of the Activity and Human Components

To this point in the chapter, we have treated the activity and human elements of the HAAT model as if they have been relatively distinct. Ignoring the work of machines for the moment, activity does not exist if someone is not performing it. In this section, we explore the intersection of the activity and the human to gain a better appreciation for humans doing activity.

Meaning of an Activity

The performance of an activity holds meaning to an individual. When you think about all the activities a person performs in a typical day across the span of a week or on special occasions, some will quickly come to mind as very important, and some will seem so insignificant that they may be difficult even to recall. Humans perform a vast number of activities daily; some such as brushing hair take almost no time at all, but others take long periods of time, such as driving between two distant points or reading a book. Humans give meaning to each of these activities.

The human-centered aspect of meaning is the self-determined perspective of an activity or the personal, pre-existing "lens" through which a person views an activity (Reed & Hocking, 2013). Personal meaning is drawn from previous experience with doing an activity along with the "in the moment" feelings generated by engaging in an activity. The sense of competence or accomplishment and the perceived challenge of an activity similarly contribute to personal meaning. The blending of previous and current experiences of an activity invoke a dynamic, fluid nature of self-perceived meaning of activity.

The occupation of riding a bike is used to illustrate the different meanings that can be ascribed to the same activity. A novice bike rider might perceive bike riding as something scary and uncomfortable because her lack of skill will not prevent her from falling. Alternately, a novice bike rider might perceive the activity as a sign of growing up, performing an activity that is demanding. With experience and competence in bike riding, the perception of the activity changes, becoming something that is fun, freeing, or providing a sense of adventure. The perception may change further if riding becomes cycling and a form of exercise or if it becomes transportation, an alternative to driving a vehicle. Although the essential activity is the same, bike riding in this example, the meaning attributed to it is not static, changing with the development and skill acquisition of the rider and with the purpose for the use of the bicycle (e.g., exercise versus transportation).

This discussion conveys, in part, the danger of making assumptions about the meaning an activity holds for an

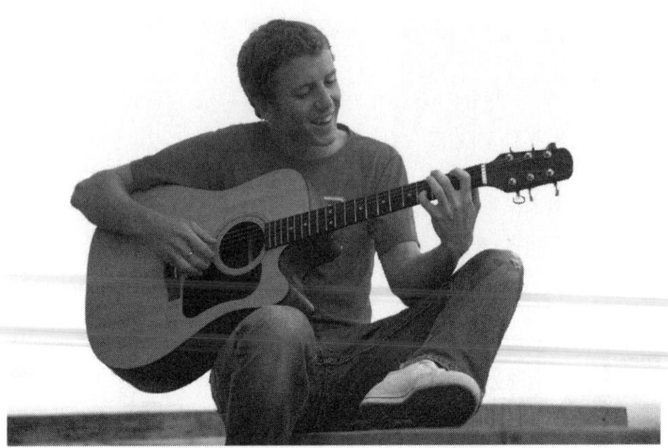

FIGURE 3-7 The activity of playing a guitar incorporates many different human functions and capabilities.

individual. An activity that might be considered work for one person is considered leisure for another. One person might view an activity such as reading as something he is forced to do, for homework as an example, but another seeks out reading as a desired activity. Understanding the meaning participation in an activity holds for an individual is useful knowledge for the clinician when determining the necessary, important, and desired activities to be enabled through AT use.

Occupational performance describes how a person does an occupation (AOTA, 2002; Chapparo & Ranka, 2005; Townsend & Polatajko, 2013). The manner in which the occupation or activity is completed, where, when, the frequency, and other temporal aspects discussed earlier are important to occupational performance. Performance of an occupation can be described in terms of the physical, sensory, cognitive, communicative, and affective elements that are used or required. For example, when a person plays a guitar, we can describe the gross and fine motor behaviors necessary to sit or stand, hold the guitar, and coordinate the actions of both hands to play desired chords. Auditory sensory feedback helps the player determine whether the chords are correct or not.

Communication is important when the guitar player is performing with others. Cognitive elements of memory for the fingering of the chords and the chords that make up the music and executive functions that help the player perform at the correct tempo, timing, and in coordination with other players are examples of the cognitive abilities that are used in this occupation. Affective aspects depend on the context in which the music is being played (Figure 3-7).

The level of skill and skill acquisition affect occupational performance. A novice is bound by procedures and rules as he develops the skills necessary to perform an occupation. Complex motor tasks may be under cognitive control as the performer learns how to complete them. Returning to the example of a guitar player, a novice player may need to think about the fingering needed to play a specific chord or use music to provide cues for finger placement. The tune is played as it is set out in the musical score. As the player gains expertise, the ability to play chords becomes much easier, no longer requiring cognitive control. The player gains confidence to deviate from the musical score to change how the tune is played. With expertise comes a degree of freedom allowing the person to experiment, take risks, and perform the occupation in novel ways.

Occupational performance is influenced by personal preferences and habits. Preferences may be expressed temporally (when and how frequently an occupation is performed), spatially (in a certain location), and through the manner in which an occupation is completed (Baum & Christiansen, 2005; Kielhofner, 2007). Habits are behaviors, usually physical but including mental, that are performed at a preconscious level as a result of experience and repetition (Christiansen, 2005).

Some have indicated that habitual actions free the individual to perform more complex and creative occupations. For example, when an individual is learning to type, concentration and physical effort are required to hit the correct keys to input the correct, desired characters. When typing becomes habitual, the individual is free to compose her thoughts as she types without the need to pay attention to the keys she must hit.

An individual who is motivated to perform an occupation may have a higher level of performance than if he was not motivated. Motivation comes from both internal sources (e.g., a student who chooses to study because he is interested in learning the material) and external sources (e.g., a student who studies to get a good grade and gain recognition from others). Self-determination and self-efficacy are related to motivation. An individual's sense of self-determination affects whether he perceives himself as capable of engaging in an activity and completing it with a degree of competence (Deci & Ryan, 2008).

Self-efficacy is the personal sense of how well one can perform an activity in an anticipated situation (Bandura, 1977). An individual may feel efficacious in certain situations but not in others. For example, a person may feel very comfortable speaking in front of a large group of people when she is reading from a script but less efficacious about speaking in front of a similarly sized group when she is speaking impromptu. A person who believes she is competent to perform an occupation generally is more motivated to perform the occupation than someone who has less confidence or direction.

Occupational satisfaction is derived from performing an activity. It describes the affective aspect of occupational performance (Townsend & Polatajko, 2013). Satisfaction is derived from the perceived level of performance, a sense of accomplishment and support received for the performance. The ability to choose the occupation and control the context in which it is performed affect satisfaction, with greater satisfaction gained when an occupation that is chosen is performed in a context or manner over which the person has some control (Miller Polgar, & Landry, 2004). This statement does not imply that satisfaction cannot be achieved from performance of occupations that are dictated (e.g., work tasks, educational tasks) or those that are performed in a prescribed manner because there is not a control–no control or choice–no choice dichotomy to occupational performance.

Rather, there is a continuum from a high degree of choice and control to less choice and control. Greater satisfaction is achieved when an individual perceives a higher level of choice and control.

Changes in skill level can affect satisfaction with occupational performance. An individual who has lost skill because of trauma or illness may experience less satisfaction with his occupational performance because he is unable to perform at a previous level of competence, which may result in discontinuing the occupation or changing how it is performed, depending on the meaning of the occupation held by the individual.

Social and cultural contexts influence the perception of satisfaction with performance. A person who excels at an occupation that is highly valued by society (e.g., professional athletes or actors) constantly has his performance critiqued in public forums.

An athlete with strong internal motivation and high self-efficacy will be less influenced in terms of satisfaction with performance than one who is more externally motivated, with lower self-efficacy. The intersection of the personal belief in self and social expressions of performance or ability contributes to satisfaction with performance.

Another concept related to occupational performance is **occupational engagement**, which refers to the degree to which a person is engaged with or involved in a particular occupation (AOTA, 2002; Townsend & Polatajko, 2013). Most people can think of times when they have participated in an occupation but have not been particularly engaged in it. Perhaps they have accompanied a friend to a movie or sports event that does not really interest them. Perhaps they are participating in a meeting that has gone on for too long. In these situations, a person is physically present, performing the activities that comprise the occupation, but is not actively engaged in the occupation, perhaps daydreaming or doing something else like responding to emails on a smart phone or tablet. Depending on the context, lack of engagement might not have much effect on the person, although if she does not engage in a meeting that results in work responsibilities or in a learning environment, the consequences of lack of engagement may be significant. Similarly, driving while distracted has major consequences.

There are some situations in which a person is not given a choice to participate in an occupation. A child may be pushed to learn a musical instrument that does not interest him. An older adult living in a long-term care facility may be taken to a group activity that is not of his choosing. These kinds of situations affect engagement with the occupation. The child required to take music lessons may put forth little effort to practice, which can lead to a limited acquisition of necessary skills and low satisfaction with performance of the musical occupation, which can then further decrease engagement.

To summarize, the intersection of the ideas of activity and human enriches our understanding of the person doing something. Although we can describe an activity in the absence of any knowledge of the person doing it, what remains is simply a mechanical description of a task. When the human is incorporated into the activity, the level of complexity is raised. The human attributes meaning to the activity as his performance expresses his identity and provides a sense of accomplishment.

Many of the occupations that we perform are not done individually. Theorists describing children's play have suggested a continuum that includes solitary play, parallel play (doing the same activity without interaction), and cooperative play, which engages more than one child (Ferland, 2005). Occupational scientists have studied groups of individuals working together in a common occupation such as meal preparation. These types of occupations are termed *shared occupations* when they involve two or more people acting together (Pierce, 2003). We now turn to a particular shared occupation, co-occupation.

Co-occupation

The concept of **co-occupation** is a recent idea that describes an occupation in which two or more people are involved that cannot be done by one person alone. For example, a conversation requires at least two people who interact with each other and take turns speaking and listening. It helps us understand the complexity of engagement in occupations and requires us to think about the shared occupations of a collective. Pierce describes co-occupations as highly interactive, reciprocal with each partner making an equal contribution (Pierce, 2011). Pickens and Pizur-Barnekow (2011) extend these ideas by discussing the implications of shared physicality, emotionality, and intentionality in the performance of co-occupations. Participants have reciprocal motor actions, are responsive to the emotional tone of others, and understand the roles others play in completing the occupation as well as their purpose for engaging in it. Shared meaning (Bruner, 1990) comes about through this confluence of shared physicality, emotionality, and intentionality achieved through co-occupation.

Many examples of co-occupations can be described. A simple example is a father reading to his child and asking the child to point out certain items in the book being read. In response to the verbal request to point out an item, the child makes the necessary movement. If the reading occurs at bedtime, the father may be attempting to create a quiet space and mood to prepare the child to sleep. His quiet tone is, hopefully, perceived and shared by the child. Both the father and child understand this shared bedtime routine.

Assistive technology's role in engagement in co-occupations is to facilitate one or both partner's participation. In this example, a child who is unable to use reliable auditory communication may use a communication device to indicate his response to the father's request.

A Paralympic sports game is an example of a complex co-occupation involving multiple players with multiple roles. Think about a football or soccer game. Each team has a goalie, team members who are forwards who advance the ball to the other team's net, members on defense who attempt to keep the ball away from their own goal, and midfielders who move the ball. Referees ensure that the game is played according to established rules. Coaches and managers are on the sidelines, and supporters are in the stands. Players respond to the physical actions of others on the field, attempting to take the ball away from opposition players and to keep the ball when it is in their team's possession. Emotions of elation, defeat, support, aggression, or frustration are exhibited and perceived by others. Intentionality is expressed in the desire to win or to support the team to win.

The concept of co-occupation contributes to our understanding of doing with AT by articulating conditions of performance of shared occupations. In the earlier example of reading at bedtime, Braille enables a partner with a visual impairment to read or identify names of objects in the book, a seating system supports upright positioning, and a hearing aid supports the child's ability to hear the father's request or the father's ability to hear the child's response. These examples demonstrate how the introduction and use of AT change the dynamics of co-occupations by changing how one or more partners complete the occupation.

Light's Model of Competence

Light (2003) describes several types of competence associated with AT use. She originally developed her categories for AAC systems (see Chapter 16), but most of the concepts apply more broadly. The first level of competence to be achieved is called **operational competence**. Operational competence is the ability to use the AT for the intended purpose. Included in this category are basic operations such as understanding how to use a joystick on a powered wheelchair to drive. Turning the device on and off, recharging batteries, and general maintenance are all part of operational competence.

After the basic operation of a device is mastered, it is necessary to develop **strategic competence** (Light, 2003). This category includes more subtle elements of using an AT device. For the wheelchair example, it might include developing skill at selecting the appropriate speed for an empty hallway versus a crowded restaurant and techniques for navigating a snowy sidewalk. For a manual wheelchair user, it might be learning how to jump curbs when there is no cut available. These strategies come with training and practice. They are part of what we call soft technologies.

The third type of competence is **social competence** (Light, 2003). This category applies more to certain types of ATs than others. For a user of AAC, social competence is required when selecting what vocabulary to use. For example, the words and formality of a conversation with a best friend are not the same as with a teacher or parent. Likewise, a user of a cognitive AT device may need training in the social expectations of using such a device.

Light also includes **linguistic competence** (Light, 2003). Although this competence was originally proposed to describe the process of developing sufficient vocabulary to use an AAC system, it can also apply to other ATs as well. A novice wheelchair user needs to have vocabulary that describes spatial concepts and operational concepts such as speed, acceleration, and force for a manual wheelchair. Users of cognitive AT devices need to have sufficient vocabulary to operate the devices and to understand their output. For example, a device for navigation in the community requires understanding of the language concept for it to be used successfully. The use of these four categories of competencies can be helpful in developing training programs, in helping new users develop strategies and social awareness, and in ensuring that the language concept necessary for understanding device use are available to the individual.

CONTEXT

The HAAT model uses the term *context* rather than *environment,* which is the term other similarly constructed models (e.g., WHO ICF, Canadian Model of Occupational Performance and Engagement and the Person-Environment-Occupational Performance Model) use to describe the contextual components that influence doing. The term *context* was deliberately chosen to convey a broader understanding of the external influences on a person doing an activity using AT. The word *environment* has the popular connotation of natural, physical elements and spaces, often related to pollution and climate change. This meaning does not capture the complexity of this element of the HAAT model and may result in exclusion of social, cultural, and institutional aspects that influence doing. By explicitly including these latter elements as components of the context, the HAAT model recognizes their contribution to doing with AT. The contextual influence on doing with AT can be understood from the perspective of how participation is enabled by physical, social, cultural, and institutional means and how that participation is sustained over a length of time (Mirza, Gossett Zakrajsek, & Borsci, 2012).

Over the past several decades, the models used to describe disability and the disablement process have changed dramatically (Whalley Hammell, 2006; McColl & Jongbloed, 2006). In the 1950s, the "problem" was seen as something intrinsic to the person with a disability that prevented him from participating in work, play, education, and ADLs. This problem was "in the person," that is, it was strictly the result of the impairment, which was then used as a rationale to exclude persons with disabilities from many different aspects of life.

More recently, there has been an increasing awareness that the difficulties experienced by individuals with disabilities result as much from contextual factors as from the impairment itself. Initially, this contextual focus was limited to the physical or built environment, with much effort to make curb cuts, install elevators, and so on. As individuals with disabilities began to participate more fully in society, it became evident that the social and attitudinal barriers were just as great as the physical ones. A "minority group model" of disability emerged in which the attention was shifted away from the impairment to the social, political, and environmental disadvantages forced on people who have disabilities (Whalley Hammell, 2006; Jongbloed & Crichton, 1990).

Bickenbach and colleagues (1999) conceptualized disability in a different way. In their view, disability is a universal experience if a person lives long enough. Contrary

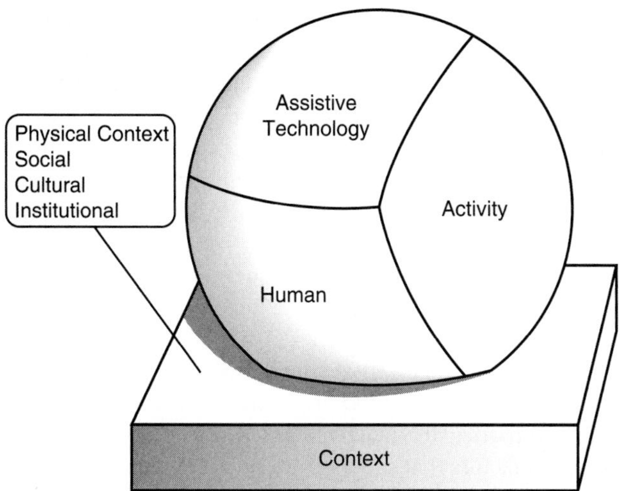

FIGURE 3-8 The Human Activity Assistive Technology (HAAT) model with elements of the context identified.

to the minority group model, which advocated for special status for individuals with disabilities, the universalism concept advocated for broader social justice and policies that were inclusive of persons with disabilities, actions that benefit a broader segment of society. From this perspective, problems of societal participation were no longer attributed to the impairment of the person with a disability. Rather, lack of participation in society was viewed as resulting from limitations in the social, cultural, institutional, and physical environments. The emphasis on participation in the ICF is indicative of the move away from a "problem in the person" concept to a "problem in the environment" model. When AT is viewed from this perspective, its purpose is reframed from minimizing personal limitations to minimizing restrictions that are created by the context in which a person lives and functions (Borg, Lindstrom, & Larsson, 2011).

In the HAAT model, we have captured these external influences in the *context.* As shown in Figure 3-8, the context includes four major considerations. These are the (1) physical context, including natural and built surroundings and physical parameters; (2) social context (e.g., with peers, with strangers); (3) cultural context; and (4) the institutional context, including formal legal, legislative, and sociocultural institutions such as religious institutions. The **contexts** in which the human carries out the activity can be determining factors in whether the person successfully uses an AT system. The supports and barriers in these environments are important considerations in the selection and evaluation of these systems.

One further distinction is important in the consideration of context—the level of environment. Three levels of environments have been described in the literature: micro environment, meso environment, and macro environment (Fougeyrollas & Gray, 1998; Townsend & Polatajko, 2002). The microenvironment refers to the closest, most intimate environments in which a person functions such as her home, school, or work setting. Here the person and her abilities are known, roles are defined, and rules and expectations are understood. The meso environment describes settings in which a person functions less frequently and includes various community facilities such as community centers, shopping malls, and churches. The macro environment refers to the broader social and cultural contexts that impose a legislative and moral behavioral framework on the person (Townsend & Polatajko, 2002). Each of these environments influences the use of AT systems. It is important to understand how each aids or hinders the use of technology.

Physical Context

Perhaps the easiest environmental component to understand is the **physical context**. This context involves the physical attributes of the environment that enable, hinder, or affect performance of daily activities, either with or without AT. This is the physical context that limits individuals with disabilities from engaging in occupations because they cannot access the places, materials, or persons to do so.

A distinction is made between the built and natural environment, which simply refers to human-made and non-human-made environments. Accessibility features can be integrated and legislated into human-made structures. The AT assessment process identifies the need for a device to be used in both natural and built environments. The device design process specifies whether a device can be used in both types of environments.

Assessment of the physical context for selection or evaluation of AT begins with articulation of the activities the person wants or needs to do in key contexts. Within buildings, people need to enter and exit the building; access various locations, possibly move between levels; and perform a variety of daily activities, such as using the toilet. Some of the physical aspects of the environment that should be considered include the width of hallways or doorways, distances between locations people must navigate, surface (e.g., carpet, transitions, floor surfaces), and height and weight of devices and objects (e.g., door) the person must manipulate.

Physical accessibility from a visual perspective involves wayfinding in an environment and locating key pieces of information. An individual with a visual impairment is assisted with movement throughout an environment with appropriate lighting, with hallways and other areas free of clutter and with a perceptible warning of hazardous situations, such as a change in elevation (e.g., stairs), (Sanford, 2012).

Modification of the environment through the use of signage that is perceptible by an individual with a visual impairment such as through the use of Braille or using an appropriate color contrast enables function in that environment. Access to visual information in an environment with the use of a low vision aid is a further consideration.

From a cognitive perspective, accessibility means signage that is easy to interpret, using simple symbols whose meaning is readily understandable. Providing signage or other forms of marking that indicate paths in large buildings is another way the physical context can be modified to support someone with a cognitive impairment. For example, some hospitals use colored lines to mark a path from a main entrance to select locations (Sanford, 2012).

Physical safety is an important consideration when assessing the environment. In the event of an emergency, the physical environment must support the ability of people with disabilities to safely move away from a dangerous situation and quickly exit the building, if needed. Such safety measures include strategies to assist people with mobility or visual impairments to move from one floor to another when elevators cannot be used or providing an alternate alarm system for deaf individuals who cannot hear an audible alarm.

Three commonly measured parameters of the physical environment—heat (related to temperature), sound, and light—most directly affect the performance of ATs. Many materials are sensitive to temperature and are affected by excessive heat or cold. For example, the properties of foams and gels used in seat cushions can change under conditions of very high or very low temperatures. Liquid crystal displays are affected by temperature, as well as by ambient (existing) light.

Ambient light in classrooms or work environments can affect the use of ATs. Some displays emit light and are better in conditions of reduced ambient light, but others reflect light and are better used in bright light. For example, direct sunlight often renders reading from screens on phones, tablets, and computers difficult, if not impossible. Low light conditions also affect the ability to read a screen and can affect the function of devices designed to assist persons with low vision.

Ambient sound (including noise) can interfere with the function of voice-activated devices or AAC systems with speech output when ambient noise levels are high. Sounds generated by such devices as printers, power wheelchairs, voice output communication aids, and auditory feedback from computer programs can be disruptive to others.

Often a person wants or needs to use the same assistive device in multiple contexts. In some cases, a device will work in one context but not in another. Voice recognition software is an example of a device that does not readily transfer from one context to another. In the relative quiet of an individual's home, voice recognition software may be an excellent alternative to direct input of computer keystrokes. However, it may not work in an office environment where noise interferes with the software, and its use may interfere with the work of colleagues in close proximity to the individual. Another example is an individual who propels his wheelchair in both a natural and built environment. Wheelchair tires that are appropriate for indoor use are often much less useful when used in outdoor conditions, particularly when propelling over grass or through sand or snow. Transportation of the device is another consideration when it is used in multiple contexts.

Social Context

The **social context** refers to individuals and groups who interact with the individual using AT, either directly or indirectly. This context can be understood from two perspectives. The first perspective involves individuals with whom a person interacts in contexts that are usually more familiar, local, and frequented. These occur in the micro and meso environments that were identified earlier. Contact with individuals in these environments tends to be direct rather than indirect. The second perspective is the larger, societal one, the macro environment that tends to have an indirect effect on the individual through the expression of societal mores, values, and practices. It is closely related to the institutional context.

Hocking (2011) poses several questions that inform the understanding of the social contextual influences on a person's doing an activity. She asks: (1) in a social context, who else is involved and do these others enable or hinder participation in activities? (2) Do disparities exist in terms of who is able to participate in activities, and who is not? What are the social factors that support or reduce these inequities? (3) What specific practices, societal norms, and traditions affect the ability to perform activity? These questions will be used to guide the discussion of the social context.

Who Is in the Social Context?

If you think about the people with whom you come into contact on a regular basis (daily, weekly), you can cluster these individuals into different groups, for example, family, friends, peers at school and work, or service providers (e.g., a personal trainer at a gym, religious leader, personal support worker). For the most part, these are people with whom we are very familiar. This familiarity results in certain mutual expectations for behavior, knowledge, attitudes, and so on. These individuals will have a direct influence on participation in activities. Some, such as family members, close friends, teachers, and co-workers, will have a more significant influence on participation but others such as service providers less so. Individuals with whom interaction is regular and frequent strongly influence what a person does through their knowledge and expectations of that person.

Individuals with whom interaction is direct but less frequent include service providers such as store clerks, extended family members and acquaintances who are not seen frequently, and others engaged in group activities such as a choir or fitness class where the group is doing an activity in parallel with minimum interaction among the group members.

A framework that is helpful in categorizing direct interactions is based on the circle of friends concept (Falvey et al., 1997). There are five circles surrounding the individual. The first circle represents the person's lifelong social partners. This group consists primarily of immediate family members. The second circle includes close friends (e.g., people who you tell your secrets to). These are often not family members. Acquaintances such as neighbors, schoolmates, co-workers, distant relatives (e.g., aunts and cousins), bus drivers, and shopkeepers are included in the third circle. The fourth circle is used to represent paid workers such as a physician, speech-language pathologist or a physical or occupational therapist, teacher, teacher assistant, or babysitter. Finally, the fifth circle is used to represent those unfamiliar partners with whom the person has occasional interactions. This circle includes everyone who does not fit in the first four circles. Thus, the familiarity with partners decreases as we move from circle one to five. One implication is that the modes of communication required to communicate with people in each circle will vary (see Chapter 16).

Indirect contact involves individuals who are physically present in a context but are separated from others, perhaps by position or practices that support the separation. Examples here include the president or executive members of a large company, a school president, or the executive director of a professional organization. These individuals exert power in the context in which they function; however, they do not come into direct contact with all of the other members in that context. A last group includes individuals with whom there is no expectation of direct interaction but whose actions have significant influence over the activities of others. This group includes people in positions of authority (WHO, 2001) such as politicians and policy makers who create and enforce legislation and administrators who create policies and procedures for organizations. The actions of this group have widespread influence over others in their social contexts.

How Do They Influence Participation and Use of Assistive Technology?

The beliefs and values, actions, and attitudes of others affect behavior and engagement in activity. Here, beliefs are considered to be worldviews, deeply held values that are foundational to how a person lives. The ICF defines attitudes as "the observable consequences of customs, practices, ideologies, values, norms, factual beliefs and religious beliefs " (WHO, 2001, p. 190). Actions are what others in social contexts do. Knowledge is influential on each of these constructs.

Attitudes and actions are rooted in a person's beliefs, which are viewed as higher order, more entrenched viewpoints. Beliefs express how a person understands his position in the world relative to others. For example, someone who believes all persons are equal will express very different opinions and actions than another person who believes that the possession of certain traits make one group of people better or worse than other.

Similarly, deeply held values may lead one person to believe that all people have the same rights and responsibilities, but another believes the opposite. Considering the different groups described in the previous section, it is apparent that as others become further removed from the individual, the influence and consequences of their beliefs on that individual are related to the power they hold in the social context. At all levels, there is great potential to enable or hinder the activities of persons with disabilities and their access to and use of AT.

Inclusive attitudes of others support activity participation and the use of AT. These attitudes recognize the person with a disability for attributes that may have little to do with the presence of an impairment. For example, the person is recognized as a child, a parent, or a teacher or as someone with a good sense of humor or perhaps a less desirable trait such as a quick temper. The point here is that the presence of the impairment does not define the person for these individuals with whom they interact. The presence of the impairment does not influence their behavior toward that person.

Awareness and acceptance of alternate ways of doing is another expression of an inclusive attitude. Breaking with societal traditions, etiquette, and practices supports doing with AT. Recognition that use of a communication aid is just another way to talk or use of a wheelchair as just another way to move leads to actions and behaviors that make it possible for persons using these devices to engage in their communities and desired activities.

On the other hand, exclusionary attitudes and prejudices limit the capabilities (Nussbaum, 2011; Sen, 2009) of persons with disabilities. As Fougeyrollas (1997) points out, social influence on individuals is related to what is considered normal or expected. Individuals who have disabilities may be stigmatized because of their disability. A frequent comment by persons with disabilities is that it is often the social environment, the attitude of others, that creates more of a disability than the physical barriers in the environment. When policies and practices do not recognize the needs of individuals with disabilities, these individuals are excluded from social participation in the areas they govern. For example, when a building is constructed with accessibility features that support the needs of persons with mobility impairments only, individuals with other impairments that affect movement in that building (e.g., a person with low vision) are excluded, preventing them from accessing the services in that building. Public transportation that does not provide options for individuals with cognitive impairments denies them community mobility.

A paternalistic perspective attitude conveys to the person with a disability that she needs to be protected, that she is not capable of looking after herself or making decisions about her own life. Policies and procedures that restrict the choices of a person with a disability often derive from a paternalistic perspective. This perspective is apparent in health care practices when treatment is recommended without regard to the person's lifestyle or when the view of patient means decisions are made for someone (Jongbloed & Crichton, 1990). Often persons with disabilities or chronic illness are referred to patients even in nonmedical spheres, so the protective and diminishing attitudes pervade past discharge from any medical care. First-person narratives by persons with disabilities frequently recount interactions in which the behaviors of others suggest that they see the presence of a disability as generalizing to other capacities. The possession of one trait that limits performance in one body function is generalized to performance of other functions (Whalley Hammell, 2006). Two common examples are when others speak louder to a person with low vision or with a communication impairment thinking that increased volume will facilitate the conversation or when others assume a cognitive impairment goes along with the use of a wheelchair. These generalizations can result in one partner assuming diminished capacity in the other and acting accordingly.

Actions of Others in the Social Context

Participation in activities and in the community is supported or hindered by the actions of others based on their understanding of their role in enacting this participation. Two actions that support participation are enabling performance and advocating for inclusion.

In the first instance, enablement is achieved by fostering a social context that supports participation of individuals with disabilities doing activity with technology. This enablement includes meaningful partnership with individuals with disabilities to determine that the needs identified are relevant and that solutions created are useable. For example, the need for accessible washroom stalls is met with the creation of such stalls, but if someone who needs to use the stall cannot access them because the door to the washroom is heavy or the path to the stall is not clear, then the accessible stall is not useable.

Advocacy involves championing for the right to full participation for all members of a community or society. However, if advocacy occurs without the participation of members of groups who are excluded or marginalized, then resulting changes may not truly be inclusive. Rather than advocating *for* a person or group, advocating *with* the person or group achieves a more inclusive result. Advocacy on a large scale involves championing full participation for a group; for example, current advocacy efforts in some countries to ratify the United Nations Convention on the Rights of Persons with Disabilities (UN, 2006). Advocacy on a smaller scale might involve a single person; for example, a mother who advocates for the opportunity for her child to go outside for recess at school.

Relationships with others in the environment affect the use of technology. Those close to the individual, such as family, friends, teachers, or coworkers, have a better understanding of the person's capacities, so use of technology is often easier. With unfamiliar people, technology use may be more complex because expectations and the understanding of how the technology works differ. For these reasons, it is important to determine who provides assistance to individuals using AT in various environments, but most important in key environments such as homes, schools, and workplaces.

The acceptance or rejection of the use of AT by others in the social context and their knowledge of the purpose and need for the AT influence whether or not the individual will be successful with their technology use. As mentioned above, if use of AT is considered as simply another way of performing an activity by others, its use is promoted. An individual may limit or stop using a device when its use is seen as a sign the user is lazy (e.g., pushing a person to walk rather than use a wheelchair).

The actions of others in the social environment is a source of **stigma**, which is defined as a mark of shame; an attribute that discredits the person who possesses it (Goffman, 1963). Certain devices such as hearing aids and power wheelchairs seem to convey greater disability than others such as eyeglasses or manual wheelchairs. Consequently, persons with disabilities may choose not to use a particular AT in a social environment because of the stigma it conveys. Consider an office worker, Ted, who has the capacity to use a manual wheelchair but who might choose to use a power chair because of the energy savings it affords. The behavior of certain colleagues in the office suggests that they perceive Ted to be less competent in performing his job tasks than he actually is. Ted's reaction may be to minimize the appearance of his disability through use of a manual wheelchair, although this choice might result in negative consequences such as excessive energy expenditure and fatigue in the short term and shoulder injury in the long term.

Cultural Context

Culture is an intangible concept that can be cumbersome to define. Wade Davis suggests that it can be understood as:

> *a unique and ever-changing constellation [that] we recognize through the observation and study of . . . language, religion, social and economic organization, decorative arts, stories, myths, ritual practices and beliefs and a host of other adaptive traits and characteristics. The full measure of a culture embraces both the actions of a people and the quality of their aspirations. No description of a people can be complete without reference to the character of their homeland, the ecological and geographical matrix in which they have determined to live out their destiny (Davis, 2009, pp. 32-33).*

This rich description of culture highlights the influence of the collective on the individual's perception and use of AT, that is, the shared beliefs that influence the client's worldview will similarly influence his readiness to incorporate AT into his daily occupations. It further suggests that in addition to beliefs, aspects such as collective aspirations, time, place, and space are all relevant to the AT design, selection, and use. These far-reaching philosophical ideas may seem quite far removed from the selection of AT. Yet cultural beliefs can be a major factor in the acceptance and use of a device, particularly when the client and clinician do not share cultural beliefs and experiences.

Consider a clinician who was raised and educated in southern Canada who assumes a clinical position in the far north of that country. The cultural beliefs and experiences of this clinician and her clients are not shared for common occupations. In the south, travel from one location to another is most commonly accomplished with a car on paved roads. In the far north, vehicles such as an automobile are not as effective, and movement from one location to another is easier in the winter when the land is frozen to allow use of snowmobiles or dog sleds. Play for a child in the north is less dependent on electronics than it is in the south because of access issues. Food preparation and other household occupations differ. Indeed, access to many amenities such as a reliable source of electricity or fresh, affordable food is limited in many remote communities in the north (MacLachlan, 2010).

The clinician is not able to rely on her own cultural experiences but must accommodate her clinical reasoning to ensure that the recommendations made will be meaningful and appropriate for the cultural (and other) context in which she practices. In simpler form: clinical recommendations that are appropriate in the **cultural context** in which she was raised and educated may be highly inappropriate in the context in which she practices.

What are some of the cultural aspects that may influence the readiness to use and accept technology? Beliefs about independence versus interdependence have implications for how the client accepts assistance. Western culture places high value on independence, which might either reinforce use of technology or restrict it. If the technology use is interpreted by the client and others as a sign of disability, vulnerability, or some other undesirable attribute, the device is more likely to be rejected or abandoned. On the other hand, technology that is valued, is seen to enable independence, or that, in the eyes of the user and others, confers a positive status is more likely to be accepted and used.

Cultural beliefs that value interdependence may cause the client to accept assistance from others and consider technology as unnecessary. Of course, it is not usually this black and white; many clients use a mix of technology and personal assistance in addition to using their own abilities (Miller Polgar, 2010).

Beliefs about disability, occupational or social justice, and the rights to choice and control over occupational engagement, also influence technology selection and use. A client and others who hold the view that a disability is some form of punishment and that those with a disability do not have the right to engage in or are not included in community or civic activities may not see the need for technology that enables these occupations. Views about personal space may influence the acceptance of technology, such as a wheelchair or some electronic aids to daily living, that place a physical barrier between the client and others in her environment. Culture, although a somewhat nebulous construct, is an important aspect in the consideration of appropriate AT. Time spent understanding the cultural beliefs and experiences of the client and significant others is necessary to facilitate the most appropriate AT recommendation.

An example that illustrates cultural aspects of independence and family roles involves Frank, who has amyotrophic lateral sclerosis (ALS) (Murphy & Cook, 1985). Before his disability, Frank was dominant as head of his family. He was fiercely independent and valued his role as provider. As he lost the ability to speak because of his ALS, he used a small typewriter-like device to interact with his family. It allowed him to retain his head-of-household role. He used his communication device to make investment decisions, plan legal affairs, and make shopping lists. His family provided the legwork to carry out his directions. As his ALS progressed, his motor control deteriorated until he could only raise his eyebrows. A new communication device, which used this limited movement, was obtained for him, but he was not interested in using it. After repeated unsuccessful attempts to provide support for the use of this new device, those working with Frank began to realize that his role in the family had changed. Because of his dependence on aids and the difficulty in communicating with the new device, he lost all interest in his family role. His wife became the family leader, and she began to make decisions that had always been reserved for him. These changes in the family, a difficult concept for Frank because of his cultural perception of family roles, led to his withdrawal and the failure of the ATs to meet his needs.

Institutional Context

The **institutional context** refers to larger organizations within a society that are responsible for policies, decision-making processes, and procedures. Institutional aspects of legislation, regulation and policy, funding at a state or provincial level, and policies at more local levels, such as municipalities, school boards, health care institutions, or other community agencies, are of particular importance to provision of AT. The Canadian Model of Occupational Performance and Engagement includes economic, legal, and political components, such as government-funded services, legislation, and political regulations and policies in the institutional element (Townsend and Polatajko, 2002). The Person-Environment-Occupational Performance model situates similar concepts in the external environment in the social and environment systems (Baum & Christiansen, 2005).

The ICF chapter that categorizes similar aspects is labeled *services, systems, and policies* (WHO, 2001). *Services* are "benefits, structured programs and operations in various sectors of society" that meet the needs of individuals (WHO, 2001, p. 192). *Systems* are the administrative and organizational layer at all levels of government or other authorities that plan, implement and monitor services. *Policies* are "rules, regulations, conventions and standards" that regulate systems and, again, exist at all levels of government or other organizations (WHO, 2001, p. 192).

Legislation

Legislation in many countries establishes laws, policies, and regulations that enable persons with disabilities to engage in activities in various contexts within their local communities and beyond. Other legislation specifically addresses AT provision and service delivery. These laws specifically comment on environmental access issues; modifications required in employment, educational, and other community settings; and the responsibility of the employer or educational system in providing accommodations for eligible individuals, including the provision of AT. It is not possible to review all of the primary legislation that influences AT use, provision, and service delivery, so a sample is provided here.

Hocking (2011) again offers key questions that guide understanding and critique of how the institutional context influences participation in activities. She poses the question of how policies and legislation affect participation and directs us to identify the sectors and institutions that explicitly or implicitly affect participation. When considering the institutional context of legislation and policy, it is useful to identify the aim or purpose of a piece of legislation or policy, key definitions (e.g., definition of a person with a disability, AT), conditions of enactment of the legislation, and related regulations. Furthermore, it is useful to identify not only what is included in legislation, regulation, or policy but also what is not. For example, in the funding area, often items such as wheelchairs or communication aids are included, but other devices such as electronic aids to daily living are not.

Rehabilitation Act of 1973 (Amended)

The Rehabilitation Act of 1973 established several important principles on which subsequent legislation has been based. The most far-reaching of these principles are nondiscrimination and **reasonable accommodation**. Section 504 of the Rehabilitation Act prohibits any activity receiving federal funds from discriminating solely on the basis of disability. To remedy discrimination, federally funded activities and programs must offer reasonable accommodations to facilities, programs, and benefits to ensure that people with disabilities have equal access and equal opportunity to derive benefits. As a result of the wide reach of federal funding, the nondiscrimination provisions of the Rehabilitation Act of 1973 architectural changes to reduce barriers such as ramps and curb cuts were made to accommodate people who use wheelchairs, and voice and Braille labels were added to signs to provide access for persons with visual impairments.

The Rehabilitation Act was amended in 1986 (PL 99-506), 1992 (PL 102-569), and 1993 (PL 103-73). Together these amendments include several provisions involving AT. First, the amendments require that each state include within its vocational rehabilitation plan a provision for AT. Because this plan is the basis by which states receive federal funding for vocational rehabilitation, there is a strong incentive to provide these technology-related services.

The Rehabilitation Act also requires that provision for acquiring appropriate and necessary AT devices and services be included in Individualized Written Rehabilitation Programs (IWRPs), renamed in the 1998 amendments as Individualized Plans for Employment (IPEs), which are written for individuals with disabilities.

A third Rehabilitation Act provision with important AT implications is Section 508. This section was developed to ensure access to "electronic office equipment" by persons with disabilities who work for the federal government. Although restricting the provision of the Act to the federal government may seem to severely reduce its impact, because the federal government is such a large purchaser of computers and other office technology, several manufacturers included in the basic designs of their computer systems technology increasing access outside of government departments.

The major intent of Section 508 is that electronic and information technology developed, procured, maintained, or used by the federal government be accessible to people with disabilities. It covers access to electronic office equipment and electronic information services provided to the public by the federal government. This measure ensures that users with disabilities (1) have access to the same databases and application programs as other users, (2) are supported in manipulating data and related information resources to attain equivalent end results as other end users, and (3) can transmit and receive messages using the same telecommunication systems as other end users.

Americans with Disabilities Act of 1990

The Americans with Disabilities Act (ADA, PL 101-336) prohibits discrimination on the basis of disability in employment, state and local government, public accommodations, commercial facilities, transportation, and telecommunications. To be protected by the ADA, an individual must meet the following ADA definitions of disability: a person who has a physical or mental impairment that substantially limits one or more major life activities, a person who has a history or record of such an impairment, or a person who is perceived by others as having such an impairment. The ADA does not specifically name all the impairments that are covered. The ADA has four main titles: Title I (employment), Title II (state and local government agencies and public transportation), Title III (public accommodations), and Title IV (telecommunications), all of which affect the application of AT.

The prohibition of employment discrimination on the basis of disability stated in Title I of the ADA requires employers with 15 or more employees, including religious entities with 15 or more employees, to provide qualified individuals with disabilities an equal opportunity to benefit from the full range of employment-related opportunities available to others. For example, it prohibits discrimination in recruitment, hiring, promotions, training, pay, fringe benefits, and other privileges of employment. It restricts questions that can be asked about an applicant's disability before a job offer is made. Many employment activities involve the use and application of AT because Title I of the ADA requires that employers make reasonable accommodation to the known physical or mental limitations of otherwise qualified individuals with disabilities unless it results in undue hardship. The application of Title I to employee fringe benefits protects employees with disabilities and family members with disabilities from discrimination in the provision of health insurance benefits, which is an important funding source for ATs.

Title II covers all activities of state and local governments regardless of the government entity's size or receipt of federal funding. Title II requires that state and local governments give people with disabilities an equal opportunity to benefit from all their programs, services, and activities (e.g., public education, employment, transportation, recreation, health care, social services, courts, voting, and town meetings). These opportunities are achieved through modification of the physical environment and use of devices to support communication of individuals with hearing, vision, or speech impairments.

The transportation provisions of Title II cover public transportation services, such as city buses and public rail transit (e.g., subways, commuter rails, Amtrak). Public transportation authorities may not discriminate against people with disabilities in the provision of their services. They must comply with requirements for accessibility in newly purchased vehicles; make good faith efforts to purchase or lease accessible used buses; remanufacture buses in an accessible manner; and unless it would result in an undue burden, provide accessible transportation options where they operate fixed-route bus or rail systems.

Title III covers businesses and nonprofit service providers that are public accommodations, privately operated entities offering certain types of courses and examinations, and privately operated transportation and commercial facilities. Public accommodations are private entities that own, lease, lease to, or operate facilities such as restaurants, retail stores, hotels, and movie theaters; private schools; convention centers; physicians' offices; homeless shelters; transportation depots; zoos; funeral homes; day care centers; and recreation facilities, including sports stadiums and fitness clubs. Transportation services provided by private entities are also covered by Title III.

Title IV addresses telephone and television access for people with hearing and speech disabilities; this section has wide AT implications because emerging and developing technologies in the telecommunications and television fields are changing at a rapid pace. Title IV requires common carriers (telephone companies) to establish interstate and intrastate telecommunications relay services (TRS) 24 hours a day, 7 days a week. TRS enables callers with hearing and speech disabilities who use text telephones (TTYs) and callers who use voice telephones to communicate with each other through a third-party communications assistant. The Federal Communications Commission (FCC) has set minimum standards for TRS services. Title IV also requires closed captioning of federally funded public service announcements.

Individuals with Disabilities Education Act, Amendments of 2004

The Education for All Handicapped Children Act (EAHCA) of 1975, PL 94-142, later amended by the Individuals with Disabilities Education (IDEA) Act of 1990 and the IDEA Amendments of 1997 (IDEA 97), PL 105-17, establish the right of every child with a disability to receive a **"free and appropriate public education" (FAPE)**. Before this law, more than 1 million children with disabilities were excluded from American public schools.

The centerpiece of the IDEA is an **individualized education plan (IEP)** that describes each student's current educational performance and outlines the program of specially designed instruction (special education) and supplemental (related) services each child with a disability is to receive as part of his or her FAPE. IEPs also state specific educational goals to be achieved by the student, both short and long term (by the end of the school year). Assistive devices and training in their use have long been recognized as components of an FAPE. In the 1997 IDEA Amendments PL 105-17, schools were directed to consider the AT needs when formulating every IEP for students with disabilities.

Other important provisions of the EAHCA and IDEA are the requirement that children with disabilities are educated with their nondisabled peers to "the maximum extent appropriate." This is known as the **"least restrictive environment"** principle. Children with disabilities are to be removed from the regular class environment "only when the nature or severity of the disability is such that education in regular classes cannot be achieved satisfactorily."

The impact of this law has been far reaching. Devices ranging from sensory aids (visual and auditory) to AAC devices to specialized computers have been used to provide access to educational programs for children with disabilities. Lack of local services or lack of funds is not sufficient reason to deny services or devices justified in the IEP. If the IEP goals are not met or if there are differences over what should be included in the IEP, a fair hearing process may be pursued.

The focus of IDEA 97 is on improving results for children with disabilities. One major portion of the original act invited states to expand and improve services to infants and toddlers with disabilities and their families (Part H, the Infants and Toddlers with Disabilities Program). In 1997, Part H became Part C of IDEA 97.

Assistive Technology Act of 1998

Designated as PL 105-394, the Assistive Technology Act replaced the Technology-Related Assistance for Individuals with Disabilities Act of 1988 (PL 100-407) and the amendments to that law (PL 103-218) enacted in 1994. The Assistive Technology Act extends funding to the 50 states, the District of Columbia, Puerto Rico, and outlying areas (Guam, American Samoa, US Virgin Islands, and the Commonwealth of the Northern Mariana Islands) that received federal funding under the Technology Act. The purposes of the Assistive Technology Act include the following:

1. Support states in sustaining and strengthening their capacity to address the AT needs of individuals with disabilities
2. Support the investment in technology across federal agencies and departments that could benefit individuals with disabilities
3. Support microloan programs to individuals wishing to purchase AT devices or services

The Assistive Technology Act is divided into three parts: Title I, State Grant Programs; Title II, National Activities; and Title III, Alternative Financing Mechanisms.

Title I provides grants to states to support capacity building and advocacy activities designed to assist the states in maintaining permanent, comprehensive, consumer-responsive, statewide programs of technology-related assistance. These include public awareness, interagency coordination, technical assistance, and training to promote access to AT and support to community-based organizations that provide AT devices and services or assist individuals in using AT. Title I also provides legal protection and advocacy services; funding for technical assistance, including a national public Internet site; and technical assistance to the states.

Title II provides for increased coordination of federal efforts related to AT and universal design. It authorized funding for multiple grant programs from fiscal years 1999 through 2000, including grants for universal design research, Small Business Innovative Research grants related to AT, grants to commercial or other organizations for research and development related to universal design concepts, grants or other mechanisms to address the unique AT needs of urban and rural areas and of children and the elderly, and grants or other mechanisms to improve training of rehabilitation engineers and technicians.

Title III requires the Secretary of Education to award grants to states and outlying areas to pay for the federal share of the cost of the establishment and administration of or the expansion and administration of specified types of alternative financing systems for AT for people with disabilities. These alternative-funding mechanisms may include a low-interest loan fund, an interest buy-down program, a revolving loan fund, a loan guarantee or insurance program, and others (RESNA Technical Assistance Project, 1999).

The primary changes in the 2004 amendment include the repeal of the provision that allows the law to expire on an annual basis. It includes the provision of AT for individuals of all ages and attempts to make the provision of AT and access to AT services more consistent across the states and other US jurisdictions (Association of Assistive Technology Act Programs, www.ataporg.com/states.html).

The Developmental Disabilities Assistance and Bill of Rights Act

The developmental disabilities program was originally enacted as Title I of the Mental Retardation Facilities and Construction Act of 1963 (PL 88-164) and has been amended eight times since then. This program provides grants to states for developmental disabilities councils (DD councils), university-affiliated programs (UAPs), and protection and advocacy activities for persons with developmental disabilities (PADDs). Grants to UAPs include grants for training projects with respect to AT services for the purpose of assisting UAPs in providing training to personnel who provide or will provide AT services and devices to PADDs and their families. Such projects may provide training and technical assistance to improve access to AT services for PADDs and may include stipends and tuition assistance for training project participants.

The Australian Disability Discrimination Act, amended in 2012, is designed to eliminate discrimination on the basis of disability in the workplace, educational setting, and other facilities in the provision of goods and services, the administration of federal programs, and in existing legislation and seeks to promote acceptance of individuals with disabilities and recognition of their fundamental rights. Similarly, the Disability Discrimination Act in the United Kingdom, amended in 2006, protects the right of individuals with disabilities to be free from discrimination in the provision of goods and services, in the employment and education sectors, and in interactions with national public organizations.

In Canada, the province of Ontario is the only one that has legislation promoting accessibility of individuals with disabilities. The Accessibility for Ontarians with Disabilities Act (2005) legislates accessibility in the provision of goods and services in provincial, public, and private sector organizations. It includes access to transportation, education, information, and communication.

Funding Regulations

Funding policies and regulations establish who is eligible to receive assistance for the purchase of devices, which devices are supported in funding schemes, and who (i.e., which professional group) serves as the funding gatekeepers.

Medicaid

Medicaid is a US federal program created in 1965 and codified as Title XIX of the Social Security Act (42 U.S.C. §§1396. et. seq.). The primary goal of Medicaid is to provide medical assistance to persons in need and to furnish them with rehabilitation and other services to help them "attain or retain capability for independence or self-care" (42 U.S.C. §1396). The federal regulations provide further that "each service must be sufficient in amount, duration and scope to reasonably achieve its purpose" (42 C.F.R. §440.230[b]). It is an income-based or "means-tested" program, so eligibility depends on a person's income level. Medicaid is an example of a program of joint federal and state responsibilities, called "cooperative federalism." These programs are noted by joint or shared responsibilities for financing and administration. The federal government guarantees no less than 50% funding for state outlays for their Medicaid programs, with the amounts increasing as the relative wealth of the state's population decreases. The federal government, through the Centers for Medicare and Medicaid Services (CMS), also establishes broad criteria for people who must be eligible for Medicaid, the services Medicaid programs must offer, and the way those services must be delivered; states then additionally make choices about who is eligible, which services are offered, and how they are delivered. States also are responsible for day-to-day program administration.

Medicaid is not a federally mandated program. Instead, states must elect to participate and express their desire to do so by submitting a "state plan for medical assistance" to CMS. Every state participates in Medicaid. The state plan is an acknowledgement that the state will follow all federally established Medicaid requirements and identifies all the choices the states will make regarding individual eligibility and covered services. The Medicaid program neither provides services directly nor pays cash assistance directly to individuals who need medical care. Rather, the program provides payment to providers (e.g., hospitals, rehabilitation centers, therapists, and durable medical equipment [DME] suppliers) for covered supplies and services rendered to qualified recipients.

Medicaid programs are the largest funding source for ATs—both devices and services—in the United States. However, its program vocabulary was established decades before the phrase *assistive technology* was coined, so reference to AT in Medicaid means access to items of DME or prosthetic devices. Reference to services means access to occupational, physical, or speech-language pathology or audiology services. An individual who seeks Medicaid funding for any of these items or services must generally meet a three-part test: (1) the individual must be eligible for Medicaid, (2) the specific device or service requested must be one that is covered by the Medicaid program, and (3) the individual must establish that the device or service requested.

Persons with disabilities who are seeking to use Medicaid as a source of funding for AT must navigate an often cumbersome process that usually requires both their specific conditions and needs to be expressed in language designed to fit program criteria. With very few exceptions, the Medicaid law and its implementing regulations do not identify specific types of treatment or devices that are covered, only broad categories of health care. This situation imposes an interpretive obligation on state program administrators who must decide whether the specific item or service requested "fits" or is "covered" by one of the state's Medicaid services. Although access to many ATs—both devices and services—is readily provided, these interpretive duties have proved a breeding ground for dispute about coverage and medical need. Many states have sought to avoid these disputes by adopting item- or service-specific clinical or coverage criteria. The most common items that are the subject of these criteria are communication devices and wheelchairs.

Medicare

The Medicaid and Medicare programs, created together in 1965, are codified as Title XVIII of the Social Security Act. Although Medicaid is focused on the needs of those who lack the financial means to meet the costs of necessary health care, Medicare initially was focused on the needs of elderly adults, defined as individuals age 65 years and older. It was believed that this population was less wealthy and less healthy and had access to less health insurance than younger individuals and therefore needed assistance meeting the costs of their health care needs. Medicare subsequently was expanded to serve individuals with disabilities who are younger than age 65 years.

Medicare is administered by the federal government, and the rules are the same for every state in the nation. Medicare is another major funding source for AT. Similar to Medicaid, however, its program vocabulary characterizes devices as either DME or prosthetic devices. It also covers occupational and physical therapy and speech-language pathology services. Medicare is a health insurance program for four groups: (1) individuals age 65 years or older; (2) people of all ages who meet the standards of disability under the Social Security Act; (3) the disabled children of persons who had been working and who became disabled themselves, died, or retired at age 65 years; and (4) people with end-stage renal disease.

It is divided into two parts. Part A, known as "hospital insurance," covers inpatient services, postdischarge care in skilled nursing homes, hospice care, and home health care. Home health care includes DME, occupational and physical therapy, and speech-language pathology services. Part B, known as "supplemental medical insurance," covers, among other items, DME, rehabilitation services, and home health care for beneficiaries not covered by Part A. Access to ATs for Medicare recipients is overwhelmingly through the Part B benefit.

The Medicare program operates like a federally subsidized insurance program. Beneficiary contributions include cash deductions and coinsurance requirements under Parts A and B and monthly premiums for Part B. Medicaid programs can assume the Medicare portion of the cost-sharing requirements for individuals who are poor and who qualify for both Medicare and Medicaid. Also, similar to many insurers, Medicare is a cost reimbursement program, meaning that Medicare recipients must first obtain an item or service and then seek Medicare reimbursement for their outlays.

Some AT devices are covered by Medicare as items of DME or as prosthetic devices. Medicare defines DME as equipment that (1) can withstand repeated use, (2) is primarily and customarily used to serve a medical purpose, (3) generally is not useful to a person in the absence of illness or injury, and (4) is appropriate for use in the home. Medicare also has a unique limitation among benefits and funding programs that applies to mobility aids. It claims that Congress has directed that it consider only a person's mobility-related ADLs that arise in the person's home, as opposed to all typical mobility needs regardless of environment, which is the generally accepted and long-standing professional standard for mobility aid assessment.

Medicare reimbursement for items or services is based on the same three factors as were stated for Medicaid: individual eligibility, coverage, and medical necessity. Medicare uses the phrase "reasonable and necessary" as a synonym of medical necessity. To be eligible for Medicare reimbursement, a covered item or service must be reasonable and necessary for the treatment of an illness or injury or to improve the functioning of a malformed body member. Medicare guidance further describes the concept of "reasonableness": although an item may be medically necessary, it may not be reimbursed by Medicare if (1) the cost of the item is disproportionate to the therapeutic benefits derived from its use, (2) the item is more expensive than an appropriate alternative, or (3) the item serves the same purpose as equipment already available to the beneficiary.

Similar to most insurance policies, Medicare excludes many items for coverage, including hearing aids and eyeglasses. Other exclusions apply to items or services deemed related to "convenience," "personal comfort," or "custodial care." Because these terms are subjective and the general acceptance of certain medical procedures changes over time, Medicare has established procedures for reexamining these conclusions.

Funding in Other Jurisdictions

Across the globe, funding for provision of assistive devices varies widely, with no funding provisions in some jurisdictions. Again, a sample of funding support is given here. In the United Kingdom, the Personal Independence Payment (PIP) is a new funding scheme that is currently transitioning to replace the Disability Living Allowance. Under this new scheme, individuals with disabilities, or their caregivers, are provided with a funding allotment after an assessment process. These funds are intended for use to offset some of the additional expenses incurred as the result of the disability. These funds are not directed to any specific product or service. The recipient determines how they will be distributed, within the parameters of the program.

A longstanding program in Ontario, Canada, is the Assistive Devices Program (ADP). Under this program, the provincial government covers a percentage of the cost of a device. A number of different categories of devices are included, such as seating, mobility, communication, computer access, and vision and hearing products. A set process is established that requires the individual seeking the device to be assessed by an ADP authorizer (someone with health care credentials who has completed the necessary process to become an authorizer) and receive a recommendation for a category of technology, which is then reviewed at the provincial level before approval and funding.

The governments of the Nordic countries of Denmark, Finland, Iceland, Norway, and Sweden promote the view that inclusion of individuals with disabilities is a public responsibility. Government funding for AT exists in each of these countries, although the structure varies. The governments of Denmark, Norway, and Sweden fund 100% of the programs that support the provision of AT. Finland and Iceland use a combination of public and private monies for this purpose. AT provision is centralized in Norway and Sweden and provided at the level of local councils in Denmark. These countries promote voluntary inclusion and accessibility rather than through legislative means (Nordic Centre for Rehabilitation Technology, 2007).

A final influence of the institutional environment on AT is legislation and standards that govern product design, function, and safety standards. For a product to be marketed and for it to be included as a device for which funding assistance is provided, the developers or manufacturers must ensure that testing and other measures have been undertaken to ensure that the product meets certain technical standards. The International Standards Organization (ISO) and the American National Standards Institution (ANSI)/RESNA organization develop these standards. Standards for individual types of ATs are discussed in later chapters.

INTEGRATING THE HUMAN DOING IN CONTEXT

To this point, the HAAT elements of activity, human, and context have been discussed as well as the interaction of the human and the activity. Activity can be understood from self-care, productivity, and leisure categories. The WHO's ICF provides additional classifications of activities and participation that are influenced by AT use. For the purposes of output of ATs, this book focuses on communication, cognitive function, manipulation, mobility, and sensory functions of audition and vision.

It is not sufficient to simply categorize activity to understand its role in a person's life; capturing information on how an activity is performed, where, when, with whom, and frequency is also necessary when considering the influence of AT on activity performance.

On a basic level, the human can be understood from the perspective of body structures and functions. However, this mechanistic view ignores the individual and collective characteristics of humans that influence why and how they do an activity. Ideas of level of expertise, meaning held of an activity, individual roles, and lifespan perspectives affect activity performance and AT use.

The human actor brings meaning to the activity. Ideas from occupational therapy and occupational science illuminate this idea of a human doing an activity. Occupational performance describes the doing, and occupational satisfaction introduces the human element of the perception of the performance. Occupational engagement brings awareness to the varying degree to which a human is actively involved in the performance of an occupation and how some occupations or activities become rote and scaffold more complex ones.

The institutional elements of physical, social, cultural, and institutional contexts all influence the human's performance of activity. The context can enable or hinder human activity via the structure of the physical context, the attitudes, knowledge, and behaviors of others in the social context, through cultural values and mores and with institutional legislation, policies, regulations, and funding.

Now we consider how these three elements interact before revisiting ideas about AT that were introduced in Chapter 2. We will describe how AT enables the human doing an activity in context.

Meaning at the Intersection of Activity, Human, and Context

Again, we return to the idea of meaning, this time considering the contextual influences, primarily social and cultural, on a person's activity participation (Reed & Hocking, 2013). Meaning is informed by everyday experiences, including transactions and engagement with others, both direct and indirect, whose actions and opinions affect the perception of a situation and a person's action as well as with objects in the context (Dewey, 1922). Similarly, past experiences influence meaning and perception of a current situation. A person comes into a situation with an established "lens" (Reed & Hocking, 2013), forecasting his expectations in that situation (Dewey, 2008). The transactional perspective suggests that the situation is dynamic and fluid such that several individuals coming together in a common situation all arrive with an existing personal lens and have the potential to shape the perspective of each other and change the meaning of the situation.

What do these ideas mean for our discussion of the activity, the human, and the context? Let's consider the experience of a person who uses an aid for oral communication who is eating at a restaurant. First, let's think about the situation when she is eating a meal with friends. The meaning that she brings to this situation, based on past interactions with these friends, might be that she will enjoy a good meal and good conversation with friends and that her use of a communication aid is simply recognized as how she talks to her friends. However, she and her friends are not alone in the restaurant. The wait staff may be unaccustomed to the use of a communication aid and ignore the woman, asking others at the table what she would like to eat. It is possible that other patrons may not accept the use of the communication aid, perhaps commenting that the quality or the volume of the auditory output of the device affects their ability to enjoy their meal. The meaning of this initially pleasurable experience shifts, perhaps becoming stressful or producing anger as a result of the behaviors and attitudes of others in the restaurant. This example demonstrates the dynamic and fluid nature of a context and its ability to affect the perception of an experience.

Meaning is constructed through our engagement with different contexts, people, and objects in the world (Reed & Hocking, 2013). Context influences the meaning of doing; this meaning may change in different contexts. Doing may be more satisfying in one context than in another, or it may feel more comfortable in one context than another. A bird watcher who is at a park with a group of other "birders" probably feels very comfortable wearing clothes that designate her as a birder, carrying binoculars and cameras around her neck, looking up into the trees or in the bushes for birds, and talking about exciting sightings. In this situation, the bird watcher feels like she belongs. If we change the context slightly, the same person dressed as a bird watcher displaying similar behaviors but now in a park or on a beach where others are doing other activities such as swimming, sunbathing, or playing beach volleyball. In this context, the bird watcher's behavior is uncommon, perhaps considered odd, which then changes her perception to feeling like an outsider. Doing the activity of bird watching might be less satisfying in a context where the person feels she does not belong.

Occupational Justice

Occupational justice is defined as "the promotion of social and economic conditions to increase individual, community, and political awareness, resources and equitable opportunities for diverse occupational opportunities that enable people to meet their potential and experience well-being" (Wilcock, 2006, p. 343). This idea is built on the social justice perspective of equitable distribution of resources (see Chapter 4 for further discussion of this idea). It is also linked to the ideas of capability theory (Sen, 2009; Nussbaum, 2003, 2011) through the notion of choice. Recognizing that none of us is free to choose what we want to do at all times, occupational justice and **capability theory** suggest the idea that individuals should have the choice to engage in an occupation and the freedom to choose how, when, and where it will be enacted. An occupationally just world enables individuals to participate in desired and necessary occupations; it identifies the barriers and limitations to this participation and seeks to eliminate them.

Occupational injustice includes barriers and limitations to occupational engagement caused by segregation, deprivation, alienation, imbalance, and marginalization (Townsend & Wilcock, 2004; Wilcock, 2006). These are interpreted from the perspective of an individual with a physical, cognitive, or sensory impairment in the following way. Segregation separates the individual from others, preventing engagement in occupations with other groups. **Occupational apartheid** further develops the theoretical ideas of segregation and is considered to be "segregation of persons or groups, through the restriction or denial of access to dignified and meaningful participation in occupations of daily life" (Kronenberg & Pollard, 2005, p. 67). The practice of segregation of students with disabilities is an example in which the physical or sensory abilities of the student were considered ahead of their cognitive abilities in terms of class or school placement when sociopolitical forces determined the educational and other occupational experiences of these students.

Occupational deprivation occurs when individuals are denied the right to participate in occupations or prevented from engaging in occupations because of circumstances out of their control (Wilcock, 2006). Whiteford (2005) describes occupational deprivation of political refugees whose lives are disrupted and consequently spend hours in detention with little to occupy themselves and little ability to meet their essential needs. A similar situation occurs for older adults who are hospitalized in an acute care setting for lack of skilled nursing accommodation. The acute care setting does not typically provide activities for these individuals, resulting in the common situation of older adults sitting in wheelchairs, lined up in the hallway, doing nothing.

Occupational alienation results when individuals or groups are denied full participation in occupations and thus become alienated from their community and society, feeling powerless and without control (Wilcock, 2006). An example of occupational alienation is seen for a person with a hearing impairment attempting to engage in occupations with others who do not have the ability to communicate with this individual. The inability to communicate can result in the withdrawal by the person with a hearing impairment if the communication difficulties are perceived as too great. Withdrawal leads to alienation as the person becomes farther and farther removed from the context of his own community.

Occupational imbalance occurs when a person focuses on one area of her life to the detriment of others or when external pressures shift the balance of occupational performance to one particular area (Christiansen, 2005; Wilcock, 2006). We all experience occupational imbalance at some point in our lives—students who are studying for final exams experience a time when they do not have free time to engage in leisure activities. Another common example is when individuals spend great amounts of time on work activities to the detriment of activities in the self-care, family, and leisure realms.

The opposite often occurs for individuals with disabilities who are overrepresented in under-or unemployment situations. Occupational imbalance does not refer to a balance of occupation in the short term, but rather challenges arise when this situation exists in the long term.

Marginalization exists when the needs of individuals for participation in occupation are not considered or not addressed. This situation results in the denial of the rights of individuals with certain characteristics for full participation in occupation. It implies that these individuals are at the margins of society and therefore not powerful enough to be included in collective occupations (Wilcock & Townsend, 2000). A recent discussion by the WHO focuses on the needs of individuals with disabilities in emergency situations. Too frequently, plans are not made to safely evacuate individuals who cannot react in emergency evacuation situations or independently (for mobility, cognitive, audition, or vision reasons). Marginalization occurs because their needs are not included when making these plans.

BRINGING IN ASSISTIVE TECHNOLOGY

Key ideas related to AT are discussed in Chapter 2 (Figure 3-9). Although formal definitions of AT state that it is technology designed specifically for individuals with a disability, one of the key themes of Chapter 2 is the blurring of mainstream technology, that is, technology designed and marketed to a broad spectrum and AT. Increasingly, products that are produced for general consumption are usable by individuals with varying abilities.

Assistive technology was described on a continuum of products ranging from mainstream products to items that are designed and created for a single individual. A second continuum describes providing the minimum amount of technology that is needed by the user. AT can support the individual with a disability or another person such as a parent, child, spouse, or other caregiver.

The last major theme of Chapter 2 identifies issues of ethical and sustainable service provision. These ideas are presented in greater detail in Chapter 4.

Meaning and Assistive Technology

When we introduce the use of AT into the doing, the meaning may be influenced in detrimental ways when the context does not support the use of technology, through physical, social, cultural, or institutional structures. In these situations, the meaning of doing with AT becomes an important consideration.

Assistive technology use is characterized as either an enabler or a hindrance to participation in activities. Miller Polgar (2010) identified several themes illustrating the meaning individuals with disabilities have for their use of AT. As an enabler, AT was simply seen as a tool, just another way of doing an activity. AT was seen as a way of "leveling the playing field," of eliminating or in some situations masking a disability. Commonly, this latter idea was related to computer access and other electronic technology in which the abilities of the user are not apparent to others.

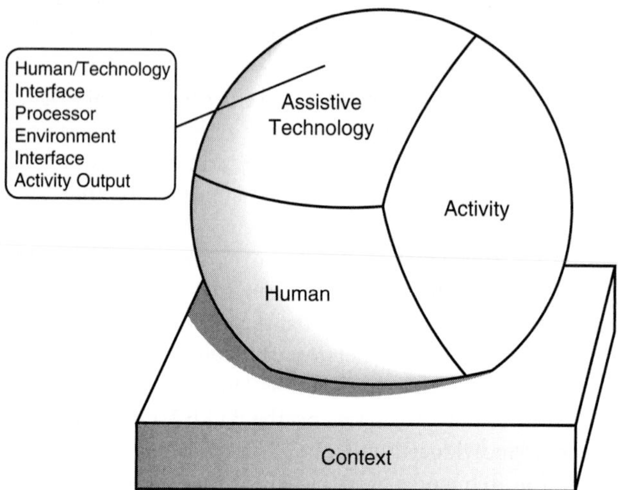

FIGURE 3-9 The Human Activity Assistive Technology (HAAT) model with elements of AT identified.

In contrast, AT was seen as a barrier, in some cases a physical barrier, and as a contributor to stigma. Equipment such as a wheelchair or communication devices mounted on a wheelchair create a physical barrier between the AT user and others. Similarly, the arrangement of AT can cause a physical barrier, as when a computer is placed so that it creates a barrier between the user and others in an environment such as a classroom.

These situations show how AT can create a physical separation. Commonly, AT use is seen as a visible sign of disability. Indeed, signage that designates accessible facilities typically features a wheelchair. Rather than a physical barrier, AT as stigma creates a social barrier, an "othering" that makes it difficult for someone using an assistive device to feel a sense of belonging and worth.

REASSEMBLING THE HAAT MODEL

In the introduction to this chapter, the order of the discussion of the HAAT elements was made explicit to mirror the order of their consideration when the model is applied for product development and design, client assessment, and outcome evaluation. Each of these three purposes of the model will be described as we conclude this overview of the HAAT model.

Product Design and Development

The ability to create a product should not be the driving force for its development; rather, the identification of a functional need, an activity, that supports the ability of a person is the starting point. Products that are designed without a function that meets a human need tend to be underused or discarded. All stages of the process are most effective when end users are part of the discussion to identify the need and how and where the device is to be used. Keeping contextual elements in focus, in particular institutional considerations such as liability and funding, is useful for the development of a product that will be accessible.

Who the intended user is affects the design of the product. A multidisciplinary team is particularly useful at this stage; engineers and industrial designers contribute their expertise for the technical design and testing aspects, and intended users and health care professionals provide expertise on how individuals with different abilities might use the device—and what would prevent them from using it. The ideas discussed earlier concerning lifespan issues and meaning affect this part of the process.

Contextual elements about physical aspects of the environment that affect device use and social and cultural elements that support or hinder use and institutional factors influence the design process, particularly in the initial conceptual stages. Designs that result in expensive technology with limited opportunity for funding support to the end user may never make it out of the design lab.

Consideration of sustainability is highly relevant in the design process. The WHO recommends that as much as possible, devices are made from materials sourced from the country of intended use, that they are manufactured in that country, and that resources are available to maintain the products as needed. Elements related to cost of the product and method of distribution are contextual influences for the design and development process (Owen & Simonds, 2010).

Client Assessment and Outcome Evaluation

The service delivery process includes both assessment for the provision of AT and evaluation of the outcome of AT use. Chapter 5 describes AT service delivery in detail. Here an outline of the process is given. The assessment starts with discussion of what the person wants and needs to do. This discussion includes others who are key individuals such as parents, children, or spouses who will also use or maintain the device. As described earlier, not only are the activities identified but further information about how, where, and temporal aspects are considered.

Assessment of the individual is the next step of the process. Relevant cognitive, sensory, motor, communication, and emotional components are assessed. During this assessment, a discussion about the meaning of the technology and concerns about the use of technology is beneficial to identify less tangible factors that will affect whether a device will be used and under what circumstances.

Consideration of the contextual elements includes identification of where the device will be used and the implications of the physical context on device use. Knowledge of who is in the contexts in which the device will be used helps determine which aspects of device use a client needs to be able to fulfill independently and which can be completed with assistance. Aspects of the institutional context such as funding, ownership, responsibility for maintenance and transportation, and any limitations on device use are additional considerations related to context.

The information that is gathered in the assessment is synthesized and results in a recommendation for a device that is communicated to the client (see Chapter 5). Part of the synthesis is the formulation of goals to be met using the device (client goals are also considered as part of the data gathering phase of the assessment process). These goals are translated into outcomes for the purpose of outcome evaluation.

Formal and informal measures of outcomes are possible; a combination of both provides evidence for the use of the device as well as context about the place of the device in the life of the user. Chapter 5 describes a number of evaluation methods that are useful for general AT device use. Outcome measures that are specific to particular devices are described in the relevant chapters. Outcome evaluation serves two purposes: evaluation of the outcome for an individual provides evidence for change in his life, and outcome evaluation for a group provides evidence for the effectiveness of a device more broadly and often forms part of the justification needed for funding, regulation changes, and further research.

SUMMARY

This chapter has described in detail three elements of the HAAT model—activity, human, and context—that influence AT design, provision, and evaluation. Although each of these elements has been described individually, their interactions have also been identified and discussed. When considered in isolation, some information is gained about influences on AT use. However, when the confluence of these ideas is recognized, the collective impact becomes evident.

When designing, prescribing, or evaluating AT, focus on the technology is the last stage of the process. Technology that is designed or prescribed without consideration of what function it serves, who will use it, and the contexts in which it will be used has a greater possibility of misuse or abandonment. The HAAT model articulates influential factors, their interactions, and a process that are posited to enable a person to engage in satisfying activities in relevant contexts.

STUDY QUESTIONS

1. What are the four basic performance areas included in the HAAT model? Give an example of each.
2. Describe the purpose of a human factors analysis and an activity analysis. How does the combined information from these types of analyses contribute to the understanding of AT use?
3. What are the six ICF body structures and function classifications that are relevant to AT use? Give an example of each.
4. What are the meanings of the terms *novice* and *expert*? How do they affect the use of AT?
5. Describe two issues that are important considerations when recommending AT for a child and for an older adult.
6. Define the construct of role. Discuss the implications of roles for the use of AT.
7. Describe the four elements of the context included in the HAAT model. Give an example of how each affects AT acquisition and use.
8. Describe the key parameters of the physical context and their relationship to AT.
9. Describe the different types of people in the social environment and how they support or hinder AT acquisition and use.
10. Discuss the influence on culture for the acquisition and use of AT.
11. Identify and describe four key considerations that are important when interpreting legislation concerning AT service delivery.
12. Describe the concept of meaning and its implications to AT use.
13. Define relevant constructs of occupational justice and their importance to AT acquisition and use.

REFERENCES

Accessibility for Ontarians with Disabilities Act (AODA): S.O. 2005, Chapter 11.

American Occupational Therapy Foundation: The occupational therapy practice framework, *Am J Occup Ther* 56:609–639, 2002.

Americans with Disabilities Act of 1990, 42 U.S.C. §§ 12101 et seq.

Assistive Technology Act of 1998, as amended, PL 108-364, §3, 118 stat 1707, 2004.

Bandura A: *Social learning theory*, Englewood Cliffs, NJ, 1977, Prentice-Hall.

Baum C, Christiansen C: Person-environment-occupation-performance: An occupation-based framework for practice. In Christiansen CH, Baum CM, Bass-Haugen J, editors: *Occupational therapy: Performance, participation, and well-being*, Thorofare NJ, 2005, SLACK, pp 242–267.

Bickenbach J, Chatterji S, Badley EM, et al.: Models of disablement, universalism and the international classification of impairment, disabilities and handicaps, *Soc Sci Med* 48:1173, 1999.

Borg J, Lindstrom A, Larsson S: Assistive technology in developing countries: A review from the perspective of the Convention on the Rights of Persons with Disabilities, *Prosthet Orthot* 35:20–29, 2011.

Bruner J: *Acts of meaning*, Cambridge, MA, 1990, Harvard University Press.

Chapparo C, Ranka J: Theoretical contexts. In Whiteford G, Wright St-Clare V, editors: *Occupation and practice in context*, Sydney, 2005, Elsevier AU, pp 51–71.

Christiansen C: Time use and patterns of occupation. In Christiansen C, Baum C, Bass-Haugen J, editors: *Occupational therapy: Performance participation, and well-being*, Thorofare, NJ, 2005, SLACK, pp 70–91.

Davis W: *The wayfinders: Why ancient wisdom matters in the modern world*, Toronto, ON, 2009, House of Anansi Press.

Deci EL, Ryan RM: Self determination theory: A macrotheory of human motivation, development, and health, *Can Psychol* 49:182–185, 2008.

Developmental Disabilities Assistance and Bill of Rights Act, as amended, PL 106-402, 114 stat 1677, 2000.

Dewey J: *Human nature and conduct: An introduction to social psychology*, New York, 1922, H. Holt and Company.

Dewey J: In Boydston JA, editor: *John Dewey: The later works, 1925-1953: vol. 3: 1927–1928, Essays, reviews, miscellany, and "impressions of Soviet Russia,"* Carbondale, IL, 2008, Southern Illinois University Press.

Disability Discrimination: *Act of 1992, as amended 2012, Act 169 of 2012, Canberra*, NSW, AU, 2012, Office of Parliamentary Counsel.

Disability Discrimination: *Act of 2005, c. 13*, London, UK, 2005, National Archives.

Ervin RB: Prevalence of functional limitations among adults 60 years of age and over: US, 1999-2002, *Advance Data from Vital Health Statistics*, 375. Atlanta, 2006, Centers for Disease Control and Prevention. Available from http://www.cdc.gov/nchs/data/ad/ad375.pdf.

Falvey MA, Forest M, Pearpoint J, Rosenberg R: *All my life's a circle: Using the toolds of circles, MAPS and PATHS*, Toronto, ON, 1997, Inclusion Press.

Falvey M, et al.: *All my life's a circle: Using the tools of circles, MAPS and PATHS*, Toronto, ON, 1994, Inclusion Press.

Ferland: *The Ludic model: Play, children with physical disabilities and occupational therapy*, Ottawa, ON, 2005, CAOT Publications ACE.

Fisk AD, Rogers WA, Charness N, Szaja SJ, Sharit J: *Designing for older adults: Principles and creative human factors approaches*, ed 2, Boca Raton FL, 2009, CRC Press.

Fougeyrollas P: The influence of the social environment on the social participation of people with disabilities. In Christiansen C, Baum C, editors: *Occupational therapy: Enabling function and well-being*, ed 2, Thoroughfare, NJ, 1997, SLACK, pp 378-391.

Fougeyrollas P, Gray DB: Classification systems, environmental factors and social change. In Gray DB, Quantrano LA, Lieberman ML, editors: *Designing and using assistive technology: The human perspective*, Baltimore, 1998, Paul H. Brookes, pp 13–28.

Goffman E: *Stigma: Notes on the management of spoiled identity*, New York, 1963, Simon & Schuster.

Hersch GI, Lamport NK, Coffey MS: *Activity analysis: Application to occupation*, ed 5, Thorofare, NJ, 2005, SLACK.

Hocking C: Public health and health promotion. In MacKenzie L, O'Toole G, editors: *Occupation analysis in practice*, Hoboken, NJ, 2011, Wiley-Blackwell, pp 246–263.

Individuals with Disabilities Education Act, as amended, PL 108-446, 104 stat 1142, 2004.

Jongbloed L, Crichton A: A new definition of disability: Implications for rehabilitation and social policy, *Can J Occup Ther* 57:32–38, 1990.

Kielhofner G: *Model of human occupation: Theory and application*, ed 4, Philadelphia, 2007, Lippincott, Williams & Wilkins.

King G, Brown E, Smith L: *Meaning and resilience in life: Learning from turning points of people with disabilities*, Westport CT: 2003, Greenwood Publishing Group.

Klingbeil H, Baer HR, Wilson PE: Aging with a disability, *Arch Phys Med Rehabil* 85(suppl 3):S68–S73, 2004.

Kronenberg F, Pollard N: Overcoming occupational apartheid: A preliminary exploration of the political nature of occupational therapy. In Kronenberg F, Simo Algardo S, Pollard N, editors: *Occupational therapy without borders: Learning from the spirit of survivors*, London, 2005, Elsevier, pp 67–86.

Light JC: Definition of communicative competence. In *Communicative competence for individuals who use AAC: From research to effective practice*, Baltimore, 2003, Paul H. Brookes Publishing Co, pp 3–40.

MacLachlan J: Remote Canadian occupational therapy: An "outside the box experience," *OT Now* 12:5–7, 2010.

McColl MA, Jongbloed L: *Disability and social policy in Canada*, Concord, ON, 2006, Captus University Press.

Miller Polgar J: The myth of neutral technology. In Oishi MMK, Mitchell IM, Van der Loos HFM, editors: *Design and use of assistive technology: Social, technical, ethical and economic challenges*, New York, 2010, Springer, pp 17–23.

Miller Polgar J: Landry J: Occupations as a means for individual and group participation in life. In Christiansen C, Townsend E, editors: *Introduction to occupation*, Saddle River, NJ, 2004, Prentice Hall, pp 197–220.

Mirza M, Gossett Zakrajsek A: Borsci S: The assessment of the environments of AT use: Accessibility, sustainability and universal design. In Federici S, Scherer MJ, editors: *Assistive technology assessment handbook*, Boca Raton, FL, 2012, CRC Press, Taylor Francis Group, pp 67–81.

Murphy JW, Cook AM: Limitations of augmentative communication systems in progressive neurological diseases. In *Proceedings of the 8th Ann Conf Rehabil Technol, Washington DC: RESNA*, pp 120–122, 1985.

Nordic Centre for Rehabilitation Technology: *Provision of assistive technology in the Nordic countries*, ed 2, Helsinki, 2007, Nordic Cooperation on Disabilities Issues (NSH).

Nussbaum M: Capabilities as fundamental entitlements: Sen and social justice, *Fem Econ* 9:33–59, 2003.

Nussbaum M: *Creating Capabilities: The human development approach*, Cambridge MA, 2011, The Belknap Press of Harvard University Press.

Owen J, Simonds C: Beyond the wheelchair: Development of motorised transport for people with severe mobility impairments in developing countries, *Disabil Rehab Assist Tech* 5:254–257, 2010.

Pickens ND, Pizur-Barnekow K: Co-occupation: Extending the dialogue, *J Occ Ther* 16:151–156, 2011.

Pierce D: *Occupation by design: Building the therapeutic process*, Philadelphia, 2003, F.A. Davis.

Pierce D: Co-occupation: The challenge of defining concepts original to occupational science, *J Occup Sci* 16:203–207, 2009.

Reed K, Hocking C: Resituating the meaning of occupation: A transactional perspective. In Cutchin M, Dickie V, editors: *Transactional perspectives on occupation*, New York, 2013, Springer, pp 39–49.

Reed KL: An annotated history of the concepts used in occupational therapy. In Christiansen C, Baum C, Bass-Haugen J, editors: *Occupational therapy: Performance participation, and well-being*, Thorofare, NJ, 2005, SLACK, pp 567–626.

Rehabilitation Act of 1973, as amended, PL 93–112, §701, 87 stat 355, 1993.

Rosen L, Ava J, Furumasu J, Harris M, Lange ML, McCarthy E et al: RESNA position paper on the application of power wheelchairs for pediatric users., Assist Technol 21:218–225, 2009.

Sanford J: *Universal design as a rehabilitation strategy: Design for the ages*, New York, 2012, Springer.

Sen A: *The idea of justice*, Cambridge, MA, 2009, The Belknap Press of Harvard University Press.

Shoenborn CA, Heyman KM: Health characteristics of adults aged 55 years and older, US, 2004-2007, *National Health Statistics Reports* Atlanta, 2009, Centers for Disease Control and Prevention. Available from http://www.cdc.gov/nchs/data/nhsr/nhsr016.pdf.

Stanton NA: Hierarchical task analysis: Developments, applications, and extensions, *Appl Ergonom* 37:55–79, 2006.

Statistics Canada: *Physical activity and limitations survey 2006: Analytical report, Catalogue no. 89-628-XIE, No. 002*, Ottawa, ON, 2007, Ministry of Industry. Available from http://www.statcan.gc.ca/pub/89-628-x/89-628-x2007002-eng.pdf.

Townsend E, Polatajko HJ: *Enabling occupation II: advancing occupational therapy vision for health, well-being and justice through occupation*, Ottawa, ON, 2002, CAOT Publications ACE.

Townsend E, Polatajko HJ: *Enabling occupation II: Advancing occupational therapy vision for health, well-being and justice through occupation*, ed 2, Ottawa, ON, 2013, CAOT Publications ACE.

United Nations: *Convention on the rights of persons with disabilities*, New York, 2006, UN. Available from www.un.org/disabilities/convention/conventionfull.shtml.

Whalley Hammell KW: *Perspectives on disability and rehabilitation: Contesting assumptions; challenging practice*, Edinburgh, 2006, Churchill Livingstone Elsevier.

Whiteford G: Understanding the occupational deprivation of refugees: A case study from Kosovo, *Can J Occup Ther* 72:78–88, 2005.

Wilcock AA, Townsend E: Occupational justice: occupational terminology interactive dialogue, *J Occup Sci* 7:84, 2000.

Wilcock AA: *An occupational perspective of health*, ed 2, Thorofare, NJ, 2006, SLACK.

World Health Organization: *International classification of functioning, disability and impairment*, Geneva, 2001, WHO.

CHAPTER 4

Ethical Issues in Assistive Technology

CHAPTER OUTLINE

LEARNING OBJECTIVES

On completing this chapter, you will be able to do the following:

1. Describe the five types of ethical principles typically applied in health-related studies.
2. Understand the major ethical issues involved in the application of assistive technologies (ATs).
3. Describe the ethical considerations involved in monitoring and surveillance.
4. Describe the ways that ATs affect social stigma for people with disabilities.
5. Discuss the tradeoffs between privacy and security.
6. Describe the ethical considerations associated with the development and application of ambient environments.
7. Understand professional ethics and standards of practice.

KEY TERMS

Ambient Environment
Autonomy
Beneficence
Distributive Justice
Ethics
Fidelity
Informed Consent
Justice
Nonmaleficence
Privacy
Professional Ethics
Security
Stigma
Surveillance

INTRODUCTION

Why study ethics in an assistive technology (AT) book? Technologies are becoming increasingly more pervasive (see Chapter 2) and consequently have a greater and greater impact on the ways people with disabilities live and interact with the world around them. The intent of AT applications is to increase independence and maximize full societal participation for individuals with disabilities.

Unfortunately, the pervasiveness of technology can also compromise **privacy** and limit independence. In particular, the increasing use of monitoring of individuals with cognitive limitations caused by intellectual disability or dementia raises important questions regarding privacy. The ethical principal of **autonomy** becomes important in these cases. ATs are often distributed, or made available, through public funding. The availability and distribution of AT are not always based on need. Government policies and societal values and resources play major roles in access to AT. Considerations of fair and equitable allocation of AT can also be informed by ethical principles. The argument is often made that distribution should be based solely on available financial resources. However, other factors are important as well. Cultural factors such as those resulting from underresourced areas such as rural parts of the developed world and many parts of the developing world play an important role in equitable distribution of ATs. These issues will take us into a discussion of the ethical principle of **distributive justice**.

Choices of ATs for a specific individual must be done in the context of the ethical principles of **nonmaleficence** and **beneficence** (i.e., help the individual and do no harm). Finally, clinical practice in AT must be carried out with honesty, integrity, and trustworthy behavior. These concepts are encompassed in the ethical principle of **fidelity**. Ethical principles provide a framework with which to evaluate AT impact from the point of view of the person who uses the AT and those with whom they interact. As we discuss in this chapter, there is more debate than agreement on most ethical topics involving AT. Differing points of view, vested interests, and health policies all lead to the need for trade-offs that are often viewed differently by consumers, families, clinicians, and care provider organizations.

Some argue that ATs are inherently neutral in an ethical sense (Cash, 2003). Others point out that the impact of AT may not be neutral because its application in clinical or community contexts may generate complex care scenarios that have ethical implications (Martin, Bengtsson, & Dröes, 2010). The coupling of the AT device to its application leads to the conclusion that the end result obtained by the application of AT cannot be easily separated from the means used to generate that result (Niemeijer, Frederiks, Riphagen, Legemaate, Eefsting, & Hertogh, 2010). The ways in which AT systems are designed and built and the information provided to the end user regarding operation and use can also raise ethical issues; for example, the technical design of many devices "include[s] characteristics affecting the rights of the users that cannot be removed because they are substantially rooted in the conception of the application" (Niemeijer et al., 2010, p. 1138).

THE ETHICAL CONTEXT

Ethics can be described as "the constructed norms of internal consistency regarding what is right and what is wrong" (Martin et al., 2010, p. 65). "Professional ethics is a code values and norms that actually guide practical decision when they are made by professionals" (Airaksinen, 2003, p. 2).

These characteristics apply to the AT service delivery process, including assessment, recommendation, delivery and setup, training, and follow-up. AT public policy and funding levels and restrictions also have ethical implications when they impact accessibility and participation for people with disabilities. There are choices made in the design characteristics of AT that can affect the degree of independence, privacy, and participation that are possible. These also have ethical ramifications. Ethical principles may be in conflict with other factors such as performance measures for which health care managers are responsible (Coeckelberg, 2010), changes in the magnitude of need such as the growing seniors' population (Eccles, 2010), and cultural issues in underresourced areas (Alampay, 2006; Borg, Larsson, & Östergren, 2011).

Kitchner (2000) describes five types of ethical principles: autonomy, fidelity, beneficence, nonmaleficence, and justice. The ethical principle of *autonomy* is encompassed in the major goal of AT application to maximize independence for people with disabilities.

There are cases in which ATs can actually compromise an individual's autonomy if they are not thoughtfully applied. The clinical decision-making process leading to the choice of particular ATs for a given individual must also be true to the principle of autonomy by focusing on the freedom of action and choice of the individual consumer. Honest and trustworthy behavior is described by the principle of *fidelity*. This is the cornerstone of professional practice. Ensuring that actions lead to good results that benefit others is at the heart of all of AT development and application and is captured in the concept of *beneficence*. Beneficence also includes the identification of potential consequences of AT application and the balancing of positive and potentially harmful aspects to maximize benefit to the individual. Not causing harm to others directly and avoiding actions that risk harming others is encompassed by the principle of *nonmaleficence*. Fairness in individual, interpersonal, organizational, and societal contexts is described by the ethical principle of justice. In this chapter, we will describe these areas of ethics and show how their application can ensure that we maintain our focus on a person-centered approach to the application of AT principles.

Autonomy

Autonomy means the right to self-determination and freedom from unnecessary constraints, interference, or loss of privacy. Autonomy as perceived by user versus caregiver versus funders differs. For example, one area that has been studied extensively is the use of monitoring and **surveillance** AT with people who have dementia. For some, using AT in this way could indicate respect of their autonomy because it enables them to participate in everyday activities while respecting their disabilities (Zwijsen, Niemeijer, & Hertogh, 2011). For example, most older people would prefer to stay in their own homes for as long as possible. Sometimes this preference is only accepted by care staff and family if monitoring and tracking technologies are used. When the ability to stay in one's home is only possible in the presence of monitoring technologies, concern about the person's safety or behavior leads to a reduction in the person's autonomy and independence (Perry, Beyer, & Holm, 2009).

Zwijsen et al. (2011) reviewed the literature related to the use of AT in the care of elderly people living in the community. They found that the ethical reasoning with regard to autonomy (but also issues of privacy and stigmatization) was motivated by political theory that views the individual as independent and self-sufficient with relationships being secondary. An underlying assumption in this approach is

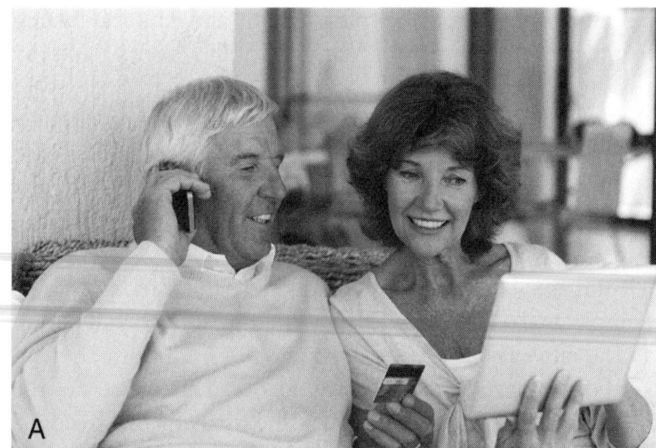

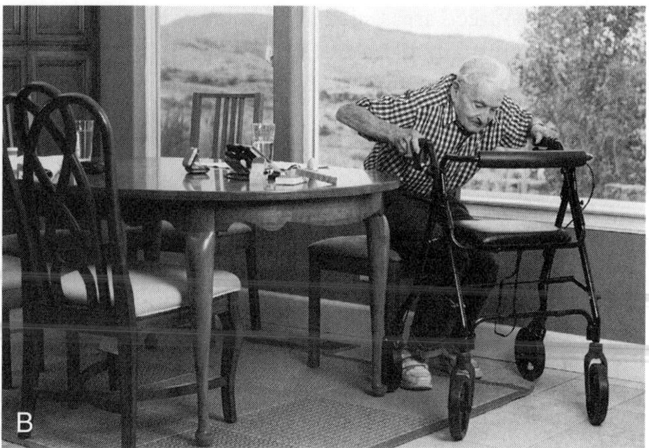

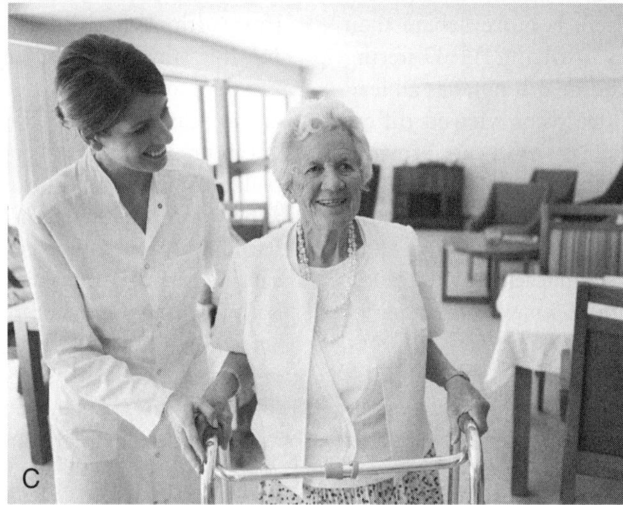

FIGURE 4-1 There are many levels of independence and dependence in the older population. Some individuals are able to function completely independently and require no assistance. They are fully autonomous (A). Other require some assistive technology assistance, but are independent with effort (B). Others require more intense assistance from a caregiver (C).

that people are self-determining individuals who make decisions for and about themselves. However, the variability of physical and cognitive function in people with disabilities and elderly adults is large (see Figure 4-1). AT can promote independence, and it can limit it. It is therefore questionable whether people, especially frail elderly people, meet the assumption of being totally self-determined or self-sufficient with or without the use of AT (Zwijsen et al., 2011). It is also questionable whether any of us are *totally* self-determined or self-sufficient given our dependence on others and on technologies (e.g., mobile phones and computers) for our daily functioning and survival.

In considering ethical issues such as autonomy, it is important to understand the underlying considerations that inform the ethical debate. Such areas as cost and funding, policy, family and caregiver concerns, and individual need may be in conflict and affect the ultimate autonomy of the individual being served. There are also differing views of what is meant by autonomy for people with intellectual disabilities and seniors in particular. Some want lots of attention to know that someone is looking out for them and are happy to have their privacy "invaded" by monitoring. Others are more concerned about privacy and want to take the risk of safety and **security** rather than be monitored constantly. The key areas where issues of autonomy arise are intellectual disability, cognitive disability in general, and aging.

Informed Consent

One of the biggest challenges when working with individuals who have a cognitive disability is to obtain **informed consent** for any intervention, including AT (Cash, 2003; Perry et al., 2009). Consent has two aspects: (1) not subjecting the individual to control by others without their explicit consent and (2) respectful interaction when presenting information, probing for understanding, and attempting to enable autonomous decision making. "Employing surveillance technologies without consent is considered by certain authors as either a civil wrong, illegal and/or tantamount to assault" (Niemeijer et al., 2010, p. 1135).

The need to obtain consent also has implications for presenting material in accessible formats, including written, oral, and nonverbal. Often a person with dementia is left out of decision making because it is presumed that he or she is unable to understand and respond. Seeking consent to use AT from a person with dementia requires ensuring that

". . . staff are trained in a range of communication methods; otherwise the person with dementia has been denied their rights" (Martin et al., 2010, p. 69).

Obtaining consent using augmentative communication technology (see Chapter 16) is difficult when the person has not yet used the technology and may not understand its implications such as what the consequences are for privacy (Martin et al., 2010; Zwijsen et al., 2011). This places additional demands on the assessment process to find innovative ways of informing prospective users of AT about the capabilities and characteristics of various options and what the implications are for privacy and autonomy as well as the potential benefits and hazards. Eccles (2010) also questions whether the assessment process is sensitive enough to evaluate ethical issues. These requirements create an obligation on care providers who are planning to use AT to be certain that staff are trained in a variety of communication methods. If not, then the person with dementia will have been denied his or her rights (Martin et al., 2010).

Perry et al. (2009) give some strategies for explaining AT and choices of technology. They point out that using pictures is of limited value because the dynamics of operation cannot be easily grasped. Videos of the AT in action are more useful, and actual trials of the technology are most useful in ensuring that informed consent is obtained. Martin et al. (2010) suggest using scenarios to describe the AT and its implications to the consumer and family, as well as for staff training.

Informed consent that requires the ability to answer questions reliably during the assessment can also be a problem, and it is important to be aware of response bias such as selecting the last option offered. The evaluator should not take answers at face value. It is also easy to influence the answers by being too enthusiastic about a particular approach and unintentionally coercing the consumer. Perry et al. (2009) discuss the trade-off between rights to privacy and the need to monitor where consent is important. It is also important to explicitly point out to the consumer and his or her family that AT cannot prevent people with dementia from all problems and risks that are a consequence of the disease (e.g., dangerous behavior, falls, wandering at night, disorientation). There are checklists to assist using technology with people who have dementia, including staff, developers, and researchers (Martin et al., 2010).

Many ethical considerations are based on informed consent and cognitive understanding of the implications of the AT. If the person's mental capacity does not allow informed consent, AT use may still be judged by the care provider to be in the best interest of the person. An alternative means of obtaining consent is through a legally designated conservator (often a family member). Even in the absence of informed consent, use of AT for surveillance may be initiated because it is in the best interests of the person or because the individual will be better off living in supported housing in the community (for example) rather than in institutional care or because she will be safer from harm (Martin et al., 2010).

Paternalism

The lack of ability to give informed consent can lead to "paternalism," which is the interference of a state or individual in relation to another person, either against his will or when the interference is justified by a claim of better protection for the individual (Martin et al., 2010, p. 71). Paternalism assumes that safety is more important than freedom of choice and that it is important to protect people from themselves. "It is conceivable that a paternalistic approach emerges as the predominant ethos within a technology enriched supported living option for people with dementia, if attempts are not made to establish the individuals' beliefs and values in relation to living in this type of care model. How then can the care provider clearly demonstrate application of the four principles of medical ethics [autonomy, beneficence, nonmaleficence, and justice]. . . ?" (Martin et al., 2010, p. 71).

Fidelity

The principle of fidelity requires faithful, loyal, honest, and trustworthy behavior (Kitchner, 2000). Purtilo (2005) lists five expectations associated with what patients might reasonably expect in terms of fidelity in the health care context:

1. That you treat them with basic respect
2. That you, the caregiver or other health care professional, are competent and capable of performing the duties required of your professional role
3. That you adhere to a professional code of ethics
4. That you follow the policies and procedures of your organization and applicable laws
5. That you will honor agreements made with the patient

Fidelity is perhaps the most common source of ethical conflict. In any particular situation, health care professionals may find themselves at odds between what they believe is right, what the patient wants, what other members of the health care team expect, what organizational policy dictates, or what the profession or the law requires. The case study describes one such ethical dilemma involving augmentative communication.

Fidelity requires being loyal to the patient. Issues of conflict of interest can arise that may compromise fidelity. For example, if a physician runs a company that manufactures wheelchairs for elderly adults, is this activity one of supplying a medical benefit, or does his recommendation of his brand of wheelchair constitute a conflict of interest? This extension of the clinician's role to include AT provision broadens the consideration of fidelity. Some AT companies employ therapists as field representatives who have a dual role. They can be very valuable in explaining features of a product during an assessment, helping with fitting of the device if necessary and generally supporting the clinician. However, they also represent one manufacturer and have a role of sales representative. Keeping these roles clearly distinct and ensuring that the patient and treating clinician understand the dual role is essential to meeting the requirements of ethical fidelity.

The principle of fidelity also applies to manufacturers of ATs because it can be difficult for a consumer to clearly

CASE STUDY

Supporting Function via Assistive Technology: Promoting Beneficence or Avoiding Nonmaleficence?

A 38-year-old Portuguese man with amyotrophic lateral sclerosis was provided with an augmentative and alternative communication (AAC) device for communication (see Chapter 16). The man used his communication device to say two things: "I would rather choke on a piece of good cod fish [very popular in Portugal] than have a GI tube" and "I do not want to be put on a mechanical ventilator at any time." He made the second statement despite the knowing that the end stage of the disease results in the inability to breathe independently. As AT practitioners, consideration of beneficence—that is, what must be done to meet obligations—leads to the conclusion that it is clearly within both our capabilities and our obligation to provide this individual with a means of communication.

Are we obligated to continue to provide additional AT as the patient's needs change as a result of the degenerative nature of the disease? Yes, within the capabilities of existing assistive technologies, we are obligated to continue to meet this man's communication needs. For example, we need to provide technology that will detect the last voluntary movements of which our patient is capable. When such technologies are unavailable, our obligation under the principle of beneficence ceases.

A more difficult question is raised by the principle of nonmaleficence. Based on this young man's two statements, have we done harm or created the possibility of harm by providing independent communication through the use of the AAC device? If my colleague had not provided the AT in the first place, would the individual's choices (willing to risk choking for the pleasure of cod fish and refusing ventilator assistance) have been articulated? Now that they have been provided, what is the obligation to follow them?

What is the role of the AT and its provision in this situation? For example, my colleague indicated that the use of the AAC device by the patient rather than his normal speech to make the two requests cast doubt on whether the statements were a valid representation of his views. For example, his limited motor capability could have resulted in errors in choosing vocabulary from the device. The device could have malfunctioned and provided the wrong output.

The validity of the utterances is established as a part of the obligation of beneficence, and failure to provide an accurate and reliable system would result in nonmaleficence. If we accept the fact that the obligation relative to the AT extends only to the establishment of reliability and accuracy, then we are left with the conclusion that the AT is neutral in the dilemma created by the patient's two requests: the patient's autonomy has been aided by the availability of the communication device. His utterances should be treated as if he would have used his natural voice. Conversely, if the communication device malfunctions in a way that generates a message that the user did not intend, then the technology itself may not be neutral. What is the role of the AT practitioner in this case? Is she guilty of nonmaleficence because of providing a defective device?

This case illustrates challenges associated with the claim that avoiding harm has priority over doing well. In many AT clinical circumstances, it is not feasible to separate beneficence and nonmaleficence. Application of either or both of these ethical principles may also conflict with personal autonomy. As this case illustrates, beneficence cannot be reduced to obligations of nonmaleficence.

understand the functioning of an AT product. AT can at times appear to be a quick and easy solution to a problem (Martin et al., 2010). An AT manufacturer or distributor has an ethical responsibility to ensure the production of a quality controlled product and the completion of necessary testing to ensure the product meets required standards. It is also a manufacturer's responsibility to ensure that the proper operation, potential benefits, and possible associated risks of the use of the product are fully described to those considering purchase. Clinical staff must be trained to understand the use and implications of technology based on the information provided by the manufacturer. This training is often provided by a distributor or by more experienced clinicians.

Beneficence

In everyday understanding, the term *beneficence* connotes acts of mercy, kindness, and charity. In ethics, the concept is broadened to effectively include "all forms of action intended to benefit or promote the good of other persons . . . helping them to further their important and legitimate interests . . ." (Beauchamp, 2008). The Care Services Improvement Partnership (CSIP) in Scotland argues that an understanding of beneficence "involves finding the balance between risk tolerance and risk aversion" (Eccles, 2010).

The principle of beneficence carries obligations such as being responsive to the needs of others. This includes universal needs such as the integrity of life and limb, disease and disability, and the necessities of human sustenance; other needs are more context dependent (Herman, 2001). Both social deficiencies and natural deficiencies can result in deficits in welfare. Social deficiencies result in injustice, which must be rectified. Rectifying natural deficiencies is a matter of beneficence and is voluntary. AT applications are natural deficiencies included in "the range of things a person might require to be an effective member of her community: from literacy to clean and presentable clothes" (Herman, 2001, p. 231). Many ATs described in this book and mainstream technologies, such as personal digital assistants (PDAs), smart phone apps, and tablets, are used to address needs across a broad spectrum of activities that address "natural deficiencies" and provide benefit to people with disabilities.

Nonmaleficence

Nonmaleficence refers to the principle of not causing harm to others directly or through avoidance of actions that risk harming others (Kitchner, 2000). This concept is fundamental to clinical practice including that focusing on ATs. The Scottish CSIP program advises that "non-malfeasance, involves a balance between avoiding harm and respecting decisions about dignity, integrity and preferences" (Eccles, 2010).

Causing harm through ATs is not something that is overtly done. Rather, there are hazards that need to be avoided. For example, the design and application of mobility and orientation aids for blind individuals (see Chapter 13) requires that obstacles be avoided to prevent injury. If the device fails to notify the user that a drop off is in her path (e.g., while walking along an elevated sidewalk), then we have not "prevented harm," and the principle of nonmaleficence has been violated. Because technologies can inherently be harmful if improperly applied, AT practice requires adherence to the principle of nonmaleficence, including adequate education and training in the use and maintenance of the technology.

Stigma

A negative outcome of the use of ATs is **stigma**. Stigma can be defined as a sign of social unacceptability because there is shame or disgrace associated with something that is socially unacceptable (Perry et al., 2009). Stigma is related to a number of social processes, including the separation of people into categories that bear labels that are negative. This identification can lead to stereotypes and discrimination. The use of AT can imply weakness or less ability, which can produce a stigma associated with the use of the AT. Stigma associated with AT use can cause harm. Conversely, AT that is based on mainstream technologies can decrease the stigma. Look at Figure 4-2. In part A the wheelchair could be stigmatizing, calling attention to a disability. In Figure 4-2-B the person is using a tablet as well as a wheelchair. Is the stigma less? In Figure 4-2-C the user is clearly disabled, but the tablet creates a positive impression of capability. Harm may result from reluctance to use the device because of the image portrayed, therefore limiting benefit from the support that AT will provide.

Harm can also be psychological, impacting self-esteem. The relationship of AT use to stigma also leads to the negative stereotype that "disability is bad; let's hide it." The degree of stigma varies for different types of AT. The situation is most important for AT devices in which the esthetics call attention to the individual's disability and increase the stigma associated with perceived weakness. For example, hearing aids carry more stigma than glasses. Hence, much effort goes into making hearing aids unobtrusive and making glasses into fashion statements (Pullin, 2009). Individualization of devices (e.g., bright colors on wheelchairs for children) can reduce stigma through person-centered planning. Universal

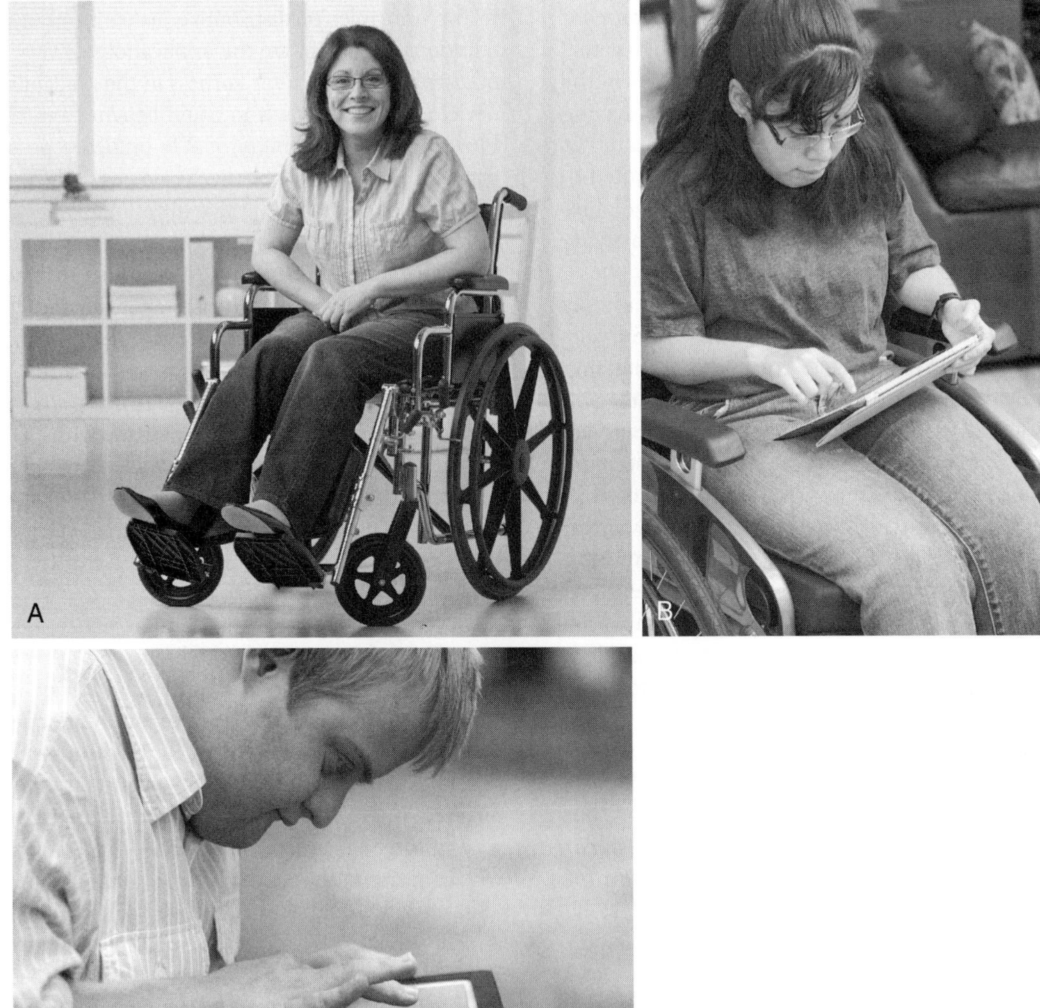

FIGURE 4-2 The type of AT used can add to or reduce stigma as these three examples show (see text).

design reduces stigma by making invisible the modifications to the environment that make it more accessible (Sanford, 2012). Careful attention to AT design and functionality can reduce stigma.

Abandonment of AT devices has also been shown to be related to stigma. The personal meaning attributed to assistive devices can influence integration of AT into the user's daily life. Users of ATs want their identification to be as individual persons and not to be stigmatized by AT use that brands them as disabled and detracts from their autonomy (Pape, Kim, & Weiner, 2002). Unfortunately, the negative perception of people with disabilities can be exacerbated by the use of ATs creating a stigma that calls attention to the disability rather than to the capability of the individual (Parette & Scherer, 2004). Elderly people are specifically concerned that the use of AT can stigmatize by making them appear less functional and more vulnerable. They and their caregivers report that they believe that AT is meant for frail and dependent elderly people and not for healthy and independent people (Zwijsen et al., 2011). The device becomes a symbol of frailty and dependence. When the costs of using a device in terms of stigma and negative identity outweigh the benefits of AT use for the individual, device abandonment can result. The reduced level of comfort may be due to actual perceived danger because of vulnerability portrayed by the type of AT, or it can be an embarrassment because of having to depend on AT for function. The need to be monitored or tracked may be taken to reflect the social value attributed to that group. There is the danger that surveillance technologies marginalize individuals with dementia by overtly identifying them as incapable of managing their own lives.

The use of surveillance technologies is an increasingly dangerous special situation that can result in stigma. Surveillance and monitoring AT may be particularly stigmatizing because the individual may believe that she has been "tagged" (Niemeijer et al., 2010). However, some types of tags are more acceptable than others. For example a GPS-based surveillance transmitter mounted unobtrusively in a shoe may be more acceptable than a wrist or ankle bracelet to a person with dementia (see Chapter 15). Likewise, a monitoring app loaded into an iPod carried by a teenager with a developmental disability may be more acceptable while providing the same surveillance as a more conspicuous monitoring device.

Another perspective on the stigma that results from the use of surveillance technology is that the large-scale implementation of monitoring in seniors housing is promoted based on being cost effective. Because this technology is applied to all residents, any individual resident does not experience a greater degree of stigma than other resident (Zwijsen et al., 2011). Such an argument is questionable for two reasons: it ignores the aspect of personal choice to be monitored or not and does not recognize the stigma associated with living in a specialized facility.

Justice

The ethical principle of justice deals with the issue of fairness in individual, interpersonal, organizational, and societal contexts (Kitchner, 2000). Justice and beneficence both focus on human welfare, but they each have distinct domains of concern (Herman, 2001). The distinction between obligations of social justice and obligations of social beneficence is small (Beauchamp, 2008). When discussing need, questions of injustice overwhelm other issues. In this chapter, we focus on how the functionality and availability of AT is affected by the concept of distributive justice.

Distributive Justice

"Principles of distributive justice are normative principles designed to guide the allocation of the benefits and burdens of economic activity" (Lamont & Favor, 2008, p. 10). There are three principles of distributive justice: (1) What is subject to distribution (e.g., income, wealth, opportunities, jobs, welfare)? (2) What is the nature of the subjects of the distribution (natural persons, reference classes, e.g., persons with disabilities)? and (3) What should the basis of the distribution be (e.g., equality, maximization according to individual characteristics, according to free transactions)? These can be applied to considerations regarding the distribution of ATs. In this chapter, we relate the current understanding of AT devices and services to the principles of distributive justice to examine two basic questions. (1) What are the implications of varying principles of distributive justice for fairness in the availability of assistive devices to individuals who could benefit from them? and (2) How does the availability of ATs influence principles of distributive justice, both negatively and positively? Although many principles of distributive justice differ in a variety of ways, ATs have an impact in two broad areas, egalitarian and difference principles (Lamont & Favor, 2008). There are a number of different formulations of both egalitarianism and difference.

In strict egalitarianism, the simplest form, each person should have the same level of material goods and services. This approach also assumes equal need, a concept that is clearly violated in the case of persons with disabilities, and individual disabling conditions can lead to significantly different needs for support from technology (e.g., the use of a cane, manual wheelchair, or powered wheelchair for mobility). Thus, strict egalitarianism is not useful as a basis for considering distributive justice for AT.

Several principles of distributive justice focus on difference. One of the most widely discussed of these is the Rawls difference principle (as cited in Lamont & Favor, 2008). Here, each person has an equal claim to a fully adequate scheme of equal basic rights and liberties. Rawls assumes that his representative "person" is rational and able to rationalize his or her own self-interest. This approach negates the rights of citizens who might be deemed "irrational." The notion that someone who is rational should decide for those deemed "irrational" (e.g., an individual with cognitive or intellectual disabilities) is problematic when considering persons with disabilities and the distribution of ATs. Cook (2009) discusses distributive justice in relation to AT application.

In the next section of this chapter, we discuss the ways in which ATs can reduce perceived and real differences in capabilities and functions. We will also discuss how ATs, if applied improperly, can lead to greater difference between people with disabilities and mainstream society and decrease the perception of capability and participation by persons with disabilities.

The initial point of reference when discussing distribution of AT devices and services is typically the device (i.e., hard technology) or service (i.e., soft technology) that is viewed as the commodity to be distributed (see Chapter 2). We include both hard and soft technologies because success depends as much on the support received by the individual as on the appropriateness of the device itself (Scherer et al., 2007).

It is really the functional outcomes of the distribution of AT devices and services that is important. By shifting our emphasis to outcomes, we can broaden the question of "What is distributed?" to one of "What is accomplished?" The most meaningful outcomes are those that lead to the greatest independence and provide the greatest opportunity for community participation. This perspective also changes the "what" is distributed from a focus on the device and service to consideration of the AT as the vehicle for participation. Peterson and Murray (2006) noted that:

> *In all of our discourse, it is important to remember that ethical AT service provision is not the ultimate outcome of all our collaborations, but a vehicle to help achieve more noble goals, including client skill and competency development, maximum independence, full participation in society, and integration into local communities. Success in these areas results in increased quality of personal and professional spheres of life for people with disabilities using AT service (Peterson & Murray, 2006, p. 66).*

This concept is grounded in a key ethical principle that it is really "capabilities" that should be distributed, attributed to Sen (1999) and Nussbaum (2006): "The freedoms of individuals are viewed as the basic building blocks to development, as well as "the expansion of 'capabilities' of persons to lead the kinds of lives they value—and have reason to value" (Sen, 1999, p. 18). If one views ATs as enabling and leading to expanded independence, then they in effect may be seen as contributing positively to the capabilities of a person with disabilities (Hansson, 2007). Short of being equated to capabilities, ATs can surely be viewed as enablers of capabilities for people with disabilities. As Hansson concludes:

> *. . . there is no doubt that [Nobel laureate] Amartya Sen's capability approach . . . [applied to] assistive technology would therefore lead to priority-setting practices that are continuous with well-established ethical criteria for the distribution of resources for therapeutic technologies (p. 263).*

Sen's own words describe the capability approach to distributive justice: "the evaluative focus of this 'capability approach' can be either on the realized functionings (what a person is actually able to do) or on the capability set of alternatives that she has (her real opportunities). The two give different types of information—the former about the things a person does and the latter about the things a person is substantively free to do" (1999, p. 75). The capability approach says that individual differences, capabilities, and choice play roles in whether people make use of resources, how they apply them, and how they are valued (Alampay, 2006). It further suggests that distribution of resources and rights is insufficient when an individual is not able to act on or use them and that the individual should be able to exercise choice to act rather than being restricted in the capability to act.

Distributive justice based on capability has two levels (Remmers, 2010). First, is the requirement to meet basic needs. Second, to meet these needs, fair distribution of the "returns of social cooperation" must be guaranteed. "The aim of the capability approach is to guarantee the minimum conditions to cooperative citizens so that they may participate in a social, economic, and cultural life. A further goal is to enable people to follow their own life's plan" (Remmers, 2010, p. 205).

Nussbaum (2006) has defined the central human capabilities based on the principle of human dignity:

1. Life: "Being able to live to the end of a human life of normal length; not dying prematurely, or before one's life is so reduced as to be not worth living."
2. Bodily health (includes nourishment and shelter)
3. Bodily integrity: free movement, freedom from sexual assault and violence, having opportunities for sexual satisfaction
4. Being able to use your senses, imagination, and thought; experiencing and producing culture, freedom of expression, and freedom of religion
5. Emotions: being able to have attachments to things and people
6. Practical reason: being able to form a conception of the good and engage in critical reflection about the planning of one's life
7. Affiliation: being able to live with and toward others, imagine the other, and respect the other
8. Other species: being able to live with concern to animals, plants, and nature
9. Play: being able to laugh, play, and enjoy recreational activities
10. Control over one's environment: political choice and participation, being able to hold property, and being able to work as a human being in mutual recognition (Nussbaum, 2006, pp. 76-78)

We can use this list of capabilities as criteria to evaluate and understand the role ATs have for persons with disabilities. ATs, by contributing to participation in the World Health Organization's (WHO's) International Classification of Functioning, Disability and Impairment sense (see Chapters 1 and 3), can play a major role in the achievement of basic capabilities by individuals with disabilities. For example, an individual who has difficulty with speech production can benefit from the use of an alternative and augmentative communication device that synthesizes speech production (see Chapter 16). Such a device augments the central human capabilities identified by Nussbaum and listed earlier, but more important, it gives the user a choice to speak or not, enhancing his freedom to participate as he chooses.

APPLICATION OF ETHICAL CONCEPTS IN ASSISTIVE TECHNOLOGY

Now that we have introduced some basic ethical concepts, we will apply them to the application of ATs in this section. The ethical topics included here are those that have received the most attention in research and clinical practice settings. We have chosen particular examples of AT applications to illustrate the relationship of AT practice to the ethical principles described earlier. These examples represent a subset of all of the possible ethical concerns in the application of AT, but they have been chosen to capture the most pressing current ethical concerns related to AT use. Specifically we discuss monitoring and surveillance, ambient environments, supporting function, and the equitable distribution of AT. Many, but not all, of the ethical issues address the use of AT with individuals who have cognitive or intellectual disabilities. Other types of disability lead to different ethical concerns. We discuss some of these in later sections.

Assistive Technology for Monitoring and Tracking

The application of ATs has very different ethical considerations than other clinical interventions. Perry et al. (2009) summarized the differences:

> *It is important to recognise that the introduction of AT&T [assistive technologies and telecare or remote monitoring] is not like any of the decisions that are made in the normal course of providing support. The introduction of AT&T involves a transfer of control from staff, or the person themselves, to a technological system. This involves a change in the normal decision making processes for the person, and potentially a change in the normal safeguards that having staff directly involved brings. It is clear that significant thought is needed in the new situations (p. 86).*

One of the most ethically challenging areas in AT application is the use of monitoring and tracking technologies with vulnerable populations, particularly those with cognitive disabilities. There are significant risks, including injury and death, to individuals with cognitive disabilities and frail elderly individuals from wandering and falls (Martin et al., 2010). The use of monitoring technology can reduce these risks, and often considerations focus on the balance between risk taking and risk aversion.

Some ATs intended to aid individuals with dementia are "low tech" (Cash, 2003). These devices can be used in the existing home of the person with dementia, are readily available for purchase, and do not require the installation of sophisticated computer equipment. They can also be easily removed or adapted as the needs of the person with dementia change or if the person moves to a new residence.

Assistive technology cannot prevent all problems and risks that are a consequence of the cognitive disability, but monitoring systems can assist in several ways. Drug dispensing units not only tell the person what pill to take and when, but they also report to family or caregivers if the person does not take her required medication. Radio or GPS tags are attached to individuals who wonder so that they can be tracked. Technology can also alert the care provider if the person is approaching an exit to leave the building or to locate an individual if he is unattended in a monitored area. Video monitoring can check individuals to make sure they are safe, that they have not fallen, and that they are responsive. So-called smart homes monitor physiological signals, have pressure mats to detect when someone has gotten out of bed in the middle of the night, sense doors, and generally watch all activity in the house. During the night, AT can alert a caregiver to offer support to a resident who goes to the bathroom (Martin et al., 2010). We discuss some of these technologies in Chapter 15.

These are just a few examples of surveillance techniques using various types of AT. Although all of these are intended to create greater independence for people by allowing them to stay in their own homes or to go out without a caregiver, serious ethical questions arise when these technologies are used. The most obvious of these is protection of autonomy and privacy. In all cases, "surveillance technologies should not replace human contact or personal care" (Niemeijer et al., 2010).

Trading Autonomy and Independence for Security and Privacy

When considering AT for monitoring and surveillance, there is an apparent conflict between the autonomy (or rights) of the resident and the duty of care by the staff (Martin et al., 2010). When AT is applied to keep people in their homes, autonomy is interpreted to mean self-control, freedom of choice, or "self-rule" for the resident traded off against beneficence and nonmaleficence of the care staff in the form of providing more security for residents of supported living situations (i.e., safeguarding the residents). Autonomy is also often viewed as the right to self-determination (Zwijsen et al., 2011).

Consideration of monitoring technology in relation to dementia care can produce different reactions. As Cash (2003) notes, "For some, technology is a saviour, the way to paradise; others are deeply suspicious of technology and scrutinize its proponents carefully for any tell-tale marks of the Beast" (Cash, 2003, p. 213). Many possibilities for AT could provide a completely monitored and supervised life within an elderly person's own home. For example, AT can be used as support for informal caregivers or as a potential solution to shortages in professional care. It can also support individuals with health problems such as dementia in meeting their everyday needs. Because AT has the potential to allow elderly people, including people with dementia, to live at home it is often promoted as a means of retaining autonomy and quality of life (Zwijsen et al., 2011). Monitoring can result in an increase in independence for individuals, reassurance for caregivers and family members, and the potential to release costs from social care budgets by reducing staffing requirement (Eccles, 2010).

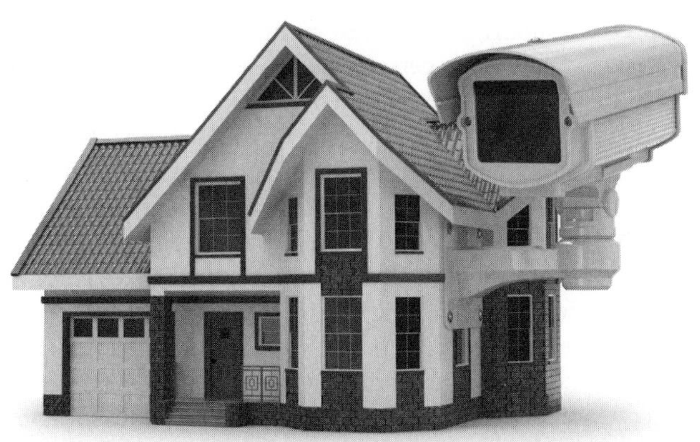

FIGURE 4-3 For some individuals being monitored is like having a giant camera that watches every move and report it to someone.

In a review of the literature around community-based living supported by AT, Zwijsen et al. (2011) found that AT is often considered the lesser of evils for individuals wishing to remain in their own homes. Living at home with AT is preferable to living in a group home with human caregivers. The loss of privacy through monitoring at home is perceived to be less than its loss by institutionalization in a group residence. Individuals also viewed AT as a least restrictive environment compared with locked doors or physical restraints. Despite this perspective that AT is the least bad solution vis-à-vis privacy, it does not mean it is automatically ethically sound. For some individuals, using AT respects their autonomy by enabling them to participate in everyday life by supporting their abilities. For example, tracking technology can enhance the feeling of autonomy by influencing the sense of security felt by a user and a caregiver when the user chooses to venture outside (Zwijsen et al., 2011). They also found that some authors believe that wandering off and getting lost is the main concern of the caregiver rather than the person with dementia. Thus, it appears that some devices meet the needs of the caregiver, not the person with dementia (Zwijsen et al., 2011).

For other individuals, the use of monitoring AT is an intrusion into their privacy that is unacceptable. They may view it as shown in Figure 4-3: a giant camera viewing everything they do and reporting it to someone (usually a family member or care provider) like "big brother." When monitoring is rejected because it interferes with independence rather than promoting it, other questions arise. The ethical principle of nonmaleficence requires assurance that being left alone does not mean that the individual will fail to thrive and eventually suffer because of lack of care. Technology can decrease isolation for some people through greater connectedness or increase it for others through reluctance to use the technology or the loss of human contact when technology is used (Eccles, 2010).

Although privacy is one of the ethical principles that should guide the design and use of ATs, it is not the only one or necessarily the most important one (Coeckelberg, 2010). "If the technology restores my communication with others (partner, family, friends, but also medical professionals), if it allows me to participate in the community, and if I am in such a condition that without constant monitoring of my bodily functions, my life expectancy decreases dramatically, then it is not clear why privacy should be the sole or overriding principle" (Coeckelberg, 2010, p. 186). Coeckelberg points out that the concerns about privacy are not new or unique to the use of AT. Being bathed by a human nurse is not very private either.

These different perspectives require person-centered planning to deal with different perceptions of privacy, autonomy, beneficence, and nonmaleficence (Zwijsen et al., 2011). The Human Activity Assistive Technology (HAAT) model (see Chapter 1) application starts with an individual who has a disability doing something (an activity) within a particular context (physical, social, cultural, or institutional) supported by technology. Thus, the perspective described here supports and is supported by the HAAT model. "The ethical implications of the use of such devices remain underexposed. With the subsequent implementation of specific monitoring devices, ethical values such as privacy, autonomy and independence appear to be at risk" (Zwijsen et al., 2011, p. 419). In general, ethical considerations lag technological development.

Another risk to ethical values is the huge potential cost that an aging population represents. This situation inevitably leads to cost as a driver of care approaches, including the use of surveillance technologies, "but technology continues to be also rather seductive to bureaucrats and policymakers as a way of addressing complex social change despite past evidence of failure and expense" (Eccles, 2010, p. 47). Currently, ethical considerations play a relatively minor role in the development and implementation of client service delivery for individuals with cognitive disabilities.

An Industry Perspective: One Company's View

A few technology companies also address ethical issues on their websites. One example is the Just Checking Company. This system, similar to many others, includes small, wireless sensors that are worn by the individual to detect movement around the home. The sensor data can be uploaded to a server via a website or mobile phone. The uploaded data are triggered as a person moves around their home. The sensor data are sent by the controller, via the mobile phone network, to the Just Checking web server. Families and professionals log on to the password-protected Just Checking website to view the chart of the activity. The website retains all the historical data for each service user and provides statistical information about when the equipment was used.

The Just Checking Company has this take on ethical principles and how they apply to this system (www.JustChecking.co.uk):

- **Nonmaleficence** means doing no harm. In the case of the Just Checking system, the system is passive and requires no physical interference, nor the wearing of any device.
- **Beneficence** means doing what is good for others. It is the basis of Western medical ethics. If it is the intention to provide care services that meet the needs of a person

and then monitoring to establish those needs and to check if the change is beneficent.

- **Autonomy** means the right to self-determination and freedom from unnecessary constraints or interference or loss of privacy. Most older people would prefer to stay in their own homes for as long as possible, but sometimes concern by relatives or neighbors about a person's safety or behavior means that a person's autonomy and independence are undermined prematurely.

The Just Checking system can enable the person to stay at home and provide a relative or caregiver with the reassurance that a loved one is capable of continuing to live in their own home for the time being. It prevents unnecessary visiting or telephoning, which may undermine autonomy, and enables the caregiver to plan more meaningful visits. Sensors can be sited to log activity without undue invasion of personal privacy, and there are no cameras. Installation of the system may afford greater privacy than caregivers calling in several times a day.

Justice is treating people fairly. Fairness includes providing the services that a vulnerable person needs to carry out his daily life. The Just Checking system helps to establish what the person is doing for himself and when he needs care. It enables family caregivers and care professionals to plan and deliver care when it is most needed rather than undermining independence.

Residential Care: Moving Out of the Home

As in the support of individuals in their own homes, community dwelling care in group residential settings often involves surveillance via AT monitoring systems (Niemeijer et al., 2010). As in other applications, AT for dementia in this setting serves two purposes: (1) support in activities of daily living and (2) monitor and safeguard residents from (self-inflicted) harm. The second includes tagging and tracking devices and has more ethical implications.

Niemeijer et al. (2010) conducted a literature review of the ethical and practical aspects of surveillance technologies in the residential care focusing on people with dementia and intellectual disability. They looked at three perspectives: that of the (1) institution, (2) resident, and (3) care relationship. Not surprisingly, these perspectives differed in terms of ethical concerns.

The institutional perspective focused on the reliability of the technology and the likelihood that its use might increase security or reduce risks while addressing staff burden. Although several reports claim increased safety and reduction of serious incidents, not much evidence is presented to substantiate this claim. There were also reports of increased staff job satisfaction after technological support. The technology does not remove risk completely, and staff can develop a false sense of security regarding patient safety. If repeated false alarms occur, then "alarm fatigue" can set in. Video surveillance can also protect residents from staff abuse.

The themes identifying considerations that need to be made relative to the resident focused on the resident's freedom (of movement) and how surveillance technologies will impact autonomy and human rights and whether it will respect the resident's personhood, privacy, and dignity. The three major subthemes reported in the literature are freedom and consent, privacy, and dignity and stigma. Surveillance technology may be viewed as a more suitable form of restraint than physical restraints, including locked doors, but freedom is still curtailed. For care providers, safety concerns are often used use to justify the use of restraints (including surveillance and monitoring).

For care providers, there is an ethical dilemma of duty of care versus autonomy of the resident and whether technology would substitute for human care. The autonomy of the patient, described as self-control, freedom of choice, or "self-rule" of the resident, is weighed against duty of care as beneficence and nonmaleficence when using surveillance technologies.

Professional care givers are more concerned about safety than family members (Niemeijer et al., 2010). In a residential setting, the safety issue is broadened to include not being a safety risk to other residents. If residents share a room, then the situation is made more complicated if one individual consents to the use of surveillance technologies that are meant for all residents but her roommate withholds consent.

As discussed elsewhere in this chapter, the substitution of surveillance technology for human care can lead to reduced staff involvement and an increase in social isolation for the residents. Niemeijer et al. (2010) describe the following ongoing ethical debate. On the one hand is the view that "the demands of work can make staff feel anxious and stressed, leading them to become very task focused, instead of person focused. A reduction in staff stress through the use of surveillance technologies could then lead to more person-centered care" (p. 1136). An alternative view claims that technology can decreases person-to-person interaction and thereby "denies personhood" in the care setting.

Because individual preferences, values, and needs vary, surveillance techniques should be individualized. There has been no consensus on whether or not surveillance technologies are an ethically viable option in the formal care of people with dementia or intellectual disability (Niemeijer et al., 2010). "The ethical debate centers not so much around the effects of this technology . . . but rather around the moral acceptability of those effects, especially when a conflict arises between the interests" (Niemeijer et al., 2010, p. 1138). In some cases, the design of the technology itself contains features that affect the rights of users and cannot be removed because they are fundamental to the technological operation. The cost of these technologies can be high, and that creates an additional ethical concern: that of distributive justice, which was discussed further earlier in this chapter.

Privacy and Security

Privacy and security of people and data are fundamental to creating an environment in which the autonomy of individual consumers is sustained. When monitoring is used in community- or residential-based care, privacy and security become critically important. Security is best viewed as a process, not a product of the technology (Martin et al., 2010). Tavani (2007) summarizes three views of privacy as:

1. Accessibility privacy, which is physically being left alone or being free from intrusion into your physical space
2. Decisional privacy, which relates to the freedom to make personal choices and decisions
3. Informational privacy, which is control over the flow of personal information, including the transfer and exchange of information

It would seem that privacy is not possible if there is real-time surveillance monitoring, but monitoring is not always an invasion of privacy if permission is granted or if the user can turn it off. "Most elderly people state that the needs for the devices overrule any possible privacy concerns, and as long as there is an appropriate balance between needs and privacy, they do not feel like their privacy is violated" (Zwijsen et al., 2011, p. 421).

The process by which privacy will be protected for the user of AT, the aim of the relevant AT, and the way it is used by service providers or care organizations should be captured in a privacy statement available from the care provider. This statement should also describe explicitly how personal data will be handled by care personnel and processed electronically. Martin et al. give some guidelines for the privacy statement in AT (2010):

> *The privacy statement should include the name and function of the person who has final responsibility for the daily processing of the personal data; the location where the data are stored in paper and/or electronic form; the specific aim, content and usage of the data and the person(s) who informs the user about this; the person(s) that can be contacted if personal data prove to be incorrect; and measures that are taken to prevent inspection, mutation or removal of data by unauthorised persons (p. 67).*

Many jurisdictions have privacy laws that require this kind of document or statement about the use and storage of information deemed private. Many have gone past the guidelines stage to policy implementation.

The ethical goal of autonomy requires attention to both security and privacy for computer-based AT systems. Assurance of both privacy and security is only possible if the AT system meets functional goals and needs of the user and operates reliably (i.e., does not have security weaknesses in its design) (Martin et al., 2010). One aspect of security that is critical is the storage of personal information about the user. In general, the guideline is to store personal data in the AT device only as long as necessary (Martin et al., 2010). For monitoring and surveillance systems, this would mean storage of personal data on the monitoring device only if necessary for the goal of assistance or care and then deleting them or transferring them to a secure central location. Some AT will, by its functional design, have personal data stored on it. For example, augmentative communication systems routinely include such data, and there are ways of protecting the data from unauthorized use by others (see Chapter 16). Likewise, some cognitive AT devices include personal data in order to facilitate community participation, and care must be taken to protect the user from inadvertently sharing this information with strangers (see Chapter 15).

One approach to security is to use passwords to protect access to personal data. This can present problems for individuals with cognitive disabilities such as dementia or intellectual disability. In these cases, automated authentication methods such as wearing a wireless authentication badge or face recognition must be considered. Privacy also requires that information security be part of the technology characteristics to ensure confidentiality (privacy), data integrity, availability, and accountability. All security and privacy methods and procedures must be informed by an ethical framework that is included in organizational policies and procedures (Martin et al., 2010).

AMBIENT ENVIRONMENTS, ARTIFICIAL INTELLIGENCE, AND ROBOTS: IMPACT ON CARE

Computing and communication systems are no longer just contained in a desktop computer that is used for work. Rather, virtually every electronic device used on a regular basis has both computing power and is linked to other devices through local networks (e.g., Wi-Fi) or the Internet. This is referred to as the **ambient environment**. The concept of embedded computing and communication among devices is known as ambient intelligence (Cook, Augusto, & Jakkula, 2009). This computer and communication capability is embedded in familiar objects such as home appliances (e.g., washing machines, refrigerators, and microwave ovens) and devices that travel with us outside the home (e.g., mobile phones and PDAs, cars and GPS navigation).

The degree to which the ambient intelligence approach has become pervasive in many aspects of our lives has led some to suggest that. ". . . information and communication technology for design of environments for ageing is of high social relevance, with respect of the quality of life of broad parts of the population" (Remmers, 2010, p. 200). There is potential for technically equipped private homes for people who are in need of care. This technology use may be viewed as socially valuable but only if a high amount of independence can be retained in a familiar home environment. It is essential that adequate consideration of enhancing the quality of life even in the presence of chronic illness or impairment be prominent (Remmers, 2010).

Rather than just compensating for lost function, ATs should contribute to growth and independence for persons with disabilities and seniors. The challenge is to balance the potential benefits of ambient environments, artificial intelligence (AI), and technologies such as robotics with ethical concerns of autonomy and privacy, but the stakes are higher because of the pervasive nature of the technology (Remmers, 2010). A fundamental concept is self-determination, including enlisting the help of others as needed. Independence does not mean doing something entirely on one's own. Rather, self-determination refers to the opportunity to make a choice on how and when daily functions such as taking a shower, bathing, dressing and undressing, using the toilet, and eating are carried out as well as completing activities such as shopping, cleaning, preparing meals, and taking care of financial affairs. The ethical principles of beneficence, nonmaleficence, and justice need to be applied to considerations of these technologies as well.

One of the areas of potential AT application is the provision of care by devices that extend the sensing role played by monitoring to clinical decision making based on sensing and AI. These devices may serve as coaches for activities of daily living (LoPresti et al., 2004) or they may be developed in the form of robots, often referred to as "carebots." Figure 4-4 illustrates a system designed for coaching individuals with cognitive disabilities such as dementia while they are doing tasks of daily living such as hand washing. A camera in the bathroom ceiling monitors the actions of the user. An artificial intelligence-based computer program determines if the appropriate steps are being taken by the user. If not, a verbal prompt is presented to the user via speakers in the ceiling. The user's performance can also be recorded for later analysis by care providers.

Much of the discussion around these devices is in terms of ongoing research, but there are also some clinical applications under way. From an ethical point of view, there are two distinct approaches: replacement of human care by ATs and care assisted by AI technologies but without replacing human care. The latter is far less controversial than the former (Coeckelberg, 2010). In this section, we will discuss both the current clinical application and the possible future implications for this type of care because the ethical issues

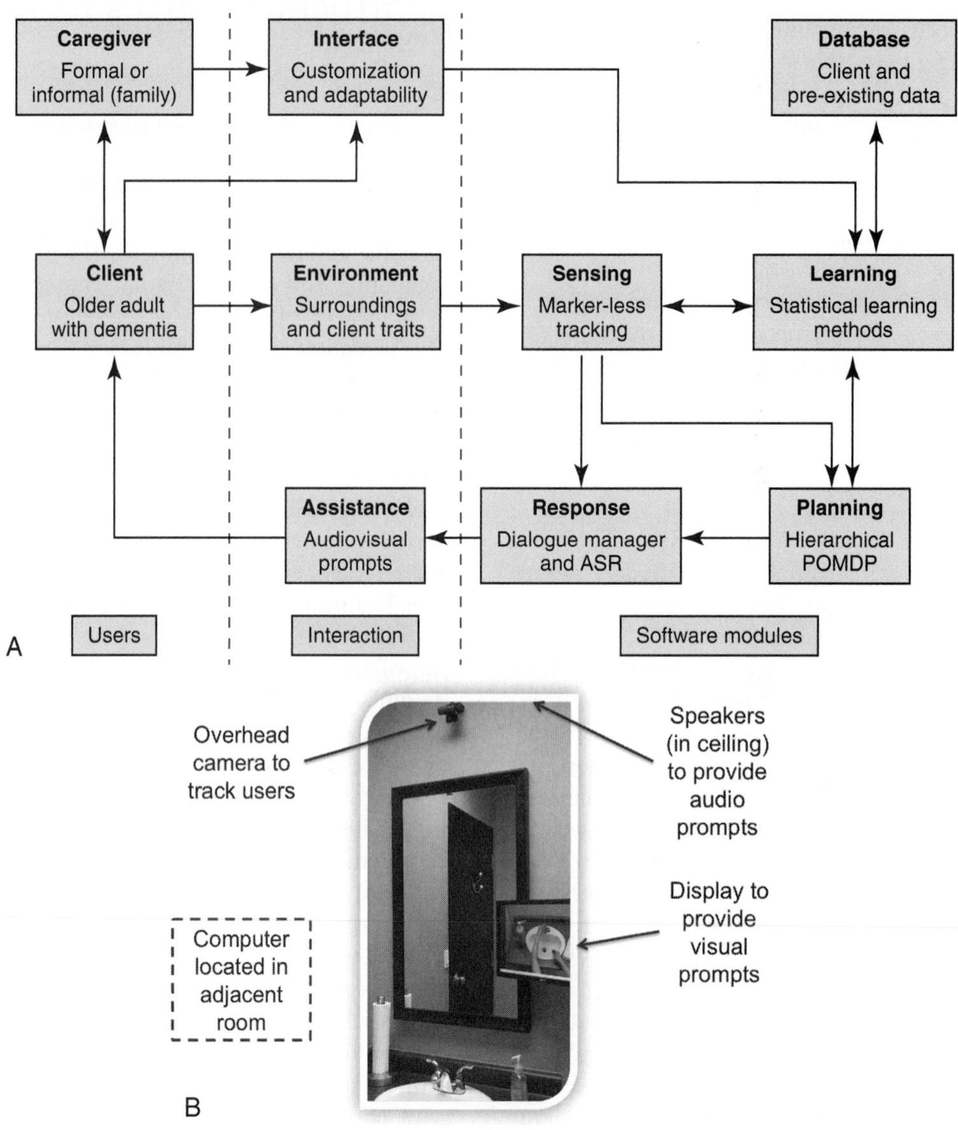

FIGURE 4-4 The COACH system has been designed to prompt individuals who have difficulty washing their hands (see text). A: Schematic diagram. B: Setup showing key components. Courtesy of Alex Mihailidis.

raised are far reaching and could impact future AT application in general.

Coeckelberg (2010) defines care in which AT provides functional gain but does not really emotionally relate to the person as "shallow care." In contrast, "deep care" is care that includes feeling for the person that is reciprocal. It is the area of deep care that causes the major ethical controversy. "The problem is not the technologies themselves, not replaceability as such, and not the (potential violation of) the principles of privacy or autonomy alone, but the question of what good care and the good life are for us as humans, for us in this context, and for us as the unique persons that we are" (Coeckelberg, 2010, p. 190). Coeckelberg describes "good care" as meeting the social and emotional needs of patients. This description leads many to argue that AT alone is not satisfactory for replacing human care (e.g., nursing care for seniors). Among the potential objections are (Coeckelberg, 2010):

1. An AI robot or an AI monitoring system is able to deliver care, but it will never really care about the human.
2. AI technologies cannot provide "good care" because that requires contact with humans who have social and emotional needs.
3. Even if AI ATs do provide good care, they will violate the fundamental principle of privacy in doing so, which is why they should be banned.
4. AI assistive robots provide "fake" care, and they are likely to "fool" people by making people think they are receiving real care.

Coeckelberg also cautions us not to "... set the standards of care too high when evaluating the introduction of AI ATs in health care, since otherwise we would have to reject many of our existing, low-tech health care practices" (2010, p. 181).

Artificial Intelligence in Assistive Technology Applications

When the AI is used as an assist to care rather than to replace human care providers, then the ethical concerns are different and may be less difficult to resolve. However, with AI or computer-based ATs (which are very often the case), there is not a binary choice between replacement of function completely and assistance provided to the user. Rather, there are varying degrees of device operation that are under the control of the user. Interestingly, computer scientists and robotic engineers refer to autonomy not from the point of view of the person as we have been discussing but from the point of the technology. So, when we are dealing with AI-based systems, we are trading off the autonomy of the technology for the autonomy of the person. This is captured in Box 4-1, which shows levels of autonomy for the technology and the corresponding role for the human user. Decision making is still by the human caregiver or at least the decision-making algorithms are informed by the care provider. The algorithms are "invisible" to the operator and may make functional operation decisions based on sensing. For example, a power wheelchair may adjust to an increasing incline and increase the motor speed to compensate for the incline. The user would have no knowledge of this change in operation. At a higher level of device autonomy, the wheelchair might be "smart" and have features that enable navigation to avoid obstacles or learning an environment so as to move around from room to room without out user control (Simpson, 2005). Here the wheelchair has greater autonomy, the user has less, and there are concerns about safety because the lack of user control could cause injury more readily. Of course, a human user can also take actions that result in injury when using a power wheelchair. The levels of autonomous device control still takes decision making out of the hands of the user. Do they reduce the user's autonomy from an ethical point of view, or are these levels of control more appropriately considered in relation to beneficence and nonmaleficence?

Robots can be programmed to exhibit different levels of autonomy with respect to the user (Parasuraman, Sheridan, & Wicke, 2000). At one end of the spectrum, the robot can accept high-level commands and accomplish a complete task (e.g., get a glass of milk). The robot performs the task without any operator intervention. This is called fully autonomous from the point of view of the robot, but it provides no autonomy to the person. The other end of the scale is called teleoperated. Here the user has direct control over the robot's movements and has to direct each step in the completion of a task. The user or operator of the robot is now fully autonomous. These levels also require different amounts of cognitive ability by the user.

The major ethical concerns with AI systems are beneficence and, especially, nonmaleficence more than autonomy because of the degree to which the technology can take over some decision making regarding the course of action of the technology. In some cases, the decision making is strictly functional. This could be the next step in an activities of daily living task (e.g., sensing a glass vs. a plate) or selecting the best the best route in a navigation plan for a blind user. Alternatively, the decision making could have medical implications (e.g., prompting someone to take her medications). Ethical issues arise based on how the technology is used. Many AI systems, especially those that include motor actions such as mobility or manipulation, are extensions of

BOX 4-1 Sheridan's Levels of Robotic Autonomy

1. Computer offers no assistance; human does it all.
2. Computer offers a complete set of action alternatives.
3. Computer narrows the selection down to a few choices.
4. Computer suggests a single action.
5. Computer executes that action if human approves.
6. Computer allows the human limited time to veto before automatic execution.
7. Computer executes automatically and then necessarily informs the human.
8. Computer informs human after automatic execution only if human asks.
9. Computer informs human after automatic execution only if it decides to.
10. Computer decides everything and acts autonomously, ignoring the human.

From Parasuraman R, Sheridan TB, Wicke CD: A model for types and levels of human interaction with automation, *IEEE Transactions On Systems, Man, and Cybernetics—Part A: Systems and Humans*, 30(3):286-297, 2000.

monitoring but with added coaching or prompting capabilities. Issues of surveillance and invasion of privacy still exist because of storage of personal data and the surrendering of autonomy with some devices. Justice issues related to things such as the availability of broadband coverage, which is often not available in rural areas or less developed countries but required for some AI AT (Eccles, 2010). Fiscal constraints are also important (Canning, 2005).

Socially Assistive Robots

Socially assistive robotics (SARs) has the goal of automating supervision, coaching, motivation, and companionship in one-on-one interactions with individuals (Feil-Seifer & Matarić, 2011). These robots are distinguished from assistive robots that provide assistance with physical tasks under the user's control. Target populations for this type of assistance include stroke survivors, elderly adults and individuals with dementia, and children with autism spectrum disorders, among many others. It is significant that a common thread for these populations is cognitive disability, opening up a range of ethical concerns. Benefits of an ethical treatment should exceed the risks if the ethical principles of beneficence and nonmaleficence are followed. There are both benefits and risks associated with SARs. These robots are not in clinical use, but there have been research studies with potential client groups.

If a user becomes emotionally attached to the robot, it can cause a significant ethical dilemma (Feil-Seifer & Matarić, 2011). If the robot is removed because of lack of adaptation in the robot software or electronic or software failure, then the emotional contact benefit is lost, and there can be a sense of loss by the user, especially if the user cannot understand the causes for the robot's removal. For example, research with SARs has shown that elderly users and users with Alzheimer's disease engage with robots and miss them when they are removed. Because there is a demonstrated emotional attachment, the question: "Is there deception inherent in the personification of a robot by a user or a caregiver?" has been proposed (Feil-Seifer & Matarić, 2011, p. 8). A number of factors relate to the personification of roots. The actual design of the robot may or may not be purposefully manipulated to alter the perceptions of the user toward therapeutic goals (Feil-Seifer & Matarić, 2011). The physical appearance, including human-like features, can influence how the robot is perceived. Larger robots are more fearsome, and smaller ones are perceived as more friendly. How the robot is dressed and the type of voice also affect user response. Feminine voices are more soothing, and the presence of a lab coat could indicate authority. As other features such as gestures, coordinated body movements, and facial expressions are added, the personification is increased.

Different groups have different reactions to SARs (Feil-Seifer & Matarić, 2011). Although some participants interacting with robots can correctly distinguish between robot activities and the equivalent capabilities in a person or pet, other users formed emotional attachments to the SARs, leading to misconceptions about the robots' emotional capabilities. One danger in this type of attachment is emotional loss (e.g., one participant thought the robot would miss him when he was not there, something the robot could not do). Another risk is that the user might believe that the robot could assist him as a human would do (e.g., telling the robot about symptoms that should be told to a clinician).

This deception has been viewed negatively because our interests are not likely to be served by illusions. In considering the potential ethical impact of SARs, Sparrow and Sparrow (2006) wrote: "What most of us want out of life is to be loved and cared for, and to have friends and companions, not merely to believe that we are loved and cared for, and to believe that we have friends and companions, when in fact these beliefs are false" (p. 155). Their concerns are on several levels. First, they believe that it is unethical to intend to deceive others even for their own subjective benefit. They also are concerned that people will be deceived when they are given AI assistive systems that have human or animal-like features. They consider these deceptions to be unethical, especially when the result of the deception could harm the individual who is being deceived. Others disagree "since in practice most of the time people are very much aware that a certain AI autonomous system such as a robot is not really human, even if the robot has a human appearance and even if they respond to the robot as if it were human" (Coeckelberg, 2010, p. 187). This discussion reinforces the patient-centered concept discussed earlier.

Sparrow and Sparrow (2006) do acknowledge that robots may have a part to play in roles when they might physically assist an individual but not replace human caregivers. But even this more limited role proposed for robots to provide care of sufficient quality to replace human care providers also leads to a concern for the overall reduction in human social interaction for this vulnerable population (Sparrow and Sparrow, 2006). Even physically assistive robots that carry out tasks of daily living might deprive a person of human contact. For some individuals living at home with care provided to them, the only human contact they have is with the cleaning staff members who come weekly because all other care can be provided remotely. If a robot cleaning system, currently available (see http://robot-vacuum-review.toptenreviews.com/ for examples), is used to vacuum their house, then even the weekly appearance of a human cleaning assistant might disappear.

EQUITABLE ASSISTIVE TECHNOLOGY DISTRIBUTION OF ASSISTIVE TECHNOLOGY: WHO GETS WHAT?

Sen (1999) relates capabilities to the outcomes achieved by considering functionings:

> *. . . the assessment of capabilities has to proceed primarily on the basis of observing a person's actual functionings, to be supplemented by other information. There is a jump here (from functioning to capabilities), but it need not be a big jump, if only because the valuation of actual functionings is one way of assessing how a person values the options he has" (Sen 1999, p. 131).*

The focus on function and outcome makes the link between capabilities and ATs more direct.

In much of his writing, Sen is concerned with economic growth and the disparity between the rich and poor, but he also established the relationship between distribution of income and the "inequality in the distribution of substantive freedoms and capabilities" (Sen, 1999, p. 119). This magnifies the problem of inequality. He is concerned with the ability that people in poverty have of converting income to capabilities, especially if they are also disabled or old. Poverty is compounded by disability. Individuals with disabilities are less likely to attend school, which limits their potential to earn an income as adults. Adults with disabilities are more likely to be unemployed or underemployed (i.e., working at a job that is not commensurate with their skill level), and when employed, they are more likely to earn a lower income than their nondisabled peers (WHO, 2011). Individuals with disabilities and their families are poorer than their peers who earn a similar income because of the extra expenses they incur related to medical costs, technology costs, and costs related to paying for assistance as well as loss of income incurred by a family member who is unable to be employed as a result of care requirements. Sen refers to these situations as "conversion handicap" (Sen, 2009).

Individuals who live in poverty have a heightened risk of acquiring a disability as a result of living conditions that result in food insecurity and unsafe housing, lack of medical care, lack of clean water and sanitation, and unsafe work conditions. Similarly, lack of access to medical care and rehabilitation can magnify the effects of an existing disability (WHO, 2011).

The personal income inequality may tend to be magnified by this "coupling" of low incomes with disabilities in the conversion of incomes into capabilities. Access to ATs can aid in the development of capabilities and help to address this conversion. Distribution of ATs cannot be a goal unto itself if the potential benefits of achieving full societal participation are to be achieved; rather, they are a means to the ultimate end of increased capabilities.

A major assessment of capabilities requires an understanding of how AT devices, services, and policies have helped people recognize new functionings and provided them with capabilities to act. When they are given choice regarding AT implementation, it is important to determine if they have taken advantage of the ATs to make them real in their lives. When AT is supplied, people have the freedom to choose whether to apply it in their lives or not. The AT supplied must work for the individual in her context.

As described by the HAAT model, it is also important that the AT supplied works for the individual in her context. The local culture must be taken into account. For example, in some distribution models AT is supplied by charitable organizations, and the devices may be cast-offs from the country of origin of the host organization. These devices that may provide functional support very well in the originating country but not in the country where the people receiving them live.

One of the challenges for individuals with significant disabilities is how resources that are available get converted into capabilities (Sen, 1999). People with disabilities may need more income to achieve the same functional outcomes as nondisabled persons (e.g., to hire attendants and pay for AT and home modifications). In Sen's words, "This entails that 'real poverty' (in terms of capability deprivation) may be, in a significant sense, more intense than what appears in the income space" (Sen, 1999, p. 88). Because ATs can increase functional capabilities, they can also augment the ability to convert resources into capabilities and functional outcomes and address capability deprivation. Applying these concepts to the distribution and use of ATs can also change perceptions of value added and make the outcome measures more human centered.

One criterion for the distribution of hard AT that is often used is medical necessity. In this scenario, funding for technology is prescribed by therapeutic need only, not by social needs for employment, education, or relationships (Canning, 2005). Medical necessity applied to AT distribution is often focused on finding the least expensive technology. This focus can be in conflict with an individual's needs considering Nussbaum's central human capabilities that are based on the principle of human dignity (Nussbaum, 2006). Independence and function are not necessarily related to medical necessity.

One example is based on the funding of wheelchairs by the US Medicare system. Medicare will not fund a powered wheelchair that is necessary for mobility in the community (including employment) if the person can use a manual wheelchair in the home (Canning, 2005). Thus, the device recommendation from a wheelchair evaluation will be driven by funding criteria in the first instance, not the needs of the individual. What an individual gets, the distributive justice ethical perspective, will also be determined by the type of funding source the individual has. For example, the outcome can be dramatically different depending on the funding available to the individual (Canning, 2005). Two scenarios are described by Canning (2005) in which the need of two individuals is nearly identical, but one has public funding and one has private insurance. Both have the same need, but the interpretation of medical necessity is different based on the funder.

The individual with private insurance will get or have access to more AT than the individual who depends on public insurance. If ATs are related to the distribution of capability, then this situation clearly violates the principle proposed by both Sen and Nussbaum because it ignores family goals and lifestyle preferences and focuses on meeting therapeutic needs with a minimum of public expenditures.

Summary

Some areas of current AT policy implementation warrant scrutiny (Eccles, 2010). These areas include the limited policy discussion of alternative models of care, the limited ethical frameworks currently in use, and performance measurement criteria that may encourage less than optimal practice. For example, care mangers may be rewarded for cost savings or safety records without consideration for the impact on autonomy or justice.

Eccles (2010) also questions whether the biomedical principles of autonomy, beneficence, nonmaleficence, and justice provide enough basis for understanding ethical issues in complex community care settings. These four principles may not be sufficient given the different cultural and contextual considerations that can impact ethical decision making, including the attitude of local staff, consumers, and managers. In the next section, we consider two other ethical constructs proposed by Eccles.

PROFESSIONAL ETHICS

Professional ethics address the behavior expected of an individual when practicing in a specific discipline. As we have seen, the ethical principle of fidelity applies directly to professional practice. Eccles (2010) proposes two other ethical constructs, ethic of care and intuitional ethics.

The ethic of care describes the interaction between professions and service users in a rehabilitation or long-term care setting based on a relationship developed and sustained over a long period of time (Eccles, 2010). This approach to care is in contrast to acute medical settings where the care is more episodic and for shorter periods of time. Acute care is based on the four bioethical principles of autonomy, beneficence, nonmaleficence, and justice. Eccles questions whether these same four principles apply to long-term care where the emphasis is on contextual relational approaches that are not necessarily uniform in their approach because they are specific to a given patient–care provider relationship. The ethic of care concept positions care as a "moral activity based on complex array of obligations and reciprocities" (Eccles, 2010, p. 51). The ethic of care varies by consumer—some want lots of human interaction, but others feel demeaned and find human care invasive.

To make monitoring meaningful, the data must be interpreted in terms of the HAAT model social context. Care workers themselves may derive satisfaction from their relations with a client. When they have developed strong relations with service users, this relationship may prompt an unreasonable reluctance on their part to use technology. Eccles (2010) concludes by asking, "If technology is viewed as an imperative in managing the demands thrown up by demographic change, how are relationships and contextual sensitivity to be recognized without more complex ethical frames of reference and enquiry?" (p. 52).

Intuitionism describes the ethical judgments that might result from different types of care, especially that provided face-to-face and that provided by telecare using distance delivery methods. "Intuitive responses to right and wrong courses of action in the face of immediate human dilemmas are less likely to be played out when the ethical dilemmas are more remote or abstract" (Eccles, 2010, p. 52). There are concerns about whether the perception of care by the consumer is the same in face-to-face situations as with remote monitoring. A major concern is whether there will be a filtering of the urgency of immediate needs because of the remoteness of the care. Intuitionism is a product of clinical experience, personal relationship with the consumer, and the application of ethical and professional practice principles.

Ethics and Standards of Practice

When applied to a field of professional endeavor such as AT delivery or a discipline such as occupational therapy and occupational therapy assistant, physical therapy and physical therapy assistant, or speech-language pathology or speech-language pathology assistant, the ethical conduct of practitioners is embodied both in a code (or canons) of ethics and in standards of practice. Standards of practice differ from codes of ethics in that they describe more specifically what is and is not considered to be good practice in a given discipline. All AT providers must comply with the code of ethics for his or her discipline. The code of ethics for a discipline is typically developed by the professional association serving it. As we have discussed, AT personnel have responsibilities in AT service delivery that are not specified by their individual discipline's code of ethics. For this reason, it is important to have a code of ethics that addresses the specific issues related to the application of ATs. Much of AT service delivery is interdisciplinary, and professional ethics may have differences across professions (e.g., assessment approaches, ethical frameworks used).

RESNA Code of Ethics for Assistive Technologies

The Rehabilitation Engineering and Assistive Technology Society of North America (RESNA) (www.resna.org) is an interdisciplinary professional association whose activities focus on ATs. Its members come from many disciplines and a variety of settings, and their activities involve the full scope of AT applications. In 1991, the RESNA Board of Directors adopted the code of ethics shown in Box 4-2. This code is similar to those of other disciplines involved in rehabilitation and is based on several of them. However, it includes issues related to the provision of technology. It is presented as a reminder of the obligations that practitioners in the AT industry have to their consumers, others who work with and care for them, the general public, and the profession as a whole.

SUMMARY

Because ATs are used in ways that can dramatically affect the lives of those who use them, important ethical questions must be considered. The ethical areas of autonomy, fidelity, beneficence, nonmaleficence, and justice need to be used as a frame of reference when applying ATs. AT applications that impact vulnerable populations such as those with dementia or intellectual disabilities raise additional questions around concepts such as informed consent, privacy, and security of data. The embedded environment and the development of technologies using AI principles have large potential benefits in terms of functionality and potential risks regarding autonomy and beneficence. The ethical principle of fidelity underlies professional ethics and standard of practice.

BOX 4-2 RESNA Standards of Practice for Assistive Technology Practitioners

These Standards of Practice set forth fundamental concepts and rules considered essential to promote the highest ethical standards among individuals who evaluate, assess the need for, recommend, or provide assistive technology. In the discharge of their professional obligations assistive technology practitioners and suppliers shall observe the following principles and rules:

1. Individuals shall keep paramount the welfare of those served professionally.
2. Individuals shall engage in only those services that are within the scope of their competence, considering the level of education, experience and training, and shall recognize the limitations imposed by the extent of their personal skills and knowledge in any professional area.
3. In making determinations as to what areas of practice are within their competency, assistive technology practitioners and suppliers shall observe all applicable licensure laws, consider the qualifications for certification or other credentials offered by recognized authorities in the primary professions which comprise the field of assistive technology, and abide by all relevant standards of practice and ethical principles, including RESNA's Code of Ethics.
4. Individuals shall truthfully, fully and accurately represent their credentials, competency, education, training and experience in both the field of assistive technology and the primary profession in which they are members. To the extent practical, individuals shall disclose their primary profession in all forms of communication, including advertising, which refers to their credential in assistive technology.
5. Individuals shall, at a minimum, inform consumers or their advocates of any employment affiliations, financial or professional interests that may be perceived to bias recommendations, and in some cases, decline to provide services or supplies where the conflict of interest is such that it may fairly be concluded that such affiliation or interest is likely to impair professional judgments.
6. Individuals shall use every resource reasonably available to ensure that the identified needs of consumers are met, including referral to other practitioners or sources which may provide the needed service or supply within the scope of their competence.
7. Individuals shall cooperate with members of other professions, where appropriate, in delivering services to consumers, and shall actively participate in the team process when the consumer's needs require such an approach.
8. Individuals shall offer an appropriate range of assistive technology services that include assessment, evaluation, recommendations, training, adjustments at delivery, and follow-up and modifications after delivery.
9. Individuals shall verify consumer's needs by using direct assessment or evaluation procedures with the consumer.
10. Individuals shall assure that the consumer fully participates, and is fully informed about all reasonable options available, regardless of finances, in the development of recommendations for intervention strategies.
11. Individuals shall consider future and emerging needs when developing intervention strategies and fully inform the consumer of those needs.
12. Individuals shall avoid providing and implementing technology, which expose the consumer to unreasonable risk, and shall advise the consumer as fully as possible of all known risks. Where adjustments, instruction for use, or necessary modifications are likely to be required to avoid or minimize such risks, individuals shall make sure that such information or service is provided.
13. Individuals shall fully inform consumers or their advocates about all relevant aspects, including the financial implications, of all final recommendations for the provision of technology, and shall not guaranty the results of any service or technology. Individuals may, however, make reasonable statements about prognosis.
14. Individuals shall maintain adequate records of the technology evaluation, assessment, recommendations, services, or products provided and preserve confidentiality of those records, unless required by law, or unless the protection of the welfare of the person or the community requires otherwise.
15. Individuals shall endeavor, through ongoing professional development, including continuing education, to remain current on all aspects of assistive technology relevant to their practice including accessibility, funding, legal or public issues, recommended practices and emerging technologies.
16. Individuals shall endeavor to institute procedures, on an on-going basis, to evaluate, promote and enhance the quality of service delivered to all consumers.
17. Individuals shall be truthful and accurate in all public statements concerning assistive technology, assistive technology practitioners and suppliers, services, and products dispensed.
18. Individuals shall not invidiously discriminate in the provision of services or supplies on the basis of disability, race, national origin, religion, creed, gender, age, or sexual orientation.
19. Individuals shall not charge for services not rendered, nor misrepresent in any fashion services delivered or products dispensed for reimbursement or any other purpose.
20. Individuals shall not engage in fraud, dishonesty or misrepresentation of any kind, or any form of conduct that adversely reflects on the field of assistive technology, or the individual's fitness to serve consumers professionally.
21. Individuals whose professional services are adversely affected by substance abuse or other health-related conditions shall seek professional advice, and where appropriate, withdraw from the affected area of practice.

RESNA, Rehabilitation Engineering and Assistive Technology Society of North America.

STUDY QUESTIONS

1. List the five types of ethical principles.
2. For each of the five types of ethical principles, identify an AT application to which that principle applies.
3. Why do we say that fidelity is perhaps the most common source of ethical conflict?
4. The concept of fidelity can be applied at several levels in the AT process. Describe how it applies to the clinician, the distributor, and the manufacturer.
5. What do we mean by the statement that the understanding of beneficence involves finding the balance between risk tolerance and risk aversion?
6. What does the principle of nonmaleficence refer to and how does it affect AT practice?
7. How is stigma related to nonmaleficence?
8. List at least three ways that ATs can contribute to stigma.

9. List three major benefits and the major ethical concerns associated with surveillance and monitoring applications.
10. We state that ATs can both reduce the differences between those with disabilities and increase those differences. Explain how this can happen.
11. List Nussbaum's (2006) central human capabilities. How do these apply to the use of ATs?
12. Discuss, in terms of the technology options available and their ethical concerns, the tradeoffs for someone who wishes to stay at home rather than go to a group setting.
13. How does the application of ATs relate to the three types of privacy described by Tavani (2007)?
14. What role does informed consent play in the ethical practice of AT delivery?
15. What are the major ethical considerations associated with the application of ATs based on the ambient environment?
16. Remmers (2010) stated that the challenge is to balance the potential benefits of ambient environments, AI, and technologies such as robotics with ethical concerns of autonomy and privacy, but the stakes are higher because of the pervasive nature of the technology. What does this mean in terms of ethical principles?
17. Coeckelberg (2010) raises four objections to the use of AI-based devices (including robots). What are they? Do you agree or disagree with this analysis? Why?
18. For intelligent technologies, we can view the concept of autonomy from the point of view of the device or the person. What ethical principles are implicated by the levels of autonomy shown in Box 4-1?
19. What is a socially assistive robot?
20. What ethical concerns are raised about the use of socially assistive robots with frail elderly individuals?
21. What is distributive justice?
22. What is the capability approach, and why is it proposed as an appropriate distributive approach for ATs?
23. What is meant by the "ethic of care," and how does it apply to AT service delivery?
24. What is meant by the term "intuitionism," and how does it apply to remote monitoring?
25. Read the RESNA ethical principles of practice (Box 4-2). Do you agree with them? Are there any that should be added or changed based on the ethical concepts presented in this chapter?

REFERENCES

Airaksinen T: The philosophy of professional ethics. In *Institutional Issues Involving Ethics and Justice, Vol. 1, UNESCO encyclopedia of institutional and infrastructural resources*, Paris, 2003, UNESCO-EOLLS Joint Committee Secretariat, pp 1–21.

Alampay EA: Beyond access to ICTs: Measuring capabilities in the information society, *IJEDICT* 2(3):4–22, 2006.

Beauchamp T: The principle of beneficence in applied ethics. In Zalta EM, editor: *The Stanford encyclopedia of philosophy,* 2008. Available from http://plato.stanford.edu/archives/fall2008/entries/principle-beneficence/.

Borg J, Larsson S, Östergren P: The right to assistive technology: For whom, for what, and by whom? *Disabil Soc* 26(2), 2011.

Canning B: Funding, ethics, and assistive technology: Should medical necessity be the criterion by which wheeled mobility equipment is justified? *Top Stroke Rehabil* 12(3):77–81, 2005.

Cash M: Assistive technology and people with dementia, *Rev Clin Gerontol* 13:313–319, 2003.

Coeckelberg M: Health care, capabilities, and AI assistive technologies, ethic, *Theory Moral Pract* 13:181–190, 2010.

Cook A: Ethical issues related to the use/non-use of assistive technologies, *Dev Disabil Bull* 37(1-2):127–152, 2009.

Cook DJ, Augusto JC, Jakkula VR: Ambient intelligence: Technologies, applications, and opportunities, *Pervasive Mob Comput* 5:277–298, 2009.

Eccles A: Ethical considerations around the implementation of telecare technologies, *J Technol Hum Serv* 28:44–59, 2010.

Feil-Seifer DJ, Matarić M: Ethical principles for socially assistive robotics, *IEEE Rob Autom Mag* 18(1):24–31, 2011.

Hansson SO: The ethics of enabling technology, *Cambridge Quarterly of Healthcare Ethics* 16(3):257–267, 2007.

Herman B: The scope of moral requirement, *Philos Public Aff* 30(3):227–256, 2001.

Kitchner KS: *Foundations of ethical practice, research, and teaching in psychology*, Mahwah, NJ, 2000, Lawrence Erlbaum Associates.

Lamont J, Favor C: Distributive justice. In Zalta EM, editor: *The Stanford encyclopedia of philosophy*, 2008. Available from http://plato.stanford.edu/archives/fall2008/entries/justice-distributive.

LoPresti EF, Mihailidis A, Kirsch N: Assistive technology for cognitive rehabilitation: state of the art, *Neuropsycholl Rehabil* 14:5–39, 2004.

Martin S, Bengtsson JH, Dröes RM: Assistive technologies and issues relating to privacy, ethics and security. In Mulvenna MD, Nugent CD, editors: *Supporting people with dementia using pervasive health technologies, advanced information and knowledge processing*, London, 2010, Springer-Verlag.

Niemeijer AR, Frederiks BJM, Riphagen II , et al.: Ethical and practical concerns of surveillance technologies in residential care for people with dementia or intellectual disabilities, An overview of the literature, *International Psychogeriatrics* 22(7):1129–1142, 2010.

Nussbaum MC: *Frontiers of justice: Disability, nationality, species membership*, Cambridge, MA, 2006, Belknap Press of Harvard University Press.

Pape TL, Kim J, Weiner B: The shape of individual meanings assigned to assistive technology: A review of personal factors, *Disabil Rehabil* 24(1/2/3):5–20, 2002.

Parette P, Scherer M: Assistive technology use and stigma, *Educ Train Dev Disabil* 39(3):217–226, 2004.

Parasuraman R, Sheridan TB, Wicke CD: A model for types and levels of human interaction with automation, *IEEE Trans. Syst. Man Cybern. Part A Syst. Humans* 30(3):286–297, 2000.

Perry J, Beyer S, Holm S: Assistive technology, telecare and people with intellectual disabilities: Ethical considerations, *J Med Ethics* 35:81–86, 2009.

Peterson D, Murray GC: Ethics and assistive technology service provision, *Disabil Rehabil Assist Technol* 1(1-2):59–67, 2006.
Pullin G: *Design meets disability*, Cambridge, MA, 2009, MIT Press.
Purtilo R: *Ethical dimensions in the health professions*, Philadelphia, 2005, Elsevier Saunders.
Remmers H: Environments for ageing, assistive technology and self-determination: Ethical perspectives, *Informatics for Health & Social Care* 35(3-4):200–210, 2010.
Sanford JA: *Universal design as a rehabilitation strategy*, New York, 2012, Springer.
Scherer M, Jutai J, Fuhrer M, et al.: A framework for modelling the selection of assistive technology devices (ATDs), *Disabil Rehabil Assist Technol* 2(1):1–8, 2007.
Sen A: *Development as freedom*, Westminster, MD, 1999, Alfred A. Knopf.
Sen A: Economic development and capability expansion in historical perspective, *Pacif Econ Rev* 6(2):179–191, 2001.
Simpson R: Smart wheelchairs: A literature review, *J Rehab Res Dev* 42(4):423–435, 2005.
Sparrow R, Sparrow L: In the hands of machines? The future of aged care, *Mind Mach* 16(2):141–161, 2006.
Tavani H: *Ethics and technology: Ethical issues in an age of information and communication technology*, ed 2, New York, 2007, John Wiley and Sons.
World Health Organization: *World report on disability*, Geneva, 2011, World Health Organization. p. 10.
Zwijsen SA, Niemeijer AR, Hertogh CMPM: Ethics of using assistive technology in the care for community-dwelling elderly people: An overview of the literature, *Aging Mental Health* 15(4):419–427, 2011.

CHAPTER 5

Delivering Assistive Technology Services to the Consumer

CHAPTER OUTLINE

LEARNING OBJECTIVES

On completing this chapter, you will be able to do the following:

1. Describe the principles related to assessment and intervention in assistive technology (AT) service delivery.
2. Describe the methods used to gather and analyze information during AT assessment and intervention.
3. Identify and describe key areas to target in the assessment phase of the service delivery process.
4. Identify and describe each of the steps in AT service delivery.
5. Describe key strategies to enable AT use.
6. Describe the methods of formal and informal evaluation of AT service outcomes.
7. Describe different types of funding sources of AT and considerations to make when determining eligibility for funding.

KEY TERMS

Activity Output
Aesthetics
Assessment
Auditory Function
Client-Centered Practice
Clinical Reasoning
Cognitive Skills
Criteria for Service
Criterion-Referenced Measurement
Cultural Context
Device Characteristics
Evaluation Phase
Environmental Interface
Feedback
Follow-Along
Follow-Up
Formal Evaluation
Funding
Implementation Phase
Informal Evaluation
Institutional Context
Language Skills
Needs Identification
Norm-Referenced Measurements
Outcome Measures
Operational Competence
Performance Aid
Physical Construction
Physical Context
Physical Properties
Physical Skill
Quantitative Measurement
Qualitative Measurement
Referral and Intake
Reliability
Sensory Functions
Service Delivery
Social Context
Somatosensory or Tactile Function
Strategic Competence
Technology Abandonment
Validity
Visual Skills
Visual Perception

INTRODUCTION

Service delivery involves all facets of the process that starts with the identification of the client's needs for assistive technology (AT) and culminates with the ongoing outcome evaluation of their use of acquired technology. Scherer defines an AT service in the following manner:

> *Any service that directly assists an individual with a disability in the selection, acquisition, or use of an assistive technology device, including...evaluation of the needs of an individual... ; purchasing, leasing or otherwise providing for acquisition ... of an assistive device; selecting, designing, fitting, customizing, adapting, applying, maintaining, repairing, or replacing assistive technology devices; . . . Training and technical assistance (Scherer, 2002, p. 6).*

This chapter describes the process by which consumers obtain AT devices and services based on the Human Activity Assistive Technology (HAAT) model. It identifies and describes several principles of assessment and implementation of AT use. Information on the full range of service delivery aspects is provided, highlighting elements in which the clinician has a primary role. To effectively provide these services to the client, the clinician should be knowledgeable in the following areas:

1. The principles related to assessment and intervention and methods of gathering and interpreting information
2. The service delivery practices used to determine the client's needs, evaluate his skills, recommend a system, and implement the system
3. The measurement of outcomes of the AT that indicate whether the identified goals have been achieved and the aggregate outcome of the use of specific technology by many clients in order to form and enhance the existing evidence base related to outcomes of AT use and service delivery
4. The identification and attainment of funding for services and equipment
5. Legislation, policies, and regulations that affect service delivery and acquisition of AT

PRINCIPLES OF ASSISTIVE TECHNOLOGY ASSESSMENT AND INTERVENTION

The AT intervention begins with an **assessment** targeting the client's goals and needs, activities, knowledge, skills and abilities, and the contexts in which the AT will be used including social, physical, and institutional elements. Through this assessment, information about the consumer is gathered and analyzed so that appropriate ATs (hard and soft) can be recommended and a plan for intervention developed. The assessment also yields information regarding the consumer's ability to use ATs. Based on the assessment results, a plan for intervention is developed. This plan includes recommendation and implementation of the system, follow-up, and follow-along. Basic principles that underlie assessment and intervention in AT service delivery are listed in Box 5-1.

BOX 5-1 Principles of Assessment and Intervention in Assistive Technology

Assistive technology assessment and intervention should consider all components of the HAAT model: the human, the activity, the assistive technology, and the context.

Assistive technology service delivery is enabling.

Assistive technology assessment is ongoing and deliberate.

Assistive technology assessment and intervention require collaboration and consumer-centered approaches.

Assistive technology assessment and intervention require an understanding of how to gather and interpret data.

Assistive technology assessment and intervention are conducted in an ethical manner.

Assistive technology intervention is conducted is a sustainable manner.

Assistive technology assessment and intervention are informed by evidence.

Assistive Technology Assessment and Intervention Should Consider All Components of the HAAT Model: Human, Activity, Assistive Technology, and Context

Often AT assessment focuses on the AT only, which can lead to later rejection or abandonment of the technology. One way to reduce the probability of abandonment or misuse is to consider systematically all four parts of the HAAT model. Needs and goals are often defined by a careful consideration of the activities to be performed by the individual. However, it is rare that the activity will be performed in only one context, so it is important to identify the influence of the physical, sociocultural, and institutional elements in the contexts in which the activities will be performed (see Chapter 3). Thus, the careful evaluation of the activities to be performed and the contextual factors under which that performance will occur are keys to success. After the goals have been identified, an assessment of the skills and abilities of the human operator (the consumer) must be identified. Only after consideration of these three components (activity, context, and human) can a clear picture emerge of the AT requirements and characteristics. The assessment process must also include an assessment of the degree to which these characteristics match the consumer's needs (Scherer, 2002). Chances of success in implementation of an AT system are enhanced by attention to all four parts of the HAAT model during the service delivery process.

Assistive Technology Service Delivery Is Enabling

The *primary* purpose of AT intervention is not remediation or rehabilitation of an impairment but enablement of activity performance and participation through provision of hard and soft technologies. This principle places the focus on functional outcomes. Client goals for activity performance and participation are identified through the application of the HAAT model. These goals are subsequently evaluated to measure the functional outcomes of the AT use.

Approaching service delivery from this perspective requires that the team determines the individual's strengths and capitalizes on them instead of focusing on deficits or impairments. For example, consider the functional activity of computer input. If we were to use a rehabilitation approach, the goal would be to improve hand and finger control sufficiently to allow for input, with the intervention focusing on exercises and activities for the fingers and hands. From an AT perspective, however, the objective becomes enabling the person to perform the functional activity of computer input using her available motor abilities. The impairment in the hands and fingers that causes the disability is not necessarily addressed. The disability of being unable to use a computer keyboard is what is addressed in the AT approach. Through the use of AT, alternatives to the typical way of using the fingers for input are considered, such as using a mouth stick, head pointer, or speech recognition system.

The use of AT is only one means to support the client to achieve her goals. It is used in combination with other interventions and strategies such as improving specific function (e.g., strength, coordination, or articulation) or environmental modification that collectively enhance activity performance and participation. Some individuals who have a severe physical disability may never have had the opportunity to develop their motor skills, and training to develop these skills can take months or years (Cook, 1991). A common example is an individual whose evaluation shows that she is able to use her head to activate a single switch to make simple choices on a computer. With training and a period of experience in using this switch, her head control may improve to the point where she can use a head-controlled mouse to make direct choices with a dedicated communication device. The latter means of control provides access that is faster and much less demanding cognitively.

Assistive Technology Assessment Is Ongoing and Deliberate

Although assessment is typically considered a discrete event in the direct service delivery process, it is actually an ongoing process. AT assessment entails a series of activities linked together and undertaken over time. The activities that occur and the decisions that are made during the intervention are deliberate rather than haphazard. Information is gathered and decisions are made from the moment of the initial intake referral through follow-along.

Progression toward the goals of the intervention plan is ongoing, with revisions to the plan as necessary. For example, during training, observation may reveal that the client can access the control interface more effectively if it is positioned at an angle instead of flat. This observation will result in adjustment to the position of the computer interface. The ideas of **client-centered practice** (Canadian Association of Occupational Therapists [CAOT], 2002) highlight the importance of involving the client at all stages of assessment, from the initial framing of the activities in which the client wishes to engage to the recommendation of an AT system. The client refers to the individual and others in his environment such as family and caregivers (CAOT, 2002). Assessment is ongoing not only while the client is actively involved in the service delivery process but also potentially throughout the client's life. Because many individuals have lifelong disabilities, they will be in need of AT throughout their lives. It is important not only to recommend AT that enables the individual today but also to anticipate the technology that will be necessary to enable him in the future. The components of the HAAT model change over each individual's lifetime. Changes may occur in the individual's skills and abilities, life roles, and goals; the capabilities of technology; and the context in which the ATs are used. Using the HAAT model as a framework, the team can predict some of these changes and plan for the client's future technology needs.

Assistive Technology Assessment and Intervention Require Collaboration and a Consumer-Centered Approach

Given the nature of AT and its impact on the consumer's activities of daily living, it is essential that the assessment and intervention be a collaborative process. McNaughton (1993) defines a collaborator as "one who works with another toward a common goal" (p. 8). Furthermore, she states that collaboration requires that (1) all participants be equal partners; (2) a problem-solving attitude be shared by all participants; (3) there be mutual respect for each other's knowledge and the contributions each person can make, as opposed to the titles he or she holds; and (4) each participant have available the information necessary to carry out his or her role (McNaughton, 1993). These ideas are supported in the ideas of client-centered practice (CAOT, 2002).

Several people are key collaborators in the assessment and ongoing evaluation process. Central to this group is the client who will be the primary user of the technology and her caregivers or family who will be assisting with care and use of the technology on a regular basis. Other collaborators include teachers, vocational counselors, employers, therapists, physicians, nurses, rehabilitation assistants, device suppliers, technicians, and representatives from the funding source. The AT assessment and intervention are more successful when these significant others are identified and involved at the beginning of the process.

There is a delicate balance between the "opinion" and "expertise" of the team (based on technical knowledge and experience with a variety of people) and the "opinion" and "expertise" of the client and family relating to the specific needs and goals of the person. The client and family come to the assessment process with expertise in their daily lives, including the activities in which they need and want to engage as well as modifications and strategies they use in the performance of these activities. The role of the team is to educate the client on the choices available to him so that he can make decisions related to the AT in an informed manner. The challenge for the clinician is to do so without unduly influencing his choice. As identified earlier, AT is one component of the process of enabling activities. However, it may not be the consumer's preferred method of performing activities. Beukelman and Mirenda (2013) discuss the importance of building consensus among the user, family members, and other team members. Negative consequences, such as a lack of vital information for intervention; lack of "ownership" of the intervention, resulting in poor follow-through with the recommendations; and distrust of the service provider, may result if the process of consensus building is not begun during the initial assessment. Initiating this process early on helps to avoid problems in the future with regard to the acceptance and utilization of a device.

A last group of people whose actions affect AT acquisition and use are individuals who create and enact policy relevant to AT (Samant et al, 2013). Typically, this group is not considered part of the collaborators who effect AT service delivery, yet their actions have increasingly important consequences for individuals who use AT to enable their daily activities because their policies and management in the health care system affect the ability to acquire devices and subsequent funding of these devices. Policy makers also influence the process of AT acquisition and the professionals required to effect that process.

Assistive Technology Assessment and Intervention Require an Understanding of How to Gather and Interpret Data

The assessment process (either initial or ongoing) involves determination of what needs to be assessed and the most effective method of completing the assessment. It occurs in both formal and informal manners using a variety of methods. Commonly, formal assessments involve use of standardized instruments, following the protocol established by the instrument developers (Miller Polgar, 2009). Informal assessment tends to occur on an ongoing basis, often involving observation or interview as the client is engaged in daily activities. Assessment includes gathering information on the client's physical, sensory, and cognitive skills emotional state; performance in functional activities; and the details of the setting in which these activities occur, including physical accessibility issues, social support, and institutional elements such as funding and policies around AT use and maintenance in these settings. Interpretation of assessment findings involves application of clinical reasoning, interpretation of the findings, and use of evidence to inform the conclusions that are made.

Assistive Technology Assessment and Intervention Are Conducted in an Ethical Manner

Ethical standards and positions that guide AT service delivery are described in Chapter 1. Here we discuss the ethical use of assessment instruments and ethical practice for interpretation of assessment findings, including actions that result from conclusions drawn from these findings. In the first instance, ethical use of an assessment instrument involves (1) use of a test that has established measurement properties, (2) use of the test for its intended purpose, (3) administration of the assessment in the standardized manner, (4) ensuring that the selected assessment is appropriate for use with the specific client, and (5) ensuring that the clinician has the necessary qualifications to use the assessment and that its administration is within her scope of practice.

BOX 5-2 Common Steps of Test Construction

Define the purpose of the test and the scope of the construct to be measured.

Develop the table of specifications or test blueprint that identify the components of the construct to be measured and their relationship to each other.

Initial development of test items, response format, administration procedures, and scoring procedures.

Evaluation of test items, response formats, administration procedures, and scoring procedures. Investigation of test measurement properties. Assembly of test materials for distribution.

From American Educational Research Association, American Psychological Association, National Council on Measurement in Education: *Standards for educational and psychological testing*, Washington, DC: AERA, 1999.

Measurement properties include information about the test development, establishment of norms for interpretation of results, reliability, and validity estimates. We will only provide basic information about each of these properties; more details are available from other sources (e.g., American Educational Research Association [AERA], American Psychological Association [APA], & National Council on Measurement in Education [NCME], 1999; Law, Baum, & Dunn, 2001; Miller Polgar, 2009). Box 5-2 shows the steps that are commonly undertaken in the construction of a test. The process of test construction should be recorded in the test manual for every well-established test. Review of this information is necessary to ensure that the test is appropriate for its planned use by the clinician.

Two aspects of the measurement properties that are particularly crucial are reliability and validity. **Reliability** is an estimation of the consistency of a test when administered in different circumstances (e.g., over time, by different raters, or with different populations) (AERA, APA, & NCME, 1999). When a test is consistent, a client's scores are anticipated to be similar over administrations when the trait being measured is considered to be stable or to change in some predicted way when the trait is considered to change. Sources of error affect the stability of the client's scores, which results in the view that any given score is made up of the client's "true" score and an error component. Sources of error include those associated with the test itself (internal sources), errors of administration, and other external errors as well as random error. A test that is well constructed will have minimal internal error and provides sufficient information to minimize error sources related to administration (Miller Polgar, 2009).

Validity refers to the conclusions that are drawn from interpretation of the test results and the confidence that is derived from these conclusions. After a test is scored, the clinician is responsible for interpreting the findings using a combination of clinical reasoning, information from the test manual, and other evidence. Conclusions relevant to AT include interpretation of the client's skills, abilities, and knowledge that affect her ability to use a device; aspects of the context that affect device use; and ultimately recommendation of specific devices that the team determines best suits the client's stated goals and needs. From a validity perspective, these conclusions are based on evidence that the test measures the construct it was designed to measure (i.e., construct validity).

Multiple sources of evidence demonstrate construct validity, including the relation of a test to a "gold standard" measurement, congruence of the test structure with that of the proposed theoretical structure of the construct of interest, representation of the construct of interest by the test items, and lack of irrelevant items that limit performance on the test (Miller Polgar, 2009).

The test manual describes the intended purpose of the test as well as a description of the construct it intends to measure. Ethical test use requires the clinician to only use a test for its intended purpose. Failure to do so results in conclusions that may be invalid and may prevent the client from accessing necessary services or devices. For example, a test that is intended to measure aspects of visual perception, such as right–left discrimination, figure ground, and form constancy, may be very useful to the understanding of the ability to perform visual tasks that use these skills but may be of no use to understand or predict the ability to maneuver a power wheelchair. Interpretation of the results of such a test to support the acquisition of a power wheelchair may lead to a client who is unsafe when driving his chair because the test was not designed to provide information that would allow prediction of the ability to be a safe driver.

A third aspect of ethical test use is compliance with the standardized administration and scoring of the test. This compliance requires the clinician to be familiar with the test administration and to follow it precisely. When nonstandardized procedures are used, the validity of the resulting conclusions comes into question. When the clinician gives the client more time to complete an item, provides some intended or unintended clue that indicates whether a correct response has been given, or otherwise alters how the client responds to an item, the established measurement properties are no longer applicable, which then prevents the clinician from making a valid interpretation of the test results. For example, if a clinician is assessing a client's ability to identify a target picture from several options and allows the client to give a verbal response when a motor response is the standardized procedure, she can no longer be certain that the client can identify the target if an incorrect response is given. Under the standardized procedure, an incorrect motor response can be interpreted with some level of confidence because that is how the test was developed and the measurement properties were established. When a client gives an incorrect verbal response, the clinician cannot reliably differentiate between recognition of the correct target and the inability to name it, which are different constructs.

Some test manuals specify ways in which test administration can be altered. These changes might be in time allotted for a response, setup of the testing environment and materials, alternate ways of providing a response, or alternate ways of presenting a test item (Miller Polgar, 2009). For example, an older adult may need test materials to be presented in a larger font because of visual changes. Such a modification is appropriate when identified in the test manual or other test materials. Another modification might be the use of probes that can be used to give the client cues if she has difficulty forming a response.

The fourth ethical aspect ensures that the test is used for the intended population. The test manual provides details about the sample. The test manual provides details about the intended population and characteristics of the samples used to establish norms, scoring interpretation, and measurement properties. When a clinician uses a test with a client who differs from the intended population in some way, the conclusions drawn from the results are suspect. The results of a test that is developed and normed for children will not provide useful information if that test is administered to an adult. Although this comment sounds quite logical, this situation is a common occurrence.

Tests that are developed in one geographical location may not be useful in another. The context of questions may not generalize from one geographical location to another. For example, a question that requires the client to have some experience with snow will not reliably assess a client who has never seen or experienced it. Language differs across locations. United States English and United Kingdom English are not the same. When a test item requires knowledge of the meaning of a specific word, a client who does not share the same meaning of that word will get the answer incorrect. Similarly, some aspects of tests that are heavily language dependent become obsolete over time, making interpretation difficult. Words and technology change, affecting the client's ability to correctly respond to an item. Rotary phones were common a few decades ago but are rarely seen today. A test that presents a rotary phone as the correct option when the client is asked to point to a phone may limit his ability to indicate the correct response, not because he does not know what a phone is but because he does not recognize a rotary phone as the same technology.

The last ethical consideration requires the clinician to have adequate training and qualifications to administer a test and to practice within her scope of practice. It is the responsibility of the clinician to ensure that she has prepared adequately to administer the test in order to minimize errors that will affect the reliability and validity of the interpretation of the test results. Some tests require a clinician to have specific academic qualifications (e.g., an occupational therapy degree or a psychology doctorate) before use of their use. Commonly, the acquisition of these tests is restricted to those individuals who can demonstrate the necessary qualifications. However, if these tests are present in a clinical setting, professional ethics requires all who use them to have the required qualifications.

Assistive Technology Intervention Is Conducted in a Sustainable Manner

The United Nations (UN) Convention on the Rights of Persons with Disabilities (UN, 2006) makes the provision of

AT and access to services for acquiring, training, and maintenance of devices explicit in several articles (see Box 5-1). Similarly, the World Health Organization's (WHO's) *World Report on Disability* (WHO, 2011) and the *WHO Guidelines on the Provision of Manual Wheelchairs in Less-Resourced Settings* (WHO and US AID from the American People, 2011) make the argument for provision of AT services in a sustainable manner. General ideas about sustainability are discussed in Chapter 1. Here, the focus is on assessment and intervention, which includes sustainability aspects of access to services and equipment that meet the needs of individuals in their own context.

Both well-resourced and less resourced regions face issues of accessibility to AT services and devices. Well-resourced countries have greater access to services such as assessment, some aspects of intervention, and public funding of certain ATs for eligible clients. As health care funding becomes scarcer in these countries, the eligibility criteria are becoming more stringent, the amount of public funding is becoming smaller, fewer devices are supported, and clinical services are more restricted. It is common for a clinician to be able to perform an initial assessment and usually a fitting or setup visit but then be unable to follow up or evaluate outcomes when the technology is provided in the community.

In less resourced countries, individuals with disabilities may have limited to no access to AT services and devices. Sometimes the devices that are provided are not appropriate for their context (e.g., provision of a device that requires periodic recharging of a battery to a person who lives without electricity). The WHO guidelines for the provision of manual wheelchairs suggests that best practice includes assessment of the contextual elements that are included in the HAAT model to determine the most appropriate technology as well as the needs of a country for AT service delivery and products. Sustainable intervention means that devices that are recommended or provided meet an established standard for quality, something that both the UN and the WHO advocate (UN, 2006; WHO, 2011; WHO and US AID from the American People, 2011).

Sustainable intervention in less resourced countries also means that infrastructure is present in the setting to support training in the use of the device, maintenance of the device, and an environment that supports the use of the device (e.g., presence of inclusive environments that support function of individuals with a variety of abilities).

In all settings, sustainable intervention considers the needs of clients who live in remote areas, such as the far north or remote rural settings, where access to services is not available on a regular basis. Provision of equipment that is supported by local infrastructure, including maintenance and use of delivery methods such as telehealth technologies, contribute to sustainable AT intervention in these regions.

Assistive Technology Assessment and Intervention Are Informed by Evidence

The final principle of assessment and intervention in AT requires the clinician to use evidence to inform his practice.

BOX 5-3 Levels of Evidence from Evidence-Based Medicine

Randomized controlled trials (RCT)
Systematic review of RCTs
Individual RCT
Cohort studies
Systematic review of cohort studies
Individual cohort study
Case control study
Systematic review of controlled studies
Individual case control study
Case series
Expert opinion

From Phillips B, Ball C, Sackett D, et al: *Levels of evidence (March 2009)*, Oxford Centre for Evidence-based Medicine, 2009. Available from: www.cebm.net. Accessed January 2, 2014.

Box 5-3 shows levels of evidence, as defined by evidence-based medicine. The reality for AT service delivery and practice is that very few high level sources of evidence (systematic reviews of randomized controlled trials [RCTs] or individual RCTs) exist. The few that have been conducted are included in the relevant technologies chapters that follow. It is more common for clinicians to base their decision making on evidence that consists of cohort studies, outcome studies, and expert opinion. In addition, clinicians have different types of literature reviews available to support their decision making, including critical literature reviews (Whittemore & Knafl, 2005) and scoping reviews (Arksey & O'Malley, 2005). In the first instance, the literature is reviewed from a critical lens to describe existing evidence. The second form of literature review is used to identify existing knowledge and gaps in the literature. Depending on the format used, these reviews may or may not evaluate the quality of the literature that is reviewed. In addition to peer-reviewed literature, scoping reviews can include "grey" literature in the form of policy documents and trade journals.

An additional type of evidence to support clinical practice is found in best practice guidelines. Several of these exist to support various aspects of AT service delivery, including assessment practice and intervention in specific areas such as pressure ulcer prevention and management (e.g., Houghton et al., 2013). When well constructed, these guidelines involve a systematic review of the evidence to support different aspects of clinical practice in a specific area, provide an evaluation of the strength of the evidence that supports practice, and make recommendation for practice in a given area. When appropriate, these guidelines have been incorporated into relevant chapters. It is the clinician's responsibility to maintain currency in his practice area and to incorporate the best available evidence to guide his decisions and practice.

OVERVIEW OF SERVICE DELIVERY IN ASSISTIVE TECHNOLOGY

Figure 5-1 illustrates a basic process by which delivery of services to the consumer occurs. The first step is **referral and intake**. Referral can be initiated by many different people,

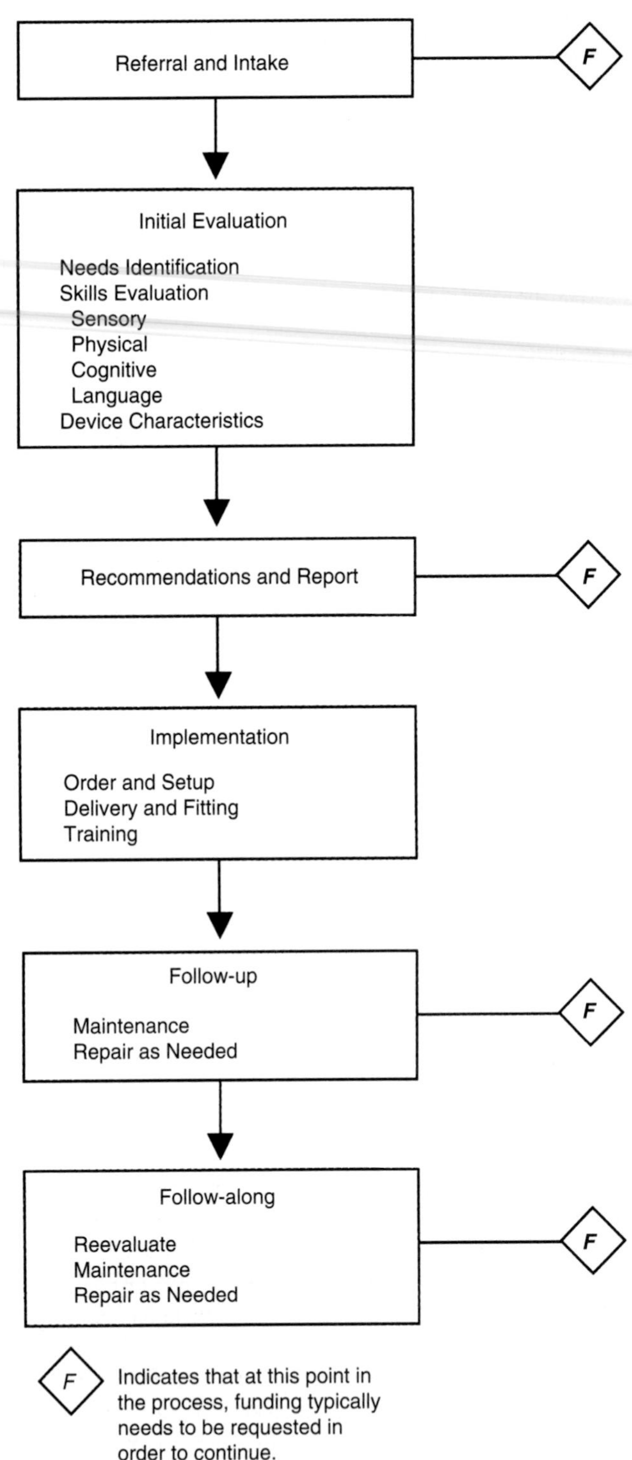

FIGURE 5-1 Steps in the service delivery process.

depending on the service delivery context. The consumer or family member, a physician or another health care professional, or teacher or other professional may make a referral for an AT assessment. The service provider gathers basic information and determines whether there is a match between the type of services she provides and the identified needs of the client.

After the criteria for intake have been met, the **evaluation phase** begins. The first step involves an interview with the client and relevant others to identify the concerns they have about engagement in daily activities, which results in *needs identification.* After a thorough identification of the client's needs, the client's sensory, physical, language, and cognitive skills are evaluated. Technologies that match the needs and skills of the consumer are identified, and ideally, a trial evaluation of these technologies takes place. The evaluation results are summarized, and *recommendations* for technologies are made based on consensus among those involved. These findings are summarized in a written *report,* which is used frequently to justify funding for the purchase of the AT system.

When funding is secured, the client proceeds with the intervention in the **implementation phase**. During this phase, the equipment that has been recommended is ordered, modified, and fabricated as necessary; set up; and delivered to the client. Initial training on the basic operation of the device and ongoing training of strategies for using the device also take place during this phase.

After the device has been delivered and training has been completed, we need to know whether the system as a whole is functioning effectively. This step normally occurs during the follow-up phase, in which we determine whether the client is satisfied with the system and whether the goals that have been identified are being met. The follow-up phase actually closes the loop by putting in place a mechanism by which regular contact is made with the consumer to see whether further AT services are indicated. When further AT services are required, the client returns to the referral, and the intake phase and the process is repeated. Building this final phase into the service delivery process ensures that the client's needs are considered throughout her lifespan. Now let's take a more in-depth look at each of these steps.

Referral and Intake

The purpose of the referral and intake phase is to (1) gather preliminary information on the consumer, (2) determine whether there is a match between the needs of the consumer and the services that can be provided by the clinician, and (3) tentatively identify services to be provided.

The client or the person making the referral on the client's behalf recognizes a need for AT services or devices, which triggers the referral to the clinician. These identified needs are called **criteria for service,** and they define the objectives for the intervention. A third-party funding agency, such as a state vocational rehabilitation agency, may be involved at this stage. The agency will have a set of policies and procedures that governs who is eligible to seek AT intervention and what devices and services are covered. Depending on the policies of the service provider, referrals are accepted from a variety of sources. These sources include the consumer, a family member or care provider, rehabilitation or educational professional, or a physician. At this time, information regarding the client's background and perceived AT needs is gathered for the initial database. This information includes personal data (e.g., age, place of residence), medical diagnosis and health information, and educational or vocational background. Information related to the individual's medical diagnosis and health information that may guide the assessment includes whether or not the condition is expected to remain stable, improve, or decline. The appropriateness of the referral is viewed from the perspective of both the clinician and the referral or funding source. When exchanging information about the client's needs and the services provided by the clinician, each party can determine whether there is a match. For example, the needs of a client with complex seating and mobility needs may not match the services provided by the clinician if he does not have the necessary expertise. For the consumer's benefit, this mismatch should be acknowledged and the client referred to another source who can more appropriately address her needs. The clinician should have, within the organization's mission statement, a policy that establishes what services are provided and who is eligible to receive services. For example, some AT service providers specialize in certain disabilities (e.g., visual impairment), and others focus on specific technologies (e.g., seating technologies). Professional codes of ethics and standards of practice (see Chapter 1) require that clinicians practice within their specialization and not try to provide services outside of this realm.

The other outcome is that there is a match between the needs of the client and the services provided by the clinician. In this case, plans are made to move forward with the initial evaluation, starting with a thorough identification of the client's needs. In some jurisdictions, funding must be secured before the initiation of the evaluation. From the information provided, the clinician also determines the level of service that would be most beneficial to the consumer. There are a number of scenarios. First, is the individual who has never used or been evaluated for ATs, which could be an individual who is newly disabled or someone with a long-standing disability. An individual with a long-standing disability who may not have previously received AT services may now be able to access assistive devices because of recent advances in technologies. In this situation, an in-depth assessment is warranted. Referrals may also be received from consumers who have used technology for some time and would like to evaluate current commercially available technologies. If this person's functional status has remained stable, it may not be necessary to conduct a complete evaluation. In some cases, the AT is not working or has been abandoned by the client, and he is seeking a referral to see if modifications to the system can aid in making it more functional. Sometimes the consumer may only require further training or reevaluation of how she is using her current system to see whether training in new strategies would be beneficial. Similarly, there may be a new care provider who needs training or technical assistance.

Initial Evaluation

Through a systematic evaluation, the clinician gathers information and facilitates decisions related to eventual device use. Because of the cost of the AT to the client (or third-party funding source), it is essential that the team is able to assist the consumer in making informed decisions in the selection of a device. Current knowledge of the available technology and use of a systematic process facilitate the decision-making process. This section focuses on the type of information gathered and the procedures used during the evaluation. We start with some background information on measurement.

Quantitative and Qualitative Measurement

Information gathered by the team throughout the AT intervention can be by either **quantitative measurement** or **qualitative measurement**. The philosophies of qualitative measures and quantitative measures are quite different. Quantitative measures assign a number to an attribute, trait, or characteristic (Nunnally and Bernstein, 1994). The assumption of quantitative measures is that the construct of interest can be measured in some meaningful way. For example, a test can be constructed that measures the joint range of motion (the construct) that an individual has available to her to control a computer access device. Joint range is expressed as degrees of motion, and a common understanding exists regarding what is meant when a specific joint range of motion is described. Here the construct can be assigned a number that is meaningful to individuals using and interpreting the test. Alternatively, a test can be constructed that intends to measure boredom. It is possible to develop a scale and have individuals rate their boredom on a 4-point scale (for example). But what does a score of 4 mean on such a scale? We can assign a number, but it does not carry any meaning.

Qualitative assessments assume that each individual has a different experience and that it is important to provide the opportunity to capture that experience. There is no attempt to measure a particular construct. Rather, the purpose is to describe and understand the user's experience with the technology. Qualitative assessments may include observation, either directly or via videotape, or interview with the client and others. Qualitative assessments often capture experiences that cannot be directly quantified or for which quantification holds little meaning. They provide the client with the opportunity to identify issues, experiences, or goals that may not be previously identified on a quantitative measure.

Both qualitative and quantitative assessment formats are important in the AT assessment process and for evaluation of the outcomes of AT use. Quantitative measures allow comparison of experiences of a large number of individuals, and a well-constructed instrument is essential in building evidence to support the efficacy of AT use. Qualitative methods provide a rich description of the experiences of AT use, which may not be readily apparent from the use of quantitative instruments alone. Together these methods can provide strong support for AT use, both on an individual and collective basis.

Norm-Referenced and Criterion-Referenced Measurements

Two commonly used standards are used for measuring performance (for both the human and the total system): norm referenced and criterion referenced. In **norm-referenced measurements,** the performance of the individual or system is ranked according to a sample of scores others have achieved on the task. Norm-referenced measures usually produce a percentile rank, a standardized score or a grade equivalent that indicates where the individual stands relative to others in the representative sample (Witt and Cavell, 1986). It is important to review how the norms were developed when selecting a norm-referenced test for use. Norms need to be relevant to the population with which the instrument is being used. They need to be recent and representative (Wiersma and Jurs, 1990). In other words, the characteristics of the sample used to develop the norms must be similar to those of the client group with which the assessment is being used. The items that form the instrument need to be relevant to the client group. For example, assessing visual-perceptual skills using blocks is not relevant for most adults. Similarly, use of outdated questions or materials will not give an accurate picture of the client's abilities. For example, testing keyboarding skills on a typewriter will give some information on keyboarding skills but does not cover the full range of skills required to use a computer (Miller Polgar, 2009). An alternative way to assess human or system performance is to rate the performance according to a specified criterion or level of mastery, which is referred to as **criterion-referenced measurement,** and the person's own skill level in using the system is used as the standard. Criterion-referenced measurement requires that different degrees of competence of the functional ability to be measured can be expressed. One standardized method of achieving this description is through Goal Attainment Scaling (GAS) (King et al., 1999). This method involves a consensus-driven process in which a target behavior is identified and five levels of competence are clearly articulated. These are coded on a 5-point scale from -2 to +2. The zero point on the scale represents basic or minimum competence.

The points below zero represent inadequate performance, and those above zero are better than expected performance. Goals are specific, measureable, and time specific. Benefits to GAS are that it is flexible, identifies performance over time, and is individualized to the client. However, it is time consuming, and because it is individualized, may not easily capture a range of functional activities. An example of GAS goals is shown in Box 5-4.

When we use the criterion-referenced approach to measurement, we accomplish two desirable goals. First, we base our assessment of progress on the person's unique set of skills and do not attempt to relate this performance to a normalized standard. Second, we have a way of measuring progress.

BOX 5-4 An Example of Goal Attainment Scaling Goals

Target behavior: Client will be able to self-initiate a wheelie with his manual wheelchair and hold the position momentarily.

+2: Client is able to self-initiate a wheelie with his manual wheelchair and propel the chair forward for a short duration. [Client achieves target behavior and demonstrates a high level of competence.]

+1: Client is able to self-initiate a wheelie with his manual wheelchair and hold the position for 1 minute. [Client achieves the target behavior and demonstrates a moderate level of competence.]

0: Client is able to self-initiate a wheelie with his manual wheelchair and hold the position momentarily. [Client achieves target behavior.]

−1: Client is able to hold a balanced wheelie position for 1 minute if another person assists him to assume the wheelie position. [Client does not achieve the target behavior but is successful with a somewhat less difficult skill.]

−2: Client is unable to hold a balanced wheelie position when another person assists him to assume the wheelie position. Client is unable to self-initiate the wheelie position. [This level is often the client's starting skill level.]

Needs Identification

Through the **needs identification** process, we determine the individual's needs and goals, which provide the basis for the AT intervention. Identifying the needs of the consumer is the most critical component of the service delivery process and is completed at the onset of evaluation. The information collected during needs identification is the cornerstone for measuring the effectiveness of the final outcome. Therefore, it is important to take this step seriously and ensure that there is a consensus among those involved as to the nature and scope of the problem to be addressed by the AT intervention and the goals identified to target these problem areas.

Information gathered during the needs identification phase is also used by the clinician to justify purchase of services and equipment. Third-party payers who fund services and equipment want to know what the problem or need is and how the equipment is going to address the need. Finally, the needs identification process results in the development of a plan for completing the remainder of the evaluation, which includes composition of the evaluation team, determination of needed evaluation tools and devices, and identification of further information required (either through evaluation of the consumer or by request from outside sources).

The purpose of the initial interview is to establish the needs and goals of AT intervention. In this interview the consumer or caregivers frame the performance issue that brings them to the AT service. The clinician guides this interview to determine the activities of self-care, work, and leisure in which the client wishes to engage and identify aspects of performance for which AT has potential benefit. Information is secured about the consumer's medical information, daily activities, settings in which these activities occur, and current or past experience with AT. Information is also gathered about current or potential sources of funding. Depending on the service delivery process, a more in-depth assessment will be conducted during the same session as this initial interview. Alternately, this initial interview serves to determine the appropriateness of the referral, and then funding is required to proceed with further stages of the intervention process. The components of an in-depth assessment are described in the chapters discussing specific types of AT.

BOX 5-5 Assessments Associated with the Matching Person with Technology Model

Matching Assistive Technology and CHild (MATCH) (Scherer, 1998): Assessment used for infants and children up to the age of 5 years old. Its purpose is to assist with the identification of appropriate ATs and to identify areas requiring further evaluation.

Survey of Technology Use (Scherer, 1998): Assessment is suitable for all ages. Asks clients to identify technology that they use and their level of comfort with adoption of new technologies. It also identifies activities in which the client engages and assesses personal characteristics of the client. It establishes the client's sense of well-being and self-esteem related to technology use (Brown-Triolo, 2002). This assessment is not specific to AT.

Assistive Technology Device Predisposition Assessment (Scherer, 1998): Assessment is suitable for adolescents and adults. It formalizes client input into the device selection process. Areas of consideration include device characteristics, psychosocial aspects of the client, psychosocial aspects of the environment, and personal characteristics associated with the client's disability (Brown-Tirolo, 2002). Related components focus specifically on the educational or the work environments.

The information for the needs assessment can be derived from an interview through a written questionnaire completed by the client or his representative or with a standardized tool. The suite of assessments associated with the Matching Person and Technology (MPT) model (Scherer, 1998) is useful to assist the clinician to identify the areas of the individual's needs and his predisposition to use AT. The MPT model indicates that aspects of the person, the technology, and the context, or milieu, are necessary considerations for AT recommendation and satisfactory use (Brown-Triolo, 2002). The MPT assessments include several different instruments that are completed jointly by the client or caregiver with the clinician. These instruments identify issues that affect the client's likely use of AT, including psychosocial aspects of the client, characteristics of the technology, issues related to the disability, and the psychosocial milieu where the technology will be used (Scherer, 2002). Assessments are available for children and their families as well as adults. Box 5-5 lists the different MPT assessments and the purposes of each.

If the information is gathered through a written questionnaire before the provider actually meets the consumer, it should be reviewed at the time of the first meeting with the consumer. The purpose of reviewing this material at the first meeting is to ensure that all of the necessary information has been provided and to analyze the information to develop the goals. In addition, the provider needs to ascertain that the consumer understands the questions that were asked. The total team should also be present at this meeting, and everyone's input regarding the needs and goals of the consumer can be discussed and a consensus reached.

After the client has clarified her activity needs, a more detailed evaluation of specific components follows. This evaluation includes assessment of basic skills, including sensory, physical, cognitive, affective (emotional) and communication, performance in functional activities, and relevant aspects of the context in which the client engages in activities. Some of the evaluation data are gathered from reports of other professionals, such as assessment of visual function by an optometrist or ophthalmologist. Other data are gathered by a collaborative effort of the team.

Skills Evaluation: Sensory

The clinician needs to understand the **sensory functions** that are available to the client when using ATs. If the primary disability is sensory, an alternative sensory pathway may need to be used, and the provider needs to know what the consumer's sensory capabilities are. For example, in the case of a consumer who is blind and who needs to read, the clinician evaluates tactile and auditory skills that can substitute for vision during reading.

In other cases, a client may have a sensory disability secondary to either a physical or cognitive limitation. For example, if a client is hard of hearing, the clinician needs to know how this impairment will affect interaction with technology, including everything from hearing auditory feedback when a computer error is made to understanding voice synthesis on a communication device. The chapters that describe AT for specific activity outputs discuss the implications of sensory limitations for use of the technology and how modifications can be made to accommodate for these limitations.

Evaluation of Functional Vision

The most critical **visual skills** needed for AT use are visual acuity to see objects in the environment and components of the technology interface; adequate visual field to capture visual information across the environment; and quality of vision (WHO, 2001), including light sensitivity and contrast sensitivity to distinguish objects in the environment. These functions are described in more detail along with common visual impairments in Chapters 3 and 13. During the initial interview, known visual problems should have been identified. A visual evaluation by a vision care professional will provide information about the following visual functions.

A *visual field deficit* can be experienced in two ways: loss of peripheral vision or central vision. Peripheral vision loss results in a narrowing of the visual fields, commonly an age-related deficit (Quintana, 2002; Scheiman, 2002). This type of loss makes it increasingly difficult to see objects to the side, with the potential to cause difficulties when maneuvering a wheelchair through a crowded environment. A central field loss has more significant functional implications because the individual loses the ability to see something they are looking at directly. Age-related macular degeneration and diabetic retinopathy are two common central field deficit disorders.

Visual acuity refers to the clarity with which a person can see objects in the environment (Quintana, 2002). This visual function is probably the best understood because it occurs so frequently in the population. There are three types, myopia or nearsightedness, farsightedness, and presbyopia or the inability to focus on a near object and is an age-related visual change. All of these functions result from an inability to focus the image on the retina. In most cases, functional vision is restored with the use of corrective lenses (glasses or contact lenses) or laser surgery. Chapter 13 discusses AT to assist individuals with low vision or blindness, for whom these common interventions are inadequate.

Visual tracking refers to the ability to track a moving object with the eyes; for example, tracking the movement of a cursor on a computer screen (Eby, Molnar, & Pellerito, 2006; Quintana, 2002). Evaluation of visual tracking includes the coordination of both eyes, tracking ability in vertical and horizontal planes, smoothness of the movements, delay in the initiation of visual tracking, and ability to track without moving the head. *Visual scanning* refers to the ability to scan the environment to gather visual information. In this situation, the object does not move; the eyes are moving (Eby et al, 2006). Visual scanning is most commonly used when reading text. Clients who have had a stroke may have a visual scanning impairment if they also have a neglect of one side of the body. In this situation, the eyes do not move past midline so visual information on the affected side of the body is not detected.

Visual contrast is required to differentiate a figure from its background, commonly used during reading and in retrieval of information from a display (Scheiman, 2002). With age and other visual impairments, contrast needs to be enhanced for the user to detect the information. *Visual accommodation* is the ability of the eyes to refocus when shifting attention between different locations (Quintana, 2002); for example, shifting attention from the board to a notebook when taking notes during class or shifting attention from the road to displays on the vehicle instrument panel while driving. This function requires coordination of the small muscles of the eye.

Evaluation of Visual Perception

Visual perception is the process of giving meaning to visual information. Visual perceptual skills that need to be considered during the AT assessment include depth perception, spatial relationships, form recognition or constancy, and figure-ground discrimination. Visual perception is an important consideration when considering the client's ability to interpret information presented in a visual display or safely navigate a mobility device in his environment. Formal testing of the consumer's visual perception may have been completed before the AT assessment, and results of this evaluation can be gathered during the initial interview. Many standardized assessments of visual perceptual abilities exist; for example, the *Motor Free Visual Perception Test,* 3rd edition (Colarusso & Hammill, 2003).

Figure-ground perception refers to the ability to discriminate between an object in the foreground and the background on which it rests. For example, recognizing that a white sock is different from the white sheet on which it rests is an indicator of intact figure-ground perception. Vision is certainly a key element of this skill, but other aspects such as recognition of the object and form constancy affect the ability to differentiate an object from the background. Figure-ground perception is also an element of hearing and refers to the ability to discriminate a sound from background or ambient noise.

Spatial relations involve understanding basic concepts such as up/down and right/left as well as understanding the relationship of objects to each other, such as on top of or in front of another object. This perceptual function is key to safe movement in the environment.

Form constancy or recognition involves the understanding that an object does not change despite being viewed from different perspectives, either as the object itself is moved or as the person moves around the object. For example, intact form constancy allows a person to recognize the size and shape of objects in the environment and to recognize that an object has not changed despite viewing it from various perspectives.

Evaluation of Auditory Function

Formal evaluation of **auditory function** is conducted by an audiologist. Any significant auditory impairment that has been previously diagnosed should be identified in the initial referral or during the needs assessment. In cases of suspected hearing loss, referral should be made to an audiologist. She will determine *auditory thresholds*, including *frequency* and *amplitude*. The amplitude of sound is measured in decibels (dB). This minimum threshold is equivalent to the ticking of a watch under quiet conditions at a distance of 20 ft.

The typical range of frequencies that can be heard by the human ear is 20 to 20,000 hertz (Hz) (Bailey, 1996). However, the ear does not respond equally to all frequencies in this range. A combination of frequency and amplitude determines the auditory threshold. Pure tone audiometry presents pure (one frequency) tones to each ear to determine the threshold of hearing for that person. The intensity of the tone is raised in 5-dB increments until the stimulus is heard. It is then lowered in 5-dB decrements until it is no longer heard. The auditory threshold is the intensity at which the person indicates that he hears the tone 50% of the time (Ballantyne, Graham, & Baguley 2009).

Evaluation of Tactile Function

Somatosensory or tactile function enables the individual to perceive information through touch, either via actively touching something or passively receiving touch (Dunn, 2009). There are three particular circumstances in which attention needs to be paid to the evaluation of tactile sensation. These occur during seating and positioning assessments, when evaluating tactile input for the use of control interfaces, and when considering the use of tactile alternatives to vision or hearing.

Tactile functions that are included in a somatosensory protocol include one-two point discrimination, perception of light touch versus deep pressure, perception of temperature, joint position sense (or proprioception), and localization of tactile stimulation. *One-two point discrimination* involves the ability to detect a single tactile stimulus from two points that are applied simultaneously. Areas such as the fingertip are able to detect two points that are quite close together because of requirements for manipulation, but other areas such as the back only detect two points when they are quite distinct (Dunn, 2009). *Perception of touch* varies from the ability to detect a stimulus that is featherweight to deep pressure, which can be harmful. This tactile function is particularly important in seating. *Temperature* perception allows the individual to detect hot and cold. This function is particularly important to assess for someone with a spinal cord injury. Serious harm can result if the individual is not able to detect hot temperatures.

Pain perception refers to the ability to detect and respond to a noxious stimulus (Dunn, 2009). Commonly, the stimulus is either sharp (e.g., pinprick) or dull (deep pressure). Finally, proprioception or joint position sense refers to how the joint or limb is positioned in space. Receptors in the muscles, tendons, and joints provide information about where the limb is in space and how it is moving through space.

Skills Evaluation: Physical

The overall goal of the **physical skills** evaluation is to determine the physical capacity of an individual to perform an activity and the most functional position or positions in which to conduct that activity related to gross motor function and manipulation and device access related to fine motor function. At a very basic level, physical skills include range of motion, muscle strength, and muscle tone and the presence of obligatory movements. Many protocols exist for evaluation of range of motion (e.g., Flynn et al., 2007; Kohlmeyer, 2003; Killingsworth & Pedretti, 2006a). Both passive and active range of motion are assessed. Range of motion is important when considering positioning needs for function and the amount of movement available to access a device or perform a task. Related to range of motion is muscle strength. Again, many protocols are available for testing muscle strength (e.g., Flynn et al., 2007; Killingsworth & Pedretti, 2006b). Muscle strength is graded in a range from unable to move independently, moves with gravity eliminated, able to move against gravity, and moves against different degrees of resistance. The presence of a neurologic disorder such as cerebral palsy, stroke or traumatic brain injury (TBI) will affect both range of motion and muscle strength. Typical protocols for testing these components are not generally useful for these populations because the position of the individual affects her muscle tone and subsequently range of motion and muscle strength. For example, a child with cerebral palsy may seem to have limited flexion range of motion in her lower extremities when lying supine. However, when turned on her side, the ability to flex the legs is much easier. In supine, the influence of the tonic labyrinthine reflex increases extensor tone. This influence is not present in side lying, making flexion much easier.

Muscle tone and the presence of obligatory movements are important considerations for individuals with neurologic disorders. As described earlier, the position of the individual affects the movements that are available. Muscle tone is assessed in various functional positions, particularly prone, supine, sitting, and standing. Obligatory movements, or reflexes, are assessed to determine how they might affect function. Key reflexes or obligatory movements include the asymmetrical and symmetrical tonic neck reflexes, tonic labyrinthine, extensor thrust, bite, and grasp reflexes.

The ability to right the head when moved out of a vertical alignment, either lateral or in the anterior-posterior plane, is another component. Postural control is a related component that refers to the ability to maintain the trunk in a vertical alignment. When completing an assessment to determine function in various positions, it is important to handle the client and to challenge his balance and postural control to determine the degree of support he will need to work in a given position and the movement available in that position.

Sitting and standing balance are additional considerations. The ability to maintain balance in these positions is determined through observation of the ability to maintain the position independently and the response to challenges to balance in these positions. Sitting balance is described as hands free, in which the individual can maintain her balance and function without using her hands to support herself; hands dependent, in which she needs to support herself with one or both hands to maintain sitting; and propped or dependent sitting, in which she cannot sit without external support (Tredwell & Roxborough, 1991). Sitting balance is an important component of a seating and mobility assessment (Chapters 9 and 10).

Gross and fine motor assessments generally test higher level motor skills. Gross motor skills include balance on one foot, performing symmetrical and asymmetrical movements of the upper and lower extremities, coordinating one side of the body, lifting and carrying objects, rapidly alternating movements, running, skipping, and hopping. The Bruininks-Oseretsky Test of Motor Proficiency (Bruininks & Bruininks, 2005) is an example of a comprehensive motor evaluation appropriate for children. The Gross Motor Function Test (Russel et al., 2002) is designed specifically for children with neurologic impairments. Again, if a neurologic condition is present it is important to remember that function is dependent on the client's position. The Assessment of Motor and Process Skills (Fischer, 2003) is a standardized test of motor control in adults.

Fine motor assessment includes rapidly alternating finger movements, performance of isolated finger movements, manipulation of objects of different sizes, and performance of specific fine motor tasks. Examples of fine motor evaluations include the Erhardt Developmental Prehension Assessment (Erhardt, 1994), the Jebsen-Taylor Hand Function Test (Bovend'Eerat et al., 2004), and the Minnesota Rate of Manipulation Test (Lafayette Instrument, 1998).

Motor planning is a higher order motor function that involves executive planning of complex motor skills. Motor planning is key to the successful use of all AT. Assessment of motor planning involves asking the client to demonstrate how he would use a common device (e.g., a pen or a hammer) with and without the actual implement present. A client may also be asked to describe how to use a particular implement or device. The ability to detect and repair errors made during the execution of a motor act is another aspect of motor planning (Toglia et al., 2009).

Skills Evaluation: Cognitive

Assessment of **cognitive skills** is important when determining whether the client will be able to learn how to use the technology as well as whether she has the capacity to use it effectively in the long term. The main cognitive dimensions to be assessed include orientation, attention, memory, and executive functions. *Orientation* refers to orientation to self, place, and time. In other words, the client is asked who he is, where he is (home, hospital, or a specific location in a facility such as the geriatric day hospital), and a temporal question (e.g., day and month). This function is very basic and usually is intact in most people except those experiencing severe dementia.

There are many aspects to *attention*. The simplest component is the ability to attend to a stimulus when it is presented (e.g., looking at a picture when it is presented on a display). Selective attention refers to the ability to focus on a desired stimulus and filter out any extraneous input. For example, selective attention is involved when we pay attention to a communication partner while in a crowded room. Sustained attention refers to the ability to focus on a task for a length of time, which varies depending on the age of the individual (young children have a short attention span), and the presence of an impairment that affects the ability to attend (e.g., developmental delay or TBI). Divided or shifting attention refers to the ability to alternate focus on different stimuli. For example, a driver exhibits divided attention while driving her vehicle and conducting a conversation with a passenger at the same time (Toglia et al., 2009).

Memory involves working memory, which is recall of information immediately after it is received (Toglia et al., 2009). Long-term memory refers to recall of information that was learned or experienced in the recent or distant past. Memory involves three processes: (1) encoding or input of information, (2) storage of information, and (3) retrieval of information (Toglia et al., 2009). Memory impairment can occur because of interruption of any of these processes.

Finally, *executive functions* refer to higher order cognitive abilities. They refer to abilities such as judgment, insight (or self-awareness), problem solving, planning and organizational skills, and self-monitoring. Clients who exhibit impairment of executive function may have difficulty planning a task (e.g., figuring out the proper sequence of steps to make a bed) or may not recognize functional limitations (Toglia et al., 2009). A common example involves drivers who are no longer safe because of a cognitive impairment but who do not recognize that they are no longer safe drivers and may exhibit impulsive behaviors such as attempting to cross a busy intersection when it is not safe.

Skills Evaluation: Language

The evaluation of **language skills** required for the use of AT devices focuses on both expressive and receptive abilities. In addition, the abilities to sequence items, use symbol systems, combine language elements into complex thoughts, and use codes are important in operating various types of ATs. Whereas the most extensive language evaluation is carried out for augmentative communication system recommendations (see Chapter 16), language skills and use are also important in using other assistive devices such as cognitive aids (see Chapter 15), mobility systems (see Chapter 10), or systems for manipulation (see Chapter 12). Language and hearing are closely coupled, and ATs intended for persons with hearing impairments must address language, as well as auditory skills (see Chapter 14).

Specific areas that are evaluated include categorization, sequencing, matching, social communicative skills (e.g., degree of interaction), receptive language skills (e.g., recognition of words or symbols, understanding of simple commands), motor speech skills, and pragmatic language skills. Advanced language capabilities (e.g., syntax and semantics) are also evaluated when possible. The evaluation of these skills for augmentative communication device use is discussed in Chapter 16.

Past Experience with Assistive Technology

The consumer's history with technology should also be discussed as part of the assessment process. Useful information can be gathered from the consumer's previous success or failure with using AT. Has he had experience in using technology before, and if so, what technology was used and was the experience successful? If not, why not? For example, a student attempted to turn the pages of different books with the use of a mouth stick, which turned out to be unsuccessful. It is important to identify and discuss reasons why the mouth stick did not work out for the individual. Perhaps the mouth stick was cumbersome and uncomfortable to use for any extended period, or perhaps he could physically perform the task with the mouth stick but did not like the aesthetics of it.

Evaluation of the Context

Evaluation of the context includes consideration of physical, social, cultural, and institutional elements (see Fig. 3-8). When possible, an assessment in the client's home is critical to determine how the AT will be used and integrated into the home setting. When an actual home visit is not possible, then a discussion needs to occur during the assessment. Although an assessment of the home is critical for mobility devices that might not physically fit into the home, it is equally important to have knowledge of how other devices such as communication aids, computers, and electronic activities of daily living (EADL) devices will be set up and accessed in the home.

The **physical context** includes consideration of the physical aspects in the setting and transportation between settings. The clinician and team need to identify the settings in which the device will be used. Typically, there will be a primary setting where the device is used most of the time (e.g., home, work, school) and other settings where it is used less often (e.g., a community setting). Within the primary setting, it is important to determine access into and out of the building; access through the building, including through doorways; travel within a room, the need to go up or down stairs; and access to key features in the home such as the toilet, shower, and so on. Attention is given to safety issues in the home such as clutter that might result in a fall.

Physical elements in the setting that affect the use of technology include light, temperature, and noise. Light affects the use of devices that have a display. The brightness of light in a room, from either artificial or natural sources, may make it easier to see a display. However, too much light might cause a glare on a screen. Temperature in a setting is often not extreme enough to affect the performance of a device, although where the device is stored (e.g., garage or shed) might expose the device to temperature extremes. Ambient noise in the setting might affect the ability to use some devices. For example, the reliability of a voice recognition system may be diminished if other conversations or noise is present. Similarly, the user may not be able to hear auditory output if there is too much noise in the background.

Transportation is considered here because it is an important consideration for portable devices and in particular for mobility devices. How a device is to be transported needs to be determined to ensure integration of the device with the transportation method. For example, some configurations of a powered wheelchair will not fit into an adapted van (e.g., wheelchairs for clients who are obese may be too wide to fit into the opening of a side-loading van). Who will be transporting the device is also important if she needs to load and unload the device from the vehicle.

The **social context** refers to who is in the setting and the type of interaction they will have with the user. Individuals in the setting, such as family members, caregivers, staff in a supported nursing facility or group home, teachers, classmates, and coworkers, may have regular and close contact with the user. Other individuals, such as an employer, facility administrator, or school principle, have less frequent interaction. However, their actions and attitudes can have a significant effect on the access and use of AT. The social context is particularly important for sensory aids, augmentative communication, and cognitive ATs.

In the social setting, it is important to consider who is available to assist the user, as needed, and the skills and abilities of these other individuals. For example, an older adult who has had a stroke and relies on others to assist with mobility or cognitive activities may have a caregiver who is also an older adult, typically a spouse. The caregiver is also likely to have some form of age-related functional change that poses a challenge to providing assistance. An older spouse may not be physically capable of assisting with the use of a mobility device or may not have the knowledge to assist with the use of a device that supports cognitive skills.

Beukelman and Mirenda (2013) discuss the need to identify actual or potential "opportunity barriers" and "access barriers" for the consumer. Although their model specifically targets consumers with augmentative communication needs, it also holds true for other area of AT. *Opportunity barriers* are imposed by individuals or situations that are not under the consumer's control. Generally, the provision of AT does not result in the elimination of these barriers. Beukelman and Mirenda (2013) identify five types of opportunity barriers: policy barriers, practice barriers, attitude barriers, knowledge barriers, and skill barriers.

Policies and practice barriers are described under the institutional context later in this chapter. In the social context, attitude, knowledge, and skill barriers apply to individuals with whom the consumer interacts and on whom the effective use of the device depends. If the consumer's job supervisor has a negative attitude regarding the use of automatic speech recognition because it is distracting to other workers, it is an attitude barrier that prevents the consumer's participation in that job. Alternatively, the supervisor may have insufficient knowledge or skill regarding a device characteristic such as automatic speech recognition to ensure that it is effectively installed and made available to the consumer.

Access barriers are barriers related to the abilities, attitudes, and resource limitations of the client or his support system (Beukelman and Mirenda, 2013). Known constraints related to user and family preferences and the attitudes of communication partners are other access barriers that should be identified. A potential barrier to accessing technology, one commonly seen during augmentative communication assessments, is resistance on the part of parents to pursue an augmentative communication device because they are worried that the use of such a device will inhibit the child's development of natural speech, a concern that is not supported by current research. As we discuss later in this chapter, the ability to find funding for AT systems and services may also pose a barrier.

Cultural context refers to the client's cultural background and the implications to acceptance and use of technology. In particular, the assessment should consider the cultural perspective of disability and how it influences the family's view of the individual. For example, the family may believe that a person with a disability should not be expected to be independent so might reject technology in favor of providing assistance from another person for daily activities. A culture that values independence highly may similarly reject technology, viewing its use as a sign of weakness or laziness.

Cultural views of acceptance of outside help will also influence whether support will be sought for an AT evaluation. The role of the user of the AT in the home may also affect whether it is accepted or used. The clinician and team need to be sensitive to how the provision and use of AT affects the perception of the user relative to her position in the family.

The **institutional context** components are similar to policy barriers defined as legislative, regulative, or agency policies that govern situations in which consumers find themselves (Beukelman and Miranda, 2013). For example, regulations in some school districts restrict the use of school-purchased AT to use in the school, preventing it from being taken home. Practice barriers refer to routine activities that are not dictated by policy but that constrain the use of ATs.

If the school's policy does not *require* that the device stay in the school but the local teacher or principal has the practice of keeping the devices in the school, the result is the same as if it were a policy. Legislative barriers refer to laws that govern access to AT (e.g., who is eligible to receive technology, what technology is provided, who pays for the technology, where it can be used another aspects that govern the use of the technology) as well as laws that govern access to services and physical structures.

Matching Device Characteristics to the User's Needs and Skills

The assessment process we have described to this point provides the basis by which the AT service delivery team carefully defines the goals to be accomplished and determines the skills the consumer has available for AT system use. It is necessary to systematically transform these goals and skills into characteristics of AT devices. We use the term **device characteristics** to refer to general properties of the technology. A *feature* is a particular implementation of a characteristic. Characteristics of automobiles include, for example, engine, color, size, performance (acceleration, gas mileage), and doors. Features for these same characteristics might include four-cylinder engine, blue color, compact size, 35 miles per gallon, and two doors. As consumers, we have certain needs and preferences, and we match these to general characteristics and specific features. We also have skills that apply to our selection. For example, we may not be able to use a standard manual transmission and choose only automatic transmission cars for consideration. Life roles also play a part in our selection decision. For instance, parents with small children may choose a minivan rather than a compact car. Context also influences device selection; for example, a vehicle with four-wheel drive is more useful than a sports car for someone living in a remote area who travels on unserviced roads.

In AT service delivery, we can use a similar matching process to choose features that match the consumer's needs and skills. In some areas of AT applications (e.g., augmentative communication), this process is referred to as *feature matching*. This systematic approach is superior to using trial and error with all the possible devices that *may* work and then trying to pick one. To use this approach, however, we must first define a set of characteristics to be considered. A generic set of AT device characteristics is listed in Box 5-6. The categories in this box parallel those used in Figure 3-9 to describe the components of the AT portion of the HAAT model. These characteristics are discussed in greater detail in Chapter 2.

BOX 5-6 Assistive Device Characteristics

Human/Technology Interface
Physical properties
User feedback
Number of inputs
Selection methods
Selection set

Processor
Commands
Control parameters
Data or information processing

Activity Output
Magnitude
Precision
Flexibility

Environmental Interface
Range
Threshold

Physical Construction
Mountability
Portability
Packaging

The Human/Technology Interface

The human/technology interface (HTI) is the portion of the device with which the consumer directly interacts. Examples of an interface include a keyboard, joystick, control unit for an EADL, access switch, and seating system. The most general human/technology characteristics, applying to all devices, are the **physical properties**. These include the size and weight of the interface, its texture and hardness, the size and brightness of the display, loudness of any auditory feedback, and the force required to use the interface. The HTI provides **feedback** to the user. Feedback can be visual, auditory, or tactile. In some cases, the feedback is a direct consequence of the interface. For example, comfort of a seat cushion is a type of feedback that is only determined over time as the client uses the seat. In other cases, the user feedback is intentionally built into the device to provide specific information to the user, such as a flashing light indicator on a television control or a tactile display on a reading device for a person with total visual impairment. Feedback is described in terms of the characteristics of magnitude, type, and origin. The *magnitude* of a visual display is the brightness of the light. The *types* of HTI feedback are other characteristics and include visual, auditory, and tactile varieties. The *origin* refers to the source of the feedback, such as that provided by a seat cushion or the voice output provided from the screen reader.

The next three characteristics listed in Box 5-6 apply to HTIs used with electronic assistive devices (including power mobility). The *number of inputs* required to operate any device is a characteristic. The selection method is how the user indicates her choice from response options presented. The options presented and their configuration comprise the selection set. The most appropriate control interface for any given consumer is largely determined by the physical and interface assessments that are described Chapter 8.

The Processor

Recall that the processor is the element of the AT device that links the HTI to the other components. Sometimes this is simply a mechanical linkage (e.g., in a reacher); in such cases, there are not many choices in characteristics because the device performs a very limited number of operations.

However, processors for electronic devices have several characteristics. The first of these is the basic set of *commands* that are necessary to operate the device. For example, in a powered wheelchair system, the basic commands are forward, backward, left, and right. In a communication device, some basic commands include printing a document and speaking. In an EADL, the commands may include lights on and off, TV channel selection, and telephone dialing. The greater the number of commands, the more flexible the system is to the user. However, this greater number creates complexity in the use of the device. Consequently, part of the assessment process includes determination of the number of concepts (e.g., on/off, forward/backward) the client can understand and thus control on the device. With training, the client will often be able to increase the number of commands he can use.

A second characteristic of the processor is the *control parameters.* In contrast to commands, control parameters allow adjustments to be made to the system; they are nice to have but not always essential. Control parameters include such things as variable speed for forward and reverse for a powered wheelchair or adjustment of pitch, voice type, and rate of speech output. A control parameter also provides the ability to switch between different applications for multiple activity outputs. For example, it is possible to operate an EADL, communication device, and computer access system from a powered wheelchair controller. As is the case with the number of commands, the greater flexibility of control parameters results in greater complexity of the use of the device. The assessment process determines the most effective balance between flexibility and simplicity (think of ease of use) for the client's use of the device.

The final general processor characteristic is *data or information processing.* In this case, the device processes information internally rather than dealing with commands or control signals. Here information is entered into the device, either by the client in the case of a control interface or captured by the device in the case of a sensory aid that receives relevant input from the environment, processed by the device, without action by the client, and then some form of output results.

Activity Output

The **activity output** is what the system accomplishes for the consumer (e.g., communication, mobility, manipulation, cognition). The first characteristic that describes the activity output is its *magnitude.* This includes the volume for a speech synthesis system, the force or torque generated by a powered wheelchair, and the brightness of a video screen display. *Precision* is a measure of how accurately the system performs the functions and how exactly it accomplishes its task. For example, a reacher may be able to pick up a cup but not a button. A *flexible* output can be used in different contexts or can be used to accomplish different goals for the consumer. Flexibility can be an important factor when the consumer has many tasks that she wishes to perform or needs to use the device in different contexts.

The Environmental Interface

The **environmental interface** is the portion of the AT system that is used to take in information from the external world for use in a sensory substitution system. For example, when a person has a visual limitation, we use a camera, and when a person has an auditory impairment, we use a microphone. Characteristics that apply to this element include the *range* of the input signal (i.e., how big or small the signal can be and still be detected). The smallest signal that can be discerned from background noise is the *threshold.* As an example of how these characteristics can be applied, consider the two problems of reading and mobility for persons with severe visual impairments. For reading, the device needs very little range because only one letter or line of text needs to be viewed at a time. However, for mobility, the environmental sensor needs to take in a variety of sizes (e.g., from a dish to a tree). For reading, the threshold is low (a letter in fine print), but for mobility, the threshold can be much higher.

Physical Construction

The final category of characteristics is **physical construction.** This category refers to the properties of the device that allow it to be mounted or positioned so that the client has reliable access to it, the portability of the device, the size and weight, and its aesthetics (appearance and color). No matter how well a system works in an assessment session, it will not be effective in everyday use unless the person has access to it at all times. This feature is determined primarily by the *mountability* of the system. The device might be mounted to a piece of furniture, such as a desk, or to another assistive device, as in the case of mounting a communication system on a powered wheelchair. In the latter case, consideration must be given to the compatibility of the two devices. The ability to remove the device when finished with its use is another mountability consideration.

Portability is a measure of the degree to which the device can be moved from place to place. This characteristic includes a consideration of size, weight, and power source. For electronic devices, portability often requires that the device be battery operated and that it be small and lightweight enough to be carried or attached to a wheelchair. If the person is ambulatory, her ability to carry the device needs to be assessed. Battery size, weight, and charge duration influence portability. A device with a large, heavy battery is less likely to be moved from one setting to another. Similarly, a device is likely to be left at home if the duration of charge is short, resulting in concern that the device will become in operable. Portability for mobility devices involves consideration of how they will be transported and who is responsible for lifting them in and out of a vehicle.

A final consideration involves the **aesthetics** of the device, including this characteristic is often overlooked in the design of the system, yet it carries a significant meaning to the user (Miller Polgar, 2010). The look of the device may convey an unintended meaning of vulnerability, frailty or stigma. A device that is aesthetically appealing is more likely to be used than one that is not.

Evaluating the Match Between Characteristics and the Consumer's Skills and Needs

Skills and Needs

At this point in the evaluation process, information has been gathered about the activities, the human (the client), the context, and the elements of the technology. These are the components that drive the decision rather than a specific device. The team can now identify different technologies and determine the match between the consumer's skills and needs and the characteristics of the device. There are two primary ways in which the team can evaluate specific technologies for use by the consumer: (1) trial using the actual device and (2) simulation of device characteristics.

Ideally, the consumer will have the opportunity to try the devices being considered and evaluate their usefulness before a recommendation is made. However, because of the expense, availability of trial equipment, and institutional or funding policies, this option is not always available. It is beneficial for the team to have available a set of devices that represents a broad range of characteristics. The service delivery program typically has a range of devices that can be used for assessment purposes, or a manufacturer's representative may provide equipment to trial. Other manufacturers and service delivery programs lease devices for this purpose. If these devices are available, it is helpful to demonstrate the various features to the consumer and have the consumer try them. There may be two or three devices being considered, and, if possible, each device should be tried and evaluated by the consumer. The trial period should be sufficiently long to give the consumer the opportunity to use the device in a variety of situations and for different purposes. For example, a communication device should be trialed with different communication partners and in different settings. Similarly, a wheelchair should be used in different settings to determine access. A number of device use aspects should be considered during the trial, including (1) how easy the device is to use and to learn to use, (2) the ability of the consumer and family to transport the device as necessary, (3) relevant positioning aspects, (4) comfort when using the device, and (5) a preliminary determination of whether the device is assisting the consumer to meet his goals.

In lieu of having the actual device available, the clinician can simulate device characteristics. Simulation requires that the team members be knowledgeable about the characteristics and features available for specific ATs. For computer-based products, the AT adaptations are often software based, and demonstration disks can be obtained from manufacturers or downloaded from a manufacturer's website. These demonstration programs illustrate the essential features of the software, but they are not fully functional, and their use is time limited. To position a control interface for simulation during assessment, universal mounting systems that can be adjusted and placed in various positions can be used. This step is important to ensure that the control interface is in a functional position for the consumer and remains stable during the assessment.

Decision Making

The team is now at the point where the assessment is complete and the client has had some opportunity to trial the equipment (or at a minimum has had some hands-on experience with it). A recommendation for a specific technology is made at this stage. The most important principle in this process is the relationship between the tasks that the client will use the AT device to accomplish, the skills and abilities of the client, and the characteristics that must be present in the device for those tasks to be accomplished. Each goal may be accomplished only if a set of essential characteristics is included in the AT system. For example, the goal may be mobility, and the characteristics of the type of cushion, wheelchair type, and color all contribute to the accomplishment of this goal.

It is important to recognize that the features that are most limiting must be considered first followed by those that are less restrictive. For example, in an augmentative communication system, the type of symbol system is often the most limiting characteristic. If a consumer requires pictures as a symbol, many devices are eliminated immediately. In contrast, spoken output as a characteristic is not as limiting because most devices have speech output. For each type of AT, it is important for the team to identify a set of general characteristics (or features) that fit within the categories of Box 5-6. The major advantage of the assessment methods described here is that they are based on a consideration of the consumer's goals and skills and the contexts in which the technology will be used first and a consideration of AT system characteristics second. Thus, the system is matched to the consumer (within the limits of current technology) rather than the consumer being forced to adapt to the system. Without a structured approach like the one presented here, however, it is very difficult to meet consumer's goals.

The decision-making process is also guided by the **clinical reasoning** of the professionals involved. Four types of clinical reasoning have been identified in the literature: procedural, interactive, conditional, and narrative (Doyle Lyons & Blesedell Crepeau, 2000; Mattingly, 1994; Mattingly & Fleming, 1994). Procedural reasoning considers the influence of the condition that resulted in the need for AT. For example, using procedural reasoning, the professional understands the influence of cerebral palsy on the ability to sit, move, speak, and manipulate objects. Interactive reasoning engages the actual client. This type of reasoning builds on the procedural reasoning by understanding the individual client with cerebral palsy and his specific situation and needs. Conditional reasoning engages the collective clinical experience of the professional (or the team). This type of reasoning draws on past experience to guide the decision making in the moment. For example, if a particular type of communication device has been beneficial for clients with a similar level of function and needs in the past, then conditional reasoning leads the clinician to consider this type of device in the present situation. Finally, narrative reasoning is the ongoing relationship of the consumer and the team and their joint understanding of the goals of the client. Collectively, these forms of clinical reasoning support the decision-making process.

Recommendations and Report

The recommendations summarize the information gathered during the evaluation and suggest a design for the AT system. At the conclusion of the assessment, everyone involved should sit down to review it and come to a consensus regarding the final recommendation. A written report is prepared that details the assessment and recommendations for an AT system. The written report synthesizes the assessment process and starts out by defining the needs and goals that have been addressed. A summary of the consumer's skills applicable to device use is provided, with a description of generic characteristics to be incorporated into a device. This summary is followed by specific recommendations for equipment, including descriptions, part numbers if applicable, manufacturer's name, any modifications that need to be made, and cost. Recommendations for soft technologies are also included in the written report. These may include recommendations for developing skills that are necessary before purchase of a device, training after the device has been purchased, and strategies for incorporating the technology into the individual's context. Finally, a plan for implementation of the recommendations is provided. This plan includes logistics such as seeking funding from the appropriate sources and who will take responsibility for implementing the recommendations.

Often the written report is aimed at various individuals, thus presenting a unique challenge for the professionals writing it. The report, first of all, needs to be geared toward the consumer, who may not be familiar with medical or technical jargon. Rehabilitation or educational professionals working with the consumer may also be receiving the report and its recommendations. These professionals typically need information on the consumer's skills when using the technology and what skill areas they may need to address to facilitate the use of the device. Some of these professionals may be very knowledgeable in AT, but for others, this experience may be their first. The contact person for the funding source will also be reading the report, and his or her interest is typically in the "bottom line," or what it is going to cost. This person wants evidence that the system recommended is going to meet the consumer's needs at the lowest possible cost. When writing a report for a third-party funder, it is critical to know its criteria and requirements and to follow them accurately to avoid unnecessary delay or denial of AT acquisition.

Implementation

After the recommendations have been made and funding is obtained, the implementation phase begins. This aspect of the delivery process consists of ordering specified equipment, obtaining commercially available equipment or fabricating custom equipment, making needed modifications, assembling or setting up equipment, thoroughly checking it as a system, fitting the device to the consumer, and training the consumer and caregivers in its use.

Ordering and Setup

Many recommended interventions have components from several manufacturers, and these must be integrated into a total system. Some of these may be mainstream commercially available components, and others may be commercial ATs. These devices are ordered from the manufacturer or equipment supplier and may take a significant time to be received after ordering. The recommendation may have also included a custom device or devices that require an adaptation. Examples of custom modifications include mounting a switch to a wheelchair or table, making a cable for connecting two devices together (e.g., a communication device and an EADL), programming a device for unique vocabulary, setting up a wheelchair to provide the appropriate degree of stability and mobility, and adapting a battery-powered toy so it can be controlled with one switch. The design and fabrication of these system components can occur during the waiting time for the delivery of the commercially available technologies. After all of the individual devices and adaptations are available, it is necessary to assemble them into a total package. For example, a wheelchair obtained from one source and a seating system from another will need to be interfaced to each other. The complexity of this assembly process varies widely, and some systems require much more effort than others.

Delivery and Fitting

After the equipment has been obtained, modified, or adapted as necessary and integrated into a system, the system is ready to be delivered to the consumer. This aspect may occur in a clinic setting, in a school or at a job site, or in the consumer's living setting. The choice of locations depends on the nature of the equipment, the ease of transport of the consumer, and the complexity of the system (i.e., technicians and tools that are needed). We refer to all system deliveries as a "fitting" because we are interfacing the human (consumer) with the rest of the system. In some cases, such as custom seating systems, the process resembles a fitting for an orthotic or prosthetic device. In other cases, the fitting focuses on installation of the system, mounting the control interface and the device to a wheelchair, and interconnection of the various components. The fitting phase may also include some amount of assessment as adjustments are made to optimize the consumer's ability to use the system. An example is the use of head switches to control a powered wheelchair. The head switches must be attached to the wheelchair and wired into the controller unit. The initial attachment is done before the fitting, and during the fitting, the location of the head switches (e.g., how close they are to the consumer's head) is adjusted to maximize performance. As much as possible, the fitting should be accomplished by a clinician and technician who can make adjustments. When a significant amount of time has elapsed between ordering and receiving the equipment, changes may have occurred in the client's function or body size. The fitting session must therefore assess whether the recommendations made at the time the device was ordered still work. If not, adjustments are made during the fitting session.

The complexity of many AT systems may require more than one session to obtain all the proper adjustments, mountings, and fittings. Frequently, the need for adjustments is only recognized after the client has used the device for a period of time and has become accustomed to its function. The clinician should be prepared to continue making adjustments and adaptations in the system until the consumer's goals and needs are met, although in reality, this part of the service delivery process is often not funded when services are provided in the community. This phase of the delivery process often involves some reassessment, but its success is directly related to the quality of the initial assessment and recommendations.

Facilitating Assistive Technology System Performance

A major concern of everyone involved in the delivery of AT services is whether the device recommended is going to meet the stated goals. It *cannot* be assumed that intervention ends with the delivery of the device. Most users of technology, even those with previous technology experience, require assistance in facilitating their performance with the device. The clinician is responsible for developing the plan for facilitating the client's performance. It is commonly the rehabilitation assistant who implements that plan. This section discusses three general strategies that can be used to facilitate development of skills in the use of the AT: training, performance aids, and written instructions (Bailey, 1996). Training engages the client as well as her family and caregivers. Performance aids are soft technologies that aid the use of a device, including things such as stored phone numbers in a telephone controller. Written instructions can be provided in multiple formats, and we present some considerations in the development of these instructions.

Training

Training in the use of an AT has been identified as one of the most crucial factors that predicts continued use and acceptance of a device. Yet training is often the element that is either missing or inadequate because of funding issues that drive practice. Clients who receive a device while they are in a clinical setting are more likely to receive training than those who receive the device after they have returned to the community. What we discuss here is considered to be an ideal situation.

Training typically occurs in a face-to-face situation, either individually or in a group. A client who is new to the use of the device is most likely to receive individual training. Clients with some experience with device use are more likely to benefit from group sessions because they are already familiar with the basic functions of the device. Wheelchair "camps" that teach specific wheelchair skills or drama programs that involve children who use communication devices are two examples of group training methods. Online instructional strategies and resources are other options for providing training when a face-to-face opportunity is not possible.

BOX 5-7 Training Strategies for the Implementation of Assistive Technology

Familiarize the client with the basic functions of the device.
Identify the different controls of the device.
Show the client what the device does.
Start simple and build to complex.
Do not assume that the client has prior knowledge with this type of device; start with a task that involves minimal control steps.
Add complexity and need for problem solving as the client gains skills with the device.
The rehabilitation assistant is responsible for safety in the clinical environment.
Build in success; know the client's skill level and work at or just above that level. Provide a level of challenge that maintains motivation but does not result in frustration.
Start with an activity that is of primary importance to the client.
Involve the client and caregivers in establishing goals and plans at all stages.
Build in informal evaluation throughout the process.

We will describe six strategies that can be implemented in training: (1) familiarize the client with the basic functions of the device, (2) start simple and build to complex, (3) build in success, (4) start with an activity that is of primary importance to the client, (5) involve the client (and caregivers) in establishing goals and plans at all stages, and (6) build in informal evaluation throughout the process (Box 5-7). These strategies were derived from a review of suggested training strategies for AT (Kirby et al., 2005; Light, 1989).

Familiarizing the client with the features of the device and how they work is an important first step. AT use is not an activity that is common, so a client receiving a device for the first time does not have prior knowledge of its use from observing others. For example, scanning as a selection method is not a common means of controlling commercial devices. A client first using scanning needs to learn about the scanning pattern, control of the speed, and how to make a selection. Similarly, a client first receiving a manual wheelchair needs to know how to apply the brakes, propel the wheels to go in a straight line or make a turn, and how to remove the foot and armrests to complete a transfer. Knowing how the device works is a first step toward successful use. This aspect of the training has been called **operational competence** (Light et al., 2003).

Clinical reasoning guides the determination of a simple activity that can be used to initiate training and ensure success (Doyle Lyons & Blesedell Crepeau, 2000). For example, use of a single switch that turns on a toy or TV when pressed once and off when pressed a second time teaches the client the basic function of a switch. Providing an environment that is free of obstacles so a client can freely propel a wheelchair allows him to safely move the chair without the need for accuracy. Interactive and conditional reasoning are used in the implementation of a training program to assist with the identification of activities that pose the right degree of challenge to the client and enable his success in the use of the device. Training that facilitates the client's use of the AT in increasingly complex situations and that incorporates his problem solving in unfamiliar situations is termed **strategic competence** (Light et al., 2003).

As with all of the other steps in the service delivery process, training involves understanding the goals of the client and involving her in the planning and decision making of the process. Working with the client on her goals ensures that training is a collaborative process and engages the client. For example, a client who has a spinal cord injury that has resulted in limited physical function will be more engaged in learning to use an electronic aid to daily living if it allows her to control a music device if listening to music is important to her. Similarly, a client who enjoys being outside and walking with her spouse will engage in wheelchair skills training if the training involves activities that enable her to resume this activity with her spouse.

Informal evaluation of the client's performance needs to occur throughout the process. Initial work in uncovering clinical reasoning in rehabilitation revealed tacit (or subconscious) reasoning that occurred during intervention as the clinician was constantly adjusting the activity in response to the client's performance or feedback (Mattingly & Fleming, 1994). These adjustments might include knowing when to provide assistance versus stepping back when the client is successfully using the device, making necessary positioning adjustments or adjustments to device controls, or modifying or changing the activity to accommodate the needs of the clients. Often these adjustments happen without conscious thought during the session. It is during the record keeping or charting that occurs after the session that these adjustments, the rationale for them, and their outcome come to the forefront. It is important to reflect on the session and record the information to document the progress and guide the next steps.

Performance Aids

A document or device containing information that an individual uses to assist in the completion of an activity is called a **performance aid**. By decreasing the amount of information to be remembered, the performance aid reduces the amount of cognitive processing required to complete an activity. With a performance aid, the user does not have to rely as much on long-term memory, which results in reduced errors, increased speed for certain tasks, and a reduced amount of training required. Performance aids do not necessarily have to be written; picture symbols can also be effective for individuals who cannot read. Bailey (1996) describes five quality standards for performance aids: (1) accessibility, (2) accuracy, (3) clarity, (4) completeness and conciseness, and (5) legibility.

Performance aids are commonly used with individuals who have memory deficits as a result of damage to the brain. One type of performance aid is simple step-by-step instructions that assist the user in carrying out a sequence of tasks. For example, Tim is a young man who has sustained a head injury. He uses a computer to complete school assignments but has problems remembering the sequence of steps to get into his computer word processing program. The steps to complete this task have been simply written and are posted next to his computer. Because Tim also has visual acuity problems, the instructions are printed in large, bold letters. For Tim, this simple performance aid has meant the difference between success and failure in using his computer.

Another type of performance aid assists in remembering several items of information. An example of this type of aid is a printed list of codes with their meanings, which an individual may have stored in her augmentative communication system. Often such a list such is attached to the side of the device so the user can view it easily as needed. Sometimes codes and their meanings are built into software programs and presented on the screen each time the user selects a letter.

Instructions

Instructions should be considered an integral part of the system and be available to the user at the time of the system delivery. These are available in many different formats, including print and digital media. Instructions are helpful when step-by-step directions with detailed information are required or when graphic information needs to be presented. The clinician must not assume that the instructions provided by the manufacturer are going to be adequate. Instructions provided by the manufacturer of the system may include too little or too much information, they may assume a basic knowledge level, or they may be difficult to follow by the user. It is recommended that instructions from the manufacturer be reviewed and supplemented as needed. When the manufacturer's documentation is overwhelming, the clinician can review the documentation and condense it into a quick reference sheet that provides simplified and frequently used information.

The clinician should consider a few factors when developing performance aids or supplementing the manufacturer's instructions. Consideration should be given as to the most useful format for the client. As the case of Tim illustrated, a picture system might be most appropriate. Some clients may not be comfortable reading instructions from a computer or tablet screen, necessitating the translation of instructions in electronic format to print format. Other clients may need oral rather than visual instructions. In some cases, multiple sets of instructions are necessary to meet the needs of the client, the family, and other caregivers.

The accessibility and usability of instructions are determined with the client. Information that is presented via print material should be analyzed for reading level and clarity of instructions. Font size and color contrast are important for clients and caregivers who have vision limitations. In this instance, simpler is better—black letters on a white background, or reverse, are the easiest to read. Consideration should be given to alternate delivery modes when the user has a visual impairment that limits her ability to read. Usability of the instructions should be checked with the client and other users to determine whether she understands the instructions that are presented.

Follow-Up and Follow-Along

After the system has been implemented, it is tempting to think that the intervention has been completed. This perception, however, is totally false; the delivery of the system marks the beginning of the time of use, and it therefore signals the beginning of the evaluation of system effectiveness. We use the term **follow-up** to refer to activities that occur during the period immediately after delivery of an AT system and that address the effectiveness of the device, training, and user strategies. The term **follow-along** is used to describe activities that take place over a longer period. This phase addresses factors such as changes in needs or goals, availability of new devices, and other concerns.

We include a formal follow-up phase in our delivery process for several reasons: (1) assistive devices can seldom be used right out of the box without ever needing to be adjusted; (2) electronic devices may need adjustment after an initial period of use; (3) training programs may provide preliminary knowledge of device use, but expertise in use comes with prolonged experience and use in multiple situations; and (4) perceived device failures can be the result of operator error caused by a lack of device understanding. A carefully developed follow-up program will identify these problems easily and address them quickly.

Repair and maintenance are often conducted during the follow-up phase. *Repair* refers to action taken to correct a problem in a system. *Maintenance,* on the other hand, is a systematic set of procedures that is aimed at keeping the device in working order. Examples of maintenance functions are proper battery charging, cleaning, tightening mounting hardware, and lubrication of moving mechanical parts. A regular schedule will ensure that necessary maintenance takes place. AT system failures result in a major disruption of the consumer's life. For example, a consumer depends on his powered wheelchair for mobility. If it fails, he may have a manual wheelchair as a backup, but his independence is significantly reduced. Repair of ATs is most often carried out either through manufacturer's representatives or directly through the manufacturer. In the latter case, the device must be returned to the factory for repair, and the consumer may be without it for several days or even longer. Prompt attention to repair needs of consumers is an important part of follow-up.

As part of a formal follow-up program, contacts with the consumer (via telephone, email, on the job site, in the home, or in the clinic) are desirable on a regular basis after delivery. These contacts occur whether there is a perceived problem or not, and they are in addition to other activities such as training and repair. This regularly scheduled contact is important because there may be unnoticed problems, or more often there are underused features that are discovered during the follow-up sessions. As we have defined it, follow-along has a much longer time frame than follow-up. Whereas follow-up typically covers the first year of operation of an AT system, follow-along is carried out over the individual's lifetime. Consumers may return for service after a period of years for several reasons. They may have found that the device is not working as they would like and is not meeting their functional goals. Another reason is to obtain information about advances in technology since they obtained their device. In other cases, the consumer may have changed in significant ways. This change is often seen in children who have grown significantly and need a revision in their seating system. Change can also be the result of a degenerative condition such as amyotrophic lateral sclerosis, and in these cases, the device may need to be altered to accommodate decreased physical function. In other cases, the change in consumer condition is a result of the development of new skills that make it possible to consider new device features. For example, a consumer who has sustained a TBI may initially receive a communication device that is based on very simple replay of sentences. As he recovers, his ability to spell effectively may improve, and a device with this capability should be considered.

There are other reasons for follow-along. One of the most important of these is a change in the life roles and context of the consumer. For example, Martin, who has severe cerebral palsy and has used an augmentative and alternative communication (AAC) device for several years, decides to move into an apartment on his own. The success of this transition could depend heavily on the availability of ATs. An EADL would allow him to control lights and appliances, answer and dial the telephone, and control the television and other entertainment devices. Reevaluation is dictated not by changes in his condition but by changes in his life roles and the context in which he will be using his technology.

The Effects of Errors in Assistive Technology Systems

Identification of errors and determination of their source is another component of the process of evaluating the match between the device characteristics and those of the consumer. Two types of errors are of concern in AT systems. *Random errors* are infrequent and are generally chance occurrences. An example of a random error is the inability to understand a voice synthesizer because of high amounts of ambient noise. If the noise is not present, there is no error, and even if there is noise, it may not lead to an error in interpretation. It is only the random co-occurrence of the need to use the voice synthesizer, the presence of noise, and a listener who does not understand the output that creates the error. Random errors may reoccur, but they are not consistently present in the system. We can do very little to avoid this type of error in the AT system design process.

Of greater concern are *periodic,* or regular, *errors,* which occur under predictable conditions. These errors may also be infrequent, but they are foreseeable. As an example, many letter-to-speech software programs make mistakes in pronunciation when used with voice synthesizers. The mispronunciation always occurs whenever the particular word is entered. This type of error can be dealt with in the design process. There are several effects of errors on AT system performance, including loss of information, injury, and embarrassment. All three of these can occur in the same system, and they may be due to the human, the activity, the context, the AT, or the interaction of all of these components. For example, a power wheelchair will not function if the user does not regularly charge the batteries. The user must somehow cause the action that results in the batteries maintaining a charge, and the power wheelchair system must provide accurate information about the degree to which the batteries are charged. Error-free function here relies on the successful integration of the human with the technology.

Loss of information is a common effect associated with augmentative communication systems (see Chapter 16) and sensory aids (see Chapters 13 and 14). Loss of information refers to an interruption in the output of the system, whether that is auditory or visual as in a voice output communication aid or physical as in the power to propel powered wheelchair. It can occur because the human operator makes an error in motor, sensory, or cognitive performance or as a result of a device error. Although the net effect on system performance of either of these errors (human or device) may be the same, it is important to distinguish between them to correct the problem.

When the human operator makes the errors, the distinction needs to be made as to whether the cause is lack of capacity (e.g., inability to control excessive tremor, resulting in erroneous selections or visual limitations in reading a display) or lack of skill (inadequate experience or practice in using the device). If the problem is the capacity of the user, then modifications must be made in the system (e.g., using a keyguard to prevent erroneous entries or an enlarged display screen to improve visibility). If the problem is one of skill, training may help reduce the number of errors.

Physical injury is a more serious effect of a system error. This type of error can occur in a mobility system (see Chapter 10) if, for example, a braking system fails or a motor fails to turn off. Consideration of this type of error leads us to the concept of "failsafe" design. This approach attempts to anticipate the types of errors and to ensure that if they do occur the probability of injury is minimized. For example, if a powered wheelchair controller fails, it should fail in the off state. If it fails in the full on state, the user may be injured because the chair cannot be controlled. Similar to loss of information, the capacity or the skill of the user can cause physical injury. Another example is the failure of a mobility aid for a person who is blind. If the device fails to identify an obstacle or a hazard such as a drop off, the individual could sustain a serious injury.

A final general effect of AT system errors is embarrassment. This effect is somewhat unique to ATs, and it is a direct result of the role that AT systems play in the daily life of the user who has a disability. Because the tasks being performed cannot be accomplished without the system, its use is continual throughout the day. Over a long period, system errors leading to embarrassment are inevitable. The embarrassment may be relatively minor, such as a manipulation system dropping a spoonful of food. In other contexts, it may be much more significant. For example, an augmentative communication device may fail and produce the wrong utterance. If the context is a presentation in an important meeting and the mistaken utterance is an obscenity, the consequences are potentially very negative. To place the importance of this type of error in perspective, recall that the device is often perceived by both the user and other people as being a part of the user. Thus, the user is held responsible for an inappropriate utterance just as if she had used her own voice to produce it.

The errors and their resulting effects may arise from any of the components of the AT system or their interaction. The human error may be related to capacity or skill. The device may malfunction, in which case the error is related to the design. The context may cause an error. For example, the pressure relief properties of a wheelchair cushion may be impaired if the cushion is exposed to extremely cold environments for a prolonged time and the cushion materials freeze. An example of an error that is caused by the interaction of the components of the HAAT model relates to devices that have many functions, with complex commands required for successful activation. In part, the error is caused by the capacity of the user to learn how to operate the device. It is also caused by the design of the device that requires complex actions for successful operation. Some of the concepts related to the client's perception of the use of AT, described in Chapter 3, are relevant here.

It is clear from this discussion that identification and reduction of errors can occur at several points in the AT process. Initially, incorporating a design and accompanying soft technologies that are congruent with inclusive design principles can minimize errors. Errors can be identified and possibly corrected through use of a thorough evaluation that leads to a suitable device recommendation, coupled with a trial period. Finally, errors in the AT system are identified and reduced through follow-up with individual users and after market research into the effectiveness of the system.

EVALUATING THE EFFECTIVENESS OF ASSISTIVE TECHNOLOGY SERVICES AND SYSTEMS

Evaluation of the effectiveness of AT services and systems is important for many reasons. First and foremost, it provides the team with an indication of the benefits of the AT service to the individual client and her family. It can provide the client with a measure of her improved function and quality of life. Formal outcome evaluation may be a condition of the funder—both in terms of outcomes for the individual client and for obtaining funding in the future. In the latter case, cumulative documentation of positive outcomes of device use, with formal assessment instruments, provides justification that the device makes a difference and thus supports provision of the device to other clients in the future. In this section, we provide information about formal assessments, which are typically completed by the clinician, and a framework for informal assessment, which is completed on an ongoing basis.

Fuhrer et al (2003) suggest that a comprehensive conceptual framework will guide the development of useful outcome measures. They describe a model that will help researchers and clinicians identify assumptions, variables, and populations when developing, considering, and implementing AT outcome measures. Outcome of device use is considered to be the frequency and duration of device use.

The model considers different time frames when evaluation is important: initial procurement of the device and the introductory period leading to short- and long-term outcomes. Three aspects are considered when a device is obtained: (1) the need for the device, (2) the type of device, including its intrinsic and extrinsic properties, and (3) the services involved when obtaining the device (Fuhrer et al., 2003). A number of constructs are considered in evaluating short- and long-term outcomes, including effectiveness, efficiency, satisfaction with the device, psychological function, and subjective opinion of the contribution of the device to the client's well-being (Fuhrer et al., 2003). If the user is not satisfied with the device, it may be abandoned in either the short or the long term. The constructs related to the International Classification of Functioning, Disability and Impairment (ICF; WHO, 2001) are mediating factors in the short and long terms.

The effectiveness of AT systems in meeting the needs of consumers is related to many factors. Sackett (1980) identifies three attributes of outcome evaluation that are relevant to AT service delivery: effectiveness, efficacy, and efficiency. Evaluation of device *effectiveness* determines whether the device does what it is intended to do (i.e., does it work?). Effectiveness is measured in terms of the impact of the product on the consumer's life and needs. Outcome measurements of effectiveness must begin with and focus on the consumer and the results of the AT intervention. These outcomes allow us to determine the *efficacy* of the service delivery structure and process. Efficacy is the ability to produce a desired result or effect in an efficient manner. This aspect is what is measured in evaluation of a service delivery structure and process. It provides useful information on how services are being delivered so that necessary revisions can be made.

A recent article by Lenker et al (2013) gathered consumer perspectives on AT outcomes research. The research involved adult users of AT who participated in focus groups. The participants indicated that they valued AT for the effects it had on their independence, their ability to participate at work and school, and its influence on their perception of their well-being (Lenker et al., 2013). Furthermore, the researchers concluded that AT outcome evaluation must focus on the service delivery process because many participants reported that the process was time consuming and frustrating, with long-term consequences. A key element of the service delivery process was the inclusion of consumers and their perspectives. Subsequent research should identify additional key elements of the service delivery process. Finally, the participants indicated that the cost of AT provision was another important component of AT research (Lenker et al., 2013).

Formal Evaluation

Formal evaluation of AT service delivery consists of **outcome measures** that evaluate general function and those that evaluate specific components of AT use. Outcome measurement in AT has gained more attention over the past decade. Instruments are being developed that enable outcome measurement related to use of specific technology such as communication devices and wheelchairs. Examples of these assessments are described in following chapters that discuss these types of technology. Box 5-8 lists some common measures of general function that are designed to be used at the initial assessment and then again at the end of service delivery to determine change in function after the implementation of the device. These assessments are the Canadian Occupational Performance Measure (Law et al., 2005), the Functional Independent Measure (Uniform Data System for Medical Rehabilitation, 1997), the WeeFIM (Uniform Data System for Medical Rehabilitation, 1993), and the Pediatric Disability Inventory (PEDI) (Haley et al., 1998).

Three further instruments are specific to AT, intended to evaluate psychosocial outcomes. These are the Psychosocial Impact of Assistive Devices Scale (PIADS) (Day & Jutai, 1996), the Family Impact of Assistive Technology Scale (FIATS) (Ryan et al., 2006, 2007), and the Quebec User Evaluation of Satisfaction with Assistive Technology (QUEST) (Demers et al., 1996). The PIADS and FIATS evaluate the psychosocial outcomes of AT use, and the QUEST evaluates clients' satisfaction with device use.

The PIADS (Day & Jutai, 1996; Jutai & Day, 2002; Day, Jutai, & Campbell, 2002) measures the outcome of AT use on psychosocial health and well-being. It is a 26-item self-rating scale composed of three subscales:

1. Competence, which measures the effects of a device on functional independence, performance, and productivity
2. Adaptability, which measures the enabling and liberating effects of a device
3. Self-esteem, which measure the extent to which a device has affected self-confidence, self-esteem, and emotional well-being (Day & Jutai, 1996)

The PIADS evaluates outcome of use of a variety of ATs. The original study focused on eyeglass and contact lens wears (Day & Jutai, 1996). Subsequent studies have used it to evaluate the psychosocial impact of EADLs on the lives of users (Jutai et al., 2000), contact lenses (Jutai et al, 2003), video relay services (Saladin & Hansman, 2008), push-rim activated, power-assisted wheelchair push rims (Geisbrecht et al., 2009), and speech recognition software (DeRosier and Farber, 2005). It has been translated for multiple cultures, including Taiwan (Hsieh and Lenker, 2006), Puerto Rico (Orellano and Jutai, 2013), and Japan (Inoue et al., 2011). The instrument has been used with adults with a variety of disabilities, including physical (Jutai et al., 2000, 2003; Giesbrecht et al, 2009), deaf and hearing impaired (Saladin and Hansman), and visual impairments (Jutai et al., 2003).

The QUEST (Demers et al., 1996) is a measure of the client's satisfaction with his use of AT. It is founded on five premises: (1) user satisfaction is multidimensional; (2)

BOX 5-8 Common Assistive Technology Outcome Measures

General Performance Measures—not Specific to Assistive Technology

Canadian Occupational Performance Measure (COPM) (2005)

The COPM measures the client's perception of the importance of self-identified occupational performance goals and their satisfaction with that performance. Goals are identified for self-care, productivity, and leisure. The COPM is designed to be used both pre- and postintervention.

Functional Independence Measure (FIM) (1997)

The FIM instrument is a widely used rehabilitation outcome measure that measures performance under the categories of self-care, bowel and bladder management, transfers, locomotion, communication, and cognition. An individual who uses AT cannot receive the maximum score, which is awarded only to individuals who perform the activity unaided. It is used pre- and postintervention. A child's version (WeeFIM) is also available.

Pediatric Evaluation of Disability Inventory (PEDI) (1998)

The PEDI is used to evaluate functional abilities and performance in infants and children (6 months to 7.5 years) with a variety of disabilities. Children older than 7.5 years whose development level is at or less than 7.5 years can also be evaluated with the PEDI. Performance is evaluated in three target areas: self-care, mobility, and social function. Results of the PEDI provide information on the child's performance, the need for assistance from caregivers, and modifications required to enable the child to perform different functions (including child-oriented modifications, use of rehabilitation equipment, and extensive modifications).

Assistive Technology–Specific Performance Measures

Psychosocial Impact of Assistive Devices Scale (PIADS) (1996)

The PIADS measures three psychosocial constructs related to the use of AT. These constructs include competence (functional independence, performance, and productivity), adaptability (the enabling and liberating effects of a device), and self-esteem (extent to which a device has affected self-confidence, self-esteem, and emotional well-being).

Quebec User Evaluation of Satisfaction with Assistive Technology (QUEST) (1996)

The QUEST involves three parts. The first provides the context in which the satisfaction with the AT is evaluated. The second part asks the user to rate the importance of a number of different variables. The third part organizes the results of part 2 into three global categories: environment, person, and AT. The final part enables to determine areas of low satisfaction with device use.

Family Impact of Assistive Technology—AS (FIATS-AS) (2006) and—AAC (FIATS-AAC) (2012)

The FIATS assesses the impact of AT use on the health and well-being of children who use AT and their families as well as the activities and participation of the children who use AT. The initial instrument was designed to assess the impact of adaptive seating use. An adaptation is used to assess the impact of augmentative and alternative communication devices.

Law M, Baptiste S, Carswell A, et al: *Canadian Occupational Performance Measure,* ed 3, Toronto: CAOT/ACE Publications, 2005.
Uniform Data System for Medical Rehabilitation (UDS): *WeeFIM,* version 4.0, Buffalo, NY: State University of New York at Buffalo, 1993.
Uniform Data System for Medical Rehabilitation (UDS): *Functional Independence Measure,* version 5.1, Buffalo, NY: Buffalo General Hospital, State University of New York, 1997.
Haley SM, Coster WJ, Ludlow LW, et al: *Pediatric Evaluation of Disability Inventory,* Boston: Trustees of Boston University, 1998.
Day H, Jutai, J: Measuring the psychosocial impact of assistive devices: The PIADS, *Can J Rehabil,* 9:159-168, 1996.
Demers L, Weiss-Lambrou, R, Ska, B: Development of the Quebec User Evaluation with Assistive Technology (QUEST), *Assist Technol,* 8:1-3, 1996.
Delarosa E, et al: Family Impact of Assistive Technology Scale: Development of a measurement scale for parents of children with complex communication needs, *Augment Altern Commun,* 28:171-180, 2012.
Ryan S, Campbell KA, Rigby P, et al: Development of the Family Impact of Assistive Technology Scale, *Int J Rehabil Res,* 29:195-200, 2006.

satisfaction is related to context, the human, and aspects of the device; (3) user satisfaction is highly variable and is unique to the individual; (4) the user must feel free to express her opinion about device use during the interview process; and (5) the instrument must be easy to understand and administer (Demers et al., 1996).

The instrument has three steps. The first step collects demographic information about the individual, the context in which he uses his device, and the device characteristics. The second step is composed of 27 items considered to represent factors most likely to affect satisfaction. These items are scored on a scale ranging from very important to not important. The client has the opportunity to add additional items reflecting satisfaction at this point. The final step involves only items scored as important or very important, which are then rated on a 6-point scale ranging from very dissatisfied to very satisfied. The end score is considered to represent global satisfaction with device use.

The QUEST has been used to measure user satisfaction with eye-tracking communication devices for users with ALS (Caligan et al., 2013), electronic mobility aids for deaf and blind individuals (Vincent et al., 2013), computer task performance (Danial-Saad et al., 2012), push-rim activated, power-assisted wheelchair (Geisbrecht et al., 2009), mobility devices (Karmarkar et al., 2009; Samuelsson, 2008) face-to-face communication devices for deaf individuals (Vincent et al., 2007), and speech recognition software (DeRosier and Farber, 2007). It has been translated for use in Taiwan (Mao et al., 2010), the Netherlands (Demers et al., 2011), and Denmark (Brandt, 2005).

The FIATS is a new instrument with ongoing development. It is intended to measure the influence of assistive device use on the health and well-being of children who use AT and their families and the activities and participation of these children (Ryan et al., 2013). The original version (Ryan et al., 2006, 2007) was developed as a measure of the impact of adaptive seating on the lives of children and their families. It consists of eight subscales covering the two broad domains (child and family health and well-being, child activity and participation) mentioned earlier. Each item is scored on a 7-point Likert scale, ranging from strongly disagree to strongly agree, with higher scores indicating a more positive influence of the device (Ryan et al., 2006, 2007). The instrument has been used to evaluate the outcome of AT use for families of children who use these devices who are between the ages of 1 and 17 years, 11 months (Delarosa et al., 2012; Ryan et al., 2009, 2013).

BOX 5-9 Informal Evaluation of Assistive Technology Use

Use of Assistive Technology

- What activities are completed with the device?
  - What affects the consumer's choice of these activities?
- When is the device used?
  - What affects the consumer's choice of when to use the device?
- Does the AT do what it is supposed to do?
- How long does the consumer use the device?
  - Can she use it for the duration of the intended activity?
  - Does she become fatigued when using the device? Is there some aspect of the device use that is causing the fatigue?
- What assistance does the consumer need to set up the device?
- Is the consumer independent in completion of the activity after the device is set up?
- Can the device be easily transported from one location to another? Within a setting? Across settings?

Human/Assistive Technology Interface

- Is the device properly positioned so the consumer can access it easily?
- Can the consumer see necessary components of the device (e.g., visual display, control switches)?
- Can the consumer hear auditory output of the device?
- Does the consumer have the physical strength, range of motion, and dexterity to use the device?
- Is the consumer comfortable when using the device over the long term?
- Can the consumer detect and repair errors when using the device?
  - Is the error a result of consumer capacity or skill?

The FIATS has been modified for use with AAC devices for children with complex communication needs (FIATS-AAC; Delarosa et al., 2012). The original instrument is now referred to as the Family Impact of Assistive Technology Scale—Adaptive Seating (FIATS-AS) and has been used to evaluate the outcome of adaptive seating for young children (Ryan et al., 2009, 2013). A Turkish version of the FIATS (FIATS-tr) is in preliminary development (Simsek et al., 2012).

Informal Evaluation

Box 5-9 lists two primary areas related to AT use that comprise an **informal evaluation** of the AT outcome. Many of these elements will have been evaluated, formally and informally, during the initial assessment process as well as during the implementation aspect of the service delivery process. These elements can be determined through observation and interview with the consumer during regular interactions. Although these elements are described separately, the process of gathering information about each of them is integrated. They are only separated here to achieve greater clarity.

The first element to consider is the actual use of the technology. What activities are completed with the device? The needs assessment and implementation process were based on client-determined goals that in part identified activities that would be completed using the device. During the evaluation, the clinician determines whether the consumer is using the AT for those activities. If not, what are the reasons that the device is not being used? What affects the consumer's choice of these activities? Perhaps he has not mastered the use of the device and finds it is easier to ask for assistance from another person or to complete the activity himself.

A related consideration is when the device is used. Time of day is a consideration here because the device might only be used when the person feels alert and able to operate it or alternately, uses it to support function when she is fatigued. Another aspect of when the device is used involves the social aspect. Does the client only use the device in settings when she is alone or with other, familiar people? Does she choose not to use the device in a setting with unfamiliar people? If so, the clinician needs to uncover the meaning of the use of the device because feelings of embarrassment or vulnerability may be associated with device use, limiting function in certain settings (Miller Polgar, 2010).

An important consideration, which seems obvious, is whether the device does what it is supposed to do. Is the device reliable? Does the device enable the function as it is intended? This observation should have been made during the trial period and initial implementation phase.

The clinician should document how long the consumer uses the device, what support is required to set up and use the device, and any changes in these elements as the consumer becomes more proficient with the device use. Similarly, any issues with transportation of the device within the setting or across settings should be documented. As mentioned earlier, transportation may be affected by the physical effort needed to move the device from one place to another as well as institutional policies that limit the device from being removed from one setting and used in another (e.g., some schools do not allow students to take technology from the school to their homes).

The second major aspect of this informal evaluation is the consideration of the HTI. Here, the clinician considers whether the device is properly positioned so the client can access it (e.g., use controls on a communication device or the joystick control of a wheelchair). In addition to positioning of the device for control access is positioning of the device for comfort. Consider whether the consumer is comfortable using the device (or sitting in a seating system) for the length of time needed to complete necessary activities.

The physical and sensory aspects of the HTI include observation and documentation of whether the consumer can see the controls and the display during use; whether he can hear the output or feedback from the device; and whether he has the necessary strength, range of motion, and dexterity to use the device. Although each of these components was evaluated during the initial assessment, the client's abilities may have changed between recommendation and receiving the technology. Furthermore, the client's functional abilities may change over time if he has a progressive condition. A child's growth, either physical or developmental, may change the skills or needs for the use of the AT.

Finally, the clinician should note errors the client makes when using the device. These errors may be due to the client's capacity (e.g., her strength may have declined, so she no longer has the physical capacity to exert sufficient force to use the technology). Alternately, the errors may be due to the client's skill level, suggesting that further training is required. Further note is made of whether the client can detect errors she makes and repair them. For example, if she initiates a turn too soon when propelling her powered wheelchair, does she recognize this error and make adjustments to avoid hitting the wall? Does she learn from this error and initiate the turn at the proper time when making subsequent turns?

Assistive Technology Abandonment

One of the most tangible indicators of lack of consumer satisfaction is when the consumer stops using a device even though the need for which the device was obtained still exists. We call this situation **technology abandonment,** and it is useful to look at some of the factors that lead to it. Phillips and Zhao (1993) surveyed more than 200 users of ATs and identified four factors that were significantly related to the abandonment of ATs: (1) failure of providers to take consumers' opinions into account, (2) easy device procurement, (3) poor device performance, and (4) changes in consumers' needs or priorities.

More recent research examined personal and social factors that predict AT abandonment. Pape et al (2002) conducted a review of the literature related to AT abandonment to look at how the personal meaning attributed to assistive devices influences their integration into the user's daily life. They found that psychosocial and cultural variables were primary factors in determining the meaning individuals assigned to AT. In particular, their expectations of how the device would function, the social costs of using the device (i.e., cost/benefit ratio of device use), and an outlook that disability did not define themselves as a person were the primary factors that contributed to whether a person integrated AT into his life or not (Pape et al., 2002). Reimer-Weiss and Wacker (2000) examined factors that predicated AT use in individuals with disability. They found that the relative advantage of the AT in the user's life and the user's involvement in the device selection process were predictors of device use or discontinuance.

Scherer and colleagues (2005) found that personal characteristics related to mood, self-esteem, self-determination, and motivation and psychosocial characteristics related to friend and family support (as examples) were significant predictors of device use (Scherer et al., 2005). Collectively, the earlier studies such as the one by Phillips and Zhao (1993) and the more recent work of Pape et al (2002), Reimer-Weiss and Wacker (2000), and Scherer et al (2005) provide evidence that characteristics of the device, the person, and his environment predict whether he will use a device or abandon it.

A FINAL WORD ABOUT FUNDING

Assistive technology is expensive. If the consumer and her family had to bear the full cost, it would result in a significant burden. In many jurisdictions, **funding** is available for certain types of AT. This section will familiarize the clinician with the different sources of funding for AT and will include a list of factors that need to be considered regarding third-party funding.

The utility of mainstream technology for clients with disabilities affects funding in both positive and negative ways. Because mainstream technology is typically less expensive than technology produced specifically for individuals with disabilities, it is easier to procure and available at a lower cost. However, these technologies are rarely included in funding programs, which means the client bears the full cost of their acquisition.

Public Funding

Governments in many jurisdictions provide full or partial funding for some devices. Funding may come from national (federal), state (provincial), or municipal governments. It may target particular groups, such as veterans, children, seniors, first nation groups, or individuals who are receiving some form of social assistance. Public funding may also be specific to a setting such as an educational or work setting. Funding is often based on medical necessity and medical necessity. Examples of public funding include Medicaid and Medicare in the United States; the Assistive Devices Program in Ontario, Canada; and the Program of Appliances for Disabled People in New South Wales, Australia. These programs are described in greater detail in Chapter 3.

Private Funding

Private Health Insurance

Private health insurance is obtained in two ways: as an employment benefit or through direct purchase by an individual. Although insurance policies may vary considerably, benefits such as durable medical equipment (see definition of assistive devices in Chapter 1) are often included. In some situations, private health insurance can be used to "top up" the funding that is received from a government source.

Other Sources of Funding

Alternative sources of funding that are not included in public funding or private insurance include service clubs, private foundations, and volunteer organizations. Various community service clubs (e.g., Kiwanis, Rotary Club) may be sources of funding for a local individual who has no other means of funding. In addition, foundations related to specific disability groups directly supply equipment and services to individuals with that particular disability.

Determining Eligibility for Funding

It is important to determine eligibility requirements when determining appropriate funding sources. The clinician must be familiar with both the requirements and the process to ensure that both are followed. Some of these requirements include the age of the client, functional status, or ability to perform specific skills. For example, some programs require that the client be able to propel a wheelchair independently for a certain distance to be eligible for funding support. Eligibility may be limited to specific settings. Some programs will only fund devices used in the school or work settings. Most funding programs list eligible device categories; for example, Medicare in the United States only funds durable medical equipment, as defined in Chapter 3. Some funding organizations define a specific timeframe in which the client is expected to use the device in order to be eligible for funding. For example, a client who has had a total hip replacement and is only expected to need a walker for 6 weeks is not likely eligible for funding to support the purchase of the walker because of the temporary nature of its use. The information required includes who is responsible for each aspect of the funding process and the support materials that are necessary for funding approval.

SUMMARY

This chapter describes the principles of assessment and intervention and the service delivery process to the consumer. The steps in the process include referral intake, needs assessment, evaluation, recommendation, implementation, follow-up, and follow-along. A framework for structuring observations of the client when using AT is described.

STUDY QUESTIONS

1. Describe the principles for AT assessment and intervention.
2. Distinguish between quantitative and qualitative assessment procedures.
3. List the steps involved in AT service delivery and write a brief description of each one.
4. List the four major categories of skill evaluation and provide two examples of each category.
5. List four considerations of the context relevant to the AT assessment.
6. Describe the difference between opportunity barriers and access barriers. Give an example of each.
7. List six training strategies and give an example of each.
8. Describe considerations that are important when determining whether written instructions are useful to the client and caregivers.
9. Discuss the four factors that influence whether an AT will be used or abandoned.
10. Describe the difference between formal and informal evaluation.
11. Describe two main elements of an informal evaluation of AT use and give two examples of each element.
12. Describe three sources of AT funding.
13. Discuss aspects that need to be considered when determining a client's eligibility for funding.

REFERENCES

American Educational Research Association: American Psychological Association, National Council on Measurement in Education: *Standards for educational and psychological testing*, Washington, DC, 1999, AERA.

Arksey H, O'Malley L: Scoping studies: Towards a methodological framework, *Int J Res Methodol* 8:19–32, 2005.

Bailey RW: *Human performance engineering*, ed 3, Upper Saddle River, NJ, 1996, Prentice Hall.

Ballantyne JC, Graham J, Baguley D: *Ballantyne's deafness*, ed 7, Chichester UK, 2009, Wiley Blackwell.

Beukelman DR, Mirenda P: *Augmentative and alternative communication, supporting children and adults with complex communication needs*, Baltimore, 2013, Paul H Brookes.

Bovend'Eerat TJH, Dawes H, Johansen-Berg H, Wade DT: Evaluation of the modified Jebson Hand Function Test and the University of Maryland arm questionnaire for stroke, *Clin Rehabil* 18:195–202, 2004.

Brandt A: Translation, cross cultural adaptation and content validation of the QUEST, *Technol Disabil* 17:205–216, 2005.

Brown-Triolo D: Understanding the person behind the technology. In Scherer MJ, editor: *Assistive technology: Matching device and consumer for successful rehabilitation*, Washington DC, 2002, American Psychological Association.

Bruininks RH, Bruininks BD: *Bruininks-Oseretsky Test of Motor Proficiency*, ed 2, Circle Pines MN, 2005, American Guidance Service Publication.

Caligan M, Godi M, Guglielmetti S, et al.: Eye-tracking communication devices in ALS: Impact on disability and quality of life, *Amyotroph Lateral Scler Frontotemporal Degener* 14:546–552, 2013.

Canadian Association of Occupational Therapists: *Enabling occupation: an occupational therapy perspective*, ed 2, Ottawa, ON, 2002, CAOT Publications/ACE.

Colarusso RP, Hammill DD: *Motor free visual perception test manual*, ed 3, Novato, CA, 2003, Academic Therapy Publications.

Cook AM: Development of motor skills for switch use by person with severe disabilities, *Dev Dis Spec Int Sec Newsletter* 14(2), 1991.

Danial-Saad Weiss PL: Schreuer N: Assessment of computer task performance (ACTP) of children and youth with intellectual and developmental disabilities, *Disabil Rehabil Assist Technol* 7:450–458, 2012.

Day H, Jutai JW: Measuring the psychosocial impact of assistive devices: The PIADS, *Can J Rehabil* 9:159–168, 1996.

Day H, Jutai JW, Campbell K: Development of a scale to measure the psychosocial impact of assistive devices: Lessons learned and road ahead, *Disabil Rehabil* 24:31–37, 2002.

Delarosa E, et al.: Family Impact of Assistive Technology Scale: Development of a measurement scale for parents of children with complex communication needs, *Augment Altern Commun* 28:171–180, 2012.

Demers L, Weiss-Lambrou R, Ska B: Development of the Quebec User Evaluation of Satisfaction with Assistive Technology (QUEST), *Assist Technol* 8(3):1–3, 1996.

Demers L, Wessels R, Weiss-Lambrou R, et al.: Key dimensions of client satisfaction with assistive technology: a cross validation of a Canadian measure in the Netherlands, *Assist Technol Res Ser* 27:250–258, 2011.

DeRosier R, Farber RS: Speech recognition software as an assistive device: a pilot study of user satisfaction and psychosocial impact, *WORK* 25:125–134, 2005.

Doyle Lyons K: Blesedell Crepeau E: The clinical reasoning of an occupational therapy assistant, *Am J Occup Ther* 55(5):577–581, 2000.

Dunn W: Sensation and sensory processing. In Blesedell Crepeau E, Cohn ES, et al.: *Willard and Spackman's occupational therapy*, ed 11, Philadelphia, 2009, Lippincott Williams & Wilkins.

Eby DW, Molnar LJ, Pellerito JM: Driving cessation and alternative community mobility. In Pellerito JM, editor: *Driver rehabilitation and community mobility: Principles and practice*, St. Louis, 2006, Mosby.

Erhardt RP: *Erhardt Developmental Prehension Assessment*, Maplewood, MN, 1994, Erhardt Developmental Products.

Fischer AG: *Assessment of motor and process skills*, Fort Collins, CO, 2003, Three Star Press.

Flynn NA, Trombly Latham CA, Podolski CR: Assessing abilities and capacities: Range of motion, strength, and endurance. In Radomski MV, Trombly Latham CA, editors: *Occupational therapy for physical dysfunction*, ed 6, Philadelphia, 2007, Lippincott, Williams & Wilkins.

Fuhrer MJ, Jutai JW, Scherer MJ, DeRuyter F: A framework for the conceptual modelling of assistive technology device outcomes, *Disabil Rehabil* 25:1243–1251, 2003.

Giesbrecht EM, Ripat JD, Quanberry AC, Cooper JE: Community participation and pushrim-activated, power-assisted wheels versus power wheelchairs, *Disabil Rehabil Assist Technol* 4:198–207, 2009.

Haley S, Coster WJ, Ludlow LW, et al.: *Pediatric Evaluation of Disability Inventory (PEDI)*, Boston, 1998, Trustees of Boston University.

Hsieh YJ, Lenker JA: Psychosocial Impact of Assistive Devices Scale: Translation and psychometric evaluation of a Chinese (Taiwanese) version, *Disabil Rehabil Assist Technol* 1:49–57, 2006.

Houghton P, Campbell K: Canadian Practice Guidelines Panel, *Canadian best practice guidelines for the prevention and management of pressure ulcers in people with spinal cord injury: A resource handbook for clinicians*, Toronto, ON, 2013, Neurotrauma Foundation.

Inoue T, Kamimura T, Sasaki K, et al.: Standardization of J-PIADS, *Assist Technol Res Series* 28:49–54, 2011.

Jutai JW, Rigby P, Ryan S, Stickel S: Psychosocial impact of electronic aids to daily living, *Assist Technol* 12:123–131, 2000.

Jutai JW, Day H: Psychosocial Impact of Assistive Devices Scale, *Technol Disabil* 4:107–111, 2002.

Jutai JW, Woolrich W, Strong G: The predictability of retention and discontinuation of contact lenses, *Optometry* 74:299–308, 2003.

Karmarkar AM, Collins DM, Kelleher A, Cooper RA: Satisfaction related to wheelchair use in older adults in both nursing homes and community dwelling, *Disabil Rehabil Assist Technol* 4:337–343, 2009.

Killingsworth AP, Pedretti LW: Joint range of motion. In Pendleton HM, Schultz-Krohn W, editors: *Pedretti's occupational therapy: Practice skills for physical dysfunction*, ed 6, St. Louis, 2006a, Mosby.

Killingsworth AP, Pedretti LW: Evaluation of muscle strength. In Pendleton HM, Schultz-Krohn W, editors: *Pedretti's occupational therapy: Practice skills for physical dysfunction*, ed 6, St. Louis, 2006b, Mosby.

Kirby RL: *Wheelchair Skills Program*, version 3.2, 2005. Available from: http://www.wheelchairskillsprogram.ca.

Kohlmeyer K: Sensory and neuromuscular function. In Blesedell Crepeau E, Cohn ES, Boyt Schell BA, editors: *Willard and Spackman's occupational therapy*, ed 10, Baltimore, 2003, Lippincott Williams & Wilkins.

King GA, McDougall J, Palisano R, et al.: Goal attainment scaling: Its use in evaluating pediatric therapy programs, *Phys Occup Ther Pediatr* 19:31–52, 1999.

Lafayette Instrument: *Minnesota Rate of Manipulation Test, Test Manual,* revised, Lafayette IN: Lafayette Instrument, 1998.

Law M, Baum C, Dunn W: *Measuring occupational performance: Supporting best practice in occupational therapy*, Thorofare, NJ, 2001, SLACK.

Law M, Baptiste S, Carswell A, et al.: *Canadian Occupational Performance Measure*, ed 3, Toronto, 2005, CAOT/ACE Publications.

Lenker JA, Harris F: Taugher M, Smith RO: Consumer perspectives on assistive technology outcomes, *Disabil Rehabil Assist Technol* 8:373–380, 2013.

Light J: Toward a definition of communicative competence for individuals using augmentative and alternative communication systems, *Augment Altern Commun* 5:137–144, 1989.

Light J, Beukleman DR, Reichle J, editors: *Communicative competence for individuals who use AAC: From research to effective practice,* Baltimore: Paul H. Brookes, 2003.

Mao H-F, Chen WY, Yao G, et al.: Cross-cultural adaptation of the QUEST 2.0: The development of the Taiwanese version, *Clin Rehabil* 24:412–421, 2010.

Mattingly C: The narrative nature of clinical reasoning. In Mattingly C, Fleming MH, editors: *Clinical reasoning: Forms of inquiry in a therapeutic practice*, Philadelphia, 1994, FA Davis.

Mattingly C, Fleming MH: *Clinical reasoning: Forms of inquiry in a therapeutic practice*, , Philadelphia, 1994, FA Davis.

McNaughton S: Connecting with consumers, *Assist Technol* 5(1):7–10, 1993.

Miller Polgar J: Critiquing assessments. In Blesedell Crepeau E, Cohn ES, Boyt Schell BA, editors: *Willard and Spackman's occupational therapy*, ed 11, Philadelphia, 2009, Lippincott Williams & Wilkins.

Miller Polgar: J: The myth of neutral technology. In Oishi MMK, Mitchel IM, Van der Loos HFM, editors: *Design and use of assistive technology: Social, technical, ethical and economic challenges*, New York, 2010, Springer.

Nunnally JC, Bernstein IH: *Psychometric theory*, ed 3, Toronto, 1994, McGraw-Hill.

Orellano EM, Jutai JW: Cross cultural adaptation of the Psychosocial Impact of Assistive Devices Scale for Puerto Rican users, *Assist Technol* 25:194–203, 2013.

Pape TL, Kim J, Weiner B: The shape of individual meanings assigned to assistive technology: A review of personal factors, *Disabil Rehabil* 24(1/2/3):5–20, 2002.

Phillips B, Zhao H: Predictors of assistive technology abandonment, *Assist Technol* 5:36–45, 1993.

Quintana LA: Assessing abilities and capacities: Vision, visual perception, and praxis. In Trombly CA, Radomski MV, editors: *Occupational therapy for physical dysfunction*, ed 5, Baltimore, 2002, Lippincott Williams & Wilkins.

Reimer-Weiss ML, Wacker RR: Factors associated with assistive technology discontinuance among individuals with disabilities, *J Rehabil* 66(3):44–50, 2000.

Russel DJ, Rosenbaum P, Wright M, et al.: *Gross Motor Function Measure*, Cambridge, 2002, Cambridge University Press.

Ryan S, Campbell KA, Rigby PJ: Reliability of the FIATS for families of young children with cerebral palsy, *Arch Phys Med Rehabil* 88:1436–1440, 2007.

Ryan S, Campbell KA, Rigby P, et al.: Development of the Family Impact of Assistive Technology Scale, *Int J Rehabil Res* 29:195–200, 2006.

Ryan S, Campbell KA, Rigby PJ, et al.: The impact of adaptive seating devices on the lives of young children and their families, *Arch Phys Med Rehabil* 90:27–33, 2009.

Ryan S, Sawatzky B, Campbell KA, et al.: Functional outcomes associated with adaptive seating interventions in children and youth with wheeled mobility needs, *Arch Phys Med Rehabil*, 2013.

Sackett DL: Evaluation of health services. In Last JM, editor: *Mosley-Roseneau's public health and preventive medicine*, ed 11, New York, 1980, Appleton-Century-Crofts.

Saladin SP, Hansman SE: Psychosocial variables related to the adoption of video relay services among deaf and hard of hearing employees at the Texas School for the Deaf, *Assist Technol* 20:36–47, 2008.

Samant D, Matter R: Harniss M: Realizing the potential of accessible ICTs in developing countries, *Disabil Rehabil Assist Technol* 8(1):11–20, 2013.

Samuelsson K, Wresssle E: User satisfaction with mobility assistive devices: and important element in the rehabilitation process, *Disabil Rehabil* 30:551–558, 2008.

Scheiman M: *Understanding and managing vision deficits: A guide for occupational therapists*, ed 2, Thorofare, NJ, 2002, SLACK.

Scherer M: *Matching person and technology: A series of assessments for evaluating predispositions to and outcomes of technology use in rehabilitation, education, the workplace and other settings*, Webster, NY, 1998, The Institute for Matching Person & Technology.

Scherer MJ: Assistive technology: Matching device and consumer for successful rehabilitation, Washington DC, 2002, American Psychological Association.

Scherer MJ, Sax C, Vanbiervliet A, Cushman LA, Scherer J: Predictors of assistive technology use: the importance of personal and psychosocial factors, *Disabil Rehabil* 27(21):1321–1331, 2005.

Simsek Simşek IE, Ryan SE, et al.: The Turkish version of the Family Impact of Assistive Technology Scale: A validity and reliability study, *Scand J Occup Ther* 19:515–520, 2012.

Toglia JP, Golisz KM: Goverover Y: Evaluation and intervention for cognitive perceptual impairments. In Blesedell Crepeau E, Cohn ES, Boyt Schell BA, editors: *Willard and Spackman's occupational therapy*, ed 11, Philadelphia, 2009, Lippincott Williams & Wilkins.

Tredwell S, Roxborough L: Cerebral palsy seating. In Letts RM, editor: *Principles of seating the disabled*, Boca Raton, FL, 1991, CRC Press.

Uniform Data System for Medical Rehabilitation (UDS): *WeeFIM* version 4.0, Buffalo, NY, 1993, State University of New York at Buffalo.

Uniform Data System for Medical Rehabilitation (UDS): *Functional Independence Measure,* version 5.1, Buffalo, NY, 1997, Buffalo General Hospital. State University of New York.

United Nations: Convention on the rights of persons with disabilities, New York: UN, 2006. Available from: www.un.org/disabilities/convention/conventionfull.shtml

Vincent C, Deaudelin I, Hotten M, et al.: Pilot on evaluating social participation following the use of an assistive technology designed to facilitate face-to-face communication between deaf and hearing persons, *Technol Disabil* 19:153–167, 2007.

Vincent C, Routhier F, Martel V, et al: Electronic mobility aid devices for deafblind persons: Outcome assessment, *Assist Technol Res Serv* 33:559–564, 2013.

Whittemore R, Knafl K: The integrative review: Updated methodology, *J Adv Nurs* 52(5):546-553, 2005.

Wiersma W, Jurs SG: *Educational measurement and testing*, ed 2, Boston, 1990, Allyn and Bacon.

Witt JC, Cavell TA: Psychological assessment. In Wodrich DL, Joy JE, editors: *Multi-disciplinary assessment of children with learning disabilities and mental retardation*, Baltimore, 1986, Paul H Brookes.

World Health Organization: *International Classification of Functioning, Disability and Health*, , Geneva, 2001, World Health Organization.

World Health Organization and US AID from the American People: *Joint position on the provision of mobility devices in less-resourced settings*, Malta, 2011, World Health Organization.

World Health Organization: *World report on disability 2011*, Geneva, 2011, World Health Organization.

CHAPTER 6

Making the Connection: User Inputs for Assistive Technologies

CHAPTER OUTLINE

LEARNING OBJECTIVES

On completing this chapter, you will be able to do the following:

1. Describe the elements of the human/technology interface and its role within the assistive technology component of the Human Activity Assistive Technology model.
2. Describe the ways that various anatomic sites can be used to control assistive technologies (ATs).
3. Identify and define the basic selection methods.
4. Describe the means by which the user's physical control can be enhanced.
5. Describe the major approaches to electronic speech generation used in ATs.
6. Discuss the outcomes that can be achieved through implementation of a motor training program and how technology can be used to improve motor response.

KEY TERMS

Abbreviation Expansion
Acceptance Time
Automatic Scanning
Coded Access
Command Domain
Control Interface
Control Sites
Continuous Input
Digital Recording
Direct Selection
Directed Scanning
Group-Item Scanning
Indirect Selection
Inverse Scanning
Linear Scanning
Prosodic Features
Rotary Scanning
Row-Column Scanning
Scanning
Selection Methods
Selection Set
Speech Synthesis
Step Scanning
Text-to-Speech Programs
Word Completion
Word Prediction

The human/technology interface (HTI) is a major part of the assistive technology component of the Human Activity Assistive Technology (HAAT) model (see Chapter 1). Bailey (1996, p. 173) defines an interface as "the boundary shared by interacting components in a system" in which "the essence of this interaction is communication or the exchange of information back and forth across the boundary." The HTI is the boundary between the human and the assistive technology (AT) across which information is exchanged. In practice, the HTI describes the way in which the human controls the device.

If the individual has good fine motor control, she may use a keyboard or mouse to control a computer or AT device. This control would also let her drive a powered wheelchair using a joystick. If another individual has poor fine motor control, it may be necessary to find alternative ways for him to control ATs or mainstream devices such as computers or cell phones using gross motor movements.

In this chapter, we discuss the possible movements that can be used to control an assistive or mainstream technology electronic device and the most common ways of accommodating for lack of motor control in electronic devices.

ACTIVITY: ENABLING PARTICIPATION

Electronic assistive devices play a major role in supporting participation by individuals who have disabilities. Assistive device control interfaces devices enable users to interact with other technologies. As discussed in Chapter 2, these technologies may be mainstream devices such as phones and tablets (see Chapter 8) or specialized ATs such as electronic aids to daily living (EADLs) (see Chapter 12), power wheelchairs (see Chapter 10), cognitive ATs (see Chapter 15), or communication devices (see Chapter 16). Each of these technologies can contribute to productivity in work or school, support recreation, and enable social participation on a broad basis. None of these benefits can occur without a well-designed and well-implemented HTI that links the user to the technology.

HUMAN: ANATOMIC SITES FOR CONTROL OF ASSISTIVE TECHNOLOGIES

The HTI for ATs described by the HAAT model links two major components, the human and the technology. In this section, the variety of required human capabilities that can be accommodated by control interfaces is described.

Control interfaces are typically used by individuals who have reduced fine motor control that makes it difficult to use common HTIs such as computer keyboards, pointing devices such as a mouse, or touch screens (see Chapter 8); light switches; controls on entertainment devices such as TVs or DVD players; and similar everyday items (see Chapter 12). Control interfaces are also useful to people who need to use a powered wheelchair (see Chapter 10) or use adapted controls to drive a vehicle (see Chapter 11).

Figure 6-1 shows the body sites that can be used to control a device. These are called **control sites.** Control sites include the hand or finger, arm, head, eye, leg, foot, and mouth (for switches based on respiration or phonation). Each control site is capable of performing a variety of movements or actions. When the interaction between a person with a disability and an assistive device involves relatively fine control, the hand and fingers are the preferred control sites because they are typically used for manipulative tasks. Even if hand control is limited, control interfaces can accommodate for limitations in fine motor control. It is also possible to improve the existing function by using control enhancers (described later in this chapter).

If fine motor control limitations prevent hand use, then the use of the head as a control site is preferred. It is possible to obtain relatively precise control using head movements such as tilting side to side, horizontal rotation, and linear forward and backward movement. Very few functional head movements are purely horizontal, vertical, or rotational.

If both hand and head control are poor, then control interfaces, generally switches, can be used to detect movements of the shoulder, elbow, forearm, hand, or finger. The use of the arm or leg is less desirable for precise tasks because these represent naturally gross movements controlled by large muscle groups, limiting their usefulness for manipulative functions such as keyboard use. Shoulder movements include elevation, flexion, extension, abduction (away from the body), and adduction (toward the body). The movements of the elbow are flexion and extension. The movements of the forearm consist of pronation (turning the palm down) and supination (turning the palm up). The wrist can flex or extend or move from side to side (radial deviation or ulnar deviation). The fingers can individually flex and extend or, together, perform a grasp and release movement. The thumb can flex and extend, abduct and adduct, and oppose each of the fingers. Each of these types of movements can be detected by an appropriate control interface.

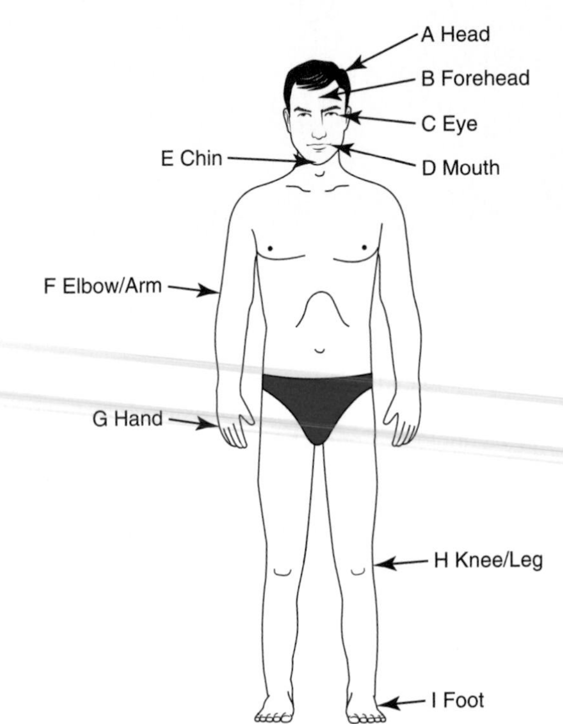

FIGURE 6-1 Anatomic sites commonly used for control of assistive technologies. (From Webster JW, Cook AM, Tompkins WJ, Vanderheiden GC: *Electronic devices for rehabilitation,* New York, 1985, John Wiley and Sons, p. 207.)

Another control site is foot movement. For fine manipulative tasks, the foot is less desirable than the hand or head because visual monitoring can be difficult, and the foot is generally not as finely controlled as the hand. However, some individuals are able to develop fine control of their feet for typing (Figure 6-2). Control movements used in the lower extremities include raising and lowering of the leg at the hip (e.g., hip abduction and adduction, knee flexion and extension) foot plantar flexion (toes point down) or dorsiflexion (toes point up), and foot inversion or eversion (rotary movement, similar to pronation and supination). Switches of various types can be controlled by these movements.

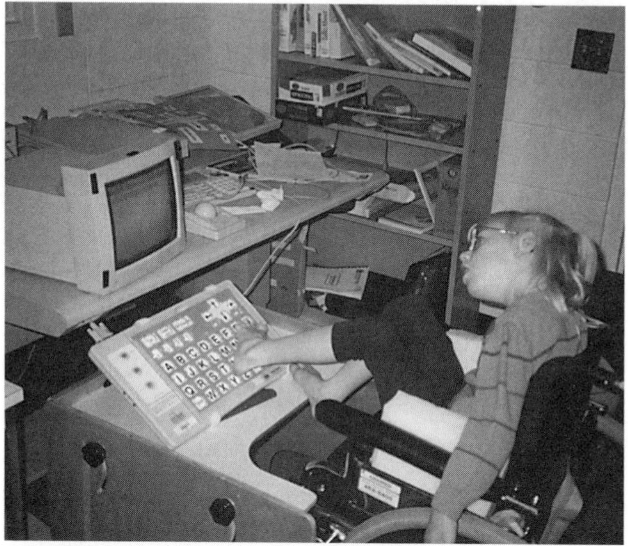

FIGURE 6-2 Child using her foot to control an expanded keyboard.

Finally, respiratory air flow can be detected and used as a control site by sip (inhaling) or puff (exhaling) to access switches. *Phonation* may produce sounds (including whistling) or speech. Control interfaces that can detect sound and speech recognition can also be used as a control interface. Tongue movements can also be used for control.

Muscle tone (high or low), strength, endurance, range of motion, the presence of tremor, and the type of tremor can all lead to reduced motor control that would require specialized HTIs. Disabilities that affect fine motor control can result in conditions that limit fine motor control (Case Study 6-1).

> **CASE STUDY 6-1**
>
> ***Comparative Evaluation***
>
> Max is an 18-year-old young man who has cerebral palsy. He lives in a residential facility and attends a work program through United Cerebral Palsy. Max has been referred to ABC Assistive Technology Center for a communication device. He currently communicates with others using a manual communication board and eye blinks for yes and no.
>
> Through evaluation of Max's range and resolution, it has been determined that his best control sites are his right hand and his head. However, he does not have fine enough control at either site to use direct selection. You decide to perform comparative interface testing using a tread switch with his hand and a lever switch at the side of his head. Data collected during the comparative testing phase of the evaluation show that Max is more accurate and faster activating the switch with his head (versus his hand). However, Max has indicated a preference for using his hand instead of his head.
>
> **Questions**
>
> 1. Given Max's limited verbal communication, how would you gather information from him regarding his opinion on the hand and the head switches?
> 2. What type of subjective information would you want to gather from Max regarding his use of and preference for each of these two switches?
> 3. Your data indicate that Max is faster and more accurate using the head switch. However, Max has indicated to you that he prefers the hand switch. What would your recommendation be and why?

ASSISTIVE TECHNOLOGY: CONNECTING THE USER TO THE TECHNOLOGY

Elements of the Human/Technology Interface

Three technology elements of the HTI contribute to the operation of a device: the control interface, the **selection set,** and the selection method. These three elements are interrelated, and careful attention must be given to each element to have an effective HTI.

Control Interface

The **control interface** is the hardware by which the human in the AT system operates or controls a device. It is sometimes also referred to as an *input device.* Examples of control interfaces include a keyboard, one or more switches, a touch screen or touch pad, a mouse, and a joystick.

Selection Set

Each control interface allows the user to choose one or more items that provide input to the AT device or control its operation in some way. The group of items available from which choices are made is called the **selection set** (Lee & Thomas, 1990). For example, if a person wants to use a power wheelchair, the selection set might be forward, back, left, right, and stop. For typing on a computer with a special control interface, the selection set would be the entire computer keyboard. Selection sets can be represented by traditional orthography (e.g., written letters, words, and sentences), symbols used to represent ideas, computer screen icons, line drawings, or pictures. The modalities in which the selection set is presented can be visual (e.g., letters on the keyboard or icons on the screen), tactile (e.g., braille), or auditory (e.g., spoken choices in auditory scanning).

The size, modality, and type of selection set chosen are based on the user's needs and the desired *activity output* (see Chapter 1). Activity outputs in the HAAT model include communication (replacing or augmenting speech or writing), mobility, manipulation (e.g., things we would normally do with our hands and arms), and cognition (assisting with mental activities). An EADL (see Chapter 12) or a power wheelchair (see Chapter 10) typically has fewer choices in the selection set than an augmentative communication device (see Chapter 16) or computer (see Chapter 8). The size of the selection set may also vary according to the user's skills and age. For example, an individual who spells and has good physical control has the skills to use the selection set of a standard keyboard, which consists of all the letters and function keys. Another individual who is working on developing language and communication skills may have a selection set consisting of only two picture symbol choices displayed on a lap tray.

Selection Methods

There are two basic **selection methods** that an individual with a disability can use to make selections with a control interface, direct selection and indirect selection. Direct selection methods generally have one interface for each selection that can be made. For example, each letter on a keyboard has a separate key. Indirect selection methods include **scanning,** directed scanning, and coded access.

The Processor: Connecting the Control Interface to the Desired Activity Output

When the control interface is activated by the user, information is sent via a signal to the *processor.* The processor interprets the information and generates two signals that are converted to (1) feedback to any display that is being used and (2) an activity output, depending on the functions of the AT system. For example, a power wheelchair (see Chapter 10) joystick is typically set up so that the signal for the UP input is transformed into forward movement of the wheelchair, DOWN into reverse movement, LEFT into movement to the left, and RIGHT into movement to the right. That same joystick can be used to control a television set (see Chapter 12) in which the same four movements of UP, DOWN, LEFT, and RIGHT control television volume up, volume down, channel up, and channel down, respectively. The *selection set* must include an element corresponding to each function of the device.

Direct Selection

Direct selection allows the individual to use the control interface to randomly choose any item in the selection set. The person indicates her choice by using voice, finger, hand, eye, or other body movement. In this method of selection, the user identifies a target and goes directly to it (Smith, 1991). At any one time, all of the elements of the selection set are equally available for selecting. Typing on a keyboard or picking a flower from the garden is direct selection. Direct selection is the most difficult method physically because it requires refined, controlled movements. Because there is an immediate, direct result from the selection made, it is more intuitive and easy to understand, and the cognitive demands are not great. Figure 6-3 shows the input that is made using direct selection to obtain the letter *S.* The various types of control interfaces that allow the individual to use direct selection are described later in this chapter.

Indirect Selection

When an individual's physical control does not support direct selection, indirect selection methods are considered. **Indirect selection** involves intermediary steps to make a selection. The most common indirect selection methods are scanning, directed scanning, and coded access. Most electronic AT devices can be accessed by more than one type of control interface and selection method. The selection set on most devices also can be varied to match the user's needs. From a manufacturing perspective, the versatility of a device allows it to be applicable to a wider population, which helps to contain the cost of the device and makes it possible to adapt to changing user needs and skills.

Scanning

With scanning, the selection set is presented on a display, and each item in the selection set is sequentially lighted or indicated by sound or speech. When the particular element that the individual wishes to choose is presented, the user activates a control interface to select that item. The control interface used for scanning is typically a single switch or an array of two or more switches. Depending on the needs of the user, scanning can vary in the format (type of symbols and the way they are presented). The way that the control interface signal is used to make the selection can also vary. Scanning requires good visual tracking skills, a high degree of attention, and the ability to sequence. The advantage of scanning is that it requires very little motor control to make a selection.

Because scanning is inherently slow, there have been a number of approaches used to make it more efficient and faster for the user. The major method for improving scanning efficiency is to use techniques that are efficient in that they allow the user to select groups of entries (e.g., letters) as opposed to entering them singly. Approaches that do this are called *rate enhancement,* and they are discussed later in this chapter.

A major challenge in scanning is maximizing the scan rate. If the rate is too fast, users will not be able to make accurate selections because they cannot respond fast enough. If the rate is too slow, the text entry rate (TER) will be slower than necessary and cause the user to be slower at generating input than is necessary. A reliable and systematic method for selecting the most appropriate scan rate for single-switch

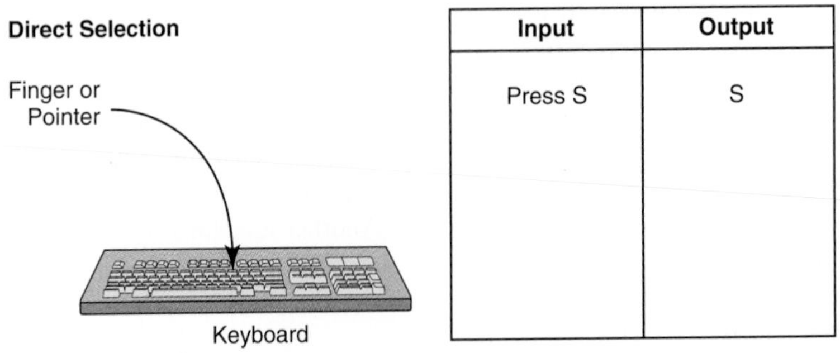

Direct Selection

Finger or Pointer

Keyboard

Input	Output
Press S	S

FIGURE 6-3 This figure shows the input required to obtain the letter *S* using direct selection. (From Smith RO: Technological approaches to performance enhancement. In Christiansen C, Baum C, editors: *Occupational therapy: Overcoming human performance deficits,* Thorofare, NJ: SLACK, 1991.)

scanning that avoids excessive trial and error is provided by the "0.65 rule" (Simpson et al., 2006). The 0.65 rule is based on data showing that the ratio between a user's reaction time and an appropriate scan rate for that user is approximately 0.65. The clinical implication is that if the consumer's reaction time can be measured, then dividing this number by 0.65 will give a scanning rate in scan per seconds that is likely to be the optimal rate for that person. For example, if the reaction time is 1 second, then the scan rate would be 1/0.65, which equals about 1.5 scan steps per second. Simpson et al. (2006) carried out a study with six individuals with significant physical disabilities secondary to cerebral palsy (CP) who used scanning for their typical data entry. The participants made entries using their own system, and the results with scan rate determined by the 0.65 rule were compared with the results with a self-selected scan rate. The data supported the hypothesis that a scan rate recommended by the 0.65 rule yielded speed and accuracy performance that was as good as or better than performance with subjects' self-selected scan rates for this group of participants.

Directed Scanning

Directed scanning is a hybrid approach in which the user activates the control interface to select the direction of the scan, vertically or horizontally. There is typically one switch for each direction of movement, typically four directions, but it can be as many as eight. The user first selects the direction in which he wishes to scan. The cursor continues to move in the selected direction by the user holding down the switch. When the switch is released, the cursor stops, and the user either waits for an **acceptance time** interval or hits an additional switch. The acceptance time is actually a slight delay between the time the selection is made and the time it is sent to the device. It allows the user to make a choice by merely waiting for the acceptance time to expire. The selected item is sent to the device.

A joystick or an array of switches (two to eight switches) is the control interface used with directed scanning. Figure 6-4 gives an example of the input required to select the letter *S* using directed scanning with a four-position joystick. Directed scanning requires more steps than direct selection but fewer steps than single-switch scanning. The user needs to be able to activate and hold the control interface and to release it at the appropriate time. If the individual can produce the movements required to use this method, the outcome is faster entry of the desired selections into the device.

Selection Techniques for Scanning

The action required by the user to activate the control interface to make a selection during scanning and directed scanning usually can be varied to accommodate the user's skills. Table 6-1 lists the three scanning techniques and the level of motor skill required by the technique. This table is helpful in matching the scanning technique to the user's skills. For example, some techniques depend more on the ability to react quickly to activate a switch. Others require vigilance and the ability to wait until a choice appears. Still others require the user to hold a switch until the choice appears and then release.

Automatic scanning continuously presents items that the user may choose. The rate of presentation (scan rate) can be set and adjusted according to how fast the user can respond.

TABLE 6-1 Selection Techniques for Scanning and Directed Scanning

	Automatic Scanning	Step Scanning	Inverse Scanning
Wait	High	Low	Medium
Activate	High	Medium	Low
Hold	Low	Low	High
Release	Low	Medium	High
Motor fatigue	Low	High	Low
Sensory/cognitive vigilance	High	Low	High

Modified from Beukelman D, Mirenda P: *Augmentative and alternative communication,* ed 3, Baltimore: Paul H. Brookes, 2013, p. 151.

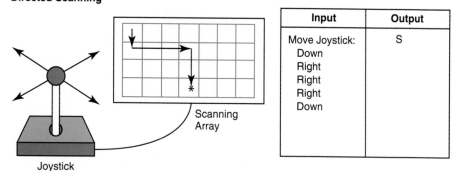

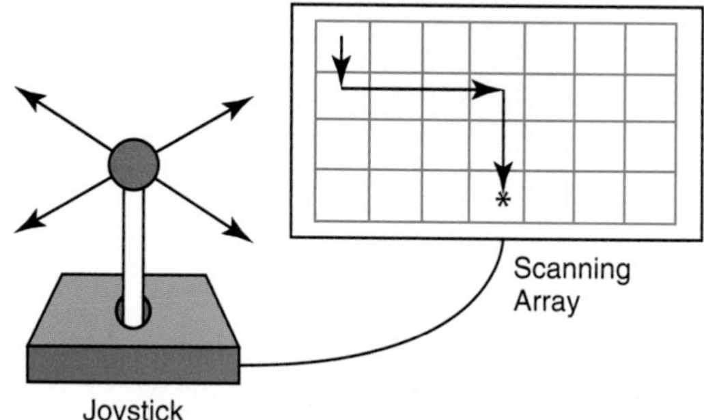

Input	Output
Move Joystick: Down Right Right Right Down	S

FIGURE 6-4 Directed scanning showing the input required to select the letter *S*. The user selects the direction of the scan, and the items in the selection set are scanned sequentially by the device. When the desired item is reached, the user makes the selection. (From Smith RO: Technological approaches to performance enhancement. In Christiansen C, Baum C, editors: *Occupational therapy: Overcoming human performance deficits,* Thorofare, NJ: SLACK, 1991.)

When the desired selection is presented, the user selects the choice by activating the control interface and stopping the scan. Automatic scanning requires a high degree of motor skill by the user to wait for the desired selection and to activate the control interface in the given time frame. It also requires a high degree of sensory and cognitive vigilance for attending to and tracking the cursor on the display.

In **step scanning**, the user activates the control interface once for each item to advance through the choices in the selection set. When the user comes to the desired choice, there are two possibilities for selecting it. Either an additional control interface is used to give a signal to select that choice or an acceptance time is used. Step scanning allows the user to control the speed at which the items are presented. The ability to wait or pause is not required for the scan, but it may be for the acceptance of the selection. The ability to activate the control interface repeatedly, however, is important for step scanning. Motor fatigue can be high because of repeated control interface activation.

Inverse scanning is initiated by the individual activating and holding the control interface closed (e.g., keeping a switch pressed). As long as the control interface is held down, the items are scanned. When the desired choice appears, the individual releases the control interface to make the selection. Inverse scanning requires holding the control interface and releasing it at the proper time. Inverse scanning may be easier for some people than automatic scanning, which requires activation of the control interface within a specified time frame. For individuals who require lots of time to initiate and follow through with movement, inverse scanning can be helpful. Similar to automatic scanning, motor fatigue is reduced over step scanning because of fewer control interface activations; however, sensory and cognitive fatigue are higher because of the vigilance required to attend to the display.

Automatic scanning can be difficult for individuals with spastic CP, and step scanning is difficult for those with athetoid CP (Davies et al., 2010). There is no conclusive evidence regarding the best method for each group.

Selection Formats for Scanning

There are a number of formats in which the items in the selection set can be presented to the user for selection in scanning (Box 6-1). In a **linear scanning** format, as shown in Figure 6-5, the items in the selection set are presented in a vertical or horizontal line and scanned one at a time until the desired selection is highlighted and selected by the user. Circular, or **rotary, scanning** (Figure 6-6) presents the items in a circle and scans them one at a time.

To increase the rate of selection during scanning, **group-item scanning** can replace the singular-item scan. In this case, there are several items in a group, and the groups are sequentially scanned as a whole. The individual first selects the group that has the desired element. After the group has been selected, the individual items in that group are scanned until the desired item is reached. When there are a large number of items, a *matrix* scan can be used. In this type of scanning, the *group* is a row of items and the *items* are located in columns, and it is called **row-column scanning.** In row-column scanning, there may be several rows of items, and each complete row is highlighted sequentially. The row with the desired item is selected; then each column in that row lights up until the desired item is selected. Figure 6-7 shows the input required using a single switch with row–column scanning to produce the letter *S*.

There are other ways that scanning formats can be adapted to increase the user's rate of selection. *Halving* is a group-item

BOX 6-1 Scanning Formats

Selection Set Formats
Linear
Circular
Matrix

Adaptations to Formats for Increasing Rate of Selection
Group item
Row–column
Halving
Quartering
Frequency of use placement

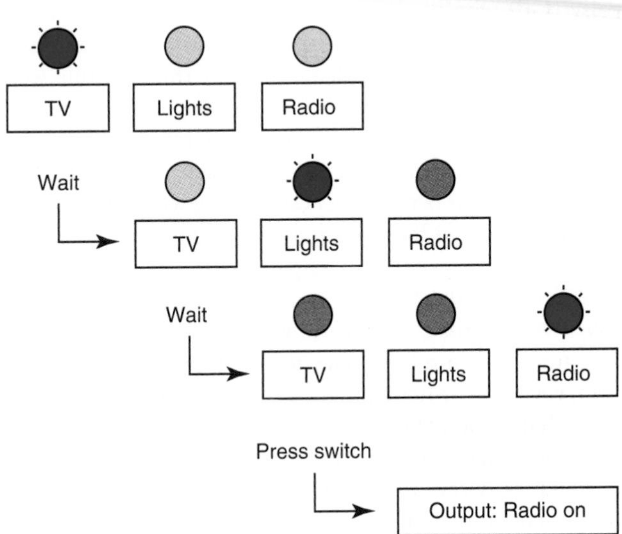

FIGURE 6-5 In linear scanning, choices are presented vertically or horizontally one at a time.

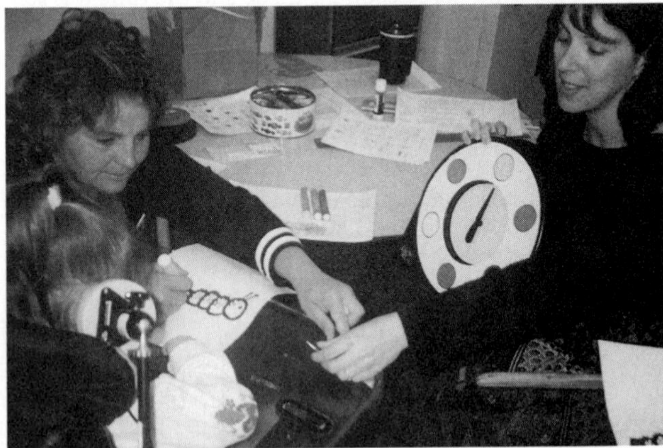

FIGURE 6-6 In rotary scanning, choices are presented one at a time in a circle. Here a child is choosing the color she wants to use by pressing her S which when the pointer is aimed at her choice.

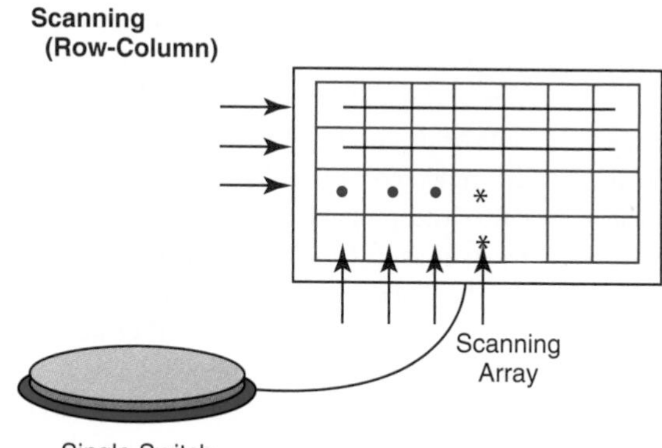

Input	Output
Press Switch	S
Wait	
Wait	
Press Switch	
Wait	
Wait	
Wait	
Press Switch	

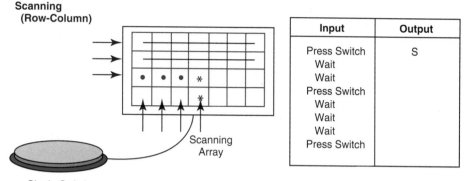

FIGURE 6-7 Row–column scanning showing the input required for selecting the letter *S*. The rows are first scanned and the user selects the row with the desired item. Then each item in that row is scanned until the desired item is selected. (From Smith RO: Technological approaches to performance enhancement. In Christiansen C, Baum C, editors: *Occupational therapy: Overcoming human performance deficits,* Thorofare, NJ: SLACK, 1991.)

approach in which the total array is divided in halves. Each half is scanned until the user selects the desired half. The scanning then proceeds in a row–column format as described until the desired item is reached. This same concept can be used in a *quartering format* in which the array is divided into fourths.

Another method used to increase rate of selection is to place the selection set elements in the scanning array according to their frequency of use. For example, if letters are being used as the selection set, placement of *E, T, A, O, N,* and *I* (the most frequently used letters) in the upper left positions of the scanning array results in an increase in rate of selection (Simpson, 2013). The application of these principles to augmentative communication is discussed in Chapter 16.

Choosing Scanning Setups for Individual Users

Scanning involves a number of variables that can affect user performance. Scan rate as described earlier is only one. The 0.65 rule is helpful for setting an initial scan rate, but there are still many options such as the arrangement of the selection set and the choice of selection method that need to be chosen for an individual. If a trial and error approach is used, it can be very difficult to obtain a configuration that yields optimal performance. "Often, so much time is spent just identifying a reliable switch site and a basic scan layout appropriate for the user's needs that very little time is left to properly adjust the remaining options" (Simpson et al., 2011, p. 2).

Models that predict performance under different configurations provide one way to choose the most appropriate configuration for a particular client (Bhattacharya et al., 2008; Simpson et al., 2011). Most of the models that have been developed assume error-free performance by the user (e.g., Bhattacharya et al., 2008). These models do not generally provide predictive performance that is closely matched to actual user results in clinical trials. Simpson et al. (2011) developed an approach that models errors and includes several types of error correction commonly applied in scanning systems when an incorrect switch activation is made by the use. The error correction methods evaluated by Simpson et al. included (1) setting a fixed number of times for the scanning to loop through the row or column or the array before starting over at the beginning (fixed loop count), (2) a stop scanning selection at the end of each row, (3) activating the switch for an extended time, and (4) selecting an (incorrect) item within the row. In addition to these errors of commission, there is the error of omission in which the user fails to make a choice in a row. Two methods of correcting for this type of error were modeled by Simpson et al.: (1) a fixed loop count as earlier and (2) a "continue scanning" item at the end of the row that is selected to restart the scanning through the row.

Using configuration options from 16 commercially available scanning systems, Simpson et al. (2011) modeled performance with varying probabilities of errors for each type described earlier. Based on their model results, they concluded that the best approach for clinicians is to: (1) use a frequency-arranged matrix, (2) avoid extra "bells and whistles" such as stop scanning or reverse scanning items, and (3) keep error rates as low as possible by focusing on development of switch skill as we describe later in this chapter.

Mankowski et al. (2013) carried out a clinical trial with five users of scanning systems to validate the error-free model developed by Simpson et al. (2011). There were five participants who were all single-switch scanning users. Scanning rate was selected using the 0.65 rule with a comparison with the participant's current scan rate.

The Simpson et al. model was used to calculate the projected TER, and this was compared with the actual TER obtained by the users transcribing a set of sentences. Alphabetic and frequency of occurrence scanning arrays were used by all participants. The predicted and actual TERs were within 10.49% averaged over all participants. For a model assuming error-free performance, the model error was 79.7%.

Mankowski et al. discuss clinical applications of this model that allow consideration of factors that will increase TER while also minimizing the chance of error.

Coded Access

Another form of indirect selection is **coded access** in which the individual uses a distinct sequence of movements to input a code for each item in the selection set. Similar to the other two methods of indirect selection, intermediate steps are required for making a selection.

The control interface used is a single switch or an array of switches configured to match the code. Morse code is one example of coded access, wherein the selection set is the alphabet but an intermediate step is necessary in order to obtain a letter. Each letter in the alphabet has a code consisting of short (dot) or long (dash) entries. The required sequence of movements for obtaining the letter *C* is dash, dot, dash, dot. Figure 6-8 shows the steps required for obtaining the letter *C* using two-switch Morse code.

In single-switch Morse code, the system is configured so that a quick activation and release of the switch results in a dot, and holding the switch closed for a longer period before releasing it results in a dash. Letter boundaries are distinguished by a slightly longer pause than between dots and dashes within one letter. As long as the user holds one of the switches, it continues to send dots or dashes. In two-switch Morse code, one switch is configured to represent a dot and the other switch a dash. This can make the entry of codes much faster, but it requires motor control sufficient to activate and release a switch quickly enough to avoid extraneous dots or dashes to be entered. The rate at which dots or dashes are repeated is usually adjustable. The computer automatically interprets the code as a letter or other character and treats it as if it had been typed.

The user must enter a series of long or short switch presses to access a letter or other keyboard entry (e.g., space bar, number, special symbol such as $ or #). Morse code was developed to be very efficient by assigning the most frequently used letters the shortest codes, (e.g., E is one dot, T is one dash). Figure 6-9 shows the symbols for international Morse code. This efficiency can be useful in written or conversational communication. In addition, Morse code does not require that a selection set be displayed as in scanning. The codes are usually memorized, although visual displays, diagrams, or charts can be used to aid in recalling the codes (Figure 6-10).

Similar to scanning, coded access requires less physical skill than direct selection. The advantage of coded access over scanning, however, is that the timing of the input is under the control of the user and is not dependent on the device. For example, the user decides how long a dot and dash last and how long to hold the switch to generate each one for Morse code, but in scanning, she has to wait for the correct choice to be presented, so the device controls the timing. The disadvantage is that coded access takes more cognitive skill, especially memory and sequencing, than direct selection.

Because codes are typically memory based, they do not require a selection display (a set of characters on the

Input	Morse code	Output
Press Switch 1	—	
Press Switch 2	•	
Press Switch 1	—	
Press Switch 2	•	C

FIGURE 6-8 The input required for selecting the letter *C* using Morse code.

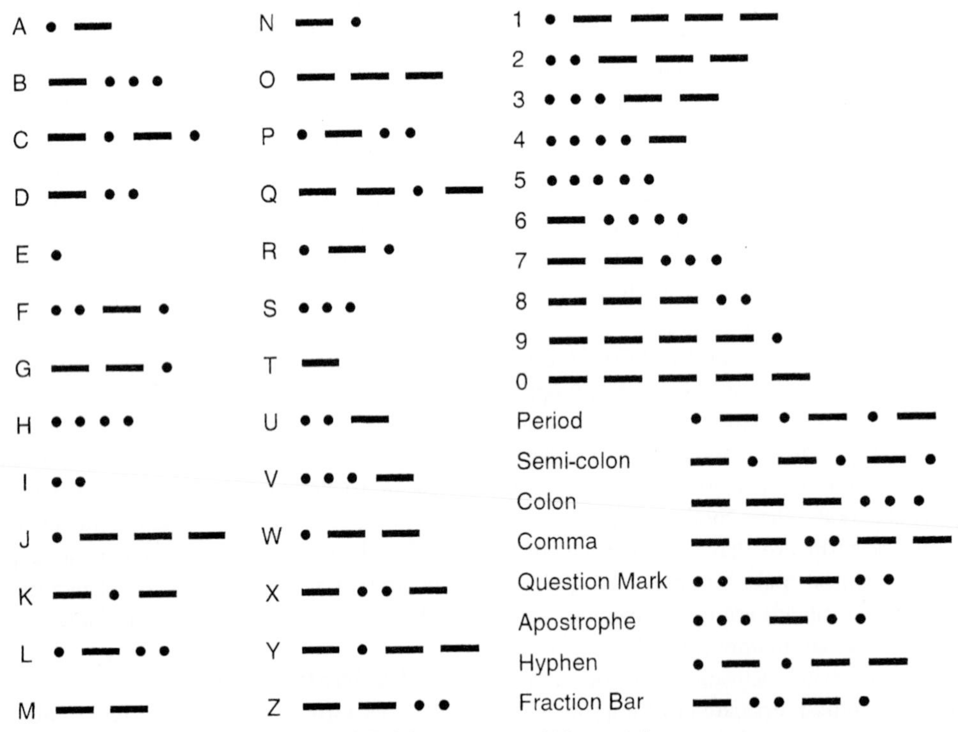

FIGURE 6-9 International Morse code.

screen) as is needed for an on-screen keyboard or scanning array. This method allows the entire screen to be used for the application software being run. It can also be used by people who have visual impairments. Original Morse code (letters and numbers only) did not include other computer items such as ESC or RETURN keys or characters such as punctuation or \ /@#$%. The absence of standardized codes for anything other than alphanumeric characters has resulted in different AT Morse code systems having different codes for these characters. Examples of codes developed for computer use by several different manufacturers are listed in Table 6-2.

Note that in some cases, the codes for the same characters are different for the two systems, and in other cases, they are the same. After the set of codes is learned and the motor patterns developed, it is very difficult to change to a new set of codes, and changing from one system to another can be both time consuming and frustrating for the consumer.

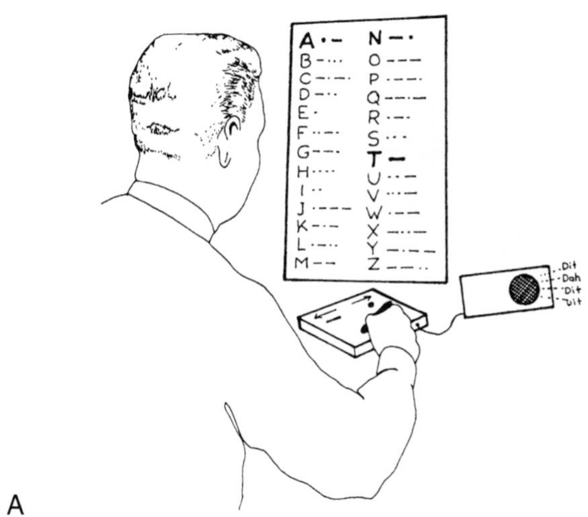

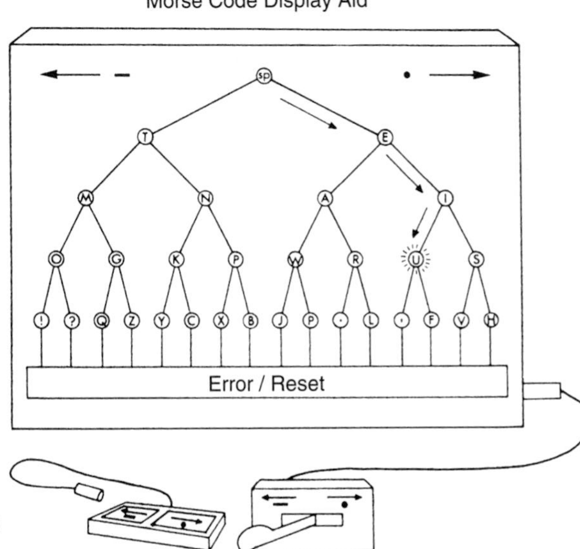

FIGURE 6-10 Encoding systems may be either chart based (**A**) or display based (**B**). (From Blackstone S: *Augmentative communication*, Rockville, MD: American Speech Language Hearing Association, 1986.)

Rate Enhancement

Rate enhancement refers to all approaches that result in the number of characters generated being greater than the number of selections the individual makes. For example, using "ASAP[space]" for "As soon as possible [space]" saves 16 keystrokes. Because an increased level of efficiency is obtained, the user has to make fewer entries, and the overall rate is increased. Rate enhancement goals and approaches differ for direct selection and scanning. In direct selection, the goal is to reduce the number of keystrokes while increasing the amount of information selected with each keystroke. In scanning, the goal is to optimize the scanning array to reduce the time required to make a desired selection. Specific approaches are discussed later in this section. Rate enhancement is used for many electronic AT applications, including augmentative communication (see Chapter 16), computer access (this chapter), cell phone access (Chapter 8), and EADLs (see Chapter 12). Many mainstream software applications use some form of rate enhancement, also called input acceleration. For example, users of email will be familiar with the list of options that appear after a few letters of an address are typed. These represent the email addresses that the program has "learned" from previous entries. This application had its origin in AT word prediction applications. Similar functionality is present in many cell phones.

Effective rate enhancement requires that the motor task become automatic (Blackstone, 1990). Motor patterns become more automatic as they are practiced. One familiar motor pattern is that of entering a commonly used phone number. Sometimes we cannot actually remember the digits of the number, but we can enter it just by the stored motor pattern (e.g., remembering the number by looking at the keypad).

TABLE 6-2 Nonstandardized Morse Codes Used for Computer Access‡

Character	Comax*	Darci Too†
ESC	..-..	..-..
ENTER	.-.-	.-.-
DELETE	-..-.	-..-.
TAB	-.--.	-.- -.
period.	.-.-.-	.-.-.-
!	.-..--	.-..- -
$	-...-.	-...-.
SPACE	..--	..- -
Comma	--..--	- -..- -
".	-- --	- -.- -
(	...--.	...- -.
)	-..--.	-.. - -.
UP ARROW	----..	- ---..
DOWN ARROW	------	------
LEFT ARROW	----.-	-----.
RIGHT ARROW	-----.	- -.-.-.

*http://comax.software.informer.com/
†http://www.westest.com/.
‡Standard alphanumerical Morse code characters are shown in Table 6-2.

TABLE 6-3 Modes (Memory, Chart, Display) of Presentation of Codes to the User

Type	Memory-Based	Chart-Based	Display-Based
Memory required	Recall	Recognition	Recognition
Advantages	Can be used by those with visual limitations	Can be seen by both user and partner	Can be updated (dynamic display), giving many stored items
Disadvantages	Limited to 200 to 300 items for most people	Must have chart in visual field; chart can become separated from device	Requires attention to display; can slow down text selection because of split attention

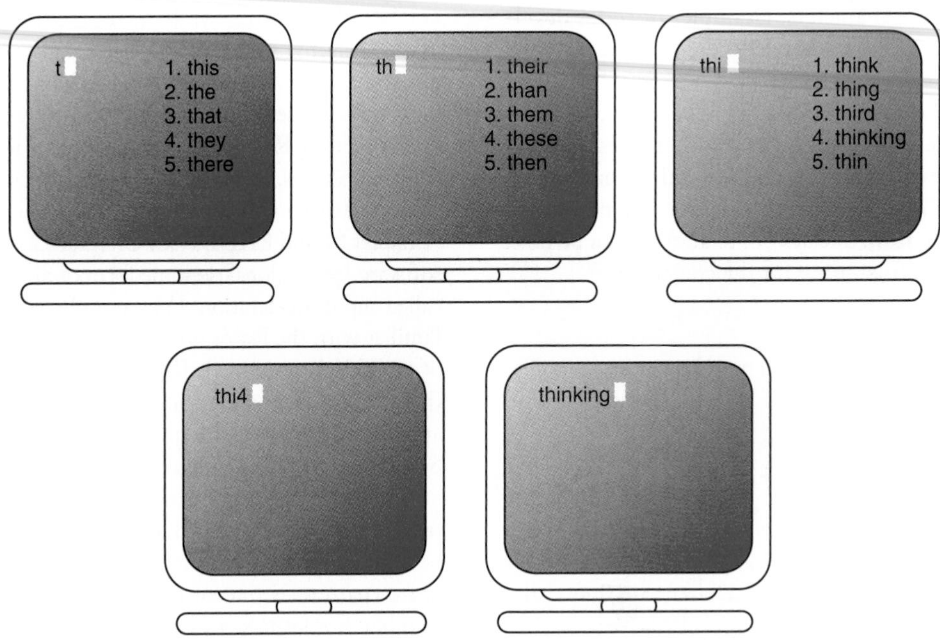

FIGURE 6-11 Word completion systems present a series of choices based on previous letters entered.

As the skills improve, motor and cognitive tasks become more automatic, and the user becomes an "expert." As Blackstone points out, after these motor patterns are established, even small changes in the task may result in dramatic *decreases* in rate. This effect on efficiency is why it is important to keep menu items or selection set items in the same place even as new items are added.

Rate enhancement techniques fall into two broad categories: (1) encoding techniques and (2) prediction techniques. Vanderheiden and Lloyd (1986) distinguish three basic types of codes: memory based, chart based, and display based. These are compared in Table 6-3.

A memory-based technique requires that both the user and his partner know the codes by memory or that the user has the codes memorized for entry into his device. Chart-based techniques are those that have an index of the codes and their corresponding vocabulary items. This can be a simple paper list attached to an electronic device or a chart on the wall (e.g., two eye blinks = "call nurse"; three eye blinks = "please turn me"; eyes up = "yes"; eyes down = "no"). Figure 6-10 illustrates both a chart-based and display-based approach for Morse code (Vanderheiden & Lloyd, 1986). In each device, two switches are used. The right switch produces dots, and the left one produces dashes.

CASE STUDY 6-2

Word Prediction Vocabularies

Assume that one college student is taking a course in assistive technologies and another student is taking a course in world religions. If both students have word completion/prediction systems, compare the word lists you might expect to be used for writing homework assignments for each course. Would most words be the same, or would they be different for the two applications? How would the word lists vary in (1) an adaptive system and (2) a nonadaptive system? What words would you start with as a basic vocabulary in each case?

Word prediction or **word completion** approaches use a window on the screen that displays an ordered list of the most likely words based on the letters entered. In word completion, the user selects the desired word, if any, by entering its code (e.g., a number listed next to the word) or continuing to enter letters if the desired word is not displayed (Figure 6-11) (Case Study 6-2). Word prediction devices offer a menu of words based on previous words entered. (e.g., "*computer*" leads to list of "software," "system," "program," and "keyboard"). The most important advantage of this approach is that the user needs only recognition memory, not recall. It also eliminates the need for memorizing codes. Word prediction (or completion) approaches require that the user

TABLE 6-4 Types of Speech Output Used in Assistive Technologies

Type of Speech Output	Major Features	Typical Assistive Technology Applications
Digital recording	Uses actual voice and can easily be child, male, or female Speech is limited to what is stored Relatively low cost	Augmentative communication
Speech synthesis	Very high quality for single words or complete phrases Intelligibility decreases for unlimited vocabulary with text to speech Unlimited vocabulary with text to speech Moderate intelligibility with letter-to-sound rules only Highly intelligible with morphonemic rules Cost depends on text-to-speech approach	Speech output for electronic aids to daily living Augmentative communication Screen readers for blind users Speech output for users with learning disabilities Speech output for phone communication by persons who are deaf

redirect the gaze from the input (keyboard keys or scanning array) to a list of words after each entry to check for the presence of the desired word, which can reduce the item selection rate compared with letter-by-letter typing. This reduction in selection rate is due to "cognitive or perceptual load" that can offset the benefits achieved in keystroke savings and result in an overall decrease in text generation rate (Hortsman & Levine, 1989). There are also cognitive demands placed on the user by the way in which the rate enhancement is implemented.

If the word lists are placed on the screen at the point in the document where the typed letters appear, then the user does not need to redirect his gaze to check the word list while typing. This approach can result in significantly fewer control interface activations in scanning. One application of this approach, called Smart Lists (Applied Human Factors Helotes, TX, http://www.ahf-net.com), can be used with either keyboard or scanning entry. Smart Keys (also Applied Human Factors Helotes) is similar to the Minspeak icon prediction (see Chapter 16). After each entry, only the keys that contain a prediction based on that entry are left on the on-screen keyboard, which can make scanning significantly faster because only the relevant keys need to be scanned.

Predictive approaches may be fixed or adaptive. Fixed types have a stored word list based on frequency of use that never changes. This method is anticipated and consistent for the user and can help in the development of motor and cognitive patterns for retrieval. Adaptive vocabularies change the ordering of words in the dictionary list by keeping track of the words used by the person. The words are always listed in frequency-of-use order customized to the individual user and are more directly matched to the user's needs and recent usage.

Current technologies may include combinations of abbreviation expansion and word prediction. **Abbreviation expansion** is a technique in which a shortened form of a word or phrase (the abbreviation) stands for the entire word or phrase (the expansion). The abbreviations are automatically expanded by the device into the desired word or phrase. Abbreviations are more direct because the user can merely enter the code and immediately get the desired word, and they allow complete phrases and sentences. Predictions are easier to use because they do not require memorization of codes. These two techniques are actually very similar for fixed predictive systems. For example, in Figure 6-11, the entry for "thinking" is the sequence *thi4 [keystroke t-h-i followed by #4 when word selection pops up]*.

SPEECH: A HUMAN/TECHNOLOGY INTERFACE OUTPUT

Speech is the auditory form of language, and electronic ATs that provide language output rely on artificial speech. The three major AT applications are screen readers and print-material reading machines for persons who are blind (see Chapter 13), voice output augmentative communication devices (see Chapter 16), and alternative reading formats for persons with cognitive disabilities (see Chapter 15). Issues unique to these applications are discussed in the relevant chapters. Synthetic speech is also used in many mainstream mobile technologies see Chapter 8). The two types of speech output are digital recording and speech synthesis. They differ in the manner by which the speech is electronically produced. Table 6-4 lists the features and the typical AT applications for the two approaches.

Digital Recording

Digital recording stores human speech in electronic memory circuits so it can be retrieved later. The speech to be stored can be entered at any time by just speaking into a built-in microphone. Even a few seconds of speech takes a great deal of memory. For example, 16 seconds of speech may take up to 1 megabyte of memory for storage without signal processing and compression. Current memory technologies are similar to those used for audio music and speech recordings, and they can store large amounts of vocabulary. The major advantage of digital recording of speech is that it allows any voice to be easily stored in the device and played back. For example, if the person who is using the AAC system (see Chapter 16) that uses digital recording is a young girl, we can use another young girl's voice to store the required messages.

Speech Synthesis

Speech synthesis generates the speech electronically instead of storing the entire signal. This approach reduces the amount of memory required. Speech output can be created from any electronic text, including that sent to the screen of a computer or mobile device. A mathematical model of the human vocal system is used to synthesize the speech. One example of a vocal tract model is shown in Figure 6-12. There are two types

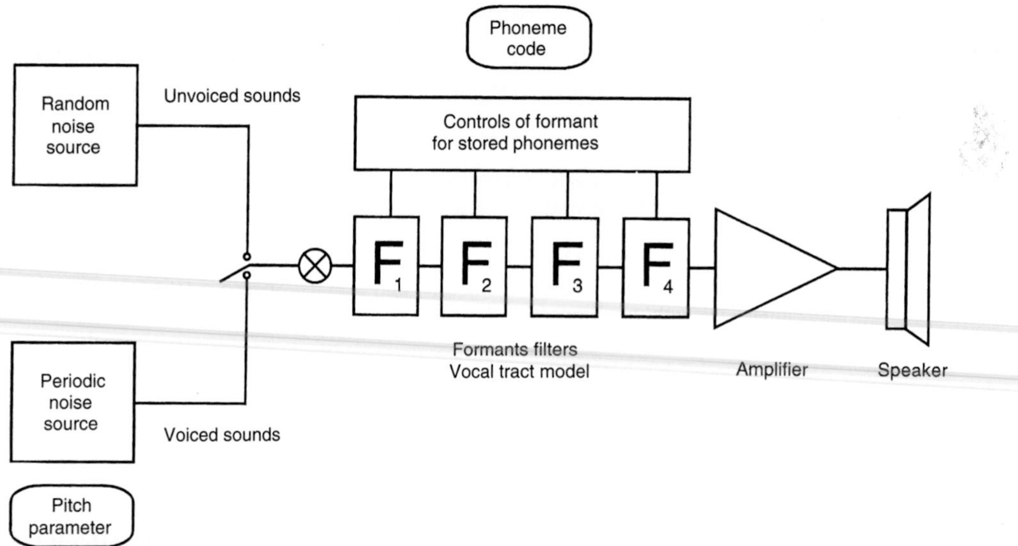

FIGURE 6-12 Speech synthesis systems are often based on a vocal tract model. Sound sources for both voiced (periodic noise) and unvoiced (random noise), as well as a computational model of the vocal tract characteristics, are included.

TABLE 6-5 Types of Text-to-Speech Systems Used in Assistive Technologies

Type of Text-to-Speech System	Major Features	Advantages and Disadvantages
Whole word look-up	Speech pattern for each word stored in memory Look up of words as they are typed	Requires large memory for even modest vocabulary size Very high intelligibility for words stored Vocabulary limited to words stored
Letter-to-sound conversion	Text is matched to sounds letter by letter according to a set of rules Can use phonemes, allophones, or diphones Limited prosodic features	Unlimited vocabulary with very low memory requirements Relatively low intelligibility Rules have many exceptions, and overall quality depends on sophistication of rules
Morphonemic text-to-speech conversion	Relies on combination of stored morphs and letter-to-sound rules Can use phonemes, allophones, or diphones Includes prosodic features	Unlimited vocabulary with moderate memory requirements Relatively high intelligibility Much higher cost than letter-to-sound rules alone

of sounds in speech, voiced and unvoiced (a hissing sound similar to unvoiced sounds such as *s* or *f*), and both these types of speech sounds must be included in the vocal tract model. These signals are then fed into a model of the vocal tract that is varied to produce the speech in a manner similar to the variation of the tongue, teeth, lips, and throat during human speech. Speech synthesizers can generate any word if the correct codes are sent to them in the correct order.

Prosodic features, which give speech its human quality, are generated by changes in three parameters: (1) amplitude, (2) pitch, and (3) duration of the spoken utterance. Human speech consists of both these basic or segmental sounds and prosodic or suprasegmental features. These features allow us to stress a phrase or word, to emphasize a point, or to generate an utterance that portrays a particular mood (e.g., angry or polite or happy). They are also responsible for the inflection changes that distinguish a yes/no question (rising pitch at the end of the sentence) from a statement (falling pitch at the end). For example, the statement, "He is going to dinner" has a falling inflection at the end. However, the inflection in the sentence, "Is he going to dinner?" rises at the end. Murray et al. (1991) developed software, called Hamlet, that used DECTalk (Fonix Corporation, Sandy, UT; http://www.fonix.com) speech synthesizer voice quality to provide vocal emotion effects to the synthetic speech.

Text-to-Speech Programs

The smallest meaningful units of language are called morphemes. Free morphemes are complete words that may stand alone (e.g., run); bound morphemes must be coupled to another morpheme (e.g., -ing) to form a complete word. Words are articulated sounds or series of sounds that are used alone as units of language; they symbolize, communicate, and have meaning. In computer use, words consist of text characters (one per letter), each of which has a specific numeric code. **Text-to-speech programs** convert text characters into the codes required by the speech synthesizer by analyzing a word or sentence. When the speech synthesizer receives these codes, they are combined phonetically into the word the user wants to say. Several approaches can be taken to generate speech from text input. Table 6-5 lists the major approaches and their features. The most common approach is to break words into syntactically significant groups called *morphs*, store sound codes associated with each morph, and match the morph to the letters typed.

Approximately 8000 morphs can generate more than 95% of the words in English. To break words down into morphs and then match the morphs to the speech sounds requires the development of a text-to-speech system.

The commonly used system, DECTalk, uses morphonemic principles of speech synthesis (Bruckert, 1984). This speech synthesizer uses a 6000-entry lexicon that contains basic pronunciation rules similar to those of MITalk-79. The emphasis of this type of system is on maximizing the use of prestored pronunciation rules and relying on letter-to-sound rules only for uncommon or user-specific words (e.g., proper names or technical terms).

There are seven built-in voices and one user-definable voice. The latter allows the user to pick fundamental frequencies, speech rate, and other parameters to create any voice (e.g., Mickey Mouse or a robot). These built-in voices include children, women, and men with different features. A small (150-word) user-defined dictionary that can contain words unique to the individual user is also included. Many augmentative communication systems now include this speech output system. The DECTalk has also been used in computer screen readers for individuals who are blind and in automated reading systems (see Chapter 13). Bruckert (1984) describes DECTalk in greater detail. A portable version, Multivoice, is also available. DECTalk and some other commercial speech synthesizers are also available in Spanish, French, and some other European languages (e.g., German, Swedish, and Italian).

Most AAC devices (see Chapter 16) and screen readers for the blind (see Chapter 13) use DECTalk, Eloquence or Vocalizer (Nuance, Peabody, MA; http://www.nuance.com/index.htm#eti), AT&T Natural Voices (AT&T, http://www.research.att.com/~ttsweb/tts/index.php), IVONA (http://www.ivona.com/us/), Acapela (http://www.acapela-group.com), or a proprietary text-to-speech system. TMA Associates (Tarzana, CA; http://www.tmaa.com/) provides listings and analysis of text-to-speech and other related products. Aaron et al. (2005) provide an excellent overview and tutorial on speech synthesis.

Audio Considerations

The intelligibility and sound quality of any speech synthesis system are dramatically affected by the quality of the amplifier and speaker used to provide the final speech output. Many commercial systems use low-power amplifiers and small, low-fidelity speakers. This technology can reduce the quality of the sound and therefore make it more difficult to understand. However, in most AAC applications, the speech synthesis system must be portable. Higher power output amplifiers require larger batteries, and larger speakers that have greater fidelity are heavier than lower-quality speakers. Both of these factors affect weight and therefore portability. The most important rule that applies here is that "you don't get something for nothing"; higher quality in speech sound output is obtained only at the cost of increased weight and reduced portability.

Telephone Use

Telephone lines have a narrower bandwidth (frequency range), which affects the amount of distortion and the quality of the speech. The use of speech synthesis and the intelligibility of speakers with dysarthria are therefore reduced over the telephone (Drager et al., 2010). Adult listeners heard mildly (90% intelligible) dysarthric spoken speech and synthesized speech in both face-to-face and telephone contexts. In the face-to-face situation, there are additional cues such as facial expressions, and the acoustic signal is not limited as it is over the telephone. Listeners found the quality of the speech synthesis equivalent to that of natural speech. Over the telephone, speech quality is degraded more for the natural dysarthric speaker than for the speech synthesis, and the listeners clearly preferred the synthetic speech.

CONTEXT

Three contexts affect the HTI as we have described in this chapter. In the social context, the use of ATs can be stigmatizing for the individual using it. It is possible that some control schemes will lead to greater stigma than others. For example, the use of scanning can significantly increase the time it takes to make choices, control a device such as a phone or tablet, or create an utterance on a communication device. The slow speed may significantly change the social interaction a person has. It can also make it difficult to effectively use system features, including mainstream applications such as texting or Internet access. These limitations can call attention to the individual's disability rather than facilitating his or her participation.

Artificial speech can also be stigmatizing. Synthetic speech can sound robotic or cartoon-like. The sound can bring unwanted attention to the user of systems that use such speech, especially in public environments such as restaurants.

In the institutional context, HTI devices can be expensive, and the process of obtaining funding can be complex. Often significant paperwork is required, and delays of weeks or months may occur between assessment and actual delivery of the required technology.

The physical context can also provide challenges. All selection systems that rely on visual displays are sensitive to ambient light conditions, especially bright sunlight.

Speech output devices are harder to understand in noisy environments. The physical space and ability of the space to support proper positioning for access is another physical context issue. Educational and work settings do not always have sufficient space to locate the system nor do they have a support surface that accommodates a functional position that facilitates access to it. All of these factors must be taken into account before a device is recommended for an individual user.

ASSESSMENT

The control sites that can potentially be used by the consumer to operate a device are shown in Figure 6-1. The various movements that each control site is capable of performing were described earlier in this chapter.

Functional Movement Evaluation

The overall goal of the physical skills evaluation is to determine the most functional position for the individual and evaluate his or her ability to access a device physically. At a very basic level, physical skills include range of motion, muscle strength and endurance, muscle tone, and the presence of primitive reflexes and reactions. Many protocols exist for evaluation of range of motion (Latella & Meriano, 2003). Both passive and active ranges of motion are assessed. Range of motion is important in consideration of positioning needs for function and the amount of movement available to access a device or perform a task (see Chapter 9 for a discussion of seating and positioning).

Related to range of motion is muscle strength. Again, many protocols are available for testing muscle strength. Muscle strength is graded in a range from unable to move independently, moves with gravity eliminated, able to move against gravity, and moves against different degrees of resistance. It is important to note that the presence of a neurologic disorder such as CP, stroke, or traumatic brain injury will affect both range of motion and muscle strength. Typical protocols for testing these components are not generally useful for these populations because the position of the individual affects muscle tone and subsequently range of motion and muscle strength. For example, a child with CP may seem to have limited flexion range of motion in the lower extremities when lying in supine. However, when turned on the side, the ability to flex the legs is much easier. In supine, the influence of the tonic labyrinthine reflex increases extensor tone. This influence is not present in sidelying, making flexion much easier (Nichols, 2005).

Muscle tone and the presence of obligatory movements are important considerations for individuals with neurologic disorders. The position of the individual affects the available movement. Muscle tone is assessed in various functional positions, particularly prone, supine, sitting, and standing. Obligatory movements, or reflexes, are assessed to determine how they might affect function. Key reflexes or obligatory movements include the asymmetrical and symmetrical tonic neck reflexes, tonic labyrinthine, extensor thrust, bite, and grasp reflexes. The ability to right the head when moved out of a vertical alignment, either lateral or in the anterior-posterior plane, is another component. Postural control is a related component that refers to the ability to maintain the trunk in a vertical alignment. When completing an assessment to determine function in various positions, it is important to handle the client and to challenge his or her balance and postural control to determine the degree of support he or she will need to work in a given position and the movement available in that position. Figure 6-13 illustrates proper positioning for use of a keyboard. Sitting and standing balance are additional considerations (see Chapter 9).

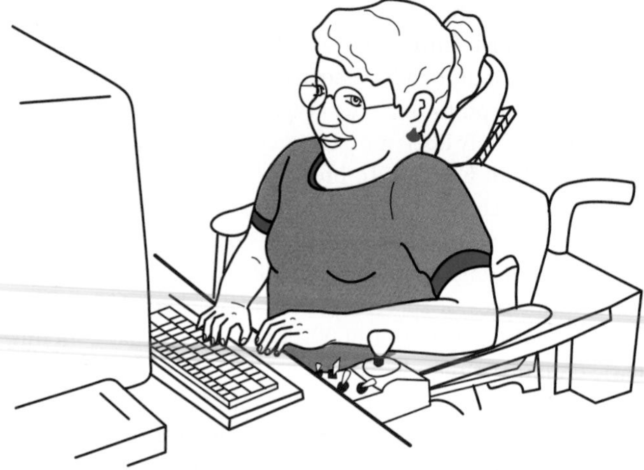

FIGURE 6-13 A proper sitting posture can promote independence and allow the child to function efficiently in the manipulation of objects or the activation of switches. (Courtesy www.Lburkhart.com.)

Gross and fine motor assessments generally test higher level motor skills. Gross motor skills include balance on one foot, performing symmetrical and asymmetrical movements of the upper and lower extremities; coordinating one side of the body; lifting and carrying objects; rapidly alternating movements; and running, skipping, and hopping. Fine motor assessment includes rapidly alternating finger movements, performance of isolated finger movements, manipulation of objects of different sizes, and performance of specific fine motor tasks. The Bruininks-Oseretsky Test of Motor Proficiency (Bruininks & Bruininks, 2005) and the Movement ABC (Henderson et al., 2007) are two examples of comprehensive motor evaluations appropriate for children. The Gross Motor Function Measure (Russell et al., 2002) is designed specifically for children with neurological impairments. Again, if a neurologic condition is present, it is important to remember that function depends on the client's position.

Simulation of functional tasks is used to evaluate the types and quality of movement an individual possesses. Functional tasks are chosen for evaluation because they are often more meaningful to the consumer than physical performance components such as strength and joint range of motion. They also provide the clinician with an opportunity to gather qualitative information regarding the consumer's movements, and results of such tasks are more likely to reflect the consumer's true abilities.

A Clinically Based Framework for Determining Optimal Anatomic Sites for Accessing a Control Interface

The hands, being the control site of choice, are the first to be assessed. Basic hand function can be observed and rated by using a "grasp module" (Figure 6-14) that includes a total of seven functional grasp patterns. The consumer's ability to complete each grasp pattern is rated (unable, poor, fair, or good). Notations are also made regarding how the consumer completed the movement and the factors that made it successful or not. For example, did the object need to be positioned in a

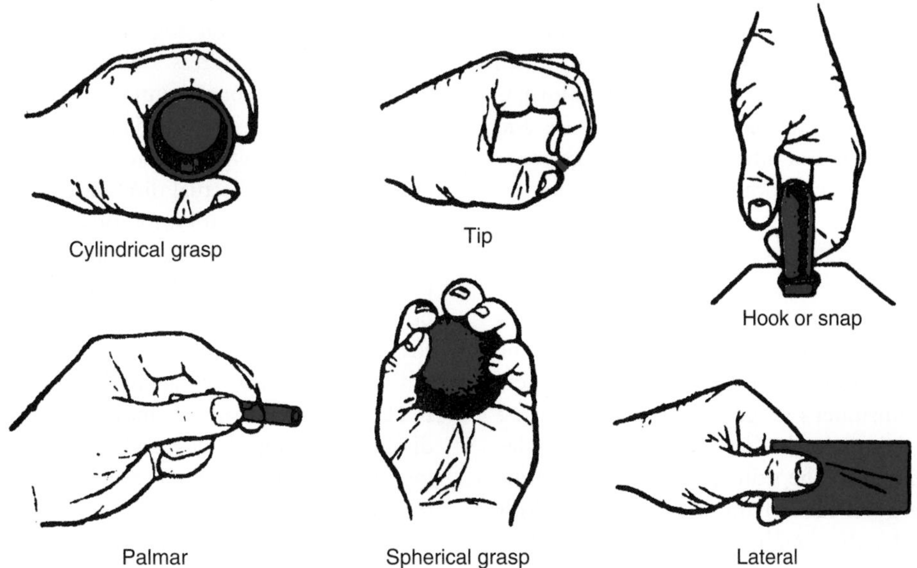

FIGURE 6-14 Functional grasp patterns for evaluating hand use.

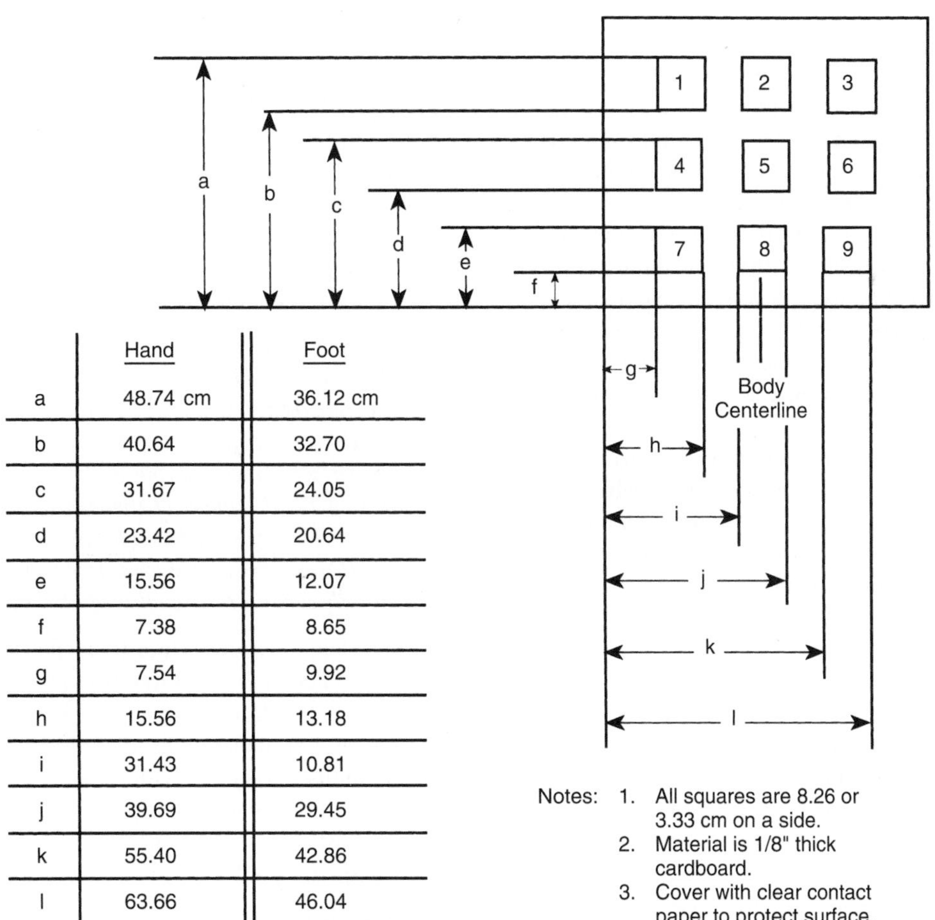

	Hand	Foot
a	48.74 cm	36.12 cm
b	40.64	32.70
c	31.67	24.05
d	23.42	20.64
e	15.56	12.07
f	7.38	8.65
g	7.54	9.92
h	15.56	13.18
i	31.43	10.81
j	39.69	29.45
k	55.40	42.86
l	63.66	46.04

FIGURE 6-15 Range and resolution board used for evaluating the ability to hit a target using a given control site.

particular way for the consumer to grasp it? Was there a delay in initiating the movement? Did the consumer have difficulty releasing the object? Was the movement pattern isolated or synergistic in nature? Did the consumer appear to have problems with depth perception when reaching for the object?

If the consumer has the potential for reliable hand use, it is then necessary to determine the minimal and maximal arm range within a workspace and the resolution in hitting a target. A range and resolution board, as shown in Figure 6-15, can be used to measure both of these. If possible, the consumer is asked to use the thumb or a finger to point to each corner of each numbered square. If the consumer is unable to point to the corners, he or she is asked to touch each square with the whole hand. This provides information regarding the approximate size of the workspace and the best locations for a control interface and a rough measure of accuracy of movement. Both arms are evaluated as appropriate.

If the hands are eliminated as a control site, other anatomic sites must be considered. For example, we can also measure range and resolution for the foot and head. With a range and resolution board of smaller dimensions, the same task can be used to evaluate foot range and targeting skills and the consumer's range and resolution with a mouth stick, light pointer, or head pointer. After completion of this component of the skills evaluation, the clinician should have a good idea of the user's physical skills and the anatomic sites that can best be used to control an interface

OUTCOMES

Optimal Control Sites

The outcome of the assessment process will be a determination of the available control sites for an individual. There may be several or only one, depending on the motor capability of the individual. The initial evaluation may only indicate *potential* control sites that may be developed with practice or anatomic sites that are easily controlled without additional training and practice. Because it is also possible that the person's skills may decrease over time in the short term during the day because of fatigue or in the longer term because of a degenerative disease, identifying a "back-up" control site is a useful strategy when possible.

In most cases, control of individual sites will improve because of repetition of any motor act. It is possible that the quality and speed of movement may improve, and even the number of movement patterns (e.g., head movement and hand movement) available may increase.

Development of Skills for the Use of Control Interfaces

Assistive technology provides many individuals who have physical disabilities with their first opportunity to perform a motor act to access communication, mobility, and environmental control or perform cognitive functions. Without these technological options, individuals with severe physical disabilities had few or no opportunities to use their existing motor movement. For this reason, there are many instances in which an individual may have a control site and the ability to activate a single switch, but the ability to activate this control interface is not consistent enough to justify the purchase of an assistive device such as a wheelchair, computer, or augmentative communication system. The intervention then becomes one of improving the individual's motor control so she will be able to reliably activate the control interface.

Skill development varies greatly across different input devices depending on cognitive load, mastery, speed, and user characteristic. Cress and French (1994) evaluated the use of different control interfaces in three groups: adults without disabilities who had computer experience, typically developing children between 2.5 and 5.0 years of age, and children with intellectual disabilities (mental age, 2.5 to 5.0 years). Adults without disabilities were able to master all of the devices (touch screen, trackball, mouse, locking trackball, and keyboard) without training. About 50% of typically developing children were able to master all devices except the locking trackball without training. After training, 80% of the typically developing children mastered all devices. The trackball was the easiest to master. Children with intellectual disabilities averaged between 0% and 46% mastery (depending on the device) without training and less than 75% mastery with training.

Adults were able to use the devices faster than the children, and the typically developing children used most devices slower than the children with intellectual disabilities. This result is probably related to the greater chronological age of the children with intellectual disabilities. An exception to the general result was the touch screen, which was used faster by the typically developing children. Performance by typically developing children was related to age and gross motor abilities. In addition to these, performance of children with intellectual disabilities was also related to pattern analysis skills, and the individual input devices showed distinctly different relationships to cognitive and motor development than for the typically developing children. Li-Tsang et al., 2005 stated:

> *This study showed that the IT competency of people with ID was poor and that there is a barrier for people with ID to get into the world of IT. Intensive, organized, systematic training seems to be the way forward. This study has shed light on how to set training goals for people with ID for learning IT. A number of limiting factors regarding access to technology were found for people with ID. If people with ID could have access to modern technology, this would hopefully enhance their quality of life (p.133).*

Selection of control interfaces for a given individual depends on cognitive and motor requirements presented by a particular interface as well as the skills of the individual in these areas. Extrapolation from successful use by adults without disabilities or typically developing children to children with disabilities is not appropriate. The amount of training required for successful use is also generally greater for children who have disabilities than it is for typically developing children or adults.

Findlater et al. (2013) and Ng et al. (2013) compared performance between older adults and younger adults using four desktop and touch screen tasks: pointing, dragging, crossing and steering, and pinch to zoom (touch screen only). Age and input device type both had significant effects on both seed and number of errors. Older adults were generally slower than younger adults, but the gap was less using the touch screen than for the mouse, and the error rate was also

TABLE 6-6 Sequential Steps in Motor Training for Switch Use

Goal	Tools Used to Accomplish Goal
1. Time-independent switch used to develop cause and effect	Appliances (fan, blender) Battery-operated toys or radio Software that produces a result whenever the switch is pressed
2. Time-dependent switch used to develop switch use at the right time	Software that requires a response at a specific time to obtain a graphic or sound result
3. Switch within specified window to develop multichoice scanning	Software requiring a response in a "time window"
4. Symbolic choice making	Simple scanning communication device Software allowing time-dependent choice making that has a symbolic label and communicative output

less (Findlater, et al., 2013). However, older users preferred a trackball to either the touch screen or mouse, and age-related performance differences were not completely compensated for by the use of the touch screen (Ng et al., 2013).

A graded approach using technology as one of the modalities for improving the individual's motor skills can and should be implemented. Table 6-6 illustrates some general steps and tools involved in such an approach. The technology then becomes a tool to meet short-term objectives aimed at reaching the long-term goal of participation in an activity using AT. It is important that this outcome and goal be kept in mind so that the clinician reevaluates the individual at periodic intervals and allows her to move beyond the use of this technology as a tool and into functional device use.

Training and Practice to Develop Motor Control

When an individual has limited upper extremity fine motor control, it is necessary to use alternative anatomic sites such as head movement or gross arm, hand, or leg movements. The efficient use of a control interface requires the equivalent of fine motor control regardless of the anatomic site. Because these alternative sites have not been used for fine motor control, a combination of training and practice is required to develop the necessary skills. For example, to be effective at activating a switch by head rotation, an individual will need to develop skills through practice. What are initially chosen as the best control site and method for an individual may not necessarily remain constant over time.

An individual may have the prerequisite motor skills to use a specific anatomic site but lack sufficient skill to control the recommended control interface. She will require training to refine her skills. Refining these motor skills may result in an increased rate of input, fewer errors, or increased endurance for using the control. For example, a person may be able to select directly but need training to learn to use a specific keyboard layout to reduce fatigue or increase speed (Case Study 6-3).

CASE STUDY 6-3

Motor Training to Enhance Function

Mrs. Bennett is a patient at the skilled nursing facility where you work. She sustained a stroke and has recently been transferred to your facility. To get her involved in using her right side, you have been asked to develop a motor training program that will engage her in using a joystick. How would you proceed?

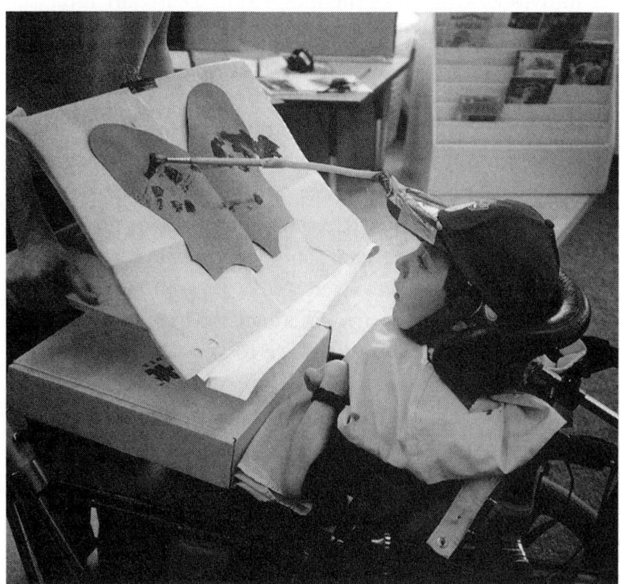

FIGURE 6-16 For assistance with painting in art class, we can attach the paintbrush to a head-pointing stick or baseball cap. The type of activity can help children develop motor skills for head pointing.

Refinement of motor skills for mouse use, especially if an anatomic site other than the hand and fingers is used, will also require training and practice. Many software programs and apps are available that have been developed to gradually improve a person's ability to use a mouse or an alternative pointing device, including the gestures required for tablets and smart phones (e.g., swipe, pinch, tap). These programs include activities for developing targeting skills and mastering point-and-click and click-and-drag skills.

Use of mechanical and electronic pointers worn on the head typically requires substantial training to gradually build the consumer's tolerance. Activities such as painting using a brush attached to head pointer (Figure 6-16) add enjoyment to the task of developing a motor skill. Effectiveness in using control enhancers such as typing stick, key guards, and mouth sticks (see Chapter 7) also requires practice. Similarly, strengthening of the person's existing neck, facial, and oral musculature and a gradual development of tolerance for the mouth stick should take place before having him perform tasks such as writing or typing. Playing simple board games, painting, or batting a balloon are examples of activities that can be used to develop skills for mouth stick or head pointer use. Many games can also be adapted so that a person using a light pointer practices using the interface through play activities. For example, a game of tag in which tagging is getting "hit" with the light from the pointer can make learning to use the light pointer more fun.

The development of motor skill for the operation of one or more control interfaces can also have carryover into more general motor skill development. Three outcomes can be achieved by a motor training and practice program: (1) the individual can broaden his repertoire of motor capabilities and the number and type of inputs that can be accessed; (2) the individual can refine the motor skills she has in using an interface to increase speed, endurance, or accuracy; and (3) the individual who lacks the motor skill to use any interface functionally can develop these skills.

A multiple baseline study with two participants, age 1 year 10 months and 5 years, taught children with severe multiple disabilities switching skills in different environments (multiple sensory room and home) (Moir, 2010). The participant's frequency of switching (number of times in each session that the participant activated the switch), response to stimuli, communication via eye gaze, and vocalization all improved over time. Three questions were asked of parents: (1) Has the switching activity made any difference to your child? (2) Has the switching made any difference to you and your family? and (3) How important has it been for your child to participate in the switching program? Parental responses indicated significant changes to the child's behavior that also produced a positive effect on the families. This limited sample study supports some interesting results in terms of related psychosocial performance that supports future investigation in this area.

Developing Scanning Skills

Table 6-6 lists four steps that can be used to develop motor skill sufficient for scanning control of an assistive device (e.g., a communication device, computer access, or EADLs). The steps in Table 6-4 are only strategies intended to meet short-term objectives. The long-term goal is participation in an activity using AT. Research on scanning has resulted in useful information regarding training and practice (Box 6-2).

Hussey et al. (1992) documented the progress of two young women after the implementation of a motor training program similar to the one described in Table 6-6. Initially, both Janice and Marge lacked the head control to activate even a single switch. After extensive training, Janice and Marge were able to directly select on an augmentative communication device using a light pointer worn on the head. These two cases illustrate that individuals can gain motor skills for a functional activity from a systematic training program.

Scanning requires cognitive skills that are not intuitive, especially for a person with significant motor limitations. The cognitive skills required are causality, ability to wait, vigilance to the task to be ready when the desired choice is presented, and reaction time to respond quickly enough to select the desired item. If an individual has difficulty with scanning, it can be challenging to determine if the difficulty is due to motor limitations or cognitive understanding of the task. Therefore, the systematic approach (see Table 6-6) starts with evaluating *causal understanding* (sometimes called cause and effect) and providing training at that level as needed.

BOX 6-2 Tips for Teaching Scanning

Piché and Reichle (1991) identified these steps for teaching scanning in either manual (i.e., no-tech) or technologically assisted systems:

- Selecting a signaling response
- Learning to use the signaling response conditionally (i.e., to indicate an item)
- Learning to use the signaling response with a larger array of items
- Learning to use the signaling response in different types of array (e.g., vertical, horizontal, row–column, circular)

Jones and Stewart (2004) surveyed 56 OTs and SLPs who were experienced in teaching scanning to determine how they carried out this training. This study yielded four themes:

- The process of training scanning is progressive and parallel.
- Clients must be considered on an individual basis when developing a training program. Training scanning is inextricably linked to functional goals.
- It is important to train both the child and the primary caregivers using a collaborative approach.

They also found that:

- Parallel training with the OT using scanning games on the computer and other activities and the SLP developing scanning skill on an AAC device was often used. This is especially true when a new mode or device is added to an existing, effective mode.
- A general progression from linear to row column takes place by using branching arrays.
- OTs were involved in all phases of scanning training with the SLPs being more involved in later stages.

AAC, Augmentative and alternative communication; *OT*, occupational therapist; *SLP*, speech-language pathologist.

Adapted from Dowden P, Cook AM: Choosing effective selection techniques for beginning communicators. In Reichle J, Beukelman D, Light J, editors: *Exemplary practices for beginning communicators*, Baltimore: Paul H. Brookes, 2002, pp. 395-432.

Causal understanding refers to the ability of the individual to understand that he can control things in his environment and can make something happen (den Ouden et al., 2005). It encompasses the prerequisite skills of attention and object permanence. The individual must be able to attend to and be aware of his environment and the permanence of objects in that environment. Information can be gathered on the individual's ability to understand cause and effect through the use of a single switch.

Some tips for preparing for this type of training are shown in Box 6-3. At the first step in Table 6-6, the goal related to AT use is for the individual to be able to activate the switch at any given time and associate the switch activation with a result. The individual is asked to use a control site to activate a single switch that is connected to some type of reinforcer. Caregivers and those working with the individual can provide initial information on what the individual enjoys and finds reinforcing. Objects that can be adapted for switch input that may be of interest include battery-operated toys, a radio, a blender, or a fan. The child shown in Figure 6-17 is using a switch with a battery-operated toy as the reinforcer. Typically, the individual who is aware that she has generated an effect will show some type of response, such as smiling, crying, or looking toward the reinforcer.

BOX 6-3 Tips for Preparing a Learner for Motor Skill Development

Before engaging the learner in early scanning activities, make sure there is:

- At least one comfortable position for an engaging activity
- An appropriate control site and switch has been identified for learner's motor control
- A well-positioned and stable switch
- Movement to activate the switch is easy for the learner
- Nearly 100% accuracy in the learners switch activation upon stimulus or cue without scanning
- The scanning method matches the learner's motor a (see Table 6-1)

Investigators have discovered that the ratio between a user's reaction time and an appropriate scan rate for that user is approximately 0.65, which we refer to as "the 0.65 rule" (Lesher et al., 2000; Simpson et al., 2006).

The learner is not rewarded for inappropriate activations (e.g., during stimulus)

- There are empty spaces (foils) in the scanning array in addition to targets.
- The scanning pattern is simple: linear or circular.
- The presentation of the options is highly salient to the learner (McCarthy et al., 2006).
- The cue or stimulus should be in the same modality as the selection set items (e.g., for visual scanning, the cue should be visual, and for auditory scanning, the stimulus should be audible).
- "Use natural cues" and prompts such as "Which toy do you want" rather than unnatural ones such as "Hit the switch now."
- For visual scanning, be sure the learner is able to look at the display continuously.
- The feedback upon selection is salient and reinforcing (McCarthy et al., 2006).

Adapted from Dowden P, Cook AM: Choosing effective selection techniques for beginning communicators. In Reichle J, Beukelman D, Light J, editors: *Exemplary practices for beginning communicators,* Baltimore: Paul H. Brookes, 2002, pp. 395-432.

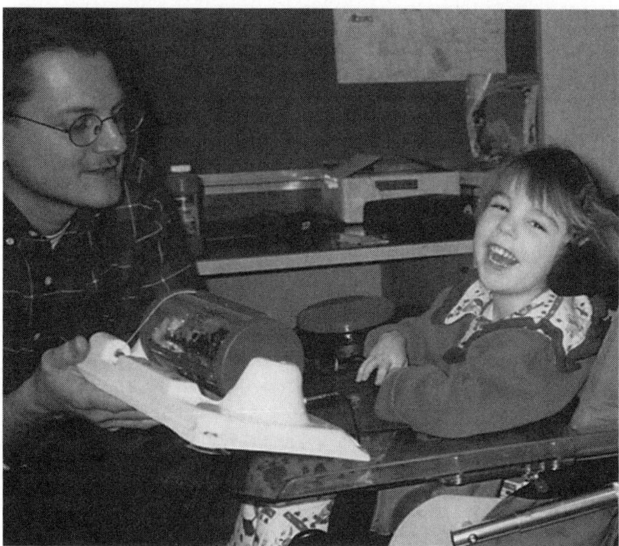

FIGURE 6-17 Child using a single switch with a battery-operated toy as a reinforcer.

If there is success with these activities, computer software programs can be used as an alternative type of reinforcement. These programs provide interesting graphics, animation, and auditory feedback each time the switch is activated. Individuals of all age groups find the programs enjoyable. Data can be collected for each switch activation, including (1) time from prompt to activation, (2) whether the individual activates the switch independently or whether verbal or physical prompting was needed, and (3) the consumer's attention to the result. There are a number of companies that sell software programs to be used at the different stages described in this section.

At the second step in Table 6-6, the goal is for the individual to activate his switch consistently at a specific time. Vigilance, ability to wait, and the ability to activate the switch at the correct time are important at this step. With some computer games, the individual needs to activate the switch for an object to move or to carry out an action such as shooting a basket, hitting a target, and so on. With some programs, as long as the individual successfully activates the switch, the movement of objects on the screen speeds up.

This approach can also be considered one-choice scanning, in which the switch is either hit or not—choice making at its most fundamental level. For example, with some computer games, the individual needs to activate the switch for an object to move or to carry out an action such as shooting a basket, hitting a target, and so on. With some programs, as long as the individual successfully activates the switch, the movement of objects on the screen speeds up. Any data provided by the program (e.g., speed, number of correct hits, errors) and data regarding the individual's success in activating the switch at the correct time and whether prompts have been needed are recorded.

Linda Burkhart has many suggestions for computer-based and non–computer-based activities that can be used for motor training (see also htpp://www.lburkhart.com). One suggestion for a non–computer-based activity is to use a battery-operated toy fireman that climbs a ladder as long as the switch is activated. To make this a time-dependent activity, a picture of a reinforcer is attached somewhere along the ladder, and the individual is asked to release the switch to stop the fireman at the picture and receive the reinforcement.

The third step of the scanning training program adds a "time window," and the individual is asked to use the switch to choose from two or more options. The skills involved at this stage include vigilance, waiting, and reaction time as in step two. The additional required skill is the understanding that a choice is only available during a "window" in which the item to be selected is highlighted. Toys, appliances, and computer software programs can also be used at this stage.

The goal is to gradually increase the number of choices from which the individual is to select. The increase in the number of choices is important if scanning is to be used for communication or environmental control. One approach is to highlight locations on the screen in sequence. When the switch is hit on a highlighted item, the program provides an interesting result. In some programs, the highlighted areas can be limited so that only one is correct, which helps the consumer develop scanning selection skills in the absence of language-based tasks. In addition to the data that have been collected in the previous stages, data on the minimal scan rate the individual can successfully use are recorded.

BOX 6-4 Tips for Teaching Scanning

The following tips can be used while teaching early switch control to emerging communicators:

- Cues to the AAC user should always be natural environmental cues (e.g., silence in the middle of a song). Using explicit commands such as saying, "Hit the switch" will keep the learner dependent on that prompt and impede learning.
- The learner must not repeatedly or continuously activate the switch in anticipation of the right moment. This would prevent him or her from learning to wait for the right moment (and later the cursor in scanning).
- It is unfair to expect communicative use of the switch or selection method before ensuring that the individual has reliable control (operational competence) over the interface itself.

AAC, Augmentative and alternative communication.
Adapted from Dowden P, Cook AM: Choosing effective selection techniques for beginning communicators. In Reichle J, Beukelman D, Light J, editors: *Exemplary practices for beginning communicators,* Baltimore: Paul H. Brookes, 2002, pp. 395-432.

If the need is for power mobility, then the next step is to use software specifically designed for developing skills in using a joystick. Alternatively, scanning training software aimed at single-switch or dual-switch wheelchair use can be used for training at this stage.

The final training phase shown in Table 6-6 is intended to add communicative intent to the task. At this stage, the cognitive skill of symbolic representation is added to the choice making. Development of the individual's language skills may have been taking place in parallel with the motor skills training (Box 6-4), and this linguistic step may follow naturally. The amount of training required for successful use is also generally greater for children who have disabilities than it is for typically developing children or adults. A summary of research that is relevant to the development of motor skills for AT use is shown in Box 6-5.

Selection of symbol systems is discussed in Chapter 16. Through this phase, the individual makes the transition from object manipulation (environmental control) to concept manipulation (communication). Greater resources are available at this stage to convey needs, wants, and other information. Simple scanning communication devices or multiple choice computer programs can also be used for further skill development as a precursor to a scanning communication device.

BOX 6-5 Research on Developing Motor Skills for Assistive Technology Use

What Does the Research Say?: Developing Skills with Switches and Other Control Interfaces

Jagacinski and Monk (1985) evaluated the use of joysticks and head pointers by young nondisabled adults. The task involved moving from a center point to one of eight lighted targets as fast as possible. The skill in using these devices for this task was acquired with some difficulty over many trials. Based on a criterion of less than 3% improvement in speed over 4 consecutive days, proficient joystick use required 6 to 18 days, and head pointer use required 7 to 29 days of practice for nondisabled, young, highly motor-skilled participants.

Jones and Stewart (2004) surveyed 56 OTs and SLPs experienced in teaching scanning to determine how they carried out this training. They indicated that:

- The time taken to achieve reliable results varies widely among children.
- Most children received parallel training from an OT using scanning games on the computer while developing scanning skills on a communication device.
- OTs were involved in all phases of scanning training with the SLPs being more involved in later stages.

Angelo (2000) reported 11 essential elements of a single-switch assessment as identified by experienced OT: reliability of movement, volitional nature of movement, safety, easily performed movement, use of activities in which learners participate regularly, efficiency of movement, previous successful movements, ability to perform a timed response within a time frame, and time required between switch activations is appropriate to child's reaction or response time.

Cress and French (1994) found that skill development varies greatly across different input devices (touch screen, trackball, mouse, locking trackball, and keyboard).

- Three groups: adults without disabilities, typically developing children between 2.5 and 5.0 years, and children with intellectual disabilities (mental age 2.5 to 5.0)
- Adults without disabilities mastered all of the devices without training.
- About 50% of typically developing children were able to master all devices except the locking trackball without training.
- After training, 80% of the typically developing children mastered all devices. The trackball was the easiest to master.
- Children with intellectual disabilities averaged between 0 and 46% mastery (depending on the device) without training and less than 75% mastery with training. The locking trackball was significantly more difficult to master than the other devices.
- Adults were able to use the devices faster than the children, and the typically developing children used most devices slower than the children with intellectual disabilities (probably related to the greater chronological age of the children with intellectual disabilities).
- Performance by typically developing children was related to age and gross motor abilities.
- Performance of children with intellectual disabilities was also related to pattern analysis skills, and the individual input devices showed distinctly different relationships to cognitive and motor development than for the typically developing children.
- Selection of control interfaces for a given individual depends on cognitive and motor requirements presented by a particular interface as well as the skills of the individual in these areas.
- Extrapolation from successful use by adults without disabilities or typically developing children to children with disabilities is not appropriate.

OT, Occupational therapist; *SLP,* speech-language pathologist.
Adapted from Dowden P, Cook AM: Choosing effective selection techniques for beginning communicators. In Reichle J, Beukelman D, Light J, editors: *Exemplary practices for beginning communicators,* Baltimore: Paul H. Brookes, 2002, pp. 395-432.

Integration of the selection set into daily activities can be evaluated in a number of ways. Goal Attainment Scaling (GAS), a criterion-referenced, individualized objective measure (Kiresuk et al., 1994), can be as used to evaluate the effectiveness of a training program. For example, Cook et al. (2005) used GAS to identify of individualized goals for children using a set of switches to control a robot in a functional task.

Individualized goals were developed for switch-controlled operation of the robot for each child in the study. For each individual goal set for the child, a scoring hierarchy is established in which a score of zero indicates achievement of the goals. Negative scores of -1 or -2 indicate degrees of failing to achieve the goal. Scores of +1 or +2 indicate that the child exceeded the goal. For each of the five scores, a task is described. For the robot task, typical goals were based on the number of prompts required (Cook et al., 2005). A score of zero meant that the switches were successfully hit without prompting. Scores above zero indicated successful completion of increasingly complicated tasks. Scores below zero indicated that either hand-over-hand (-2) or verbal (-1) prompting levels were required. There are also standardized outcome measures that are described in Chapter 5. For example, the Psychosocial Impact of Assistive Devices Scale (PIADS) and Quebec User Evaluation of Satisfaction with Assistive Technology (QUEST) can be used to evaluate outcomes for individuals using particular selection methods.

SUMMARY

In this chapter, we have defined the elements of the HTI and their relationship to the other components of AT. The elements of the HTI include the control interface, the selection method, and the selection set. The selection set encompasses the items in the array from which the user can choose. There are two basic methods by which the user makes selections, direct selection or indirect selection. Indirect selection encompasses a subset of selection methods known as scanning, directed scanning, and coded access. Each selection method applies to a different set of consumer skills. The development of motor and cognitive skills for scanning requires a thoughtful and well-designed approach.

STUDY QUESTIONS

1. Define the elements of the HTI and how they are related to the processor and the output.
2. What are the major anatomic sites that are used for control of ATs?
3. Describe the available movements for each anatomic site.
4. What is the order of preference in considering alternative anatomic sites? Why is this order used?
5. What are the major challenges for a person using head control for a fine motor task such as typing?
6. What is a selection set?
7. What is a control interface?
8. What are the two basic selection methods used with control interfaces?
9. What are the scanning formats that can be used to accelerate scanning?
10. What is "directed scanning"? Why is it useful?
11. Why is coded access an indirect selection method? What is the selection set for Morse code?
12. Examine Table 6-2. Which Morse codes listed in the nonstandard section are the same for both example systems? Why do you think these particular codes happen to be the same, given that there are no standards? Why do you think that the other codes are different for different systems?
13. Describe the three different selection techniques used with scanning and directed scanning. Which one provides the user with more control and why?
14. What are the relative advantages and disadvantages of the three common scanning methods? Select a client profile that would benefit from each type.
15. What are the cognitive skills necessary to use scanning?
16. What do we mean by the "processor" in an AT system? What does it do?
17. What does "rate enhancement" mean? What are the two main types?
18. What memory skills does a person need to use word prediction or word completion?
19. What is "abbreviation expansion"? What cognitive skills are required to use it?
20. What outcomes can be achieved through the implementation of training programs for the development of motor skills?
21. Describe the steps taken in a training program to develop motor control.
22. Why is it recommended that selection skill (e.g., scanning) be developed with games or other activities before the person uses it for a functional task?
23. Assume that you are asked to train a person to use scanning. How would your approach differ for:
    a. A 60-year-old man who has recently sustained a stroke
    b. A 5-year-old child with cerebral palsy
    c. A 45-year-old woman with multiple sclerosis
24. If you are the person tasked with making a new system work with an individual, how would you determine if the selection system was the correct one for that person?

REFERENCES

Aaron A, Eide E, Pitrelli JF: Conversational computers, *Sci Am* 292(6):64–69, 2005.

Angelo J: Factors affecting the use of a single switch with assistive technology devices, *J Rehabil Res Dev* 37(5):591–598, 2000.

Bhattacharya S, Samanta D, Basu A: Performance models for automatic evaluation of virtual scanning keyboards, *IEEE Trans Neural Syst Rehabil Eng* 16(5):510–519, 2008.

Bailey RW: *Human performance engineering*, ed 2, Upper Saddle River, NJ, 1996, Prentice Hall.

Blackstone S: The role of rate in communication, *Augment Commun News* 3(5):1–3, 1990.

Bruckert E: A new text-to-speech product produces dynamic human-quality voice, *Speech Technol* 4:114–119, 1984.

Bruininks RH, Bruininks BD: *Bruininks-Oseretsky test of motor proficiency: Examiners manual*, ed 2, Circle Pines, MN, 2005, AGS Publishing.

Cook AM, Bentz B, Harbottle N, et al.: School-based use of a robotic arm system by children with disabilities, *IEEE Trans Neural Syst Rehabil Eng* 13:452–460, 2005.

Cress CJ, French GJ: The relationship between cognitive load measurements and estimates of computer input control skills, *Assist Technol* 6:54–66, 1994.

Davies TC, Mudge S, Ameratunga S, Stott NS: Enabling self-directed computer use for individuals with cerebral palsy: A systematic review of assistive devices and technologies, *Dev Med Child Neurol* 52:510–516, 2010.

den Ouden HEM, Frith U, Frith C, Blakemore SJ: Thinking about intentions, *NeuroImage* 28:787–796, 2005.

Dowden P, Cook AM: Choosing effective selection techniques for beginning communicators. In Reichle J, Beukelman D, Light J, editors: *Exemplary practices for beginning communicators*, Baltimore, 2002, Paul H. Brookes, pp. 395–432.

Drager KDR, Reichle J, Pinkoski C: Synthesized speech output and children: A scoping review, *Am J Speech-Lang Pathol* 19:259–273, 2010.

Findlater L, Froehlich J, Fattal K, et al.: Age-related differences in performance with touchscreens compared to traditional mouse input, *Proceedings of CHI*, 2013. Paris, April 27-May 2, 2013.

Henderson SE, Sugden DA, Barnett AL: *Movement assessment battery for children*, ed 2, London, 2007, The Psychological Corporation.

Hortsman HM, Levine SP, Jaros LA: Keyboard emulation for access to IBM-PC-compatible computers by people with motor impairments, *Assist Technol* 1:63–70, 1989.

Hussey SM, Cook AM, Whinnery SE, et al.: A conceptual model for developing augmentative communication skills in individuals with severe disabilities, *Proc RESNA Int 92 Conf* 287–289, 1992.

Jagacinski RJ, Monk DL: Fitts' Law in two dimensions with hand and head movements, *J Mot Behav* 17(1):7–95, 1985.

Jones J, Stewart H: A description of how three occupational therapists train children in using the scanning access technique, *Aust J Occ Ther* 51:155–165, 2004.

Kiresuk TJ, Smith A, Cardillo JE, editors: *Goal attainment scaling: Applications, theory and measurement*, Hillsdale, NJ, 1994, Erlbaum.

Latella D, Meriano C: *Occupational therapy manual for evaluation of range of motion and muscle strength*, New York, 2003, Delmar.

Lee KS, Thomas DJ: *Control of computer-based technology for people with physical disabilities: An assessment manual*, Toronto, 1990, University of Toronto Press.

Lesher GW, Higginbotham J, Moulton BJ: Techniques for automatically updating scanning delays, *Annual Conference on Rehabilitation Technology (RESNA)*, Orlando, 2000, RESNA Press.

Li-Tsang C, Yeung S, Chan C, Hui-Chan C: Factors affecting people with intellectual disabilities in learning to use computer technology, *Int J Rehabil Res* 28:127–133, 2005.

McCarthy J, Light J, Drager K, et al.: Re-designing scanning to reduce learning demands: The performance of typically developing 2-year-olds, *Augment Altern Commun* 22:269–283, 2006.

Mankowski R, Simpson RC, Koester HH: Validating a model of row–column scanning, *Disabil Rehabil Assist Technol* 8(4): 321–329, 2013.

Moir L: Evaluating the effectiveness of different environments on the learning of switching skills in children with severe and profound multiple disabilities, *Br J Occ Ther* 73(10):446–456, 2010.

Murray IR, et al: Emotional synthetic speech in an integrated communication prosthesis, *Proc 14th Annu Conf Rehabil Eng*, pp. 311–313, June 1991.

Ng HC, Tao D, Calvin KL: Age differences in computer input device use: A comparison of touchscreen, trackball, and mouse, in Á. Rocha et al. (Eds.): *Advances in Information Systems and Technologies*, AISC 206, pp. 1015–1024. 2013.

Nichols DS: Development of postural control. In Case-Smith J, editor: *Occupational therapy for children*, ed 5, St. Louis, 2005, Elsevier Mosby, pp. 278–303.

Piché L, Reichle J: Teaching scanning selection techniques. In Reichle J, York J, Sigafoos J, editors: *Implementing augmentative and alternative communication: Strategies for learners with severe disabilities*, Baltimore, 1991, Paul H. Brookes, pp. 257–274.

Russell DJ, Rosenbaum PL, Avery LM, Lane M: *Gross Motor Function Measure (GMFM-66 and GMFM-88: User's manual)*, London, 2002, MacKeith Press.

Simpson RC: *Computer access for people with disabilities*, CRC Press Boca Raton, FL: 2013.

Simpson RC, Koester HH, LoPresti EF: Selecting an appropriate scan rate: The ".65 rule," *Annual Conference on Rehabilitation Technology (RESNA)*, 2006. Atlanta.

Simpson RC, Mankowski R, Koester HH: Modeling one-switch row-column scanning with errors and error correction methods, *Open Rehabil J* 4:1–12, 2011.

Smith RO: Technological approaches to performance enhancement. In Christiansen C, Baum C, editors: *Occupational therapy overcoming human performance deficits*, Thorofare, NJ, 1991, SLACK.

Vanderheiden GC, Lloyd LL: Communication systems and their components. In Blackstone S, Bruskin D, editors: *Augmentative communication: An introduction*, Rockville, MD, 1986, American Speech Language and Hearing Association.

CHAPTER 7

Control Interfaces for Assistive Technologies

CHAPTER OUTLINE

LEARNING OBJECTIVES

On completing this chapter, you will be able to do the following:

1. Describe the elements of the human/technology interface and its role within the assistive technology component of the Human Activity Assistive Technology model.
2. Describe the characteristics of control interfaces.
3. Identify technologies for direct selection.
4. Identify technologies for indirect selection.
5. Discuss a framework for control interface assessment.
6. Describe context issues related to control interface use.
7. Describe strategies for determining the effectiveness of control interfaces.

KEY TERMS

Acceptance Time
Activation and Deactivation Characteristics
Command Domain
Concept Keyboards
Control Enhancers
Control Interface
Distributed Controls
Input Domain
Integrated Controls
On-Screen Keyboard
Paralysis
Range of Motion
Resolution
Sensory Characteristics
Shield
Spatial Characteristics

ACTIVITY: ENABLING PARTICIPATION

Activities typically carried out by the use of electronic assistive technology (AT) systems include communication, mobility (e.g., a power wheelchair or scooter), cognitive processing (e.g., a navigation or memory aid), and controlling the immediate environment (e.g., turning on a light or controlling a television). Communication, mobility, and environmental control and manipulation activities are enabled by the devices that are discussed in this chapter. To accomplish tasks associated with these activities, an individual must activate a **control interface** to provide an input to operate the device (e.g., turn it on, make it move, or make it talk).

HUMAN SKILLS FOR CONTROL: CHARACTERISTICS OF CONTROLLED MOVEMENTS

The successful use of a control interface requires motor, sensory, and cognitive abilities. Control interfaces come in many different sizes and shapes, specific activities dictate the type of control interface that is chosen, and the specific device must be matched to the user's motor and cognitive skills. For a person to know that she has successfully activated the device, it is necessary for there to be sensory feedback. This usually takes place through a visual or auditory display or both. Alternative displays for people with visual or auditory impairments are discussed in Chapters 13 and 14, respectively.

Human motor, sensory, and cognitive skills vary widely. Consequently, it is necessary for control interfaces to be flexible and for there to be a wide variety of choices available that can match the user's skills. Control interfaces differ according to their spatial, sensory, and activation characteristic and the corresponding skills required to operate them.

Characterization of Controlled Movements

The movements required for control interfaces use can be characterized in several ways, as listed in Table 7-1. By defining the resolution, range, strength, and flexibility for an anatomic site, we can relate these to the skills required for the use of control interfaces.

Resolution

Resolution describes the smallest separation between two objects that the user can reliably control. For example, the spacing of individual keys on a keyboard requires relatively fine motor control. Alternatively, a 6-inch-diameter single switch used to turn on a toy requires much lower resolution on the part of the user.

Range of Motion

The maximal extent of movement possible is **range of motion** (ROM), which is defined as active range of "the arc of motion through which the joint passes when voluntarily moved by muscles acting on the joint" (Early, 2006, p. 121). Some tasks require large range, and others require small range. For example, whereas the use of push rims on a manual wheelchair requires a relatively large range of motion, the use of a computer mouse requires a relatively small range. The combination of resolution and range allows us to define the user's workspace. ROM is affected by disease or injury. For example, *contractures*, a shortening of the muscles and tendons that limits joint ROM, may occur as a result of increased tone. ROM restrictions can also be long term and only changed with difficulty, as in the case of contractures, or short term when the individual's position limits available ROM. In the latter situation, a change in position can result in greater available ROM.

TABLE 7-1 Effector Characteristics

Effector	Resolution	Range	Strength	Versatility
Fingers	High	Small	Low	Very high
Hand	Moderate	Moderate	Moderate	Moderate
Arm	Low	Large	Large	Low
Head	Moderate	Moderate	Moderate	High
Leg	Low	Moderate	High	Low
Foot	Moderate	Large	High	Low
Eyes	High	Small	NA	Moderate

NA, Not applicable.

Strength

Even if the necessary resolution and range are available, there may be insufficient strength to activate the control. In general, the upper extremities function best when precision and control are required, and the lower extremities are best suited for power and strength. AT systems may require a minimal level of strength to activate a control interface.

In some disabilities, strength is significantly reduced. For example, **paralysis** resulting from a spinal cord injury prevents the use of certain muscle groups, depending on the level of the injury (Table 7-2). In this case, the major goal is to find a movement that is not paralyzed; head or chin control may be required. Partial paralysis or *paresis* is a muscle weakness that makes it difficult to move but does not prevent movement as paralysis does. In this case, the AT control interfaces must accommodate for reduced strength. For example, an adapted door handle could be used to require less force to be applied for opening. In muscular dystrophy, fine motor control is often available, but muscle weakness results in very low levels of strength that may lead to restricted movement over large distances; however, fine movements such as those required for small keyboards may be possible.

Disabilities can also lead to changes in muscle tone that affect control interface use. Depending on the level of damage to the nervous system, impaired muscle tone can include flaccidity, spasticity, and rigidity. A reduction in normal muscle tone is referred to as flaccidity or hypotonicity. When muscle tone is increased, it is referred to as hypertonicity or spasticity. Several types of disorders can result in spasticity. Increased muscle tone is often accompanied by exaggerated reflexes and imbalances between the antagonistic muscle pairs controlling joints. With rigidity, there is an increase of muscle tone in both the antagonist and agonist muscles at the same time, resulting in resistance to passive ROM throughout the range and in any direction (Undzis et al., 1996). It is possible for a person to exhibit a mixture of types of muscle tone and for the tone to fluctuate throughout the course of a day. This fluctuation has a direct consequence on effector use and therefore on the control of ATs. In some cases, uncontrolled excessive force is generated. Too much strength can limit fine motor control. Spastic movements are poorly controlled, and they often lead to force in excess of that required for control. Because many control interfaces, such as joysticks, are designed for normal upper extremity levels of force, the excessive forces generated by spastic movements can result in damage to the AT system, as well as to poor performance.

Endurance

Endurance refers to the ability to sustain a force and to repeat the application of a force over time. In some neuromuscular disabilities, such as myasthenia gravis, initial strength may be within a normal range. However, as the individual repeats a movement, there is a continual decrease in performance until total fatigue occurs. Aspects of the AT system design can minimize the effect of fatigue in several ways by requiring low-energy expenditure for activation. An example is a joystick for a wheelchair that requires very little travel and small force. Careful consideration of the strength and endurance available to move an effector is crucial to the successful application of AT systems. The presence of pain also affects controller use. Sometimes pain is consistent; in other cases, it changes throughout the day in response to activity or medication.

Versatility

Versatility refers to the capability of anatomic control sites to be used for a variety of tasks and in a variety of different ways for the same task. For example, both the hand (fingers) and foot (toes) can be used to press a key or switch. However, the hand can also be used to grasp a handle (e.g., a joystick), making it more versatile than the foot. The quality of movement may be smooth or uncoordinated, primitive reflex patterns may dominate movement or be absent, and sensory deficits may or may not be present. All of these factors can influence the use of control interfaces.

ASSISTIVE TECHNOLOGY: CHARACTERISTICS OF CONTROL INTERFACES

Before discussing specific control interfaces, we will look at some general characteristic that are useful when matching control interfaces to the skills of specific users.

Spatial Characteristics

The **spatial characteristics** of a control interface are (1) its overall physical size (dimensions), shape, and weight; (2) the number of available targets contained within the control interface (e.g., a keyboard has more than 100 targets, a joystick may have only four, and a single switch has one); (3) the size of each target; and (4) the spacing between targets.

The target size and spacing should be matched to the individual's fine and gross motor skill as measured by range and resolution. Targets that are large and spaced far apart are useful for individuals with good ROM but limited fine motor control, e.g., someone with a coordination disorder or a tremor. For example, a single control interface has one target, and the target size is the dimension (height and width) of the control interface. A single control interface can accommodate an individual who has limitations in ROM and limited fine motor control. Small, closely spaced targets

TABLE 7-2 Motions and Functions Available at Different Levels of Spinal Cord Injury

Level of Injury	Active Motion Available*	Possible Functions
C3	Neck motion Chin control	Unable to perform personal care Directs others in transfers, personal care Uses mouth or chin control for assistive technologies, ventilator on wheelchair
C4	Neck motion Shrugs shoulder	Same as C3 except: No ventilator Shoulder switch available
C5	Some shoulder motions Flex elbow, no extension	Assistance for bathing or dressing, bladder or bowel care, transfer Uses mobile arm support for feeding, hygiene, grooming, writing, telephone (must be set up by attendant) Uses chin or mouth control for assistive technologies Can propel manual wheelchair short distances with hand rim projections
C6	Wrist extension Forearm pronation Full shoulder motions	Independent transfer, dressing, personal hygiene Manual wheelchair possible with adapted rims and hand splints for writing, feeding, hygiene, grooming, telephone, and typing
C7	Wrist, elbow, shoulder motions; no finger grasp	Independent sitting Drive with adapted controls; uses hand splints for manipulation
C8	No intrinsic hand muscles; limited sensation in the fingers	Limited hand grasp with splints
T1	Paralysis of intrinsic hand muscles; limited flexibility of hand	Weak unaided grasp
T2-T12	Full use of upper extremities; increasing lower extremity function at lower levels; increasing trunk control at lower levels	Manual wheelchair; may use reachers; trunk supports required for higher levels

*At each lower level, all of the functions of higher levels are available plus those listed for the given level.
Modified from Adler C: Spinal cord injury. In Pendleton HM, Schultz-Krohn W, editors: *Pedretti's occupational therapy: Practice skills for physical dysfunction*, ed 6, St. Louis: Mosby, 2006.

are useful for individuals with limited ROM, muscle weakness, and accurate fine motor control (e.g., in someone with muscular dystrophy).

Activation and Deactivation Characteristics

Several characteristics are related to the activation of the control interface. These include method of activation, effort, displacement, flexibility, durability, and maintainability. Deactivation or the release of a control interface also needs to be considered, and it may be different than activation.

Method of Activation

Control interfaces can be activated by a variety of methods that are shown in Table 7-3. The first column identifies the three ways the user can send a signal to the control interface: movement, respiration, and phonation; the middle column shows how each of these signals is detected by the control interface; and the right column provides examples of control interfaces.

Movements by the user can be detected by the control interface in three basic ways. The largest category is *mechanical control interfaces,* which detect a bodily movement that generates a force. Most control interfaces, keyboards, joysticks, and other controls that require movement or force for activation (e.g., mouse, trackball) fall into this category. Force is always required to activate a mechanical control interface; however, mechanical displacement may or may not occur. For example, some keyboards require very little displacement for activation.

Electromagnetic control interfaces do not require contact from the user's body for activation. They detect movement at a distance through either light or radiofrequency energy. Examples include head-mounted light sources and detectors and transmitters used with electronic aids of daily living (EADLs; see Chapter 12) for remote control (similar to garage door openers or TV remote controls). *Electrical control interfaces* are sensitive to electric currents generated by the body. One type, called a capacitive switch, detects static electricity on the surface of the body. This is similar to the game children play when they attempt to shock someone with static electricity. A common example of this type of interface is seen in the touch screen on mobile devices such as phones and tablets. The control interface requires no force and is therefore useful to individuals who have muscle weakness.

The electromyographic (EMG) signal associated with muscle contraction is detected using electrodes attached to the skin to detect. Electrodes placed near the eyes can measure eye movements and generate an electroculographic (EOG) signal based on them. Brain-computer interfaces (BCIs) detect electrical activity either on the surface of the skull or through electrodes implanted in the cortex. *Proximity control interfaces* detect movement without coming into contact with the body. Gesture recognition systems fit into this category.

The second type of body-generated signal shown in Table 7-3 is *respiration.* The signal detected is either airflow or air pressure. One common control interface based on respiration is called a sip-and-puff switch. This switch requires that the user be able to place and maintain her lips around a tube and control airflow. Sipping (drawing air in) and puffing (blowing air out) each generate different signals that can be used for control.

When sound or speech is produced by the airflow, we call it phonation, the third type of activation shown in Table 7-3. There are switches that rely on production of a clicking sound or consistent vocalization to activate. Speech recognition interfaces also rely on phonation. Individuals who have physical involvement that makes other means of activating a control interface difficult may be able to produce sounds, letters, or words consistently enough to activate a control interface. The last type of activation in Table 7-3 is direct brain signal detection, which we discuss in Chapter 8.

Effort

To activate a control interface, the individual must exert some *effort.* The effort required varies from zero for touch switches upward to a relatively large amount for some mechanical switches. An example is using a light pointer to choose from

TABLE 7-3 Methods of Activation

Signal Sent, Signal Detected	User Action (What the Body Does)	Examples
1. Movement (eye, head, tongue, arms, legs)	1a. Mechanical switch: activation by the application of a force 1b. Electromagnetic switch: activation by the receipt of electromagnetic energy such as light or radio waves 1c. Electrical switch: activation by detection of electrical signals from the surface of the body 1d. Proximity switch: activation by a movement close to the detector but without contact	1a. Joystick, keyboard, tread switch 1b. Light pointer, light detector, remote radio transmitter 1c. EMG, EOG, capacitive, or contact switch, touch screen 1d. Heat-sensitive switches, camera (detect gestures)
2. Respiration (inhalation–expiration)	2. Pneumatic switch: activation by detection of respiratory airflow or pressure	2. Puff and sip
3. Phonation	3. Sound or voice switch: activation by the detection of articulated sounds or speech	3. Sound switch, whistle switch, speech recognition
4. Brain electrical activity	4. Different thought patterns generate unique EEG signals	4. BCI

BCI, Brain–computer interface; *EEG,* electroencephalography; *EMG,* electromyographic; *EOG,* electroculographic.

an array of different items where the effort required is sufficient head movement to aim the light beam at one item and move items and enough postural stability to hold the light beam on the desired item.

Electrical interfaces require a range of user effort from zero (for a touch switch) to relatively high for muscle force activation using an EMG. Some electrical control interfaces such as the BCI also use sophisticated signal processing and require that the user develop skills through training to take advantage of the interface. Electrical control interfaces often have an adjustable sensitivity to allow the switch to accommodate for varying levels of effort. This type of adjustment can also be used to prevent accidental activations caused by a switch that is too sensitive.

The activation effort of pneumatic control interfaces is how hard (pressure) or how fast (flow) air is exhaled or inhaled. For example, some power wheelchair processors use a system in which a hard puff (large effort and high pressure generated) results in forward motion, a soft puff (small effort and low pressure generated) in a right turn, a hard sip in reverse, and a soft sip in a left turn. The difference in these control signals is based primarily on effort generated.

Phonation signals also have a level of effort related to volume or loudness. Noise-activated or sound-activated switches are similar to those found on some toys or so-called "clap switches" on lamps. For speech recognition control interfaces, the effort also includes proper pronunciation because the detection is based on identification of a particular word (see Chapter 6).

Some control interfaces, such as the touch switch, have an adjustment for the amount of effort required to activate them. This type of control can be useful for evaluation purposes or for an individual who has fluctuating endurance or a degenerative condition.

Deactivation

There is also a force required to release some control interfaces. Muscle contraction is necessary to *deactivate* an interface by removing or releasing the action that activated it. Weiss (1990) measured both activation and deactivation forces for several mechanical switches and found that force was required to release the control interface in all cases, but the deactivation force was approximately one third to half that required for activation.

Flexibility

The *flexibility* of the control interface is the number of ways in which it can be operated by a control site. There are many types of keyboards, joysticks, and switches and just as many ways in which they can be activated by the user. Individuals with physical disabilities may or may not have deficits in strength, ROM, muscle tone, sensation, or coordination. One person may push a key with a finger, another may use a thumb, and a third may use a head pointer. Control interfaces that allow for various ways of activation are termed *flexible*.

Being able to mount a control interface at the optimal position in the individual's workspace facilitates activation. Some control interfaces, such as a computer mouse, are not intended for mounting and need to be used on a table or other flat surface, but other control interfaces, such as a joystick, can usually be mounted in a variety of locations and can therefore be activated by the chin, hand, or foot. Mounting systems are discussed later in this chapter.

Durability and Maintainability

The *durability* of the control interface is important. Switches and keyboards made out of plastic, for example, may not hold up well under some circumstances. A users who have difficulty controlling the force of their movements will easily break an interface that is made out of plastic. In the long run, it may be cost effective to buy a more expensive interface that is made out of metal and will last longer.

A final consideration is the maintainability of the control interface. It is important to consider whether the interface can be easily cleaned and how it should be cleaned so as not to damage any components. Do any of its components need to be replaced periodically, and, if so, how difficult a procedure it is? For example, certain switches require a battery to operate them, and when the battery dies, it must be replaced. It also helps to know who will be able to repair the control interface if it breaks down, what repairs can be completed by the user or caregiver, which ones need to be completed by someone with specific expertise, and if it is in need of repair whether there is a loaner available for the consumer to use in the interim.

Sensory Characteristics

The auditory, somatosensory, and visual feedback produced during the activation of the control interface comprise its **sensory characteristics.** Some control interfaces (e.g., keyboards that use mechanical switches) provide auditory feedback in the form of a click when activated. Other interfaces (e.g., keyboards have a smooth membrane surface) do not provide any natural auditory feedback. Often a tone is emitted to let the user know that a selection has been made.

When the interface is within the consumer's visual field, visual data are obtained through observation of the placement and the movement of the control interface. For some individuals, the type of visual data will mean the difference between successful and unsuccessful use of a control interface. For example, someone who has difficulty attending to objects in the environment may be more attentive to a control interface that is large and brightly colored.

The eye is sensitive to colors in the visual spectrum (from violet to red), but the eye is not equally sensitive to all colors in this range. If the eye is fixed and not allowed to rotate, the limits of color vision are 60 degrees to each side of the midline. Within this range, the response of the retina to colors is not equal for all wavelengths (colors). Figure 7-1 illustrates that blue objects are visible over the entire 60-degree range, but yellow, red, and green are recognizable only at points closer to the fixed (center) point of vision. This color sensitivity limitation has a practical implication when working with individuals who rely on peripheral vision or who have difficult in moving their eyes to track objects. If a target (e.g., a switch) is green or red, its position may limit the person's ability to see the object. We can increase visibility of the switch by using blue or yellow.

Somatosensory feedback is the tactile, kinesthetic, or proprioceptive input sensed when the control interface is activated. For example, the texture or "feel" of the activation surface provides tactile data. The position in space of the body part and its movement when the user activates the control interface provides proprioceptive feedback. The displacement of the control interface when it is activated provides kinesthetic (movement) feedback, as well as tactile and proprioceptive feedbacks that are beneficial to the user. If there is small movement, as with a membrane keyboard or touch screen, the sensory feedback is less, and the individual may press harder than necessary. This extra, sustained force may result in errors because many keyboards will repeat entries if a key is pressed for more than a second or two. (This can be adjusted on most computers and many assistive devices; see Chapter 8.)

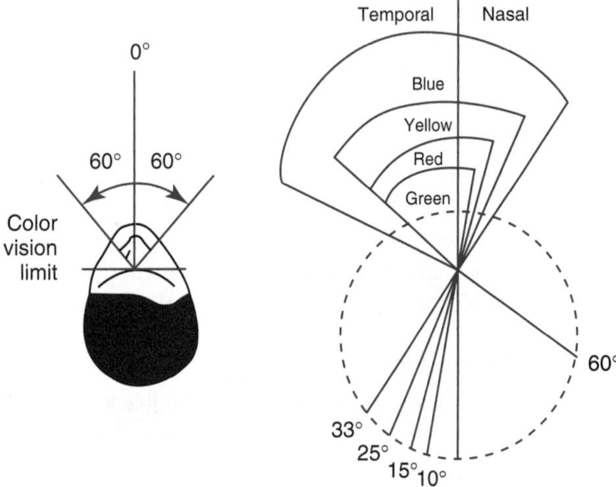

FIGURE 7-1 Color response of the eye differs with visual angle. (Modified from Woodson W, Conover D: *Human engineering guide for equipment designers,* Berkeley: University of California Press, 1964.)

Control interfaces that require more effort typically provide more sensory feedback. Likewise, switches that require very little effort provide very little sensory feedback. Some switches and touch screens are activated by an electric charge from the body. Because it is the transfer of electrical energy from the body to the interface, it requires only touch, and the activation does not provide the user with any somatosensory or auditory feedback. Many mechanical switches provide abundant feedback through the feel (tactile), an observable movement of the mechanism (visual), and an audible click (auditory).

CONTROL INTERFACES FOR DIRECT SELECTION

Direct selection (see Chapter 6) is generally preferable to indirect selection because it is faster and more efficient. For these reasons, it is often worth the effort to try to find direct selection approaches before trying indirect selection methods (scanning or encoded access). Control interfaces for direct selection include various types of keyboards, pointing interfaces, speech recognition, and eye gaze. Hand movement is the preferred control site for direct selection because of the inherent fine motor control. Many individuals also use foot or head control for direct selection, and automatic speech recognition allows a "hands-free" approach.

Keyboards

A keyboard is the most efficient means of inputting information for written communication, computer access, and smart phone or tablet input. However, many individuals with disabilities are unable to use a standard keyboard. Fortunately, there are a number of alternatives. Table 7-4 provides examples of some commercially available alternatives to the standard keyboard.

TABLE 7-4 Alternative Keyboards for Direct Selection

Category	Description	Device Name/Manufacturer
Expanded keyboards	Generally membrane keyboards that have enlarged target areas, often programmable so that key size can be customized; useful for individuals with good range and poor resolution; also useful for individuals with limited cognitive or language skills or visual impairment	IntelliKeys (IntelliTools), Big Keys LX, Clevy Keyboard, Early Learning Keyboard, Helpikeys, Jumbo XL II Hi-Visibility Keyboard, Jumbo XL II Keyboard, Jumbo XL Keyboard (Inclusive Technologies); Expanded Keyboard (Maltron)
Contracted keyboards	Miniature, full-function keyboards, typically with membrane overlay; useful for individuals with limited range of motion and good resolution	The Magic Wand Keyboard (In Touch Systems)
Touch screens and touch tablets	Activated by either breaking a very thin light beam or by a capacitive array that detects the electrical charge on the finger; the electrode array used to detect where the finger or pointer is touching is transparent; the touch screen can be placed over the face of a monitor	Touch Window for 15- and 17-inch monitors (RiverDeep); MagicTouch (Laureate Learning Systems, Inc.)
Special-purpose keyboards	Keyboards on special-purpose devices, such as augmentative communication and environmental control devices; available keys may be much more limited in number or may be specific in function compared with a standard keyboard	See Chapter 16

Data from RiverDeep, San Francisco (web.riverdeep.net/portal/page?_pageid=813,1&_dad=portal&_schema=PORTAL); Laureate Learning Systems, Inc. Winooski, VT (www.laureatelearning.com or www.magictouch.com of KeyTec, Inc.); IntelliTools (http://www.ablenetinc.com/Assistive-Technology/IntelliTools); Inclusive Technologies (http://www.inclusive.co.uk/catalogue/index.html); In Touch Systems, Spring Valley, NY (www.magicwandkeyboard.com); and Maltron-USA (www.maltron.com/keyboard-info/maltron-expanded-keyboard).

Standard Keyboards

For individuals who may have difficulty writing because of fatigue or minimally impaired motor control, a standard keyboard on a computer may be all that is needed. A standard keyboard typically has a full alphanumeric array consisting of letters, numbers, punctuation symbols, special characters (e.g., \/@#$%), and special keys (e.g., END, DEL, SHIFT, CONTROL, and ALT).

Key size, spacing, and amount of distance the keys travel vary depending on the type and manufacturer of the keyboard. Laptop computer keyboards are smaller than desktop computer keyboards, and they are often flat as opposed to the tiered key rows on a full-size keyboard. This configuration can increase difficulty for some individuals.

Ergonomic Keyboards

Standard keyboards place the hands in an unnatural position with the forearms pronated and the wrists extended and ulnarly deviated causing strain on the tendons and nerves. The term *repetitive strain injury* (RSI) can result from sustained, repetitive movements in this unnatural position (van Tulder et al., 2007). Carpal tunnel syndrome is the most common RSI.

Ergonomic keyboards attempt to reduce the strain by putting the forearms, wrists, and hands in a neutral position that is more natural and comfortable. There are three basic ways in which the standard keyboard has been redesigned. The first and most common type of ergonomic keyboard is the fixed-split keyboard (e.g., Figure 7-2 *A*). Here the keys are spaced farther apart, and the keyboard is curved, so that the hands are placed in a more neutral position. Many of these keyboards have a built-in wrist rest for support while typing.

The second basic type of ergonomic keyboard is the adjustable-split keyboard (Figure 7-2 *B*) that also splits the keyboard layout into two parts. A mechanism on the keyboard allows one or both sides of the keyboard to be adjusted horizontally and vertically from 0 to 30 degrees to the most comfortable position

The third type of ergonomic keyboard uses a concave key well design (Figure 7-2 *C*) in which the keys are arranged in a well. The principle behind this design is that finger excursion is reduced by having the keys arranged at the same distance from each of the finger joints (Anson, 1997).

Situations in which an ergonomic keyboard may be recommended for a consumer include (1) meeting the needs of a consumer with physical limitations (e.g., limits in ROM) and (2) when the consumer finds the ergonomic keyboard more comfortable to use than a standard keyboard. Manufacturers of ergonomic keyboards claim that their keyboards reduce the strain placed on the wrist and hands. However, there is limited evidence to support that ergonomic keyboards offer benefits (Amini, 2010).

Expanded Keyboards

Individuals who cannot target the keys on a standard keyboard but still have adequate control to select directly may be able to use an *expanded keyboard*. Expanded keyboards have enlarged target areas from which the individual can directly select (Figure 7-3). The minimum size of the target areas on an expanded keyboard is 1 inch square. If the person still has difficulty targeting this size of key, the expanded keyboard can be customized by grouping keys together to form larger keys. In this way, the keyboard can be redesigned to match the skills of the user.

Expanded keyboards vary in overall size and can be chosen depending on the size of the selection set needed by the individual and the key size the individual is able to target accurately. IntelliKeys (Cambium Learning Group, Dallas, www.cambiumlearningtechnologies.com) has a large surface area that can be configured for a variety of key sizes and shapes. It comes with several standard keyboard overlays, such as the one shown in Figure 7-3 *B*. This overlay is an example of a layout that has been configured with different sizes and different shapes of keys on the same keyboard. The IntelliKeys can also be customized to match specific applications by using the companion Overlay Maker software. The keys can be labeled with letters, words, symbols, or pictures. Because they can be customized, expanded keyboards are also useful with individuals who have a cognitive or visual impairment. Examples of expanded keyboards are shown in Table 7-4.

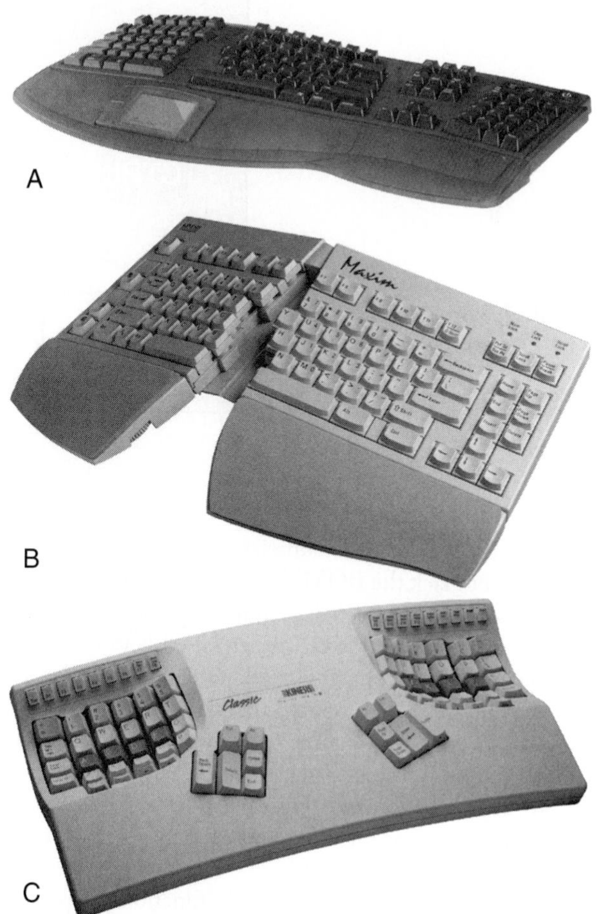

FIGURE 7-2 Ergonomic keyboards. **A,** The Tru-Form keyboard. **B,** The Maxim adjustable keyboard. **C,** The contoured keyboard. (A, courtesy Adesso, www.adessoinc.com; B and C, courtesy Kinesis Corporation, www.kinesis-ergo.com.)

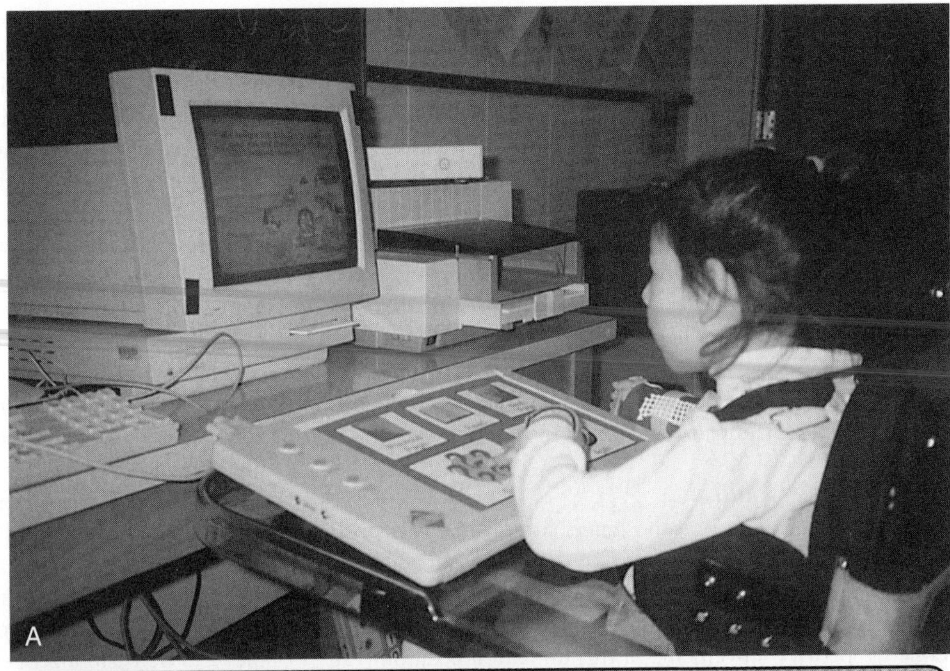

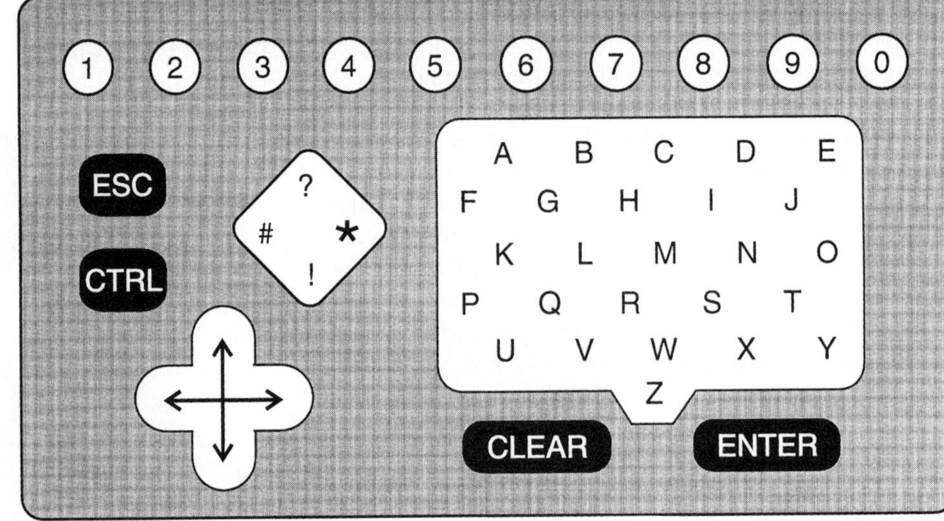

FIGURE 7-3 **A,** Consumer using an expanded keyboard with thumb. **B,** Expanded keyboard showing configuration with different sizes and shapes of keys on the same keyboard.

Contracted Keyboards

For individuals who have sufficient fine motor control to select keys but lack the ROM to reach all the keys on a standard keyboard, a contracted, or mini, keyboard may be the solution. These keyboards use either raised keys or a membrane surface. For computer use, additional modifier keys are used on contracted keyboards so that all keys of the standard keyboard are available. Figure 7-4 shows a consumer being evaluated to use a mouth stick with a USB mini keyboard. This keyboard is approximately 7.25 × 4.2 inches in overall size, with the size of each key approximately one half inch on a side.

Several of the keys have multiple functions, depending on which modifier key is pressed first. The functions corresponding to various modifiers can be colored to match the modifier key. The letter placement is based on a "frequency of use" system in which the letters most commonly used in the English language are placed toward the center, with the less commonly used letters placed in the outer edges of the keyboard to minimize the distance that the person has to move in order to make selections when typing. Persons using contracted keyboards type with a single digit, a handheld typing stick, or a mouth stick.

Smart phones (see Chapter 8) also use small or contracted keyboards. These can cause problems for individuals who have fine motor limitations.

Touch Screens

Touch screens are available on augmentative communication devices (see Chapter 16), EADLs (see Chapter 12), notebook computers (see Chapter 8), and mobile phones and tablets (see Chapter 8). The user makes selections by movements such as swiping, tapping, pinching, and multiple finger gestures that can be difficult for individuals with fine

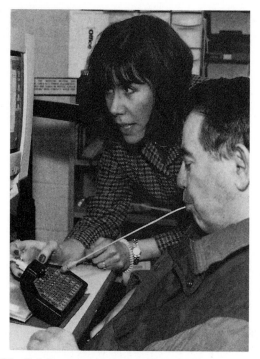

FIGURE 7-4 Consumer being evaluated using the WinMini Keyboard and a mouth stick.

motor impairments. Using a touch screen with icons makes selection cognitively easier for many users, particularly young children, because it is more direct and intuitive. A handheld pointer can help increase accuracy.

Touch screens on mobile devices use icons for selecting apps, functions, and actions. The advantage of the icons is that the children or others who cannot read text can directly touch a picture or symbol and have the device carry out a task. Touch screens are also useful for older adults who have limited experience with a computer and who find it difficult to use a mouse.

Concept Keyboards for Users with Cognitive Limitations

Concept keyboards replace the letters and numbers of the keyboard with pictures, symbols, or words that represent the concepts being used or taught. When the user presses on the picture, the correct character is sent to the computer to create the desired effect. As an example, a child who is having difficulty with monetary concepts may be more successful using a concept keyboard in which each key displayed is a coin of a particular denomination rather than the value (number) or name of the coin (letters). The child can push on the coin and have that number of cents entered into a shopping program. This approach is more motivating for some children, and it is easier to press on a key labeled with a quarter than to enter "2" and "5." Very simple apps such as children's games may require only a few keys.

Eye-Controlled Systems

Often consumers use direction of eye gaze as their only means of indicating. Manual eye-controlled communication systems have been in use for a long time (see Chapter 16). In manual systems, the user communicates yes or no through eye blinks or uses the eyes to point to letters on an alphabet board to spell utterances. This manual form of using eye movement as a means of input can be automated by electronically detecting the user's eye movements as a control interface for direct selection.

There are currently two basic types of eye-controlled systems. One type uses an infrared video camera mounted adjacent to a computer display. An infrared beam from the camera is shined on the person's eye and then reflected by the retina. The camera picks up this reflection of the individual's eye as he looks at the on-screen keyboard appearing on the computer monitor. Special processing software in the computer analyzes the images coming into the camera from the eyes and determines where and for how long the person is looking at the screen. The user makes a selection by looking at it for a specified period, which can be adjusted according to the user's needs. The EyeGaze Edge System (LC Technologies, www.eyegaze.com), Quick Glance (EyeTech Digital Systems, www.eyetechaac.com), and Tobii (Tobii-Technology, www.tobii.com) are examples of eye-controlled systems. The operating principles generally require that the user of the technology be capable of maintaining a stable head position (preferably in midline) and that she is able to focus her visual point of regard on the target for a sufficient period of time. Smooth vertical and horizontal eye movements through the majority of the range are also required.

Eye-controlled systems can be beneficial for individuals who have little or no movement in their limbs and may also have limited speech, for example, someone who has had a brainstem stroke, has amyotrophic lateral sclerosis (ALS), or has high-level quadriplegia. Some disadvantages of eye-controlled systems are that sunlight, bright incandescent lighting, and contact lenses may interfere with system tracking. The cost of such systems is still rather high in comparison with other input methods. For some individuals, however, it may be the only reliable means of voluntary movement for controlling an assistive device.

Tracking of Body Features

Another approach to cursor control is the use of a camera to track body features (Betke et al., 2002). This system uses a digital camera and image recognition software to track a particular feature. The most easily tracked feature is the tip of the nose, but the eye (gross eye position, not POG), lip, chin, and thumb have also been used. The movement of the feature being tracked is converted into a signal that controls an on-screen mouse cursor. Betke et al. (2002) describe the technical features of the system software in detail. Trials with nondisabled subjects in an on-screen game in which targets were "captured" by pointing the cursor at them showed that the camera mouse was accurate but slower than a typical hand-controlled mouse. With an on-screen keyboard used for a typing task, the camera mouse was half as fast as a regular mouse, but the accuracy obtained was equivalent on each system. Eleven persons with disabilities ranging in age from

2 to 58 years used the camera mouse. Eight of the 11 were able to control it reliably and continued to use it. With the increasing availability of built-in cameras in computers, the camera mouse requires only a software program to capture the body feature image and interpret its movement as mouse commands, which may make this approach more common.

Enhancing Keyboard Control

Keyboard control can be aided by proper positioning of both the keyboard and the individual and by the use of devices that make selection easier. We refer to the latter as control enhancers.

Positioning the Person for Keyboard Use

Both the individual and the keyboard must be properly positioned to maximize function. Proper positioning to maximize an individual's function is discussed in Chapter 9. A person's position should be observed as he or she uses a device to be sure that activation of the control interface does not result in an undesirable change in body position. The position of the control interface can also affect the person's ability to activate it, and changing the height or the angle of the control interface even slightly may dramatically improve the person's control ability.

Control enhancers are aids and strategies that enhance or extend the physical control (range and resolution) a person has available to use a control interface. In some cases, a person's control may be enhanced to the extent that he can select directly. In other cases, control enhancers can minimize fatigue. Control enhancers include strategies, such as varying the position or the characteristics of the control interface, and devices such as mouth sticks, head and hand pointers, and arm supports.

Features that enhance control are sometimes incorporated into the interface. For example, some joysticks have a feature, called tremor dampening, that allows adjustment of the joystick for people who have tremors. Tremor-dampening joysticks are able to distinguish between tremors, which are faster and smaller in amplitude, and intentional movements, which are slower and larger. The joystick is adjusted so that the tremors are disregarded and only intentional movements are detected, making it possible for an individual who has a tremor to operate a joystick to control a power wheelchair.

Head Pointers, Hand Pointers, and Mouth Sticks

For individuals who lack functional movement in their arms and hands, a mouth stick (Figure 7-5 *A*) or head pointer (Figure 7-5 *B*) can be used with head and neck movement to access a keyboard or perform other types of direct selection tasks (e.g., dialing a telephone number or turning pages in a book). A mechanical head pointer is a rod with a rubber tip that is attached to a head band. The individual can use the end of the head pointer to depress keys. Besides being able to move the head vertically and horizontally, the individual must have the ability to move the head forward to depress keys.

There are also light pointers that can be worn on the head or held in the hand to control devices. One advantage of head-controlled light pointers is that it is not necessary for the user to move the head forward or backward. Light pointers are described further in the section on pointing interfaces.

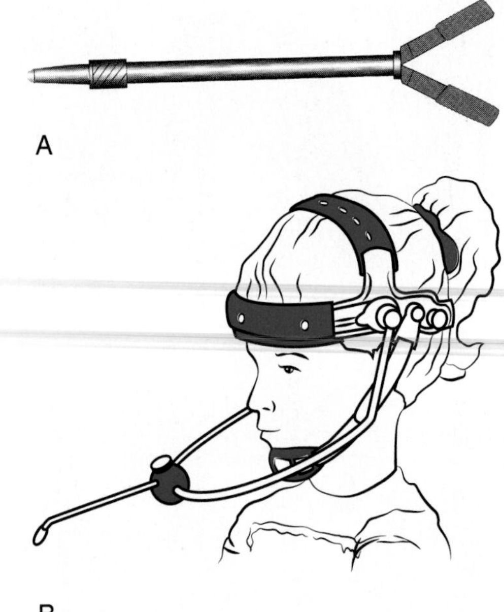

FIGURE 7-5 Control enhancers. **A,** Mouth stick. **B,** Head pointer.

Hand pointers (Figure 7-6 *A*) can be grasped with a gross hand grip. These devices include a projection with a rubber tip that can be used to press keys. These are sometimes referred to as typing aids. A pointing aid may help an individual who has the gross motor ability to move her arm and hand around a keyboard but has difficulty extending and isolating a finger to depress a key. There are commercially available aids that can be strapped onto the hand to assist in pointing, such as the typing aid shown in Figure 7-6 *B*. In some cases, it is necessary to custom fabricate a pointing aid for it to fit the consumer's hand appropriately. These custom-fabricated aids can range from complex hand splints to simple tools such as a pencil with an enlarged eraser.

Mouth sticks, a pointer attached to a mouthpiece, are often used by individuals with quadriplegia as a result of spinal cord injuries (see Figure 7-5 *A*). The user grips the mouthpiece between his teeth and moves his head to manipulate a control interfaces or other objects. The shaft of the mouth stick can be made from a wooden dowel, a piece of plastic, or aluminum. In some cases, interchangeable tips for different functions (e.g., painting, writing, typing) can be inserted into the distal end of the shaft. The mouthpiece can be a standard U shape that is gripped between the teeth or a custom-made insert. Mouth sticks are also available from several suppliers (e.g., Patterson Medical, www.pattersonmedical.com/app.aspx?cmd=searchResults&sk=mouth+stick). Use of a mouth stick requires good oral-motor control.

Mobile Arm Supports

Individuals who have weakness in the arm may not have enough strength to access the full range of a keyboard

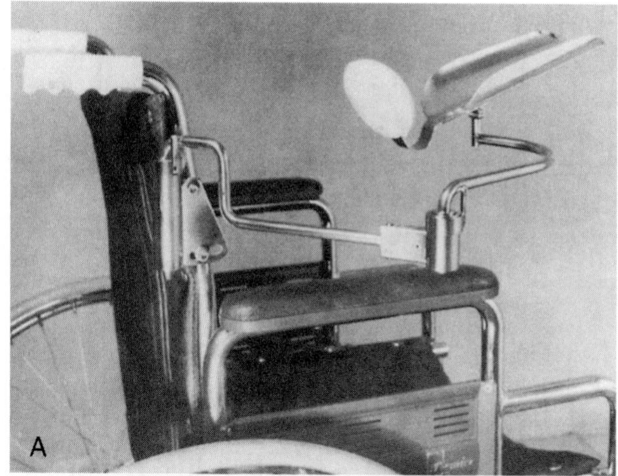

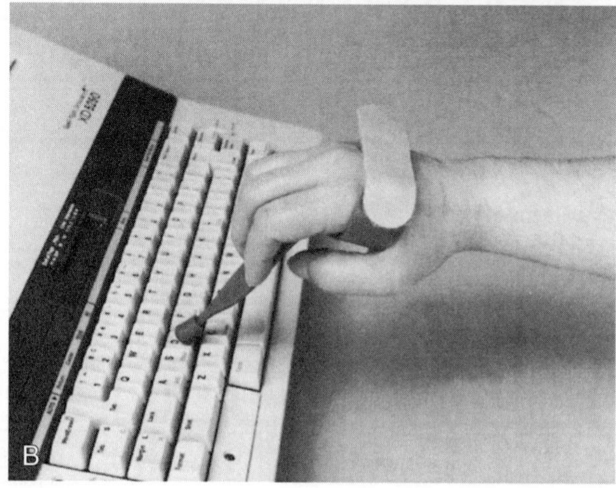

FIGURE 7-6 Control enhancers. **A,** Mobile arm support used to enhance the control in the upper extremity for accessing a control interface. **B,** Typing aid used to enhance a person's ability to point and access a keyboard. (Courtesy Sammons Preston Co., Bolingbrook, IL.)

adequately. A mobile arm support (see Figure 7-6 *A*), which props the arm and assists in arm movements by eliminating some of the effects of gravity, may then allow the individual to access a keyboard.

Keyboard Layouts

The QWERTY keyboard layout (Figure 7-7 *A*), the one most familiar to people, was originally designed more than 100 years ago to slow down 10-finger typists using a manual typewriter so the keys would not jam. The QWERTY layout requires much excursion of the fingers and assumes that two hands with 10 fingers will be used. Redefining the layout of the characters on the keyboard can reduce the amount of finger movements required by the user to access the keys and may reduce fatigue and the likelihood of an individual's incurring a RSI.

Alternative keyboard layout designs have been developed to accelerate typing speed when an individual is using only one hand or a mouth stick or another alternative access device. The definition of the keyboard layout on computer keyboards is determined by software in the computer, and the keys are labeled with the corresponding characters. The keyboard hardware (other than labeling of the keys) is not modified with any of the alternative keyboard layouts.

The Dvorak keyboard layout was designed in the 1930s to reduce fatigue and increase speed by placing letters that are most frequently used on the home row of the keyboard. On the left side of the home row are all the vowels. Five of the most used consonants are on the right side of the home row. There are three Dvorak keyboard layouts: one for two-handed typists (Figure 7-7 *B*), one for right hand-only typists (Figure 7-7 *C*), and one for left-hand-only typists (similar to that shown for right-hand-only typist but flipped). Information on how to redefine the computer keyboard as a Dvorak layout can be found in Easy Access on Windows and as an option in Apple OS X.

The Chubon keyboard is a layout pattern that was designed to be used by the single-digit or typing-stick typist (Chubon & Hester, 1988). In this layout (Figure 7-7 *D*), the letters in the English language that are used most frequently are arranged near each other in the center. This layout also places letters that are most frequently used together (e.g., *r* and *e*) in close proximity, which reduces the amount of movement required by the user for entering text and helps to increase the rate of input. For individuals who use a mouth stick or typing stick, an alternative keyboard layout that reduces the amount of travel to keys can significantly increase efficiency.

Another alternative keyboard layout is an alphabetical array. Often individuals who are nonverbal and have been using a manual communication board to spell have learned to use an array in which the letters are placed in alphabetical order. They are very familiar with this arrangement and may be very efficient in selecting characters. For these individuals, it often does not make sense to have them learn a completely new letter arrangement. In this case, the keyboard can be redefined by using software to have an alphabetical arrangement.

When selecting a keyboard pattern, several factors need to be considered. First consider whether the user is already familiar with one particular keyboard layout. If this is the case, it is important to keep in mind that the time needed for retraining to use a new keyboard pattern is estimated at 90 to 100 hours (Anson, 1997). Another factor to consider is whether the keyboard is shared with other individuals. It is possible to have the computer keyboard defined to use two keyboard patterns (e.g., QWERTY and Dvorak) and to label the keys so that the standard keys are not obscured (e.g., via a clear overlay with the new key labels on them, so when placed over the standard keys the original labels are still visible). However, this modification can be confusing to all typists. There are few data to support the claims that alternative keyboard patterns increase speed or reduce injury. Selecting an alternative keyboard, similar to other technologies, depends on the needs and skills of the user and which layout she feels most comfortable and efficient using.

Key Guards, Shields, and Templates

Some people may be able to select individual keys directly, but they may occasionally miss the desired key and enter the wrong key. For individuals who have difficulty in accurately targeting and activating keys, a key guard (Figure 7-8) placed

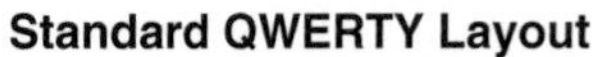

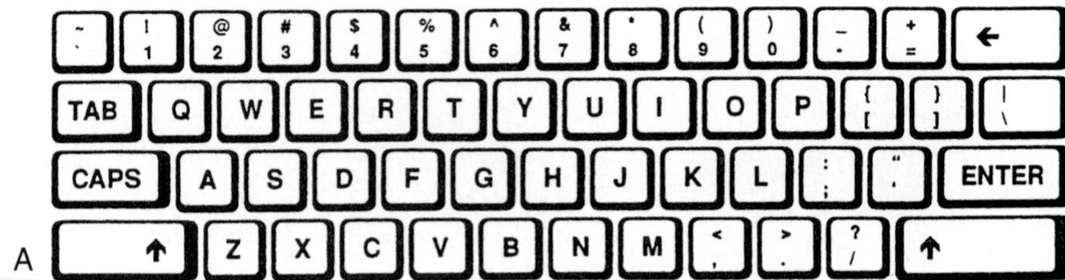

Dvorak Layout for Two Hands

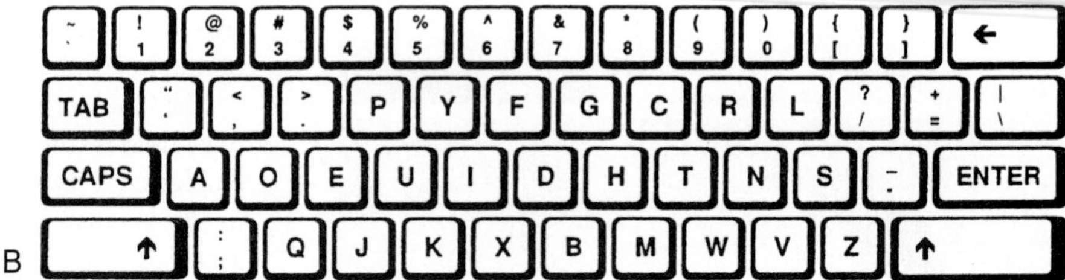

Dvorak Layout for the Right Hand

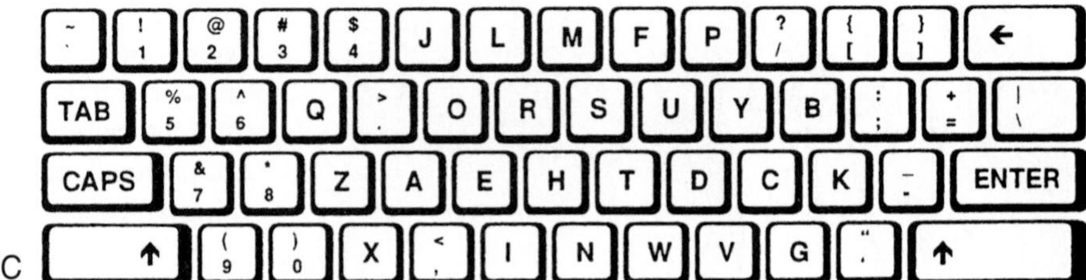

Chubon Keyboard Pattern

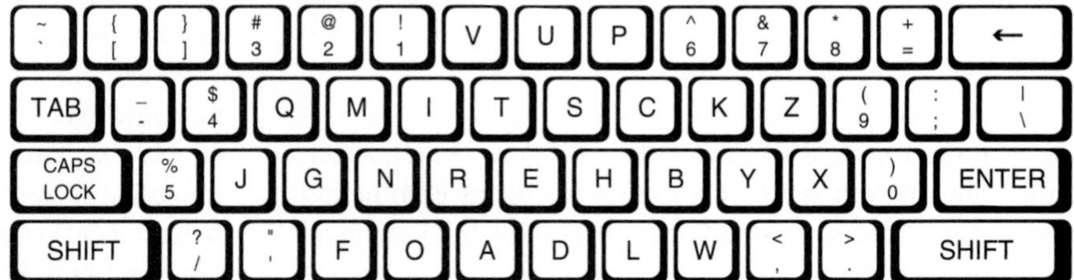

FIGURE 7-7 **A,** Standard QWERTY layout. Dvorak keyboard layouts: **B,** two-hand layout; **C,** one-hand layout, right hand; and **D,** Chubon keyboard layout for a typist who uses a single digit or a typing stick.

over the keyboard helps by isolating each key and guiding the person's movement. A key guard is also useful for individuals who have extraneous movements each time they bring their hand off the keyboard in their attempt to target a new key. Instead of moving away from the keyboard to make the next selection, the person can rest her hand on top of the key guard without activating any keys and make relatively isolated, controlled (and thus faster) selections. Although key guards have been shown to increase the user's accuracy, speed is typically compromised (McCormack, 1990). In nearly all situations, a clear key guard is preferred, so that there is minimal obstruction of the labels on the keys. The position of the keyboard with a key guard needs to be assessed to ensure that the key labels are not being obstructed from the user's view. Key guards are commercially available for common computer keyboards. When an individual uses a special terminal in a work setting and would benefit from a key guard, a custom key guard can be fabricated out of clear plastic.

Similar to the use of a key guard is the use of a **shield** on the keyboard to block out certain keys. This modification is typically done with children who are just beginning to use computers and are using software programs that only require the use of a few select keys. To guide the child to the correct keys and increase her chances of success with the program, a shield is placed over the keys that are not being used.

Technologies for Reducing Accidental Entries

Many keyboards produce multiple entries of characters by prolonged pressing of the key called *key repeat.* Although this feature is useful to nondisabled users (e.g., to obtain multiple

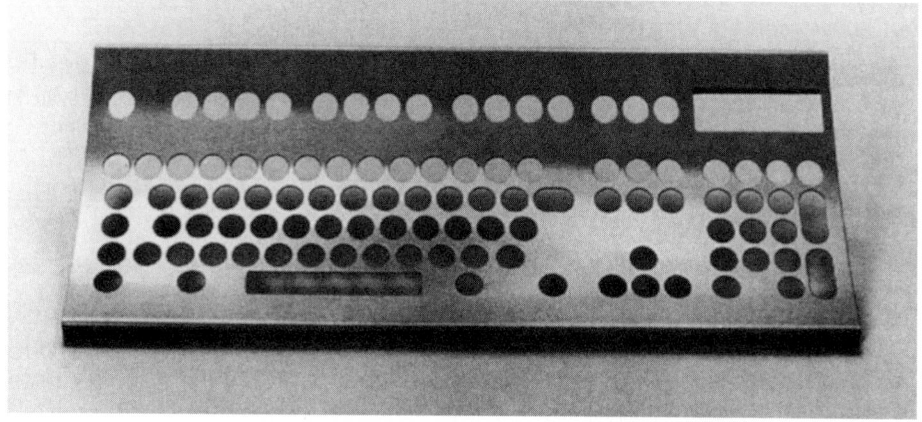

FIGURE 7-8 Keyguard. (Courtesy TASH, Ajax, Ontario, Canada.)

spaces or underlines), it can present a problem for persons with disabilities who may not be able to release the key fast enough to prevent double entry. There are a number of ways this can be avoided.

Certain types and sensitivities of keyboards may increase or decrease double entries, and auditory feedback (e.g., a beep) when a key is activated may also cue the user to release the key in a timely manner. Both of these are sensory characteristics of control interfaces (described earlier in this chapter) that need to be considered as part of the overall assessment. Sometimes the presence of a key guard helps to diminish the double entries. If the double entries remain a problem, features built into current operating systems can be used (see Chapter 8).

Positioning the Keyboard for Use

It is always important to position the keyboard so that it can be easily accessed by the user. Most keyboards are connected with a cable to the computer, which allows some latitude in positioning them so they are accessible. Other keyboards are wirelessly linked by Bluetooth so they can be more flexibly positioned and mounted (e.g., to wheelchairs). Keyboards can also be placed on stands that raise them (e.g., for mouth stick use) or easels that tilt them (e.g., for easier hand access or foot access).

> **CASE STUDY**
>
> *Larry*
>
> Larry was 25 years old when he sustained a traumatic brain injury in a car accident. That was 2 years ago. He attends a day program. He wants to get a job, but all the jobs that he can do require him to use a computer. Unfortunately, his intention tremor makes it difficult for him to type. What types of keyboard modifications would you suggest that Larry try? Why did you choose them?

STANDARD AND ALTERNATIVE ELECTRONIC POINTING INTERFACES

The other commonly used control interface for direct selection in general-purpose computers is a *mouse.* There are also alternative pointing interfaces that can replace the mouse, such as a trackball, a head sensor, a continuous joystick, or the use of the arrow keys on the keypad called *MouseKeys* (see Chapter 8).

Selection by a pointing interface involves two steps: (1) moving a cursor to a desired location, called the target, and (2) holding the cursor on the target long enough for it to be selected. Selection is usually by another action, typically “clicking” using a button on the pointing device. Some pointing interfaces also allow selection via holding on a target. Holding the cursor on the target is often called “dwelling.” There are also alternative ways for a user to carry out other mouse selection methods such as dragging a cursor or double clicking to select. These are described in Chapter 8.

Mouse

As the mouse moves, the computer screen shows a pointer (also called a cursor) that follows the mouse movement. The GUI (graphical user interface) is used as the selection set. In this type of selection set, the screen contains a list of options, either written words or icons. If the mouse is moved to the option and a button is pressed (usually called *clicking*), then that item is chosen. Two rapid clicks are used to run, or execute, the program related to the icon. If the mouse button is held down while the mouse is pointing to a menu item and then the mouse is moved down the list (called *dragging* the mouse), a new list of choices appears. The GUI reduces the number of keystrokes and provides a prompting display for the user.

The mouse is ideally suited for functions such as drawing, moving around in a document, or moving a block of text. The mouse can be a useful tool for individuals with disabilities who cannot otherwise draw with a pen or pencil. However, mouse use requires a high degree of eye–hand coordination and motor coordination and a certain amount of ROM. The standard computer mouse is available in many different shapes and sizes.

If a consumer is having difficulty using the mouse that came with the computer, the solution may be as simple as finding a mouse that fits his or her hand better. The standard

TABLE 7-5 Alternative Electronic Pointing Interfaces

Category	Description	Device Name/Manufacturer
Keypad mouse	Mouse movement is replaced by keys that move the mouse cursor in horizontal, vertical, and diagonal directions. One or more keys perform the functions of the mouse button (click, double click, drag). The ATEC Computer Switch Interface allows connection of up to five switches to a USB port and is the lowest priced of all the standard interfaces. It even remembers your settings when you turn the computer off! In addition to the usual settings found on other devices, the ATEC Computer Switch Interface adds a setting for mouse control. The user can use five switches to move the mouse up, down, left, right, and click.	ATEC Computer Switch Interface (Adaptivation, Inc.)
Trackball	Looks like an inverted mouse; a ball is mounted on a stationary base. Included on the base are one or more buttons that provide the functions of the standard mouse buttons. The base and hand remain stationary, and the fingers move the ball. Requires minimal range of motion and less eye–hand coordination.	Big Track, n-Abler (Inclusive Technology, Trackman Marble Mouse and Wireless Trackball M570, Logitech); EasyBall (Microsoft); Roller Plus and Roller II Trackball (Traxsys Computer Products)
Continuous input joysticks	Joysticks (continuous input and switched) are used as direct selection interfaces for powered mobility. For computer use, movements are similar to wheelchair control; easy to relate cursor movement (direction, speed, and distance) to joystick movement.	Jouse2 (Compusult Limited); Roller Plus Joystick, Roller II Joystick, and EasiTrax (Traxsys Computer Products); JoyStick-C and JoyStick-C lite (Inclusive Technology); all manufacturers of power wheelchairs have their own joysticks, which are supplied with the wheelchair
Head-controlled mouse	An interface controlled through head movement; the user wears a sensor on the head, which is detected by a unit on the computer. Movement of the head is translated into cursor movement on the screen.	HeadMouse Extreme (Prentke Romich Co. & Origin Instruments Co.); TrackerPro (AbleNet); SmartNAV-4 (Inclusive Technology)
Light pointers and light sensors	These devices either emit a light beam that can be used to point to objects or as a control interface, or they receive light and provide an output when the light is reflected from an object or the light beam is interrupted.	(Laser light pointers can be used if the precautions shown in Box 7-1 are followed.)

Data from Ability Research, Inc., Minnetoka, MN (http://www.abilityresearch.net/); Adaptivation, Sioux Falls, SD (www.adaptivation.com); Compusult Limited, Mount Pearl, Newfoundland (www.jouse.com/html/about.html); Logitech, Fremont, CA (www.logitech.com); Inclusive Technology (http://www.inclusive.co.uk/catalogue/index.html); Microsoft, Redmond, WA (www.microsoft.com); Origin Instruments, Grand Prairie, TX (www.orin.com); Traxsys Computer Products (assistive.traxsys.com/staticProductListing.asp); and Prentke Romich Co., Wooster, OH (www.prentrom.com).

mouse requires a great deal of motor control, however, and many individuals with disabilities find that the use of a standard computer mouse is difficult or impossible. Simpson (2013) describes the major problems people with disabilities encounter when using a mouse. These problems include difficulty grasping and manipulating the mouse, problems executing long or straight movements of the cursor, difficulty positioning the cursor inside a target on the screen, problems with single or double clicking, and problems with clicking and dragging.

The basic operating system allows the speed of mouse movement, the trail left by the mouse, and other features to be adjusted. For individuals with severe motor impairments, the built-in adjustment of mouse speed, cursor size, and so on are not sufficient to allow use of the mouse or other pointing device. Commercial products extend the range of these adjustments and add other features such as wrapping the cursor around the screen when it reaches one side (i.e., when the cursor hits the right edge of the screen, it appears again on the left side).

Another option is to try a different control site for mouse use. If the consumer has better control of his feet than his hands, his foot can be used with a foot-controlled mouse (www.fentek-ind.com/footime.htm#.UpyzQaNrZ30). There are also alternatives to a mouse that are easier for many persons with disabilities. Any control interface that can imitate the two-dimensional movement (up/down, left/right) of the mouse can be made to look to the computer like a mouse. Table 7-5 lists the major alternatives to mouse input and example devices. Examples of several of these approaches are shown in Figure 7-9.

Keypad Mouse

For individuals who are able to use a standard keyboard but have difficulty using a standard mouse, the first alternative to evaluate is the keypad mouse. A numerical keypad is embedded in most standard computer keyboards. MouseKeys, included in the accessibility options for Windows and in the OS operating systems, allows use of the keypad to simulate mouse movement. When the NUM LOCK key is engaged, each key on the numerical keypad functions as the number to which it is assigned (1 to 9). When the NUM LOCK key is disengaged and MouseKeys is running, these keys can perform the same functions as a mouse. The "5" key serves as a mouse click, and the surrounding number keys move the mouse in vertical, horizontal, or diagonal directions. This software interprets the keys as mouse input when MouseKeys is active and interprets them as arrow keys when

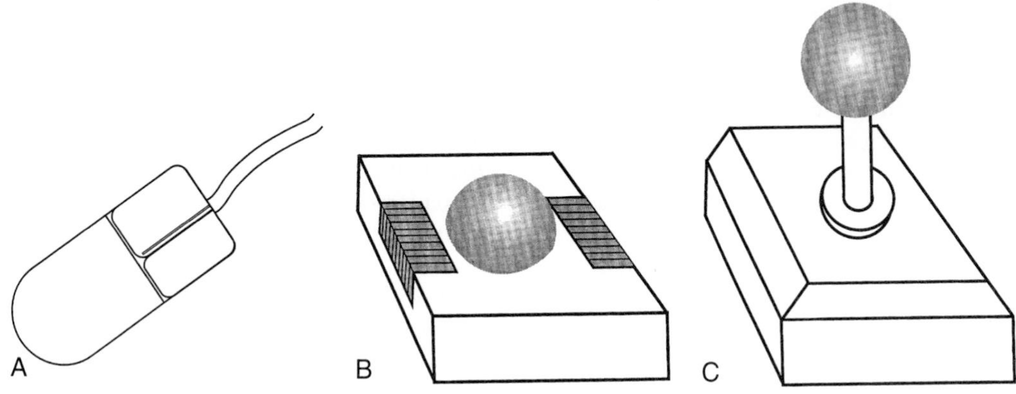

FIGURE 7-9 Pointing interfaces. **A,** Standard computer mouse. **B,** Trackball. **C,** Proportional joystick.

it is not active. MouseKeys allows adjustment of the mouse speed (distance the cursor moves with each arrow key press) and acceleration (the rate at which the cursor moves).

Trackball

Use of a trackball is one approach that was developed for the able-bodied population but has often been found to be helpful for persons who cannot use a mouse. This device looks like an inverted mouse; a ball is mounted on a stationary base. Included on the base are one or more buttons that provide the functions of the standard mouse buttons. The ball is rotated by moving the hand or finger across it, causing the cursor to move on the screen. Because the base and hand remain stationary and the fingers move the ball, this approach requires less ROM than a standard mouse and is easier for some users who have disabilities. It is also possible to use the trackball easily with other body sites such as a chin or foot. On most trackballs, the user can latch the mouse button, which allows single-finger or mouth stick users to perform "click and drag" functions without having to hold down a button while simultaneously moving the mouse. Trackballs are available in a variety of sizes, shapes, and configurations. There are trackballs (e.g., the Trackman Marble Plus, www.logitech.com/en-ca/product/trackman-marble) in which the ball is positioned on the side where it can be controlled by the thumb. There are also very small trackballs, such as the Thumbalina Mini Trackball (www.trackballworld.com/40-320.html), that fit in the palm of the hand. Allowing the consumer to try the different types of trackballs is important even if it means taking a trip to a local computer store that has different models available for demonstration.

Continuous Joysticks

A joystick provides four directions of control and is thus ideally suited for use as another alternative to a mouse. There are two types of joysticks, proportional (continuous) and switched (discrete). A proportional joystick has continuous signals, so any movement of the control handle results in an immediate response by the **command domain** in that direction. By using a proportional joystick, the individual can control not only direction of movement but also the rate of that movement. Proportional joysticks are most commonly used with power wheelchairs (see Chapter 10). The farther the wheelchair joystick moves away from the starting point, the faster the wheelchair goes. The proportional joystick is also more likely to be used as a mouse substitute because the direction and rate of cursor movement can be controlled by the user (see www.infogrip.com/products/manufacturers/traxsys/roller-joystick.html).

The Jouse 2 is a joystick-operated mouse that is controlled with the chin or mouth (http://www.jouse.com/jouse3/home). Mouse button activations can be made by using a sip-and-puff switch that is built into the joystick. Just like the proportional joystick used for wheelchair control, the joystick used for a mouse substitute will cause the mouse pointer to move faster the farther away it gets from the center position. A major difference between mouse and trackball use and the use of a joystick is that whereas the joystick is always referenced to a center point, the mouse cursor movement is relative to the current position. This difference in reference point can cause difficulties for the consumer when first using the joystick. The user must spend some time learning how to use this control interface for it to be an effective alternative to the mouse (Anson, 1997).

Casas et al. (2012) described a modification of a wheelchair joystick to allow it to be used in place of a computer mouse. Their modification is entirely external to the joystick, meaning that it does not impact the wheelchair joystick warranty. They based their design on the addition of an external biaxial accelerometer external to the joystick electronics to sense the movements of the joystick. The accelerometer is placed in a disk around the lever of the joystick and is connected to electronics that process the accelerometer signal to convert is to a mouse-like input signal to a USB port on the computer. The electronic box includes two jacks that allow external switches to be attached to function like the mouse buttons. A third switch allows selection between wheelchair control and computer control. The use of the joystick for both wheelchair control and computer access is an example of **integrated controls** that are discussed in a later section of this chapter.

Head-Controlled Mouse

For individuals who lack the hand or foot movement to operate a mouse or joystick, there are alternative pointing interfaces that are controlled with head movement (Evans et al., 2000). In general, head-controlled mouse systems operate by using a tracking unit that senses and measures head position relative to a fixed reference point. This reference point is the center of the screen for the cursor. As the head moves away from this point in any direction, the cursor is moved on the screen. The technology that is used to sense the head movement differs from one system to another; it may be ultrasound, infrared (IR), gyroscopical, or image recognition (video). Each of these relies on transmission of a signal to the sensor on the user's head and detection of a reflected signal that is sent back. An alternative approach is to locate a transmitter on the user's head with a receiver that monitors the change in head position (Evans et al., 2000). Different commercial systems implement this reflective measurement in a variety of ways. In the early versions of head-controlled interfaces, the headset worn by the user was connected with a wire to the computer, limiting the user's mobility. Most of the systems currently available have a wireless connection, which allows the user to move around more freely.

These systems are intended for individuals who lack upper extremity movement and who can accurately control head movement. For example, persons with high-level spinal cord injuries who cannot use any limb often find these head pointers to be rapid and easy to use. However, individuals who have random head movement or who do not have trunk alignment with the vertical axis of the video screen often have significantly more trouble using this type of input device.

Several devices require only a reflective dot to be placed on the user's face (usually the forehead) (Figure 7-10 *A*). A tracking unit on the computer detects the movement of the reflective dot on the head and translates it into a signal that the computer interprets as if it were sent by a mouse. By moving the head (with the dot on it), the person moves the cursor on the screen. This design eliminates the bulky head pointer used in earlier devices. (Currently available systems include Tracker, AbleNet, www.ablenetinc.com/Assistive-Technology/Computer-Access/TrackerPro; HeadMouse, Origin Instruments, www.orin.com/access/headmouse; and SmartNav, Natural Point; www.naturalpoint.com/smartnav/support/downloads.html). Several augmentative communication devices (see Chapter 16) have built-in head tracking using this approach.

Control of the mouse cursor is either relative (like a joystick) or absolute (like a mouse). With absolute devices, the mouse cursor position corresponds to the position of the device (e.g., a trackball, hand-operated mouse). To operate a relative device, the person moves the cursor by displacing the control. When the cursor reaches the desired location, the control is released. The next movement is then made from that location by displacing the control again. A joystick is an example of a relative pointing device. Because a hand-operated mouse can also be lifted and repositioned, it can act like a relative device. Users with disabilities prefer the relative technique (Evans et al., 2000).

Movement times for nondisabled individuals are greater for head-controlled cursor systems than for a conventional mouse (Taveira & Choi, 2009). Movement times are also greater for small versus large targets and for far versus near targets in both nondisabled individuals and those with cerebral palsy (CP). On the basis of reduction in average movement time as an indicator of relative learning, 15 sets of 48 trials (with one trial defined as mouse cursor movement from center screen to a randomly presented target) were sufficient to attain stable performance using both mouse- and head-operated systems in nondisabled individuals. Two participants with CP were included in this study. One participant's learning approximated that of the nondisabled control subjects. The other participant's learning was more rapid but also more variable, and both speed and accuracy of head control were dramatically affected by proper trunk stability provided through a seating system (see Chapter 9).

User operational characteristics, including satisfaction, were evaluated for five currently available mouse alternatives that were based on head tracking by gathering the subjective evaluation of the users (Phillips & Lin, 2003). The users included individuals with high-level spinal cord injuries and those with CP. Dependent variables were speed, accuracy, and distance or displacement in target acquisition tasks. Variable performance was reported for participants with CP, even when identical interfaces were used.

Three different technologies, IR with a reflective dot (Tracker), ultrasonography (HeadMaster; no longer available), and gyroscopic (Tracer, Boost Technologies, www.boosttechnology.com), were evaluated by six nondisabled subjects (Anson et al., 2003). Comparisons of speed, accuracy, and user preference were made by using a drawing task with an on-screen cursor. Each of the three approaches was fastest for one third of the subjects, and all were equally accurate. The preferred device was the Tracker. This device has only a reflective dot attached to the head, but the other two had additional hardware attached. Although results for a persons with disabilities would likely differ, this study did indicate that all head-pointing technologies can yield fast and accurate results.

The impact on performance of repeated trials of the head-controlled mouse system (Tracker) was evaluated in a series of target acquisition tasks for 12 persons with CP (Cook et al., 2005). Time to target, time to select, and distance moved to target (i.e., the screen distance traveled over the path between start and finish of a selection movement) were measured. The targets were reduced in size across four once-weekly 1-hour sessions. Nine of the 12 participants were able to achieve a smaller target at the end of the session compared with the initial target size. For the same-size targets, six participants reduced their times to target, and seven reduced the distance moved to acquire the target. However, only two participants showed a decrease in their time to select scores, which is an indication of the difficulty of holding a target for a preset dwell time. These results indicate that individuals with CP may be able to use head-controlled cursor systems if they are given sufficient practice time with a gradual reduction of target size as skill increases.

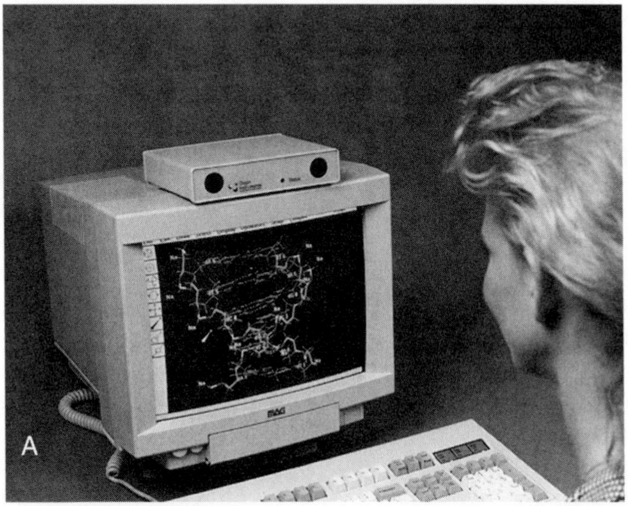

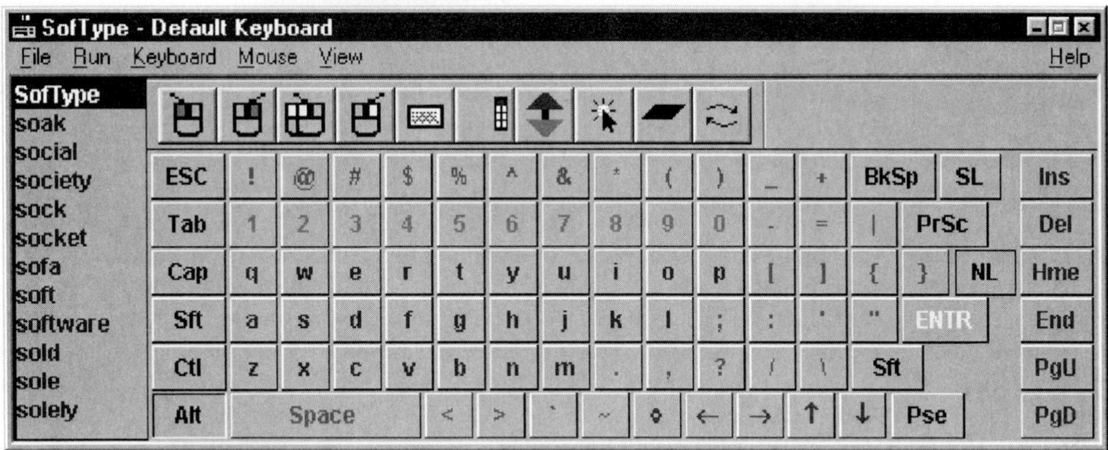

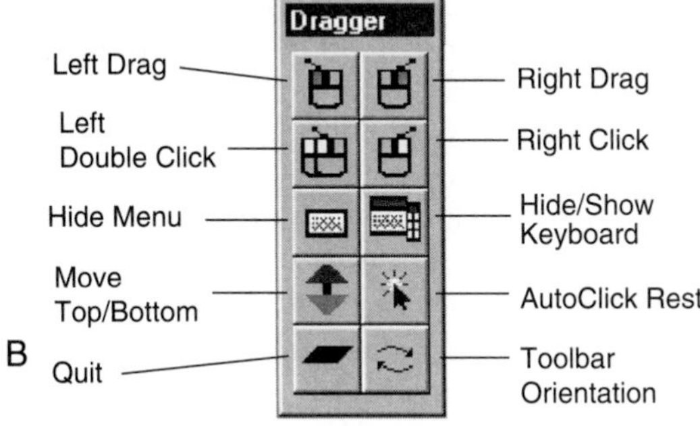

FIGURE 7-10 **A,** Head-controlled mouse. **B,** An example of an on-screen keyboard screen for Microsoft Windows. (Courtesy Origin Instruments Corporation, www.orin.com.)

Comparison of Keypad- and Head-Controlled Mouse Alternatives

When a consumer has difficulty in using a standard mouse, alternatives are considered, and it is necessary to make comparisons among different alternatives. Generally, there is little empirical evidence to guide decision making. One study that is useful in this regard compared the use of a head-controlled mouse (Tracker) and an expanded keyboard used as a key-pad mouse (Intellikeys; IntelliTools, Petaluma, CA, http://www.ablenetinc.com/Assistive-Technology/IntelliTools) (Capilouto et al., 2005). These two devices were chosen because they both require gross motor movements and would likely be considered as alternatives for a specific consumer. The two devices were tested in a target acquisition task by nondisabled university students. Each device was used to acquire a target by moving a cursor from a starting point in the center of the screen. The time to capture a target decreased with practice for both devices, but the head pointer resulted in faster performance. The time to acquire a target was longer for targets spaced further from the starting point, but this effect was less for the head-pointing device. Reaction time was less for the head-pointing device as well. All of these results are related to the necessity for sequential action in the case of the keyboard (i.e., moving from one key to another to change mouse movement direction compared with continuous movement using the head-pointing system).

USING POINTING INTERFACES FOR DIRECT SELECTION

Because direct selection involves choosing from an array of items, we can think of mouse use or other pointing as direct selection too. When using a graphic user interface (icons on a screen), the mouse is moved to the icon of choice, and we click or double click to open or run the chosen file or program. This is direct selection. There are also alternative pointing interfaces that can replace the mouse, such as a trackball, a head sensor, a continuous joystick, or the use of the arrow keys on the keypad (called *MouseKeys*).

Making Selections with a Pointing Device

Pointing devices can be used to select programs, features, or other apps just like typical mouse control for a GUI. To provide text input on the screen using a pointing device, an **on-screen keyboard**—a video image of the keyboard on the video screen—is used together with a cursor (see Figure 7-10 *B)*.

To make a selection, it is necessary to direct the pointer to the desired item on the screen (the target) and stay fixed on the target while executing the action needed to make a selection (e.g., clicking or double clicking or clicking and holding to drag the item). These all imply that the targeted selection is accurate. The person may be able to get to a target area on the screen, but the size of the target may affect her ability to maintain that position while selecting it. Any location on the screen can be a target, and these can be of different sizes. Depending on the software app, the size of the target may be fixed, or it may be possible to modify the size to meet the user's needs.

The functions of the mouse button(s) can also be replaced for those unable to hit them or for the use of the head-controlled interface that only includes pointing, not clicking. Selecting an icon or text character, opening a window, and clicking and double clicking are done by using either a switch or an acceptance (or dwell) time (which can be adjusted to meet the user's needs). When a switch is used, it is often a puff-and-sip switch that is attached directly to the headset (e.g., Origin Instruments, www.orin.com/access/sip_puff). The person generates a single puff to click and two puffs to double click. To perform the drag function, the user must produce sustained pressure on the puff switch, and some individuals may not have sufficient breath control. Switch selection provides good control for the user, but it also requires additional user motor control to activate the switch.

In the **acceptance time** *or dwell time selection,* the user pauses at the selection for a predetermined period (which is adjustable). At the end of the acceptance time period, the device automatically executes whatever function was selected (e.g., click).

On-screen displays give the user the option of various mouse functions. Commercial programs allow the user to select what mouse button function (click to select, double click to open and run the application, or drag to move) is activated with the third control interface press. In some cases, the selected function is implemented only after an acceptance time. If an additional control interface press occurs before the acceptance time (less than 1 second, typically), the selection is cancelled, which allows for error correction before an entry is made. Scan rate, scanning line width, dwell time before rest or selection, and other characteristics are adjustable on most commercial products. Some of these parameters are discussed in Chapter 6.

The particular app for mouse selection varies by manufacturer. One is called Dragger (Origin Instruments) (see Figure 7-10 *B*). The dwell selection function in Dragger is called AutoClick. When AutoClick is active, every time the pointer comes to rest, a left click will occur for the dwell time. This single-switch closure can result in a double click, right click, or left and right drag using the Dragger toolbar. Similar approaches are used in other systems (e.g., dwell click in Smart Nav and Dwell Clicker 2 (AbleNet or Sensory Software, http://sensorysoftware.com/more-assistive-tecthnology-software/dwell-clicker-2/). The latter can be downloaded free.

For consumers who only have enough motor control for a single or dual switch, there are several general approaches to scanning for emulation of these mouse functions (Blackstein-Alder et al., 2004). One approach is Cartesian scanning in which pressing a switch causes a line to move slowly down the screen intersecting various on-screen icons. A second switch press causes a pointer or vertical line to move across the screen. When the pointer or vertical line is located over the desired screen icon, a third switch press selects that icon as though the mouse button had been pressed. This function is similar to matrix-type row column scanning except that the scan is continuous rather than moving discretely between choices. A second approach is similar except that the movement of the lines is in discrete steps rather than continuous. This is easier for some users to follow and gives them a specific target time during which they must hit the switch. This method more closely approximates typical row column scanning.

A third approach is rotational scanning that involves two steps, pointing toward a target, and then moving the mouse pointer toward the target. When the user activates the control interface once, a scan line is drawn from the center to the right-hand side of the computer screen. This scan line rotates about the center at a continuous speed counterclockwise around the screen similar to a radar display. When the line intersects an on-screen target, the user activates the control interface a second time to stop the rotational scanning. This line remains visible, and a second perpendicular line begins scanning outward from the center. When this line intersects the desired target, the user hits the control interface a third time to make the selection.

Another approach to mouse emulation is the creation of on-screen "hot spots" in software applications. These are scanned sequentially. This approach optimizes the scan to only the parts of the screen that are active during an application. For example, in a child's reading program, the hot spots could be characters that speak during a story. Many setups are available for popular programs and are stored for a particular application. A variety of scanning selection techniques (e.g., automatic, inverse, and step) can be used to scan the hotspots with one or switches. Several commercial products provide for mouse functions during scanning (Dragger, Origin Instruments, Grand Prairie, TX, www.orin.com; ScanBuddy, Applied Human Factors, Helotes, TX, www.ahf-net.com). An example is shown in Figure 7-10 *B*.

In general, these programs allow the user to select the mouse function following the selection of a target using any of the scanning or hotspot approaches described here. A more generic approach is one in which all interface objects in Windows are scanned as hot spots until the scan is stopped by control interface activation (WiVik, www.wivik.com). This action begins the next sequence (e.g., scanning down a list of choices in an opened menu).

Pointing interfaces vary in terms of the tactile and proprioceptive feedback they provide, which may affect the user's performance. Using a pointing interface also requires a significant amount of coordination between the body site executing the movement of the cursor and the eyes following the cursor on the screen and locating the targets. It is important to determine whether the layout of the items on the screen (the selection set) is beneficial or detrimental to the user's performance. For example, it may be easier for the user to see one part of the screen than another. It may also be more difficult to move the pointer to some parts of the screen because of motor control limitations. It is possible to rearrange the elements on the screen, to reposition the pointing device, and to change the size of the elements on the screen to compensate for these problems. The selection set and its layout vary depending on the pointing interface and the software being used. It is important to know whether the layout of the selection set can be modified for a particular pointing interface and what type of modifications will benefit the user.

Light Pointers

A visible light beam may be used as a pointing interface for direct selection. In a simple form, the light can be pointed at objects in a room or at letters on a piece of paper. The effectiveness of the light pointer is directly related to how bright and focused it is, and this in turn affects size and weight. Light pointers are most commonly attached to a band worn on the head, but they can also be held in the hand. Highly focused light sources such as laser pens may cause damage if they are shined directly into the eye (Box 7-1) (Hyman et al., 1992; Salamo & Jakobs, 1996).

CONTROL INTERFACES FOR INDIRECT SELECTION

Indirect methods of selection use a single control interface or an array of control interfaces and require that the consumer be able to carry out a certain set of skills. These controls are used with scanning and coded access discussed in Chapter 6.

BOX 7-1 Tips on Safe Use of Laser Light as a Head Pointer

Laser light sources (including laser pens) are a source of highly focused light of high intensity. Because they are focused, the energy is all concentrated on a small area—including the retina if the light is shined in the eye of another person. Lasers are grouped into five classes: I (<0.01 mw), II (0.01 to 1 mw), IIIa (1 to 5 mw), IIIB (1 mw to 0.5 w), and IV (>0.5 w). Salamo and Jakobs (1996) recommend an exposure of less than 0.0004 milliwatts (0.4 microwatts) for 1 second as the limit for safe continuous exposure as might occur in a classroom. Only class I lasers meet this criteria, and they are so dim as to not be visible in a brightly lit classroom. Laser pointers are at least class II. Because of the continuous use, the possible limitation of protective reflexes that protect nondisabled individuals from exposure to class I lasers and the uncontrolled environment (i.e., the classroom), caution should be exercised when using laser pointers for choice making and pointing.

Types of Single Switches

Numerous single control interfaces (switches) are commercially available. When selecting or evaluating the effectiveness of a control interface for an individual, it is important to consider the spatial, activation-deactivation, and sensory characteristics discussed earlier. Single-switch interfaces can be activated by body movement, respiration, or phonation. Table 7-6 summarizes the types of single-switch interfaces and gives a sampling of switches that are available.

Single switches come in many different sizes and shapes and have diverse force and sensory requirements. It is critical that the consumer has the opportunity to try out any switch being considered for a control interface. Table 7-6 summarizes the types of single-switch interfaces and gives a sampling of control interfaces that are commercially available based on the categories shown in Table 7-3. The switches that are activated by body movement detect the movement in one of four ways: mechanical, electromagnetic, electrical, or proximity. Switches that are mechanical in nature are activated by force applied by any part of the body.

Mechanical Control Interfaces

Mechanical control interfaces are the most commonly used type of single switch, and they can be of various shapes and sizes. Paddle switches (Figure 7-11 *A*) have movement in one direction. On some types of paddle switches, the sensitivity can be adjusted according to the user's needs. Wobble (Figure 7-11 *B*) and leaf switches (Figure 7-11 *C*) have a 2- to 4-inch shaft that can be activated by the user in two directions. The wobble switch makes an audible click when activated, and the leaf switch does not, making the wobble switch more desirable when the switch is out of the user's visual range, such as during head activation. Lever switches (Figure 7-11 *D*) are similar to wobble switches with the exception that they can only be activated in one direction. This type of switch usually has a round, padded area at the end of a shaft and produces an audible click, which also makes it desirable for activation by the head.

TABLE 7-6 Examples of Single-Switch Interfaces

Category	Description	Switch Name/Manufacturer
Mechanical switches	Activated by the application of a force; generic names of switches include paddle, plate, button, lever, membrane	Pal Pads, Taction Pads, and Flexible Switch (Adaptivation Corp; Big Red (now called Big Red Twist), Jelly Bean (now called Jelly Bean Twist) and Buddy Button Switches (AbleNet, Inc.); Lolly, Thumb, Lever (long and short), Leaf (long and short), and Tread Switches (Zygo Industries); Access Switch (unlimiter) Single Rocking Lever, Dual-rocking Lever, and Wobble Switch (Prentke Romich Co.); Moon, Membrane, Flexible, Wobble, Picture Plate switch (AMDi); Ultra Light Switch (Adaptive Switch Laboratories, Inc.)
Electromagnetic switches	Activated by the receipt of electromagnetic energy such as light or radio waves	Fiber Optic Sensor (Adaptive Switch Laboratories, Inc.); SCATIR (AbleNet, Inc.) Infrared, sound, and touch switch (Words+; now AAC Works)
Electrical control switches	Activated by detection of electrical signals from the surface of the body	Brainfingers 9, Cyberlink (Adaptivation Corp.)
Proximity switches	Activated by a movement close to the detector but without actual contact	ASL 204M, 204-3 Pin, 208M, 208-3 Pin Proximity Switch (Adaptive Switch Laboratories, Inc.); Proximity Switches (AMDi)
Pneumatic switches	Activated by detection of respiratory air flow or pressure	Pneumatic Switch (Adaptivation Corp); Sip, Grip and Puff Switch (Toys for Special Children); ASL 308 Pneumatic Switch (Adaptive Switch Laboratories, Inc.); PRC Pneumatic Switch Model PS-3 (Prentke Romich Co.); Pneumatic Switch Model CM-3 (Zygo Industries)
Phonation switches	Activated by sound or speech	Voice Activated and Sound Activated Switches (Enabling Devices); Infrared/Sound and Voice Switches (Zygo Industries)

Data from Ablenet Inc., Minneapolis, MN (www.ablenetinc.com); Adaptive Switch Laboratories, Inc., Spicewood, TX (www.asl-inc.com); Adaptivation Co., Sioux Falls, SD (www.adaptivation.com); AMDi, Hicksville, Northwest Territories (http://www.amdi.net/products); Emerge Medical, Atlanta, GA (www.emergemedical.com/); Prentke Romich, Wooster, OH (www.prentrom.com); Saltillo (www.saltillo.com/), Enabling Devices—Toys for Special Children, Hastings-on-Hudson, NY (www.enablingdevices.com); and Zygo, Portland, OR (www.zygo-usa.com).

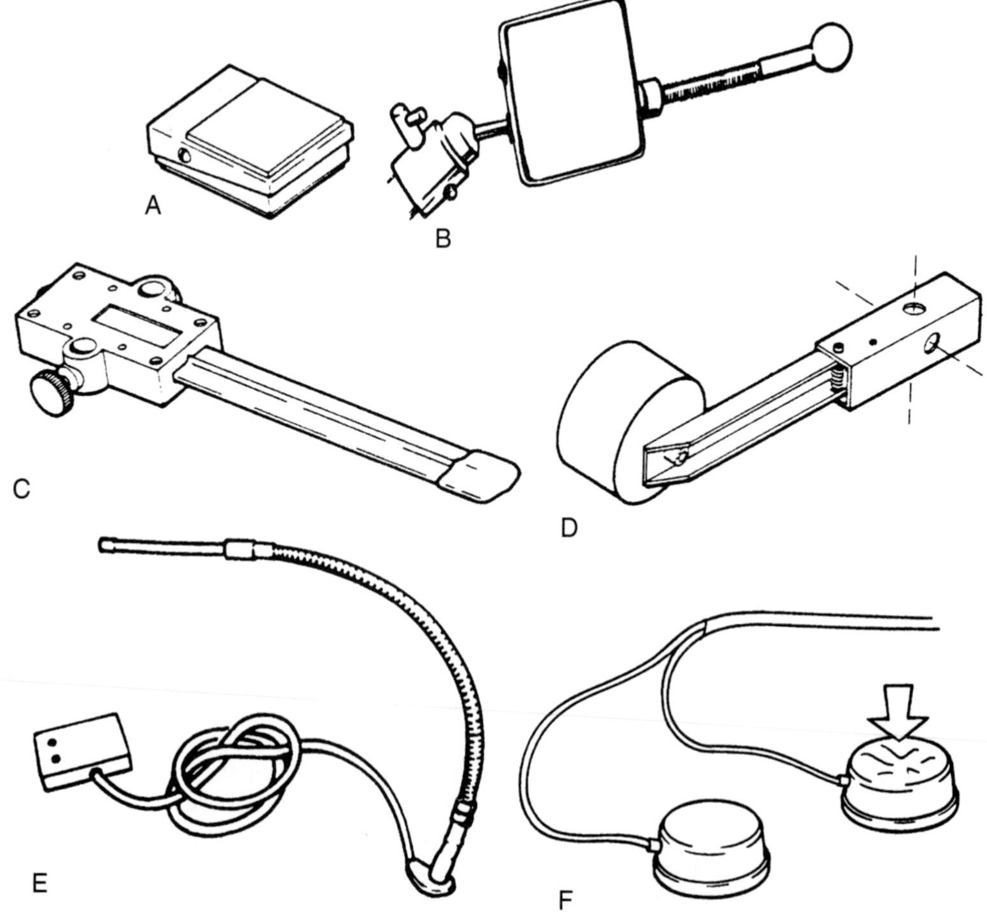

FIGURE 7-11 Examples of single switches. **A,** Paddle switch. **B,** Wobble switch. **C,** Leaf switch. **D,** Lever switch. **E,** Puff-and-sip switch. **F,** Pillow switch. (A, C, and D, courtesy Zygo Industries, Portland, OR. B, E, and F from Bergen AF, Presperin J, Tallman T: *Positioning for function: Wheelchairs and other assistive technologies,* Valhalla, NY: Valhalla Rehabilitation Publications, 1990.)

There are also various types of button switches that come in different sizes, from a large, round switch such as the Big Red switch (www.ablenetinc.com/Assistive-Technology/Switches/Big-Red), to a small button switch that can be held between the thumb and the index finger, such as the Spec switches (www.ablenetinc.com/Assistive-Technology/Switches/Specs-Switch). Membrane switches consist of a very thin pad, which requires some degree of force to activate. These pads are available in various sizes, from as small as 2 × 3 inches to as large as 3 × 5 inches. The advantages of these membrane pads are that they are flexible, can be paired with an object (by being directly attached to it), and can be used to teach the user to make a direct connection between the object and the switch. The main disadvantage of membrane control interfaces is that they provide poor tactile feedback, which can lead to extra activations or failure to apply enough force to activate the control interface. All of these control interfaces are activated by body movement that produces a force on the control interface. They are considered *passive control interfaces* because they do not require any outside power source.

Proximity Switches

There are also control interfaces that are activated with body movement but do not require force or even contact with the control interface. These are referred to as *proximity* switches (e.g., Adaptive Switch Laboratories, www.asl-inc.com; Candy Corn Switch, AbleNet, www.ablenetinc.com). Proximity switches are *active,* meaning they require an outside power source, such as a battery, to operate. The switch is activated when it detects an object within its range, adjustable from nearly touching the switch to several inches. Proximity switches are useful when controlled movements required to activate typical switches are absent (e.g., in athetoid CP).

Pneumatic Control Interfaces

Pneumatic switches are activated by detection of respiratory airflow or pressure and include puff-and-sip and pillow switches. Puff-and-sip switches (https://enablingdevices.com/catalog/capability_switches/sip-puff-breath-switches, www.ablenetinc.com/Assistive-Technology/Switches/Candy-Corn-Proximity-Sensor-Switch) (Figure 7-11 *E*) are activated by the individual's blowing air into the switch or sucking air out of it. The individual can send varying degrees of air pressure to the switch, which provides different commands to the processor. Pillow switches (Figure 7-11 *F*) respond to air pressure when a bulb or pad is squeezed

Switch Arrays, Discrete Joysticks, and Chord Keyboards

Control interfaces are commercially available in preconfigured arrays (two to eight) that have the advantages of multiple signals while retaining the requirement of low resolution typical of single switches. Any of the single switches we have discussed can be used to design a custom array to meet the needs of the consumer.

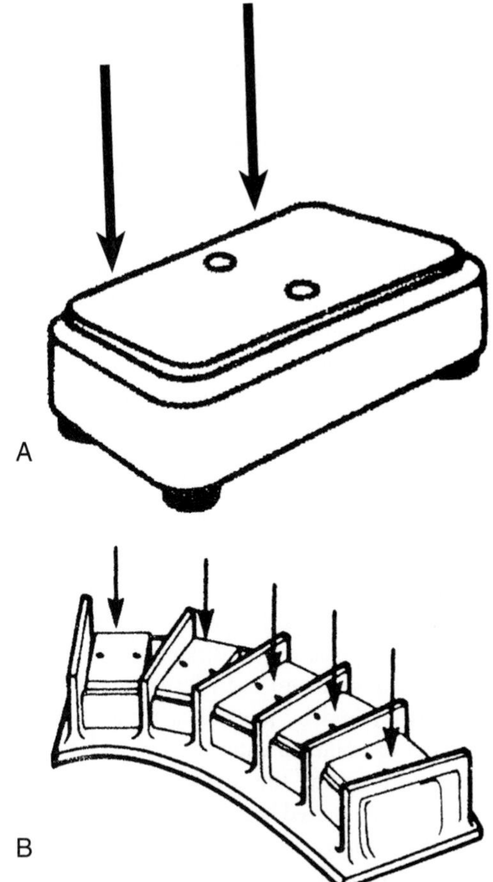

FIGURE 7-12 Examples of switch arrays. **A,** Dual rocker switch. (Webster JG, Cook, A.M., Tomkins, W.J et al., editors: *Electronic devices for rehabilitation,* New York: John Wiley and Sons, 1985.) **B,** Slot switch. (Courtesy Zygo Industries, Portland, OR.)

Paddle switches are often used in switch arrays when two to five input signals are desirable. A type of paddle switch that provides dual input from one control is called a *rocker switch* (Figure 7-12 *A*). A rocker switch is similar to a seesaw rocking from side to side around a fulcrum. This design allows the user to maintain contact with the switch and perform a rotating movement with the control site to activate each side. This type of dual-switch array is often used for Morse code input, with one side signaling dots and the other side dashes. The slot switch (Figure 7-12 *B*) is one example of a commercially available paddle switch array. Slot switches are typically used by someone who has gross motor skills and a fairly large ROM. There are other switch arrays that are mounted and activated using the head. Switch arrays are often used for power wheelchair control; we discuss them in greater detail in Chapter 10.

A discrete joystick is also considered an array of switches. It consists of four or five control interface input signals (UP, DOWN, LEFT, RIGHT, and ENTER) that are either open or closed (off or on), with nothing in between. To close the switched joystick, the control handle is moved in the direction of one of the switches. Switched joysticks require limited range but moderate resolution by the user. They are available with a variety of displacements, forces, and handles to accommodate different grasping abilities of the user. If there is a maximum of five items (e.g., directions of a power wheelchair) in the selection set, the joystick functions as an interface for direct selection. When the selection set is more than five, indirect selection is required using directed scanning. Using the joystick with this method, the individual selects the direction and the device determines the speed of cursor movement.

A chord keyboard is an array of switches or keys (typically five), each of which is intended to be pushed by a finger (e.g., the BAT keyboard, www.infogrip.com/bat-keyboard.html).[1] Two-handed versions have 10 or more switches or keys (some have multiple keys for thumb use), and one-handed versions have five or more. To make an entry, one or more (usually at least two) of the switches are pushed simultaneously. This is analogous to the playing of several notes together on a piano to make a musical chord. The most commonly used chord keyboard is the one used by court stenographers who can transcribe speech as it is spoken at more than 150 words per minute. Chord keyboards have often been proposed for rapid text entry by persons with disabilities.

With a chord keyboard each letter, number, and special symbol is entered by pressing a combination of keys (switches). For example, to enter the letter C, keys 1 and 3 may be pressed together. The codes for each selection must be learned and memorized because it is not possible to label the keys with the necessary codes. Therefore, the individual using a chord keyboard needs to have good memory skills in addition to good fine motor control and good coordination of the fingers.

Enhancing Control-Joystick Templates

A template used on a joystick to guide the individual's movement is similar to the use of a key guard for a keyboard. The template has four channels that guide the movement of the joystick. The shape of the channel may vary depending on the template. For example, an individual using the cross-shaped template in Figure 7-13 *A* may need more precise movement to move the joystick to enter the desired channel, but once in one of these channels, the joystick will be able to stay easily even in the face of tremor. The template in Figure 7-13 *B* makes it easy for the individual to enter one of the channels but difficult to stay. A compromise is shown in Figure 7-13 *C*. The template in Figure 7-13 *D* restricting the travel at the end of the channel with the star template (Figure 7-13 *B*), Table 7-7 shows control enhancers and modifications in technique that can assist an individual who has limited motor control.

Mounting the Control Interface for Use

It is also necessary to mount single switches, joysticks, and switch arrays in a convenient location. The most common mounting locations are attachments to a table, a desk, a wheelchair, a lap tray, or the person's body. There are commercially available mounting systems for table and wheelchair

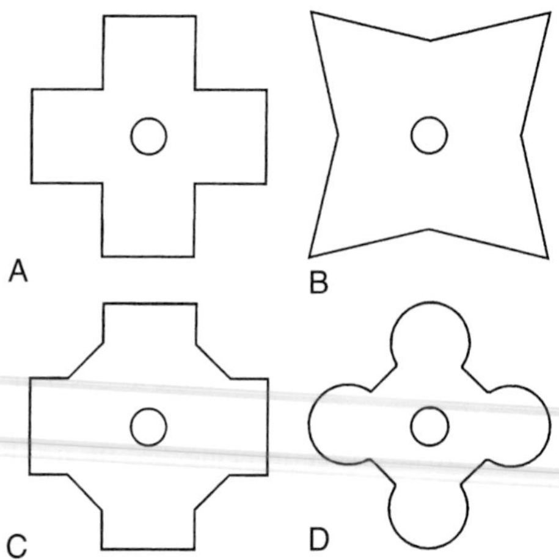

FIGURE 7-13 **A** to **D**, Four different shapes of joystick templates to maximize the user's skills.

TABLE 7-7 Control Enhancers and Technique Modifications

Control enhancers: Devices or equipment to extend or enhance motor control for direct selection (or for indirect selection where indicated by the*).

Postural Supports	At Hands or Arms	At Head
Lap tray*	Finger splint or pointer	Mouth stick
Arm rests*	Universal cuff with typing stick	Head pointer
Hip belt*	Wrist strap pointer	Head light
Chest straps*	Mobile arm supports*	Head mouse
Lateral supports*	Hand brace*	Head rest*
Abductor/adductor	Hand splint*	

Technique modifications: Changes to the selection technique to reduce the demands for direct selection (or for indirect selection as indicated by the *).

Selection Set Design	Interface Adjustments	Additional Aids
Target size*	Acceptance time*	Key guards
Spacing*	Delay until repeat*	Templates*
Array shape*	Repeat rate*	Shields*
Angle*	Cursor speed*	Hand rest*
Height*	Sensitivity*	
Order of items	Activation feedback*	

From Dowden P, Cook AM: Choosing effective selection techniques for beginning communicators. In Reichle J, Beukelman D, Light J, editors: *Exemplary practices for beginning communicators*, Baltimore: Paul H. Brookes, 2002.

mounting. Some mounting requirements are more challenging than others. For example, it is generally more difficult to position a joystick for foot or chin use than it is to place it for hand use.

There are flexible and fixed mounting systems. Flexible mounting systems (Figure 7-14) can be adjusted and placed in various positions, which is advantageous for individuals who require changes in the position of their control interface because of fluctuating skill or need. The

[1] For example, the BAT keyboard, http://www.infogrip.com/bat-keyboard.html.

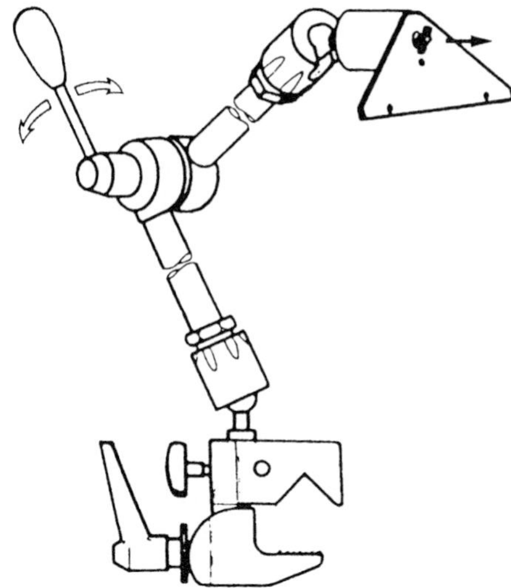

FIGURE 7-14 Flexible mounting system. (Courtesy Zygo Industries, Portland, OR.)

disadvantage of flexible mounting systems is that the position for the control interface must be determined each time it is put in place. Sometimes even a slight fluctuation in the position of the control interface can make a significant difference in the individual's ability to access it. An individual may use the same device in different positions (e.g., sitting in a wheelchair or lying in bed for EADL devices) (see Chapter 12).

Other mounting systems are fixed and are designed for use of a specific control site and control interface, making the mounting more stable and less likely to move or change position and require adjustment. It is important to know the correct position of the switch to maximize ease of use. Each time the individual is set up to use the device, the switch needs to be placed in the correct position.

The majority of control interfaces have a cable that connects them to the device being used. However, there are wireless keyboards, pointing interfaces, and switches. There are also separate wireless links that can be used with most control interfaces. Table 7-8 lists a number of switch interfaces, some of which are wireless. These links consist of a transmitter that the control interface plugs into and a receiver that

TABLE 7-8 USB Switch Interfaces

Switch interface	Features	Comments
AbleNet Hitch Computer Switch Interface*	This plug and play switch interface allows use by both Windows and Macintosh users. Hitch has five sets of functions. It has five switches at a time.	Rows of functions are chosen with a single push of a button. Hitch easily delivers up, down, left, right, and enter controls to your switches.
Crick USB Switch Box†	Four switch inputs	Works with Crick software; automatically detects which application and downloads setups
Don Johnston Switch Interface Pro6‡	Five switch inputs and four built-in scanning arrays for a variety of educational programs	No software needed; supports Clicker 6 software Scanning arrays: Row 1: Up arrow, down arrow, left arrow, right arrow, enter click, right click, double click, space, enter Row 2: space, enter, tab, shift tab Row 3: click, 1, 2, 3, 0 backspace Row 4: click, F3, F5, F7, F9
Inclusive Technologies Simple Switch Box§	Two switch inputs, defined as SPACE and ENTER	Works with any programs requiring these two keys
QuizWorks Wireless Switch Interface¶	Receiver plugs into the USB port; up to five switches plug into transmitter that can be mounted wherever the switches are	Switch inputs can be configured on the receiver; no software required
Sensory Software International Joy Box, USB¶¶	12 switch inputs for all mouse functions	Works with the Grid 2 software; the Switch Driver allows you to configure each switch independently
Sensory Software International Radio Switch** (remove tangles and wires with radio switches)	Receiver plugs into the USB port; two switches plug into transmitter that can be mounted wherever the switches are (e.g., on a wheelchair)	No drivers are needed to use the radio switches with popular software such as The Grid 2, Clicker, or Widgit software. Switch functions can be configured by any key with Switch Driver (also from Sensory Software)
PRC USB Switch Interface Box††	Six single-switch inputs	Works with the WIVIK 3 onscreen keyboards, emulates all mouse functions with two dual switch connections and a joystick connection

*webstore.ablenetinc.com/hitch-computer-switch-interface/p/10034100.
†http://www.cricksoft.com/uk/products/accessibility/usb.aspx.
‡http://www.donjohnston.com/products/access_solutions/hardware/switch_interface_pro_5/index.html.
§http://www.inclusive.co.uk/simple-switch-box-p2577.
¶http://www.quizworks.com/wireless_switch_interface.html.
¶¶http://www.sensorysoftware.com/
**http://www.sensorysoftware.com/
††https://store.prentrom.com/product_info.php/products_id/19?osCsid=g3lf6fe3g2smhghelnntjpsih5.

plugs into the device. When the control interface is pressed, the signal is transmitted to the receiver and the device. The control interface is not connected to the device by a cable, so the user has more freedom of movement. Wireless control interfaces communicate with the processor via infrared signals or Bluetooth radio signals such as those used with television remote controls.

The obvious advantages of a remote control interface are that there is one less wire for the user to become tangled in and that it looks better. In many situations, the person with a disability needs a personal attendant to assist with connecting the cable of the interface to the computer. When a wireless control interface is mounted on the person's wheelchair, it allows the person to move to or away from the device being controlled without having to connect or disconnect the interface. The use of a remotely connected control interface can reduce the need for an attendant to physically connect the control interface by plugging it in. A wireless device also makes use in different locations easier.

CONTEXT

Just as specific types of control methods can be stigmatizing for the individual using them, so can specific types of controls. Those that are most like mainstream applications, (e.g., keyboards and touch screens) are least stigmatizing. Those that are most unique to ATs such as head-pointing interfaces and switch arrays are more likely to call negative attention to the individual.

When the severity of a disability is greater, it often requires more complex and costly control interfaces such as eye pointing or automatic speech recognition. Because they are more expensive, funding for them may be more difficult or more complicated to obtain than for more common interfaces like keyboards.

Some control interfaces have the potential to be disruptive in group environments. In particular, automatic speech recognition (see Chapter 6) can be distracting to others if used in a workplace or classroom.

Environmental conditions can also affect some control interfaces. For example, some eye tracking systems are sensitive to the amount of ambient light and may work better in limited light than in full sun outdoors. The use of light pointers can also be affected by the amount of ambient light. Some touch-sensitive screens and switches are affected by the relative humidity in the air. They may work better on dry, hot days than on humid days.

ASSESSMENT

Selecting a control interface for an individual can be a complex process. Control interfaces are used to enable a range of activities, including mobility (powered wheelchair, driving), aids to daily living (e.g., electronic controls for TV, DVD, turning on lights, opening doors), communication (speech-generating device control), and cognitive ATs (e.g., for navigation, prompting systems). These activities occur in the home, in the community, in schools, and at work. Often both care providers and the individual using the AT need to access the control interface and understand its use.

Understanding the characteristics of control interfaces as described in this chapter and following a systematic process to determine the user's skills and evaluate the effectiveness of control interfaces can make the selection process easier. Figure 7-15 outlines a framework to guide the (Assisitve Technology Provider) through the decision-making process, ultimately leading to the selection of a human/technology interface (HTI) that matches the user's needs and skills. Based on information acquired from the needs identification and physical-sensory components of the evaluation process described in Chapter 5, the clinician makes a decision to pursue further evaluation on one of two paths: (1) interfaces for direct selection or (2) interfaces for indirect selection.

In general, control interfaces for direct selection typically have greater numbers of targets and require more refined resolution (e.g., fine motor skills) skills. Control interfaces for indirect selection have eight or fewer targets and are more suitable for individuals with gross motor control. To make an informed decision regarding the most appropriate control interface for a user, the ATP needs to understand the alternatives that are available and evaluate and compare the consumer's ability to operate them.

Gathering information during the assessment regarding how often the interface is to be used and the amount of force that is to be generated on the interface by the user assists the ATP in making recommendations that correspond with the durability of the control interface. If the control interface is to be used by someone who exerts a great deal of pressure on it because of uncontrolled movements, it must be constructed so it can withstand this type of use.

Applying the Outcomes of Needs Identification and Physical-Sensory Evaluations to Control Interface Selection

Figure 7-15 lists specific information related to HTI selection. Identifying the activity the consumer wants to perform provides us with information on how large an **input domain** (how many control signals) is required and therefore possible control interfaces to consider. If the consumer is in need of a powered wheelchair and is interested in using a computer, for example, it is not necessary to determine whether he can use both a joystick and a keyboard. Alternatively, he may use an integrated control for both functions. The range of activities affects the way in which we pursue selection of a control interface or multiple interfaces. We need to consider whether a different control interface for each function or a single integrated control for all the functions is to be used.

The information shown in Figure 7-15 is gathered during the physical-sensory skills evaluation that gives us a profile of the user's skills and can be used to select control interfaces. The range measurement determines the size of the individual's workspace (e.g., the overall size of a keyboard or switch array) and gives an indication of the possible locations for placement of a control interface (or interfaces). The

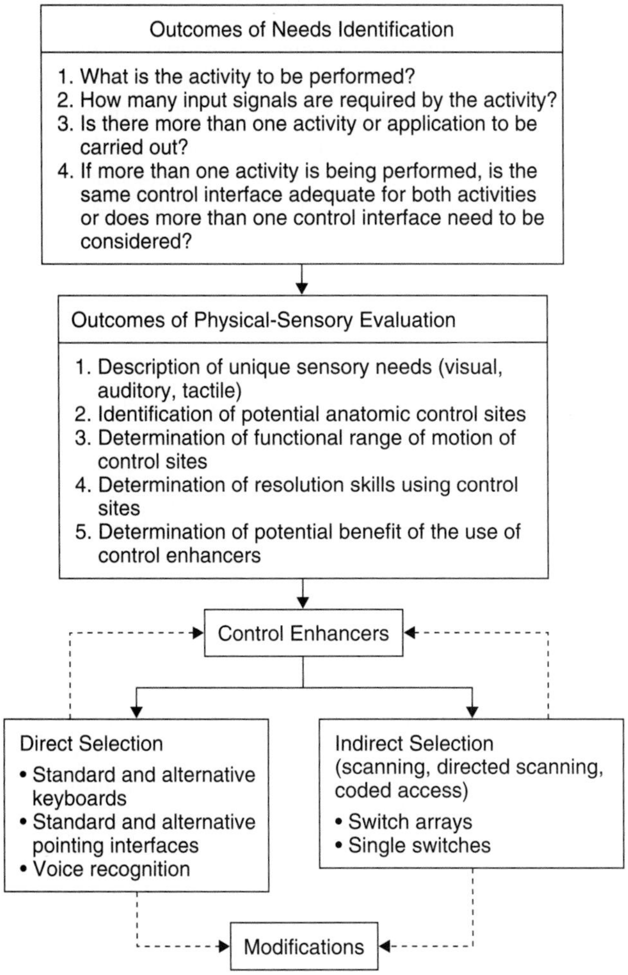

Outcomes of Needs Identification

1. What is the activity to be performed?
2. How many input signals are required by the activity?
3. Is there more than one activity or application to be carried out?
4. If more than one activity is being performed, is the same control interface adequate for both activities or does more than one control interface need to be considered?

Outcomes of Physical-Sensory Evaluation

1. Description of unique sensory needs (visual, auditory, tactile)
2. Identification of potential anatomic control sites
3. Determination of functional range of motion of control sites
4. Determination of resolution skills using control sites
5. Determination of potential benefit of the use of control enhancers

Control Enhancers

Direct Selection
- Standard and alternative keyboards
- Standard and alternative pointing interfaces
- Voice recognition

Indirect Selection (scanning, directed scanning, coded access)
- Switch arrays
- Single switches

Modifications

FIGURE 7-15 Framework for control interface decision making.

resolution measurement specifies the consumer's ability to control her movement to select a closely spaced targets (e.g., a smart phone touch screen versus an enlarged keyboard or single switch).

Potential candidate control interfaces that match the range and resolution characteristics are selected, and comparative testing is conducted. The purpose of comparative testing using the control interfaces is to determine speed and accuracy of use for each interface evaluated as well as obtaining the consumer's view on difficulty of use.

It is recommended that users develop a repertoire of control methods so they broaden the potential number of devices they can access. For example, if a child who previously used a single switch becomes proficient in the use of a joystick, both of these control options can be maintained through different activities. The joystick can be used to play computer games or activate a communication device, and the single switch can still be used to turn on music. The *parallel interventions model* (Angelo & Smith, 1989; Smith, 1991) proposes that the individual use an initial switch for accessing a device while simultaneously participating in a motor training program to maximize his ability to operate control interfaces. For example, after a period of training, the user may be able to progress from using a single switch to a switch array or from an expanded keyboard to a standard keyboard.

BOX 7-2 Critical Questions for Evaluating Keyboard Use

1. Can the consumer reach all the keys on the keyboard?
2. Are the size, spacing, and sensory feedback of the keys appropriate?
3. Is the consumer's speed of input adequate for the task?
4. Does the consumer target keys with approximately 75% accuracy?
5. Is the consumer able to simultaneously hold down the modifier key and select another key?
6. Is the consumer able to control the duration for which a key must be pressed before it repeats itself?
7. Does the consumer effectively use the standard keyboard layout?

Selecting a Control Interface

Frequently, the use of more than one body control site and candidate interface is considered for a given consumer. Using a set of critical questions for each type of interface to evaluate each pairing (control site and interface), control interface recommendations can be made.

Keyboard Evaluation

The critical questions presented in Box 7-2 can assist the ATP in determining the consumer's ability to use any keyboard. As each question is considered, a "yes" answer means that the evaluation is proceeding on the correct pathway and the ATP should continue with the next question. Affirmative responses to all seven questions indicate that the control interface by itself is likely to meet the consumer's needs. The answer to the first question is determined by asking the consumer to reach the keys at each corner of the keyboard. To obtain an answer to the second question, have the consumer press several keys located in different areas of the keyboard and marked with colored dots. The consumer's rate of input can be timed for entering characters. Accuracy can be measured by monitoring errors made during these tasks. The criterion for accuracy is subject to clinical judgment. We recommend that accuracy be determined by at least three out of four correct selections (75%).

In general, speed and accuracy are in opposition; that is, as speed increases, accuracy decreases. In some situations, speed is of primary importance (e.g., in a school or work setting). In general, speed and accuracy are in opposition. That is, as speed increases, accuracy decreases. In some cases, to be accurate, the consumer may make selections so slowly and deliberately that the use of the control interface under investigation becomes impractical. For example, if it takes several seconds to select a key, this rate may be equivalent to the use of scanning to make a selection. Because scanning takes much less physical effort, it should then be considered as an alternative to direct selection.

If the answer to any of the questions in Box 7-2 is determined to be no, then the use of a control enhancer, the

BOX 7-3 Critical Questions for Evaluating Single-Switch and Switch-Array Use

1. Can the consumer activate the switch?
2. Can the consumer wait for the appropriate selection?
3. Can the consumer activate the switch at the right time?
4. Can the consumer maintain switch activation (hold)?
5. Can the consumer release on command?
6. Can the consumer repeatedly carry out the steps necessary for the selection?

use of modifications, or a less limiting keyboard should be considered. For example, if a standard keyboard cannot be used because of a targeting problem, we may consider the following: (1) an enlarged keyboard with larger targets (less limiting), (2) a key guard (modification), or (3) a typing aid (a control enhancer). Modifications apply to all types of keyboards and are addressed after we discuss the different types of keyboards.

Indirect Selection (Switch) Evaluation

When an individual's physical control does not permit him to select directly, indirect selection methods are considered. Indirect methods of selection use a single switch or an array of switches and require that the consumer be able to carry out a certain set of skills.

Box 7-3 shows the critical questions to pose during the evaluation to determine whether the consumer has the basic set of skills for switch use. During the evaluation, it is first necessary to determine whether the user can activate the switch, which determines whether there is a match between the sensory, spatial, and activation (e.g., force) requirements of the switch and the physical-sensory skills of the user. If activation is possible, it is necessary to look at other skills related to the way the switch is to be used for indirect selection (see Table 7-3).

The first skill is waiting for the desired selection to be presented. This task requires that the consumer have sensory skills for awareness of the selections being presented. Depending on the consumer's sensory abilities, selections can be presented visually or auditorily. An inability to wait can result from problems with central processing or motor control. If the consumer is having difficulty waiting, determining the underlying cause (i.e., sensory, central processing, or motor) may make it possible to modify the task, although the cause is not always easy to determine. The consumer must also be able to reliably activate the switch at the right time (i.e., when the desired selection is presented).

Another critical condition is that the consumer be able to hold a switch in its closed position for the time it takes the signal from the control interface to register. This time may differ from switch to switch. In addition, applications such as Morse code input, inverse scanning, and wheelchair mobility require the user to hold the switch closed. Within each of these applications, the length of this hold time varies. For example, for a person using one-switch Morse code, the hold time varies from shorter to longer depending on the input signal (dot or dash). Inverse scanning (see Chapter 6) and wheelchair mobility (see Chapter 10) are other applications that require the user to hold down the switch for varying lengths of time. With inverse scanning, the switch is held until the right choice appears; for wheelchair mobility, the switch is held down until the user wants the chair to stop. If the consumer is having difficulty activating or holding the switch, the switch may require too much force or displacement for activation or the sensory feedback it provides may be inadequate. If this is the case, having the consumer experiment with less limiting switches is recommended. Releasing the switch in a timely manner is the next criterion. Inability to release the switch causes inadvertent selections. Frustration, embarrassment, and possibly serious injury in the case of mobility can result if the user cannot carry out precise holding and release of the switch. It is easier for some individuals to activate and hold the switch than to release it. Finally, it should be determined whether the consumer is able to carry out these sets of skills repeatedly.

Pointing Evaluation

It is necessary to determine whether the consumer can use the pointing interface to reach the items in the selection set (targets) and stay fixed on the target while executing the action needed to make a selection. These all imply that the selection targeted is accurate. The person may be able to get to a target area on the screen, but the size of the target may affect his or her ability to maintain that position while selecting it. Any location on the screen can be a target, and these can be of different sizes. Depending on the software program, the size of the target may be fixed, or it may be possible to modify the size to meet the user's needs. As we have described, there are two techniques to make a selection: acceptance time and manual selection. For acceptance or dwell time selection, the user must be able to hold the cursor on the target for a predetermined period (which is adjustable) and that pause signals the selection. With the manual selection technique, the user must be able to activate an additional switch to let the device know that the selection has been made. The second approach provides more control for the user, but it also requires additional user motor control.

Box 7-4 identifies the critical questions to consider when assessing an individual for using any type of pointing interface. It is necessary to determine whether the consumer can use the pointing interface to reach the items in the selection set (targets) and stay fixed on the target while executing the action needed to make a selection. The person may be able to get to a target area on the screen, but the size of the target may affect his or her ability to maintain that position while selecting it. Any location on the screen can be a target, and these can be of different sizes.

Pointing interfaces vary in terms of the tactile and proprioceptive feedback that they provide and this may affect the user's performance. Using a pointing interface also requires a significant amount of coordination between the body site executing the movement of the cursor and the eyes following the cursor on the screen and locating the targets. The

CASE STUDY

Evaluation and Selection of a Pointing Interface

David is a 21-year-old man who has muscular dystrophy. He would like to be able to access the family computer for educational and recreational purposes. David would like to play computer-based games and use drawing programs that typically require a mouse. He lacks movement in his four extremities, with the exception of wrist and finger movement. He is able to reach with each hand from within 3 inches of his body to 8 inches out from his body. With his right hand he can reach approximately 5.5 inches to the right of midline, and with his left hand, he can reach 3 inches to the left of midline. He cannot cross midline with either hand.

David tried a contracted keyboard, and he was able to point to keys in a restricted range near the middle of the keyboard. He was unable to access other areas of the keyboard without assistance for repositioning of his arms. He was able to move a continuous joystick in all four directions and use it with the on-screen keyboard software, but this was difficult for him. A trackball was also used with the on-screen keyboard software to determine whether David could use it. He could easily use the trackball as a pointing device to point to the keys shown on the screen. Using a drawing program and the trackball, he was able to direct the cursor to various parts of the screen with enough precision to draw lines and shapes. However, he was unable to hold the trackball in place with the cursor on the desired selection and simultaneously press the button on the trackball with the same hand to make his selection. The acceptance time selection technique was shown to him, and he was able to easily use this technique.

Questions

1. From the data given, should the ATP recommend a contracted keyboard for David?
2. From the information given, what would be the optimal control interface for David? What other information is needed regarding David's needs and skills that might influence the recommendation?
3. What other software will David need to operate the recommended control interface?

BOX 7-4 Critical Questions for Evaluating Use of Electronic Pointing Interfaces

1. Can the consumer use the pointing interface to reach all the targets on the screen?
2. Are the size and spacing of the screen targets appropriate?
3. Is the consumer able to complete the action needed to make a selection and perform other mouse functions required by the application software (click, drag, and double click)?
4. Is the sensory feedback provided by the control interface and the user display adequate?
5. Does the consumer use the keyboard layout effectively?

selection set and its layout will vary depending on the pointing interface and the software being used, and the ATP should determine whether the layout of the items in the selection set is beneficial or detrimental to the user's performance.

Comparative Testing of Candidate Control Interfaces

The clinician can begin evaluating the consumer's skills by using simple technology such as a switch-controlled music player or adapted battery-operated toy as an output when the switch is activated. After it is determined that the consumer can use the switch reliably to control this output, switch activation, holding, and release can be evaluated with software games designed for that purpose (www.oneswitch.org.uk/2/switch-downloads.htm).

After potential anatomic sites and candidate control interface combinations have been chosen, the consumer's ability to use these interfaces is measured. Comparative testing provides the ATP with data on the consumer's speed and accuracy in using particular control interfaces. These data can be used to compare different interfaces operated with a given site. If a control enhancer (e.g., mouth stick, head pointer) or modification (e.g., key guard) is being considered, its use should also be evaluated. Gathering quantitative information on the person's ability to use the control interface is important in making decisions regarding the selection of a control site and interface. Noting the consumer's preferences is critical during the comparative evaluation process.

Speed of response is often used to compare control interfaces. Because these measurements are typically made in the controlled setting of the clinic, they must be carefully applied to contexts outside the clinic. A second measure is accuracy of response that is often based on selecting the correct target for direct selection or switch arrays or joysticks. The standard of performance for accuracy is typically the number of correct responses out of the total number of trials. Accuracy is also based on experience and training or practice can improve accuracy dramatically. Speed of response and accuracy are generally inversely proportional to each other for novice users. The selected control interface is first placed in a position where the consumer can easily activate it. It may be necessary to try different locations before finding the position at which the consumer has the greatest control.

Computer-assisted assessment provides several useful features. First, data collection and analysis can be automated, relieving the clinician of tedious record keeping. Performance measures for each possible control site–interface pair can be obtained. The effects of different positions for the control interface or the use of control enhancers and modifications can also be measured. Because several different control site–interface combinations can be evaluated, this data collection process can facilitate the choice of interfaces on the basis of measured results. Second, the computer can provide a variety of contingent results (including graphics, sound, and speech) when the control interface is activated. This variety of results not only makes the task more interesting, but it also can allow assessment of visual and auditory capabilities. A number of tools have been developed for computer access assessment. We discuss these in Chapter 8.

Multiple versus Integrated Control Interfaces

Although generally an individual's "best" available control site is used, in some cases, more than one control site must be identified. This situation most often occurs when one person uses several types of ATs. For example, head control may be used for augmentative communication and foot control for a powered wheelchair. In other cases, such as with some neuromuscular disabilities (e.g., ALS), multiple sites need to be identified because of progressive paralysis. The course of this progression can vary from months to years.

The variation in ability to use effectors over the course of the disease makes it necessary to find flexible control interfaces that can be used with multiple control sites or to find separate control interfaces for several sites initially. Another reason for having multiple switch sites is fatigue during the day. Sometimes people need to switch to another control because the first is fatiguing and they cannot sustain its use over the course of the activity or the day.

A long-standing goal of rehabilitation engineers and other rehab therapy professionals is the integration of systems for augmentative and alternative communication (AAC), power mobility, environmental control, and computer access (Barker & Cook, 1981; Caves et al., 1991). One of the major reasons for this emphasis is to allow the use of the same control interface for several applications, called integrated control. Integration of controls can free the individual from multiple controls and can reduce the jumble of electronic devices surrounding the person.

Ding et al. (2003) reviewed applications of integrated controls in power mobility, augmentative communication, EADLs, and computer access. They also describe the Multiple Master Multiple Slave (M3S) protocol for interfacing ATs (Linnman, 1996). This protocol is an open network standard for interconnecting electronic rehabilitation devices for power mobility (see Chapter 10), EADLs and robotics (see Chapter 12), and augmentative communication (see Chapter 16). The M3S standard also includes safety features that allow rapid shutdown of electronic controls (especially wheelchair and robotics) if a failure occurs. It also provides a framework for AT interfaces that makes them more compatible and more easily combined into integrated controls.

The main or controlling device is generally only capable of operating one single function device at a time, and the user designates the mode in which he or she would like to function. For example, several power wheelchairs have processors that allow the consumer to use one interface, such as a joystick, to control many functions. By selecting the drive mode, the person uses the joystick to propel the wheelchair in all directions. The person can exit the wheelchair drive mode, select the mode designated for environmental control, and turn the lights on and off in the house. Likewise, many augmentative communication devices allow control of appliances and other electronic devices.

There is an inherent value in the simplification that can result from integration of control over separate functions; however, there are also many situations in which separate control interfaces (called **distributed controls**) and devices for each of the functions are warranted. Before deciding whether to use an integrated control or distributed controls, the implications of each method for the consumer should be carefully considered. As a guideline, Guerette and Sumi (1994) recommend that integrated controls be used when (1) the person has one single reliable control site; (2) the optimal control interface for each assistive device is the same; (3) speed, accuracy, ease of use, or endurance increases with the use of a single interface; and (4) the person or his family prefers integrated controls for aesthetics, performance, or other subjective reasons. Guidelines for using integrated controls are listed in Table 7-9.

TABLE 7-9 Guidelines for Using Integrated Controls

Integrated controls should be used when (Guerette & Sumi, 1994):	Integrated controls may not be useful when (Guerette & Nakai, 1996):
1. The person has one single reliable control site	1. Performance on one or more assistive devices is severely compromised by integrating control
2. The optimal control interface for each assistive device is the same	2. An individual wishes to operate an assistive device from a position other than from a power wheelchair
3. Speed, accuracy, ease of use, or endurance increases with the use of a single interface	3. Physical, cognitive, or visual-perceptual limitations preclude integrating
4. The person or his family prefers integrated controls for aesthetic, performance, or other subjective reasons	4. It is the individual's preference to use separate controls; identify situations where integrated control may not be appropriate
	5. External factors such as cost or technical limitations preclude the use of integrated controls (p. 64)

In some cases, the consumer may have only one body site that she can control, and she may also have limited range and resolution of this control site. Trying to position more than one control interface for use by this site could be difficult, and using the same control interface for multiple functions would be easier and more effective. The optimal way for the consumer to operate each assistive device can be important. Assume that the consumer needs to control both a power wheelchair and an AAC device. If the consumer can easily control a joystick, that would be the optimal control interface for the power wheelchair. If this is also the easiest control interface for the consumer to use for controlling an AAC device, an integrated control (the joystick) to operate both devices would be beneficial. However, if this person is able to use direct selection with an expanded keyboard for controlling an AAC device, the keyboard would be the optimal control interface for AAC. Integrating the control interfaces by using the joystick for both functions would not be optimal in this situation.

In one survey, the majority of consumers using integrated controls were either very satisfied or satisfied with

CASE STUDY

Evaluation and Selection of Switches

Mrs. Antonelli is a 30-year-old woman who has spastic quadriplegia as a result of meningitis at age 10 years. She lives with her husband and 2-year-old daughter. Mrs. Antonelli was referred for an evaluation for an augmentative communication system for conversation and writing. She has limited functional speech and communicates primarily by finger spelling with her left hand. Her husband interprets the finger spelling, but many others with whom Mrs. Antonelli would like to communicate do not understand her finger spelling. She independently uses a power wheelchair that she controls by a joystick with her left hand.

Mrs. Antonelli showed limited range using either hand, and her resolution seemed fair; therefore, her ability to use keyboards was assessed by use of a contracted keyboard with each hand. She copied words with a great deal of effort and was less than 50% accurate.

Because Mrs. Antonelli uses a switched joystick to control her power wheelchair, a switched joystick was tried with an electronic communication device in a directed scanning mode. Mrs. Antonelli used her left hand with the joystick in approximately the same position as her wheelchair joystick. She was able to move this joystick in all four directions. However, when asked to hold and release the joystick on a specific target, Mrs. Antonelli had difficulty. She was able to do this, but it required significant effort and several attempts to successfully select the desired target.

In the example of Mrs. Antonelli (see Case Study: Evaluation and Selection of Switches), it was easy for her to control her power wheelchair using the joystick with her left hand. However, this method was not the easiest method for her to use to operate the communication device. She had the option, however, of using another body site, and it turned out that the "best" way for her to access the communication device was by using a dual rocker control interface with her right hand. If the controls had been integrated and she was to use the joystick for both power mobility and AAC, her activity output for communication would have been significantly compromised. The decision was made to use distributed controls, and her performance in communication was much improved.

their integrated control device (Angelo & Trefler, 1998). The reasons the respondents gave for being satisfied with their integrated control device were an increase in independence and the ability to control other equipment such as televisions and computers using their main control interface (e.g., a wheelchair joystick or augmentative communication device).

OUTCOMES: IS IT WORKING? EVALUATING THE EFFECTIVENESS OF A CONTROL INTERFACE

After a control interface is selected and implemented for an individual, then its effectiveness must be evaluated on an ongoing basis. The evaluation of effectiveness may be at the time of initial use, after a length of time of device use, or at any point when a change has occurred. The impetus to change control method may be due to the individual (e.g., a degenerative condition that makes use of a particular control interface difficult or changes that occur as the user ages). Finally, the consumer may be experiencing difficulties (poor accuracy, excessive fatigue) using the control interface for the desired activities.

Alternatively, a change may be required because of a change in technology. For example, a new wheelchair may be acquired, and the control interfaces will have to be mounted to the chair and set up for the user or the new wheelchair may use a different control interface to operate it. A new device to be controlled (e.g., a more advanced augmentative communication system) may be introduced, requiring changes in the control interface. In all of these cases, reevaluation of effectiveness is required.

Evaluating the effectiveness of a control interface that has been selected and installed can be challenging because of the large number of factors that can be involved. Figure 7-16 shows a systematic approach to evaluation of how well a control interface is working for an individual consumer. The process includes observation of the consumer carrying out the desired tasks. The range of possible tasks for which a control interface might be used includes controlling a power wheelchair (see Chapter 10), making choices with an EADL (see Chapter 12), using an augmentative communication system (see Chapter 16), cognitive ATs (see Chapter 15), or providing input to a computer (see Chapter 8).

When observing the consumer carry out the desired activity, it is important to note whether the speed and accuracy of selection are sufficient to accomplish the desired task and the effort expended does not result in fatigue during routine use. In general, accuracy is more important than speed. If indirect selection is being used, then accuracy is measured by whether the switch (or switches) can be pressed on command. If direct selection is being used with a keyboard, then accuracy involves not only hitting a key on a keyboard or a location on a touch screen but also hitting the correct key or screen location. A consumer using an adapted mouse input could be asked to move the mouse pointer to a specific screen location and carry out other mouse functions such as click, double click, or dragging an icon to a new location. A user controlling a power wheelchair with a joystick may be asked to drive the wheelchair to a specific location or to turn in a specific direction.

The first step in evaluating the effectiveness of a control interface is to ensure that the individual is properly positioned. The chosen anatomic site must be free to move as much as possible without restriction (e.g., from a head rest, wheelchair arm, or other constraint). The next step is to be sure that the control interface is placed in a position where the consumer can easily activate it without losing body position or exerting undue physical effort.

After the individual and the control are properly positioned, it is possible to determine how accurately the

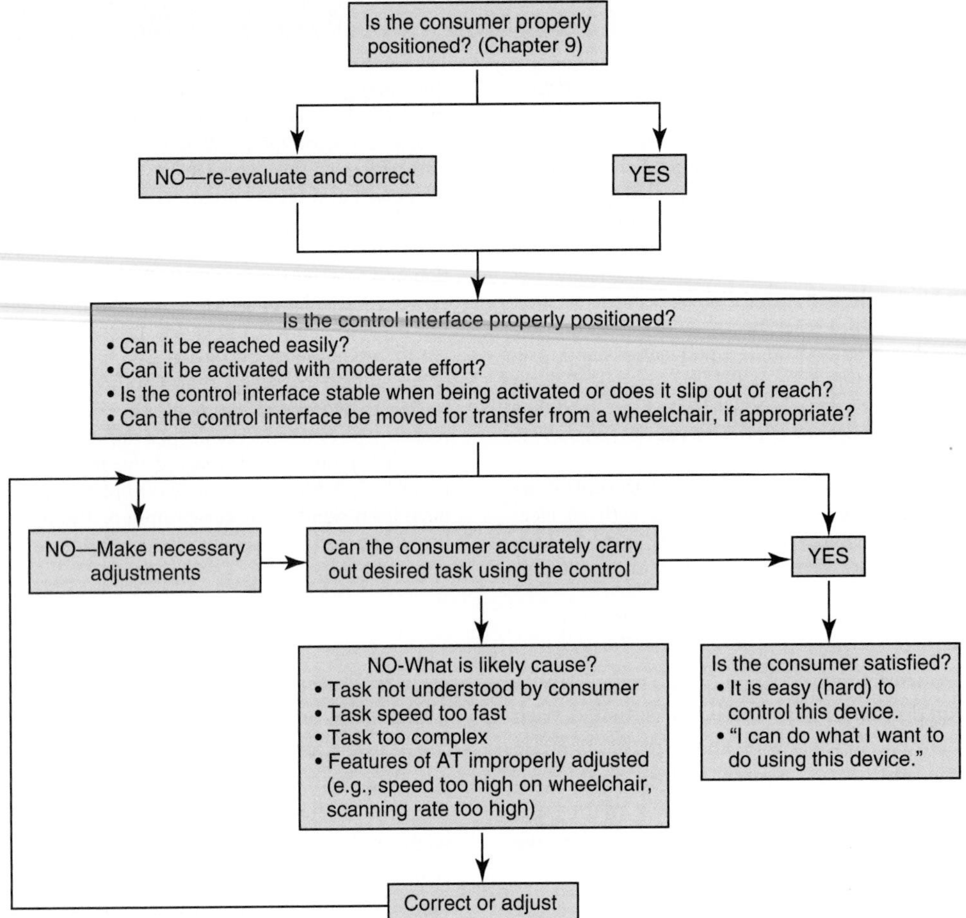

FIGURE 7-16 Evaluation of the effectiveness of a control interface in use.

consumer is using the control interface. To determine if the task was completed accurately, the observer must know what the consumer was trying to accomplish. The observer should direct the consumer to make specific selections using the control interface, keeping track of how long it takes to complete the tasks, how accurately it is done, and how much effort (both physical and cognitive) it requires.

Any limitations in accuracy or speed or high levels of fatigue require changes in the system. This may mean repositioning a control interface to make it easier to activate, choosing a control interface that requires less force or ROM to activate it, or looking for an entire new control interface–anatomic site combination that is less fatiguing. It is also important to note the consumer's evaluation of how successful the control interface–anatomic site combination is in meeting his or her needs.

SUMMARY

In this chapter, we have defined the technology elements of the HTI and their relationship to the other components of the AT. Control interfaces can be characterized by their sensory, spatial, and activation–deactivation features. Understanding these characteristics can help the clinician sort through the maze of control interfaces. This chapter also describes a framework that provides the clinician with a systematic process for matching the interface to the needs and skills of consumers. Critical questions were identified that relate to the user's skills needed to control particular types of interfaces. Addressing these questions during the evaluation can facilitate the selection of an appropriate control interface for the consumer. Evaluation of the effectiveness of control interfaces is also described.

STUDY QUESTIONS

1. What are the major activities supported by control interfaces?
2. What is the function of the control interface? Describe the difference between a discrete and a continuous input with examples for each.
3. Define the elements of the HTI and how they are related to the processor and the output.
4. What are the somatosensory characteristics of control interfaces that need to be considered when evaluating the usefulness of a control interface for a consumer?
5. List two disabilities or conditions that might lead to the need for enhanced sensory feedback from a control interface.
6. What are the two factors that determine the spatial characteristics of a control interface?
7. Describe three control interface activation characteristics.
8. List three types of ATs that use control interfaces.
9. How are sensory and activation characteristics of control interfaces related?
10. What is a control enhancer? List several examples.
11. List three types of control enhancers.
12. What type of disability or condition would require each type of control enhancer that you listed in #11?
13. Compare the user profile for a standard, an ergonomic, an expanded, and a contracted keyboard.
14. What is the major purpose of an ergonomic keyboard?
15. What are the two most common approaches to detecting eye position and movement for use as a control interface?
16. List three types of modifications to keyboards and pointing devices and give an example of the problems that each solves.
17. What are the major types of single switches in terms of how they are activated by the consumer?
18. What is point of gaze, and why is it a potential limitation in eye-tracking systems?
19. Review the description of control interface flexibility in the section on characteristics of control interfaces. Pick three control interfaces described in the text: one that is very flexible, one that is moderately flexible, and one that is not flexible. Justify your choices.
20. What factors are important when evaluating whether a control interface is working for an individual?
21. What are the steps you would use to determine if a control interface is working well for an individual consumer?
22. Describe distributed and integrated control. What are the advantages and disadvantages of each?
23. What are the major considerations in determining whether a control interface is mounted correctly for a consumer?
24. What kinds of problems can be caused by poor mounting?
25. What are the two types of mounting systems for control interfaces?
26. What role does proper positioning play in successful use of a control interface?
27. Describe distributed and integrated control. What are the advantages and disadvantages of each?

REFERENCES

Amini D: Occupational therapy interventions for work-related injuries and conditions of the forearm, wrist, and hand: A systematic review, *Am J Occup Ther* 65(1):29–36, 2010.

Angelo J, Smith RO: The critical role of occupational therapy in augmentative communication services. In American Occupational Therapy Association, editor: *Technology review '89: Perspectives on occupational therapy practice*, Rockville, MD, 1989, American Occupational Therapy Association.

Angelo J, Trefler E: A survey of persons who use integrated control devices, *Assist Technol* 10:77–83, 1998.

Anson DK: *Alternative computer access: A guide to selection*, Philadelphia, 1997, FA Davis.

Anson D, Lawler G, Kissinger A, et al: A comparison of head pointer technologies, *Proc 2003 RESNA Conf.* Available from: www.resna.org/ProfResources/Publications/Proceedings/2003/Papers/ComputerAccess/Anson_CA_Headpointers.php. Accessed June 28, 2005.

Barker MR, Cook AM: A systematic approach to evaluating physical ability for control of assistive devices, *Proc 4th Ann Conf Rehabil Eng*, June 1981, pp. 287–289.

Betke M, Gips J, Fleming P: The camera mouse: Visual tracking of body features to provide computer access for people with severe disabilities, *IEEE Trans Neural Syst Rehabil Eng* 10:1–10, 2002.

Blackstein-Alder S, Shein F, Quintal J, et al.: Mouse manipulation through single switch scanning, *Assist Technol* 16:28–42, 2004.

Capilouto GJ, McClenaghan B, Williams HG, et al.: Performance investigation of a head-operated device and expanded membrane cursor keys in a target acquisition task, *Technol Disabil* 17:173–183, 2005.

Casas R, Quilez M, Hornerol G, et al.: Mouse for computer control from the joystick of the wheelchair, *J Accessibility Design for All* 2(2):117–135, 2012.

Caves K, Gross K, Henderson K, et al: The use of integrated controls for mobility, communication and computer access, *Proc 14th RESNA Conf*, June 1991, pp. 166–167.

Chubon RA, Hester MR: An enhanced standard computer keyboard system for single-finger and typing-stick typing, *J Rehabil Res Dev* 25(4):17–24, 1988.

Cook AM, Dobbs BM, Warren S, et al.: Measuring target acquisition utilizing Madentec's tracker system in individuals with cerebral palsy, *Technol Disabil* 17:115–163, 2005.

Ding D, Cooper RA, Kaminski BA, et al.: Integrated control and related technology of assistive devices, *Assist Technol* 15(2): 89–97, 2003.

Dowden P, Cook AM: Choosing effective selection techniques for beginning communicators. In Reichle J, Beukelman D, Light J, editors: *Exemplary practices for beginning communicators*, Baltimore, 2002, Paul H. Brookes, pp 395–432.
Early MB: *Physical dysfunction practice skills for the occupational therapy assistant*, ed 2, St. Louis, 2006, Elsevier.
Evans DG, Drew R, Blenkhorn P: Controlling muse pointer position using an infrared head-operated joystick, *IEEE Trans Rehab Engr* 8:107–117, 2000.
Guerette PJ, Nakai RJ: Access to assistive technology: A comparison of integrated and distributed control, *Technol Disabil* 5:63–73, 1996.
Guerette P, Sumi E: Integrating control of multiple assistive devices: A retrospective review, *Assist Technol* 6:67–76, 1994.
Hyman WA, Miller GE, Neigut JS: Laser diodes for head pointing and environmental control, *Proc RESNA Conf* 377–379, 1992.
Linnman S: M3S: The local network for electric wheelchairs and rehabilitation equipment, *IEEE Trans Rehabil Eng* 4:188–192, 1996.
McCormack DJ: The effects of keyguard use and pelvic positioning on typing speed and accuracy in a boy with cerebral palsy, *Am J Occup Ther* 44(4):312–315, 1990.
Phillips B, Lin A: Head-tracking technology for mouse control: A comparison project. In *Proc 2003 RESNA Conf*, Washington, DC, 2003, RESNA.
Salamo GJ, Jakobs T: Laser pointers: Are they safe for use by children? *Augment Altern Commun* 12:47–51, 1996.
Simpson RC: *Computer access for people with disabilities*, CRC Press, Boca Raton, FL, 2013.
Smith RO: Technological approaches to performance enhancement. In Christiansen C, Baum C, editors: *Occupational therapy overcoming human performance deficits*, Thorofare, NJ, 1991, SLACK.
Taveira A, Choi S: Review study of computer input devices and older users, *Int J Human-Computer Interaction* 25(5):455–474, 2009.
Undzis MF, Zoltan B, Pedretti LW: Evaluation of motor control. In Pedretti LW, editor: *Occupational therapy: Practice skills for physical dysfunction*, St. Louis, 1996, Mosby.
van Tulder M, Malnivara A, Koes B: Repetitive strain injury, *Lancet* 369:1815–1822, 2007.
Weiss PL: Mechanical characteristics of microswitches adapted for the physically disabled, *J Biomed Eng* 12:398–402, 1990.

CHAPTER 8

Accessing Mainstream Information and Communication Technologies: The Technology and the Web

CHAPTER OUTLINE

LEARNING OBJECTIVES

On completing this chapter, you will be able to do the following:

1. Describe the major issues facing people with disabilities who want to use mainstream technologies
2. Describe the user interface for mainstream technologies
3. Describe the major approaches to computer keyboard and mouse emulation
4. Describe the major approaches for generating accessibility to tablet technologies
5. Describe the major approaches for generating accessibility to smart phone technologies

KEY TERMS

Accessibility Software
Android
Application Program
Bluetooth
Control Interface
Continuous Input
Ease of Access
Information and Communication Technologies (ICTS)
iOS
Keyboard
Mouse
Multitasking
On-Screen Keyboards
OSX
Raising the Floor (RtF)
Setup
Touchscreen
Universal Access
USB Port
USB Switch Connector
Windows

ACTIVITY: ACCESSING THE INFORMATION HIGHWAY

As we discussed in Chapter 2, the move from a machine-based or manufacturing economy to a knowledge-based economy is creating opportunities for people with disabilities. The new economy is heavily based on **information and communication technologies (ICTs)**. For people who have disabilities, this may mean working from home and avoiding the challenges of public transportation. It can also mean the use of the Internet for commerce, where they can participate and compete on the basis of performance that is viewed without their disability being a prominent factor in the interaction as it might be in face-to-face meetings and offices (Bowker & Tuffin, 2003).

Mainstream ICTs include desktop and notebook computers, basic cell phones, smart phones, and tablets. These technologies are pervasive in the business and personal lives of most individuals in developed countries and are increasing in underresourced countries as well. Access to them for both personal and professional use is therefore essential for people who have disabilities.

To make ICTs accessible, we need to understand the requirements for operating them. Let's look at a familiar example, the smart phone. A typical smart phone has either a keypad or a touchscreen for entering information or scrolling through menu choices, a screen that presents choices through either icons or text (or possibly spoken output), and a speaker that provides auditory information (speech and sounds such as ring tones and text alerts). Most likely, it will also have automatic speech recognition (ASR) for alternative entry of commands (e.g., speaking an address in a navigation system) The user must be able to use the input (type or speak), see the visual display and hear the auditory output, and understand the operation of the phone sufficiently to make choices, execute voice or text messaging, browse the Internet, and manage the data in the phone (e.g., contacts, Website). Most of us take these operational functions for granted because we also take the existence of the necessary skills for granted. How access to these technologies is created is the subject of this chapter.

Cell Phone Accessibility

Cell phone usage is pervasive throughout the world. In the United States, it is estimated that 75% of adults have a cell phone (Kane et al., 2009). For individual with disabilities, the use of a cell phone can contribute to increased independence. There are about 53 million consumers with disabilities in the United States (Smith-Jackson et al., 2003). This potential market for cell phones and other electronic technologies makes it important for these devices to be accessible to people with disabilities. In the United States, there is an additional reason for cell phone manufacturers to be concerned about accessibility—the US Telecommunications Act of 1996. This act is designed to ensure that the 20% of US citizens who have disabilities have equal access to cell phones and other telecommunications devices (Smith-Jackson et al., 2003). Individuals with a range of sensory and motor disabilities are included. Other countries, particularly Canada and European and Asian countries, have similar legislation and policies to ensure access for people with disabilities.

Internet Accessibility

Persons with physical disabilities who want to use the Internet require only an accessible computer, tablet, or smart phone, assuming that those technologies are accessible to them. People with disabilities have talked about Internet use as "leveling the playing field" because they can access the Internet and communicate with others through it in the same way as people who do not have a physical disability (Miller Polgar, 2010). One participant commented: "We are all give the exact same abilities in the digital environment . . . and when you are online, nobody knows you have a disability so it [the disability] never really comes into it." (Miller Polgar et al., 2009, p. 20).

The actual use of the Internet by persons with physical disabilities has not been carefully studied in general, with the exception of people who have sustained spinal cord injuries (SCIs) (Drainoni et al., 2004). A large group (n = 516) of individuals with SCI from the 16 centers in the Model Spinal Cord Injury System (MSCIS) participated in a survey of Internet use. A smaller sample, derived from the larger group, also participated in an assessment of elements of the Health-Related Quality of Life (HRQOL) instrument. The rate of Internet access was 66% compared with a rate of 43% in the general population. There were significant differences in access, however, based on race, employment status, income, education, and marital status. The most significant HRQOL impact on Internet usage was the pain interference parameter. Frequency of use varied widely from nonuse to rare to frequent. Most (81%) of the SCI respondents used the Internet at least weekly. Success in achieving desired outcomes from Internet use improved markedly from infrequent to rare use but not from rare to frequent. Primary uses were social (email, chat rooms) and information seeking (health-related information, online shopping).

Vicente and López (2010) investigated the differences between Internet users with and without disabilities in Spain. Affordability is an issue because people with disabilities have lower incomes, and they may also lack soft technologies (training, support). People with disabilities and elderly individuals have attitudes toward the Internet that can limit its usefulness to them. In general, they have a lack of interest, low motivation, and anxiety about technology use. All of these factors are dependent on socioeconomic background. Once online, factors of Internet use come into play. Digital skills decline with age and differ by gender. Enjoyment and perceived usefulness of functions such as e-banking and e-commerce are also lower for people with disabilities and elderly adults than they are for the general population. In contrast to earlier studies, Vicente and López found that online patterns of use when compared with users without disability showed no difference. Previous studies had indicated lower e-commerce, educational use, information retrieval, and email use for people with disabilities and elderly adults. These considerations should be taken into account when working to establish mainstream technology use for people with disabilities or elderly individuals. This study indicates that the situation is changing, and more people with disabilities and older individuals are increasingly finding the Internet to be useful and accessible.

Raising the Floor

To address global issue of disability, ICT access, and infrastructure for Web accessibility, an initiative call **Raising**

the Floor (RtF) has been established. Its mandate from its Website (raisingthefloor.org) is:

> *Raising the Floor (RtF) is an international coalition of individuals and organizations working to ensure that the Internet, and everything available through it, is accessible to people experiencing accessibility barriers due to disability, literacy, or age. Of particular concern are people who are underserved or unserved due to the type or combination of disabilities they have, the part of the world they live in, or the limited resources (financial or program) available to them. A central activity of Raising the Floor – International is coordination of an emerging consortium to build a Global Public Inclusive Infrastructure (GPII).*

Human: Challenges in Using Mainstream Technologies with Physical Disabilities

People with motor disabilities may be limited in their ability to use the standard **keyboard, mouse,** or **touchscreen.** Keyboard and mouse access issues are discussed in Chapter 7.

The benefits of smart phone technologies are possible, but special considerations must be taken into account to make the technology accessible, and the design of the technology assumes certain skills, abilities, and knowledge are available. The user needs enough fine motor control to tap at the right location or swipe to change pages and generate the right amount of force to activate physical keys or buttons. She must also understand the operational procedures for everything from opening a program or making a phone call to surfing the Web. The user must have sufficient motor, speech, vision, hearing, and cognitive skills if a device is to be used successfully. If any of these skills are limited, then some adaptation is necessary to create access. In this chapter, we focus on upper extremity motor limitations.

People who have upper extremity motor limitations may require alternatives for input because keyboards. Mouse pointing or touchscreen movements may be difficult. For people with visual limitations, the size, contrast, and spacing of display items may be limiting (see Chapter 13). For individuals with cognitive limitations, the complexity of operating systems and multimedia Websites may prevent or severely limit use (see Chapter 15). General issues for all people with disabilities are the compatibility of mainstream technologies and Websites with assistive technologies (ATs) such as speech-generating devices (see Chapter 16).

Individuals with SCIs have a slightly different set of problems, although physical access is still a major issue. Kane et al. (2009) describe the ideal cell phone for someone with a SCI. Among the critical factors that he cites are continuous power on because many on off buttons are small and hard to activate, touchscreen access that requires a flick of the finger rather than continuous pressing of multiple keys, synchronizing with one or more email systems, a protective case because the unit may be dropped because of limited fine motor control, and a lanyard for retrieving the phone if it does drop. Less essential but useful is a **Bluetooth** earpiece, but it is important to find one that can be easily donned and doffed.

Burgstahler et al. (2011) describe three case studies to illustrate the challenges faced by individuals with motor disabilities in accessing computers and mobile technologies. The challenges and solutions in accessing computers and mobile of three individuals with (1) high-level SCI, (2) cerebral palsy, and (3) muscular dystrophy are described. The diversity of the disabilities in these cases provides a rich picture of real-life options for school, work, and community activity through computer and cell phone access. The ongoing challenges of access (mostly described in this chapter) are also highlighted for individuals with these three conditions.

Smart phone technology also has the potential to provide assistance to individuals with chronic conditions such as stroke, Alzheimer disease (AD), congestive heart failure, and Parkinson's disease (Armstrong et al., 2009). Armstrong et al. describe the major unmet needs for AD as an example of the use of smart phones in chronic disease care. These are: "(1) the need for general and personalized information; (2) the need for support with regard to symptoms of dementia; (3) the need for social contact and company; and (4) the need for health monitoring and perceived safety" (p. 28). Some technological solutions for AD have been developed (see Chapter 15), but many needs are still unmet.

ASSISTIVE TECHNOLOGY: INPUT ACCESSIBILITY FOR MAINSTREAM TECHNOLOGIES

In several countries, including the United States, many computer adaptations are mandated by legislation such as US PL 508. The best approach to adapting a computer or other ICT for use by individuals with physical limitations is to begin with the simplest modifications designed for the most minimal of physical limitations on the part of the user. This level of accessibly might include the built-in accessibility feature, a typing aid, a key guard, or simply repositioning the computer to be in a more accessible location (e.g., to one side, higher, lower). If the minimal adaptation is not sufficient for a given user, then more complex adaptations need to be considered.

No matter how complex the adaptation is, the goal is always to make sure that (1) all of the functions of the mainstream technology are available to the user who has a disability and (2) all application software that runs on the unmodified technology runs on the adapted technology. All of the keyboard keys, including modifier (e.g., shift, control, alt) and special function keys, and all pointing functions, such as point, click, drag, swipe, or tap must be available on the adapted input system. If a program (e.g., word processor) works with the standard technology (computer, phone, tablet), then it should work with the adaptations that are provided for the individual with a disability.

Complexity in Mainstream Devices

Persons with disabilities are concerned about the complexity of current cell phones and have a desire for phones with basic features that are easily learned and can be accessed by individuals who have fine motor limitations (Smith-Jackson et al., 2003). In a study of people with a variety of sensory and motor disabilities, Kane et al. (2009) found that most of the participants did not use a cell phone with accessibility features. The 24 participants described more than 90 devices that they carried with them at least once a week. These devices included both high-tech (cell phones, computer) and low-tech (simple magnifiers) devices. Specific difficulties included using a phone while walking, using a phone in a crowded spaces, fatigue with prolonged usage, and device failure. The participants also identified strategies that helped them. Some installed accessibility software on their mobile devices, but not all of the cell phones had provision for adding software. A number of participants, especially those who depended on their phone for geographic location or other security reasons, carried a second or third device as a backup. Cell phone use by persons with visual limitation is discussed in Chapter 13.

As functions are added to devices, they become increasingly more complex with fewer buttons that have multiple functions depending on the application program and smaller screens to accommodate mobile use. For elderly individuals whose visual acuity, working memory, and fine motor skills decline with age, this additional complexity can cause problems (Leung et al., 2010). Elderly individuals have less computer and smart mobile technology experience than younger generations that have grown up with these technologies, further limiting their ability to take advantage of these technologies. These factors present significant learning and training challenges for seniors who want to incorporate modern technologies into their lives. Blogs and Websites specifically designed to assist seniors choose and use a cell phone are increasing (Pedlow et al., 2010).

One soft technology approach to addressing the problems of complexity in electronic assistive devices and the challenges of learning to use them is to develop a multilayered approach (Leung et al., 2010). In multilayered systems, novices (new users with little or no experience) first learn to perform basic tasks using a functionality–simplified version of the human/technology interface (HTI). As they master the basic functions, additional layers of functionality can be added sequentially until all necessary functions have been learned. In a controlled experiment with seniors (ages 65 to 81 years) and younger users (ages 21 to 36 years), the multilayered approach was found to be more beneficial for older than for younger individuals (Leung et al., 2010). The multilayered approach is a good example of soft technology applications.

Universal Design for Information and Communication Technologies

Hellman (2007) describes 10 guidelines for mobile device design based on the 10 universal design principles (see Chapter 2). These are navigation of functions, handling errors, criteria for easily understood search functions, alternatives for the user interface, allowing sufficient processing time for the individual to respond to prompts, characteristics of text to ensure that it is easily read and understood, the use of alternative outputs such as voice and sound, the role of graphics (not always a benefit), limiting the necessity for PIN codes and other numerical entries, and criteria for the presentation of help information. Hellman applies these 10 guidelines to a case study of a mobile phone application for interaction with the Norwegian tax authority.

CASE STUDY

The Universal Remote Console

The Universal Remote Console (URC) framework is a protocol approved by the International Standards Organization (ISO) that provides a format for specialized user interfaces (e.g., for individuals with limited fine motor control or visual limitations) that connect to a mainstream product, making it accessible. This approach combines universal design, in which the mainstream company provides user interfaces (e.g., touch pad, mouse, and visual display) that can be used by the majority of individuals as part of the product. The company also provides a way for other companies to connect its interface for use by a more limited population with the same mainstream product using the ISO standard to make sure third-party interfaces are compatible with the mainstream product. Thus, more severely disabled users can obtain the same functionality and access to apps as the rest of the population. The company that makes the specialized interface can achieve a more viable market because its product can be interfaced to a number of different mainstream products because all of them conform to the same ISO standard. Using the concept of imbedded intelligence (see later in this chapter), the specialized interface features can be downloaded from a cloud-based resource on demand. As Emilani et al. (2011) point out, this gives each player the opportunity to focus on what he does best. The mainstream company can focus on mass production that reduces cost and can include innovations because of the size of their market. The specialized interface company can focus on meeting the specific AT needs of a narrower portion of the population but can also achieve some economy of scale because their interface can be used with a range of mainstream products. "This will result in an ecosystem that allows for economically sustainable solutions for all users beyond the 5th and 95th percentile" (Emiliani et al., 2011, p 110). One potentially limiting factor in this analysis is that many large companies consider the user interface to be a part of their product branding (Emiliani et al., 2011). They may be reluctant to allow third parties to connect their specialized interfaces to the mainstream product for fear that it will change the user experience in ways that are not consistent with their business plans.

Design flaws in mobile phones may be due to the lack of accessibility issues in business plans or to the lack of experience that designers have with disability. A set of design considerations for accessible mobile phones intended to help designers who lack understanding of people with disabilities was developed corresponding to universal design guidelines (Lee et al., 2006).

An alternative approach to making mainstream technologies accessible has been used in the telecommunications industry. According to Section 255 of the US Telecommunications Act of 1996, companies are required to make telecommunications equipment and services accessible to consumers with disabilities if "readily achievable" (47 U.S.C. § 255(a)(b)(c)) (Schaefer, 2006). According to Schaefer, companies narrowly apply the "readily achievable" concept by differentiating product focusing on accessibility features that can be accomplished "without much difficulty or expense." This has been termed a "product line approach" to accessibility (Schaefer, 2006). This strategy is similar to the modular approach except that it consists of a series of products with varying levels of accessibility built in. Companies may opt for the product line approach because of cost considerations, but there are several disadvantages for people with disabilities. Because not all products are accessible, the products with the greatest functionality may not be available to people with disabilities. This can lead to complaints from consumers who have disabilities because of lack of access to needed features. From the point of view of universal design, the product line approach also has limitations (Schaefer, 2006). It may be difficult to meet the needs of individuals with more severe disabilities even with product differentiation, and AT components may be required for them to gain access to the mainstream technologies. According to Scheafer (2006, p. 122), "The definition and principles of universal design are still applicable because the concept of universal design recognizes the need to design for compatibility with a broad range of assistive technology."

Standards

A variety of technical standards relate to ATs. Appropriate standards can enhance proliferation of AT apps, especially with cross-platform interoperability as an issue (i.e., similar operating systems for computer, smart phone, and tablet), but they can also create obstacles to development, add additional costs, and result in delays in getting a product to market (Engelen et al., 2011). Some standards are regional (e.g., the European Union) or unique to a country, and others are global through the ISO. Engelen et al. (2011) give an overview of AT and universal design standards and the standard development process.

CROSS-PLATFORM ACCESSIBILITY

Some accessibility approaches are found on computers, phones, and tablets. In this section, we describe the most common of these. In later sections, accessibility features unique to a single platform are discussed.

Automatic Speech Recognition As an Alternative Input

Principles of Automatic Speech Recognition

Automatic speech recognition technology can be applied to computer access by allowing the user to speak the names of the keyboard characters or key words and have these spoken utterances interpreted by the computer as if they had been typed. This approach is appealing because human speech is so rapid and voice control is so natural. ASR systems that are extremely reliable, flexible, and easy to use are available for use as full-function keyboard and for mouse emulation. For example, if a word processing program is being run, then control functions such as delete, move, and print and the most common vocabulary the person normally uses, a greeting and ending for a business letter, and other similar vocabulary items can be used. If the user changes to a spreadsheet program, he or she can use vocabulary that contains items specific to that application. Microsoft Vista includes ASR as part of the built-in package of accessories.

> **CASE STUDY**
>
> ***Evaluation and Selection of Speech Recognition***
>
> Marilyn Abraham is a 44-year-old woman who has been diagnosed as having reflex sympathetic dystrophy (RSD) of both wrists. Apparently caused by vasospasm and vasodilation, RSD is a reaction to pain after an injury (van Tulder et al., 2007). It results in edema; shiny, blotchy skin; and pain. Ms. Abraham is a secretary in a large state office, which she shares with other coworkers. She uses the computer for much of the day. The RSD developed in her right wrist as a result of the repetitive motion she uses in performing her job. After this injury, she received retraining to transfer her hand dominance to her left hand, and the Dvorak one-handed keyboard layout was recommended (see Figure 7-7). Subsequently, she broke her left wrist in a motor vehicle accident, which also resulted in RSD. She is able to type or use the mouse for only 10 minutes before her hands and forearms swell. Ms. Abraham has tried different positions and adaptations when typing. For example, she used a pointer held by a cuff in her palm to type so that her forearm remained in a neutral position. This method still resulted in swelling and pain. She also has neck pain when she uses the keyboard.
>
> Ms. Abraham first tried using a trackball with her hand and the on-screen keyboard. After using the trackball for a short time, Ms. Abraham found that it also caused pain. Ms. Abraham next tried using her right foot with an expanded keyboard and then a trackball. There were concerns about the utility of both these approaches because of potential neck strain from looking down and the possibility that the repeated movement of her ankle to input characters using the trackball might lead to repetitive motion problems with her foot.
>
> Next Ms. Abraham tried a head-controlled interface that was worn on a band and attached to her head. She used this interface with an on-screen keyboard and acceptance time to make a selection. She was able to control this interface without difficulty but thought that after a period of use, her neck would become tired.
>
> **Questions**
>
> 1. What other control interfaces could you try with Ms. Abraham?
> 2. If you evaluate ASR for Ms. Abraham, what issues will you need to take into consideration?

Two basic types of ASR systems exist. With a *speaker-dependent system,* the user trains the system to recognize his or her voice by producing several samples of the same element. The method in which the training is handled varies among systems. The system analyzes these samples so that it can recognize variations in the user's speech and generate a computer input (e.g., enter a given letter, as string of letters, or a control key such as RETURN) corresponding to what was spoken. Even after the system has been trained with several speech samples, there likely will be times when the system does not recognize the user's speech and does not produce a response. Recognition accuracy is steadily increasing as advances are made in the computer algorithms used for analysis. Rates can be greater than 90% for general input and nearly 100% for isolated word applications (e.g., command and control, database, spreadsheet). Speaker-dependent systems can be further divided into continuous and discrete categories. Comerford et al. (1997) describe the development of ASR systems and the technical aspects of these systems.

Speaker-independent systems recognize speech patterns of different individuals without training (Gallant, 1989). These systems are developed by using samples of speech from hundreds of people and information provided by phonologists on the various pronunciations of words (Baker, 1981). The tradeoff with this type of total recognition system is that the vocabulary set is small. In AT applications, speaker-independent systems are primarily used for environmental and robotic control (see Chapter 12) and power mobility (see Chapter 10).

Discrete speech recognition systems require the user to pause between each word for recognition to occur, which is a very unnatural type of speech. There have been reports of voice problems associated with the use of discrete speech recognition systems (Kambeyanda et al., 1997). These are due to the abrupt starting and stopping of speech required for these systems coupled with the monotone quality required for good recognition, both of which are unnatural speech patterns. Continuous ASR systems allow the user to speak in a more normal manner without major pauses. The rates of input are within the range of normal rates of human speech (150 to 250 words per minute). Although the possibility of damage to the vocal folds is reduced with these systems, it is not totally eliminated. Because the discrete systems are more accurate for single-word recognition, they are sometimes used for commands and control in applications such as spreadsheets and databases. Some manufacturers (e.g., Dragon Systems, Nuance, Inc., Burlington, MA, www.nuance.com) provide both continuous (e.g., Naturally Speaking) and discrete (e.g., Dragon Dictate) ASR, sometimes bundled into the same package.

Speech recognition can be used for computer access, wheelchair control, and electronic activities of daily living (EADLs). The systems shown in Table 8-1 allow the consumer to use speech to enter text directly into a computer application program. Recognition of control words, such as "save file," used in a word processor is also trained. System vocabulary is also growing rapidly. Early systems had recognition vocabularies (the list of words the system can recognize when spoken) in the 1000 to 5000 range. Current systems have vocabularies of 50,000 words or more. The faster speech rate, larger vocabularies, and continuous recognition all place significant demands on the speed and memory of the host computer. Continuous speech recognition systems require large amounts of memory and high-speed computers. As the cost of this added computer functionality continues to decline, these additional requirements will be less important. Simpson (2013) provides a detailed description of ASR for computer access, including the major challenges in applying this technology. These include longer times for error correction because whole words reentered incorrectly rather than single letters when correcting a keyboard error keyboard. Working in environments where others are present can make ASR inappropriate because of the annoyance of others. If sensitive information is to be entered, having it overheard might compromise security.

TABLE 8-1 Speech Recognition Interfaces

Category	Description	Device Name/ Manufacturer
Speaker-dependent systems	Recognition depends on the system's learning the user's speech patterns and building a user vocabulary.	Naturally Speaking and Dragon Dictate (Dragon Systems), Via Voice (IBM), Hear-Say (Voice Pilot Technologies)
Speaker-independent systems	The operation is similar to continuous speech recognition systems, but there is no training required. Generally limited to small, application-specific vocabularies.	Used in special-purpose assistive devices for environmental control or robotic control (see Chapter 12) and wheelchair control (see Chapter 10).

Other hardware issues are important in ASR as well. Foremost of these is the microphone (Simpson, 2013). Although the microphones supplied with ASR systems are satisfactory for use by nondisabled users, they are not adequate when the user has limited breath support, special positioning requirements, or low-volume speech. Most ASR systems use a standard headset microphone. Individuals who have disabilities may not be able to don and doff such microphones independently, and desk-mounted types are often used.

Electronic activities of daily living may also use speech recognition to access their functions (see Chapter 12). In such devices, the individual can instruct the system to turn lights off and on or perform other functions by voice. The user can train the system to execute these commands with just about any sound, letter, or word.

The questions listed in Box 8-1 can be used to determine the usefulness of speech recognition for a given consumer. The key for success in using speech-activated systems is that the user be able to produce a *consistent* vocalization or verbalization. Differences in speech production are found not only among individual speakers but also within the same speaker. Variability in the user's speech can cause problems with recognition. For this reason, this type of **control interface** may not be effective for individuals who have dysarthria. Individuals who have had a SCI and have no functional use of the upper extremities yet have good speech control are potential candidates for a speech recognition system. It is important when considering a speech recognition system to determine whether the user's voice pitch, articulation,

BOX 8-1 Critical Questions for Evaluating Use of Speech Recognition Interface

1. Can the consumer consistently utter all of the sounds necessary to access the speech recognition system?
2. Is the recognition vocabulary adequate?
3. Are the consumer's voice articulation, pitch, and loudness consistent enough for accurate selection?
4. Is there likely to be background noise in the consumer's context that will interfere with the speech recognition system?
5. Would an alternative template or vocabulary be beneficial?

and loudness change or fatigue over time. Other noises or voices in the area where the speech-activated system is being used can also confuse the system, resulting in either an incorrect selection or the system having difficulty registering any selection, causing the user to repeat the vocalization several times.

Automatic Speech Recognition Built into the Operating System

Several mainstream computer and mobile technologies also includes a built-in ASR system. These include Microsoft **Windows** (Speech Recognition), Apple **iOS** (Speak Selection) and **OSX** (Dictation and Siri), **Android** (Google Voice typing), and Blackberry (Voice Recognition). These systems have adjustments of parameters such as rate of speech, blocking of offensive words, and recognition of punctuation and special characters (e.g., typing " :" and ")": causes the device to say "say smiley face"). Specific adjustments vary from system to system.

Automatic Speech Recognition as an Add-On Accessory

There are downloadable apps for the iOS, Android, and Blackberry operating systems from the appropriate stores. These apps expand the capabilities with greater adaptability and adjustability to meet the needs of specific users. Voice Finger (voicefinger.cozendey.com) is a downloadable accessory for Windows, OSX, iOS, and Android platforms. It provides complete voice control of the mouse and keyboard and does not require additional switches or keyboard access.

Brain–Computer Interface

A significant number of people cannot effectively use any of the interfaces described in this chapter. For these individuals, the brain–computer interface (BCI) may offer promise. Although this approach is still primarily in the research stage, there are promising results to date. It is likely that we will see a much greater understanding of the biological–physical interface for the control of computers in the future (Applewhite, 2004). Figure 8-1 is an overview of a typical BCI system (Schalk et al., 2004). Features or signals that have been used include slow cortical potentials, P300 evoked potentials, sensorimotor rhythms recorded from the cortex, and neuronal action potentials recorded within the cortex.

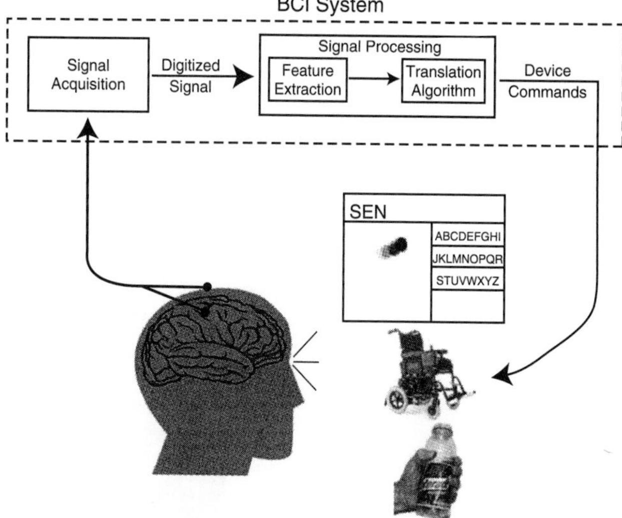

FIGURE 8-1 An overview of a typical brain control interface system. (From Schalk G, McFarland DJ, Hinterberger T, et al.: BCI2000: A general-purpose brain-computer interface (BCI) system, *IEEE Trans Biomed Eng*, 51:1034-1043, 2004.)

Principles

The success of BCI systems depends on the type of brain signal, the methods of signal processing to extract relevant features, the algorithms that translate the features into control signals (most often a mouse-like cursor movement on the screen), user feedback, and user characteristics. BCI systems may be grouped into a set of functional components (Mason & Birch, 2003). The BCI input device provides amplification, feature extraction, feature translation, and user feedback. The control interface converts this signal to those required to control the output device (e.g., power wheelchair, EADL, computer). The device controller provides the actual control signal to the target device (e.g., signals to the motors of a power wheelchair, mouse cursor movement signals to a computer). Schalk et al. (2004) give technical details of the major approaches to BCI system design. Signals are mathematically analyzed to extract features useful for control (Fabiani et al., 2004).

Because the neural signals are very low amplitude, recordings from the outside of the skull are subject to low signal-to-noise ratios and generally weaker signals. Electrodes located on the surface of the cortex have stronger and more varied signals and less interfering muscle artifact and are more stable than those attached to the scalp (Leuthardt et al., 2004). However, two main obstacles to invasive BCI systems are (1) recording electrodes become overgrown with connective tissue, resulting in their loss of electrical contact with the brain tissue and reducing their effective functional life, and (2) there is a greater chance of infection because the cables connecting the electrodes to the amplifier must pass through an aperture in the skull (Frolov et al., 2013). For these reasons, it is expected that noninvasive BCIs will be used on a large-scale basis in the near future.

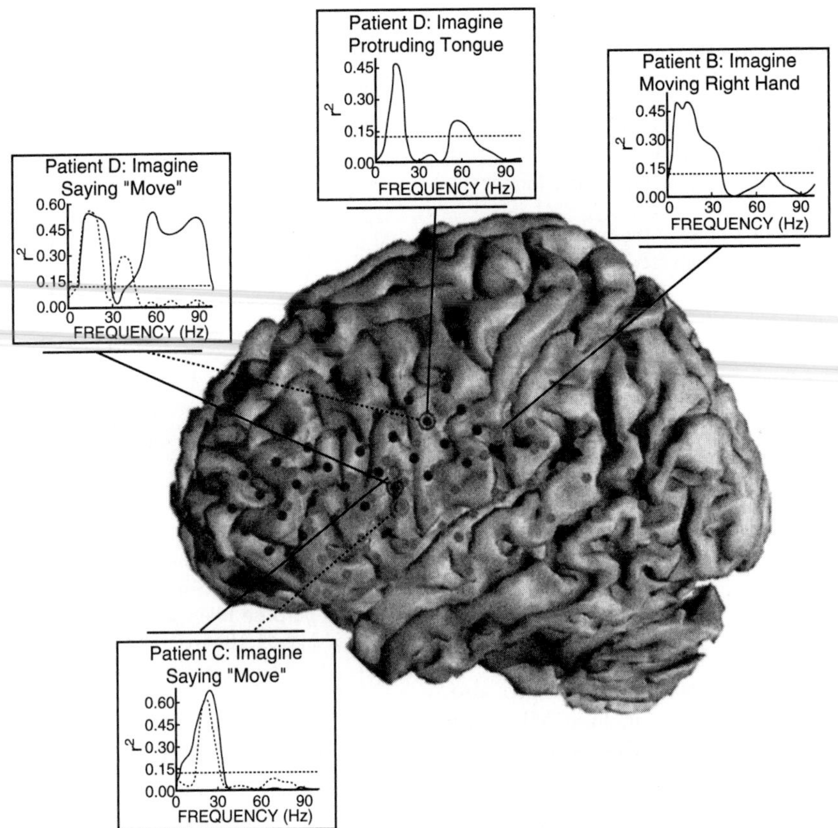

FIGURE 8-2 An example of differing signals measured on the surface of the cortex for different imagined motor acts. (From Leuthardt EC, Schalk G, Wolpaw JR, et al.: A brain-computer interfaces using electrocorticographic signals in humans, *J Neural Eng*, 1:63-71, 2004.)

One typical task for a user is to visualize different movements or sensations or images. An example of differing signals measured on the surface of the cortex for different imagined motor acts is shown in Figure 8-2 (Leuthardt et al., 2004). The unique signal patterns shown in Figure 8-2 can be used to generate control signals. The process of obtaining useful control signals is the use of a classifier that adapts to the user's response (Frolov et al., 2013). Initially, the user is instructed to perform several types of mental tasks, and those generating the most easily classified signals are identified. Then each task is associated with a unique command for an external device such as a computer mouse or TV controller (e.g., channel change or volume change). The user than must solve the corresponding mental task to generate the desired command.

An alternative approach to BCI signal processing is to use evoked response signals (Schalk et al., 2004). The P300 component of the evoked potential detects an "unexpected, rarely presented significant stimulus when it appears among frequently presented insignificant stimuli" (Frolov et al., 2013, p. 198). When using evoked response BCI to select characters from a display, one approach is simply highlighting characters, called character flashing (CF). Kauffmann et al. (2013) used a different stimulation paradigm for event-related potentials (ERPs) based on flashing characters with superimposed pictures of well-known faces, termed face flashing (FF).

The participants were 16 nondisabled BCI novices (11 women; mean age, 23.69 years; standard deviation [SD], 2.6; range, 19–33) and nine individuals with neurodegenerative diseases (eight men; mean age, 50 years, SD = 15.21; range, 26–72). All participants performed spelling tasks using CF and FF. The individuals with neurodegenerative diseases achieved considerably worse performance with CF compared with the nondisabled individuals. The group difference disappeared when FF was used and two participants who were highly inefficient with the classic CF paradigm spelled highly accurately using FF.

Clinical Evaluation

As BCI technology has evolved and has been used more, it has been possible to get reactions of patients to the technology and to begin looking at some practical issues underlying widespread clinic use of BCI (Grübler et al., 2013). Participants in an international BCI research project on noninvasive BCIs for stroke rehabilitation and AT control were interviewed. Semistructured interviews were held with 19 research subjects (15 men and four women ages 29–71 years) in two different groups. Seven were subacute individuals who had a stroke, and 12 were persons with motor impairments. This was a two-part study consisting of successful BCI training and use of BCI to control ATs of various types. All 12 of the motor-impaired participants had previous satisfying experiences with non-BCI ATs. None of the participants had experience with BCI use before the study. Improvements in hand movement occurred for most of the seven individuals who had a stroke, which led to satisfaction. Some also said they were satisfied because their expectations had not been very high initially.

The quality of recognition by different subjects is highly variable. Some struggled with the requirement for mental imagery used in this study, stating that the requirements for use were not clear. Four of the stroke patients reported improvements in function as a result of the BCI-based rehabilitation program. The requirement of prolonged attention and concentration was challenging for some. Grübler et al. (2013) concluded: "Though the engineering part of BCIs is certainly clearly understood, researchers are currently not able to predict whether a device would work with a certain individual or say why it does or does not."

Morse Code Input

Coded access, specifically Morse code input, is discussed in Chapter 6. Some of the approaches used with computers and mobile technologies are described here. Several third-party devices provide Morse code input to Windows and Macintosh computers.

The DARCI USB (ww.westest.com) provides Morse code alternative input using one, two, or three switches. It connects through s **USB port.** The Darci USB includes both a hardware component for attaching the control interfaces (switches) to the computer and software to translate the Morse code entries into keyboard commands. The MouseKeys accessibility feature must be activated for use.

Comax (osa.comax.com/index.htm) is a software application for Windows that uses Morse code to replace the keyboard. If mouse click is used for code input, no additional hardware is required. External switches can be connected for one- or two-switch Morse code using a mouse with keyjack available from Comax or other USB switch inputs (see Table 7-8). Morse features such as speed, timing of dots, and dashes are adjustable.

The Tandem Master (http://www.tandemmaster.org/home.html) is a Morse code input device designed to provide a Morse code keyboard equivalent for Windows and Macintosh computers. The device is seen as a USB keyboard and mouse while the user inputs Morse code. The Tandem Master is designed to work with the Morse-2-USB controller that provides input for switch Morse code. Templates with unique Morse sequences can be stored. Morse features can be adjusted.

Original Morse code (letters and numbers only) did not include other keyboard characters such as ESC or RETURN keys or characters such as punctuation or \ /@#$%. The absence of standardized codes for anything other than alphanumeric characters has resulted in different AT Morse code systems having different codes for these characters. Examples of codes developed for computer use in several different products are listed in Table 6-2. Note that in some cases, the codes for the same characters are different for the two systems, and in other cases they are the same. After the set of codes is learned and the motor patterns developed, it is very difficult to change to a new set of codes, and changing from one system to another can be both time consuming and frustrating for the consumer.

The Google Play store and the Apple Store have Morse input apps for phones and tablets. Some of these apps provide an alternative keyboard based on Morse code with just two enlarged keys on the screen. Other devices work with external switches.

CASE STUDY

Learning Morse Code by Jim Lubin

I'm a c2 vent dependent quadriplegic with very little head movement, so sip and puff works best for me. I've been using Morse code to access the computer for the past 22 years. I learned it when I was in rehab in 1989. The therapists had the Morse codes incorporated into pictures, and I memorized the pictures.

For example:

A = dot dash = a picture of an Arrow going toward a bull's-eye target.

B = dot dash dash dash = a picture of a Bee

H = dot dot dot dot = picture of a simple House with the dots the 4 corners of the square house

I had the paper taped above my bed so I could study when stuck in bed. I got to practice on the computer about 2½ hours a day during OT and speech therapies. I learned the letters and numbers in about 2 weeks. I was still having to think about the codes in the pictures back then. Now it is just automatic to me. I just type without thinking of the codes.

I had tried a typing tutor years ago and got to 19 wpm.

COMPUTER ACCESS

Built-In Software Adaptations to the Standard Keyboard and Mouse

Persons with disabilities often have difficulty pressing more than one key at a time because they are single finger typists. They may also have accidental key activation because of poor fine motor control. Software adaptations for these and other problems are shown in Table 8-2. These software adaptations are built into Windows (Microsoft accessibility Website: www.microsoft.com/enable) and Apple (Apple Accessibility Website: www.apple.com/accessibility) OSX operating systems. The software adaptations can be adjusted for an individual user through the control panel.

Accessibility for the Macintosh includes those features shown in Table 8-2. When StickyKeys is used, the modifier keys are converted to sequential rather than simultaneous use. This means that instead of having to press the shift key and

TABLE 8-2 Minimal Adaptations to the Standard Keyboard and Mouse*

Need Addressed	Software Approach
Modifier key cannot be used at same time as another key	StickyKeys†
User cannot release key before it starts to repeat	FilterKeys†
User accidentally hits wrong keys	SlowKeys,† BounceKeys,† FilterKeys†
User cannot manipulate mouse	MouseKeys†
User wants to use augmentative communication device as input	SerialKeys† in Windows XP or an alternative (similar to AAC Keys)
Keyboard is difficult	Touchscreen (iOS, Android, Microsoft Surface)
User cannot access keyboard	On-screen keyboard (Windows and OSX) Built-in ASR (Windows, Apple OSX and iOS, Android)

*Universal Access in Macintosh operating system, Apple Computer, Cupertino, CA; Accessibility Options in Windows XP, Microsoft Corp., Seattle, WA.
†Software modifications developed at the Trace Center, University of Wisconsin, Madison. These are included as before-market modifications to the Macintosh operating system or Windows. The function of each program is as follows:
StickyKeys: User can press modifier key and then press a second key without holding both down simultaneously.
SlowKeys: A delay can be added before the character selected by hitting a key is entered into the computer; this means that the user can release an incorrect key before it is entered.
BounceKeys: These prevent double characters from being entered if the user bounces on the key when pressing and releasing.
FilterKeys: The combination of SlowKeys, BounceKeys, and RepeatKeys in Microsoft Windows.
MouseKeys: Substitutes arrow keys for mouse movements.
SerialKeys: Allows any serial input to replace mouse and keyboard; this function has largely been replaced by USB standard devices.
Touchscreen with a touchscreen monitor: Uses a finger on the screen to move icons, point, resize windows, play media, and pan and zoom.
Multi-touch: Can use gestures on the track pad to control input, pinch, swipe, or rotate gestures (similar to iPod Touch and iPhone).

another key at the same time, the user can press the shift key, and then press another key and the second key will be shifted. StickyKeys allows either a single finger or a head pointer or a toe to be used to access all the functions on standard keyboards. FilterKeys and other designations such as BounceKeys, SlowKeys, and RepeatKeys are options designed to avoid double entries because of holding a key too long or accidentally hitting a key multiple times because of lack of fine motor control. Both Windows and Macintosh operating systems provide many options to make the keyboard and mouse faster and easier to use. In both cases, the operating system leads the user through choices based on a description of the need.

Both Windows and Macintosh have built-in **on-screen keyboards.** Two modes of entry are available when an on-screen key is highlighted by mouse cursor movement: clicking and dwelling. In the latter, the user keeps the mouse pointer on an on-screen key for an adjustable, preset time, and the key is entered. The on-screen feature also allows entry by scanning. An area of the screen can be designed as a "hot key" with text, graphics, or control functions (similar to opening a file or running a program) stored at that location. When the hotspot is selected by pressing, scanning, tapping, or other means, the stored text or function is entered into the computer. An auditory click or flashing icon or other feedback may be provided to indicate selection of a hotspot. Limited ASR capability is also included in Windows, Macintosh, and several smart phone operating systems (e.g., Android: developer.android.com/resources/articles/speech-input.html, and iOS).

Persons with disabilities often have difficulty in pressing more than one key at a time because they are single-finger typists. They may also have accidental key activation as a result of poor fine motor control. Software adaptations for these and other problems are shown in Table 8-2. These software adaptations are built into Windows and Apple Macintosh operating systems. Collectively, these are called **Ease of Access** in Windows (Microsoft accessibility Website: www.microsoft.com/enable/products/windowsxp/default.aspx) and **Universal Access** for the Macintosh (Apple Accessibility Website: www.apple.com/accessibility). They are accessed and adjusted for an individual user through the control panel. In the OSX, the accessibility features are located in "System Preferences -> Universal Access."

Easy Access features are those shown in Table 8-2. When StickyKeys is used, the modifier keys are converted to sequential rather than simultaneous use, which allows other effectors (e.g., the head and foot) to also be used to access standard keyboards. In many cases, there is also a need for StickyKeys (Windows and Macintosh) and FilterKeys (Windows) or SlowKeys (Macintosh) adaptations. FilterKeys includes the functions of BounceKeys, SlowKeys, and RepeatKeys. In Windows, a number of options can be chosen to make the keyboard and mouse faster and easier to use. Options that can be adjusted are described on the Microsoft Website (www.microsoft.com/enable/products/windowsxp/default.aspx). The Macintosh OSX operating system also includes a feature called Speakable Items that uses speech recognition to close or minimize windows, navigate menus, open and switch between apps, turn text into sticky notes, or start a screen saver (www.apple.com/accessibility/osx). This speech recognition feature does not need to be trained because there is a short list of possible choices.

An on-screen keyboard utility in Windows and Macintosh operates in a manner similar to those described in this chapter but it has only basic functionality. Two modes of entry are available when an on-screen key is highlighted by mouse cursor movement: clicking and dwelling. In the latter, the user keeps the mouse pointer on an on-screen key for an adjustable, preset time, and the key is entered. The on-screen feature also allows entry by scanning with a hot key or switch-input device. Several keyboard configurations are included, and an auditory click may be activated to indicate entry of a character. Windows combines the on-screen keyboard, Narrator, and the magnifier program and a utility manager in its accessibility menu, which is accessed through the start menu. The Accessibility Wizard guides the user through the accessibility options to configure the system specifically for his or her use.

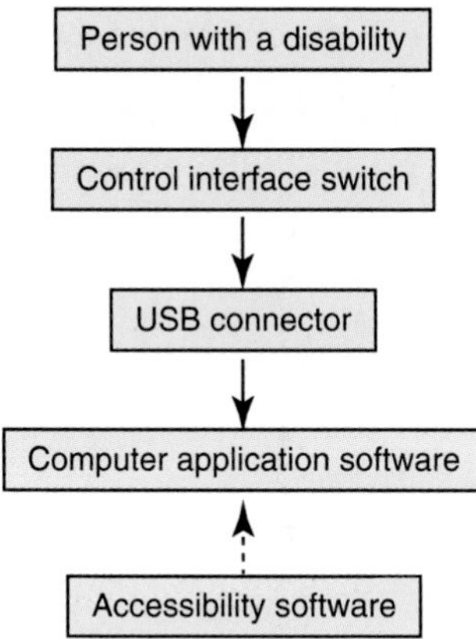

FIGURE 8-3 Major components involved in third-party accessibility options.

All Macintosh notebooks and desktop computers (using a Magic Trackpad) include multi-touch technology (www.apple.com/ca/accessibility/) that allows gestures on the trackpad to control the computer. With pinch, swipe, or rotate gestures, the user can zoom in on text, advance through a file, or adjust an image. Video demonstrations of these gestures are shown on the Apple Accessibility Website (www.apple.com/osx/what-is/gestures.html). Some require coordinated movements that may be difficult for individuals with fine motor control limitations, but most are easily achieved.

Third-Party Accessibility Options

Although the built-in accessibility features address the needs of many users, those with more severe motor limitations may require more extensive adaptations to access the computer.

Each key on the standard keyboard has a code that is sent to the computer when the key is pressed (called an ASCII [pronounced "asky"] code). If another control interface or different keyboard is to be used as an alternative input device, pressing a control interface or key must generate the same coded information that the computer expects from a mouse or keyboard. This requires that a *decoder* is added between the control interface and the computer (Anson, 1997). The term *keyboard or mouse emulator* is often used to describe devices that provide this decoding function. The emulator is just an alternative device that is made to function like a keyboard or mouse.

Figure 8-3 shows the major components involved in third-party accessibility options. Not all of the components shown in the figure are included in every system. Individual needs of the person with a disability will dictate what components are needed. The control interface may be any of those described in Chapter 7 or ASR and BCIs as described in this chapter. The most commonly used are expanded keyboard or contracted keyboards, single or multiple switches, and joysticks.

USB Switch Connectors

The control interface must have a way of connecting to the computer so that alternative approaches can be substituted for the keyboard, mouse, or both. This is accomplished using a **USB Switch connector** that connects the control interface to the computer via a USB port.

The required keyboard or mouse decoding is either built into the USB connector and supplied to the computer through the USB port or included in the accessibility software. An additional advantage of the USB port is that it supplies power to the external device from the computer, which eliminates the necessity for an external power source for USB input devices and is especially valuable for AT applications that are based on portable computers.

Many switch connectors are available for connecting single or multiple switches to the computer. Table 7-8 lists some of these together with their characteristics. Some of these emulate mouse and keyboards and some only one of them. Some of the connectors are wireless, giving more freedom of movement and reducing the tangle of wires that often surrounds a person using adapted computer access. All current commercially available devices use the USB standard for providing adapted input and are designed for either or both of the Windows-based and Macintosh computers. All have provisions for attachment of control interfaces.

The switch connector provides the interface necessary for an external control interface to control an **application program** running on the computer. The application program is just the task that the computer is to do. It could be word processing, email, social networking, or playing a video game. It could also be an educational program or software to aid rehabilitation such as cognitive retraining software. Many application programs can use a generic setup with a few features. Others benefit from more customization. As shown in Table 7-8 some of the USB connectors have options that match particular application programs. Others have specific keys associated with switch inputs. Still others have generic inputs that can be configured to meet the needs of the application program.

There are challenges involved in using the USB HID standard, and these can result in incompatibilities between AT devices and between the AT device and the host computer (Vanderheiden & Zimmermann, 2002). The existing USB HDI 1.11 document standard provides definitions for common human input devices such as keyboards, mouse pointers, joysticks, and game pads (USB Implementers' Forum, 2001). However, it does not currently have a definition specifically for AT input devices. Therefore, AT products must still emulate one of the defined devices (e.g., a keyboard or mouse) to provide the specialized input. There are no general standards defined to do this for AT developers to follow, which has resulted in different manufacturers using the USB HID in different ways. The lack of general standards results in some incompatibilities between AT products and confusion for the end users. To address this issue, the Accessibility Interoperability Alliance (AIA), has been formed by a group of leading IT and AT companies, content providers, and other key engineering organizations. Their goal is to work to create and harmonize standards for accessible technology.

Accessibility Software

General purpose keyboard or mouse emulation that allows access to all of the computer keyboard characters and mouse functions requires an additional **accessibility software** app to be loaded into the computer. This software is a key element in the emulation process.

Emulators have a general set of characteristics that allow the computer to be altered for a given application and a specific person with a disability. Some or all of these general characteristics are included in commercially available emulators. The characteristics of an emulator are customized for an individual application and user through a **setup** (also called an overlay, screen, or grid), a concept that originated with the Adaptive Firmware Card (AFC) for the Apple II series of computers (Schwejda & Vanderheiden, 1982). Emulators also use built-in synthetic speech feedback in "talking setups" that allow the user to receive auditory, as well as visual, prompting and feedback. This is useful for young children who may not be able to read, for visually impaired individuals, and as an added input modality for persons with learning disabilities.

As shown in Box 8-2, a setup consists of three basic elements: (1) an input method, (2) overlays, and (3) a set of options. Different manufacturers may use different names for these three elements, but their function is comparable across manufacturers. The features of the setup may be implemented in hardware (electronic circuits), software (a program), or both. Setups are also usually stored in memory within the emulator hardware (e.g., an alternative keyboard), or in memory on the computer. This capacity allows different setups to be available for different users of a computer (e.g., in a classroom setting); they can be loaded into the computer or the emulator as needed. As shown in Box 8-2, the setup is used with an application program. The concept of setup also applies to customization of cognitive ATs (see Chapter 15) and augmentative communication systems (see Chapter 16).

Box 8-3 lists the key steps in developing a setup for an individual. Remember that many standard setups are available for popular programs. Several examples of setups that may be used with different application programs are shown in Figure 8-4. The setup shown in Figure 8-4 *A* is intended to be used for text entry in a business environment. The on-screen keyboard could be used with any pointing device by someone who has difficulty using the keyboard. For a single-switch user, the setup includes an overlay on the screen for use as a scanning array with special characters included, as shown in Figure 8-4 *B*.

For both Figure 8-4 *A* and *B*, the application program is any that uses text entry (e.g., a word processor, a spreadsheet, a database, email). Auto capitalization automatically enters one space and latches the shift function following sentence-ending punctuation (i.e., .?!). Abbreviation expansion or word completion can enhance the rate of text entry (see Chapter 6). Macros are often used to control application program functions. For example, adding a new row into a spread sheet usually involves several mouse movements and clicking. The macro could accomplish all of these tasks with a single scanning array selection.

BOX 8-2 Major Features of Commonly Used Emulators

A setup consists of the following three parts:
1. Input method
Keyboard
- Assisted
- Contracted
- Expanded
- Virtual
- Normal

Morse code
- One switch
- Two switch

ASCII
- Parallel
- Serial

Scanning
- Linear or row–column
- Auto, inverse, or step
- Single, dual, four, or five switch
- Switched joystick

Proportional
- Mouse
- Trackball
- Joystick

2. Overlay: All three of the following may be the same or different:
User: the selection set arrangement from which the user chooses
Computer: the character or string of characters sent to the application program when the user chooses
Speech: synthetic speech used as a prompt to the user or as feedback when a selection is made
3. Options:
Abbreviations: text-based codes
Autocaps: CAP and 2 spaces after a period, exclamation point, or question mark
Key repeat rate
Levels: like a shift, can be many levels on one setup; equivalent in scanning is branching
Macros: codes can include control characters and functions
Mouse emulation: move, drag, click, and tab
Multitasking: can interrupt one mode for another
Predictive entry: previous characters determine user overlay
Rate: how fast or slow the user can input to the emulator
Screen selection display location: where on the screen the user overlay appears
Slowdown of programs

Application Program
The business, education, or recreational program being used

BOX 8-3 Tips for Creating a Setup

1. Determine the desired actions that you want the computer to carry out when a selection set element is chosen.
2. Determine the number of available motor actions from the user (i.e., a keyboard vs. a single or dual switch or mouse).
3. Determine the way in which you will present the choices to the user (e.g., graphics, words, or pictures).
4. Determine what happens when a selection is made by the user:
   a. Is there auditory feedback (e.g., "good job" or the name of the object selected)?
   b. Is there visual feedback (e.g., flashing image or change in the screen content such as a letter typed or a selection made in a program)?
   c. What does the computer do when the choice is made (e.g., run a program, turn the page of a story)?

	Method	Overlay	Options	Application
A	Virtual keyboard	User: QWERTY Layout Computer: Same Speech: No	Speed of mouse • •	Business, productivity software (e.g, word processing, spreadsheet)
B	Single-switch scanning	User: ETA Array Computer: Same Speech: No	Rate • •	
C	Expanded keyboard	User: ⟹ STOP Computer: Arrow, Return Speech: "This one," "Next one"	Speech Slowdown • •	Early education matching task with arrow and return
D	Single-switch scanning	User: ---> OK Computer: Arrow, Return Speech: "This one," "Next one"	Rate Speech Slowdown	

FIGURE 8-4 An emulator setup consists of three parts: input method, overlay, and options. **A** to **D**, Four examples of setups for different consumers and different applications are shown. ETA is the scanning array with the most frequent letters at the beginning of the array.

The setup, shown in Figure 8-4 *C* and *D*, is for a young child who is using any of a wide range of software programs that require selection of an answer by matching a cursor (pointer) location with the correct item (Figure 8-5). The task may be to match numbers, letters, shapes, words, or pictures using the RIGHT ARROW to move the cursor RETURN (ENTER) to select the one that the student believes is correct. Because the user is not likely to have learned to read yet, we use symbols and speech in the setup to help identify the choices to be made and as a reinforcer when the choice is made ("this one," "next one") in Figure 8-4 *C* and *D*. An example setup is shown in Figure 8-6. The setup in Figure 8-4 *C* is for use with an expanded keyboard, and the overlay in Figure 8-4 *D* uses scanning on the screen to make the choices.

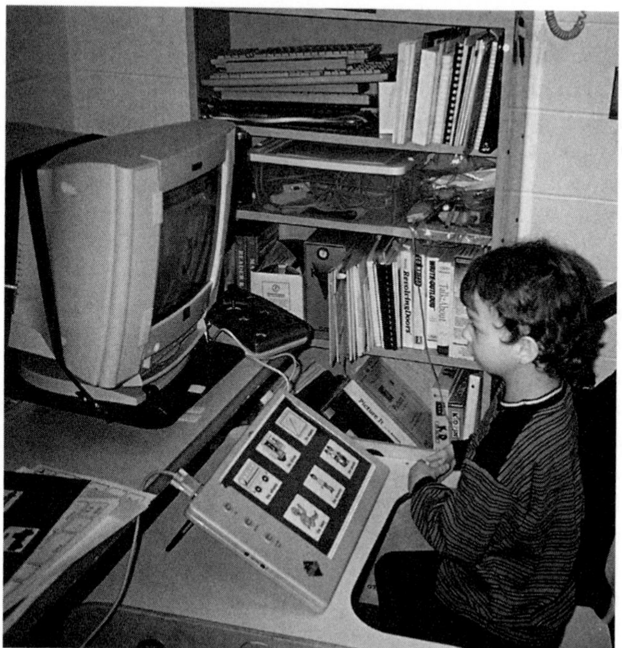

FIGURE 8-5 A symbol-based overlay for use with an expanded keyboard and an educational software program.

Many emulators allow other features, such as mouse emulation and the use of macro instructions and **multitasking** through the accessibility software. Mouse emulation substitutes a set of keys, a scanning array, or Morse code characters for mouse functions (similar to MouseKeys; see Table 8-2). Macros can be used to return the mouse cursor to a specific location based on stored information. This function can save time when scanning is the mode used for mouse emulation. All of these features can be incorporated into a setup that can be loaded when it is necessary or desirable to use the mouse. Mouse emulation is discussed in Chapter 8.

Table 8-3 describes examples of assistive software products. Often they are categorized as on-screen keyboards, but they have many features that extend beyond the simple on-screen keyboards included with the Windows and Mac OSX operating systems. All come with a set of on-screen keyboards intended for use with different programs. These are the setup we have described earlier in this chapter, also known as grids or overlays. Most of these products allow the user to make a custom setup or to modify the setups that are

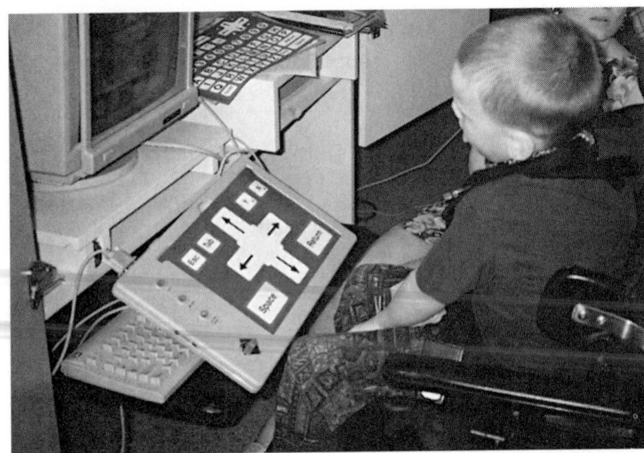

FIGURE 8-6 An overlay for cursor-controlling movement using arrows. This is being used with an expanded keyboard and an educational software program.

included with the program. Some include features that allow mouse functions of clicking, dragging, and double clicking to be emulated. A variety of control interfaces are supported by these products.

Many include single- or dual-switch scanning for making selections from an on-screen setup. A few include more extensive switch input options, as shown in Table 8-3. Macro refers to a single instruction that expands into a set of instructions when selected. Macros in a setup can open a program, cause an entry to be spoken or printed, or perform other functions such as saving a file by storing the correct key combination in one element of the setup. Macros can reduce multiple key entries or mouse manipulations to a single selection from the setup. The majority of the programs shown in Table 8-3 include word completion or word prediction (see Chapter 6).

Other features included in some programs are the capability of using photos or symbols as elements of the setup, voice output, advanced word prediction features, the capability of locating the on-screen keyboard at different locations on the screen, and the capability of making the on-screen keyboard transparent or partially hidden when no choices are being made. There are online evaluations of these programs. Look for on-screen keyboards (e.g., www.bltt.org/software/osk.htm). Several free on-screen keyboards are shown in Table 8-3. A partial listing and evaluation of free on-screen keyboards can be found at www.techsupportalert.com/best-free-onscreen-keyboard-osk.htm.

ACCESS TO PHONES AND TABLETS

Built-In Accessibility Features

Four features of cell phone technology affect access for people with disabilities: (1) increased processing power, (2) ease of downloading applications into the phone, (3) wireless connection to a worldwide network, (4) low cost and reachable by persons with disabilities because these features are built into standard cell phones (Fruchterman, 2003). Open source code refers to an operating system that is freely available to anyone. This is the feature that has led to the plethora of "apps," which are applications for a wide variety of things that can be downloaded in a smart phone or tablet. This means that new applications can be developed by lots of people without having to rely on the original owner of the software to integrate them.

Commercially available cell phones have increasing diversity of software for tasks such as text-to-speech output, voice recognition, and many other applications for particular activities or tasks. Typical tasks include business (banking, financial planning), entertainment (music, games, books and magazines), self-care (e.g., fitness or nutrition apps), travel (flight and hotel booking), and many more. Many apps are also being developed to meet the needs of persons with disabilities.

iOS Accessibility

The operating system for Apple's phones and tablet, iOS, has accessibility features (www.apple.com/accessibility/ios/# motor-skill) for the iPhone, the iPod Touch, and the iPad that are similar to those in the OSX operating system for the Macintosh computer. These include VoiceOver, Assistive Touch, and built-in ASR (called Dictation). Assistive Touch allows creation of custom gestures (e.g., converting the pinch gesture to a tap of a finger). It is also possible to use an on-screen tap for pressing the Home button if that is difficult for the user. Gestures such as rotate and shake are also available when the device is mounted on a wheelchair. Custom gestures are limited to those actions that would normally require movements that may be difficult for individuals who have motor problems (e.g., shaking the phone or rotating and locking the screen). Keyboard shortcuts are a form of abbreviation expansion (see Chapter 6). Custom shortcuts can be created for frequently used words or phrases.

Android Accessibility

The Android operating system is used for both phone and tablet applications. Android accessibility features (developer.android.com/guide/topics/ui/accessibility/index.html) include text to speech, haptic feedback, gesture navigation, and trackball and directional-pad navigation. Android application developers can take advantage of these services to make their applications more accessible. Third-party Android developers can also build their own accessibility services.

Blackberry Accessibility

The operating system for the Blackberry phone and tablet includes built-in features for accessibility (ca.blackberry.com/legal/accessibility.html#/h:/legal/accessibility/mobility.html). Predictive text and autotext (abbreviation expansion) and short-cut keys (macros) save keystrokes. Voice dialing, automatic redial, and speed dial reduce the number of entries required to make a call. The phone is made with nonslip surfaces to hold the smart phone with less effort.

TABLE 8-3 Examples of Computer Accessibility Software

Product	Platform	On-Screen Keyboard Features	Mouse emulation features	Control Interfaces	Scanning	Macros	Word Completion Prediction?	Other Features	Free?
Click-N-Type (www.lakefolks .org/cnt)	Windows	Custom design or modify existing screens	—	Mouse, trackball, touchscreen, or other pointing device	Quartering	Yes	Yes; free separate download	Autoclick allows users to perform hover delay entry	Yes
Dasher (www.inference .phy.cam.ac.uk/ dasher)	Windows Mac OS iOS Android	Zooming interface; display zooms in on letters; any point you zoom in on corresponds to a piece of text; choose what you write by choosing where to zoom		Joystick, touch-screen, trackball, or mouse; head mouse or by eye gaze			Yes; part of zooming interface		Yes
Free Virtual Keyboard (freevirtual keyboard.com)	Windows	Touchscreen access to OSK		Requires passive touchscreen					Yes
Hot Virtual Keyboard (hot-virtual-keyboard.com)	Windows	User custom design of screens (grids)		Requires passive touchscreen			Yes		No
Grid 2/Grid Player (www.sensory software.com)	Windows	User custom design of screens (grids)	Dwell Clicker 2; left click, right click, double click, or drag	Standard or modified keyboard and mouse; one to eight switches; touchscreen, head mouse eye gaze, joystick	Row–column, automatic, step	Yes	Yes	Voice output, simplified email and SMS grids; photos and symbols as grid elements	
Grid Player (www.sensory software.com)	iOS			Built-in touchscreen				Voice output; photos and symbols as grid elements	No
REACH (newsite .ahf-net.com)	Windows	Customization, themes to group such as program overlays	Mouse Assist: double clicking, dragging, or left, right clicks	Pointing interface; one or two switches	Automatic, inverse; auditory scanning; error correction	Yes	Yes	Smart keys; smart lists; advanced word prediction photos and symbols	No

Continued

TABLE 8-3 Examples of Computer Accessibility Software —cont'd

Product	Platform	On-Screen Keyboard Features	Mouse emulation features	Control Interfaces	Scanning	Macros	Word Completion Prediction?	Other Features	Free?
WiVik (www.wivik .com)	Windows	Customization resize keys; relocate keyboard on screen	Point, click, dwell	Any pointing device or one to six switches	automatic, inverse, step	Yes	Yes	Word and speech output; abbreviation expansion	No
KeyStrokes (www.assistive ware.com/ product/ keystrokes)	Mac OSX	Layout kitchen custom utility; automatically show and hide the keyboard as needed	Right and left click, double click, dragging	Mouse, trackball, head pointer, or other mouse emulator	No	Yes	Yes, US English, UK English, French, German, Dutch, Norwegian, Italian, Spanish, and Russian; photos and symbols as layout elements		No
Switch XS (www .assistiveware. com/product/ switchxs)	Mac OS X	Layout kitchen custom utility; scanning panel partially or fully transparent when no scan		One or two switches	Step, inverse, automatic		Photos and symbols as layout elements	Audio cueing; speech cueing; key repeat; mouse speed and movement	No

After-Market Accessibility Options

Smart phone and tablet accessibility for individuals with motor disabilities is accomplished through combinations of software apps and hardware interfaces for attaching control interfaces of various types. As with computer access, different approaches are used for different platforms. There are some general principles that apply, however, and we focus on those in this section. Links that have additional information are also included. We refer to these options as after-market options because some are available as add-on accessories from the manufacturer, and some are provided by third-party companies.

External Control Interface Connections for Tablets and Smart Phones

Connections of control interfaces such as switches, external keyboards, and alternative pointing devices require a physical connection to the phone or tablet. There are two basic approaches to this, hardwired via a port connector (e.g., the Apple's 30 pin or Lightning connectors or micro USB connectors on other tablets) or wirelessly through Bluetooth.

Bluetooth connections allow more physical independence between the control interface and the tablet or phone, but they consume power from the device, possibly limiting the useable time for access before recharging the tablet or phone. Also, the phone or tablet Bluetooth connection is available to connect a speaker, keyboard, mobile phone, or other device. A number of switch connectors for the Apple iPad rely on the Voice Over feature of the iOS. This may limit the applicability because not all iOS-based Apps are compatible with Voice Over. Table 8-4 lists examples of control interface connectors designed for use with tablets and phones. The devices listed are meant to be exemplary, and not all possible input devices are listed.

Accessibility Software for Phones and Tablets: "There's an App for That"

Some of the programs described in Table 8-3 have versions that run on mobile platforms. For example, Dasher (www.inference.phy.cam.ac.uk/dasher/MobileDasher.html) currently runs on Apple iOS/iPhone and Android. Dasher works as a system input method. There is also a version of the Grid (Grid Player) that runs in the iOS operating system (www.sensorysoftware.com/home.html).

A number of apps for tablets and smart phones are available from "app stores" that provide access to a large number of downloadable programs (www.apple.com/accessibility/third-party/ and play.google.com/store/search?q=accesibility&c=apps). Some of these are developed by the manufacturers (e.g., Apple, Android, Blackberry). Others are provided by other third-party vendors. Some apps address specific areas such as environmental control (see Chapter 12), vision (see Chapter 13), hearing (see Chapter 14), cognitive ATs (see Chapter 15), or augmentative communication (see Chapter 16). Other apps focus on more general aspects of accessibility to phones and tablets. We discuss those here.

Typical capabilities of apps for motor access include:

- Word completion or prediction to make typing faster
- Single-button access to programs to avoid fine motor movements
- Custom gestures (e.g., to avoid pinch, two-finger swipe, or taping) to accommodate for fine motor limitations
- Making custom keypads that are larger, have different keys, or are arranged differently
- Motor practice, usually in the form of games
- Enlarged phone buttons

MOUNTING

For persons with significant motor limitations, mounting of the device and any external control interfaces are critical for success. For example, Bryen and Pecunas (2004) describe an application in which a cell phone was mounted to a wheelchair within range of a head pointer by an augmentative communication user. They describe specific issues such as protection from moisture, provision of continuous power from the wheelchair battery to ensure continued power with the unit on all the time, and external speaker and microphone to ensure that the synthesized speech from the communication device was clearly heard over the phone. We discuss mounting of the control interface in Chapter 7.

Several companies make mounting systems for positioning computers, phones, or tablets for easy use on tables, wheelchairs, or the floor (e.g., DAESSY Mounting System, Daedalus, www.daessy.com/dms/indexm.html; Rehadapt, www.rehadapt.de/en; Blue Sky Designs, Mount'nMover, www.mountnmover.com). In addition to companies that specialize in mounting systems, many of the companies providing AT products also provide mounting systems. Mounting systems typically consist of a stand (for table or floor mounting) or a tubing clamp (for wheelchair mounting); an adjustable arm for positioning the device; and a plate for connecting the computer, phone, or tablet to the stand or positioning arm. Some models have a "swing-away" feature that allows the mounted device to be moved out of the way for transfers.

Various models include mechanisms for easy attachment and detachment from wheelchairs for self-care, transfers, and transportation. Adjustment of position is accomplished by combinations of locking joints in the moveable arm. Some of the joints are "locked" merely by tightening a clamp; others have lockable steps that can be selected. The lockable steps provide more stable operation, but they have a finite number (sometimes quite large) of locations compared with the continuously adjustable clamps. Titling of the mounted device is also available from some manufacturers (e.g., www.mountnmover.com). The Mount'nMover is designed so that the multiple locked positions can be set, and the user can make adjustments independently.

Mounting systems often have many options based on the type of device to be mounted, the location (e.g., a specific wheelchair), and the intended use. Picking the right

TABLE 8-4 External Control Interface Connection to Tablets and Phones

Product	Platform	Phone or Tablet	Connection Method	Control Interfaces	Special Considerations	Other Features
ZyBox (www.zygo-usa.com/usa/index.php?option=com_virtuemart&page=shop.browse&category_id=142&Itemid=11)	iOS	iPad	Apple 30-pin or Lightning connector	Up to six switches	Works with apps that are compatible with the iOS Voice Over (VO) commands	Automatic detection of switch connections No app or setup required; Powered from the iOS device
APPlicator (www.pretorianuk.com/ipad-access-devices)	iOS	iPad, iPod, iPhone (specific versions)	Bluetooth	Up to four switches	Switch access to apps that were developed to support switches	Programmable functions include 24 mouse and keyboard commands and full music controls Rechargeable lithium-ion battery via supplied USB connector
Switch2 Scan (www.pretorianuk.com/ipad-access-devices)	iOS	iPad	Bluetooth	Up to four switches	Access to all iPad functions, apps, music, media, iBooks, and data entry	On-screen keyboard scanning, step, and automatic modes; rechargeable lithium-ion battery via supplied USB connector
J Pad (www.pretorianuk.com/ipad-access-devices)	iOS	iPad, iPad mini, iPhone	Bluetooth	Joystick scanning interface, 2 switches	Switch access to iPad apps, music, media, iBooks, video, pictures, switch-adapted apps	On-screen keyboard entry
Hook (http://webstore.ablenetinc.com/hook%e2%84%a2-ipod-switch-access/p/10035005/)	iOS	iPod Touch, iPod Nano, iPhone 4, iPhone 3GS	Apple 30-pin or Lightning connector	Single or dual switch	Control of music playlist (music, podcasts, audiobooks)	Auditory scanned menu, motivation mode to play music for a set duration of time on switch activation
SimplyWorks integrated wireless system (www.pretorianuk.com/simplyworks)	iOS, Android,	Variety of tablets; see Website	Micro USB connector on Android-operated tablets, Bluetooth on iPad	Switches, trackball, joystick	Integrated wireless system	Mouse emulator, options
Tecla Shield (komodoopenlab.com/tecla)	iOS Android	iPhone, iPad, iPod Touch, Samsung Galaxy, and Google Nexus	Bluetooth	Up to six switch inputs, wheelchair driving controls, compatible with built-in ASR (iOS and Android)	Works with apps that are compatible with the iOS Voice Over (VO) commands Requires app for Android	Built-in rechargeable battery that lasts 4+ days Switch access to Siri 2 and Google voice assistants
Pererro (assistive-technology.co.uk/products/pererro)	iOS	iPhone, iPod touch, iPad	Apple 30-pin or Lightning connector	Single switch	Works with apps that are compatible with the iOS VO commands, step or auto scan modes	Scanning access features such as phone, messaging, email, and social networking applications
iPorta (www.dynamiccontrols.com/iportal/iportal-accessibility)	iOS	iPhone, iPod Touch, and iPad	Bluetooth	Wheelchair joystick or specialty input device, including head array	Works with apps that are compatible with the iOS VO commands and assistive touch features	Intended to provide access to iOS devices from wheelchair control

combination of parts and assembling the mount can be challenging. Rehabadapt has developed a Virtual Mounting System (VMS) approach (http://www.rehadapt.com/index.php/en/) that is designed to make the mounting selection process easier. The clinician takes digital pictures of the device positioned where she would like it to be mounted. The pictures, together with detailed information about the wheelchair, control interface, and device to be used, are emailed to the company. Rehadapt uses this input to produce a visualized proposal of the mounting system superimposed on the user's wheelchair image and a detailed list of the parts that need to be ordered to build the mounting.

CONTEXT

Social Context Connections via Information and Communication Technologies

A concern regarding Internet access is that it might reduce interpersonal contact and isolate people with disabilities from social interaction. Drainoni et al. (2004) found that the opposite was true because the use of Internet contact reduced many of the barriers faced by people who have sustained SCIs (e.g., transportation, telephone use, and need for personal attendants for outside trips). With the increase in social media, people without disabilities are also using the Internet as their primary communication medium.

The Internet has the potential to provide social interaction opportunities for children with physical and multiple disabilities such as cerebral palsy, muscular dystrophy, or acquired brain injury for making and maintaining social interactions (Raghavendra et al., 2012). These interactions can lead to friendships and inclusion in peer groups, especially for teenagers who have disabilities. Raghavendra et al. (2012) conducted a qualitative study of 15 participants with physical disabilities ranging from 11 to 18 years of age, with a mean age of 14.6 years. Typical of their generation, participants reported using home or school computers for email, social networking (e.g., Facebook), and instant messaging as well as visiting sports sites to check scores and follow players. They also used the Internet for school assignments and work. Participants reported that their use of the Internet was not significantly different from that of their peers without disabilities. Although most participants were independent in using the Internet, most reported that they had relied on friends or siblings to teach them how to use the Internet.

Family support, knowledge and skills, and the comfort level of family members with Internet use were the most important facilitators. AT was used infrequently and at a simple level. Similarly, the greatest barrier to use was limited family resources such as young people having to share access to one computer or the Internet with other family members. Internet problems such as limited download or use quotas, technical breakdowns, or lack of home Internet access and limited wireless connections (especially in rural areas) were also reported as barriers. Typing speed of those with physical disabilities was frustrating for live online interactions such as games or instant messaging.

Institutional Context

Political Infrastructure

In rural areas and throughout developing countries, the ICT infrastructure may not support wideband connectivity. This type of connectivity is required for smart phone and high-speed Internet access. Without it, access to Web-based services such as social media and embedded networks is limited or absent. The provision of these services is often based on a combination of political and economic considerations. In developing countries, a major driver for economic growth is development of broadband Internet (International Telecommunication Union, 2011). Whether this growth includes people with disabilities or not depends on the availability of the accessibility options discussed in this chapter.

Service Providers

Organizations that provide AT services can be slow in adapting technology innovations (Emiliani et al., 2011). This is primarily because innovations in the ATs may require changes in the service delivery component such as assessment, funding authorization, setup, and training of the end user. Universal design approaches are not always supported by the service delivery sector for several reasons. The most important is that mainstream technologies may not be paid for by social service agencies even if they are functionally equivalent (or more) than ATs and are much less expensive. A second concern is that provision of accessible features in mainstream technologies might make the service component less valuable because their services would not be as intense.

"Some service providers for people with disabilities have also been reluctant to exploit the full potential of ICT and AT, as their role and incentives is based on having clients come to them for evaluation and fitting of special ATs" (Emiliani et al., 2011, p. 108).

End Users

End users can be suspicious about universal design approaches based on mainstream technologies that they fear would not be eligible for the same funding as are ATs. This concern is well-founded because government agencies such as Medicare in the United States have refused to fund tablets and other mainstream technologies even though they provide the same capabilities as specialized ATs (Hershberger, 2011). However, "the relatively low cost of these solutions means that more families, school districts, and other agencies are able to consider the purchase of augmentative and alternative communication (AAC) technologies on their own; third party funding may not be necessary" (McNaughton & Light, 2013, p. 108). This change in paradigm means that individuals can play a more active role in obtaining AT if appropriate apps and necessary support services are available through service providers.

Physical Context: Ambient and Ubiquitous Computing

The goal of universal design for ICT is to have an environment with enough embedded intelligence to be easily adaptable (Emiliani, 2006). In an environment like this, there is no clearly predefined service; rather, services are reconfigured in real time to accommodate different needs in different contexts of use. Services are highly interactive, inherently multimedia, and sensory multimodal (i.e., access via auditory or visual means is equally possible). This cooperation between users or representatives of users is critical in a variety of contexts of use.

The overall goal is to have access to information involving communities of users with a wide range of motor, sensory, and cognitive skills who interact in common (sometimes virtual) spaces. The physical context for ATs includes the concept of **ambient intelligence**, which is defined as ". . . an environment where (i) technology is embedded in the physical and social environment of people; (ii) technology is context aware—employing machine perception a model of activities of people and their social and physical context can be obtained; (iii) technology is personalized—addressing each user as an individual person; (iv) technology is adaptive to context and activities of the person; (v) technology is anticipatory—predicting user's needs and taking action to support them" (Emiliani et al., 2011, p 110). These characteristics lend themselves particularly well to meeting the needs of persons with disabilities. Because the technology is embedded in the environment, is context aware, and can predict users' needs, it can benefit individuals without their having to take action to access it. For people with cognitive disabilities, this opens many options that would not otherwise be possible. For example, an AT system can detect where the person is and what he needs to do in that location (e.g., shopping or an independent living skill such as self-care) and then respond to the need by downloading appropriate software directly into their device (Lewis & Ward, 2011).

Other important characteristics of intelligent ambient environments are the ability to personalize applications and adapt to the context and activities of the individual. These features are fundamental to monitoring systems such as those that ensure seniors take medications and report to a care provider if they do not (Pape et al., 2002). The availability of stored user profiles can also enable accessibility to a variety of information environments such as ATM machines, information kiosks, and other public ICT systems by downloading the user's profile (e.g., visual or motor access features) when needed (Abascal et al., 2011). In this scenario, the special adaptations needed by an individual user would be stored and downloaded to the necessary device when needed without any request from the person being necessary. The user always has the same accessibly features available regardless of the particular ICT being used. This approach, referred to as "one size fits one," will provide the opportunity for a better fit to needs of an individual than the universal design approach of one size fits all (Emiliani et al., 2011).

The ambient environment also opens up many innovative approaches such as this to meeting the needs of people with disabilities. This environment has been called "calm, invisible and unobtrusive" (Lee et al., 2010). These characteristics are perfect for applications that assist people without their knowing they have been assisted.

So where is this "ambient environment"? It is embedded in a variety of devices such as appliances, mobile ICTs, kiosks, and other public places (Carbonell, 2007). A key element of embedded applications is the existence of networked environments including, but not limited to, the Internet (Spaanenburg & Spaanenburg, 2011). Home networks will be used composed of 25% wireless, 5% powerlines, and 70% specialized lines (e.g., phone wires). There is a worldwide trend for appliances to be connected to networks through power lines. One protocol for power line networks is X10, often used in ATs for environmental control (see Chapter 12). Because phone lines are designed for voice, it is necessary to have additional devices developed for multiplexing to three channels: audio (DC, 3.4 kHz), phone (25–1.1 MHz), and video and data (5.5–9.5 MHz) (Spaanenburg & Spaanenburg, 2011).

The embedded environment essential to AT applications incudes the concept of the "cloud," a complex of very large servers that are linked (Murua et al., 2011). Commonly used cloud services include Google Apps (www.google.com/enterprise/apps), Amazon Web Services (aws.amazon.com), and Apple's iCloud (www.apple.com/ca/icloud/?cid=wwa-ca-kwg-features-0001). With cloud computing, users on a variety of devices, including desktop computers, laptops, and mobile technologies (smart phones, tablets) can access programs, store data, and process information over the Internet using services from cloud-computing providers (Leavitt, 2009). There are also cloud-based AT service delivery systems that include special accessibility features for elderly individuals or those with disabilities (Murua et al., 2011). In these cases, the application also includes features that enable accessibility and allow a user to connect to the cloud through a variety of devices such as public servers such as ATMs, smart home appliances, and personal devices such as computers and mobile technologies (Lee et al., 2010).

ASSESSMENT

Computer Access Assessment

Scott (2006) conducted a Delphi study to determine elements that should be included in a comprehensive and valid computer access assessment. Rather than developing a specific assessment, this study aimed to formulate criteria for elements that should be incorporated into an instrument for determining AT for computer access. The Delphi electronic survey study was based on a literature review in the areas of neuroscience and rehabilitation. As a result of the Delphi evaluation involving 33 experts in computer access, Scott determined that an assessment instrument should be broad ranging, integrating both intrinsic and extrinsic factors. His study identified 25 intrinsic and 15 extrinsic elements that should be included in a computer access assessment. Many of these elements are generic AT assessment areas described throughout this book. Questions that should be answered in a computer access assessment are shown in Box 8-4 (Simpson, 2013, pp. 257–258). These questions can help to structure an assessment.

Simpson et al. (2010) classified the barriers to computer access assessment as cost (not usually reimbursed unless vocation rehabilitation funds it), changing consumer needs, and a large variety of options available. They describe nine computer access assessment tools in terms of three characteristics: (1) types of information gathered (qualitative vs. quantitative), (2) method of data collection and management (manual vs. computerized), and (3) focus of approach (assessment of ability vs. prescription of "best" device). Two of those are described here as examples of available tools for computer access assessment.

The Compass software (Koester Performance Research, www.kpronline.com) consists of four components (LoPresti et al., 2003). Skills related to keyboard use, pointing device use, text entry, and use of switches for scanning and other alternative input methods are evaluated through tests organized hierarchically to assess skills through successively more complex aspects of skills, such as the ability to press and hold a switch, and higher level skills, such as editing a sentence. The hierarchy also isolates the physical component of the test from its perceptual and cognitive aspects. Higher level tasks incorporate more perceptual and cognitive skills. Data are resented visually and in summary form. Data presentation allows clinicians, clients, family members, and case workers to examine data collected during skill tests. Compass includes summaries of client skills and comparisons of performance between control interface methods or over repeated trial across time. The overall design of Compass was informed by surveys and interviews with rehabilitation professionals.

The Assessment of Computer Task Performance includes more than 20 tasks that identify actions performed during computer use, such as keyboard input (i.e., capacity to strike each key on the keyboard and to strike two keys simultaneously) and mouse actions (i.e., ability to click, double click, and cover the length and width of the screen) (Dumont et al., 2002). The instrument was validated in a study with 24 participants with impairments and 30 participants without impairments. Test–retest reliability, internal consistency, construct validity (factor structure), and discrimination among known groups were assessed. Dumont et al. (2002) list more than 20 tasks that constitute the Assessment of Computer Task Performance. These tasks facilitate a structured instrument with clients and provide data to support therapeutic recommendations.

Phone Access Assessment

Nguyen et al. (2007) developed an approach for assessment of mobile phone access by people with physical disabilities.

BOX 8-4 Questions to Be Answered by a Mainstream Technology (Including Computer) Access Assessment

Questions Regarding the Technology and Regarding the Person

Some important questions to consider when examining products include:

- Will this device soon be outdated? Is something better on the horizon?
- Does it fit the individual?
- Is it convenient to use in the client's environment(s)?
- Does this device represent the simplest, most efficient way to accomplish the task, or is this device too complicated?
- Does it work efficiently and effectively?
- Is it easy to learn to use this device?
- Are all of the technologies compatible with each other and the computer access technologies the client already uses?
- Is the manufacturer willing to provide a loaner for an extended trial before purchase?
- Does the manufacturer provide training in using the device?
- Does the manufacturer have a local sales representative? Do company sales people seem knowledgeable and helpful?
- Is it safe to use?
- Does the device fit well into the user's lifestyle?
- Can the user operate the device independently or with a minimum of assistance?
- Does the device "stick out" too much and advertise the disability of the user?
- Does the device have the potential to increase the quantity and quality of time spent with nondisabled peers, or does the device separate the user from others?
- Do the benefits the device provides justify the cost?
- Are there less expensive devices or models that serve the purpose as well?
- Is this device the user's own choice?
- Does the client like this device and want to use it?
- Would the user have preferred some other device or means to perform the task?
- Will using the device always be a chore, or can using it become a habit?

Questions specific to hardware (e.g., keyboards, pointing devices)

- What is the manufacturer's repair policy?
- Does the manufacturer provide a warranty or a replacement when a device is being repaired?
- Are the company's service people knowledgeable and helpful?
- How long is the device guaranteed to function?
- Are repair services available? At what cost?
- How portable is the product? This includes size and weight along with the need to install drivers or other supporting software.
- How durable is the product?

Questions specific to software include:

- Is the software designed to run off of an external disk or thumb drive, or does it need to be installed on the computer in order to run?
- What is the company's update policy?
- How often are updates released?
- Are updates installed automatically?
- How often does the company charge for updates?

Modified from Simpson RC: *Computer access for people with disabilities*, Boca Raton, FL 2013, pp. 257-258.

The major components of this approach are shown in Figure 8-7. The assessment identified the participants' communication needs and accessibility problems and measured performance and frustration when accessing telecommunications equipment. The result of this process was matching of individual needs with the available solutions. This assessment methodology was evaluated with ten participants who had mild, moderate, and severe physical disabilities. An "ABA" style assessment approach was used: A was *before intervention* without equipment (before the trial), B was *during intervention* with equipment (at the end of the trial), and C was *after intervention* without equipment (after the trial had concluded and the equipment had been withdrawn for 2 weeks). The participants' performance and satisfaction relating to the problem areas they identified were measured using the Canadian Occupational Performance Measure (COPM) questionnaire (see Chapter 5). A specially designed accessibility questionnaire addressed the technical aspects of telecommunication use, including access to:

- Voice calls (using speed dialing, voice dialing, or other methods)
- Text messaging (SMS) or email (opening, creating, and sending)
- Voicemail (retrieving a message)
- Access to the information services (e.g., weather, news, sports, lotto numbers)
- Browsing the Internet

Typical problems for participants with mild physical disabilities preventing use of standard telecommunications equipment included small keys and displays and difficulties related to lifting or holding the phone for the duration of the call. Participants with moderate physical disabilities were restricted to the use of one mode of communication such as text or voice or limited use of both. Severe physical disabilities required participants to uses a switch scanning method for access to AAC, and independent use of conventional telecommunications equipment was not possible.

The features that were judged most important to participants were features such as hands-free solutions like voice dialing and speakerphones. "Car kits" that used speech recognition, a speakerphone, voice and speed dialing, and the use of a "magic word" to activate the voice dialing feature of the phone were installed on the participants' wheelchairs. Participants reported dramatic improvements in the ability to answer incoming calls and make calls. There was also substantial improvement in text messaging in the ability to compose and send a message or to open and read a message. The process also introduced participants to features of their phones that they did not know existed. They also reported decreased reliance on a third party to perform phone-related tasks.

Tablet Access Assessment

There have not been published reports of assessment protocols for tablets. As in all assessments, the starting point is to establish a clear statement of the individual's needs and goals for which the tablet might be used. The general assessment guidelines in Chapter 5 apply here as well. Specifically related to tablet use by individuals who have motor disabilities, the primary elements that should be considered are the ability to understand and use the required gestures (e.g., pinch, swipe, multiple-finger swipe) and the ability to hold the device or manipulate it to a workable position. If there are limitations in these areas, then some of the built-in and third-party accessible features described earlier in this chapter can be used.

OUTCOMES

Keeping Up with Innovations

Technology advances, especially in ICT, occur rapidly and consistently. It is important that these innovations benefit not only the general public but also people who have disabilities. Keeping up with innovations involves all of those who are involved in providing technologies for persons with

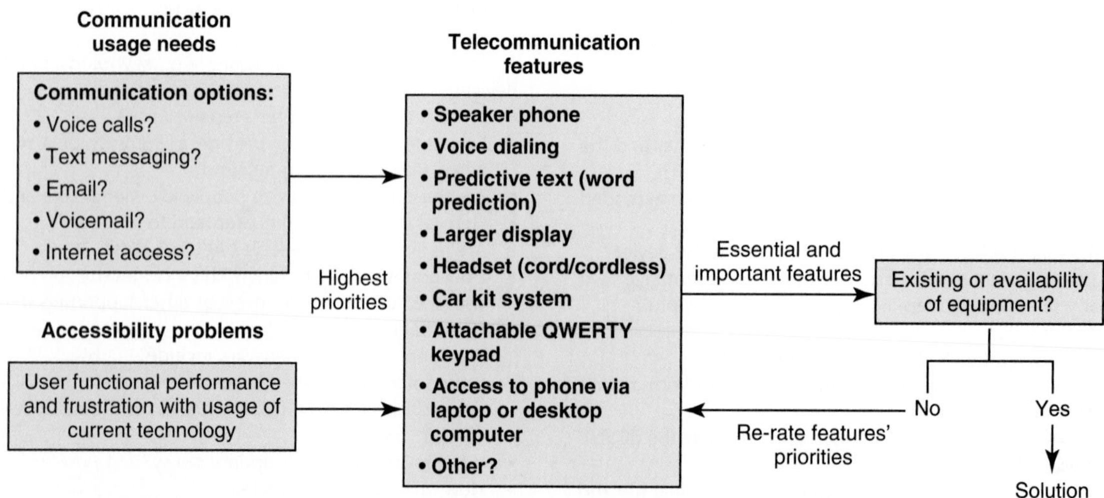

FIGURE 8-7 An assessment process for matching mobile phone characteristics to the needs of people with physical disabilities. From Nguyen T, Garrett R, Downing A, et al.: Research into telecommunications options for people with physical disabilities, *Assist Technol*, 19:81, 2007

> **CASE STUDY**
>
> *Mr. Cohen*
>
> You work in an adult residential faculty. Mr. Cohen, a resident who sustained a closed head injury about 2 years ago, is expecting a visit from his son, Bill, who lives out of town. Bill arrives with an iPad and the greeting, "This is just what dad needs to keep up with the world via the Internet!" Bill has not seen his father for a few months, and he also is not familiar with Mr. Cohen's program.
>
> **Questions**
>
> 1. What questions would you ask Bill to start the process of evaluating the usefulness of the iPad for Mr. Cohen?
> 2. What would you ask Mr. Cohen to do to see if the device might actually meet one of his needs?
> 3. How would you address Bill's concerns for his father if you reach the conclusion that Mr. Cohen cannot use the iPad?

disabilities (Emiliani et al., 2011). The primary players are industry (mainstream manufacturers and AT companies), service delivery organizations, end users, and the research community. The traditional business model based on competition in the free marketplace is altered in the case of technology for disability because it can be hard to define who the end user is (Emiliani et al., 2011).

Companies often find a niche market and focus on that; this can limit the breadth of the population served as well as the ability to innovate. Companies that specialize in ATs are often small organizations that do not have the resources to conduct research and development, and this limits innovation. Because AT products are often paid for by social service agencies, there can be a significant bureaucracy associated with reimbursement, especially for a new product. The paperwork and delays in getting approval may not be compatible with the economic sustainability of a small company. Small AT companies prefer to fill a niche by meeting the needs of customers that they know well rather than to compete more broadly (Emiliani et al., 2011).

In contrast, large companies that produce mainstream technologies (e.g., Apple, Microsoft, IBM, Oracle, SUN, HP) are aware of the needs of people with disabilities and could make their products totally accessible without additional accessibility features provided by AT companies. They tend not to design these features in precisely because the smaller companies making the accessible add-in technologies would be eliminated or as Emiliani et al. (2011) describe the situation, "They are afraid to be accused of cannibalizing the market and killing the AT industry" (p. 107). This leads to the inclusion of only the minimal adaptations necessary to meet legal guidelines.

Keeping Mainstream Technologies Accessible

Communication technologies change rapidly, and each change may result in the need to redesign accessible interfaces. Because of cooperation between computer software companies and AT developers, we are closer to the goal of having AT adaptations ready when the mainstream computer product ships, but there are still many problems with "workarounds" necessary to make mainstream operating system, productivity software, and Internet access available to people with disabilities. Often the workarounds provided by third-party suppliers become potentially incompatible with the new operating system, and they have to be redesigned. An example (courtesy of Randy Marsden) is a product that was designed to provide augmentative communication by using a mainstream laptop computer. It was necessary to include single-switch access, so the developer chose an unused memory location in the operating system for switch input. Unfortunately, the operating system was updated a few years later, and the software company decided to use the memory location as the on/off switch for the laptop. So, every time a user tried to control the communication program with her switch, it turned off the computer.

Although the manufacturers of the major operating systems (Microsoft Windows and Apple OS) now work more closely with AT companies as they make changes that will affect the AT products, the challenge of keeping apps current with mobile technology innovations continues today. Innovations are being made in mainstream ICT products such as mobile phones and tablets that affect apps and how they are implemented and controlled. This is particularly true for apps that rely on external interfacing to the mainstream technology such as for single-switch access. Because those developing the apps are generally not associated with the mainstream company, they may not be aware of changes in operating systems or hardware until the new version is released. They must then make changes in their app, and this can result in a significant delay before the mainstream technology is again available through the AT application software.

The prognosis is not good for people with disabilities unless there is considerable effort to keep them connected to ICT and thereby to commerce, employment, and personal achievement. There two fundamental approaches to this problem: (1) make mainstream technologies accessible to people who have disabilities (through universal design) or (2) design special-purpose technologies specifically for people with disabilities using ATs.

Development and maintenance of access to ICT must be driven by the needs of people with disabilities.

SUMMARY

The dramatic expansion of both the availability and capabilities of mobile technologies has created opportunities for people with disabilities to obtain devices with expanded features at lower cost than traditional specialized ATs. Unfortunately, that potential is often reduced by the lack of accessibility of mainstream technologies such as smart phones and tablets. In this chapter, we have described a variety of approaches to making computers, phones, and tablets accessible through built-in features, software apps, and third-party devices. Various aspects of context are important such as the embedded intelligent environment and issues of funding, stigma, and cost. Assessment for computer access is well developed but not so much for mobile technologies in general.

STUDY QUESTIONS

1. Define the elements of the HTI and how they are related to the processor and the output.
2. What are the accessibility features included in the OSx/iOS?
3. Explain the significance of having a USB HID specific to ATs.
4. What are the primary considerations that would lead to the choice of speech recognition as an alternative direct selection method?
5. Describe the difference between continuous and discrete speech recognition systems.
6. What is the difference between speaker-independent and speaker-dependent ASR systems?
7. Describe the major components of a BCI.
8. What are the major approaches to BCI development? Which approach do you think offers the most promise? Why?
9. There are several things about the way a computer mouse is used that can make it difficult for a person with a disability. Can you list three?
10. There are several adjustments built in to computers that can help match a user's needs to the mouse functions. What are they?
11. What is the most common way of connecting switches to a computer?
12. What are the major features of mainstream technologies (cell phones, smart phones, and pad computers) that can limit their usefulness to people who have disabilities?
13. What is included in a setup in an alternative access system for a computer or mainstream ICT device?
14. What are the relative disadvantages and advantages of software-based and hardware-based alternative access devices?
15. What does the term *transparent access* mean, and what features are used to implement it?
16. What unique considerations are there for Morse code input when it is used for computer access?
17. What are the social context implications for mainstream technology access?
18. What are the major factors that either drive or prevent innovation in the service provider, end user, and developer and manufacturer sectors?
19. What is the ambient environment?
20. What are the implications of the ambient environment for people with disabilities?
21. What are the major threats to obtaining and maintaining access to mainstream technologies for people with disabilities?
22. What are the major considerations when developing a mounting system for mainstream technologies and their control interfaces?

REFERENCES

Abascal J, Aizpurua A, Cearreta I, et al.: Automatically generating tailored accessible user interfaces for ubiquitous services, *ASSETS'11*, 187–194, 2011. October 24–26, Dundee, Scotland.

Applewhite A: 40 years: The luminaries, *IEEE Spectrum* 41(11):37–58, 2004.

Armstrong N, Nugent C, Moore G, Finlay D: Mapping user needs to smartphone services for persons ,with chronic disease, ICOST 2009, *Lecture Notes in Computer Science* 5597:25–31, 2009.

Anson DK: *Alternative computer access: A guide to selection*, Philadelphia, 1997, FA Davis.

Baker JM: How to achieve recognition: A tutorial/status report on automatic speech recognition, *Speech Technol* 36–43, 1981. Fall:30–31.

Bowker N, Tuffin K: Dicing with deception: People with disabilities' strategies for managing safety and identity online, *Journal of Computer-Mediated Communication* 8(2), 2003.

Bryen DN, Pecunas P: Augmentative and alternative communication and cell phone use: One off-the-shelf solution and some policy considerations, *Assist Technol* 16(1):11–17, 2004.

Burgstahler S, Comden D, Lee S-M, et al.: Computer and cell phone access for individuals with mobility impairments: An overview and case studies, *NeuroRehabilitation* 28(3):183–197, 2011.

Carbonell N: Ambient multimodality: An asset for developing universal access to the information society. In *Proceedings of 3rd International Conference on Universal Access in Human-Computer Interaction*, 2007. Las Vegas.

Comerford R, Makhoul J, Schwartz R: The voice of the computer is heard in the land (and it listens too), *IEEE Spectrum* 34:39–47, 1997.

Drainoni M, Houlihan B, Williams S, et al.: Patterns of internet use by persons with spinal cord injuries and relationship to health-related quality of life, *Arch Phys Med Rehabil* 85:1872–1879, 2004.

Dumont C, Vincent C, Mazer B: Development of a standardized instrument to assess computer task performance, *Am J Occup Ther* 56:60–68, 2002.

Emiliani P: Assistive technology (AT) versus mainstream technology (MST): The research perspective, *Technol Disabil* 18(1):19–29, 2006.

Emiliani P, Stephanidis C, Vanderheiden G: Technology and inclusion: Past, present and foreseeable future, *Technol Disabil* 23(3):101–114, 2011.

Engelen J, Blijham N, Strobbe C: The role of technical standards for AT and DfA equipment and services, *Technol Disabil* 23(3):149–161, 2011.

Fabiani GE, McFarland DJ, Wolpaw JR, Pfurtscheller G: Conversion of EEG activity into cursor movement by a brain-computer interface (BCI), *IEEE Trans Neural Syst Rehabil Eng* 12:331–338, 2004.

Frolov AA, Biryukova EV, Bobrova PD, et al.: Principles of neurorehabilitation based on the brain–computer interface and biologically adequate control of the exoskeleton, *Fiziol Cheloveka* 39(2):196–208, 2013.

Fruchterman JR: In the palm of your hand: A vision of the future of technology for people with visual impairments, *J Vis Impair Blindness* 97(10):585–591, 2003.

Gallant JA: Speech-recognition products, *Electronic Design News* 7:112–122, 1989.

Hellman R: Universal design and mobile devices. In *Lecture Notes in Computer Science (including subseries Lecture Notes in Artificial Intelligence and Lecture Notes in Bioinformatics)*, 4554 LNCS, Part 1. 2007, pp 147–156.

Grübler G, Al-Khodairy A, Leeb R, et al: Psychosocial and ethical aspects in non-invasive EEG-based BCI research—A survey among BCI users and BCI professionals, *Neuroethics*, 29-41, 2013

Hershberger D: Mobile technology and AAC apps from an AAC developer' s perspective, *Perspect Augment Altern Commun* 20(1):28–33, 2011.

International Telecommunication Union: *Measuring the information society*, Geneva, 2011, International Telecommunication Union.

Kane SK, Jayant C, Wobbrock JO, Ladner RE: Freedom to roam: A study of mobile device adoption and accessibility for people with visual and motor disabilities, 2009. In *ASSETS'09: Proceedings of the 11th International ACM SIGACCESS Conference on Computers and Accessibility*, 2009, pp 115–122.

Kambeyanda D, Singer L, Cronk S: Potential problems associated with the use of speech recognition products, *Assist Technol* 9:95–101, 1997.

Kaufmann T, Schulz SM, Köblitz A, et al.: Face stimuli effectively prevent brain–computer interface inefficiency in patients with neurodegenerative disease, *Clin Neurophysiol* 124:893–900, 2013.

Leavitt N: Is cloud computing really ready for prime time? *Computer* 42(1):15–20, 2009.

Lee K, Lunney T, Curran K, Santos JA: Proactive context: Awareness in ambient assisted living. In *International Conference of Aging, Disability and Independence (ICADI 2010)*, September 8-10, 2010. Newcastle, UK.

Lee YS, Jhangian I, Smith-Jackson TL, Nussbaum MA, Tomioka K, Design Considerations for Accessible Mobile Phones, *Proceedings of the Human Factors and Ergonomics Society 50th annual meeting*:2178–2193, 2006.

Leuthardt EC, Schalk G, Wolpaw JR, et al.: A brain-computer interfaces using electrocorticographic signals in humans, *J Neural Eng* 1:63–71, 2004.

Lewis C, Ward N: Opportunities in cloud computing for people with cognitive disabilities: Designer and user perspective. In Stephanidis C, editor: *Universal Access in HCI, Part II, HCII 2011, LNCS*, 6766. 2011, pp 326–331.

Leung R, Findlater L, McGranere J, et al.: Multi-layered interfaces to improve older adult's initial learnability of mobile applications, *ACM Transactions on Accessible Computing* 3(1):1–30, 2010.

LoPresti EF, Koester HH, McMillan W, et al.: Compass: Software for computer skills assessment. Presented at *CSUN's 18 Annual Conference, Technology and Persons with Disabilities*, Edinburgh, March 2003.

McNaughton D, Light J: The iPad and mobile technology revolution: Benefits and challenges for individuals who require augmentative and alternative communication, *Augment Altern Commun* 29(2):107–116, 2013.

Mason SG, Birch GE: A general framework for brain-computer interface design, *IEEE Trans Neural Syst Rehabil Eng* 11:70–85, 2003.

Miller Polgar J: The myth of neutral technology. In Oishi MMK, Mitchell IM, Van der Loos FHM, editors: *Design and use of assistive technology: Social technical, ethical and economic challenges*, New York, 2010, Springer, pp 17–23.

Miller Polgar J, Winter S, Howard S, et al.: The meaning of assistive technology use. In *Proceedings of the 25th International Seating Symposium*, 2009, Orlando, FL. p. 75.

Murua A, González I, Gómez-Martínez E: Cloud-based assistive technology services. In *Proceedings of the Federated Conference on Computer Science and Information Systems*, 2011, pp 985–989.

Nguyen T, Garrett R, Downing A, et al.: Research into telecommunications options for people with physical disabilities, *Assist Technol* 19:78–93, 2007.

Pape TL, Kim J, Weiner B: The shape of individual meanings assigned to assistive technology: A review of personal factors, *Disabil Rehabil* 24(1/2/3):5–20, 2002.

Pedlow R, Kasnitz D, Shuttleworth R: Barriers to the adoption of cell phones for older people with impairments in the USA: Results from an expert review and field study, *Technol Disabil* 22(3):147–158, 2010.

Raghavendra P, Wood D, Newman L, Lawry J: Why aren't you on Facebook? Patterns and experiences of using the Internet among young people with physical disabilities, *Technol Disabil* 24(1):49–162, 2012.

Schaefer K: Market-based solutions for improving telecommunications access and choice for consumers with disabilities, *J Disabil Policy Stud* 17(2):116–126, 2006.

Schalk G, McFarland DJ, Hinterberger T, et al.: BCI2000: A general-purpose brain-computer interface (BCI) system, *IEEE Trans Biomed Eng* 51:1034–1043, 2004.

Schwejda P, Vanderheiden G: Adaptive-firmware card for the Apple II, *Byte* 7:276–314, 1982.

Scott B: Essential elements for assessment of persons with severe neurological impairments for computer access utilizing assistive technology devices: A Delphi study, *Disabil Rehabil Assist Technol* 1(1-2):3–16, 2006.

Simpson RC: *Computer access for people with disabilities*, Boca Raton, 2013, FL.

Simpson R, Koester HH, LoPresti EF: Research in computer access assessment and intervention, *Phys Med Rehabil Clin North Am* 21(1):15–32, 2010.

Smith-Jackson TL, Nussbaum MA, Mooney AM: Accessible cell phone design: Development and application of a needs analysis framework, *Disabil Rehabil* 25(10):549–560, 2003.

Spaanenburg L, Spaanenburg H: Bringing the cloud back to home, cloud connectivity and embedded sensory systems, part 4, 239–277, in L. Spaanenburg, H. Spaanenburg, Cloud Connectivity and Embedded 239 Sensory Systems, DOI 10.1007/978-1-4419-7545-4_7, C Springer Science+Business Media, LLC 2011.

USB Implementers' Forum: Universal Serial Bus (USB): Device class definition for human interface devices (HID) (Version 1.11). Beaverton, OR, 2001.

Vanderheiden G, Zimmermann G: State of the science: Access to information technologies. In Winters JM, et al.: *Emerging and accessible telecommunications, information and healthcare technologies*, Arlington, VA, 2002, RESNA Press, pp 152–184.

van Tulder M, Malnivara A, Koes B: Repetitive strain injury, *Lancet* 369:1815–1822, 2007.

Vicente MR, López AJ: A multidimensional analysis of the disability digital divide: Some evidence for Internet use, *Inform Soc* 26(1):48–64, 2010.

CHAPTER 9

Enabling Function and Participation with Seating Technologies

CHAPTER OUTLINE

Introduction
Activity
Human
  Postural Control
  Tissue Integrity and Pressure Redistribution
  Comfort
Context
  Physical Context
  Social Context
  Institutional Context
Assistive Technologies for Seating and Positioning
  Biomechanical Principles
  Sitting Posture and Center of Pressure
Seating Technologies
  Design and Construction of Seating Systems
  Properties of Materials Used to Construct Seating Systems
  Classification of Support Surface Technologies
  Cushion Covers
Seating Assessment
  Needs Identification
  Standardized Measures
  Activity
  Human Factors
  Context Factors
  Matching Device Characteristics to a Consumer's Needs and Skills
Intervention
  Principles of Seating for Postural Control
  Principles of Seating for Tissue Integrity
  Principles of Seating for Comfort
Outcome Evaluation
  Pelvic Stabilization
  Reach
  Pressure Redistribution Cushions
Summary

LEARNING OBJECTIVES

On completing this chapter, you will be able to do the following:

1. Identify the potential outcomes of seating for postural control, tissue integrity, and comfort.
2. Describe a comprehensive seating assessment.
3. Describe key biomechanical principles related to sitting and seating technologies.
4. Describe the principles of seating for postural control.
5. Describe the factors that contribute to the development of pressure ulcers.
6. Discuss pressure mapping systems and the issues related to their use in the clinic.
7. Describe seating technologies used for tissue integrity.
8. Discuss the principles of seating for comfort.
9. Discuss the design and construction of seating technologies.
10. Describe the different characteristics of seating materials.
11. Discuss the different classifications of materials used to construct seats.
12. Describe the purpose and content of outcome measures specific to seating technologies.

KEY TERMS

Acceleration
Center of Gravity
Center of Pressure
Compression
Contour
Displacement
Dampening
Density
Envelopment
Equilibrium
Fixed Deformity
Flexible Deformity
Force
Friction
Frictional Forces
Gravitational Line
Gravity
Immersion
Kinematics
Kinetics
Linear
Line of Application
Magnitude
Mobility
Pelvic Obliquity
Pelvic Rotation
Planar
Postural Control
Pressure
Pressure Mapping
Pressure Redistribution
Pressure Ulcer
Recovery
Resilience
Restraint
Rotational

Scoliosis
Shear
Sliding Resistance
Stability
Stability Zone
Stiffness
Stress
Support Surfaces
Tension
Windswept Hip Deformity

INTRODUCTION

For a user of assistive technologies (ATs), a prerequisite to any interaction or activity is a physical position that is comfortable and that promotes function. The primary purpose of seating devices is to maximize a person's ability to function in activities across all performance areas (self-care, work or school, play or leisure). Three distinct areas of seating intervention have emerged, each serving a particular consumer need. These three categories of seating intervention are (1) seating for postural control, (2) seating for tissue integrity, and (3) seating for comfort (Geyer et al., 2003).

The first part of this chapter describes the needs served by seating systems, assessment of individuals for seating, and biomechanical principles related to seating. The remainder of the chapter provides in-depth information on each of the three categories of seating needs, including related principles and the technologies used for intervention. Seating components are interfaced with some type of mobility base. For purposes of this text, however, these two systems are separated. Mobility devices are discussed in Chapter 10.

ACTIVITY

We perform many daily activities in the seated position. Most of us do not think about what we are sitting on until we become uncomfortable or our seated position limits our activity performance. Think about sitting in a lecture hall, listening to a dull lecture. At first, you are unaware of the chair (seated support) surface. As time goes by, you become increasingly more aware of it and any discomfort to the point where you are no longer engaged with the lecture and focus on your discomfort. Consider another situation: think about being perched on a high stool and working at a workstation with shelves placed above it. Now imagine reaching for an object on a shelf that is just beyond your reach, remaining seated. The lack of support provided by the stool will most likely make you feel insecure as you reach for the object. These examples demonstrate that how we are seated affects our ability to perform activity. Appropriate seating provides a stable base, affords a proper biomechanical position, and is comfortable.

The International Classification of Functioning, Disability and Impairment (ICF) (World Health Organization [WHO], 2001) includes several classifications that are influenced by a good biomechanical and comfortable seated position. Some of these classifications can be considered foundational to other more complex occupations and include lifting and carrying in the hands (transferring an object from one place to another), fine hand use (picking up, grasping, manipulating, and releasing), hand and arm use (pulling, pushing, reaching, turning, or twisting the hands or arms, throwing, and catching) (WHO, 2001, pp. 141-143).

When combined, these foundational movements support more complex occupations that are performed in sitting. Eating a meal (and some meal preparation); writing or using a computer at home, school, or work; driving a vehicle or being a passenger; performing occupations such as sewing; assembly processes in manufacturing; and caregiving occupations such as feeding a child or adult are all performed while seated. Each of these occupations—and others that you might identify—is enabled by a stable, comfortable seating support surface.

HUMAN

Postural Control

The needs of children and adults with cerebral palsy (CP) and other neuromuscular disorders have led to the development of seating interventions for postural control. These individuals typically have abnormal muscle tone, muscle weakness, primitive reflexes, or uncoordinated movements that impair their ability to maintain an upright posture in a wheelchair without some form of support. Their impaired motor control affects their ability to participate in activities of daily living (ADLs), can compromise their general health status, and can result in skeletal deformities.

Lacoste et al. (2009) described stability and postural control issues in a sample of children with CP (n = 31). Although this study is modest in size, it provides interesting information about the nature of instability in this population that informs our understanding of seating needs for this population. Questionnaires were used to collect perceptions of parents and clinicians about the bidirectional relationship between instability and occupation. The average length of time sitting in a wheelchair for this sample was 11 hours a day. Instability in the seated position was noted after one half hour, a finding that has implications for the children's engagement in occupations over the course of the day.

Stability was defined as sliding forward in the seat or lateral or anterior trunk flexion and was influenced by activity, emotion, and the amount of effort expended in performance (Lacoste et al., 2009). Reaching, propelling a wheelchair, talking or using a communication device, eating or drinking, reading, and writing were occupations for which performance was more difficult from a position of instability and that added to the child's instability during performance.

Individuals with CP, head injury, and some sequelae of stroke experience high muscle tone in which excessive activity of the motor units is present in at least one muscle group around a joint. This high tone prevents the individual from relaxing these muscles, which results in limited movements in the antagonist muscles. Frequently, the antigravity muscles (flexors in the upper extremity and extensors in the lower extremity) demonstrate high tone in individuals with CP. In some situations, often after head trauma, excessive activity is seen in all muscle groups around a joint, which results in very restricted movement in any direction. This muscle imbalance affects the ability to sit unsupported.

The opposite situation occurs when either the motor units are lost as is the case in dystrophies or when the lower motor neuron is damaged as in a spinal cord injury (SCI). In this situation, the individual cannot actively contract his muscles to generate the power necessary for movement. Individuals with low or absent tone cannot maintain a sitting position because of loss of strength and endurance.

The dynamic nature of a motor impairment influences the ability to sit. Individuals who have sustained a stroke can expect that some or all sitting balance will return as they recover. Similarly, an individual who has had a SCI may recover some function in the initial period after the injury and will then plateau. Children will develop sitting abilities as they grow, develop, and strengthen. On the other hand, individuals with a progressive disorder such as multiple sclerosis will see their ability to sit deteriorate. As individuals age with a disability, they also often experience greater motor impairments. These changes should be anticipated during the seating assessment.

Tissue Integrity and Pressure Redistribution

Individuals who remain in bed for prolonged periods of time or who use a wheelchair and have limited ability to reposition themselves are at risk for development of pressure ulcers. In particular, individuals with SCI are at a high risk because they lack sensation and have limited movement below the level of the lesion. Persons with multiple sclerosis, cancer, or muscular dystrophy; elderly adults; and others who have limited mobility and therefore a reduced ability to relieve pressure from weight-bearing surfaces also benefit from technologies in this category.

The primary population served by the category of seating interventions for **pressure redistribution** is individuals with SCI. These individuals can have partial or complete paralysis and reduced or absent sensation below the level of their lesions. As a result, they are susceptible to breakdown of the tissue over bony prominences on weight-bearing surfaces. It is estimated that approximately one third of individuals with SCI will encounter some type of tissue breakdown during their lifetimes (Krause et al., 2001) and that approximately 25% of the health care costs associated with the consequences of a SCI are related to pressure ulcers (Krause et al., 2001).

The incidence of pressure ulcers varies across settings. Woodbury and Houghton (2004) found the following incidence rates in Canadian settings: acute care hospital, 25.1%; nonacute facilities such as rehabilitation centers and long-term care, 29.9%; mixed health care (acute and nonacute), 22.1%; and community, 15.1%. It is estimated that the cost of treating a single pressure ulcer ranges from US$50,000 to $500,000, depending on severity.

Chen et al. (2005) examined pressure ulcer prevalence in persons with SCI who were followed up through the National Spinal Cord Injury Database over the past two decades. Their sample included 3361 community-dwelling individuals with SCI who were followed up by nine centers participating in the Model Spinal Cord Injury Systems project. These nine centers were chosen because they collected continuous data throughout the duration of the study. The authors explored the relationship of risk factors and prevalence of pressure ulcer over time after the injury. Thirty-three percent of the patients had a pressure ulcer on entry to the study. The risk of pressure ulcer was relatively stable in the first 10 years after the injury. Older subjects (50 years and older) were more likely to have pressure ulcers. Other significant risk factors included male sex, African American race, single marital status, education less than high school, and presence of other comorbid medical conditions (Chen et al., 2005).

It is estimated that approximately one third of individuals with SCI will encounter some type of tissue breakdown during their lifetimes (Krause et al., 2001) and that approximately 25% of the health care costs associated with the consequences of a SCI are related to pressure ulcers (Krause et al., 2001). Other populations with a high incidence of pressure ulcers include individuals with hemiplegia caused by stroke, multiple sclerosis, cancer, elderly adults, and individuals who have had a femoral fracture.

In addition to the costs for medical care, there are social costs that have a greater effect on individuals and their families. These social costs include (1) time lost from work and school, which affects the person and his or her family; (2) time lost from other meaningful activities; (3) time away from family, which can affect the person's social development; and (4) loss of personal independence and productivity, which results in mental health issues (Allman, 1997; Cutajar & Roberts, 2005; Dorsett & Geraghty, 2004).

Mechanics of Pressure Ulcer Development

By definition, the development of a pressure ulcer occurs in the presence of pressure, considering both the magnitude and duration of its application. External compression forces applied in a perpendicular direction to a localized area are considered to be the primary cause of ulcers with a superficial origin. A pressure ulcer can develop with high magnitude over a short duration or low magnitude over long duration. Several studies using animal models have demonstrated the relationship among pressure magnitude, duration, and pressure ulcer development (Gefen, 2009; Kosiak, 1961; Linder-Ganz & Gefen, 2004; Reswick & Rogers, 1976; see also Sprigle & Sonnenblum, 2011, for a review). Gefen (2009) conducted a review of the evidence on the amount of time required for a pressure ulcer to form from clinical,

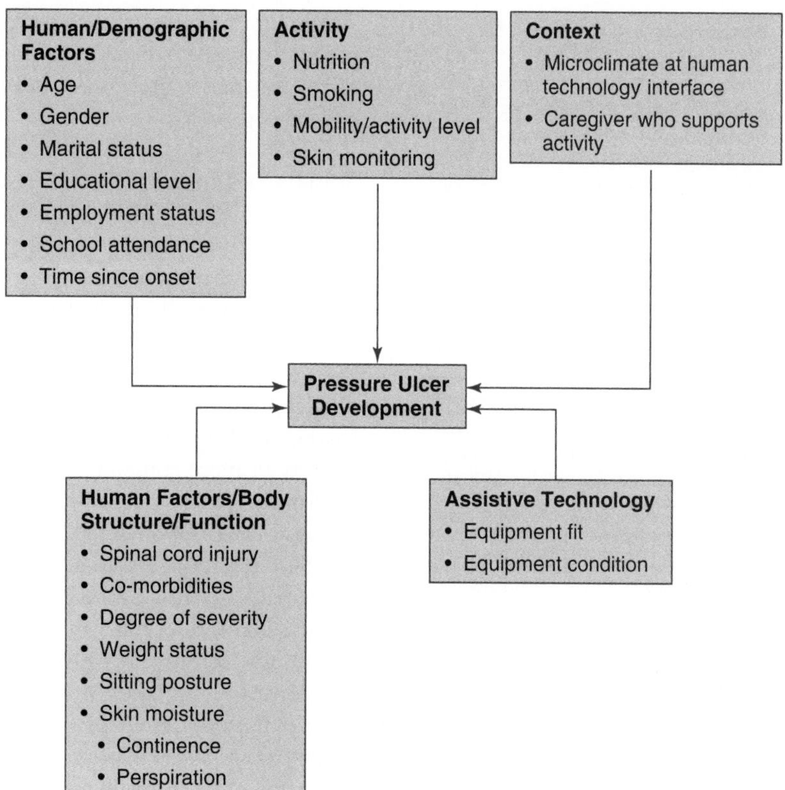

FIGURE 9-1 Pressure ulcer risk factors.

animal, and engineering models. He concluded that under sustained high pressure, deep tissue changes that might ultimately lead to a pressure ulcer were detected in the first hour after application of a load. Load on the tissue was higher in sitting than in lying, although the time to development of a pressure ulcer was not studied in the sitting position.

Movement introduces two additional forces that are implicated in the development of pressure ulcers, shear and friction. Friction is the force between two surfaces at risk or in motion. It leads to injury and ulceration of the surface of the skin. A typical friction injury to the skin occurs when the client moves across a rough surface such as bedding. Moisture, heat, and properties of materials (e.g., clothing or the wheelchair cushion material) can increase frictional forces.

Shear forces occur when a perpendicular force is paired with movement with the result that the superficial structures (e.g., skin in contact with the wheelchair seat cushion) do not move relative to each other, but the deep structures (e.g., muscle and blood vessels near the bone) do move. These deep structures are compressed and deformed, resulting in damage and the formation of a deep tissue injury that may progress upward to the surface (Linder-Ganz & Gefen, 2009). Because the origin of the pressure ulcer is deep, it might not be detected through recommended skin management regimens until the damage is significant.

A final mechanism to consider is a tissue reperfusion injury. With application of external pressure, the normal flow of blood and oxygen to tissue in that area is reduced. Typically, after the external pressure is removed, circulation to the area is restored, resulting in reperfusion of the tissues (i.e., oxygen is restored). However, if this situation is sustained and reperfusion is limited, changes occur in the tissue cells that eventually lead to cell death.

To summarize, pressure ulcer formation results from application of an external force on the body. Both the magnitude and duration of force application influence the development. Two additional forces (shear and friction) are contributing factors. Finally, recent research indicates that pressure ulcers can start at the surface, where they are detected as reddened or warm areas, or as skin abrasion, or at deep structures, where they are much more difficult to detect until the injury is advanced.

Contributing Factors

The Canadian Best Practice Guidelines for the Prevention and Management of Pressure Ulcers in People with Spinal Cord Injury (Houghton, Campbell and Best Practice Guidelines Panel, 2013) identifies several factors that are associated with the formation of pressure ulcers, classifies these factors into protective, risk, and potential categories, with evidence to support these classifications. Figure 9-1 shows these factors, classified according to the elements of the Human Activity Assistive Technology (HAAT) model. Key resources for best practice guidelines for management of pressure ulcers are listed in Box 9-1.

Protective Factors

Several factors were identified as protective factors against the development of pressure ulcers. These included being

BOX 9-1 Resources for Best Practice Guidelines for Pressure Ulcer Management

Houghton P, Campbell, K, Canadian Practice Guidelines Panel: Canadian Best Practice Guidelines for the prevention and management of pressure ulcers in people with spinal cord injury. A resource for clinicians, 2013. Available from http://www.onf.org.

Registered Nurses Association of Ontario: Risk assessment and prevention of pressure ulcers, Toronto: Registered Nurses Association of Ontario, 2005, 2011 supplement. Available from www.rnao.ca/bpg/guidelines/risk-assessment-and-pressure-ulcers.

National Pressure Ulcer Advisory Panel. International Pressure Ulcer Guidelines (available for purchase).

European Pressure Ulcer Advisory Panel and National Pressure Ulcer Advisory Panel. (2009). Pressure ulcer prevention: A quick reference guide. Washington DC: National Pressure Ulcer Advisory Panel. Available from www.epuap.org/guidelines/Final_Quick_Prevention.pdf. Accessed January 12, 2014.

Consortium for Spinal Cord Medicine: Clinical practice guidelines: Pressure ulcer prevention and treatment following spinal cord injury: a clinical practice guideline for health-care professionals, J Spinal Cord Med, 24(suppl 1):S40-S101, 2001.

Consortium for Spinal Cord Medicine: Pressure Ulcers: What you should know: A guide for people with spinal cord injury, 2007. Available from www.scicpg.org/cpg_cons_pdf/PUC.pdf.

married, being female, having a higher level of education, employment, or going to school (Houghton et al., 2013; Krause, 2001). Health promotion behaviors have the potential to be protective, but current evidence is not strong enough to classify them as such. These behaviors include maintaining a healthy lifestyle, eating a proper diet, maintaining a sufficient activity level and specific to a person with a disability, and maintaining an effective skin care and inspection regimen (Houghton et al., 2013).

Other Factors That Contribute to Pressure Ulcer Development

Mobility and Activity Level

Two aspects contribute to risk of pressure ulcer formation related to physical activity or mobility, the ability to move in order to relieve or redistribute pressure, and the amount of physical activity in which the individual engages. Moving to relieve pressure over an area is how the body typically responds to prevent tissue damage. Normally, when there is a lack of oxygen and chemical irritation, pain signals from the nerve endings trigger postural changes, and there is little tissue damage. However, when a person does not sense pain or discomfort or has limited or no mobility, she is unable to respond to these signals, which can result in remaining in a position for a long time and ultimately the development of a pressure ulcer.

Individuals who lack normal sensation, such as those who have sustained a SCI or who have spina bifida, are unable to recognize and respond to these pain signals and are particularly susceptible to the development of pressure ulcers (Chen et al., 2005). Individuals with movement limitations because of pain, muscle denervation, or neurologic impairment affecting coordination are also at risk. Mobility may also be limited by the client's personal preferences; for example, a client may wish to remain in his wheelchair for much of the day and refuse to be transferred to another support surface (e.g., bed).

Spinal Cord Injury

Individuals with SCI are at great risk for development of pressure ulcers for many reasons, including impairments of sensation and movement, changes in skin and muscle tissue that occur over a long duration, urinary and fecal incontinence, IT flattening, autonomic dysreflexia, and problems with temperature regulation resulting in greater sweating. The length of time since the initial injury, the level of injury (higher level injury results in greater risk), and the degree of severity (a more complete injury results in greater risk) are all risk factors for development of pressure ulcer (Houghton et al., 2013; Wolfe et al., 2010) The length of time since the SCI results in tissue alterations (e.g., loss of collagen, abnormal vascularity, tone changes). A related change that is particularly important to seating is the flattening of the ischial tuberosities (ITs). Over time, the loss of muscle fiber and cortical bone, coupled with pressure on the ITs, causes them to flatten (Linder-Ganz & Gefen, 2009). The resulting shape change alters the force, which then contributes to the formation of deep tissue injury. Individuals with higher level injuries and greater severity have greater sensory and mobility impairments that limit both their ability to detect pain and discomfort and to move to relieve pressure. Completion of regular skin inspection and the ability to do so are potential protection factors.

Weight Status

The body type of the individual has some effect on pressure distribution. A thin person has less subcutaneous fat to act as padding, and therefore forces per unit area of the skin are increased. An overweight individual has more padding over which to distribute pressure. However, it may be more difficult for an overweight individual to perform pressure relief exercises. Caregivers may also have more difficulty moving an overweight individual, which may make shearing and friction forces a greater possibility.

Nutrition

Inadequate nutrition is often associated with weight loss and muscular atrophy, both of which reduce the amount of tissue between the seat surface and the bony prominences. Inadequate dietary intake, which results in anemia, decreased protein levels, and vitamin C deficiency, can result in greater susceptibility to pressure ulcer formation and delayed healing of an existing ulcer (Consortium for Spinal Cord Medicine Clinical Practice Guidelines, 2001; Houghton et al., 2013). Research on the role of adequate nutrition for the prevention and treatment of pressure ulcers in older adults supports the inclusion of evaluation of nutritional status and the use of an adequate diet for individuals at risk (Houghton et al., 2013; Registered Nurses Association of Ontario, 2005/2011).

Comorbidities

Several comorbidities are risk factors for four reasons: they affect mobility, result in impaired sensation, result in impaired circulation, and affect proper nutrition. The Canadian Guidelines found sufficient evidence to identify heart, kidney, and lung diseases; urinary tract infection; deep vein thrombosis; pneumonia; and leg fracture as risk factors (Houghton et al., 2013). Diabetes and low albumin levels were considered potential risk factors because of insufficient evidence that supported their contribution to the development of pressure ulcers. Smoking, which leads to poor health conditions over time, impairs circulation, which then limits the tissue's reperfusion response when pressure is released (Consortium for Spinal Cord Medicine, 2001).

Age

As people age, the skin loses some of its elasticity and muscles atrophy, which increases vulnerability to friction or shearing. Movement during everyday activities may be sufficient to cause skin tears that, coupled with lack of mobility and other risk factors, can lead to a pressure ulcer. Loss of muscle tissue means less padding between the bone and support surface. Many of the other risk factors (e.g., lower mobility, poor nutrition, and concurrent medical conditions) are more prevalent in older adults (Consortium for Spinal Cord Medicine, 2001).

Sitting Posture

Posture and deformity can affect the pressure distribution of the seat–buttock interface and can potentially contribute to skin breakdown. Two specific postures that pose a risk for pressure ulcer formation are pelvic obliquity and sacral sitting. Pelvic obliquity, which will be discussed in detail in a subsequent section, results in increased pressure and shear under the affected lower IT and the posterior aspect of the lower greater trochanter (Hobson, 1989; Zacharkow, 1984, 1988). The loss of lumbar lordosis when sitting is another risk factor. This position occurs as a result of limited hip mobility for flexion or decreased spinal mobility for extension (Zacharkow, 1984). Consequently, a sacral sitting posture is typically assumed, which results in significant amounts of pressure being placed on the sacrococcygeal region. The Consortium for Spinal Cord Medicine identified equipment that did not fit properly or that did not properly support the user as a contributing factor (Consortium for Spinal Cord Medicine, 2001).

Microclimate

Moisture and temperature at the interface between the person and the wheelchair cushion affect pressure ulcer formation. Moist skin is more susceptible to the development of pressure ulcers than dry skin because the moisture increases friction between the skin and support surfaces. Skin moisture results from the microclimate between the body and the seating surface as well as urinary and fecal continence that are associated with a primary condition. Urinary tract infections may also contribute to pressure ulcer formation, although the Canadian Best Practice for the Prevention and Management of Pressure Ulcers in People with Spinal Cord Injury Guidelines (Houghton et al., 2013) concluded there was insufficient evidence to categorize them as a risk factor. A warm, damp environment increases the potential for bacterial growth and infection.

Comfort

The third category of seating addresses the need to improve an individual's level of physical comfort through postural accommodation. Persons in this category may or may not use a wheelchair on a regular basis and typically have normal or near-normal sensation; however, any prolonged sitting causes discomfort from which they are unable to obtain relief. Therefore, they have unique needs and are not completely served by either category described earlier. There are four distinct populations who can benefit from seating technologies for comfort: (1) wheelchair users who have sitting discomfort and pain (e.g., individuals with postpolio syndrome, amyotrophic lateral sclerosis, amputation, or multiple sclerosis), (2) older adults with limited mobility (e.g., resulting from frailty or conditions such as osteoarthritis or rheumatoid arthritis, (3) individuals whose mobility is restricted because of morbid obesity, and (4) individuals with restricted mobility because of cardiac or respiratory conditions. For individuals in any one of these populations, discomfort in seating can lead to a decreased ability to participate in ADLs. In cases of severe discomfort, the individual may be restricted to bed rest for some or all of the day, which further reduces the individual's ability to function and can lead to medical problems as well.

CONTEXT

Physical Context

Ambient temperature affects the performance of seating products that are made with a gel component. This semi-fluid material becomes less viscous at higher temperatures, which reduces the amount of cushioning this part of the seat is intended to provide. This material will also freeze if it is left in an unheated environment (e.g., vehicle or garage) in locations where the temperature is below the freezing point.

Exposure to sunlight degrades foam, which is one reason why all cushions have some form of cover. However, there are situations when a custom-built seat cushion or back is left uncovered before final fitting that ensures the proper fit. In these situations, the foam is exposed and should be protected from sunlight. Light exposure can also affect the material used to cover the cushion, affecting its properties and thus altering the function of the cushion.

Moisture is a third physical factor that affects cushion function. The microclimate at the interface between the individual and the cushion was discussed in the previous section on pressure ulcers. A cushion will be exposed to moisture when used outdoors in the rain or may have liquids spilled on it in certain situations. Foam in particular degrades when it gets wet. Bacteria can also grow in a wet foam cushion.

Social Context

The consumer may be assisted by many people during the day, including family, caregivers, and school personnel. The social context influences the instructions given to the users of the system and considerations with respect to the weight, complexity, and maintenance of the system (e.g., cleaning and ensuring proper inflation of air-filled cushions or even distribution of gel inserts). Misuse or inadequate maintenance of the system will reduce its effectiveness in meeting the client's needs. The user and the caregivers need to be familiar with proper use and care of the seating system. Adequate instruction, reinforced over time, is key to preventing misuse of the system.

Individuals who routinely lift and carry a seating system must be able to do so with good body mechanics to decrease the risk of injury. Materials used to construct seating systems have changed in recent years, in part to decrease the weight. However, some custom-made systems (e.g., foam in place, which is discussed later) can be quite heavy. Maintenance of the system is another consideration. Air-filled cushions require careful attention to ensure that they are properly inflated and free of punctures. As mentioned earlier, the properties of some materials are affected by extremes of temperatures, so whoever is responsible for maintenance of the system must take care to avoid damage to it by not leaving it in a location where it would be exposed to temperature extremes (e.g., in a car on a hot summer day or cold winter night). An individual maintaining a system should also take care not to use harsh or abrasive chemicals when cleaning the device because they can also cause damage. In some situations, the system that is most ideal for the client cannot be recommended because of the inability of the caregiver to use and care for it.

Institutional Context

Funding implications are a key institutional consideration. General considerations with respect to funding are described in Chapter 5. The clinician usually has the responsibility to provide the necessary documentation to justify and secure funding for seating devices. Consequently, it is important to remain current on funding requirements when recommending seating products. The process for obtaining funding, including who bears the responsibility for each aspect of the process and eligibility requirements of the user and device, are the main aspects of funding that require the clinician's attention.

Another type of legislation that has unique implications for seating products is the use of restraints. The Centers for Medicare and Medicaid Services (CMS) defines a **restraint** as "any manual method or physical or mechanical device, material or equipment attached or adjacent to the resident's body that the individual cannot remove easily which restricts freedom of movement or normal access to one's body." (Centers for Medicare and Medicaid Services), Certain legal jurisdictions have legislation that regulates the use of restraints with individuals residing in institutional settings. The intent of this legislation is to limit inappropriate use of restraints, such as tying an individual into a chair simply to prevent him or her from moving around when safety is not an issue. This legislation has implications for the use of straps, pelvic belts, and sub-ASIS (anterior-superior iliac spine) bars that are used in seating systems for positioning and safety reasons. The legislation typically regulates how restraints are used in institutional settings, requiring most institutions to have a plan and a documented process when restraints are used. The clinician should know if this legislation exists in her jurisdiction and the influence of this type of legislation on the recommendation of positioning belts and other equipment or setup that is considered to be a restraint.

ASSISTIVE TECHNOLOGIES FOR SEATING AND POSITIONING

Biomechanical Principles

The principles of biomechanics, the study of body position and movement, are fundamental to an understanding of the use of seating, positioning, and mobility systems for persons with disabilities. This section discusses some of the key concepts and then presents the principles of seating for each application of these technologies.

Kinematics: Study of Motion

The mobility and position of the consumer, the configuration of the seating system components, and the interaction of the person and the system affect the outcome of this intervention. **Kinematics** describe movement. **Displacement** defines the position of a body in space; a change in displacement results in a new position. For example, assisting the client to maintain a midline position of the body is a goal of seating for postural control. Achieving this goal may require *displacement* from the rest position to midline by application of an external lateral trunk support. The rate of change in displacement is called *velocity*. The speed of change of the velocity (increasing or decreasing) is called **acceleration.** One of the most common accelerations is that of gravity. The term **gravity** actually refers to the acceleration of an object toward the center of the earth. Acceleration of an object is directly related to the force generated by the object's movement.

There are two fundamental types of displacement, linear and rotational. When all parts of a body move in the same direction at the same time and for the same distance, the movement is **linear** (Low & Reed, 1996). For example, a person generates translational movement when walking. Displacements caused by external positioning components can also be translational. If the direction, distance, and time of the movement occur simultaneously but the movement is through an angle instead of in a straight line, the movement is called **rotational.** Rotational movements occur around an axis called the fulcrum. The majority of body movements are rotational, such as hip or elbow flexion and shoulder flexion or extension. Some positioning components cause rotational displacements (e.g., reclining the back of a wheelchair causes rotation at the pelvis and hip).

Kinetics: Forces

Force is a major element in biomechanics and seating for individuals with disabilities. **Force** is anything that acts on a body to *change* its rate of acceleration or alter its momentum (Low & Reed, 1996). It is described by both magnitude and direction (Sprigle, 2000). Forces can be applied to the body internally or externally. Internal forces are generated inside the body, such as muscle contractions that cause movement of the joints. Externally applied forces come from outside the body and act on it in some way, such as the forces applied by a support surface and components of a seating system such as lateral supports. The force resulting from the acceleration of gravity is another external and ever-present force that acts on the body and influences its posture and movement (Sprigle, 2000). This force on the body acts along a line called the **gravitational line,** and its effect is localized around a point in the body called the **center of gravity.** The force of the earth's gravitational field tends to pull the body toward the center of the earth and must be accounted for in designing a seating system. The center of gravity changes as posture changes from standing to sitting and in different sitting positions.

Four properties of force, which ultimately determine its result, are magnitude, direction, line of application, and point of application. **Magnitude** is the amount or size of the force measured in newtons, pounds, or kilograms. Forces are applied in some *direction,* either pushing or pulling, and are applied along a particular line of application. The force acts at a particular point on the body, called the *point of application* (Low & Reed, 1996).

Types of Forces

There are three different types of force. Each of these types produces different effects on the body, and it is important to understand these differences when designing seating and positioning systems. **Tension** forces act in the same line but away from each other (pulling apart), such as the force applied on the antagonist muscle during contraction of the agonist muscle. **Compression** occurs when forces act toward each other (pushing together), such the force of the weight of the body of the cushion when the client sits on it. Shear and friction are related concepts that occur when the forces are parallel to each other (sliding across the surfaces) (National Pressure Ulcer Advisory Panel [NPUAP], 2007). **Friction** occurs when the superficial layer of tissue moves relative to the seating surface; for example, friction occurs when the client performs a sliding transfer. **Shear** occurs when the superficial layer is stationary relative to the support surface, but the deep structures move (NPUAP, 2007). For example, during a low-range movement to shift weight, the client's skin may not move, but the muscles and bones deep in the area do, which results in pressure and deformation of the deep soft tissue. Each of these types of forces can also be applied externally to the body, such as the force exerted by a seating surface on the ITs (compression), the force exerted by lateral supports to extend the trunk (tension), or the force exerted on the deep tissues in the buttocks when a seat back is reclined (shearing).

Stress

Stress is the resulting molecular change inside biologic (e.g., soft tissue and bone) or nonbiologic (e.g., metals, plastics, or foams) materials. Stress is caused by the same three types of forces—tension, compression, or shear—and can result in damage to the biologic tissue or other material if it is prolonged. For example, a shear force applied to a foam seat cushion can result in tearing of the foam. This is a change in the molecular structure of the foam caused by an externally applied force. Likewise, a piece of connective tissue that is subjected to severe or prolonged compression loading by sitting (e.g., under the ITs) may be damaged by crushing of the tissue. This externally applied force results in compression inside the tissue, causing a change in the structure of the biologic material.

Pressure

Every force is applied over a surface area. For example, with a postural support system, the force of each component is applied to an area of the body. **Pressure** is defined as force per unit area, which means that a force applied over a very small area generates more pressure than the same force applied over a larger area (NPUAP, 2007). Imagine a 10-lb cat lying on a surface such as your stomach. The force generated by the cat is applied over the entire surface of its body, and the pressure is uniform. Now imagine the same cat standing on your stomach. The force of the cat is the same, but the pressure at each of the cat's paws is much greater (and it hurts more) because the areas of application (the paws) are much smaller than when the force is distributed over the whole surface area of the cat. This basic concept of distributing pressure by increasing the area of application is applied extensively in seating and positioning systems.

Newton's Laws of Motion

The English scientist Sir Isaac Newton formulated three laws relating to forces on bodies at rest and in motion. Newton's third law is the one most applicable to seating and positioning systems. This law states that if one body exerts a force on another, there is an equal and opposite force, called a reaction, exerted on the first body by the second (Low & Reed, 1996). This law is applied to seating systems with the assumption that every force exerted by the human body while sitting in a wheelchair or a seating system is balanced by an opposite force exerted by the sitting surface on the person (Sprigle, 2000). The force generated by the body is equal in magnitude and opposite in direction to the force generated by the seating system, which is often referred to as **equilibrium.** When a body is at rest and all internal and external forces are balanced, the body is in a state of static equilibrium. When forces are balanced around a body during movement, resulting in a constant velocity, it is described as dynamic equilibrium. Both types of equilibrium are important in seating and positioning systems.

Friction

Throughout this discussion, it has been assumed that ideal circumstances exist. For example, a shear force applied to a body causes it to move across a surface, and ideally it encounters no resistance to movement from that surface. In reality, of course, this is not true because frictional forces exist between two bodies in contact moving in opposite directions (Sprigle, 2000). Two types of friction are defined, static friction and dynamic friction. *Static friction* is the force that must be overcome to start a body in motion. Static friction is proportional in magnitude to the perpendicular (compression) force holding the two bodies together. Static friction is independent of the area of contact between the two bodies. When motion is initiated, the resistive force is generally smaller, and it takes less force to keep the bodies moving relative to each other than to start movement. Friction during movement is called *dynamic friction.* Both of these frictional forces are affected by surface conditions such as moisture, heat, texture, and lubricants, and both are important considerations in the recommendation and design of seating surfaces.

Sitting Posture and Center of Pressure

Stability and mobility are two related dimensions of seated postural control. Stability allows an individual to maintain an upright seated position, and **mobility** allows movement that enables function; for example, mobility allows the individual to lean forward to reach to shake a friend's hand. Seating interventions for postural control must achieve an optimal balance between stability and mobility.

Two constructs are important to consider when discussing postural control, center of gravity, and center of pressure. The location of the center of gravity is fairly well defined in standing. Its location is described as passing through the mastoid processes of the jaw, a point just in front of the shoulder, a point just behind the center of the hip joints, a point just in front of the center of the knee joints, and approximately 5 to 6 cm in front of the ankle joints (Figure 9-2). In this posture, the pelvis is in a neutral position, and there is a natural lordosis of the lumbar spine (Zacharkow, 1988). The location in sitting is more difficult to determine, but it is usually considered to be lower, with the buttocks and thighs forming the base of support. The individual must maintain the center of gravity over the base of support to maintain an upright posture in either sitting or standing. Seating interventions for postural control assist the client to keep the center of posture within the limits of the base of support.

It is not practical to measure or monitor the center of gravity in the clinic because it is defined by three-dimensional coordinates (anterior-posterior, lateral, and vertical). The **center of pressure** is described only in the horizontal plane, which makes it a much more clinically useful outcome. Its location in the frontal and lateral planes can be identified and monitored in the clinic by using a pressure mapping system.

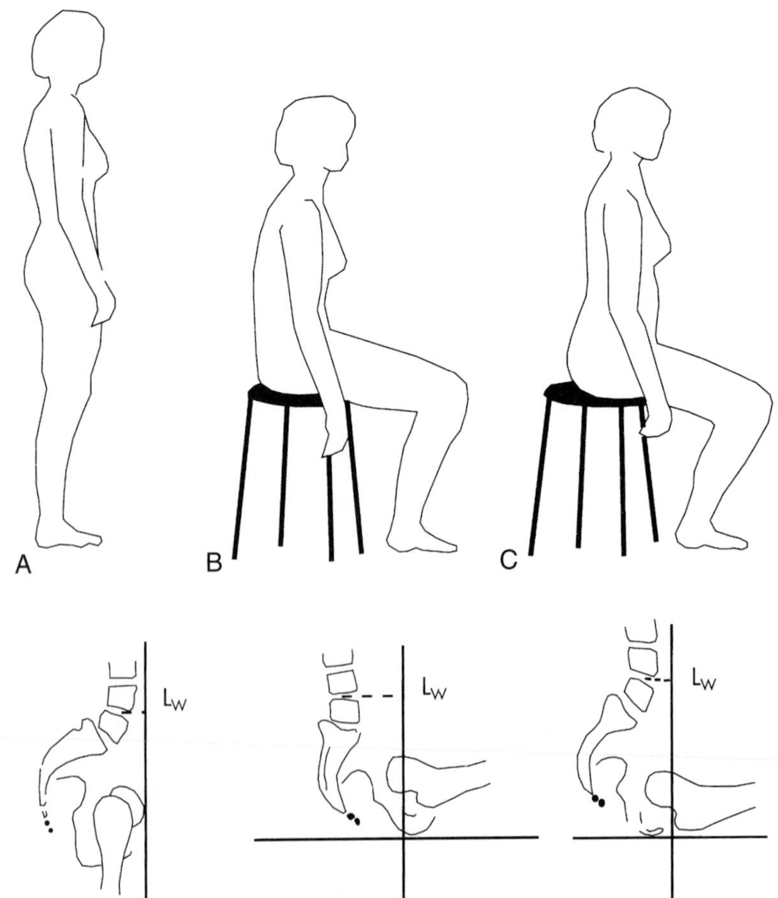

FIGURE 9-2 Center of mass in sitting. **A,** Line of gravity in erect upright standing. **B,** Relaxed unsupported sitting resulting in backward tilt of the pelvis and flattening of the lumbar lordosis. **C,** Erect sitting with reduction in backward pelvic tilt and increased lordosis. *LW,* Lever arm. (From Frankel VH, Nordin M: *Basic biomechanics of the skeletal system,* Philadelphia, 1980, Lea & Febiger.)

These systems use various technologies to monitor the pressure between the individual and a support surface (i.e., between the client's buttocks and thighs and the seat cushion). They are most commonly used to show pressure distribution when pressure-relief cushions are evaluated, so their function will be described in greater detail in that section.

The ideal location of the center of pressure is midway between the ITs. Dunk and Callaghan (2005) found that the location of the center of pressure in the frontal plane varied between men and women. They studied various sitting postural parameters of university students engaged in computer activities while sitting on different office chairs. They found that the center of pressure was behind the center of mass of the chair for men and ahead of it for women. This finding has interesting implications for seating intervention, although it has not been explored.

Parkinson et al. (2006) describe the **stability zone** or limit, which they define as the balance limits for a person either sitting or standing. A seat back and laterals or armrests will affect the stability limits in sitting. The authors initially hypothesized that the stability was limited laterally by the ITs and posteriorly by the coccyx in the absence of these system features. The thighs provide support when the individual is reaching forward. Age, strength, and range of motion were identified as additional factors that affected the stability zone. They quantified the center of pressure during a lateral reaching task with a sample that included both young and older individuals and subjects with a body mass index that ranged from underweight to obese. The greater trochanter, rather than the ITs, was found to be more indicative of the stability zone because subjects shifted their weight laterally as they reached. Stability during reach was also affected by age, reach direction (lateral and forward reach were greater than rearward), and hip breadth (Parkinson et al., 2006).

The center of pressure is an interesting phenomenon that has been explored recently, primarily in a nonclinical population. The studies described above suggest that differences exist in parameters related to center of pressure between men and women (Dunk & Callaghan, 2005), body mass, and age (Parkinson et al., 2006). These studies did not include individuals with disabilities, so the implications of the findings to this group are not clear. Further study is needed to explore the relationship between center of pressure and function and the effect of various seating interventions on this relationship.

SEATING TECHNOLOGIES

There is considerable overlap between the technologies used to address goals related to postural control, tissue integrity, and comfort. Furthermore, many clients require seating that addresses two or more of these goals. Box 9-2 shows some of the potential goals or outcomes of seating technology use. Seating technologies in general will be discussed, with identification of their specific application to these goals where appropriate. This section is divided into two components: the design and the construction of the seating system and the properties of the materials used to construct it. The evaluation process described in this chapter guides the selection of the most appropriate system. The client should be allowed a trial period of use of the system because comfort and functional issues will become evident with use of the system over time.

The NPUAP defines **support surfaces** as "a specialized device for pressure redistribution designed for management of tissue loads, micro-climate, and/or other therapeutic functions (i.e., any mattresses, integrated bed system, mattress replacement, overlay, or seat cushion, or seat cushion overlay)" (NPUAP, 2007, p. 1). Wheelchair cushions are discussed in this chapter.

Design and Construction of Seating Systems

The design of the seating system refers to the degree of contouring present in the seat and back and the degree of adjustability that is present in the components. These technologies range from systems that are relatively flat without any contouring that matches the shape of the body segments they support to custom-contoured systems that are constructed to match as closely as possible the body contours of the user. In most setting, prefabricated technologies are available so that the clinician no longer needs to construct the components in the seating system.

Planar

The simplest construction is a **planar** cushion. These technologies are flat surfaces that rely on the properties of the cushion material to conform to the body's shape. In general, they are appropriate for individuals who require minimal support or who do not use a seating system for long periods of time. Other positioning components can be added to this basic structure if additional support is required. Planar foam cushions, as shown in Figure 9-3, are designed from flat blocks of foam, which can involve a single layer of foam or more than one type of foam layered for a different form of support. Commonly, higher density foam is used on the bottom of the cushion for support with lower density foam placed on top to envelop the body. Air-filled cushions also have a planar construction.

Prefabricated planar components are made in standard sizes to fit a wide range of individuals. The backs are constructed with a plastic shell to which foam is attached. A solid seat pan on the wheelchair typically provides a base of

BOX 9-2 Potential Outcomes of Proper Seating and Positioning

Facilitation of optimal postural control to enable engagement in functional activities

Provision of an optimal balance between stability and mobility in the seated position

Maintenance of neutral skeletal alignment

Prevention of skeletal deformities; where fixed deformities exist, minimize their influence on body functions and performance of activities of daily living

Maintenance of tissue integrity and pressure redistribution

Maintenance of a position of comfort

Provide a comfortable, supportive position that reduces fatigue experienced by user while sitting

Enhance respiratory and circulatory function

Facilitate caregiver activities

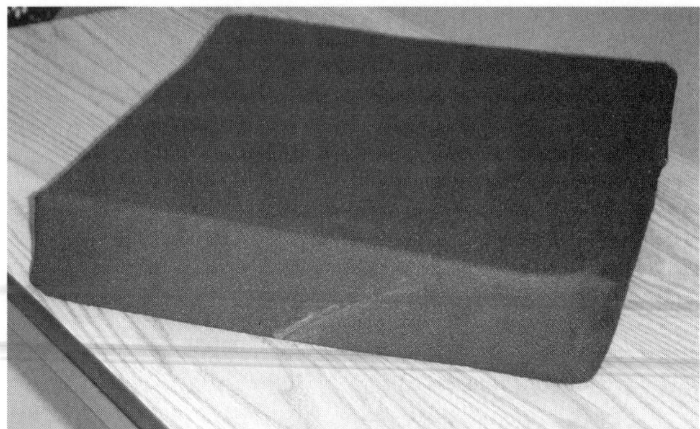

FIGURE 9-3 Planar cushion.

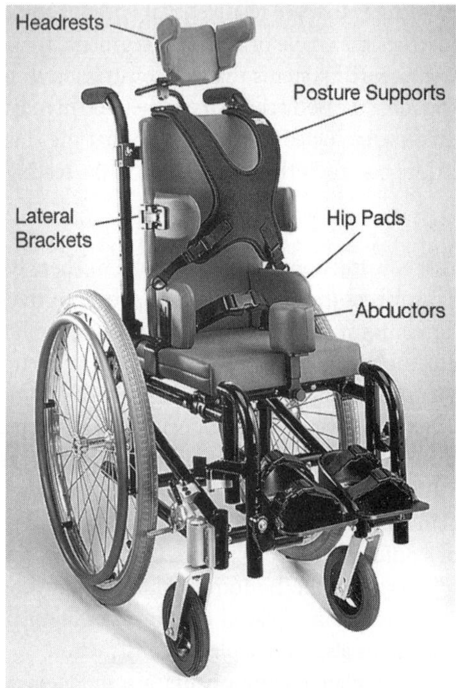

FIGURE 9-4 Planar seating system including lateral and pelvic support components. (Courtesy of Adaptive Engineering Lab, Inc, www.aelseating.com).

support for a seat cushion. Other positioning components are attached with hardware to the seat or back (Figure 9-4). The seat and back are attached to the wheelchair frame with interfacing hardware. Much of the hardware that interfaces the various components can be adjusted for angle, width, and depth to accommodate positioning needs and provide flexibility for growth or postural changes.

Custom-fabricated planar systems are made of similar materials and designs as prefabricated systems, but the dimensions of the seating system components are customized to fit the individual. These systems can be fabricated on site directly with the consumer, or specifications of the consumer's measurements can be sent to a manufacturer for fabrication. The density of the foam pieces can also be selected to accommodate the needs of the individual. Lateral supports, headrests, and other components are added to the basic foam and plywood (or plastic) structure. This approach is highly labor intensive and is being replaced at many sites as a result of the advent of a large array of off-the-shelf technologies.

Contour Cushions

Most seat cushions on the market at this time are contoured. These technologies are useful for individuals with moderate seating and positioning needs for postural management or who are at risk for pressure ulcer development. These technologies use curved surfaces that more closely match the shape of the human body. Commonly, a **contour** cushion has an anterior shelf to support the thighs. This shelf may be further contoured to help maintain femoral alignment. The back of the seat has a depressed pelvic loading area where the pelvis "sits" into the cushion. The front of the cushion is frequently beveled to provide more comfort behind the knees and allow increased knee flexion if needed. Greater support and control are gained by increasing the degree of contouring. The Matrix is one example of a standard contoured cushion (Figure 9-5).

Custom Contoured Cushions

The cushion that provides the greatest amount of body contact and therefore the most support is one that has been shaped, or custom contoured, to the individual's body. A

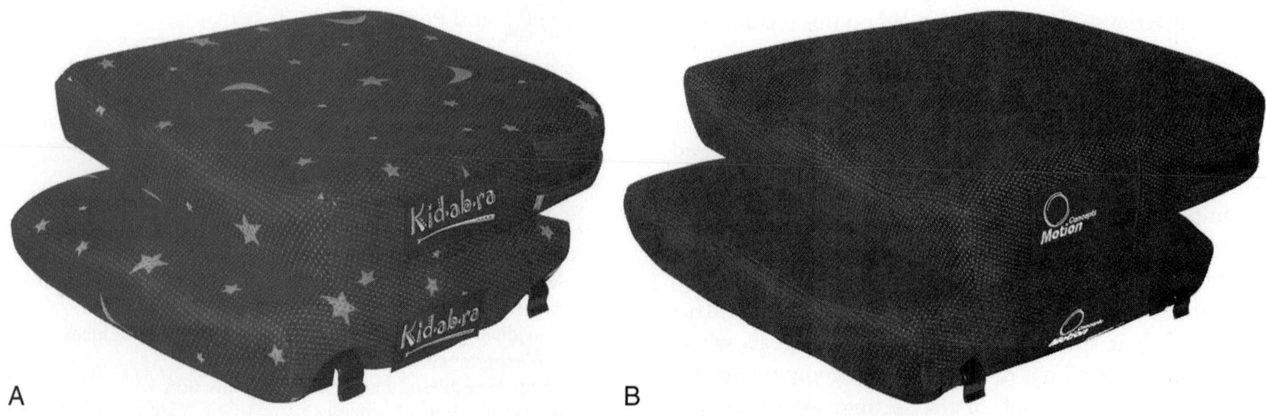

FIGURE 9-5 Matrix cushion. **A,** Child version. **B,** Adult version. (Courtesy of Invacare Corp, www.invacare.ca).

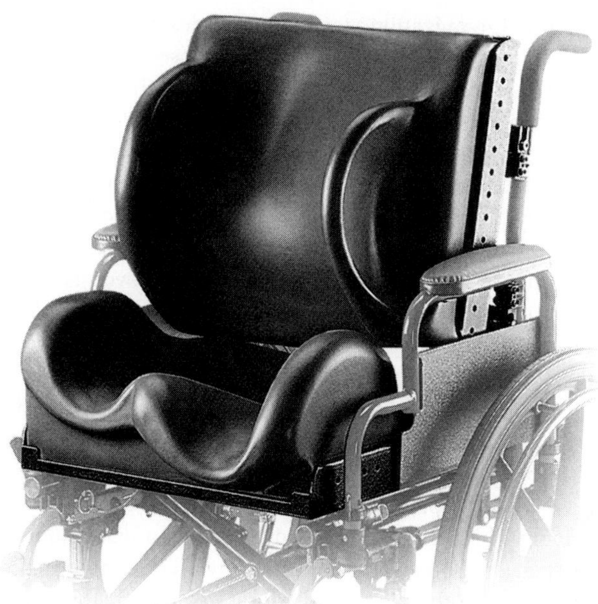

FIGURE 9-6 Custom-contoured seating system. (Courtesy of Invacare Corp, www.invacare.ca).

number of technologies are available to achieve a custom-contoured system. One example is shown in Figure 9-6. These types of systems differ primarily in terms of the fabrication techniques used and whether the fabrication is completed on site or in a central location. The disadvantages of custom-contoured support surfaces are that transfers to and from the system are more difficult; the system is static and has no dynamic properties, thus limiting the individual to one fixed position; and there is limited ability within the system to allow for growth of the individual. Box 9-3 describes the common custom contoured construction methods.

Prefabricated Backs

Prefabricated backs can be adjustable or not. These components usually have a hard shell to provide support with foam layered on top to maximize body contact with the support surface for positioning, pressure redistribution, and comfort. Typically, this seating component is attached between the upright canes of the wheelchair, with quick release hardware for easy removal if the seating and mobility system must be transported. Figure 9-7 shows an example of a prefabricated back that is not adjustable. Adjustable prefabricated backs provide a large degree of adjustability that can be accomplished in the clinical setting. Figure 9-8 is an example of an adjustable back. The clinician can make adjustments on the basis of an optimal seated position determined by a mat assessment. These backs allow the clinician to adjust the height, depth, and width, back angle, and placement of the laterals. Some of these systems allow the clinician to create a biplanar back in which the upper and lower segments of the back are set at different angles. This configuration is often used to provide specific postural control. Although the pivot point can be placed at any spinal level, when placed at the level of the posterior superior iliac spine, it can assist with control of the pelvis. Studies have investigated the effect of pelvic stability on function (Miller Polgar et al., 2000; Rigby et al., 2001), but no clinical studies have evaluated the effect of this particular back configuration on postural control and subsequently function.

BOX 9-3 Examples of Custom-Contoured Construction Technologies

Foam in place

- The client sits in position of comfort and function in frame with flexible covering.
- Covering is shaped to conform to the client's body contours.
- Foam is added, which expands to match the client's shape.
- The client is transferred from the frame.
- Foam hardens over several hours.
- After the foam has hardened, further contouring is done by hand.
- When a satisfactory fit is achieved, the foam is covered, attached to a firm base, and mounted on the client's wheelchair.
- This type of contour cushion can be made on site.

Vacuum Consolidation

- The client sits in a position of comfort and function on a latex bag filled with beads, which is placed either on his or her wheelchair or a fitting chair.
- The bag is then contoured to match the shape of the client.
- A vacuum is used to draw air out of the bag, consolidating the beads.
- The cushion is then made by making a negative and then positive mold.
- This type of cushion is either made on site or sent to a commercial manufacturer.

Seating Simulators

- The client sits in a position of comfort and function in a simulator chair.
- The simulator chair can be adjusted in many ways (e.g., seat depth, width, seat-to-back angle).
- The simulator chair maps the contours of the client's body, and the mapping is transferred to a data sheet.
- A molding bag is then used to capture the optimal shape of the cushion.
- This shape is then captured and then transmitted to a company that makes the system.
- The Shape Sensor system by Invacare (www.invacare.com) is an example of this technology.

Computer-Aided Design

- Digitizing technology is used to capture the client's body shape and measurements.
- These data are transformed to create a virtual image.
- This virtual image is then used to guide the seating system construction.
- Precision carving (computer guided) is one method of fabrication.
- Vacuum forming is another fabrication method used.
- The Ottobock Shape System is an example of this technology (www.ottobock.com).

Properties of Materials Used to Construct Seating Systems

An understanding of the properties of the materials used in seating technologies will assist in the selection of appropriate cushions. Key material properties include density, stiffness

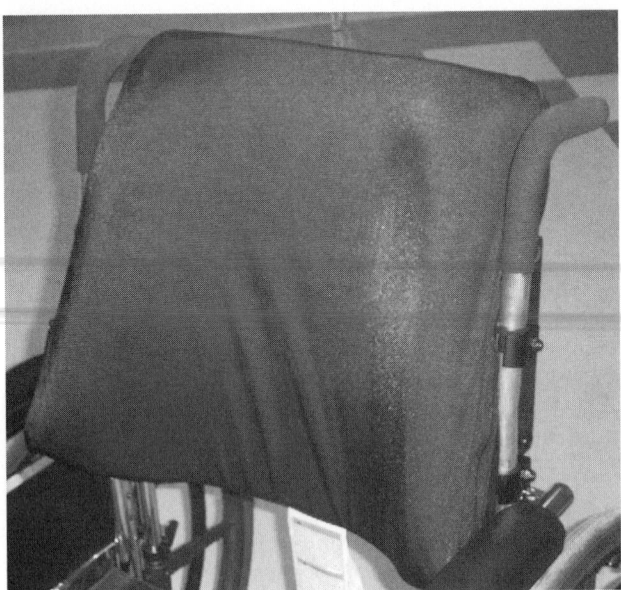

FIGURE 9-7 Commercial back.

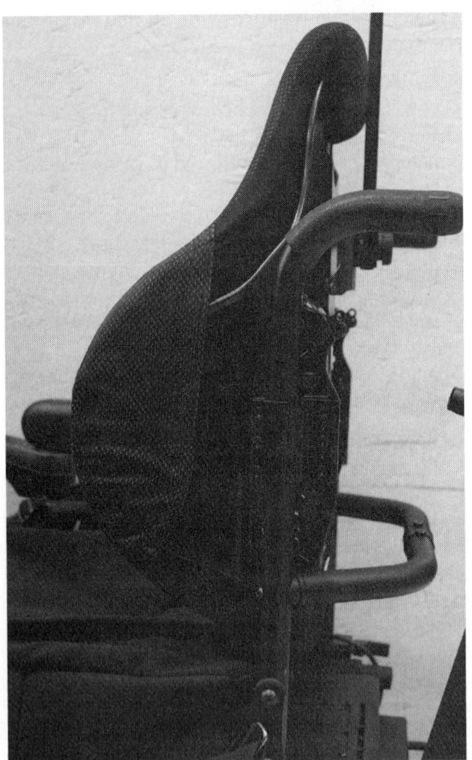

FIGURE 9-8 Prefabricated adjustable back.

or immersion, envelopment, resilience, and dampening (Brienza & Geyer, 2000, NPUAP, 2007; Sprigle, 2000).

The **density** of a material is the ratio of its weight to its volume. A greater density generally means a more durable material but not always. Low-density materials will fatigue faster than high-density ones under the same loading conditions. The **stiffness** or immersion of a material describes how much it gives under load. In a cushion, this is the distance that the person sinks into the cushion. Soft materials may bottom out, but failure to compress can also lead to an increase in seating pressures and tissue breakdown. The International Standards Organization standards also describe lateral and forward stiffness that describes the response of the cushion to a lateral force. It is easier to slide on a cushion with low stiffness, but the shearing forces are higher, resulting in a cushion with less stability. **Sliding resistance** is a cushion property related to friction. A cushion with high resistance limits how much the user slides, helping to support upright posture, but consequently makes transfers more difficult.

Resilience is the ability of a material to recover its shape after a load is removed or to adjust to a load as it is applied. Short-term resilience is the immediate recovery when a load is altered, such as when someone shifts weight on a seat cushion. Long-term resilience is the overnight recovery of a cushion that has been loaded and then unloaded. **Dampening** is the ability of the cushion to soften on impact; it is best observed by dropping a relatively heavy object on the material. If the object sinks into the material, then dampening is occurring. If it bounces off or if the material does not react to the object, then the material is poorly dampened. This is the "shock absorber" feature of cushion materials and is important in minimizing the transmission of forces from the ground to individuals as they travel over rough surfaces or obstacles. **Envelopment** is the degree to which the person sinks into the cushion and the degree to which the cushion surrounds the buttocks. Good envelopment promotes stability and helps reduce peak pressures. **Recovery** refers to the degree to which a cushion returns to its preloaded state when a load is removed.

Classification of Support Surface Technologies

The NPUAP defines four categories of support surfaces that are important to this discussion: reactive and active support surfaces, powered and nonpowered (NPUAP, 2007). A reactive support surface, which may be powered or nonpowered, responds only when a load is introduced (e.g., a foam cushion retains its shape until the user sits on it, at which time it conforms to the user's shape). In contrast, the load distribution characteristics of an active support surface change in the presence or absence of a load. A nonpowered support surface does not require any external energy source, but a powered support surface does (NPUAP, 2007).

Sprigle et al. (2001), Brienza and Geyer (2000), and the NPUAP (2007) describe uniform terminology for classification of the material used to construct wheelchair cushions. They described the following categories of cushions: (1) made from cellular materials, (2) containing fluid (Sprigle et al.) or cell or bladder construction (NPUAP), and (3) other constructions (e.g., elastomer, gel [NPUAP]). Table 9-1 summarizes these types of materials and their characteristics.

Cushion Covers

Selection of a cover for a seat or back cushion can be as important as the determination of the material used to make the cushion because an improper cover can negate some of the benefits of that material (Tang, 1991). The cover selected should conform integrally to the cushion's contours, particularly in nonplanar systems. It should not interfere with the envelopment properties of the cushion nor add to shearing

TABLE 9-1 Classification of Cushion Technologies

Description	Advantages	Disadvantages
	Cushions Made from Cellular Technologies	
Foam		
Most common material used to make seat back cushions Come in variety of thicknesses and densities Open cell foams have interconnected, perforated cells that allow airflow (e.g., polyurethane and latex) Closed cell foams are composed of individual cells encased in a membrane (e.g., Ethafoam)	Inexpensive Lightweight Compress with weight so have good envelopment Open cell foams allow better ventilation Less dense than closed cell foams, so they weigh less Lightweight Easy to shape Provide a good base for other, softer foams	Foam that is too soft will "bottom out" so that the client is in contact with the underlying support structure Tendency to trap heat Prone to deterioration with moisture and light Lose resilience over time Absorb moisture, making them difficult to clean Tend to break down quicker than other foams Tend to be rigid, so they do not provide much envelopment, which provides less postural stability Will break down with moisture and heat Airflow is restricted to provide less ventilation
Viscoelastic Foam or Matrix (Figure 9-9) Examples: Sunmate, T-foam, and Tempur-Med		
Originally developed for space travel Very dense foam that is distinguished by its ability to retain its shape for a length of time Sometimes called "memory foam" Available in different densities	Accommodate slowly to a constant load Have a "memory" that delays their return to their original shape Provide good envelopment, which provides a stable base for posture Good thermal properties (conduct heat away from the body)	Degree of envelopment can increase the sliding resistance Resilience and dampening are variable depending on the density
Flexible Matrix (Figure 9-10) Example: Stimulite cushion from Supracor		
Honeycomb structure composed of thermoplastic material Arranged in layers of interconnected open cells that flex when pressure is applied Available in both planar and contoured versions	Conform to user's body providing pressure redistribution Open cells allow airflow for ventilation, limiting accumulation of moisture from sweat or urine Good resiliency	Less envelopment than viscoelastic products
	Cushions Containing Fluid	
Air Filled (Figure 9-11) Example: ROHO		
Consists of a sealed receptacle that holds air May be a single compartment or, more commonly, have multiple compartments	Good long- and short-term resilience Pressure distribution properties tend to be good but depend on maintenance Many models allow the cushion to be inflated to different degrees, providing pressure redistribution as needed Lightweight Materials do not deteriorate over time	Must be properly inflated: overinflation results in poor postural stability and lack of envelopment; underinflation results in "bottoming out" of the cushion Users with poor sensation may not detect inadequate inflation High maintenance, prone to tears and punctures, and need to monitor inflation level
Viscoelastic Fluid (Figure 9-12) Examples: Jay cushions, Action cushions		
Viscosity refers to the degree to which fluid molecules move across each other: low-viscose fluids move easily (e.g., water) Most cushion materials in this category have high viscosity	Good dampening and thermal properties Provide a stable base	Poor envelopment, short- and long-term resilience Affected by temperature; will freeze in cold weather Fluid will shift, allowing user to sit on hard surface Require kneading to ensure uniform distribution of the gel
	Other Constructions	
Hybrid Cushions (Figure 9-13) Examples: Otto Bock Cloud, Jay Cushions, Invacare Infinity Cushions		
Combination of materials described in other categories Most common is closed-cell foam base with membrane that contains gel, viscous fluid, or air on top or inserted into a cutout	Good envelopment, thermal properties, and pressure redistribution Good postural support	Weight varies depending on material Maintenance varies depending on material and configuration of components

Sources: Brienza & Geyer, 2000; Sprigle et al., 2001; Tang, 1991.

FIGURE 9-9 Viscoelastic foam. (Courtesy of Sunmate, www.sunmatecushions.com).

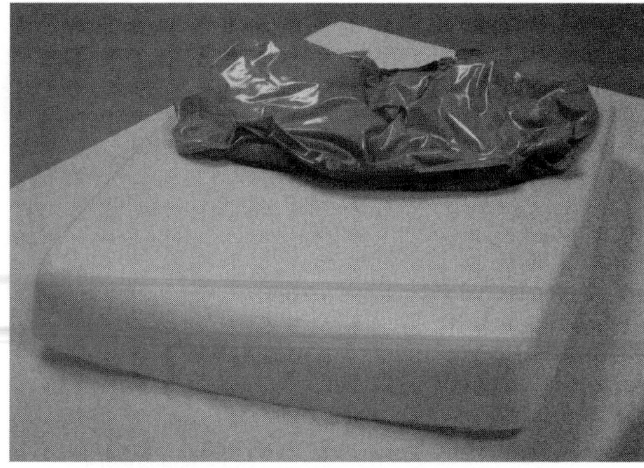

FIGURE 9-12 Viscoelastic fluid–filled cushion.

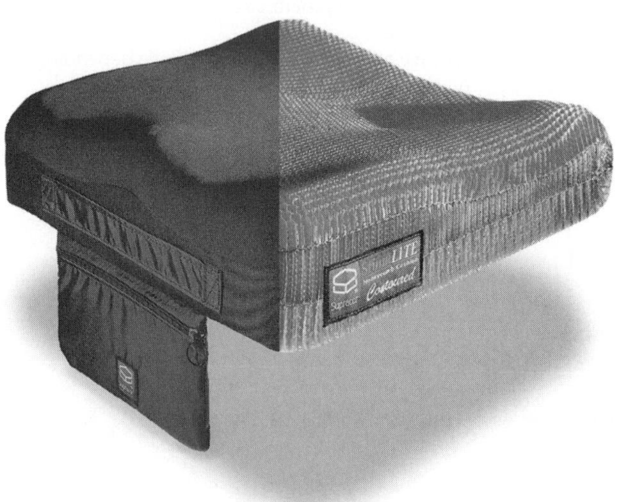

FIGURE 9-10 Flexible matrix cushion. (Courtesy of Supracor Inc., www.supracor.com).

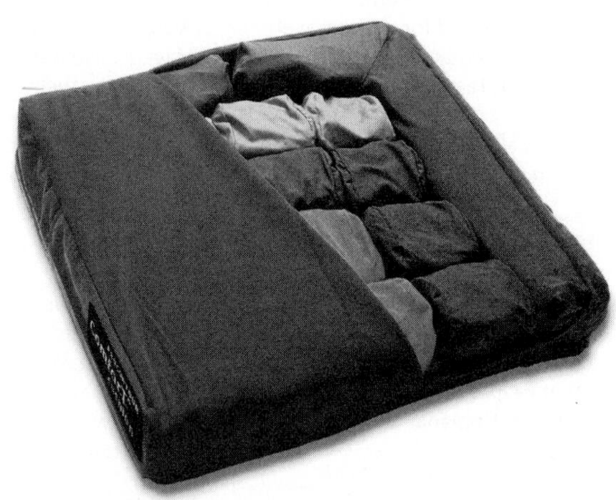

FIGURE 9-13 Hybrid cushion. (Courtesy of Ottobock, www.ottobock.com).

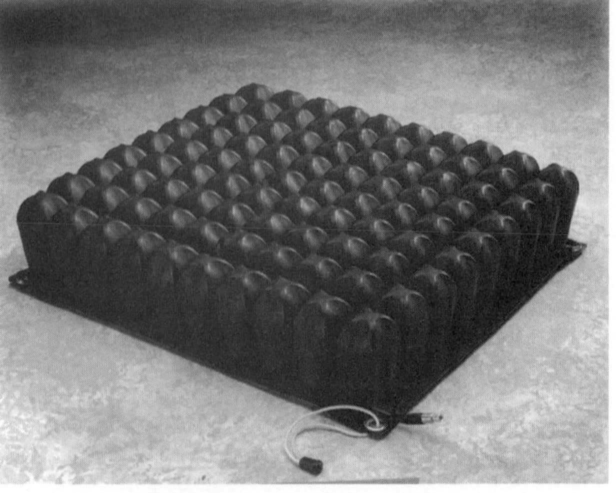

FIGURE 9-11 Air-filled cushion.

and friction. A cover that is too tight will prevent the client from sinking into the contours of the cushion. One that is too large will wrinkle, creating additional pressure points.

The clinician should know how the fabric handles moisture, either as a result of incontinence or perspiration. Most cushions will be used in hot, humid conditions for at least part of the year, so perspiration is an issue even when incontinence is not a concern. Many technical fabrics, blending Lycra and polyester, wick moisture away from the body, which is an important consideration when prevention of pressure ulcers is a goal. Options for covers typically include a simple stretch cover, one that has a moisture barrier for use when incontinence is an issue and covers that use technical fabrics, as mentioned earlier. The cushion cover should be easy to remove and clean.

SEATING ASSESSMENT

In practice, a single assessment is used to gather information to make a recommendation for seating and mobility technologies. This process will be described and applied to seating here and then applied to mobility technologies in the succeeding chapter.

The process of assessing individuals for the purpose of recommending seating and technologies requires a systematic method that includes consideration of many factors. Chapter 5 describes a general process for evaluation of AT needs and intervention. Figure 9-14 outlines a framework to guide AT professionals (clinicians) through the decision-making process and ultimate selection of seating and positioning technologies that match the needs and skills of the user.

As with other areas of AT, the process of delivering seating services involves a transdisciplinary team. The client, including the person who will use the seating system and caregivers or family, are central to this team. Their needs, goals, abilities, and lifestyle drive the assessment. Occupational and physical therapists typically provide expertise in physical, cognitive, and affective performance; ADLs; and environmental factors that enable or hinder daily activities or seating and mobility use. The physician provides relevant medical information such as whether surgery or other medical procedures are planned and what effects these procedures may have on the consumer's seating. Some jurisdictions also require that the physician makes or approves the seating recommendation. AT suppliers often provide knowledge of available technologies and their application to meet specific goals. Sometimes a rehabilitation engineer provides this service. When the consumer's need cannot be met by commercial products, the rehabilitation engineer or seating technician can design and build a custom system. This discussion of seating and mobility assessment assumes that the clinician already knows the institutional and regulatory requirements necessary to justify and gain approval for funding of eligible, recommended equipment.

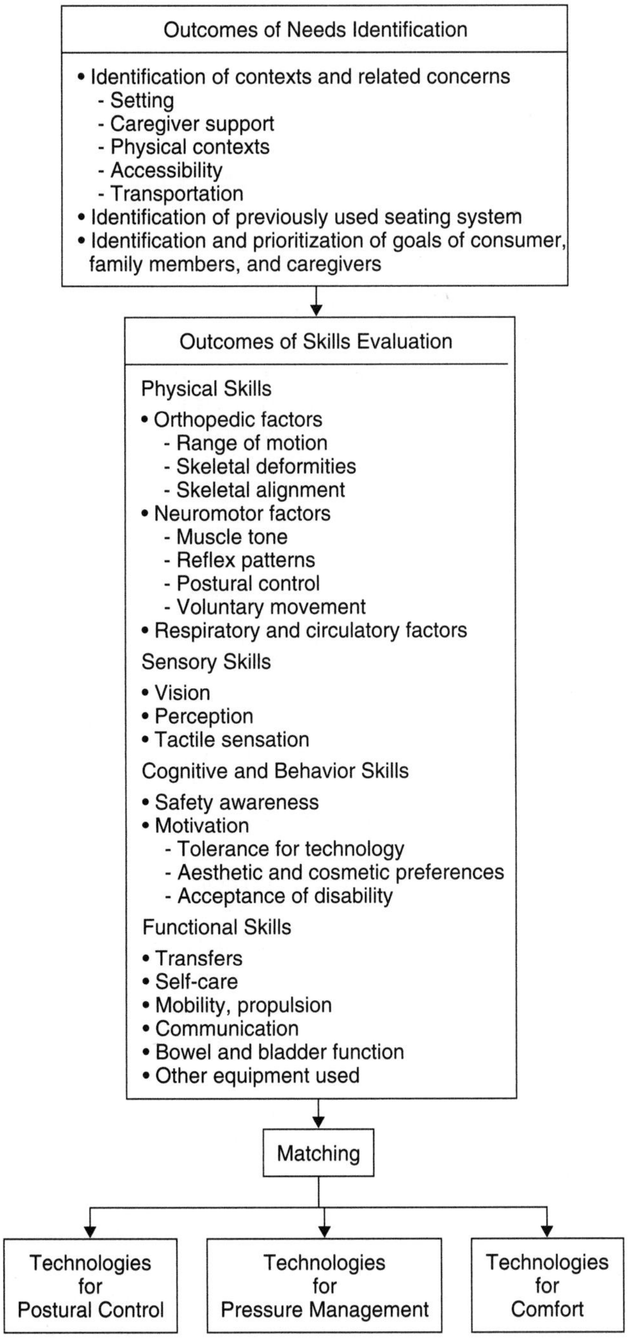

Outcomes of Needs Identification

- Identification of contexts and related concerns
  - Setting
  - Caregiver support
  - Physical contexts
  - Accessibility
  - Transportation
- Identification of previously used seating system
- Identification and prioritization of goals of consumer, family members, and caregivers

↓

Outcomes of Skills Evaluation

Physical Skills
- Orthopedic factors
  - Range of motion
  - Skeletal deformities
  - Skeletal alignment
- Neuromotor factors
  - Muscle tone
  - Reflex patterns
  - Postural control
  - Voluntary movement
- Respiratory and circulatory factors

Sensory Skills
- Vision
- Perception
- Tactile sensation

Cognitive and Behavior Skills
- Safety awareness
- Motivation
  - Tolerance for technology
  - Aesthetic and cosmetic preferences
  - Acceptance of disability

Functional Skills
- Transfers
- Self-care
- Mobility, propulsion
- Communication
- Bowel and bladder function
- Other equipment used

↓

Matching

↓

Technologies for Postural Control	Technologies for Pressure Management	Technologies for Comfort

FIGURE 9-14 Seating assessment framework.

Needs Identification

Box 9-2 lists the desired outcomes of the seating intervention. It is the clinician's responsibility to facilitate the identification and prioritization of these goals in collaboration with the client. Design of a seating system sometimes involves compromising the various goals. For example, desired biomechanical alignment may not be possible for a person with severe postural deformities when the resulting properly aligned position is too uncomfortable.

Standardized Measures

Measures that provide a general assessment of function of individuals with disabilities are described in Chapter 5. General assessments that are useful for seating and mobility include the Gross Motor Function Measure (Russell et al., 2013) and related Classification System (Palisano et al., 2008), and the Chailey Levels of Ability (Pountney et al., 1999). Field and Livingstone (2013) conducted a systematic review of clinical measures of postural control. They identified 19 such measures and concluded that none of them is robust in their current state of development. They found that clinical utility was limited by the need for special equipment needed and the lack of consideration of participation, contextual, and familial elements (Field & Roxborough). The measurement properties of most are quite limited. Interrater reliability is commonly determined, but other types of reliability are either not established or not done in a rigorous manner. Validity studies are particularly lacking for this area; when they have been done, they examine validity related to content of the measure but not that related to construct, which is the more important validity consideration (Messick, 1980).

Three that assess postural control are the Seated Postural Control Measure (SPCM) (Fife et al., 1991, 1993) and Seated Postural Control Measure—Adult Version (SPCMA) (Gagnon et al., 2005) and the Posture and Postural Ability Scale (PPAS) (Rodby-Bousquet et al., 2012). The Tool for Assessing Wheelchair disComfort (TAWC)

(Crane, 2004, 2005, 2007) provides a means of quantifying comfort when sitting for prolonged periods of time, typically in a wheelchair and seating system.

The SPCM and SPCMA each have three components: the Level of Seating Scale, alignment while seated, and alignment after an activity. The Level of Seating Scale provides a description of current sitting abilities, providing a description of the amount of support a person needs to maintain a sitting position and when independence in sitting is possible, the postural stability the person has. It uses an 8-point ordinal scale. The alignment portions include pictures depicting alignment at different anatomical sites (e.g., head, trunk, pelvis) that enable the clinician to describe postural alignment in a static situation and following movement (Fife et al., 1991).

The Posture and Postural Ability Scale was developed to assess adults with CP. It uses a 7-point ordinal scale to quantify postural ability in supine, prone, sitting, and standing, with a score of 1 indicating lower ability. Quality and symmetry are assessed with a yes/no scale through observation from frontal and sagittal perspectives (Rodby-Bousquet et al., 2012).

The TAWC (Crane, 2004, 2005, 2007) provides a means to quantify the level of discomfort experienced by a person after a prolonged period of time sitting, commonly in a wheelchair. It has three components: a demographic section to gather information about wheelchair and seating use, position, and activities; a general discomfort assessment that enables a description of the perception of discomfort (e.g., pain, temperature); and a rating scale (discomfort intensity rating) that quantifies discomfort overall and at different anatomical sites. General discomfort is rated on a 7-point scale with strongly disagree and strongly agree as the anchors.

Activity

Any assessment with the goal of identifying seating needs and recommended technology starts with discussion of the activities the user wants and needs to complete while using the seating system. A general measure such as the Canadian Occupational Performance Measure (Law et al., 2005) provides a systematic means of discussing key activities in the area of self-care, productivity, and leisure.

The level of assistance an individual requires to use the seating system is an important consideration in the assessment. Consideration must be given to whether an individual can transfer to the system and fasten any straps independently when he or she expects to use the seating system independently. The complexity of the system and the ease of access influence the demands placed on an individual providing assistance with a transfer.

Functional skills, including transfers to and from different surfaces (e.g., bed to wheelchair, car to wheelchair), self-care skills (e.g., feeding, dressing), wheelchair mobility, written and verbal communication skills, and bowel and bladder care, should be evaluated. What equipment the person will use while in the seating system needs to be taken into consideration. For example, respiratory equipment and augmentative communication devices are frequently mounted on the wheelchair and need to be in a position that is functional for the user.

It is important that the individual's ability to perform functional activities be evaluated both in the existing system and in a simulation of the proposed system. By observing the consumer performing functional activities from his or her existing system, the clinician learns two things. First, the clinician can determine the consumer's level of independence and areas where function is impeded. The clinician can also learn what strategies the individual currently uses to complete functional activities. By using the methods described in this chapter, the clinician can then simulate different positions with the consumer. The clinician can have the individual perform functional tasks while in these simulated positions. Changing the sitting position will affect the person's ability to perform certain activities. It is important to select a system that maximizes the person's function and does not interfere with the use of strategies that have proven to be beneficial. For example, a teenager who uses an abnormal asymmetrical tonic neck reflex to operate a single switch should not be prohibited from doing so unless another movement can be found that accomplishes this task. It will sometimes be necessary to trade an ideal seated posture for a posture that allows the individual to be more functional.

Human Factors

Physical Skills or Mat Assessment

The physical evaluation includes assessment of orthopedic factors, postural control, and respiratory and circulatory factors. It is recommended that evaluation of physical skills take place with the person both in a sitting position and supine on a flat surface such as a mat.

Orthopedic Factors

Orthopedic evaluation involves measurement of joint range of motion and assessment of skeletal deformities and skeletal alignment to determine optimal angles for sitting. Obtaining information regarding limitations in range of motion and deformities is necessary to determine whether the goal of the seating system will be to prevent deformities, correct deformities, or accommodate deformities (Trefler et al., 1993).

Starting with the consumer supine on the mat, mobility of the lumbar spine and pelvis are assessed, followed by *range of motion measurements* of the hips, knees, ankles, upper extremities, and neck. Once these measurements are made, the consumer assumes a seated position. Joint angle and body measurements as shown in Figure 9-15 can be made at this time. Alignment of the individual's head, shoulders, and trunk with the pelvis is determined next (see SPCM discussed earlier). Range of motion and skeletal alignment should also be assessed with the individual in a sitting position to determine how the body parts are affected by gravity. Details of the measurement methods and evaluation of postural alignment are available from a number of sources (c.f., Buck, 2009; Waugh & Crane, 2013)

It is important to determine whether any skeletal deformities present are fixed or flexible. In a **fixed deformity**, permanent changes have taken place in the bones, muscles, capsular ligaments, or tendons that restrict the normal range of motion of the particular joint. Fixed deformities affect the skeletal alignment of the other joints and typically require a

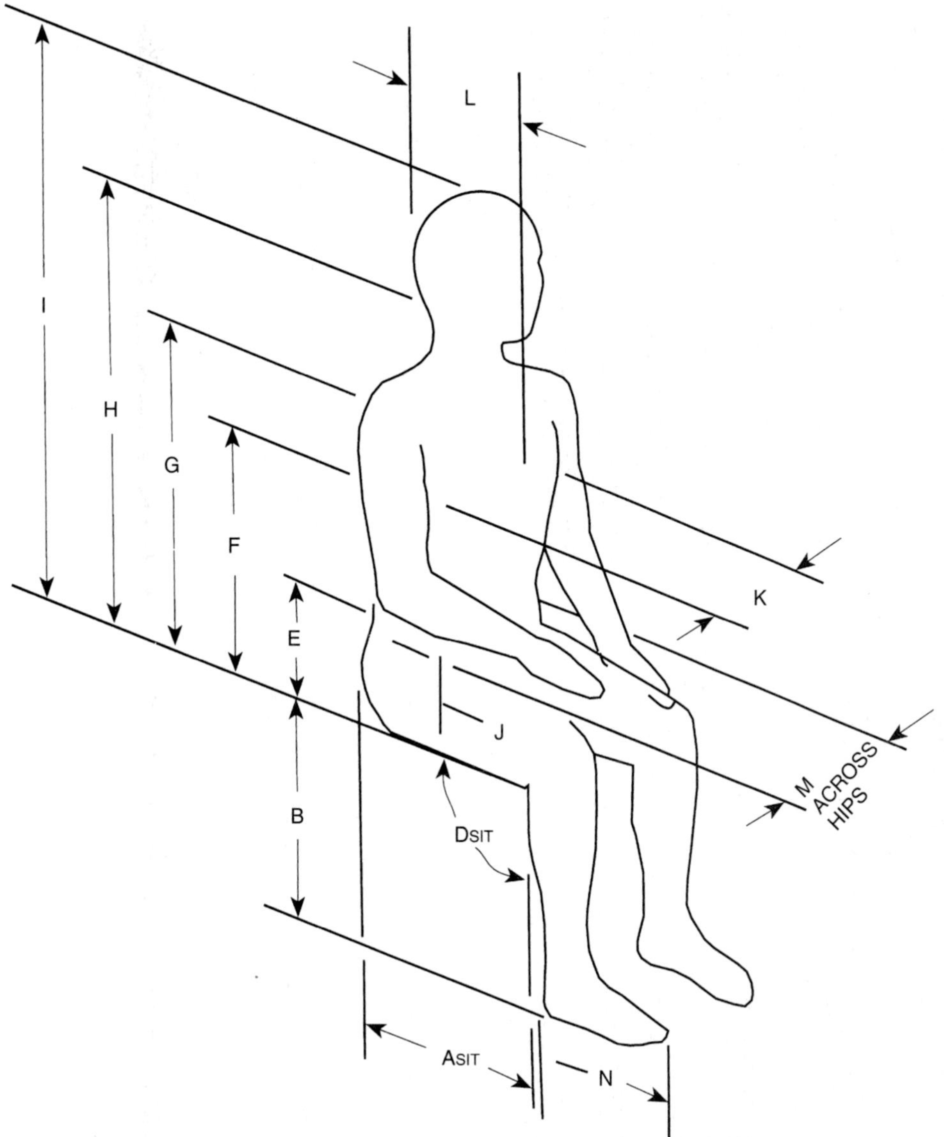

FIGURE 9-15 Joint angle and body measurements taken during a seating evaluation. ASIT(R and L), behind hips/popliteal fossa; B (R and L) popliteal fossa/heal; DSIT, knee flexion angle; E sitting surface/pelvic crest; F sitting surface/axilla; G sitting surface/shoulder; H sitting surface/occiput; I sitting surface/crown of head; J sitting surface/hanging elbow; K width across the trunk; L depth of trunk; M width across hips; N heel/toe. (From Bergen AF, Presperin, Tallman T: Positioning for function: wheelchairs and other assistive technologies, Valhalla, NY, 1990, Valhalla Rehabilitation Publications).

seating system that is designed to accommodate the deformity. Often, increased tone and muscle tightness cause persons to assume certain postures, and they may appear to have a deformity. With externally applied resistance (passive stretch) in the opposite direction, however, it is possible to move the joint and reduce the deformity. The person is then considered to have a **flexible deformity** at that joint. Depending on the situation, the seating system may be designed to correct a flexible deformity. Specific deformities and their effects on sitting posture are described in the section on seating principles for postural control.

Some individuals have had surgery to correct one or more deformities. The clinician should be aware of any surgery the consumer may have undergone and be knowledgeable about the implications it has for seating intervention. In other cases, the team may decide during the evaluation that surgical or orthotic intervention should be considered before seating intervention takes place. If this is the situation, referral to the appropriate medical professional is necessary. Letts (1991) examines surgical interventions related to the seated position.

Postural Control

The user's **postural control** is a key element to assess, particularly for children developing motor control, individuals recovering motor function after a neurologic injury such as traumatic brain injury, or someone losing motor control as a consequence of a progressive illness. Two important aspects should be considered: the individual's ability to control the posture in a sitting position (i.e., how much support is required to maintain a comfortable sitting position with a reasonable amount of effort) and the response to various positional changes. The most effective way to assess these aspects is with the client seated on a mat.

The ability of an individual to control his or her posture during sitting is determined with the client seated on a mat with the feet supported. The client's sitting ability is described by the amount of support required to maintain a seated position. Whereas hands-free sitters are those who do not need to use their hands to support themselves to maintain sitting, hands-dependent sitters do need to use their hands. These individuals could not perform a seated activity using their hands without some type of external support. A dependent sitter does not have sufficient motor control to support herself in sitting at all. Postural control tends to be less than in those in the other two categories. The Levels of Sitting Scale is also useful for determining the amount of support required to maintain a seated position (Field & Roxborough, 2011, 2012).

The amount of external control required to assist an individual to maintain a seated position is an important determination. Kangas (2000) recommends provision of the minimal amount of external support. Support may vary with the activity. Less support may be needed when the individual is engaged in a sedentary activity such as watching television. Alternatively, more support is needed when the individual is using his hands for an activity and the focus of attention is on the activity. The individual should not need to divert attention to the maintenance of posture when engaged in an activity.

Finally, the clinician needs to determine the individual's response to various postural changes. Primarily, the clinician should assess the effect of changes of pelvic position on the client's postural control. What happens when the pelvis is positioned in a neutral, anterior-tipped, or posterior-tipped position? Similarly, what effect does change of spinal alignment or lower limb position have on postural control? The client's response to these position changes will influence the configuration of the seating system and whether any dynamic elements need to be provided.

Respiratory and Circulatory Factors

The person's *respiratory* status and *circulation* are other factors addressed during the evaluation. With skeletal deformities, pulmonary and cardiac function can be compromised. It is important to know whether certain positions enhance or limit respiration. Circulation, particularly in the lower limbs, needs to be considered as well. Some individuals may have a condition that predisposes them to circulatory problems; particularly for these consumers, positions that impair circulation should be avoided.

Sensory and Perceptual Skills

Vision and visual perception contribute to a person's balance and sitting posture, and deficits in these areas need to be considered during the evaluation. The configuration of the seat can affect the user's line of vision. For example, an individual with poor postural control who is unable to maintain spinal extension with consequent neck flexion may not be able to maintain the head in an upright position if the seat-to-back angle is set at 90 degrees. The user's line of vision will be downward in this seating configuration. A person's awareness of body position *(proprioception)* in space also influences body posture.

Tactile sensation is another factor to consider. Some individuals may react defensively to the touch of certain textures or positioning components on the body. Other individuals lack tactile sensation, which can contribute to skin breakdown. The clinician should determine whether there is any known decrease in sensation, particularly in the buttock area, and whether there is a history of pressure ulcers. The condition of the person's skin on weight-bearing surfaces (including areas on the trunk that are braced by lateral supports) should be checked for evidence of skin breakdown, circulation, color, smoothness, sensation, and moisture (Tredwell & Roxborough, 1991).

CASE STUDY

Jillian

Jillian is a happy 5-year-old girl with CP resulting in severe motor impairment. Jillian is nonverbal and uses a smile or an eye blink to indicate yes. She is very alert and aware of her environment. She will be attending kindergarten in the fall. She does not have a wheelchair and has never been evaluated for a seating system. Her parents carry her from place to place or use an umbrella stroller for her as needed. She receives therapy with a neurodevelopmental treatment approach three times a week. When they made the initial phone referral, Jillian's parents stated to you that they have put off getting a seating system for Jillian because they did not want her to "look handicapped." With Jillian soon to be attending school, they have decided it is time to get her a wheelchair and seating system.

Jillian has mixed tone. Her lower extremities, particularly her ankles, have increased tone. The tone in her upper extremities is increased as well. Her trunk and neck are hypotonic. She exhibits a startle reflex and the symmetrical tonic neck reflex. She does not have any apparent orthopedic deformities. She is unable to keep her head up for any length of time unless she is reclined back slightly. Jillian can use a switch with her right hand when her head is held upright. She can also use the touch screen on the computer, but she needs help with sitting. Jillian is dependent for mobility and all other functional activities.

Questions

1. From the information you have so far, what might be the goals of seating for Jillian?
2. Write a list of interview questions you would ask of her parents and therapists.
3. How would you proceed with a seating evaluation for Jillian?
4. On the basis of the information you have about Jillian at this time, what technological approaches would you consider for her and why? What type of positioning accessories would you consider and why?
5. List potential funding sources for Jillian's seating system. How would you justify her system to the funding source (refer to Chapter 5)?

BOX 9-4 Pressure Ulcer Risk Assessments

Common Scales for Assessing Risk of Pressure Ulcer Formation

Braden Scale (Bergstrom et al., 1987)

Components

- Sensory perception
- Moisture
- Activity
- Mobility
- Nutrition
- Friction and shear

The first four items are scored on a scale of 1 to 4. The last item is scored on a scale of 1 to 3 with higher numbers denoting lower risk. A score of less than or equal to 9 suggests a very high risk. (Braden, 2001)

Norton Scale (Norton et al., 1975)

Components

- Physical condition
- Mental condition
- Activity
- Mobility
- Incontinence

Items are scored on scale of 1 to 4 with lower number suggesting a higher risk.

Waterlow Score (Waterlow, 1985; revised 2005)

Components

- Build and weight for height
- Skin type visual risk areas
- Sex and age
- Malnutrition screening tool
- Continence
- Mobility
- Special risks
  - Tissue malnutrition
  - Neurologic deficit
  - Recent surgery or trauma

Each component is scored on either a 0 to 3 or 0 to 5 scale. A score of 10+ indicates at risk, 15+ high risk, and 20+ very high risk for pressure ulcer formation.

Individuals whose ability to reposition themselves or whose activity is limited to bed or chair should be assessed for the risk of pressure ulcer development. Scales are available to determine the magnitude of risk by measuring the degree to which mobility and activity levels are limited. Three commonly used scales that assess these factors are the Norton Scale (Norton et al., 1975), the Waterlow Scale (Waterlow, 1985 [revised 2005]), and the Braden Scale (Bergstrom et al., 1987). In addition to mobility, these scales also assess other factors that place a person at risk for development of pressure ulcers, such as incontinence, impaired nutritional status, and altered level of consciousness. Individuals should be assessed with a validated systematic risk assessment tool. Box 9-4 summarizes pressure ulcer risk assessment instruments.

Cognitive Skills

Cognitive skills such as problem solving and motor planning are not as much of an issue in seating as in mobility. However, a few areas require consideration. Individuals with poor safety judgment may not be aware of the need to keep a positioning belt fastened, and special considerations may be necessary. When the seating system is complex, understanding the client's cognitive abilities will aid the decision to teach the client or the caregiver about the proper use of the system. Knowing the individual's language and communication skills (see Chapter 16) will help determine how the clinician gathers information during the evaluation. For example, if a person relies on an augmentative communication device or on yes/no responses, these modes of communication should be used during the evaluation process. If it is known that the consumer is not reliable in his or her responses, then the clinician should seek assistance from a caregiver in interpreting the consumer's responses to the seating system.

Psychosocial Factors

The meaning that technology holds for the individual is an important factor to explore with the user, although it is more significant for the mobility component of a seating and mobility system. Many clients prefer technology that does not draw attention to a disability. This preference will be a factor in the selection of a seating system. Esthetics is an important factor in acceptance and rejection of the technology (Pape et al., 2002). Behavioral problems, such as an agitated person who throws himself against the back of the chair, can also present a safety problem that needs to be addressed. Working together with the consumer and the caregiver to address these concerns is essential.

Context Factors

Physical Context Assessment

The seating assessment should determine in which environments the seating system will be used (e.g., home, school, workplace, and vehicle and whether it is necessary for the system to be used in different environments). Knowledge of where the seating system will be used helps the clinician determine whether the system will be removed and reinstalled in the mobility device or other devices. For instance, an individual who transfers to the car seat when traveling from home to school will remove the seating system when the mobility device is stored in the vehicle and replace it on arrival at the destination. Many seating devices designed for young children are intended to pair with different bases (e.g., the system may be used in a stroller, high chair, or floor sitter).

The clinician should determine the extent to which the seating system will be used outdoors. Temperature is an important factor to consider when designing a seating system. Extreme heat or cold will affect the function of many materials, limiting their ability to meet the goals set for use of the system. Exposure to light sources may affect some materials used to cover a system component, altering its properties and again, affecting the function of the system.

Social Context

The clinician must know who is available to assist the consumer with the use of the system when it is used in multiple settings. This knowledge influences the instruction given to the users of the system and influences considerations with respect to the weight, complexity, and maintenance of the system. Many clinicians who recommend seating products have seen situations in which a simple seat cushion is placed backward in a mobility device, causing great discomfort to the user. The risk of misuse is much greater with complex seating systems. Consequently, the clinician must ensure that the user and any caregivers are familiar with proper use of the seating system. Adequate instruction is key to preventing misuse of the system.

Institutional Context Assessment

Funding implications are a key institutional consideration. General considerations with respect to funding are described in Chapters 3 and 5. The clinician has the responsibility of providing the necessary documentation to secure funding but may rely on others, such as the client, family, or rehabilitation assistant, to provide important information about function to include in the documentation.

Some legal jurisdictions have legislation that regulates the use of restraints with individuals residing in institutional settings. The intent of this legislation is to limit inappropriate use of restraints. The legislation typically regulates how restraints are used in institutional settings, requiring most institutions to have a plan and a documented process when restraints are used. Box 9-5 provides information on what to look for in an institution's guidelines and care plan concerning restraint use. The clinician should be familiar with the restraint use policies of the institution, how these policies affect her practice, and what is required in all parts of the service delivery process when the client's seating system includes elements listed that are considered to be restraints.

Restraints are frequently used to prevent falls. However, there is little evidence to suggest their use actually does result in any significant reduction in the incidence of falls. The clinician should monitor the client for any adverse outcomes associated with the use of restraints. These outcomes include agitation if the client becomes upset by the restriction of movement, redness, skin abrasion or pressure ulcer formation, or undue limitation of functional activities if the client's movement is overly restrained by the seating components.

BOX 9-5 Considerations for Use of Restraints with Clients in Institutional Settings

Restraint Guidelines

- The least restrictive device should be used.
- The client's response to the restraint should be reassessed frequently because being retrained can increase agitation.
- The client should be reassessed frequently to determine whether continued restraint is required.
- Restraints should be removed periodically.
- The facility's guidelines for documenting use of restraints need to be followed.
- Depending on jurisdiction, a physician's order is required at regular intervals for continued use of restraints.

Care Plan

- Reposition the client frequently; monitor the client's position to ensure that he is not at risk of injury because of his position nor at risk for a pressure ulcer from immobility caused by the restraint.
- Perform skin care routine on a regular basis, including observation of the skin for areas of redness that might indicate formation of a pressure ulcer.
- Perform range of motion exercises (active or passive as the client is able) frequently during the day.
- Provide assistance with activities of daily living; if the client remains in a restraint during these activities, ensure that the restraint is not limiting her performance.
- Ensure ongoing assessment by the team to monitor the need for continued use of the restraint.

Alternative Strategies

- Observe the client to determine if behavior that prompted the use of the restraint is triggered by something in the environment, such as:
  - Another person in the environment may trigger agitated behavior, so limiting the interaction may be calming.
  - If restraints are used to prevent falling out of bed, lower the bed and use mats to reduce the risk of injury in the event of a fall.
  - Provide stimulating activities that engage the client to encourage calmer emotions.
- When possible, include the individual in a group so he can be observed and assisted on an ongoing basis.
- Be aware of the effect of your style of communication and interaction on the client's emotion because these may increase agitation.
- Use a positioning alarm on bed that alert the staff if a client tries to climb out of bed.
- Enhance exercise programs.
- Ensure that staff is familiar with the client, his needs, and his abilities.
- Ensure that the client is comfortable in bed.

References: Collins et al., 2009; Registered Nurses Association of Ontario, 2012.

Matching Device Characteristics to a Consumer's Needs and Skills

The information that has been gathered regarding needs and skills provides a profile of the user. The primary seating need (postural control, tissue integrity, comfort) can then be determined, which allows identification of potential technologies and evaluation of their effectiveness in meeting the consumer's needs.

The next step is to actually simulate with the consumer one or more of the alternatives. The clinician can observe the effects of changes in body position and materials by having the consumer try variations of the positioning system. Trial positioning is also helpful for assessing the person's ability to use control interfaces such as the joystick of a power wheelchair. Changes in position can be made to see whether they have beneficial or adverse effects on the person's ability to control a device or perform other functional skills. Simulation makes it easier to document the need for and effectiveness of a particular system so that funding can be obtained. If specific cushions or positioning components are being considered for a consumer, it helps to have her try the actual product and determine whether she likes it. In some instances, it may be desirable for the consumer to take the system home for a trial period, which allows her to use the system over a longer period and in her natural environment.

BOX 9-6 Critical Questions to Inform a Seating Recommendation

Does the seating system meet the consumer's goals and needs (e.g., postural control, pressure redistribution, comfort)?

Does the seating system provide stability and allow for maximal performance in functional activities (e.g., transfers, weight shifts, activities of daily living)?

Is the seating system durable enough to meet the consumer's needs for a reasonable period?

Is the seating system sufficiently flexible to meet the consumer's changing needs (e.g., change in functional abilities, growth changes)?

Are there resources available to ensure appropriate maintenance of the seating system?

Can the consumer or third-party payer finance the cost of the seating system?

Several critical questions can help the clinician evaluate the effectiveness of the technologies that have been simulated and to select an appropriate seating system for the consumer. These questions, which summarize the needs evaluation, the skill assessment, and the simulation, are shown in Box 9-6. The primary concern is whether the simulated seating system meets the goals identified during the needs assessment. The clinician should consider the extent to which the system achieves the desired goals with respect to positioning, support of function, and comfort. The caregiver's ability to lift, carry, and maintain the seating system is a further factor to consider. A system that does not meet these goals to the satisfaction of the client or the caregiver will not be used.

INTERVENTION

Principles of Seating for Postural Control

Children and adults who have irregular tone, muscle weakness, abnormal reflex patterns, shortening of a muscle group, or skeletal deformity are likely to require external positioning devices to control their posture and prevent deformities. Within this category, some individuals have mild impairments and require only minimal support, but other individuals have severe physical impairments and require extensive postural support. The components that make up a seating system can provide support to the body to improve skeletal alignment, normalize tone, prevent deformities, and enhance movement. Box 9-7 summarizes guidelines for implementation of seating for postural control.

Guidelines for Postural Control

The most important principle related to postural control is that proximal stabilization, near the center of the body, facilitates movement and control of the head and the extremities (e.g., function). During normal development, an infant achieves stability in the proximal joints before using the distal limbs for manipulation. For example, before a baby can successfully reach out and grab a toy while sitting, he must have mastered the ability to maintain a balanced sitting posture

BOX 9-7 Guidelines for Positioning for Postural Control

1. Proximal stabilization (i.e., a stable pelvis) is important for trunk and head control and use of the upper and lower extremities.
2. Sitting is a dynamic activity. Seating for postural control should enable the client's movement rather than restrict it.
3. The pelvis is a key point of control because its position affects posture in the rest of the body.
4. The lower extremities should be in a neutral position with respect to internal and external rotation, abduction, and adduction.
5. The trunk should be upright and in a midline position (i.e., limited lateral flexion and rotation).
6. The head should also be in a midline position with a neutral neck position (for neck flexion and extension, rotation, and lateral flexion).
7. The shoulders should be down and forward with a neutral position with respect to internal and external rotation and abduction and adduction. The elbows should be supported at about a 90-degree angle.

BOX 9-8 Levels of Postural Control in Sitting

The Hands-Free Sitter

Can sit for prolonged periods without using the hands for support

Seating system is designed primarily for mobility, to provide a stable base of support, and to be comfortable

The Hands-Dependent Sitter

One or both hands are used to maintain support while sitting

Seating system is designed to provide pelvic or trunk support to free the person's hands for functional activities

The Propped Sitter

Lacks any ability to support self in sitting

Seating system provides total body support

(Bertenthal & Von Hofsten, 1998; Hadders-Algra et al., 1998, 1999; Savelsbergh & Van der Kamp, 1994). Otherwise the hands must be used to maintain balance, which limits their use for manipulation. Seating for postural control provides external positioning components for an individual who does not have internal mechanisms to control body posture. Tredwell and Roxborough (1991) present a classification scheme (Box 9-8) that is useful in describing the amount of control a person exhibits in sitting. Each category is matched with a brief description of the recommended degree of support provided by the seating system.

When any type of external support is provided, care needs to be taken so that the individual is not excessively positioned. We need to keep in mind that sitting is a *dynamic activity*. We often associate sitting with relaxation and lack of activity and movement, when in fact many activities are performed while sitting, such as writing, driving, talking on the phone, and typing. Even during quiet sitting, an individual frequently shifts weight to maintain comfort. It is not uncommon to see individuals "properly" positioned to the point that they are no longer able to use the motor movements they have used in the past to complete functional tasks. The *fewest* restraints necessary to optimize function should be used (Kangas, 2000). This section presents a set of general guidelines for proceeding with the development of a postural seating system for an individual.

Pelvis and Lower Extremities

We have described the important role of the pelvis in relation to the center of gravity and sitting. The pelvis is a key point of control, and its position affects the posture of the rest of the body. Therefore, alignment and stabilization of the pelvis are normally the first areas addressed in positioning an individual. A position with the pelvis in neutral or in a slight anterior tilt is desired (Mayall & Desharnais, 1995). The pelvis should be level and in midline.

A position of hip flexion at approximately 90 to 100 degrees is recommended frequently for individuals with neuromotor impairments (Bergen et al., 1990; Trefler et al., 1993; Tredwell & Roxborough, 1991). However, there are several situations in which this position is not optimal. Hip angle is guided by the postural responses of the client during the mat assessment. A 90- to 100-degree angle of hip flexion is intended to inhibit extensor tone and reduce the posterior tilt of the pelvis, thus keeping the individual positioned back in the seat. In some instances, it is necessary to increase the amount of hip flexion (thus reducing the angle to less than 90 degrees) to further inhibit extensor tone. Alternately, in some instances, 90 degrees of hip flexion is not achievable (because of deformity) or is not the most appropriate position. Some individuals are not able to maintain an upright position when placed in a position of 90 degrees of hip flexion. Similarly, tight hamstrings may prevent achievement of 90 degrees at the knees. The clinician needs to determine the effect of deformities and muscle tone on both function and comfort in the sitting position during a mat assessment to determine the most appropriate position of the pelvis, hips, and lower extremities.

Asymmetrical postures that may be present in the pelvis and hips include pelvic obliquity, pelvic rotation, pelvic tilt, and windswept hips. These postural asymmetries are often interrelated. They may be flexible postures or fixed bony deformities that restrict the mobility of the pelvis and limit the attainment of the recommended pelvic position.

An individual with a **pelvic obliquity** has one side of the pelvis higher than the other when viewed in the frontal plane (Figure 9-16 *A*). The obliquity is named for the side that is lower; for example, with a left pelvic obliquity, the left side is lower than the right. This deformity is often accompanied by **pelvic rotation,** in which one side of the pelvis is forward of the other side (Figure 9-16 *B*). **Windswept hip deformity** manifests itself with one hip adducted and the other hip abducted. This deformity has usually been found to be the end stage of a sequence that proceeds as follows: hip subluxation and dislocation, pelvic obliquity, scoliosis, and windswept hip deformity. Typically, all of these components are present in this deformity. The hip on the high side is typically dislocated, and the opposite hip may or may not be dislocated (Letts, 1991). When fixed deformities such as these are present, the seating system should be designed to accommodate them rather than to attempt to correct them (Mayall & Desharnais, 1995).

Support to the pelvis can be provided under, behind, in front, or from the sides. At the very least, a firm seating surface for the individual to sit on will level and stabilize the pelvis. Individuals with moderate to severe involvement typically need more support for stabilization. This support can be provided by contours around the buttocks and up into the lumbar area. Alteration of the seat-to-back angle may be required when the individual has severe extensor tone. During the mat assessment, with the person in sitting, the therapist should move the client through different hip ranges to determine which hip angle achieves the most postural control (Houghton et al., 2013). This optimal angle can then be replicated in the seating system, bearing in mind that the actual angle of the hip (femur to acetabulum) will be more acute than the seat-to-back angle of the seating system. A seat with a pelvic loading area (i.e., a depression at the back of the cushion into which the pelvis sinks) will support the pelvis in a neutral position and prevent forward movement. Supports to prevent lateral shifting of the pelvis or external rotation of the hips can be provided either by contouring the seat to provide channels that position the thighs or with some form of lateral support at the pelvic level.

Pelvic positioning belts or bars support the pelvis from the front. The placement of the belt is important to effectively maintain pelvic position. Depending on the person's pelvic mobility, comfort, and positioning needs, the pelvic positioning belt is placed at an angle ranging from 45 to 90 degrees to the seating surface, as shown in Figure 9-17. In

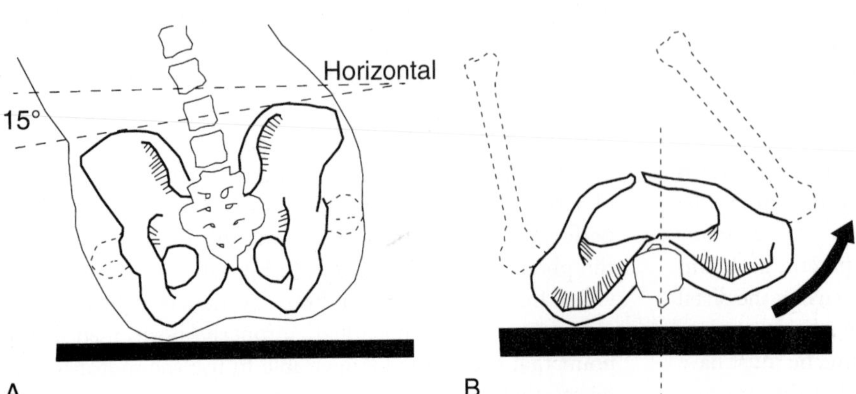

FIGURE 9-16 A, Pelvic obliquity viewed in the frontal plane, **B,** Pelvic rotation (From Siekman A: The biomechanics of seating: a consumer guide, Action Dig March/April:8-9, 1992).

most cases, a belt with an angle of pull at 45 degrees sufficiently maintains the pelvis in position. If there is excessive hip extension or a need for anterior pelvic mobility, positioning the belt at a 90-degree angle of pull is more effective. Pelvic positioning belts can be soft and flexible (e.g., webbing or padded vinyl) or rigid when more support is required. A rigid pelvic positioning device, also called a sub-ASIS bar (Figure 9-18), is typically a close-fitting, padded metal bar that is attached to the wheelchair frame or seat insert to position the pelvis below the individual's ASIS. It is designed to be used in conjunction with a complete seat and back system for individuals who require greater control to maintain the neutral position of the pelvis and to prevent pelvic rotation. Handling of the client to determine the effect of pressure, or control, around the pelvis (e.g., at the ASIS or posterior-superior iliac spine) during the mat assessment will help determine optimal placement of any pelvic stabilizing devices.

Adequately positioning the lower extremities helps to maintain the pelvic and hip positions. The positions of the legs and feet affect the position of the pelvis and therefore need to be addressed simultaneously. It is recommended that the legs be positioned so that the femurs are neutral with respect to abduction and adduction and rotation and with approximately 90 degrees of knee flexion, although there are some exceptions that will be noted below. Some form of sculpting is frequently used in the seat to keep the femurs in a neutral position and to limit adduction and internal rotation (Figure 9-19). A frequently encountered problem in the lower extremities is hamstring tightness, which may or may not result in flexion contractures of the knees. Recall that these muscles originate on the pelvis. Attempts to position the individual to stretch these muscles and reduce the knee flexion contracture will result in a pull on the pelvis, tipping it into a posterior pelvic tilt. The client may then slide forward in the chair into a sacral sitting position. It is best to accommodate this problem by modifying the seating surface (shortening the seat depth or undercutting the front edge) so that the legs are allowed to flex under the seating surface. This contouring maintains the correct pelvic position. If there is fixed knee extension, the lower leg must be completely supported with pads or troughs that match the range of motion in the knee.

Support for the feet is important for maintaining hip and knee position, for preventing deformities in the ankles, and for distributing pressure. If the feet are left to hang or are positioned too low, pressure increases under the anterior thigh area, which can cut off blood flow. Positioning the feet too high places excess pressure on the ITs and the sacrum, which can cause formation of a pressure ulcer. It is recommended that the feet be positioned flat and with 90 degrees of ankle flexion (Mayall & Desharnais, 1995). Support surfaces for the feet can be one or two platforms and in different sizes, depending on the person's needs. Increasing the thickness of the foot support under the shorter leg serves to accommodate unequal lower leg length. Foot platforms can be angled to accommodate fixed plantar flexion contractures of the ankle. Various strapping systems can be used to maintain the desired ankle position, including straps over the top of the foot, behind the heel, and enclosing the ankle (Figure 9-20).

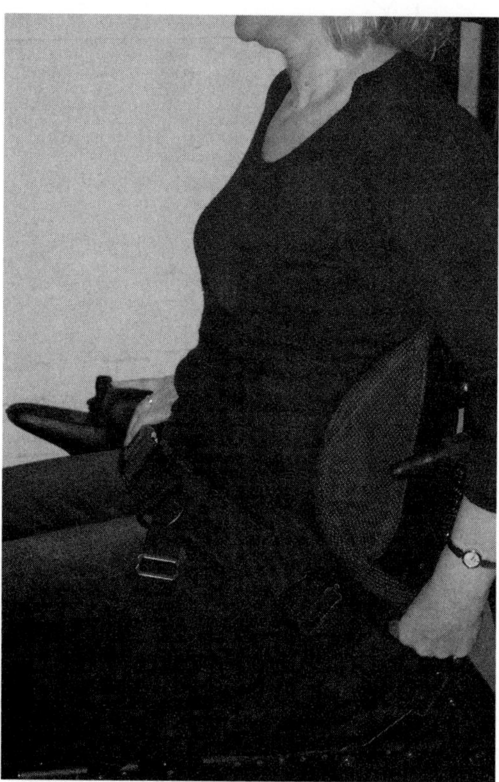

FIGURE 9-17 Proper placement of a pelvic belt.

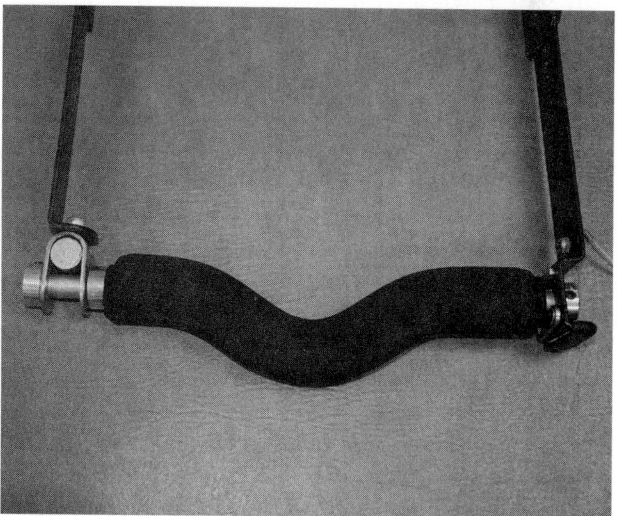

FIGURE 9-18 Sub-ASIS (anterior-superior iliac spine) bar.

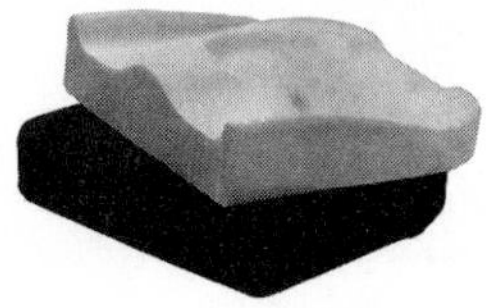

FIGURE 9-19 Sculpted foam cushion demonstrating sculpting to control the pelvis and align the femurs. (Courtesy of Invacare Corp, www.invacare.com).

Trunk

After the desired position in the pelvis and lower extremities has been obtained, the trunk is considered. An upright position with the trunk aligned in midline is desirable. This position may not be attainable if the individual has fixed deformities. Possible spinal deformities are scoliosis, lordosis, kyphosis, or a combination of these. **Scoliosis** of the spine occurs when there is lateral curvature or rotation of the vertebral column. Scoliotic curves are further defined according to the anatomical site in the vertebral column that is involved, that is, cervical, thoracic, or lumbar. Compensatory (or secondary) curves develop as a result of the head's attempting to maintain its upright position (Figure 9-21 *A*) (Cailliet, 1975). Figure 9-21 *B*, shows an uncompensated curve with the spine unbalanced and the head lateral to the center of gravity. Rotation of the vertebrae is also frequently found in scoliosis and can cause greater respiratory difficulty than lateral curving (Cailliet, 1975).

The amount of trunk support required depends on how much control over the trunk that the individual has and is determined during the mat assessment with the client in sitting. As in the pelvis, trunk support can be provided from behind, at the side, or in front. The amount of support provided from behind is related to back height and contouring. The height of the back can be varied, depending on the amount of upper body support needed. Someone who requires minimal support can use a lower backrest height; a higher backrest is necessary for the individual with a need for greater support. Contouring accommodates to the individual's body shape and provides optimal support. If the person has kyphosis, the back needs to be recessed so that he or she is not pushed forward in the seat. For lordosis, lumbar support can be added to bring the seat back in contact with the person. Contouring of the back at the shoulder level can reduce shoulder retraction that is present.

When a person has difficulty maintaining a midline position (side to side) of the trunk, lateral support is provided. The positioning of the lateral supports depends on how much control the person has, again, determined in the seated position during a mat assessment. Lateral supports placed high on the trunk and close to the body provide greater control than those placed lower on the trunk (Buck, 2009; Houghton et al., 2013; Mayall & Desharnais, 1995). Because the forces placed on the body by the lateral supports can be great, care should be taken in placement of these components and selection of materials (well padded) to prevent tissue damage. Figure 9-4 shows laterals attached to the wheelchair to provide trunk support.

Tilting the seating system back slightly can eliminate some of the effects of gravity for individuals with spinal deformities, low tone, decreased strength in the trunk, or poor head control and can also help the individual maintain a more symmetrical posture. The force of gravity is reduced in the tilt position, making it easier to maintain the trunk in midline and increasing the comfort of the laterals. The positive effects of tilt on trunk position must be evaluated by the

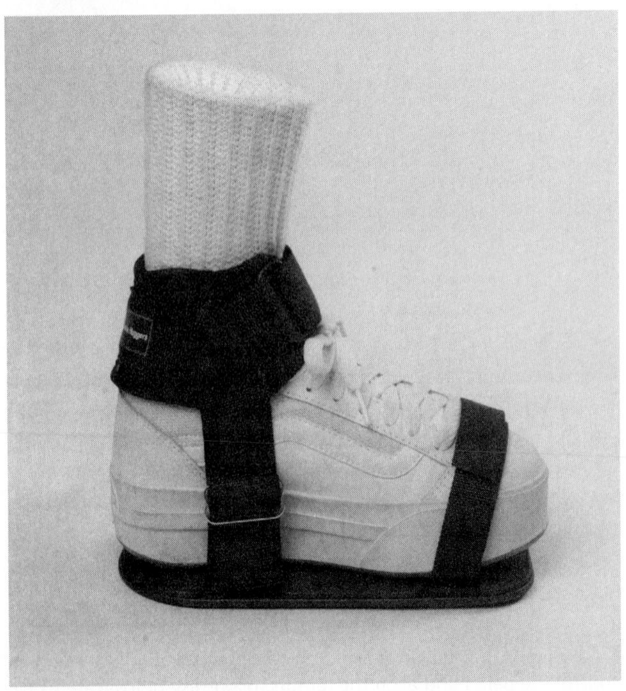

FIGURE 9-20 Ankle hugger. (Courtesy of Bodypoint Designs Inc, www.bodypoint.com).

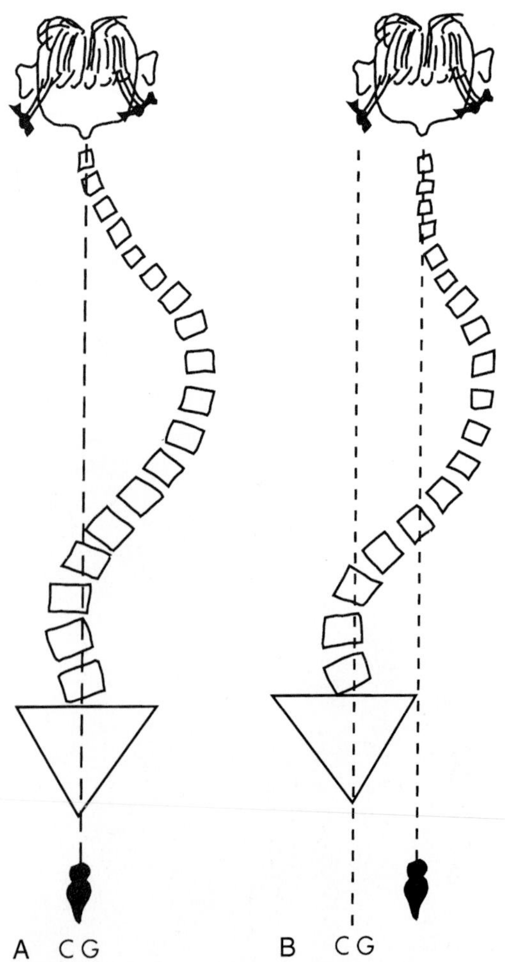

FIGURE 9-21 **A,** Development of compensatory curve in scoliosis; **B,** Uncompensated scoliotic curve, CG, Center of Gravity. (From Cailliet R, Scoliosis: diagnosis and management, Philadelphia, 1975, FA Davis Co.).

limitations this position can place on function. Vision, the ability to eat, use of equipment on a tray, and social engagement are just some activities that can be compromised when the wheelchair seat is tilted. Tilt systems will be discussed in greater detail in the next chapter on mobility technologies.

When control is required to prevent forward trunk flexion, anterior supports can be used. This type of support is necessary for individuals who need to be in an upright position for a functional or therapeutic activity but who do not have the ability to maintain this position independently. The most common approaches used are straps, chest panels, and rigid shoulder supports. One simple approach is to use straps that are attached to the seat back below shoulder level, come up over the shoulders, and attach to the seating system near the hips (Figure 9-22). The chest restraint must be well maintained because it poses a safety concern if the lower attachment becomes loose, allowing the strap to constrict around the neck (Trefler et al., 1993).

Head and Neck

With the pelvis, lower extremities, and trunk positioned, head and neck positions are considered next. The position of the head is important in inhibiting abnormal reflexes and maximizing the visual skills of the individual. In some cases, a headrest is necessary only part of the time, for example, when the individual becomes fatigued or during transportation. The most common problems leading to the need for positioning of the head include hyperextension of the neck, weak neck musculature, lateral neck flexion, and neck rotation. In addition, support is required for the head when the person is either reclined or in tilt. As in the positioning of other body segments, posterior, anterior, or lateral components are used for support. Figure 9-23 shows examples of different headrest configurations. Posterior support can range from a high backrest (for those requiring minimal support) to headrests of different types. With any posterior head support, it is important to avoid triggering extension or pushing the head forward into flexion. Anterior support may be provided by headbands, which are used in conjunction with posterior head supports, although supervision is required when these are in use. The Nodstop Special Needs system (www.nodstopspecialneeds.com) is an example of such an anterior support. It consists of a band that is covered in a soft material, with Velcro strapping. The band attaches to a hat, such as a baseball cap, and the system is then attached to the headrest of the seating system.

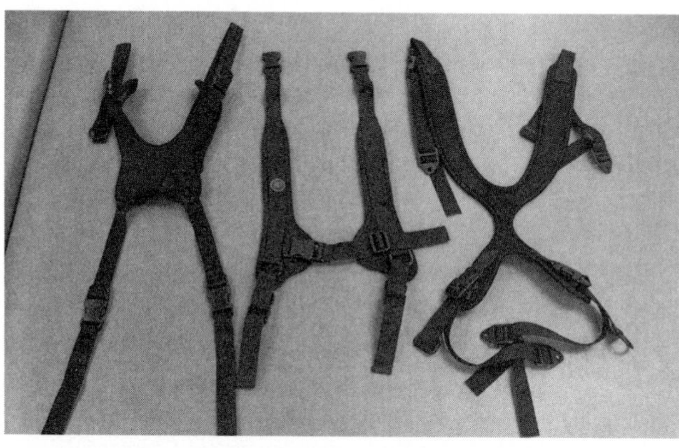

FIGURE 9-22 A variety of chest strap configurations used to assist the client to maintain an upright trunk position.

Upper Extremities

Support of the upper extremities is an essential component of the seating system. A lack of support for the arms can adversely affect head and neck position. Additionally, arms that are left to hang can sustain injury if caught on something or can acquire subluxation of the glenohumeral joint of the shoulder. The most common upper extremity support is the armrests of the wheelchair, which are discussed in the next chapter. Using an upper extremity support surface, such as a lap tray, helps with positioning of the head and neck, reduces the likelihood of damage to the arms and shoulder joints, and places the hands in a midline position that facilitates bilateral manual activities. The height of the lap tray depends on the needs of the consumer. Commonly, the tray is mounted so that it allows the forearms to rest on it with the elbows bent at a 90-degree angle. Some individuals do not want a lap tray but still require positioning of the upper extremities. For these situations, individual arm troughs Figure 9-24 mounted to the armrests of the wheelchair are available, which provide channeling and support for the arms.

Principles of Seating for Tissue Integrity

A second major goal of seating interventions is pressure redistribution. The emphasis in this area is to distribute pressure at the wheelchair cushion–human interface and maintain the

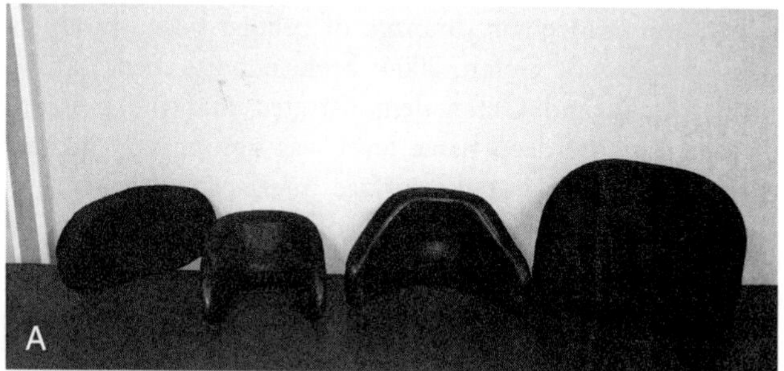

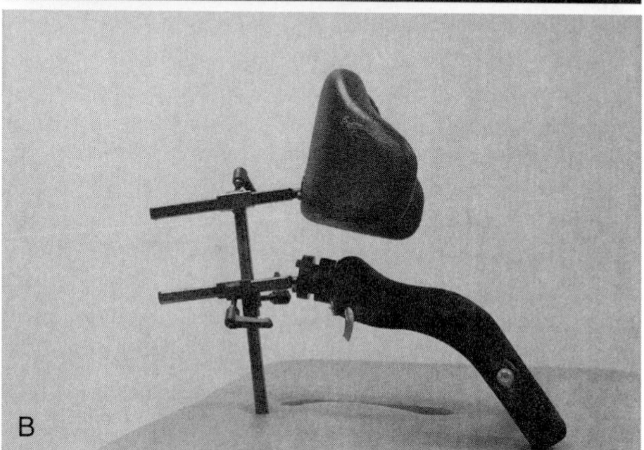

FIGURE 9-23 Different headrest configurations. **A,** A variety of headrest configurations showing different sizes and depths. **B,** Headrest and rigid shoulder support combination.

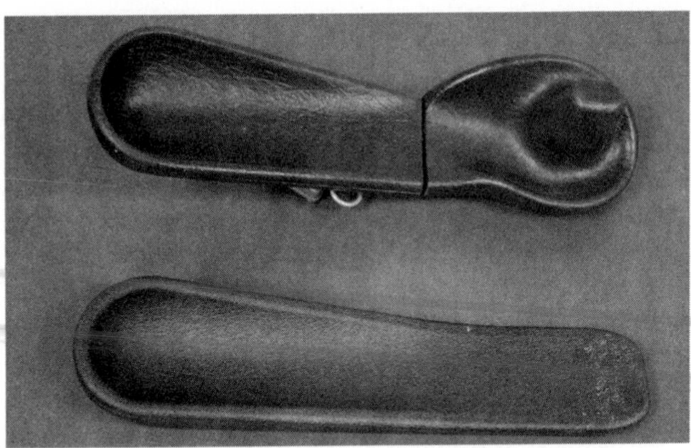

FIGURE 9-24 Arm troughs.

skin in a healthy condition so that pressure ulcers are prevented. A **pressure ulcer** is "localized injury to the skin and/or underlying tissue usually over a bony prominence, as a result of pressure, or pressure in combination with shear" (NPUAP, 2009). The sacrum, coccyx, ITs, trochanters, external malleoli, and heels are the most commonly affected areas. The NPUAP engaged in an extensive consultation and consensus-building process, engaging international experts, to develop a strategy to identify different stages or categories of pressure ulcers. These stages and categories are listed in Table 9-2.

Pressure Measurement

Pressure ulcers result from sustained compression of soft tissues, particularly under bony prominences. The predominant hypotheses concerning the pathogenesis of pressure ulcers include localized tissue ischemia, sustained deformation of the cells, impaired nutritional flow to the cells, reperfusion injury, and inadequate drainage of cellular waste products (Linder-Ganz & Gefen, 2004; Stekelenburg et al., 2006). Linder-Ganz and Gefen demonstrated that the pressure measured at the deep tissue level was significantly greater than that measured at the surface interface, although they could not predict a specific relationship. The prevalence of pressure ulcers and the resulting costs underscore the need to measure the forces applied to the muscle in an attempt to prevent prolonged exposure to high loads. Many sophisticated pressure measurements systems have been developed, including near-infrared tissue spectrophotoscopy, Raman spectrography, and indwelling sensors. However, these systems are not feasible in the clinical situation.

In the clinic, **pressure mapping** systems are the primary means of quantifying pressure. These systems quantify pressure at the buttock–seat interface, allowing a comparison among various cushions. They can also be used to quantify asymmetries in sitting and the effect of cushion configuration in promoting symmetry. The three most common pressure mapping systems are the Force Sensing Array (Vista Medical, www.pressuremapping.com), Body Pressure Management System (www.tekscan.com), and Xsensor (Xsensor Technology Corporation, www.xsensor.com/wheelchair_seating_systems). Each of these systems uses a flexible matrix of pressure sensors that provide a map of the distribution of pressure at the interface between the seat cushion or back and the client's body. These sensors are arranged in a grid pattern on the pressure mat. The number of sensors and their sensitivity vary across the different systems and should be taken into consideration when considering the purchase of a system. The systems vary in the technology used to measure pressure. These technologies include capacitance sensors that measure the ability to store an electrical charge, piezoresistive sensors that measure the change in resistance when force is applied, and electrically conductive sensors that measure the change in current flow.

Two properties influence the reliability of the pressure measurements, creep and hysteresis. Creep refers to the stability of the pressure reading over time. Hysteresis refers to the change in pressure reading as the device is loaded and unloaded (e.g., as the client sits on the cushion). Each of these systems corrects for these two variables in their software, but these properties still influence the reliability of the measurement systems to varying degrees, which needs

CASE STUDY

Alex

Twenty years ago, at the age of 22 years, Alex sustained a SCI in a single-car accident. The lesion was at the T1 to T2 level, leaving him completely paralyzed below that level. After his initial hospitalization and adjustment to his disability, he returned to college and completed a master's degree in vocational counseling. He has a successful private practice as a vocational counselor, which has kept him very busy—so busy, in fact, that he did not pay attention to his skin and ended up with a small pressure sore on his left IT. After weeks of medical treatment and hours spent in bed allowing the ulcer to heal, he is ready to get back to working full time again. His doctor has referred him to the clinician for evaluation for a seating system that will manage his pressure. The physician's report states that scoliosis is also beginning to develop.

Alex currently has a lightweight manual wheelchair with a sling back and a 2-inch foam cushion with a knit cover placed on top of the sling seat. He is independent with mobility by using his upper extremities. He transfers in and out of the wheelchair to all surfaces independently, including to and from his car. He is independent in all self-care activities. He is married, and his wife is responsible for all home management activities. He does admit that he has gotten into the habit of hooking his left arm behind the wheelchair push handle for stability during certain activities. He did not realize that this could be the cause of some of his problems.

Questions

1. On the basis of the information given, what might be the goals of seating for Alex?
2. Write a list of questions to ask of Alex during the initial interview.
3. How should the clinician proceed with a seating evaluation for Alex?
4. On the basis of the information given, what technological approaches should be considered and why? What types of positioning accessories should be considered and why?
5. List potential funding sources for Alex's seating system. How could his system be justified to the funding source (see Chapter 5)?

TABLE 9-2 International Pressure Ulcer Advisory Panel Pressure Ulcer Stages and Categories

Category and Stage	Definition
Category and stage I: nonblanchable erythema	"Intact skin with non-blanchable redness of a localized area usually over a bony prominence. Darkly pigmented skin may not have visible blanching; its color may differ from the surrounding areas. The area may be painful, firm, soft, warmer or cooler as compared to adjacent tissue. Category I may be difficult to detect in individuals with dark skin tones. May indicate 'at risk' persons."
Category and stage II: partial thickness	"Partial thickness loss of dermis presenting as a shallow open ulcer with a red pink wound bed, without slough. May also present as an intact or open/ruptured serum-filled or serosanguineous filled blister. Presents as a shiny or dry shallow ulcer without slough or bruising*. This category should not be used to describe skin tears, tape burns, incontinence associated dermatitis, maceration or excoriation. *Bruising indicates deep tissue injury."
Category and stage III: full-thickness skin loss	"Full thickness tissue loss. Subcutaneous fat may be visible but bone, tendon or muscle are *not* exposed. Slough may be present but does not obscure the depth of tissue loss. *May* include undermining and tunneling. The depth of a Category/Stage III pressure ulcer varies by anatomical location. The bridge of the nose, ear, occiput and malleolus do not have (adipose) subcutaneous tissue and Category/Stage III ulcers can be shallow. In contrast, areas of significant adiposity can develop extremely deep Category/Stage III pressure ulcers. Bone/tendon is not visible or directly palpable." (Italics in the original)
Category and stage IV: full-thickness tissue loss	"Full thickness tissue loss with exposed bone, tendon or muscle. Slough or eschar may be present. Often includes undermining and tunneling. The depth of a Category/Stage IV pressure ulcer varies by anatomical location. The bridge of the nose, ear, occiput and malleolus do not have (adipose) subcutaneous tissue and these ulcers can be shallow. Category/Stage IV ulcers can extend into muscle and/or supporting structures (e.g. fascia, tendon or joint capsule) making osteomyelitis or osteitis likely to occur. Exposed bone/muscle is visible or directly palpable."
Additional Categories and Stages for the United States	
Unstageable or unclassified: full-thickness skin or tissue loss—depth unknown	"Full thickness tissue loss in which actual depth of the ulcer is completely obscured by slough (yellow, tan, gray, green or brown) and/or eschar (tan, brown or black) in the wound bed. Until enough slough and/or eschar are removed to expose the base of the wound, the true depth cannot be determined; but it will be either a Category/Stage III or IV. Stable (dry, adherent, intact without erythema or fluctuance) eschar on the heels on the heels serves as 'the body's natural (biological) cover' and should not be removed."
Suspected deep tissue injury—depth unknown	"Purple or maroon localized area of discolored intact skin or blood-filled blister due to damage of underlying soft tissue from pressure and/or **shear**. The area may be preceded by tissue that is painful, firm, mushy, boggy, warmer or cooler as compared to adjacent tissue. Deep tissue injury may be difficult to detect in individuals with dark skin tones. Evolution may include a thin blister over a dark wound bed. The wound may further evolve and become covered with thin eschar. Evolution may be rapid exposing additional layers of tissue even with optimal treatment."

Source: Available from www.npuap.org/resources/educational-and-clinical-resources/npuap-pressure-ulcer-stagescategories/.

to be taken into consideration when these systems are used clinically.

The output from each of these systems is generally similar, although care must be taken when the results of research or measurements obtained by use of the different systems are compared. As will be seen below, these systems differ in their performance. All of the systems provide a visual output (Figure 9-25) that allows a quick inspection of the pressure distribution. The visual output may show pressure distribution with a color display or as peaks and depressions. The actual pressure value for each cell can be displayed as well. Data are captured continuously at varying sampling rates. The system provides data on peak and mean pressure, number of sensors activated, minimum and maximum pressure, and the location of the center of pressure. Most systems enable multiple displays such as the pressure map on one side and a video recording on the other. Another useful feature is the ability to define a particular area of the pressure map for which the system will generate pressure statistics.

The breadth of information that these systems provide is both useful and a distraction. Although data showing peak and mean pressure seem easy to interpret, there is little consensus on what is desired pressure at the seat–buttock interface. Different ways of interpreting these data will be discussed below in the discussion of a pressure mapping protocol.

Hadcock et al. (2003) compared incremental loading, low threshold, and stability (creep) of the F-scan, FSA, and Xsensor systems under static and dynamic conditions by using planar and curved surfaces. The curved surface was cylindrical, which is quite different from a contoured seating surface, so the results of this aspect of the study must be interpreted with caution for the purposes of seating intervention. This study involved bench testing and did not include measurement with any wheelchair users. The results on a flat surface indicated that the FSA system was the most accurate followed by the Xsensor and the F-scan. Creep was similar for the Xsensor and F-Scan (17.62% and 17.23%, respectively) systems, and both were better than the FSA system (19.54%) (Hadcock et al., 2003). The Xsensor was better at detecting pressures under light loading conditions.

Pressure mapping in the clinical situation is used to make comparisons among various cushions so the clinician can

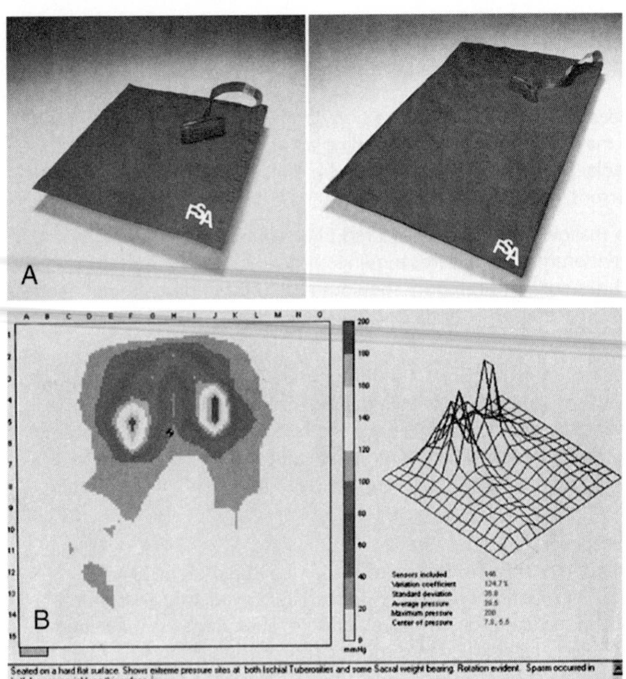

FIGURE 9-25 Pressure mapping output. **A,** Pressure mapping technology. **B,** Output from pressure mapping data collection. (Courtesy of Vista Medical, www.pressuremapping com).

rank the cushions for their ability to distribute pressure as measured by the pressure mapping systems. Sprigle (2000) suggests that pressure mapping is best used to rule out a cushion and is an adjunct to other clinical seating assessments. Swaine (2003) has developed a protocol for both obtaining and interpreting pressure measurements that is becoming more prevalent internationally. Swaine describes a consistent setup of the equipment and cushions to be evaluated, an initial check of the equipment, length of recording time, palpation of bony prominences, and documentation. She also suggests that interpretation of the results is based on peak pressure, the area of the client's buttocks that is in contact with the pressure mat, and any asymmetries of pressure distribution.

Swaine's work provides a useful basis for clinicians using pressure mapping to determine the optimal cushion for their clients' needs. Caution is still advised because questions remain about a protocol and the interpretation of the data. For example, whereas Swaine (2003) suggests that peak pressure is determined by taking the average of the four highest sensor cells around a bony prominence, Dunk and Callaghan (2005) take the average of all sensors within 10% of the cell, measuring the highest peak pressure. Swaine recommends that clients sit on a cushion for 8 to 10 minutes, but Stinson et al. (2002) suggest that 6 minutes is sufficient. Pressure gradient rather than absolute pressure has been suggested as a better indicator of risk for development of a pressure ulcer, but there is no consensus on what constitutes an acceptable gradient. These concerns suggest that although pressure mapping remains a very useful tool it augments clinical judgment, it does not replace it.

Two main technologies exist to manage pressure for persons who use wheelchairs, pressure redistribution cushions and tilt and recline components on wheelchairs. The latter is discussed in Chapter 10. Numerous studies have measured characteristics and properties of a variety of pressure redistribution cushions. The majority of investigations have used tissue interface pressure as the basis for comparing these products. Some studies have also compared changes in transcutaneous oxygen tension and capillary blood flow.

Individuals who are at risk for development of pressure ulcers can benefit from proper positioning in the wheelchair as well. In fact, it is recommended that positioning be addressed first because postural alignment often results in changes in pressure distribution (Minkel, 1990). Through postural alignment, pressure can be distributed more evenly; postural deformities, such as pelvic obliquity, scoliosis, and kyphosis, can be reduced; back pain can be alleviated; and stability can be increased. These changes will influence the individual's mobility, energy expenditure, and function.

Many of the principles described regarding sitting posture and postural control apply to individuals at risk for pressure ulcer development as well. Some of the technologies for postural control are beneficial for persons with SCIs, and new technologies that specifically address the needs of this population have been developed. Some basic strategies for positioning for postural management for this population are described.

Most wheelchairs intended for daily use have a solid seat pan that provides a solid base for a seat cushion. Commercially available backs tend to have a plastic molded shell and attached to the seat uprights with hardware. (e.g., Varilite Evolution Back or J2 Back, Sunrise Medical, Inc., www.sunrisemedical.com). (Figure 9-7 shows a commercially available back.) The seat back should be assessed for appropriate height and seat-to-back angle. It is recommended that the back be reclined approximately 15 degrees to help stabilize the trunk and prevent forward loss of balance. The back height is determined by the amount of support needed by the individual. Many persons with paraplegia have adequate trunk strength and wish to preserve mobility (particularly for sports), so they prefer lower backs on their wheelchairs and prefer not to use trunk-positioning components. Persons with C4 to C5 quadriplegia, with less trunk control, can benefit from a higher seat back that supports all or part of the scapulae, and those with C1 to C3 spared require headrests.

Principles of Seating for Comfort

Discomfort from sitting in a seating system (and wheelchair) can result in loss of function, reduced quality of life, ergonomic issues related to wheelchair propulsion, and the assumption of improper postures in an attempt to relieve pain (Crane et al., 2007). Individuals may experience discomfort after sitting for prolong periods, when exerting effort to perform an activity, the position they have assumed, and pressure. Discomfort varies according to duration, location, and intensity (Crane et al., 2007). Individuals who experience discomfort for reasons related to postural control or pressure may find relief through the application of seating principles appropriate for these populations. In other instances, combining these applications and determining the source of the discomfort are useful strategies to promote greater comfort.

Technologies to Enhance Sitting Comfort for Wheelchair Users

In a study that assessed the satisfaction of wheelchair users, comfort was rated as the most important variable for a wheelchair seating aid (Weiss-Lambrou et al., 1999). At the same time, comfort was rated as the least satisfying variable among these wheelchair users. The reasons stated for dissatisfaction related to comfort included seat cushions that caused pain and discomfort, fatigue, uncomfortable headrests and thoracic supports, sliding in the wheelchair seat caused by discomfort, and poor posture as a result of unsuitable installation. Comfort is also related to the contact surface between the seating system and the person. For example, materials that provide good air exchange, maintain an even temperature, and control moisture are more likely to provide a comfortable sitting climate.

Wheelchair users who have discomfort and chronic pain need seating systems that allow them to relieve the discomfort and participate fully in ADLs. These needs are best addressed after a thorough mat assessment that identifies the user's most comfortable seated position and the combination of technologies identified earlier that best addresses comfort needs. (Mobility technologies that provide users with the ability to adjust their positions in the wheelchair are discussed in Chapter 10). The TAWC (Crane et al., 2004, 2005, 2007) provides a measure of the intensity, duration, and site of discomfort, enabling the clinician to target the client's discomfort more directly.

Technologies That Increase Ease of Sitting for Older Adults

People are living longer, which means that the number of well older adults and those in need of supervised care is growing considerably. As an individual ages, mobility may be reduced as a result of acute illnesses or trauma, such as stroke, hip fracture, or progressive conditions such as arthritis. Consequently, it is likely that the amount of time an individual spends sitting increases. The goal of seating in this category depends on the individual's needs and skills, as it does for the other categories. Just as there is a range of needs for the elderly population, there is also a range of seating technologies. Seating technologies for the aging population can be matched to the level of functional mobility the individual has: (1) ambulatory; (2) mobile, nonambulatory; and (3) dependent mobile (Fernie & Letts, 1991). Chairs are needed that promote comfort, safety, ease of ingress and egress, and propulsion if necessary.

OUTCOME EVALUATION

Outcome of the use of a seating system is most often coupled with wheelchair use because these technologies are typically recommended together. This section will focus on work that has evaluated specifically seating technology. Evaluation of the outcome of seating and mobility technology combined will be considered in the next chapter.

There has been little research on the effectiveness of seating technologies, partly because of the challenges of conducting a rigorous, controlled study when the recommendation for a seating system and its setup are so highly individual. It is difficult to define a single intervention that is common across a large number of research participants, which is necessary in a controlled, experimental project. However, three outcomes of seating intervention have received some attention in the literature: effect of pelvic stabilization, effect of a seated support surface on reach, and efficacy of pressure redistribution cushions.

Pelvic Stabilization

Research examining the role of pelvic stability in the facilitation of function supports the assertion of starting with the pelvis when an appropriate seating system in being determined. Two studies investigated the effect of two methods of pelvic stabilization: a regular lap belt, typically using hook and pile fastening, versus a rigid pelvic stabilizer (a sub-ASIS bar in one case and the Embrace Pelvic Positioner [Body Tech NW, Mukilteo, WA, http://www.bodytechnw.com/pelvic_positioners.php] in the second) on function of children with CP (Miller Polgar et al., 2000; Rigby et al., 2001). Both of these studies compared daily function, as perceived by the participants and their families, when using the typical lap belt versus the rigid pelvic stabilizer. Results were comparable in both, with better function found with the rigid pelvic stabilizer. Significant differences were found on the Canadian Occupational Performance Measure (Law et al., 2005) before and after implementation of the rigid pelvic stabilizer. The results of these studies are limited by the small sample size, but the convergence of their findings provides evidence for the practice of controlling the pelvis in seating for postural control.

Reach

Limited published evidence has documented the effect of seating intervention on reaching ability. Aissaoui and colleagues (2001) explored the effect of seat cushions on dynamic stability during a reaching task. They measured reaching movements using a seat force platform and interface pressure mapping, comparing theses movements of participants with either paraplegia or quadriplegia, when using a Roho, contoured foam, or a planar foam cushion. In all situations, the contour foam cushion was the most effective in providing stability to support reach.

Pressure Redistribution Cushions

The evidence for the effectiveness of pressure redistribution cushions comes from four lines of inquiry: evaluation of the properties of these cushions in a laboratory using a rigid indenter (a mechanical device that is designed to mimic the shape and structure of buttocks and upper thighs), single case studies of clients after provision of a cushion, qualitative studies regarding their use, and single randomized controlled trials (RCT) comparing the outcome of use of a standard foam cushion with pressure redistribution cushions. A few systematic reviews of all interventions related to pressure ulcers have included seating technologies.

Laboratory investigations investigate properties such as reduction of shear and friction, envelopment, immersion, displacement after application of a load, and "bounce back" after the load has been removed. Aikins et al. (2011) explored the relationship between interface shear stress and displacement in several different types of pressure-reducing cushions. They found viscous fluid cushions had the least amount of interface shear stress followed by air-filled, elastic or viscoelastic, foam, and then honeycomb constructions. Ferguson-Pell et al. (2009) examined heat and moisture dissipation, comparing cushions based on material and construction (contoured or noncontoured). They proposed a matrix classification system of low heat and low moisture dissipation, low heat and high moisture dissipation, high heat and low moisture dissipation, and high heat and high moisture dissipation. They concluded that the material of the cushion affected heat dissipation but not moisture. The cushion cover material and its construction did not have an effect. Their results enabled them to fit the cushions studied into two of the four classifications (high heat and low moisture dissipation and one other that was not identified). They concluded that the classification system has potential but is not clinically useful at this time.

A small number of RCTs have been completed related to pressure redistributing cushions. Most of these were completed about 20 years ago, so they are not reviewed here because the technologies that were used at that time are not in use today for the most part. Geyer et al. (2001) and Brienza et al. (2010) conducted an RCT comparing a standard segmented foam cushion with three different pressure redistributing cushions (Roho Quadtro, J2 DEEP Contour, and the Infinity MC) in a sample of residents in a long-term-care supervised nursing facility. The outcome measure was incidence of IT or IT and sacral pressure ulcers. The incidence for both of these types of pressure ulcers was lower in the group that received the pressure redistributing cushions, which led the researchers to conclude that these cushions are effective in redistributing pressure in this population (Brienza et al., 2010).

SUMMARY

This chapter has shown the potential outcomes that can be achieved through seating in three primary areas of need: postural control, tissue integrity, and comfort. Procedures for evaluation and matching of device characteristics to the individual's needs have been presented. Basic principles of biomechanics frequently used in seating and positioning have been discussed. Different types of seating technologies and cushion classifications have been described, along with their application to the three primary goals of seating.

STUDY QUESTIONS

1. Describe the three primary goals of seating intervention. What are the key elements of a mat assessment? Describe each of these.
2. Describe three additional factors that the clinician should consider when designing a seating system.
3. Describe the influence of the physical, sociocultural, and institutional contexts on design of a seating system.
4. What are the three types of force? Why are they relevant to seating and positioning?
5. What is meant by the center of pressure, and how does it relate to seating and positioning systems?
6. Describe the basic premises underlying seating intervention for postural control.
7. Why is the pelvis the starting point when seating for postural control? Describe the major approaches used to obtain alignment and control of the pelvis.
8. List three methods used to support the trunk in postural control seating systems and describe when each method is indicated.
9. Describe how the head can be positioned posteriorly, anteriorly, and laterally. What factors lead to the use of each of these?
10. What is the major cause of pressure ulcer development? What are other factors that contribute to the development of pressure ulcers?
11. Describe Swaine's pressure mapping protocol. Describe the output of pressure mapping systems. Discuss two controversial aspects of pressure measurement.
12. What is a honeycomb cushion? What advantages does it have over other approaches?
13. How do viscoelastic fluid–filled and foam cushions differ? List an advantage and disadvantage of each.
14. What are the primary populations for whom comfort is the major goal in developing a seating system?

REFERENCES

Aissaoui R, Boucher C, Bournonnais D, Lacoste M: Effect of seat cushion on dynamic stability in sitting during a reaching task in wheelchair users with paraplegia, *Arch Phys Med Rehabil* 82:274–281, 2001.

Aikins JS, Karg PE, Brienza DM: Interface shear and pressure characteristics of wheelchair seat cushions, *J Rehabil Res Dev* 48:225–234, 2011.

Allman RM: Pressure ulcer prevalence, incidence, risk factors, and impact, *Clin Geriatr Med* 13:421–436, 1997.

Bergen AF, Presperin J, Tallman T: *Positioning for function: Wheelchairs and other assistive technologies*, Valhalla, NY, 1990, Valhalla Rehabilitation Publications.

Bergstrom N, Braden BJ, Laguzza A, Holman V: The Braden Scale for predicting pressure sore risk, *Nurs Res* 36:205–210, 1987.

Bertenthal B, Von Hofsten C: Eye, head and trunk control: The foundation of manual development, *Neurosci Biobehav Rev* 22:515–520, 1998.

Braden B: Risk assessment in pressure ulcer prevention. In Krasner D, Rodeheaver, G & Sibbald G Co-editors: Chronic wound care: A clinical source book for healthcare professionals, 3rd ed. Wayne PA, 2001, HMP Communications.

Brienza D, Geyer MJ: Understanding support surface technologies, *Adv Skin Wound Care* 13(5):237–244, 2000.

Brienza DM, Kelsey S, Karg P, et al.: A randomized control trial on preventing pressure ulcers with wheelchair seat cushions, *J Am Geront Soc* 58:2308–2314, 2010.

Buck S: *More than 4 wheels: Applying clinical practice to seating, mobility and assistive technology*, Milton, ON, 2009, Therapy NOW!. Inc.

Cailliet R: *Scoliosis: Diagnosis and management*, Philadelphia, 1975, FA Davis.

Centers for Medicare and Medicaid Services (42 CFR 483.13 (a)).

Chen Y, DeVivo MJ, Jackson AB: Pressure ulcer prevalence in people with spinal cord injury: Age-period-duration effects, *Arch Phys Med Rehabil* 86:1208–1213, 2005.

Collins LG, Haines C, Perkel RL: Restraining devices for patients in acute and long term care facilities, *Am Fam Physician* 79:4, 254–256, 2009.

Consortium for Spinal Cord Medicine Clinical Practice Guidelines: Pressure ulcer prevention and treatment following spinal cord injury: A clinical practice guideline for healthcare professionals, *J Spinal Cord Med* 24(suppl 1):S40–S101, 2001.

Crane BA, Holm MB, Hobson D, et al.: Development of a consumer driven wheelchair seating discomfort tool (WcS-DAT), *Int J Rehab Res* 27:85–90, 2004.

Crane BA, Holm MB, Hobson D, et al.: Test-retest reliability, internal item consistency and concurrent validity of a wheelchair seating discomfort assessment tool, *Assist Tech* 17:98–107, 2005.

Crane BA, Holm MB, Hobson D, et al.: Responsiveness of the TAWC tool for assessing wheelchair discomfort, *Disabil Rehabil: Assist Tech* 2:97–103, 2007.

Cutajar R, Roberts A: Occupations and pressure sore development in Saudi men with paraplegia, *Br J Occup Ther* 68:307–314, 2005.

Dorsett P, Geraghty T: Depression and adjustment after spinal cord injury: A three-year longitudinal study, *Top Spinal Cord Inj Rehabil* 9:43–46, 2004.

Dunk N, Callaghan J: Gender-based differences in postural responses to seated exposures, *Clin Biomech* 20:1101–1110, 2005.

European Pressure Ulcer Advisory Panel, National Pressure Ulcer Advisory Panel: *Prevention and treatment of pressure ulcers: Quick reference guide*, Washington DC, 2009, NPUAP.

Ferguson-Pell M, Hirose H, Nicholson G, Call E: Thermodynamic rigid cushion load indenter: A buttock-shaped temperature and humidity measurement system for cushioning surfaces under anatomical compression conditions, *J Rehabil Res Dev* 46:945–956, 2009.

Fernie G, Letts RM: Seating the elderly. In Letts RM, editor: *Principles of seating the disabled*, Boca Raton, FL, 1991, CRC Press.

Field DA, Livingstone R: Clinical tools that measure sitting posture, seated postural control or functional abilities in children with motor impairments: A systematic review, *Clin Rehabil* 27(11):994–1004, 2013.

Field DA, Roxborough LA: Responsiveness of the Seated Postural Control Measure and the Levels of Seating Scale in children with neuromotor disabilities, *Disabil Rehabil Assist Technol* 6:473–482, 2011.

Field DA, Roxborough LA: Validation of the relation between type and amount of seating support required and the Levels of Seating Scale scores for children with neuromotor disabilities, *Dev Neurorehabil* 15:202–208, 2012.

Fife SA, Roxborough LA, Armstrong RW, et al.: Development of a clinical measure of postural control for assessment of adaptive seating intervention in children with neuromotor disabilities, *Phys Ther* 71:981–993, 1991.

Fife SA, Roxborough LA, Story M, et al.: Reliability of a measure to assess outcomes of adaptive seating in children with neuromotor disabilities, *Can J Rehabil* 7:11–13, 1993.

Gagnon B, Noreau L: Vincent C: Reliability of the Seated Postural Control Measure for adult wheelchair users, *Disabil Rehabil* 27:1479–1491, 2005.

Gefen A: How much time does it take to get a pressure ulcer: Integrated evidence from human, animal, and In vitro studies, *Ostomy Wound Care* 54:10–17, 2009.

Geyer MJ, Brienza DM, Bertocci GE, et al.: Wheelchair seating: A state of the science report, *Assist Technol* 15:120–128, 2003.

Geyer MJ, Brienza DM, Karg P, et al.: A randomized control trial to evaluate pressure-reducing seat cushions for elderly wheelchair users, *Adv Skin and Wound Care* 14:120–129, 2001.

Hadcock L, Stevenson J, Morin E ,et al: Pressure measurement applications for humans, *Proceedings of Association of Canadian Ergonomists Conference*, London, ON, August 2003.

Hadders-Algra M, Brogren E, Forssberg H: Development of postural control—Differences between ventral and dorsal muscles? *Neurosci Biobehav Rev* 22:501–506, 1998.

Hadders-Algra M, van der Fits IB, Stremmelaar EF, Touwen BC: Development of postural adjustments during reaching in infants with CP, *Dev Med Child Neurol* 41:766–776, 1999.

Hobson DA: Contributions of posture and deformity to the body-seat interface variables of a person with spinal cord injury, *Proceedings of the Fifth International Seating Symposium*, Memphis, TN, 1989, pp. 153–171.

Houghton P, Campbell K: Canadian Practice Guidelines Panel: *Canadian Best Practice Guidelines for the prevention and management of pressure ulcers in people with spinal cord injury. A resource for clinicians*, 2013. Available from http://www.onf.org.

Kangas KM: Creating mobility within mobility systems, *Rehab Manag* 13:58–60, 62, 2000.

Kosiak M: Etiology of decubitus ulcers, *Arch Phys Med Rehabil* 42:19–29, 1961.

Krause JS, et al.: An exploratory study of pressure ulcers after SCI: Relationship to protective behaviours and risk factors, *Arch Phys Med Rehabil* 82:107–113, 2001.

Lacoste M, Therrien M, Prince F: Stability of children with cerebral palsy in their wheelchair seating: perceptions of parents and children, *Disabil Rehabil Assist Technol* 4:143–150, 2009.

Law M, Baptiste S, Carswell A, et al.: *Canadian Occupational Performance Measure*, Toronto, 2005, CAOT Publications ACE.

Letts RM, editor: *Principles of seating the disabled*, Boca Raton, FL, 1991, CRC Press.

Linder-Ganz E, Gefen A: Mechanical compression-induced pressure sores in rat hindlimb: Muscle stiffness, histology and compression models, *J Appl Physiol* 96:2034–2049, 2004.

Linder-Ganz E, Gefen A: Stress analyses coupled with damage laws to determine biomechanical risk factors for deep tissue injury during sitting, *J Biomech Eng*, 131:011003, 2009.

Low J, Reed D: *Basic biomechanics explained*, Oxford, 1996, Butterworth Heinemann.

Mayall JK, Desharnais G: Positioning in a wheelchair: A guide for professional caregivers of the disabled adult, Thorofare, NJ, 1995, SLACK.

Messick S: Test validity and the ethics of assessment, *Am Psychol* 35:1012–1027, 1980. 10.

Miller Polgar J, Spaulding S, Mandich A, et al: Comparison of occupational performance between two methods of pelvic stabilization, *Proceedings of the Tri-Joint Congress*, Toronto, June 2000.

Minkel JL: Seating SCI clients, *Proceedings of the Sixth Northeast RESNA Regional Conference*, Washington, DC, 1990, RESNA.

National Pressure Ulcer Advisory Panel: *Terms and definitions related to support surfaces. Ver*, January 29, 2007. Available from www.npuap.org. Accessed June 10, 2013.

Norton D, McLaren R, Exton-Smith AN: *An investigation of geriatric nursing problems in hospital*, London, 1975, Churchill Livingstone. Original work published in 1962.

Palisano R, Rosenbaum P, Bartlett D, Livingston MH: Content validity of the expanded and revised Gross Motor Function Classification System, *Dev Med Child Neurol* 50:744–750, 2008.

Pape TL-B, Kim J, Weiner B: The shaping of individual meanings assigned to AT: A review of personal factors, *Disabil Rehabil* 24:5–20, 2002.

Parkinson MB, Chaffin DB, Reed MP: Center of pressure excursion capability in performance of seated lateral-reaching tasks, *Clin Biomech* 21:26–32, 2006.

Pountney TE, Cheek L, Green E, et al.: Content and criterion validation of the Chailey Levels of Ability, *Physiotherapy* 85:410–414, 1999.

Registered Nurses Association of Ontario, Promoting safety: alternative approaches to the use of restraints, Toronto, 2012, Registered Nurses Association of Ontario.

Registered Nurses Association of Ontario: *Risk assessment and prevention of pressure ulcers*, Toronto, 2005, Registered Nurses Association of Ontario. 2011 supplement. Available from www.rnao.ca/bpg/guidelines/risk-assessment-and-pressure-ulcers.

Reswick JB, Rogers JE: Experience at Rancho Los Amigos Hospital with devices and techniques to prevent pressure sores. In Kenedi RM, Cowden JM, Scales JT, editors: *Bedsore biomechanics*, Baltimore, 1976, University Park Press.

Rigby P, Reid D, Schoger S, Ryan S: Effects of a wheelchair-mounted rigid pelvic stabilizer on caregiver assistance for children, *Assist Technol* 13:2–11, 2001.

Rodby-Bousquet E, Agustsson A, et al.: Interrater reliability and construct validity of the Posture and Postural Ability Scale in adults with cerebral palsy in supine, prone, sitting and standing positions, *Clin Rehabil* 28(1):82–90, 2012. 2014.

Russell D, Rosenbaum PL, Wright M, Avery L: *The Gross Motor Function Measure, GMFM-66 and GMFM-88 (user's manual)*, ed 2, London, 2013, Mac Keith Press.

Savelsbergh GJP, Van der Kamp J: The effect of body orientation to gravity on early infant reaching, *J Exp Child Psychol* 8:510–528, 1994.

Siekman A: The biomechanics of seating: a consumer guide, Action Dig March/April:8-9, 1992

Sprigle S: Effects of forces and the selection of support surfaces, *Top Geriatr Rehabil* 16:47–62, 2000.

Sprigle S, Press L, Davis K: Development of uniform terminology and procedures to describe wheelchair cushion characteristics, *J Rehabil Res Dev* 38:449–461, 2001.

Sprigle S, Sonnenblum S: Assessing evidence supporting redistribution of pressure for pressure ulcer prevention: A review, *J Rehab Res Dev* 48:203–214, 2011.

Stekelenburg CWJ, et al.: Compression-induced deep tissue injury examined with magnetic resonance imaging and histology, *J Appl Physiol* 100:1946–1954, 2006.

Stinson M, Porter A, Eakin P: Measuring interface pressure: a laboratory-based investigation into the effects of repositioning on sitting time, *Am J Occup Ther* 56:185–190, 2002.

Swaine J: Seeing the difference, *Rehab Manag* 16(9):26–28, 2003. 30-31.

Tang S: Seat cushions. In Webster JG, editor: *Prevention of pressure sores*, Bristol, UK, 1991, IOP Publishing.

Tredwell S, Roxborough L: Cerebral palsy seating. In Letts RM, editor: *Principles of seating the disabled*, Boca Raton, FL, 1991, CRC Press.

Trefler E, Hobson DA, Taylor SJ: *Seating and mobility for persons with physical disabilities*, Tucson, 1993, Therapy Skill Builders.

Waterlow J: Pressure sores, a risk assessment card, *Nurs Times* 81:49–55, 1985.

Waugh K, Crane BA: *A clinical application guide to standardized wheelchair seating measures of the body and seating support surfaces*, Available from, rev ed, Denver, 2013, University of Colorado/Assistive Technology Partners. www.assistivetechnologypartners.org. Accessed January 10, 2014.

Weiss-Lambrou R, Tremblay C, LeBlanc R, et al.: Wheelchair seating aids: How satisfied are consumers? *Assist Technol* 11:43–52, 1999.

Wolfe DL, Hsieh JTC, Mehta S: Rehabilitation practices and associated outcomes following spinal cord injury. In Eng JJ, Teasell RW, Miller WC, et al, editors: *Spinal cord injury rehabilitation evidence*, version 3.0, 2010. Available from www.scireproject.com. Accessed October 22, 2013.

Woodbury G, Houghton P: Prevalence of pressure ulcers in Canadian health-care settings, *Ostomy Wound Manage* 50:22–38, 2004.

World Health Organization: *International Classification of Functioning, Disability and Health*, Geneva, 2001, World Health Organization.

Zacharkow D: *Wheelchair posture and pressure sores*, Springfield, IL, 1984, Charles C Thomas.

Zacharkow D: *Posture, sitting, standing, chair design and exercise*, Springfield, IL, 1988, Charles C Thomas.

CHAPTER 10

Technologies That Enable Mobility

CHAPTER OUTLINE

Activity Component
Human Component
Disorders Resulting in Mobility Impairments
Mobility Issues Across the Lifespan
Mobility and Obesity
Context Components
Physical Context
Social Context
Cultural Context
Institutional Context
Assessment for Wheeled Mobility
Needs Assessment
Assessment of the Human Factors
Assessment of the Context
Assistive Technology
Supporting Structure
Frame Types
Propelling Structure: Manual
Propelling Structure: Powered
Specialized Bases for Manual Wheelchairs
Specialized Bases for Powered Wheelchairs
Smart Wheelchairs
Wheelchair Standards
Implementation and Training for Manual and Powered Mobility
Fitting of Mobility Systems
Maintenance and Repair of Personal Mobility Systems
Developing Mobility Skills for Manual and Powered Systems
Outcome Evaluation
Outcome Evaluation Instruments
Outcomes of Wheeled Mobility Device Use
Summary

LEARNING OBJECTIVES

On completing this chapter, you will be able to:

1. Identity the activity, human, and contextual influences on the use of wheeled mobility
2. Describe the assessment of the consumer for a mobility system
3. Describe the two primary structures of wheelchairs
4. Identify the major characteristics of manual wheelchairs
5. Describe the classifications of powered mobility systems and their characteristics
6. Understand the influence of the relationship between the center of gravity of the user and the center of mass of the wheelchair on the function of the wheelchair
8. Describe the key elements of implementation and training for the use of wheeled mobility devices
9. Identify standardized assessments that are specific to use of wheeled mobility devices

KEY TERMS

Alignment
Anti-Tip Devices
Armrests
Bariatrics
Bariatric Chair
Camber
Center of Mass
Center of Gravity
Dependent Mobility
Footplate
Front Rigging
Independent Manual Mobility
Independent Powered Mobility
Legrest
Lightweight Wheelchair
Lightweight High-Strength Wheelchair
Low-Shear Systems
Manual Wheelchair
Nonproportional Control
Powered Wheelchair
Propelling Structure
Proportional Control
Push Handles
Recline
Rigid Sport Ultralightweight Wheelchair
Scooter
Shear
Smart Wheelchair
Standard Wheelchair
Standing Frame
Standing Wheelchair
Supporting Structure
Tilt
Ultralightweight Wheelchair
Wheel Lock

Mobility is fundamental to each individual's quality of life and is necessary for functioning in each of the performance areas: self-care, work or school, and play or leisure. As we have described for other activity outputs, limitations to functional mobility can be either augmented or replaced with assistive technologies. The activity output of ambulation can be augmented with low-tech aids such as canes, walkers, or crutches or replaced by wheeled mobility systems of various types. In addition to the functional gain of increased independence in mobility, other goals such as positive self-image, social interaction, and health maintenance are achieved. In this chapter we focus on manual and powered wheelchair systems to enhance an individual's mobility. Our emphasis is on the total process of delivering these systems to those who need them, from initial need and goal setting, through assessment and recommendation, to implementation and training.

ACTIVITY COMPONENT

This chapter discusses personal mobility (i.e., the ability to move oneself from one place to another) within a building, around and outside a building, or between buildings. Personal mobility is distinguished from mobility achieved through the use of any form of transportation, private or public (see Chapter 11). The World Health Organization's Classification of Functioning identifies mobility as an activity, rather than an impairment of a body structure or function (WHO, 2001). Only one sub-classification, moving around using equipment, specifically refers to the use of mobility devices. When using the ICF for its intended purpose of classification of factors that influence a health condition, the other categories of the mobility classification exclude anyone who uses a mobility device to get around. However, for the purposes of this discussion, relevant mobility classifications will be identified to illustrate different aspects of mobility.

The ICF describes moving around inside different types of buildings, including the home and community. Moving inside a building involves getting in and out of a building, moving to different locations, moving between floors, and moving outside and around a building. The ICF mobility chapter also describes moving between buildings (i.e., leaving one building and traveling to another one).

Use of transportation to move around is also included in the ICF mobility chapter, including traveling as a passenger or as the driver. This classification explicitly excludes the use of mobility devices, for the purposes of the ICF. However, for our purposes, we think about a wheelchair used as a seat in some form of vehicle and the requirements to lift a mobility device in and out of a vehicle.

Mobility is a foundational activity for many other skills and activities. It enables a person to move to or about a location where the activity will be completed, whether that is within a building or in the community and beyond. Several authors describe the lack of access to mobility devices (Buck, 2009; Mortensen et al., 2005) as a limitation to full participation in society.

Mobility using a wheelchair is an activity itself that has received considerable attention to describe the skills that are required for competence. Measures such as the Wheelchair Skills Test (Kirby et al., 2002; Kirby et al., 2004) identify different wheelchair skills that range from basic use of the wheelchair, such as engaging and disengaging the brakes, basic maneuvers such as moving the wheelchair forward a short distance, and complex maneuvers such as climbing a curb or popping a wheelie. These skills are important when understanding the activity of mobility when using a wheelchair.

The wheelchair assessment identifies the occupations in which the individual will engage while using a wheelchair. Because the wheelchair and seating components are a unit, the occupations identified include both those for which seated support is of primary importance and those for which mobility is required. For example, in the workplace, seated support is of primary importance when considering work occupations that are completed at a desk. Mobility becomes important when the individual moves about the building to access different locations or to enter and exit. Both types of occupations influence the recommendations derived from the results of the wheelchair assessment.

The frequency of use of the wheelchair is another activity consideration. Some clients require use of their chair for most of their waking hours, perhaps transferring to another seat in the evening when they are relaxing, but otherwise using the wheelchair on a full-time basis. Alternatively, some clients may only need a wheelchair when the need for mobility over an extended time arises and fatigue or some other condition interferes. For example, some clients may use a wheelchair on a part-time basis when they go out into the community for extended times or for moving around large sites such as an airport. In other situations, such as moving about the home, a wheelchair is not required because their mobility abilities enable them to move safely in another way.

Understanding the activity of mobility also requires knowledge of how the wheelchair is used—is the client independent in all wheelchair skills or are there some instances when assistance is needed? For example, a client who uses a wheelchair on a part-time basis may not have developed sufficient skills to maneuver it safely, and so requires assistance from other persons. Another client who is developing wheelchair skills or who is unable to learn advanced skills like a wheelie, may only require assistance for specific skills. A competent wheelchair user, who uses it on a full-time basis, likely requires assistance rarely, in unusual circumstances (e.g., moving the chair across sand or snow).

Mobility, the ability to move around in and among locations, is both an activity on its own and one that supports other activities. When considering the activity component of wheelchair mobility, the clinician seeks to understand the frequency with which the wheelchair is used, the assistance required and the circumstances under which that assistance is needed, the wheelchair skills available and needed, when and how the wheelchair will be transported, and other occupations that are conducted while seated in the wheelchair.

HUMAN COMPONENT

A significant increase in the number of individuals using mobility systems, across many countries, is related to three trends: (1) the increasing proportion of older adults in many countries (WHO, 2011), (2) the rising rates of obesity (WHO, 2008, 2011), and (3) accessibility legislation. The population of most developing countries is aging, with the proportion of older individuals (65 years and older) ranging from a low of 10% in South Africa to a high of ≈40% in Japan by 2050, for OECD countries reporting these projections (Ministry of Industry, 2010). The projection for the United States is that 20.2% of the population will be over 65 years of age. The Canadian estimate is 22.1% (Ministry of Industry, 2010). The proportion of individuals reporting a disability increases substantially with age (Ministry of Industry, 2010). Age-related physical changes such as arthritis result in mobility impairments that require the use of mobility devices (Ministry of Industry, 2010).

The proportion of morbidly obese individuals is rising, particularly in North America, which has resulted in the development of mobility devices specifically designed to support the increased size and weight of these individuals (WHO, 2008). **Bariatric chairs** are now available for these individuals whose mobility is impaired by obesity and related chronic diseases.

Accessibility legislation in many countries has reduced physical and institutional barriers to community participation of individuals with disabilities, with the result that more people are using mobility devices for instrumental activities of daily living. This type of legislation affects the incidence of wheelchair use in two ways: mandating construction of physical environments that are accessible to individuals who use a wheelchair and defining funding mechanisms to support the acquisition of mobility devices. Relevant legislation is discussed in Chapter 3.

Data collected in the 2000 U.S. census indicate that 20.9 million U.S. families have at least one individual with a disability living in their household (Wang, 2005). Of these, 16.6% report a physical disability that results in a functional limitation. The Profile of Disability in Canada indicates that 13.7% of the Canadian population reports a mobility impairment (Cossette, 2002).

Kaye, Kang, and LePlante (2002) provide information on the number of Americans who use mobility devices. These data are derived from the 1994–1995 National Health Interview Survey on Disability (NHIS-D). The survey indicated that 1.6 million Americans who live outside of an institutional setting use a mobility device. The vast majority of these individuals (1.5 million) use a manual wheelchair (Kaye et al., 2002). Elderly individuals (65 years of age or older) have the highest rate of mobility use, accounting for 57.5% of manual wheelchair users and 69.7% of power wheelchair users (Kaye et al., 2002). The WHO report on the Guidelines on the Provision of Manual Wheelchairs in Less-Resourced Countries (WHO, 2008) estimates 1% of the population in developing countries requires a wheelchair.

Disorders Resulting in Mobility Impairments

There are many causes of mobility impairment. Disorders that result in mobility impairment may be neurological, musculoskeletal, or cognitive in nature. Bear in mind that not all individuals with a given diagnosis experience a similar impairment in mobility. The onset of the disorder, whether it was acquired or congenital, also affects the individual's mobility needs.

Kaye et al. (2002) present the top 10 conditions in the United States that result in use of a wheelchair or scooter. Individuals who have had a stroke are the leading group of mobility device users (11.1%) (Kaye at al., 2002). Additional neurological disorders that may result in mobility impairment include cerebral palsy, Guillain-Barré syndrome, Huntington's chorea, traumatic brain injury, muscular dystrophy, Parkinson's disease, poliomyelitis, spinal cord injury, spina bifida, and multiple sclerosis. Symptoms commonly seen in these neurological disorders are muscle weakness or paralysis, sensory deficits, and abnormal muscle tone. All these disorders can lead to limitations with joint range of motion, postural control, and mobility. The individual may also have cognitive and sensory impairments as a result of the disorder.

Orthopedic and rheumatological conditions account for another large group of mobility device users (Kaye et al., 2002). Some of the symptoms commonly seen in individuals with arthritis include painful, swollen, and stiff joints (particularly in hand and wrist); muscle weakness, muscle wasting around the affected joints, complaints of feeling fatigued, and, in later stages, joint contractures resulting in range-of-motion limitations. Other disorders that affect the musculoskeletal system and may result in mobility impairments include ankylosing spondylitis, osteogenesis imperfecta, osteoporosis, Paget's disease, and scoliosis. Individuals with a lower extremity amputation, acquired or congenital, may also use a mobility device.

Diabetes, cardiorespiratory conditions, and obesity are chronic conditions that may require the use of a mobility device. Frequently, fatigue or restrictions related to energy expenditure are the reasons for use of a mobility device with this population. Amputations resulting from complications due to diabetes may also lead to the use of a mobility device.

Disorders that affect an individual's cognitive functioning and ability to learn, such as Alzheimer's disease and cognitive impairment, can also be associated with mobility impairments. In the first instance, dementia, the adult wheelchair user may require special consideration of safety measures if the user has limited memory or insight concerning safe mobility (Mortenson et al., 2005). For example, as the cognitive impairment progresses, judgment can become impaired. A client at this stage may not recognize unsafe situations such as a stairwell and attempt to propel the chair down stairs or may not be able to control anger and use the wheelchair as a weapon and propel it into another person. In situations where cognitive impairment limits safe mobility, modifications are required to wheelchair skills training to simplify instructions and give additional wayfinding cues in familiar environments; measures such as use of seatbelts may be used for safety; and considerations given to the ability of the caregiver to push, lift, and stow the chair when this assistance is required. A wheelchair seatbelt may be considered a restraint in some jurisdictions. A summary of best practices for use of restraints is provided in Chapter 9.

Warren (1990) proposes a classification system that is useful to understand ambulation needs. The degree of limitation in mobility varies across a broad scope, as shown in Box 10-1. At one end of the range are individuals who are considered *marginal ambulators*. At the opposite end of the range are those individuals who have severe mobility limitations and are dependent in manual mobility, with powered mobility being their only option for independence.

Warren (1990) describes marginal ambulators as able to move independently in their environment but functional only at a slow rate or for short distances. Persons who have marginal ambulating skills can benefit from part-time use of a powered mobility device such as a scooter, which allows them to walk inside the home using a walker or cane and use a powered device within the home to augment ambulation. Next are individuals who are exclusive users of manual wheelchairs. They may rely on a caregiver to propel the wheelchair or they propel a manual wheelchair using one of three methods: (1) using both upper extremities, (2) using both lower extremities, or (3) using an upper and lower extremity on the same side of the body (e.g., a person who has had a stroke). *Marginal manual wheelchair users* are able to propel a wheelchair manually but have upper body weakness, respiratory problems, or postural asymmetry as a result of pushing that limits their ability to propel a manual chair for a prolonged time (Warren, 1990). Marginal manual wheelchair users may also include individuals who formerly used a manual wheelchair for their mobility needs and have sustained an overuse injury from propelling the chair. Propelling a wheelchair for any length of time depletes the energy of these individuals and compromises their productivity in other areas of life. Marginal manual wheelchair users can benefit from powered mobility on a full-time or part-time basis.

BOX 10-1 Scope of Mobility Limitations

Full ambulator: no mobility impairment

Marginal ambulator: can walk short distances; may need wheelchair at times, particularly outside the home

Manual wheelchair user: has some method of propelling a manual wheelchair, whether it is with both upper extremities, both lower extremities, or one upper and one lower extremity

Marginal manual wheelchair user: may have upper extremity injury caused by overuse, or manual wheelchair mobility may not be the most efficient means of mobility for the person; manual wheelchair is used part of the time and powered wheelchair part of the time

Totally/severely mobility-impaired user: unable to propel self independently in a manual wheelchair; dependent mobility base, or powered mobility base the only option for independent mobility

Mobility Issues Across the Lifespan

Mobility needs differ across the lifespan. In this section, we focus on two issues that warrant special attention: (1) powered mobility for young children, and (2) mobility for older adults.

The use of powered mobility by young children is an area that has received a great deal of attention in the last decade. In the past, powered mobility was deemed inappropriate for young children for a number of reasons. These concerns were related to the ability of children to operate a powered wheelchair safely, the initial cost of the wheelchair and cost of replacing it as the child grows, and possible detrimental effects on physical development if the child depends on a powered system instead of self-locomotion (Kermoian, 1998). Recent literature supports the provision of powered mobility to young children (Rosen et al., 2009; Furumasu, Guerette, & Teft, 2004; Kangas, 2010).

Opportunities for early mobility have widespread benefits to the child, not only physically, but cognitively and socially (Deitz, Swinth, & White, 2002; Jones, McEwen, & Neas, 2012; Rosen et al., 2009). Children who are able to move independently in their environment can initiate interactions with others; they don't need to wait for another person to take them where they want to go.

Most current literature suggests that affording the opportunity for mobility should occur at an appropriate developmental time. The goal of such mobility is not to learn how to control a chair, but to experience movement within the environment and to engage in relevant functional tasks, supported by mobility. As with any young child, it is the responsibility of the parent, caregiver, or clinician to ensure a safe environment in which the child can explore and experience mobility (Kangas, 2010; Rosen et al., 2009).

Some needs that are specific to the older adult wheelchair user have been identified in the literature. Comfort, safety, increased function, and a feeling of security when moving in their environment have been identified as important needs related to seating and mobility for residents of long-term care facilities (Mendoza et al., 2003; Mortenson et al., 2005; Mortenson et al., 2006). The older adult wheelchair user may depend on another person to push the wheelchair. Therefore a mobility device that can be used easily by an attendant is important (Buck, 2009; Ham, Aldersea, & Porter, 1998). Safety and security are deemed important for the user of the wheelchair, as well as for the care provider. For instance, it is important that the care provider be able to transfer a person in and out of the wheelchair safely. Both the user and the care provider will be more inclined to use a wheelchair that is comfortable, safe, secure, and easy to use.

Mobility and Obesity

Wheelchairs that target the bariatric client are a recent development in wheelchair design. **Bariatrics** is a term that describes the practice of medicine concerning individuals who are significantly overweight. It is derived from the Greek "baros" meaning weight and "iatrics" meaning medical treatment. In some situations, the client's obesity is the cause of the mobility impairment. Obesity has become a major health problem in North America. The Center for Disease Control data (CDC, 2006) report a growing trend in the prevalence of obesity (generally defined as a BMI of 30 or over). In 1995, the prevalence of obesity was less than 20% in all states. In 2000, 28% of states reported obesity prevalence of less than 20%, but by 2005 this incidence had dropped to only 4 states. The 2005 figures further indicate that 17 states report a prevalence of obesity of equal to or greater than 25% and 3 report a prevalence rate of equal to or greater than 30% (CDC, 2006).

Diabetes is a serious chronic health condition that is associated with obesity. Mobility in this population is restricted by the excessive weight, low physical endurance, cardiorespiratory complications, and complications arising from diabetes including vision impairment, circulatory and sensory impairments, and amputation. Typical wheelchairs have standard weight limits up to 300 pounds. Chairs for bariatric clients are capable of supporting weights up to 600 pounds and in some cases up to 1000 pounds. Examples of these chairs will be described later in this chapter. Clients who are morbidly obese present specific challenges when measuring for a wheelchair, as will be discussed later.

CONTEXT COMPONENTS

Physical Context

The *physical contexts* in which the mobility device is used influence the client's ability to use the chair and the type of chair recommended as a result of the wheelchair assessment. Some key considerations include: Will the device be used both indoors and outdoors? How accessible are these environments? Width of doorways, floor surfaces, bathroom layout, and access to the structure (e.g., ramp, stairs) all need to be considered. On what type of surfaces will the consumer travel when using the device outdoors? Does the user expect or need to transport the device between different locations such as home, school, or work? How will the user and the mobility device travel (e.g., will he or she use a private vehicle or public transportation)? Does the user access other modes of transportation such as trains or airplanes or school bus?

The ability to use the chair and the type of chair recommended vary if the client only uses it indoors versus when both indoor and outdoor use are required. Exclusive indoor use often means the client propels the chair on two types of surfaces—hard floors such as wood, ceramic, or linoleum or softer surfaces such as carpeting. The width of doorways and hallways and the travel space around furniture may be restricted in the home, office, or school environment. In contrast, when the client uses the chair both indoors and outdoors, different considerations for the travel surface and the type of travel are made. Outdoor surfaces vary in terms of terrain (e.g., sand, gravel, grass, concrete), and presence of slopes and potholes and other obstructions. These obstacles affect the choice of tire and the ability to maneuver both a manual and power wheelchair. Distances traveled are a factor here, affecting both the individual's endurance level and battery charge time.

Just as the climate was a factor in the recommendation concerning a seating system, it also influences the recommendation of a mobility device. A different recommendation for device may be made if the consumer lives in a climate where snow is a typical part of winter and he or she expects to use the device outdoors versus a consumer who lives in a climate where snow and cold temperatures are not a routine expectation. Additionally, when the wheelchair is used outdoors, the travel surface will be affected by rain (e.g., softening natural surfaces such as grass or creating puddles). Rain and snow also affect the durability of the wheelchair and the performance of electronic components.

Clients who live in rural or remote locations face different conditions than those who live in urban conditions. In the first instance, clients may need to travel longer distances, may have less access to accessible buildings or sidewalks, and few opportunities for accessible public transportation. These clients may not have ready access to clinicians or technicians when problems arise related to their use of the wheelchair.

Social Context

Family members, peers, and others in the social environment can influence the choice and use of a mobility device. Peers with experience with various mobility devices can be a great source of information and share their knowledge of what works and what does not. Conversely, peers and families may exert pressure in the choice of a manual versus a power wheelchair. The individual may prefer to use a power chair because it allows him or her to conserve energy for other occupations but may be viewed as lazy by others for choosing this technology. The willingness or ability of decision makers in the school, workplace, and other community environments to accommodate various types of mobility devices also needs to be considered. Lack of knowledge of necessary accommodations by an employer may result in a work environment that is not physically accessible to the client. In this instance, it is the employer's lack of information that is limiting rather than the actual physical barriers.

Cultural Context

The cultural context affects wheelchair use and recommendation in three ways: values related to cultural and societal inclusivity, availability of technology, and access to technology. A culture that values inclusivity seeks to implement strategies and programs that enable full societal and community participation by all citizens. The United Nations Convention on the Rights of Persons with Disabilities (UN, 2006) declares the rights of all persons, regardless of abilities, to full participation and identifies elements that comprise full participation. Signatories of this convention commit to establishing ways of meeting all of the goals identified in the articles that make up this convention.

Availability of technology means all residents of a given country can acquire the necessary devices. The WHO *World Report on Disability* (2011) indicates that provision of assistive technology must suit the environment and the user and provide adequate follow-up. Such provision requires the technology to fit the intended user and support the user's needs as well as be useful in his or her environment. For example, a client who lives in a remote area that does not have paved roads will have a difficult time maneuvering a wheelchair that has smooth tires over dirt paths.

The WHO document *Guidelines on the Provision of Manual Wheelchairs in Less-Resourced Countries* (WHO, 2008) lists further principles relevant to the provision of these devices. These principles include: (1) the device is acceptable to the users and others in the environment, (2) users are able to access these devices, (3) the device is adaptable to the needs of the user and the context in which it will be used, (4) devices are affordable, (5) available, and (6) the device is of high quality (WHO, 2008).

When inclusion of all citizens is valued and technology is available, the last aspect is that technology is accessible. Legislation, policy, and other programs that assist clients to acquire technology are also important components of the cultural context. Cultures that recognize the rights of all citizens take steps to establish funding mechanisms to ensure some reasonable access to technology, in this case mobility technology, to support full participation.

Institutional Context

Institutional regulations and policies influence the recommendation of a mobility device. The clinician must be aware of the criteria for funding these devices in his or her jurisdiction, including who is eligible for funding, requirements for stability of client condition, restrictions on where the device must be used, and the requirements of client performance (e.g., the ability to propel a wheelchair a specific distance without assistance). The clinician considers the client's future needs and the implications that a current recommendation will have on the ability to access an appropriate mobility device in the future. For example, some funding programs have a specified time during which replacement of an existing system is not funded. Further, some stipulate that if a person receives one type of mobility device (e.g., manual or powered wheelchair), a second mobility device will not be funded for a specified length of time.

As mentioned previously, legislation such as the Americans with Disabilities Act (ADA, 1990) defines access to environments and technology. These types of legislation define the different types of environmental accessibility features required and the conditions under which they must be implemented (e.g., new construction, renovations of buildings of a certain age). They further identify who has the responsibility to fund the construction of accessibility features. In addition, such legislation identifies conditions of employment, access to public facilities, and education that affect access to mobility devices.

Individual institutions, such as long-term care or skilled nursing facilities, frequently have policies that affect wheelchair use. Some of these policies limit the resident's ability to use a wheelchair if the resident has repeatedly demonstrated use of the chair that threatens the safety of themselves or others in the environment (Mendoza et al., 2003). Some institutions will not allow residents access to power wheelchairs due to concerns regarding maintenance and safety. Other policies establish responsibilities for daily and long-term maintenance of the chair and transportation when the user takes it between locations.

ASSESSMENT FOR WHEELED MOBILITY

Commonly, the assessment described in Chapter 9 to determine the most appropriate seating components is the same assessment that determines the wheeled mobility base. Consequently, the discussion of the assessment that was presented in Chapter 9 will not be repeated here.

Needs Assessment

The goal of wheeled mobility intervention is to support the user's ability to move in the environment (i.e., the mobility output of the activity component of the HAAT model). Consistent with the HAAT model described in Chapters 1 and 3, the evaluation to determine the most appropriate wheeled mobility base starts with an assessment of the activities in which the individual wishes to engage while using mobility technology. Will the mobility device be used primarily to move from one place to another in the community or will the individual use it as the primary means of mobility and consequently perform most activities (e.g., ADL, work, and leisure occupations) while seated in the device? The clinician determines which activities are important and necessary for the user to complete as well as those in which the user wishes to engage. Further, the level of assistance the user requires to complete these activities is determined. As mentioned earlier, the client may complete these activities independently, with the assistance of another person, or with the use of other technology. In the latter case, it is necessary to consider the interface between the wheelchair and other technology, such as a communication device, that will be used.

Assessment of the Human Factors

Box 10-2 identifies the factors that should be considered when selecting a mobility base for a consumer. Some of this information is available through the client's chart or background information. Examples of this background information include client living situation (alone, with others, and type of accommodation), diagnosis (including length of time since onset), existing technology, and age. The consumer

BOX 10-2 Factors to Consider When Selecting a Wheelchair

Consumer profile: Disability, date of onset, prognosis, size, and weight
Consumer needs: Activities, contexts of use (e.g., accessibility, indoor/outdoor), preferences, transportation, reliability, durability, cost
Physical and sensory skills: Range of motion, motor control, strength, vision, perception
Functional skills: Transfers and ability to propel (manual or powered)

profile provides background information about the client. Knowing whether an impairment is acute or long-term, relatively stable, or progressive influences the choice of wheeled mobility. A client who has a progressive impairment such as amyotrophic lateral sclerosis (ALS) will lose function over time, so the clinician should be alert to signs that the wheelchair is no longer meeting the client's needs. For example, a client whose motor function is declining may show fatigue when propelling a manual wheelchair over a distance that was easy for her or him to travel earlier. Alternatively, a client who uses a joystick to control a power wheelchair may show loss of ability to reliably stop the chair or control its speed. Clients whose cognitive abilities are declining may become lost in familiar surroundings, use their chairs inappropriately to intentionally run into people or objects, or forget how to control the chair.

Noting changes in a client's weight or posture will also provide clues that the wheeled mobility device (and seating system) is no longer adequate. The individual's physical and sensory skills are evaluated for range of motion, strength, motor control, skin integrity, vision, and perception. This assessment also includes determining the user's optimal control site and interface for propelling the wheelchair. Information on the person's weight and size is gathered to determine the size and capacity of the wheelchair. Measurements of the person's leg length, thigh length, back height to base of scapula, back height to top of shoulder, and hip breadth are taken while the person is sitting (refer to the discussion in Chapter 9). An obese person will need a bariatric wheelchair. Clients who are obese should be measured while sitting because adipose tissue spreads when they lie down, resulting in inaccurate measurements (Daus, 2003). If the consumer is a child and is expected to grow, that expected change needs to be reflected in the decision making as well.

The person's functional abilities are also evaluated. Two elements are important. The first is evaluation of different ADLs and IADLs. In addition to identifying in which occupations the individual wishes to engage, this evaluation will determine how they complete those activities. The second element involves evaluation of wheelchair skills. The Wheelchair Skills Test (WST)[1] (Kirby et al., 2002; Kirby et al., 2004) is a well-developed, standardized measure of various wheelchair skills. This test assesses the individual's ability to perform basic wheelchair skills such as removal of an armrest and application of the brakes to more complex, advanced skills such as performing a wheelie to negotiate a curb. This test is one of the few that has had extensive research in all phases of its development. In addition to the evaluation, a training program has also been developed and evaluated. Information about this test and the training program are available at www.wheelchairskillsprogram.ca.

When an individual has a severe mobility limitation, powered mobility may be the best option to gain functional mobility. These individuals often have a manual wheelchair, propelled by a caregiver, as a back-up chair. Powered mobility devices have the potential to enable the user's participation in school, work, leisure, and other community-based activities. The control interfaces (see Chapter 7) available today make it possible for someone with only one or two movements, for example lateral flexion of the head or shoulder rotation, to operate a powered wheelchair; however, perceptual, cognitive, and behavioral impairments may prevent individuals from using a powered wheelchair even if they have the necessary motor skills. For example, a client with a visual-spatial impairment may have difficulty navigating a cluttered environment if she or he cannot maintain a safe distance from people or objects in the environment. When the individual also uses an augmentative communication system or an adapted van, integration of all of these devices is considered at the time of selection of the most appropriate mobility device. All mobility device users will require a system to support their seating needs (see Chapter 9).

[1] Wheelchair Skills Test 4.1 Manual, http://www.wheelchairskillsprogram.ca/eng/manual.htm.

Assessment of the Context

Physical Context

The previous discussion on the physical context identified several questions about the context in which the wheelchair will be used that influence the recommendation. Where possible, the clinician should visit the client's home to determine any limitations this environment poses for use of the chair. Often it is not possible to visit other relevant environments, such as the work or school environment (although the latter may be possible). In this situation, the clinician uses the interview to understand the issues related to wheelchair use across environments. Similarly, the clinician asks about transportation to determine the fit between wheelchair and mode of transportation.

Social Context

As described earlier, the clinician determines who is in the environments in which the wheelchair will be used and their influence on its use. Where appropriate, the clinician identifies who the caregiver is and the issues that may affect his or her ability to support wheelchair use. For example, the clinician determines if the caregiver is able to assist with transfers, propelling the wheelchair when needed, lifting and moving the wheelchair (e.g., into and out of a vehicle), securing it in a vehicle, and providing routine care and maintenance. If multiple caregivers will assist the individual, as sometimes is the case with home care providers, the clinician and the client should identify potential aspects of the use of the wheelchair that might prove a challenge for a caregiver unfamiliar with the client and the technology. In this case, strategies for educating each caregiver are developed.

The influence of others in the environment, such as employers and school personnel, is also considered. In the work environment, the clinician determines whether any policies exist that might limit the client's ability to function in the environment with a wheelchair, for example, access to accessible washrooms or a height adjustable desk that will accommodate the chair. Similar considerations are made in the school environment related to the knowledge and attitudes of school personnel related to accommodation of a person using a wheelchair.

Institutional Context

Policies, legislation, and regulations related to funding, access, and wheelchair use were identified in an earlier section of this chapter. The clinician has the responsibility to become familiar with all of the institutional elements, particularly policies and practices that will affect acquisition and use of the wheelchair, before making a recommendation and providing the supporting documentation for funding.

ASSISTIVE TECHNOLOGY

In this section we discuss the major characteristics of manual and powered mobility systems. Table 10-1 lists the major manufacturers of personal mobility systems. Modern mobility systems are more flexible and capable of being adapted to a variety of functional tasks. These adaptations may include height adjustment, tilt, recline, axle position adjustment, and combinations of all of these.

The selection of a wheelchair is based on the evaluation discussed in the previous section and is a process of matching characteristics to the consumer's needs and skills (Scherer, 2002). To meet the varied needs of individuals with mobility impairments, there are three broad categories of wheeled mobility systems: dependent mobility, independent manual

TABLE 10-1 Major Wheelchair Manufacturers

Manufacturer	Type of Wheelchairs	Web Address
Altimate Medical, Inc. 800-342-8968	Standing systems	www.easystand.com
Amigo Mobility International, Inc. 800-692-6446	Scooters	www.myamigo.com
Bruno Independent Living Aids 800-882-8183	Adult and pediatric scooters, sedan and van wheelchair lifts	www.bruno.com
Columbia Medical 800-454-6612	Dependent mobility bases	www.columbiamedical.com
Convaid, Inc	Dependent mobility bases, transport chairs	www.convaid.com
ConvaQuip	Bariatric wheelchairs	www.convaquip.com
Etac (in the USA) Balder USA, Inc. 888-422-5337	Independent manual wheelchairs for children and adults	www.etac.com
Freedom Designs 800-554-8044	Pediatric wheelchairs, tilt-in-space wheelchairs	www.freedomdesigns.com
Invacare 800-333-6900	Manual, power, and sports wheelchairs	www.invacare.com
Levo USA, Inc. 888-538-6872	Manual and powered stand-up wheelchairs for adults and children	www.levo.ch
Mulholland Positioning Systems, Inc. 800-543-4769	A variety of standing systems, pediatric wheeled bases and tilt bases	www.mulhollandinc.com
Otto Bock 800-328-4058	Pediatric seating and positioning, adult positioning, manual and power wheelchairs	www.ottobockus.com
PDG 888-858-4422	Wheelchairs for individuals with special needs, such as bariatric chairs, high agitation, and manual tilt wheelchairs	www.pdgmobility.com
Permobil, Inc. 800-736-0925	Stand-up powered wheelchairs; powered wheelchair with elevating seat; sports wheelchairs, lightweight manual wheelchairs	www.permobil.com
Pride Mobility Products Corp. USA 800-800-8586 Canada 888-570-1113	Manual and electrically powered wheelchairs, scooters	www.pridemobility.com
Snug Seat 800-336-7684	Specialty bases for children and adults, car seats, dependent and independent mobility bases, pediatric wheelchairs	www.snugseat.com
Sunrise Medical 800-333-4000	Dependent and independent manual bases, sports wheelchairs, lightweight manual wheelchairs, powered wheelchairs, add-on power unit; adult and pediatric wheelchairs, tilt wheelchairs, and scooters	www.sunrisemedical.com
TiLite 800-545-2266	Adult and pediatric titanium wheelchairs; manual wheelchair; sports wheelchair; ASK – see power	www.tilite.com

mobility, and independent powered mobility. **Dependent mobility** systems are propelled by an attendant and include strollers and transport chairs, as well as a manual chair that is propelled by an attendant. A dependent mobility system is chosen when (1) the individual is not at all capable of independently propelling a wheelchair or (2) a secondary system is needed that is lightweight and easily transported. An **independent manual mobility** system is for those individuals who have the ability to propel a wheelchair manually. These bases have two large wheels in the back and two smaller front wheels that allow the user to propel independently. **Independent powered mobility** systems are required when the user has difficulty propelling a **manual wheelchair**. These are **powered wheelchairs** that are driven by the user.

Within each of these categories there are many commercial options available to meet the needs of the individual user. In this section we discuss the characteristics of mobility systems, starting with the wheelchair's two basic structures: a supporting structure and a propelling structure. Figure 10-1 shows the anatomy of a folding manual wheelchair. Figure 10-2 shows the anatomy of a rigid frame manual wheelchair.

Supporting Structure

The **supporting structure** of the wheelchair consists of the frame and attachments to it. Specialized seating and positioning (see Chapter 9) is often considered part of the supporting structure. Accessories to the frame (e.g., armrests, footrests) are also a part of the supporting structure. In some wheelchairs these accessories are manufactured as part of the frame. Some supporting structures are unique in that they are adjustable to allow for changes in the orientation of the user in space, including systems that provide tilt or support in a standing position.

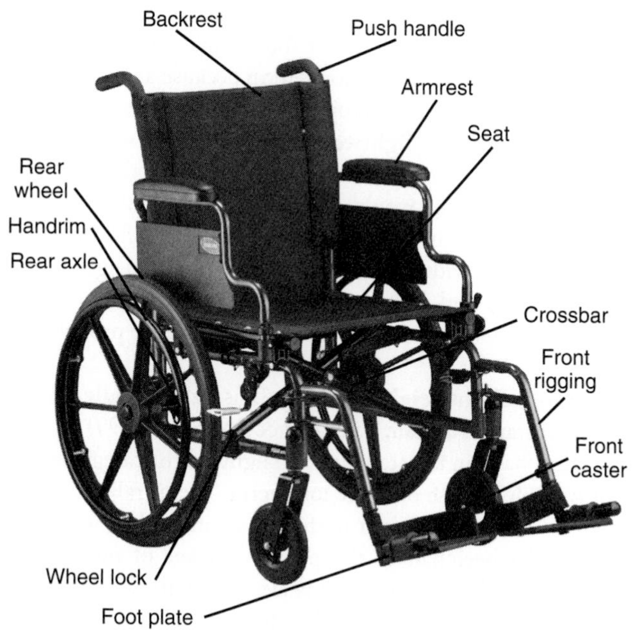

FIGURE 10-1 Manual wheelchair showing the major parts of the supporting and propelling structures.

Frame Types

Three underlying factors will be discussed before describing different classifications of manual wheelchairs: type of frame (rigid or folding), adjustability of the position of the axle of the rear wheel and material used to construct the wheelchair frame.

Frames may be either folding or rigid, and there are three common frame styles (Cooper, 1998). Rigid frames are available in a box, cantilever, and T or I frame style. Typically the box frame construction (Figure 10-3) has a rectangular shape that provides a strong and durable base to which the seat and wheels are attached. Lighter weight designs are accomplished by replacing the box with a single bar extending between the wheels, forming a cantilever structure. Upright tubes from this main support are used to attach the seat and back. The footrests are extensions of the seat rails. The T construction uses a bar similar to the cantilever

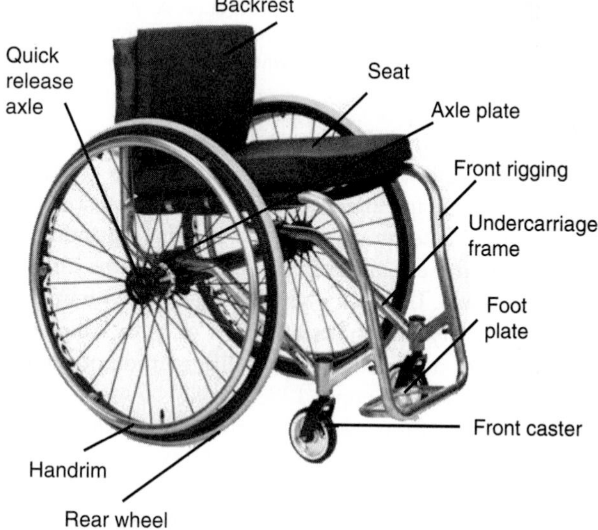

FIGURE 10-2 Rigid frame wheelchair showing the major parts of the supporting and propelling structures.

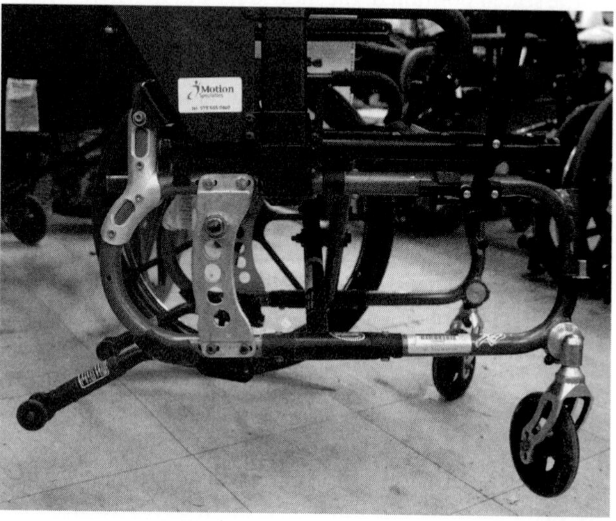

FIGURE 10-3 Rigid frame wheelchair with a box frame style.

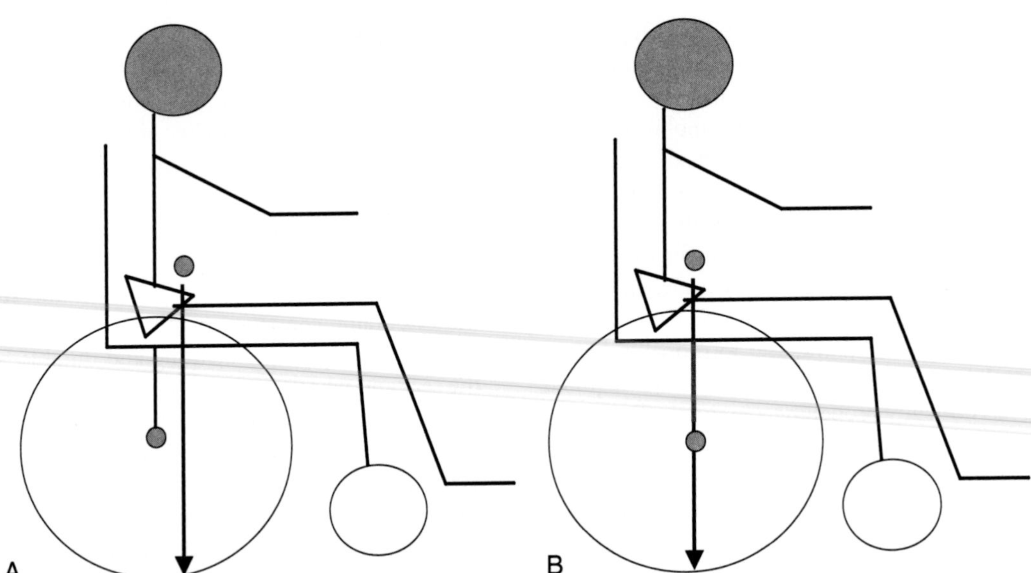

FIGURE 10-4 Relationship of the center of mass of the user to the axle of the wheel affects the mobility and stability of the chair. **A,** When the user is seated with his center of mass ahead of the axle of the wheelchair, the chair is more stable. **B,** When the user is seated with his center of mass directly above the axle of the wheelchair, the chair is more mobile.

design but has a single bar attached to the center of the cantilever that connects to a single front caster. This configuration forms a T shape under the seat. If two front casters are used, then the T becomes an I shape. For transportation, the wheels on all these chairs are removed, and in some cases the back folds down. The choice between rigid or box frame and folding frame styles involves a number of factors, including the consumer's needs, functional ability, method of transfer, and level of activity (Cooper, 1998).

The position of the axle of the drive wheel relative to the user's **center of gravity** affects the stability and maneuverability of the wheelchair. Figure 10-4 shows this relationship. The center of mass of an empty wheelchair is located under the seat, in front of the drive wheels (Engstrom, 2002). When the user is seated in the wheelchair, the center of mass moves above the seat and forward and backward depending on the seated position of the individual and the drive wheels.

When the center of mass is forward of the axis of the drive wheels, more weight is placed on the castors, making it more difficult to lift them (Engstrom, 2002). The chair is more stable but less maneuverable in this configuration. As the center of mass moves backward, closer to the axis of the drive wheel or even slightly behind it, stability decreases and maneuverability increases.

Understanding this relationship is important when setting up the chair. An active user will want a configuration that is easily maneuverable and allows him or her to perform a wheelie (i.e., lift the castors up) to clear curbs and other barriers. A less confident wheelchair user will be most comfortable with a chair that does not tip backward easily, allowing him or her to feel secure in the chair.

A recent advancement in the wheelchair industry is the material used to form the chair frame. Much of the advancement in materials comes from the cycling industry. Wheelchair frames are made from many materials, including steel, aluminum, steel/aluminum alloy, titanium, and carbon fiber composites. These materials vary in their weight, strength, cost, how they conduct vibration, method of attaching components together, and how they are formed. Wheelchairs are classified according to a number of parameters including weight, adjustability, and available options. **Standard wheelchairs** are generally useful for very short-term use such as rentals at an airport or shopping mall (Schmeler & Bunning, 1999). They are folding chairs, with very limited adjustment; in particular, the axle of the rear wheel is fixed. Features such as footrests and armrests may be fixed or detachable. There is limited choice of seat width and depth. They are the heaviest of the manual wheelchairs and therefore are not useful for long-term because as they require a great deal of energy to propel on a regular basis.

Lightweight and **lightweight high strength wheelchairs** (Schmeler & Bunning, 1999) weigh less than the standard chair, as their name would suggest. Otherwise, they tend to have similar features. These chairs offer more flexibility in choice of seat width and adjustment of back height. Both the standard and lightweight chairs are available with a lower seat-to-floor height that allows the user to propel with the feet.

An **ultralightweight wheelchair** is substantially lighter than the standard chair. Schmeler & Bunning (1999) suggest that the chairs in the standard and lightweight categories are not suitable for use over the long term. The ultralightweight chair is one they consider useful for an individual who uses a manual wheelchair as the primary means of mobility. It retains the folding frame and is available with a lower seat-to-floor height for individuals who propel with their feet. The axle of the rear wheel is adjustable relative to the center of gravity of the user.

Rigid sport ultralightweight wheelchairs (Schmeler & Bunning, 1999) are a huge growth area for the wheelchair industry. The primary difference between these and the previous categories is the rigid frame. These chairs have quick release rear wheels and the back of most folds down to facilitate transfer and storage of the chair in a vehicle. The axle of the rear wheel of these chairs can be adjusted relative to the center of gravity of the user.

A final comment will be made about the seat-to-floor height of the chair. This dimension is important for two reasons: (1) access to tables, counters, and other structures and (2) access to the floor for users who propel the chair with their feet. In the first instance, the height of the chair should allow the user to roll the chair to a table or desk, permitting the user's knees to be under the table or desk. In the second instance, the seat is lowered to provide a seat-to-floor height that allows the person to "walk" his or her feet on the floor, thus propelling the chair.

Accessories

Armrests on conventional wheelchairs may be manufactured as a fixed part of the frame, flip back out of the way, or be completely removable. Nonremovable armrests decrease the width of the wheelchair slightly, and do not get lost because they cannot be removed. In general it is advantageous to have armrests that flip back or are removable to facilitate transfers and other activities. Two lengths of armrests are available. Desk-length armrests are shorter in the front to allow the consumer to move close to a desk or table. Full-length armrests, which provide more support, extend to the front of the seat rails. Armrests may be fixed or adjustable in height.

Armrests that are height adjustable can be moved up or down to accommodate the length of the user's trunk and provide the proper amount of support for the arms. A clothing guard on the armrests prevents clothing and body parts from rubbing against the wheels.

Legrests and **footplates** support the legs and feet. Taken together, these two components are often called the **front rigging** of the wheelchair. Angle options are often available for the legrests with either 90° or 70° hangers. These options increase the comfort of the user by accommodating his or her preferred knee flexion angle but they can also add to the turning radius, which may be a factor for mobility in some environments. Legrests may be fixed (built into the frame) or removable (swing away). Styles that swing away make it easier to transfer in and out of the wheelchair. Footplates are attached to the leg rests and are available as a single plate to support both feet or as two separate units, with individual height adjustment. The height of the footplate should support the desired position of the lower extremities. The angle of the footplate can also be adjusted to accommodate ankle flexion or extension. Heel loops can be attached to the back of the footplate to prevent the foot from sliding backward (see Figure 10-1).

Wheel locks are the devices that prevent the wheels from moving during transfers and other stationary activities. They are available in a number of configurations such as push or pull to lock, with lever extensions for individuals with limited reach, under the seat mounts, hill holders (device that "holds" the wheelchair on an incline, preventing it from rolling downhill) and attendant controlled. Figure 10-5 shows some of the various brake styles. The client's preferred method of transfer, ability to access the wheel lock, the most reliable method available to manipulate the wheel lock, and the ability of the user or caregiver to maintain this component influence the selection of this component. As with the brakes of a motor vehicle, proper maintenance of the wheel locks is an important safety consideration. Wheel locks that are improperly maintained may not be in secure contact with the tire, causing instability, particularly during transfers or when holding the chair on an incline/decline.

Anti-tip devices are small wheels attached to a rod and mounted at the back of the chair. These devices prevent the chair from tipping backwards. When the drive wheels are located forward on the chair, anti-tip devices are recommended, particularly when the individual cannot safely perform a wheelie. Since these devices limit backward tipping of the chair, they can interfere with travel over some obstacles such as curbs. Anti-tip devices can be removed or rotated so they do not interfere with such travel when an attendant is pushing the chair. However, they should be returned to their original position when the user resumes propelling the chair (Engstrom, 2002). Anti-tipping devices can be seen on the back of the chair in the Figure 10-10, which shows a composite mag wheel.

Push handles are another option on a manual chair. These are the handles used by an attendant or caregiver to maneuver the chair. Some of these are height adjustable to accommodate the different heights of individuals who push the chair. Extended handles are available for pediatric chairs to avoid low-back strain for the individual pushing the chair. Push handles have different shapes and are of different materials to assist with grip and handling in difficult situations such as inclement weather or traveling up or down a hill.

The upholstery of most wheelchairs intended for regular, long-term use is designed to be used with a seating system. The option exists for most chairs to remove the upholstery completely and replace with a back or seat that is attached directly to the frame of the chair. Generally, only those chairs that are for occasional use come with hammock style upholstery attached to the frame.

Frames for Tilt and Recline

Tilt and **recline** features are available on both manual frames and power bases. Figure 10-6 *A* and *B* shows examples of these systems. These features recognize that sitting is not a static activity and that we need to provide the opportunity to change position for individuals who cannot do so independently. Tilt refers to the ability to rotate a specific seating position around a fixed axis, thus changing the orientation in space. Recline refers changing the seat-to-back angle, resulting in a seat-to-back angle greater than 90° (Lange, 2000). The seat-to-back angle typically ranges from upright to nearly horizontal. Tilt and recline have

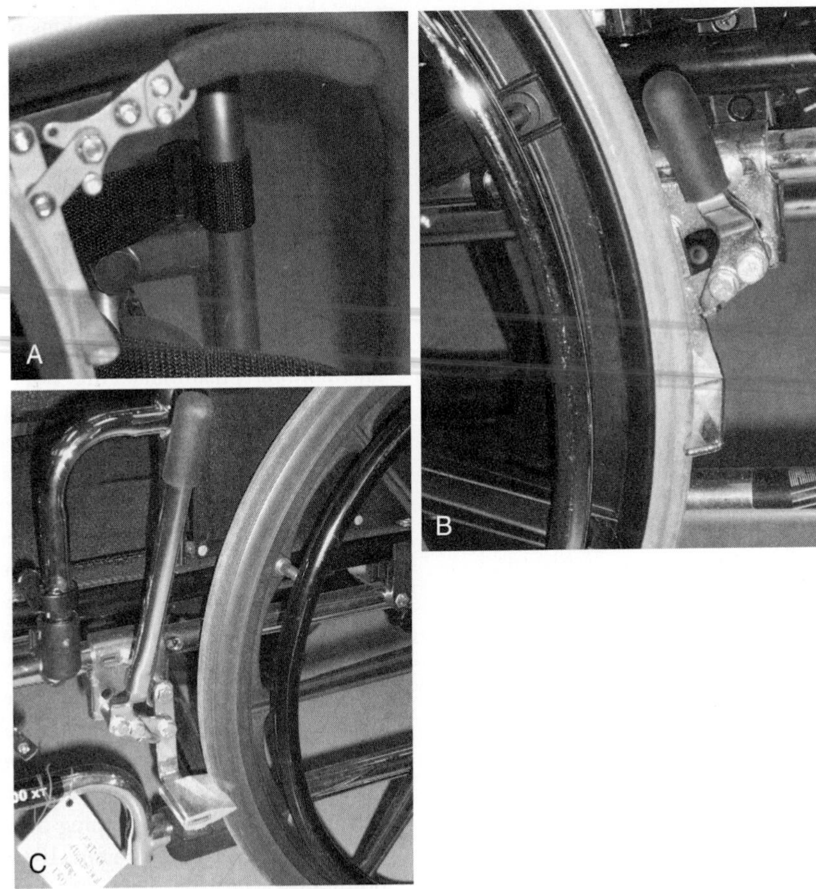

FIGURE 10-5 Wheel locks. **A,** Example of push to lock wheel lock. **B,** Examples of pull to lock wheel lock. **C,** A wheel lock with an extended handle.

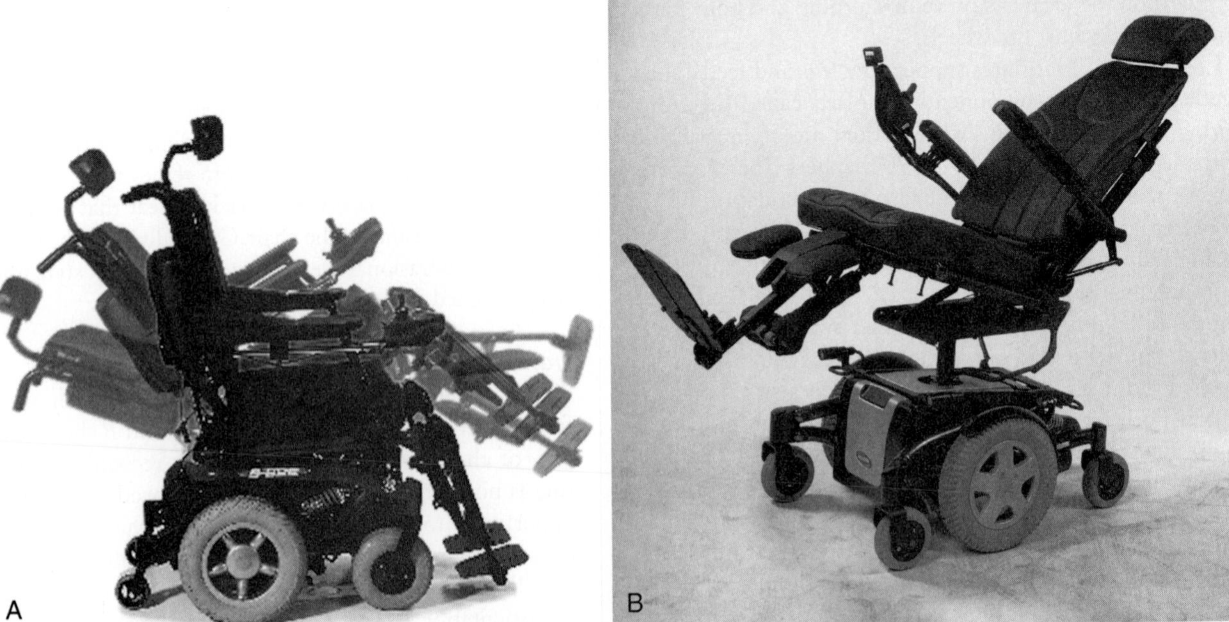

FIGURE 10-6 Tilt and recline wheelchair supporting structures. **A,** Supporting structure with tilt feature. **B,** Supporting structure with recline feature. (A, Courtesy of Sunrise Medical, B Courtesy of Motion Concepts)

some common benefits to the user. Both provide a change of position and improved circulation, thus bringing pressure relief and greater comfort (Lange, 2000; Wilson & Miller Polgar, 2005; Smith, 2004). They have the potential to improve head and postural control, providing an improved functional position and influence muscle tone (Engstrom, 2002; Kreutz, 1997; Lange, 2000; Smith, 2004). Clients with neurological problems may have difficulty maintaining postural control (see Chapter 9) in an upright position. Moderate tilt and recline positions may reduce the effects of gravity, allowing a more upright posture, thus aiding function. They have the potential to improve respiratory function, provide a better visual field, regulate blood pressure, ease transfers, and allow rest during the day (Kreutz, 1997; Lange, 2000). Recline or tilt can be used to achieve a more typical spinal alignment, for example, to reduce a thoracic kyphosis (Engstrom, 2002).

Recline is also useful for individuals who become fatigued when sitting upright for a length of time. A chair with a recline feature allows rest without the need to transfer to bed. Clients with a hip deformity that limits their ability to flex the hip will benefit from recline to achieve a comfortable seating position. It can alleviate orthostatic hypotension (Kreutz, 1997; Lange, 2000) and improve bowel and bladder function. Recline may be preferred to tilt in a work or social environment since it is considered to be less obtrusive by the user (Lange, 2000). Recline does not raise the knees during the position change, which allows the use of this position while continuing to work at a desk or table.

Recline is not a good option for some consumers. Opening the hip angle will cause excessive extensor tone in some individuals, particularly children with cerebral palsy or individuals who have sustained a head injury. Obviously, it is not useful when the user has limited hip extension range of motion. Individuals who use a custom contoured seating system should not use a recline system due to the shear forces that are inevitably present when changing the seat-to-back angle.

Shear is of concern when changing the seat-to-back angle. Recall from Chapter 9 that shear is defined as the friction that occurs when two surfaces slide across each other. Shear has the potential to tear skin, which can lead to a pressure ulcer. Most recline systems are designed to minimize shear, referred to as **low-shear systems**. These systems follow the user as the system reclines, resulting in a reduction of shear but not its elimination (Smith, 2004). Low-shear systems are available in both manual and power options.

Tilt systems are recommended when it is desirable to maintain the seating position for function or for control of other devices mounted to the wheelchair, such as augmentative and alternative communication devices (Lange, 2000). Because the whole seat pivots around an axis, shear is not as significant a concern as it is with a recline system. In addition to rearward tilt, some systems also provide lateral tilt, which again maintains the seating position but tilts the user in the saggital plane. The combination of anterior-posterior and lateral tilt gives the user control to change position as he or she wishes.

Tilt systems do pose disadvantages that recline systems do not. Most systems increase the seat-to-floor height. Further, when the user is in the tilt position, the knees are raised, sometimes higher than the level of the head. The seat-to-floor height and position may interfere with the ability to work at a table or desk and poses a risk for injury if the user attempts to move into a tilt position while seated at a desk or table. As the seat tilts and the knees are raised, the lower extremity may be impinged between a desk and the system (Lange, 2000). Since tilt maintains the hip angle (typically 90°), bladder constriction may occur, causing problems with fully emptying the bladder (Kreutz, 1997). Extreme degrees of tilt may cause the user to feel posturally insecure, which has the potential to increase muscle contraction, thus defeating the purpose of alleviating fatigue. Finally, tilt may interfere with the use of a tray: objects will slide off a tray when in tilt.

Center of mass shifts are a consideration when evaluating a wheelchair that incorporates a tilt-in-space option. The relationship of the center of mass of the seat to the center of mass of the base must be considered. The center of mass moves posteriorly as the seat tilts on some systems. This movement can cause rearward instability if the center of mass of the seat is shifted too far back with respect to the center of mass of the base. Most current wheelchair designs compensate for this concern with mechanisms that maintain the center of mass of the seat over the center of mass of the base.

Consumers who use either a tilt-in-space or a recline system frequently also have other assistive technology, and use of that technology must be integrated with these positioning options, specifically, control of a power wheelchair with a head array, use of a ventilator and/or use of an adapted van. Head array controls should be turned off when the user is in the tilt or recline position so that she or he can fully rest the head. When a ventilator is mounted on the wheelchair, care must be taken to ensure that the tilt or recline mechanism does not impinge on the unit and that the ventilator retains its proper position (Lange, 2000). Finally, evaluation of the user's method of transportation must be considered when tilt and recline options are used. Tilt increases the seat-to-floor height, which may prevent the user from transferring into an adapted van. Both have the potential to increase the overall length of the system, which may limit the maneuverability of the user and chair once in a van (Lange, 2000; Phillips, Fisher & Miller Polgar, 2005). Integration of wheelchairs with adapted vans will be considered in Chapter 11 when transportation is discussed.

Frames for Standing

We normally think of mobility in terms of wheelchairs; that is, the user is seated. There are, however, many advantages to placing an individual in a standing position (Eng et al., 2001; Eng, 2004; Mogul-Rotman & Fisher, 2002). Among the

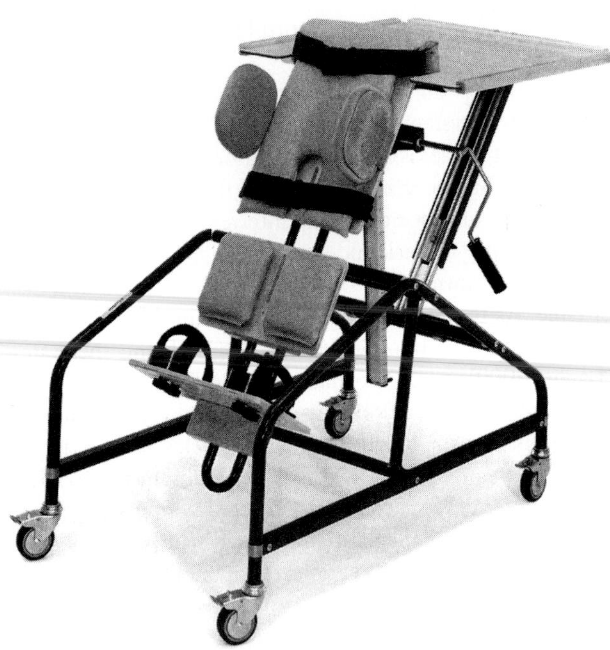

FIGURE 10-7 Large prone stander. (Courtesy of Rifton)

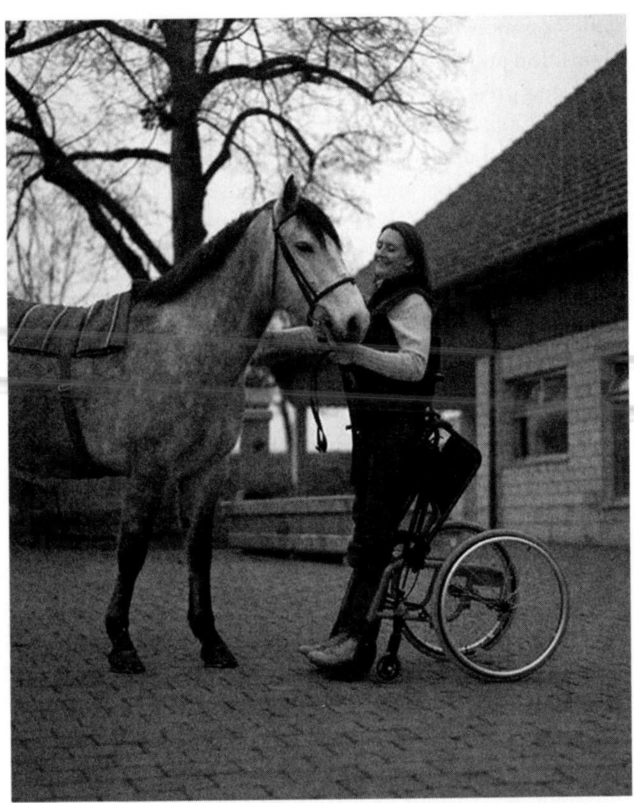

FIGURE 10-8 Stand-up wheelchair. (Courtesy of Levo AG)

positive effects of standing are physiological improvement in bladder and bowel function, alleviation of orthostatic hypotension, prevention of pressure ulcers (see Chapter 9), reduction in muscle contractures and osteoporosis, and improved circulation. In addition, there are psychological benefits from being able to interact face to face with other people. For example, the height differential between someone seated and someone standing may imply an adult–child relationship, whereas standing and interacting face to face implies a relationship among peers. Standing frames and standing wheelchairs are two types of supporting structures that allow the individual to stand.

Standing frames are categorized as prone standers, supine standers, upright standers, and mobile standers (Mogul-Rotman & Fisher, 2002). Prone standers, such as the one shown in Figure 10-7, are the most common type. They provide support on the anterior side of the body. Weight bearing on the long bones and lower extremity joints is a major benefit. Weight bearing strengthens bones and can limit advancement of osteoporosis (loss of bone density) that results from prolonged immobility and lack of weight bearing. Often a lap tray is added to the stander, which serves two purposes. First, it provides a supportive surface for the upper extremities as the user leans on it. Second, it provides a work surface for activities such as writing, playing with toys, or using a communication device. Prone standers are generally tilted forward to use gravity to assist maintenance of an upright position in the stander. Some types have fixed angles and others are adjustable. Adjustment for growth is incorporated into some designs. This type of standing frame does not give the individual the option of moving into a seated position, as does the stand-up wheelchair discussed below.

Supine standers are less common, and there are fewer options. This type of stander provides support for the posterior surfaces of the body. Because the user is leaning back, it is more difficult to use his or her hands. Line of sight will also be affected. This type of stander is useful for persons who do not have good head control, since the stander supports the head and neck. Upright standers provide for complete weight bearing on the lower extremities. People who have good upper body strength can use stationary models. Mobile versions are often sit-to-stand wheelchairs that allow changes in position from sitting to standing throughout the day. The change from sitting to standing and vice versa can be either powered or manual. When in a vertical position, these units generally function like a prone stander.

Standing wheelchairs have both functional and social benefits. Many tasks of daily living, such as cooking, are simplified with the use of a standing wheelchair. Additionally, the use of a standing wheelchair may make it possible to avoid modifications to a home or work setting. For example, a person cooking dinner while using a standing wheelchair is able to reach items in upper cabinets and reach the surface of cabinets and stoves without requiring modifications. Individuals who use a standing wheelchair report positive psychological benefits when they are at the same level as others (Eng, 2004).

Standing wheelchairs (Figure 10-8) are available in three basic configurations: manual driven with a manual lifting mechanism, manual driven with a power lifting mechanism, and power driven with a power lifting mechanism. Standing wheelchairs with manual lifting mechanisms consist of a hydraulic system that uses either a pump or a lever to raise the person to the standing position. With a powered system, the person activates a button to move into the upright position. When standing, the person is supported by padded bars at the knees and torso. Stability in the upright position is a concern with standing wheelchairs since movement into the standing position moves the client's center of gravity forward in the chair, ahead of the center of mass of the base. For this reason not all standing wheelchairs are mobile while in the upright position. Those that are designed to be mobile in the standing positioning have a wider-than-normal base of support or adjust the center of mass of the user so that it remains over the center of the drive wheels. Typically, those chairs that are not meant to be mobile in the standing position have a drive lockout.

Frames That Provide Variable Seat Height

Another available option on powered wheelchair frames is an elevating seat. The person remains in a seated position, and when the mechanism is activated, the wheelchair seat raises and lowers within a given range. A seat that lowers near the floor is particularly useful for small children. Being at floor level allows the child to play on the floor and interact at a level with children of the same age.

There are also benefits to raising the height of a seat. As with a standing wheelchair, a seat elevator can make it easier for the individual to participate in certain self-care, work, and educational activities by reducing the need for environmental accommodations. As with standing wheelchairs and tilt-in-space and recline systems, the location of the center of mass has implications to safety. Some systems have a power lockout that prevents the chair from moving when the seat is raised to a certain height. Stability when traveling around corners may be compromised if the center of mass is too high relative to the footprint of the chair.

Frames That Accommodate Growth

A major requirement of the supporting structure of the wheelchairs for children is that they accommodate growth. Two approaches are commonly used to accommodate growth (including clients with weight gain). The first of these is to design the supporting structure so that it can be adjusted directly. Kits are provided in the second option that allow replacement of various tubes on the frame increasing seat width and length, seat-to-floor height, and access to the wheels. Wheelchairs that are adjustable are now more common.

Access to the drive wheels is another consideration when recommending pediatric chairs. One strategy to improve this access is to set the drive wheels in slight camber. A second approach, for very young children, is to reverse the configuration of the drive wheels, placing them at the front of the chair with the casters at the back. Stability of the chair, rearward, must be carefully assessed with this configuration.

Push handles are a final consideration for a pediatric frame. Extended handles are available so that the caregiver does not need to lean or bend forward to grasp the push handles. This configuration greatly reduces the load placed on the caregiver's lower back by allowing an upright position during this activity.

Propelling Structure: Manual

For manual wheelchairs, the **propelling structure** consists of two main parts: (1) wheels (including tires and casters) and (2) an interface that the consumer uses to move the wheelchair (Ragnarsson, 1990). We discuss each of these components in this section.

Tires

There are three main types of wheelchair tires: solid, semi-pneumatic, and pneumatic (Robson, 2005). Solid tires require less maintenance than other types but are the least versatile. They generally perform well on smooth indoor surfaces but are less efficient when used on carpeted surfaces or other rough, uneven terrain. Solid tires typically have a smooth surface.

Pneumatic tires may have an inner tube or a flat-free insert. Although they are useful over more varied terrain than solid tires, they require maintenance to maintain proper tire pressure and can be punctured, resulting in a flat. Sawatsky et al. (2005) found that rolling resistance and energy expenditure were significantly decreased when tires were inflated to 50% of their recommended pressure. They report clinical evidence that wheelchair tires are commonly found to be inflated to only 25% of their recommended pressure. In addition to maintaining tire pressure, the user should inspect the tires regularly for any cracks or imperfections that may lead to a flat. These tires are available with different tread depths; deeper treads are useful on rough terrain but create more rolling resistance when used on smoother surfaces.

Wheels

Rear wheels are of two basic types: composite or spoke, shown in Figure 10-9 (Robson, 2005). Composite wheels tend to be more economical than spoke wheels and require less maintenance. There is less risk of the user getting a hand caught in the wheel. These wheels tend to be more rigid than spoke wheels and thus may make for a more uncomfortable ride (Robson, 2005). Spoke wheels typically require maintenance because it is more difficult to clean them and the spokes should be readjusted. These wheels tend to transmit less vibration from the surface to the user than do more rigid composite wheels (Robson, 2005). They are lighter in weight than composite wheels. High-performance wheels (such as the Spinergy wheel) are available for active users such as individuals who use their chairs to travel long distances regularly, use a wheelie to change heights as in climbing a curb, or who use their chairs most of the day, moving about their environment. These wheels use lightweight materials that provide better strength and greater shock absorption. Wheels range in size from 18 to 26 inches in diameter. Powered wheelchairs typically have 18-inch wheels and conventional manual types have 24-inch wheels.

Many wheelchairs allow adjustment of the location of the drive wheels forward or rearward on the chair. Figure 10-10

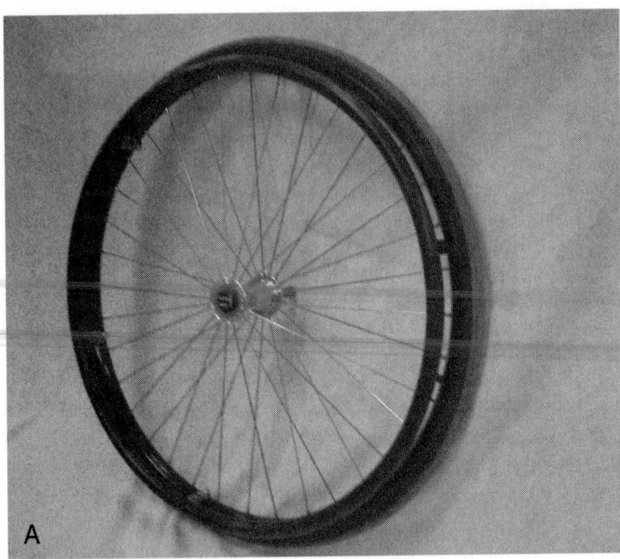

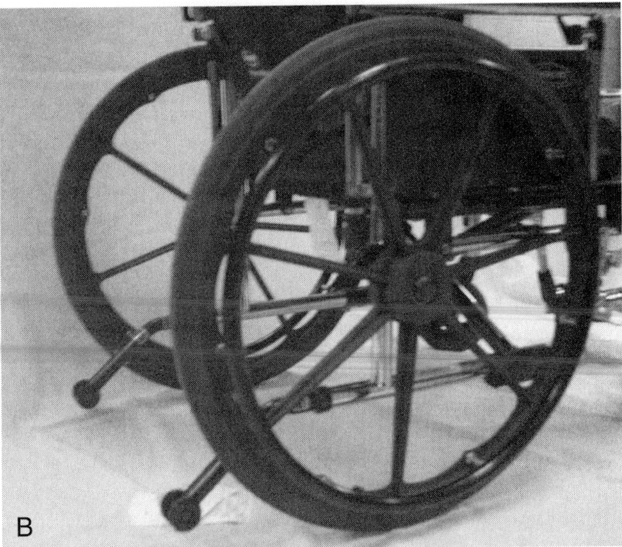

FIGURE 10-9 Types of rear wheels for a manual wheelchair. **A,** Spoked wheel. **B,** Composite mag wheel.

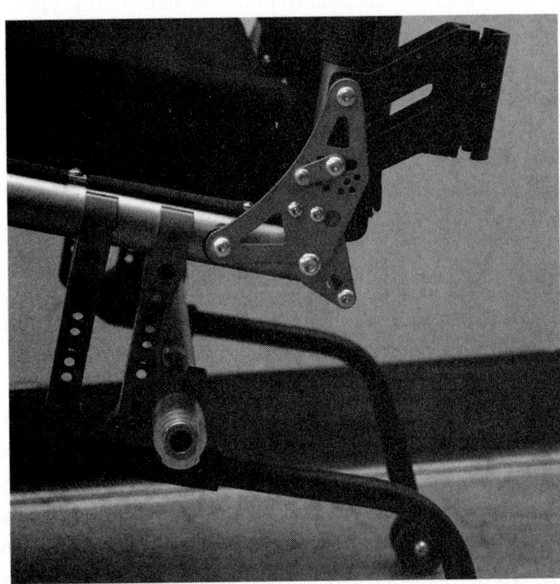

FIGURE 10-10 Axle plate of manual wheelchair that allows adjustability of the position of the rear wheels.

shows a mounting plate that allows adjustments of the position of the drive wheels. The location of the wheels relative to the center of gravity of the user affects the mobility and stability of the chair. When the axle of the wheel is located either directly under the user's center of gravity or anterior to it, the result is a more maneuverable, responsive chair—one that is desired by the active user. More novice wheelchair users or those with less control will feel most comfortable with the axis of the wheel located slightly behind their center of gravity, resulting in a more stable chair (Engstrom, 2002). Wheel camber affects the responsiveness of the chair. **Camber** refers to the degree to which the wheel is mounted off vertical, usually 1 to 4 degrees. Camber tips the wheel so the top is closer to the user's body. When the wheels are set this way the wheelchair becomes more stable and propulsion is more efficient. There is greater access to the wheels. Camber increases the overall width of the chair and lowers the rear seat-to-floor height (Robson, 2005). Wheel alignment also affects the ease with which the chair can be propelled. **Alignment** refers to the degree to which the two wheels are parallel to each other. If they are not parallel and at equal distance from each other, there is greater rolling resistance for the wheelchair.

Casters

The front wheels on wheelchairs are referred to as *casters.* They range in diameter from 2¾ to 8¼ inches (Buck, 2009). Larger casters give a smoother ride but are less responsive and can interfere with foot placement (Robson, 2005). Smaller casters are more responsive, contribute to more efficient propulsion, and allow more flexibility in the position of the feet, but these benefits are compromised by a rougher ride (Engstrom, 2002; Robson, 2005). Solid, semipneumatic casters are available. The relationship of the user's center of gravity to the chair's center of mass is important here. If the user is seated too far forward in the chair, excess weight is placed on the casters (i.e., front loading the casters), making it more difficult to propel as the force required to overcome inertia is greater (Engstrom, 2002). This situation may also result in loss of forward stability with an added risk of the chair tipping forward.

Attention to the function of the casters is important because they contribute to the overall function of the chair. Shimmy is one of the major problems with casters (Buck, 2009). This term refers to the rapid vibration that is often experienced when pushing a shopping cart. Smaller casters tend to have less shimmy than larger ones. Shimmy can result from the position of the caster fork and stem, uneven wear of the caster wheel, and the tension in the caster axle and swivel mechanism where they attach to the frame. Caster float occurs when one of the casters does not touch the floor when the wheelchair is on level ground (Cooper, 1998), which can

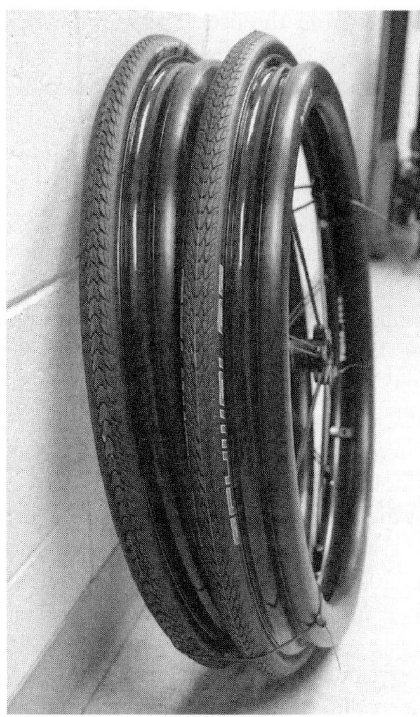

FIGURE 10-11 Hand rim showing ergonomic design.

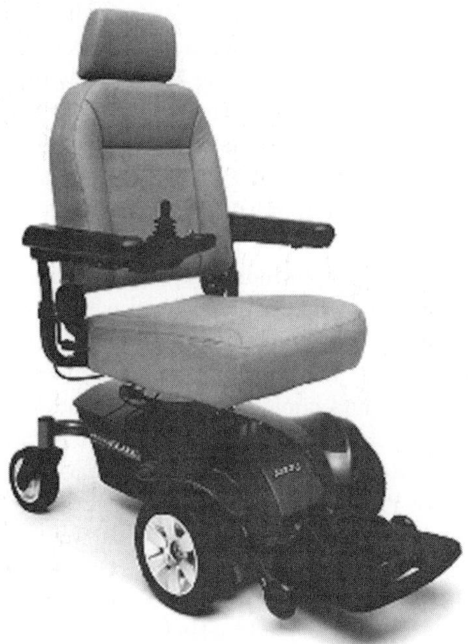

FIGURE 10-12 Powered wheelchair with midwheel drive system. (Courtesy of Pride Mobility Products Corporation)

result in reduced stability and performance. If caster shimmy is observed, it is an indication that maintenance of the chair is needed. Excessive wear on one caster or unequal camber in the rear wheels will bring about caster float. Replacing the caster, adjusting the rear wheel camber, or lowering the caster that floats with a spacer can eliminate the problem (Cooper, 1998).

Hand Rims

The human/technology interface for a manual wheelchair is most commonly a ring attached to the wheel, called a hand rim. Hand rims are made from a variety of materials including titanium, aluminum, and stainless steel. They may have a vinyl coating. Ergonomically designed hand rims use a material that spans the space between the wheel rim and the hand rim, thus allowing a natural fit with the user's palm (Figure 10-11). If an individual has the use of only one arm and hand for propelling the wheelchair, two hand rims are put on the intact side and a linkage is attached between the inner hand rim and the opposite wheel (Buck, 2009). By grasping both hand rims, the user can move forward. Turning is possible using one hand rim at a time. Often the person who uses this hand rim configuration will also use at least one leg to propel the chair.

Propelling Structure: Powered

The **propelling structure** of powered wheelchairs has more variability than do manual systems. The major components are a wheeled mobility base with a power drive to the wheels, a control interface that the consumer uses to direct the movement of the wheelchair, an electronic controller, and powered accessories (e.g., recline, tilt). This section discusses current approaches.

Drive Wheels

Powered wheelchairs have undergone a tremendous change in the last decade. The development of microprocessing capabilities enables developers of powered mobility technology to include a wide range of functions in these devices. One of the most significant developments is the change in the location of the drive wheels. Power is delivered to one pair of wheels in mobility technology with additional sets of wheels providing stability. Direct drive systems also often provide dynamic or active braking of the wheelchair by providing a voltage that stops the motor. This action offers more control than the common situation of letting the chair coast to a stop after the voltage is turned off to the motor. Powered wheelchairs are generally classified as rear-, mid-, or front-wheel drive depending on the location of the wheels that propel the chair. Rear- and mid-wheel drive chairs are the most common. In addition to castors, anti-tipping devices may also be present on a power chair. Figure 10-12 shows a mid-wheel drive powered wheelchair, with the housing for the motor and batteries located underneath the seat.

Denison and Gayton (2002) proposed an additional drive classification based on the relationship of the drive wheel to the center of gravity of the user as well as the ratio of weight on the drive wheels to that on the castors. The drive wheels of a rear-wheel drive chair are located behind the center of gravity of the user. These are well behind the center of gravity in a low-ratio rear-wheel drive. The front wheels are castors and anti-tipping wheels may or may not be present. The drive wheels of a high-ratio rear wheel drive are closer to the user's center of gravity. In addition to front castors, anti-tipping wheels are located behind the drive wheels. The drive wheels of a mid-wheel drive chair are located directly under the user's center of gravity. Castors are located both in front of and behind the drive wheels. These castors are intended to be in contact with the surface when the chair is in motion. The drive wheels of a front-wheel drive chair are located ahead of the user's center of gravity, with the high-ratio front-wheel drive wheels being closer to the center of gravity than the low-ratio. The location of the drive wheels affects the performance of the chair, making it an important consideration when recommending a chair to a client.

Evaluation of the clients' physical and cognitive abilities and examination of their mobility needs are important steps in determining which type of powered wheelchair is most suited to their needs and lifestyle. There is limited literature that evaluates the function of powered wheelchairs to assist the client and clinician in making a power mobility decision. Rentschler and colleagues from the Rehabilitation Engineering Research Center on Wheeled Mobility at the University of Pittsburgh used the ANSI/RESNA standards to evaluate five powered wheelchairs that were commonly recommended for clients in the Veterans Affairs Healthcare system (Rentschler et al., 2004). They examined two rear-wheel drive chairs, two mid-wheel drive chairs, and one front-wheel drive. While their results did not point conclusively to the benefits of one chair over another, they do give a good initial foundation with which to compare a chair's performance to the consumer's needs.

Control Interfaces for Powered Mobility Systems

There are a number of ways in which a powered wheelchair can be controlled. Two control distinctions need to be made before discussing the various technologies: proportional versus nonproportional control. **Proportional control** with 360-degree directionality means that the chair moves in whichever direction the joystick is displaced. The greater the displacement, the faster the chair moves (Lange, 2005). The joystick controls fewer degrees of movement with **nonproportional control.** Regardless of the displacement, the chair travels at a preselected speed. If the user wishes to change direction she or he must release the joystick in one direction and activate it in the direction of the change (Lange, 2005).

Many options exist that provide access to powered wheelchair controls. The initial assessment by the clinician includes the determination of movements that the client is able to make reliably. A similar process can be used to determine the most appropriate method of access, as was described in Chapters 6, 7 and 8 regarding computer and AAC access. An important difference between assessment for computer access versus powered wheelchair control is that the clinician needs to determine that the movement of the control interface used to control the powered wheelchair is safe as well as reliable (i.e., the user must be able to initiate or cease a movement as required because they are controlling a moving vehicle).

Many of the types of switches described in Chapter 8 are also useful for powered mobility control. These switches can be mechanical or electronic (Lange, 2005). Mechanical switches must be physically activated to initiate a control command. For example, they must be moved, depressed, touched, or released. Capacitive switches do not require physical contact from the user. Proximity switches activate when the user is close to the switch, but not necessarily touching it. Fiberoptic switches emit an invisible beam that initiates an action when interrupted (Lange, 2005).

The most common method of control of a powered wheelchair is direct selection through the use of a four-direction joystick. Typically, a joystick can be positioned on either side of the chair or in midline to be controlled with the hand or forearm. It can also be fixed or mounted on a swing-away plate that facilitates transfers. It can be positioned to be used with the chin, foot, leg, or head. When a chin joystick is used, an additional switch (often activated by a shoulder shrug) can be used to control a powered arm that moves the joystick into position for use and swings it out of the way for eating, talking, or mouthstick use.

Most joysticks have a ball on top. However, many types of handles are available for users with different grasping abilities (Lange, 2005). For example, a U-shaped cuff that supports the person's hand on the sides may enhance control of the joystick. Other variations include smaller or larger balls, a T-bar (shown in Figure 10-15), and an extended joystick. A new product, Touch Drive 2,[2] uses a touch screen in place of a joystick. This unit allows the client to use different access methods to control it. Movement up, down, right, or left results in corresponding movements of the chair. Speed is determined by the speed of movement on the touch pad. Maintaining contact with the touch pad in the desired direction keeps the chair moving in that direction.

Sip-and-puff switches are a common control interface for individuals with a high spinal cord lesion. A small tube is placed in close proximity to the person's mouth. The user controls the switch with either a puff (blowing air out of the mouth) or sip (sucking air into the mouth). A hard puff causes the chair to move forward while a hard sip causes it to move in reverse. A soft puff turns the chair right; a soft sip turns it left. The forward direction is latched (i.e., once the user activates forward movement, the chair will continue to travel in that direction until reverse is activated). Good oral motor control is required to use a sip-and-puff system. Figure 10-13 shows a sip-and-puff system for controlling a wheelchair.

Various head control systems are available and are arranged in a head array in a headrest. Figure 10-14 shows an example of this type of control interface. These are electronic, not mechanical, switches. Typically the user has access to three switches: moving the head backwards causes the chair to move forward, tilting it to the right moves the chair right, and the opposite initiates travel to the left. Tilting the head forward stops the chair (Lange, 2005). Control can be either proportional or nonproportional, depending on the head control of the user. Individuals who tend to move into extension when their neck is extended may not be good candidates for this type of system because they may not be able to reliably stop or reverse the chair if extensor tone inhibits forward flexion of the neck.

[2]www.switchit-inc.com.

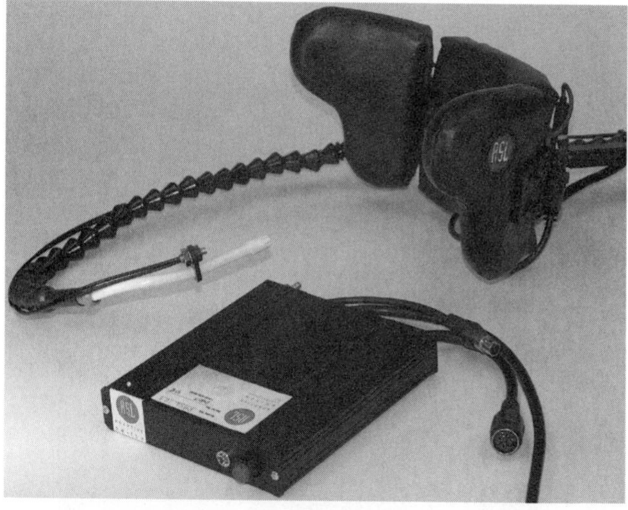

FIGURE 10-13 Sip-and-puff controller. (Courtesy of Adaptive Switch Laboratories)

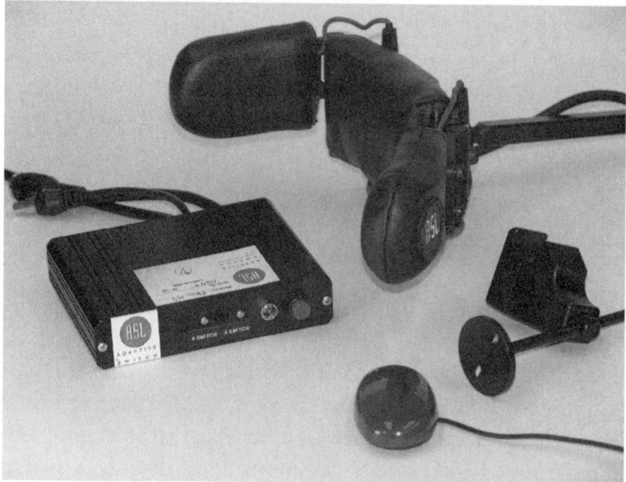

FIGURE 10-14 Head array, power wheelchair controller. (Courtesy of Adaptive Switch Laboratories)

Indirect selection using scanning is also available for consumers who can only use a single switch. In this case there are four lights, one for each direction, arranged in a cross pattern. The lights scan around the pattern until the user presses a switch. The wheelchair then moves in the direction selected. Other functions are also scanned. Single-switch scanning is time-consuming, as well as cognitively demanding, and is typically considered only after other options have been excluded. Another major issue with this approach is the tendency of the chair to wander from a straight line of travel, necessitating the inclusion of steering switches that make small corrections to the direction of travel.

Controllers

A powered wheelchair controller connects the control interface to the drive system. This component is the processor in the assistive technology component of our Human Activity Assistive Technology (HAAT) model. Figure 10-15 *A* and *B* shows a typical wheelchair controller. In a proportional drive system, the controller determines the amount of voltage supplied to the motor by the amount of deflection in the joystick. This voltage is directly related to motor speed. This type of proportionality is not obtained from a switched control interface. To allow the wheelchair to accelerate gradually (as the user with a proportional control would do), the controller provides a gradual acceleration when any direction is selected. In most controllers, the rate of acceleration can be adjusted to meet the consumer's needs. For example, an expert powered wheelchair user could have the acceleration set on the high end so that the chair is highly responsive, whereas a novice user could set the rate of acceleration slower to allow for a slower start. The rate of deceleration (braking) can also be adjusted. Deceleration is the swiftness with which the wheelchair comes to a stop once the control interface is deactivated. With these two features on a controller, it is possible to set one rate for acceleration and a different rate for braking.

Controllers also provide either momentary or latched switch control. In momentary control, the motors are activated only while the switch is pressed, which provides the greatest control for the user. Some consumers are unable to maintain switch activation, but they can press and release quickly. In this case, latched control is used. In this mode, when the switch is pressed once, the motors turn on and remain on. When the switch is pressed again, the motors turn off. It is important that the consumer be able to activate the switch reliably and rapidly when it is in the latched mode, so as to stop quickly when necessary. This feature is often used with sip-and-puff switches. It allows the user to give a hard puff once to latch the control for the wheelchair to move either forward or backward and then use soft sips and puffs to turn left or right (Taylor & Kreutz, 1997).

Most powered wheelchair controllers are programmable by the user to some extent, which gives them much more flexibility and adjustability. The clinician completes the initial programming when the chair is set up, based on his or her assessment. Forward and reverse maximal speeds can be independently adjusted. On some devices the ratio of forward to reverse speed is adjustable. It is more difficult to control the wheelchair when turning than when going straight, and the controller feature that allows turning speed to be set independently of (or as a function of) forward speed is useful.

Some consumers have difficulty controlling their movements because of tremor, which can make the use of a joystick or other wheelchair control interface difficult. To accommodate for tremor, an averaging feature is incorporated into some controllers. The averaging system effectively damps out the tremor by ignoring small rapid movements and responding to larger, slower ones (Aylor et al., 1979). The disadvantage of this approach is that the system can become sluggish, resulting in reduced capability to respond to obstacles quickly. This feature is sometimes referred to as the *sensitivity* or *tremor dampening* of the controller.

Another adjustment allowed by the controller is the ability to alter the degree of range of motion required for an individual to operate a control interface. This feature is called the *short throw adjustment* and is most commonly used with

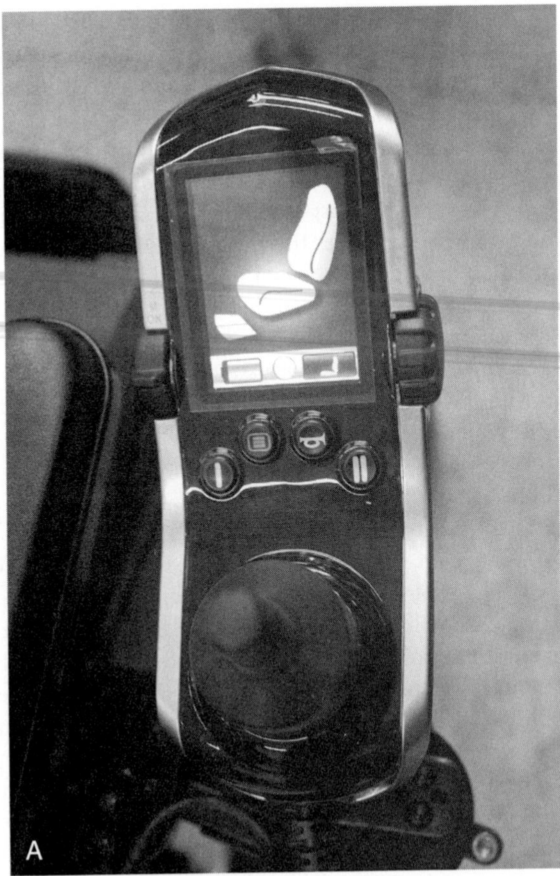

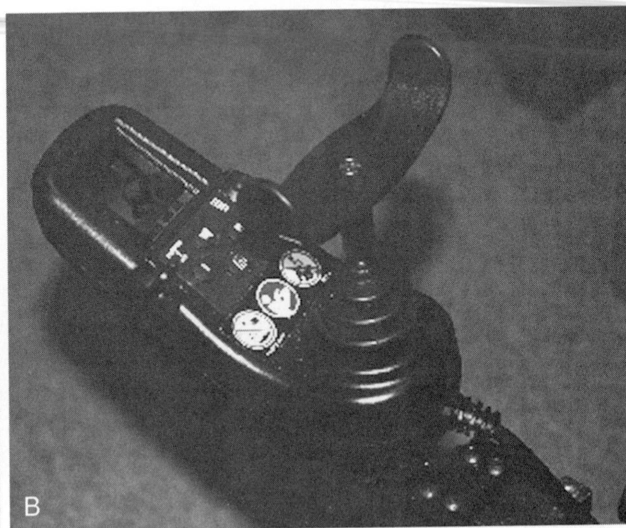

FIGURE 10-15 **A,** Powered wheelchair controller with LED. **B,** Powered wheelchair controller with T-bar joystick.

joysticks. It is useful for consumers who have limited range of motion at the control site that is being used. Many controller models have an LED display that visually represents the different functions and the results of adjustments as they are made (Figure 10-15 *A*).

Computer-based controllers allow the storage of a set of values for parameters like those described earlier. These parameters can then be recalled for use in a particular situation (e.g., outdoors on a hill or indoors on a smooth floor). A therapist working with a consumer to gradually develop driving skills can also store the setups and recall them when needed. Different configurations can be stored for each consumer in training or assessment settings where several consumers may use one powered wheelchair. Most powered wheelchair controllers also have provision for the attachment of an "attendant control," which is very useful for training. This control can override the user's control interface in an emergency situation or training.

Another feature of many controllers is the ability to operate different functions of the wheelchair or other devices with the same control interface. Generally an output from the controller is connected to the external device (e.g., an augmentative communication system or electronic aid to daily living [EADL]). Using a switch, the user is able to transfer the output of the controller from the motors to the external device. The control interface is then able to control the external device directly. A visual display identifies which function is being used. For example, if a joystick were being used for mobility, switching to communication auxiliary mode would allow directed scanning (see Chapter 7) to be used for selections on an augmentative communication device. A switch allows the user to change between these two operations.

Batteries

The power for a powered wheelchair is supplied by a pair of batteries mounted under the seat of the chair. The batteries used are rechargeable lead-acid types. Batteries differ in several ways. Automobile batteries require a high current for a short period to start the car. Wheelchair batteries, on the other hand, require smaller amounts of current for a longer time. This difference is reflected in the use of deep-cycle lead-acid batteries for power wheelchairs. These have thicker plates, which allow them to provide current for longer periods. The chemicals inside the battery may be in a liquid form, called a wet cell, or in a semisolid form, called a gel. Wet-cell batteries are less expensive and last longer; however, they are more hazardous and require more maintenance than gel batteries, so are less commonly used for powered wheelchairs. The fluid in wet-cell batteries is subject to spilling and evaporation. Replacement of the fluid with distilled water is required at regular intervals.

Gel (often called sealed) batteries will not spill, which makes them more desirable for transportation. They do not require any maintenance other than keeping them charged.

These batteries are typically allowed on public transportation systems where the wet-cell batteries often are not. They do not need to be fully discharged before they require recharging. They do not have a "memory," which means that the battery capacity is not limited by previous recharges. Battery power between charges is determined by the capacity measured in ampere-hours. At room temperature, wheelchair batteries commonly have 30 to 90 ampere-hours capacity at 12 volts (Cooper, 1998). The type of motors, environmental conditions (e.g., extremes of temperature), and amount of regular maintenance can all affect battery life and performance. Different batteries require different types of chargers, and it is imperative that the correct battery charger be used. The technology for wheelchair batteries has changed very little over the years. Smaller, lighter-weight batteries with an increase in capacity would help to decrease the weight of powered wheelchairs and increase the distance that the user can travel on one charge.

ANSI/RESNA standards identify a test method for determining the capacity of wheelchair batteries on a single charge. This test requires the chair to be driven at maximum speed around a 54.5 m track 10 times in each direction. Amperes per hour are measured and the theoretical maximum distance is calculated from this measurement (ANSI/RESNA, 1998). Rentscher et al. (2004) indicate that this test does not take into account the varying draw on battery power when the user travels up hill, in different weather conditions, or across different terrains, for example. Information on the theoretical distance of a battery is vital information since serious injury or death could result from a power wheelchair user who is stranded by a dead battery.

Ventilators

Consideration must be given to the placement and movement of a ventilator when the powered wheelchair user is dependent for respiratory support. Like many other products, ventilators have become much more compact and streamlined in recent years, yet they still affect the overall length, weight, and center of mass of the chair. Ventilators can be mounted low on the base of the chair or on a frame that is attached to the vertical uprights of the back. Mounts for ventilators can be fixed or articulating. The orientation of the ventilator is congruent with that of the wheelchair seat in a fixed mount. An articulating mount is required with a wheelchair frame that tilts or reclines. This option maintains the vertical orientation of the ventilator as the seat moves in tilt or recline modes. Further, it keeps the ventilator out of the way of the chair batteries.

Specialized Bases for Manual Wheelchairs

Having described the major wheelchair characteristics, we can now look at dependent mobility bases that have unique structural and propelling characteristics. Because an attendant or care provider is responsible for pushing the consumer in a dependent-mobility wheelchair, special attention is given to biomechanics of the caregiver during this activity. Items normally required for independent manual mobility (e.g., large rear wheels with hand rims) are often omitted in these systems. Bases for dependent mobility are commonly lighter weight and lower priced than wheelchairs for independent manual mobility (Buck, 2009).

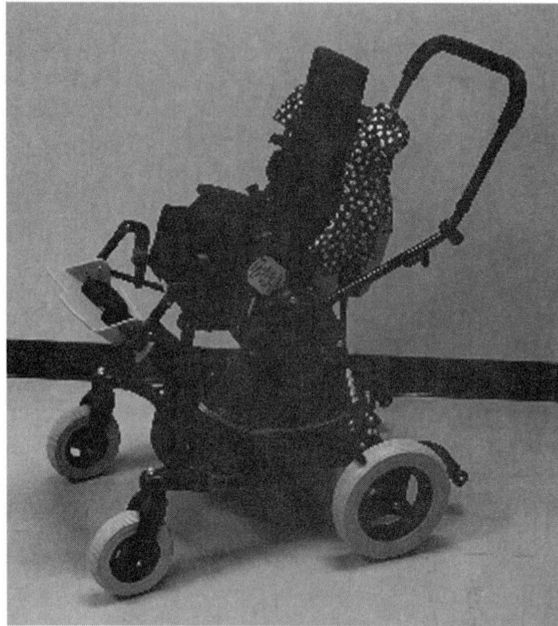

FIGURE 10-16 Firm stroller base.

Stroller Bases

Strollers, similar to those used for transporting very young children, are typically of two types: (1) umbrella folding with a sling seat and (2) full-sized units with solid seats (Buck, 2009). Although originally designed for children, there are now strollers that accommodate consumers who weigh up to 200 pounds. The umbrella type generally does not provide good sitting support, but it folds easily for storage in a vehicle. Consumers who use strollers should not be transported in the stroller unless it has been crash tested (Kemper, 1993). In North America, stroller bases that have met crash testing standards will be listed in the WC19 category, which lists all mobility devices that have been tested and are compliant with standards related to the ability to withstand a vehicle crash. These devices have attachment sites that are an integral part of the frame. A list of wheelchairs and seating products that are WC19 compliant can be found at http://www.rercwts.org/RERC_WTS2_KT/RERC_WTS2_KT_Stand/RERC_WTS2_19_Chart.html .

An attraction of stroller bases is that they resemble standard strollers in appearance, which can be appealing to parents. One feature that appeals to parents is the ease with which they can be transported. The small wheels and short wheelbase of most strollers make them easily maneuverable by an attendant. One disadvantage of the stroller is that the child or adult is often in a reclined position, which may limit his or her ability to carry out functional tasks. Strollers are sometimes purchased as a second wheelchair to facilitate transportation, with a standard wheelchair used for functional tasks. Figure 10-16 shows an example of a solid stroller base.

Transport Wheelchairs

Transport wheelchairs are designed for occasional use, often available for transporting patients in hospitals or in short-term situations such as traversing an airport or shopping mall. They typically have upholstery seating and four small wheels. They do not have any adjustability nor is it anticipated that seating systems will be used. They are lightweight, durable, and relatively maintenance-free. These chairs provide a short-term, dependent mobility option and are not intended to provide seating and positioning in the long term.

Wheelchairs for Use by Older Clients

The setup of a manual wheelchair for regular use by an older client is different from that of a younger, more active user. Age-related disabilities such as arthritis, osteoporosis (loss of bone density), and sarcopenia (loss of muscle fiber) contribute to reduced muscle strength and range of motion. Further, older clients may feel less secure in their movements. Age-related visual changes, including disorders such as age-related macular degeneration and glaucoma, are further considerations for setup of a chair for use by an older client. Care should be taken to ensure that the center of gravity ratio of the client to the axis of the drive wheel provides an optimal stability and mobility balance. Access to the drive wheels and hand rims relative to range of motion and strength in the upper extremities needs to be considered along with rolling resistance. Effects of visual-perceptual changes resulting from a cerebral vascular accident will affect the user's ability to navigate in the environment and will need to be considered when providing training in wheelchair skills.

Some manufacturers are producing chairs that have a rocking feature. Often these chairs have a tilt feature as well. A mechanism on the chair allows the user to rock the seat of the chair. This mechanism can be disengaged in some situations, such as transportation, when it is not desired. This feature is recommended for clients who become agitated, with the view that the rocking motion is calming for the client.

Wheelchairs for Bariatric Clients

Bariatric clients, those individuals with a BMI (Body Mass Index) of 30 or greater, are a population with an increasing prevalence in North America. These individuals require frames that are designed to accommodate their weight and their larger size. Most typical wheelchairs have a maximum weight capacity of 300 pounds. Chairs for bariatric clients accommodate a maximum weight of 600 pounds with some manufacturers offering chairs that will accommodate up to 1000 pounds (Daus, 2003). The location of the mechanics of electrically powered wheelchairs beneath the seat allows the use of a larger seat while still maintaining as narrow a width as possible. Some chairs provide user adjustable seat depth and width. Tilt is also an option that can be provided for the bariatric client. The Eclipse (Figure 10-17) is an example of a chair designed for bariatric clients[3]

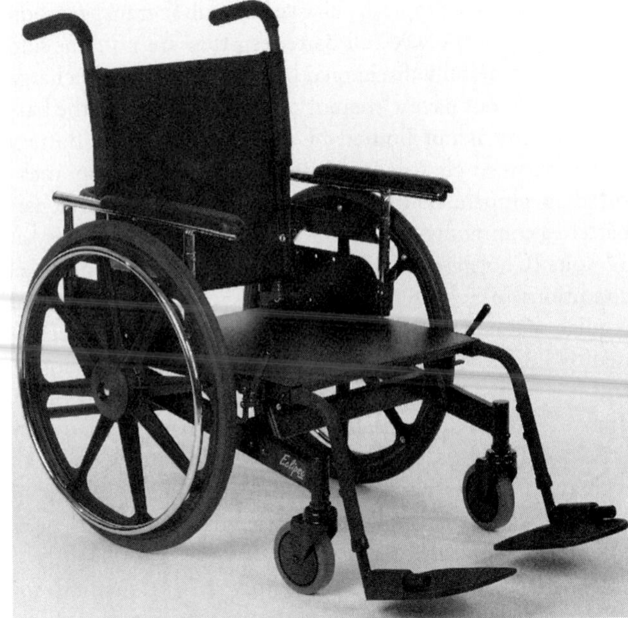

FIGURE 10-17 Eclipse wheelchair for bariatric client. (Courtesy of PDG Mobility)

Fitting a wheelchair for a bariatric client has special considerations since soft tissue distribution and accumulation vary, resulting in different body sizes and shapes (Daus, 2003). Measurement should be done in the seated position and on a firm surface. If there is significant soft tissue accumulation around the buttocks, the configuration of the seat back must be considered, since the buttocks may protrude further than the shoulders, requiring the individual to lean back if his upper back is to be in contact with the seat back. Some manufacturers produce a back that provides support along the entire back surface. A change in the width of the back from hip to shoulder to accommodate a different shape is another accommodation made by some manufacturers.

Specialized Bases for Powered Wheelchairs

Customized Powered Wheelchairs

The range and combinations of features available on powered wheelchairs is rapidly increasing. Some of these features, such as tilt, recline, elevating seats, and footrests, have been mentioned already. The Attitude™ (Figure 10-18 *A*) and the Latitude™ (Figure 10-18 *B*) systems both provide power options to enable independent transfers. The Attitude™ has a foot platform that lowers to the ground and then rises up to seat height, allowing an individual to transfer independently. To transfer into the chair, the foot platform is lowered to the floor; the user transfers onto the foot platform, raises it to seat height, and then transfers on to the seat. The Latitude system is similar, but in this case the entire seat moves forward and down to the floor.[4]

Scooters

Scooters (Figure 10-19 *A*) comprise a large proportion of the powered system market. Individuals who are marginal

[3] PDG Mobility, www.pdgmobility.com.

[4] From Motion Concepts: www.motionconcepts.com.

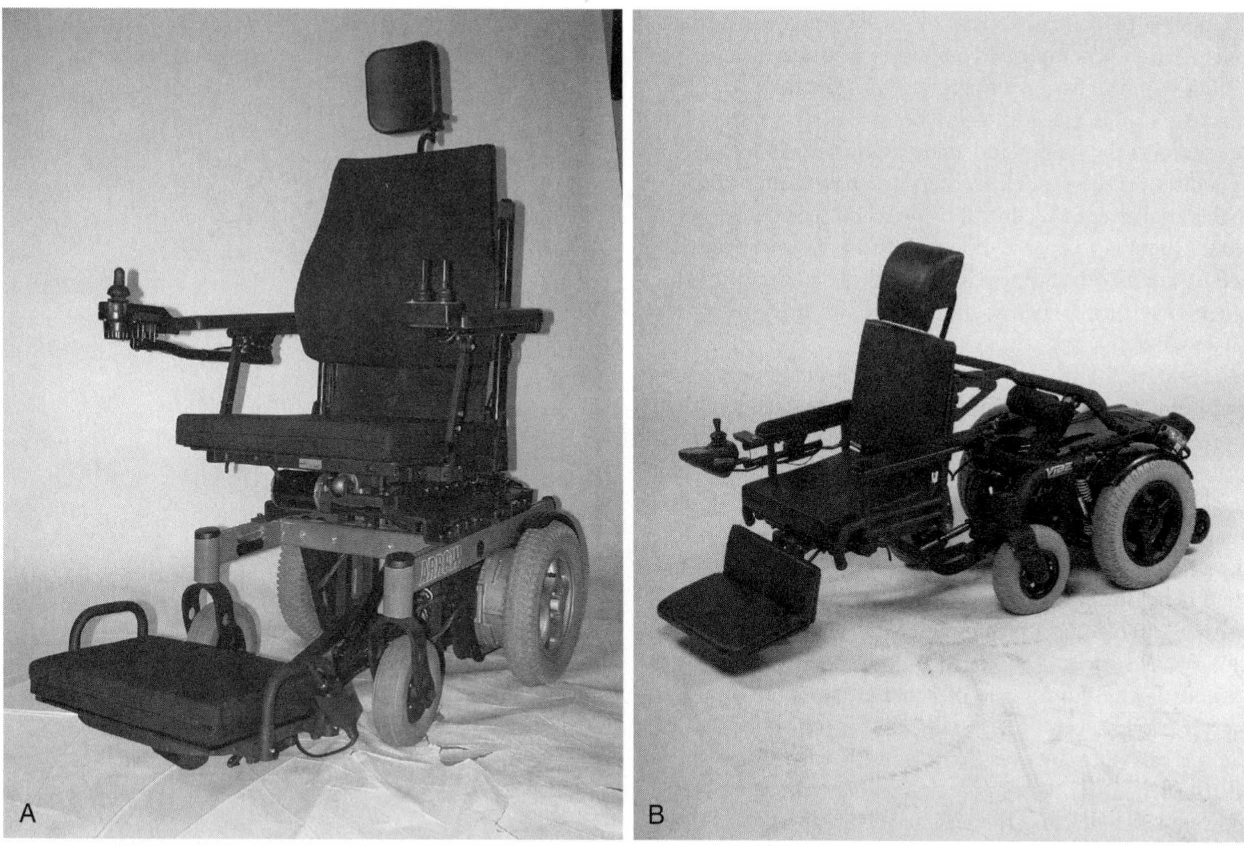

FIGURE 10-18 Attitude and Latitude electrically powered wheelchair systems that allow the user to transfer independently from the floor to the chair. **A,** Attitude. **B,** Latitude. (Courtesy of Motion Concepts)

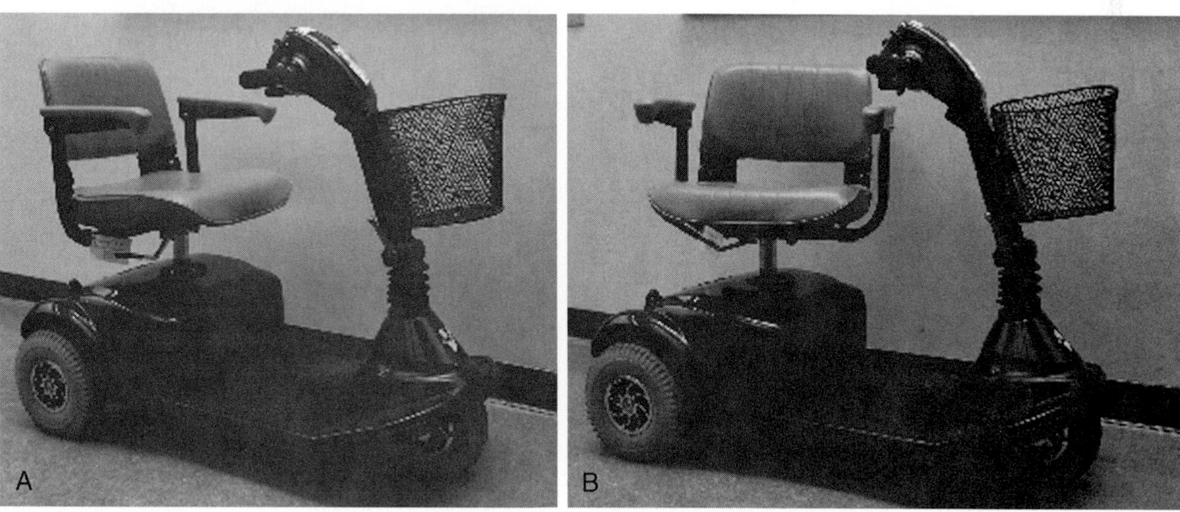

FIGURE 10-19 **A,** Scooter. **B,** Scooter with seat swiveled.

ambulators and need mobility to conserve energy most often use the scooter. For this reason, it is most commonly used by the consumer outside the home. Grocery stores and shopping malls often provide scooters for customers who may need them. The propelling structure of the scooter includes the drive train, the tires, the tiller, and the battery. There are a number of models available in either three- or four-wheel versions with front-wheel drive or rear-wheel drive. Scooters with front-wheel drive do better on level terrain and are more maneuverable. For this reason, they perform better in small spaces. In rear-wheel drive scooters, the rider's weight is positioned over the motor so there is better traction and more power. The bases of rear-wheel drive scooters are wider and longer than the other powered chairs. These scooters are better able to handle inclines and uneven or rough terrain and therefore are preferable for outdoor use.

A tiller-type control is used to steer the wheelchair and acceleration is accomplished by either grasping a lever on the tiller with the fingers or pressing with the thumb. When the accelerator is released, the scooter eases to a stop. On some scooters the height and angle of the tiller is adjustable. Depending on the model, scooters can have either proportional (variable-speed) control or switched (constant-speed) control. There is a separate control setting for adjusting the speed of the scooter. Some scooters have a dial that provides a range of settings, whereas others have a toggle switch for high and low.

The seat of the scooter is mounted to a single post coming up from the base. Typically the seat is a bucket type that has few options for seat width, depth, or back height (Buck, 2009). The seats come in padded or unpadded versions and several types of armrest styles (fixed, flip-up, or none) are available. Most scooters have a mechanism that releases the seat so it can swivel to the side and then lock in place. This feature is helpful for transfers in and out of the seat and for accessing a table surface. Figure 10-19 *B* shows a scooter with a swivel seat.

Some of the advantages of scooters are that they are lighter in weight, can be disassembled for transportation in a car, are easy to maneuver, are less costly than other powered wheelchairs, and are more acceptable than other types of powered wheelchairs. The primary disadvantage of scooters is that they do not provide flexibility in control interfaces. The consumer needs to have a fair amount of trunk and upper extremity control to operate the tiller of the scooter. Scooters also have very little flexibility in terms of speed, braking, or turning control. Finally, the seat of a scooter typically does not provide adequate postural support, and many types of seating systems needed by individuals with postural control problems cannot be interfaced to a scooter.

Power-Assist Mechanisms

Considerable attention has been given to the shoulder injuries that result from prolonged propulsion of a manual wheelchair (for example, see Boninger et al., 2002, 2005; Cooper et al., 1997b; Sawatsky et al., 2005; Veeger et al., 2002). One option for individuals with shoulder pain that limits the ability to propel a manual wheelchair but for whom a powered wheelchair is not desirable is push rim–activated power-assist wheels. These wheels are interchanged with those of a manual wheelchair. A motor is located in the hub of the rear wheels that is linked to the hand rims (Algood et al., 2005). These units supply power to the manual wheelchair as needed by the user. When the user applies force above a preset level to the hand rims, such as when going up an incline, the motors engage and help to propel the wheelchair. Propulsion and braking assistance are provided for both forward and rearward motion. The unit can also be turned off, which allows the manual wheelchair to function in the usual manner. These units add considerable weight to a manual chair, which is a consideration in their selection. Giesbrecht and colleagues (2009) found that participation in daily activities and psychosocial aspects of device use were similar across power-assist wheels and a powered wheelchair, suggesting that the former are alternatives to a powered chair in some situations. Figure 10-20 shows an example of a power-assist product.

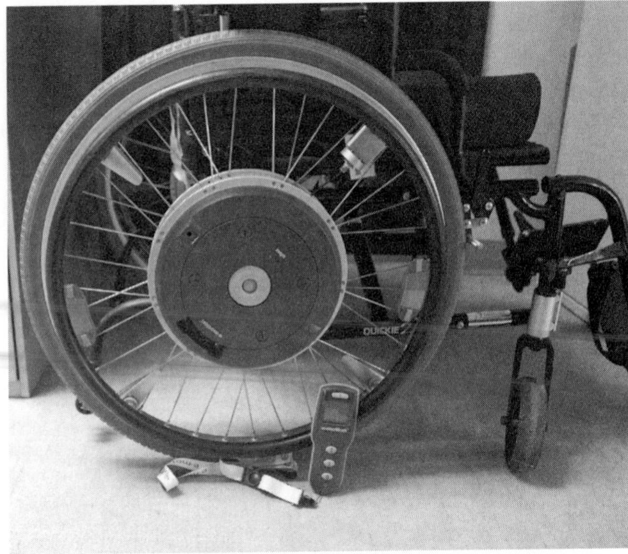

FIGURE 10-20 Push–rim activated power-assist wheels.

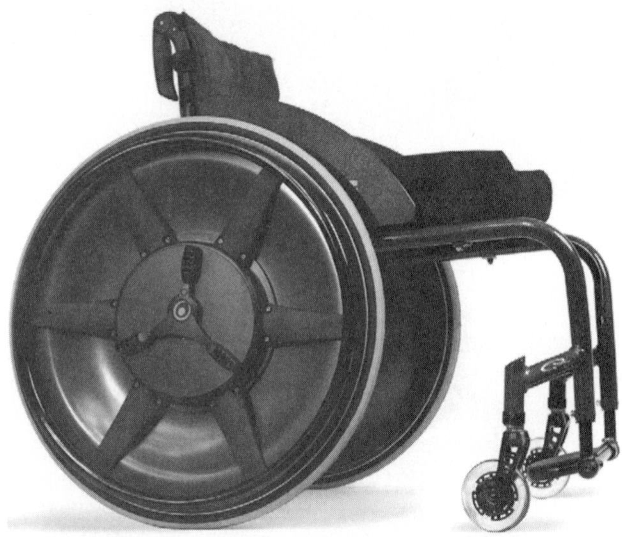

FIGURE 10-21 MagicWheels™ multigear wheels for manual wheelchair. (Courtesy of Magic Wheels, Inc.)

Another product on the market with a similar purpose is Magicwheels™, which provides geared technology for manual wheelchairs (Figure 10-21).[5] Magicwheels™ gives the user a selection of two gears, similar to the concept of bicycle gears, with the second gear providing a 2:1 mechanical advantage. The user selects the second gear by moving the housing of the gear, located on the hub of the wheel. Changing gears does not require grip or substantial strength. Magicwheels™ are most useful on inclines, where they provide assistance propelling upwards and braking when traveling down. Finley et al (2006) completed a pilot study of the

[5] From Magic Wheels Inc.: www.magicwheels.com.

effect of Magicwheels™ use on shoulder pain, length of time the user was able to sustain uphill travel, and perceived exertion during this task. An A-B-A design was used, with baseline being use of consumer's typical wheels. After 4 months of use, shoulder pain was stable or reduced and users were able to travel uphill for a longer time with no change in perceived exertion. Howarth and colleagues (2010) investigated muscle effort of healthy volunteers when ascending ramps of various grades, using Magicwheels™ and with a nongeared wheel. Trunk muscle effort was lower with Magicwheels™ as the ramp grade increased, as was shoulder flexion. Overall, use of Magicwheels™ required more sustained muscle effort because of the longer time taken to ascend the ramp. Because this study used healthy volunteers, it needs to be repeated with wheelchair users to further investigate the effects of Magicwheels™ on propulsive efforts when ascending a ramp.

SMART WHEELCHAIRS

Smart technology is being incorporated into wheelchairs to provide additional options for individuals who are unable to control a wheelchair in other ways. **Smart wheelchairs** are defined as "either a standard power wheelchair to which a computer and a collection of sensors have been added or a mobile robot base to which a seat has been attached" (Simpson, 2005, p. 424). These technologies are useful for wheelchair users who have low vision or severely restricted visual field, motor impairments such as excessive tone or tremor, or cognitive impairments that limit the ability to navigate a wheelchair safely. Smart technologies can be integrated into available power systems or built as an add-on feature (Simpson, 2005).

Smart wheelchairs typically provide two functions: collision avoidance and navigation, either along a path or through obstacles (Mitchell et al., 2014; Simpson, 2005; Wang et al., 2013). In the first instance, sensors detect an obstacle in the path of the wheelchair and will slow or stop the chair or provide some form of warning if the user doesn't perform a maneuver to avoid it (Wang et al., 2013). In the latter instance, the sensors guide the chair along a pathway that is programmed into the chair's control system or that follows an environmental path, or sensors can also guide the chair through a feature such as a doorway.

Mitchell et al. (2014) describe a shared control system, in which control of the wheelchair is shared between the user and the onboard computer. This method of control may be more acceptable to users because they retain some control and do not experience the sensation of the chair moving without their guidance. An autonomous control system is one in which the onboard computer assumes full control of the chair (Wang et al., 2013).

Four main types of sensors are used to guide the chair: infrared (see Chapter 12 for a further explanation of this type of sensor), sonar (sound wave technology), laser range finders, and computer vision (Simpson, 2005). Sensors are also categorized as contact, requiring physical contact before action is taken, or proximity, which require objects to be close to each other but not in direct contact (Wang et al., 2013).

Wang et al. (2013) conducted a qualitative study with potential users of smart wheelchairs, caregivers, and prescribers, investigating their perceptions of collision avoidance technology. Their findings were grouped into three themes: (1) potential uses of the technology, (2) concerns about the technology design, and (3) potential users of the technology. Many functions were identified that had the potential to be aided by smart technology, including maneuvering in confined spaces, backing up, avoiding moving obstacles, as an aid to learning to drive a power chair, and managing physical outdoor barriers such as curbs, potholes, and uneven or sloped surfaces. Concerns about the design included lack of confidence if full control was held by the wheelchair, recognition of the user's intentions and the immediate environment by the chair, discrimination among objects, reliability of the device (e.g., avoiding an obstacle when needed), properties of the human technology interface, and situations where the smart technology would prevent the user's intention, such as pulling up to a table or desk. Safety concerns were identified, in particular safety of others in the environment. Most participants expressed the opinion that this type of technology would be most useful for clients with visual impairments and less so for clients with cognitive impairments (Wang, 2013).

As might be anticipated, the cost of these systems is extremely high, although available "plug and play" technology is likely to reduce this cost in the near future (Mihailidis, personal communication, October, 2013). Smart technology for wheelchairs is not available on the commercial market, existing only in research settings. However, research continues to make this technology more accessible, reliable, and safe. We introduced the functions of smart wheelchairs here in anticipation that some of this technology will be available for clients in the near future.

WHEELCHAIR STANDARDS

Standards can be used to provide manufacturing guidance to ensure product quality. One area of assistive technologies in which standards have been developed is for wheelchairs. Both the International Standards Organization (ISO) and the American National Standards Institute (ANSI) and RESNA have published standards for manual and power wheelchairs, seating systems, and wheelchair use during transportation. There is considerable overlap in these standards. A comparison of the ISO and ANSI/RESNA standards is in Box 10-3.

Although these standards are voluntary, there are strong motivations for manufacturers to adhere to them. For example, the Department of Veterans Affairs (VA) has purchasing requirements for wheelchairs. As the largest purchaser of wheelchairs in the United States, the VA could significantly impact compliance with the standards shown in Box 10-3 by adopting them by reference rather than developing their own standards. Some published studies exist that have

BOX 10-3 Comparison of ISO and ANSI/RESNA Wheelchair Standards

Standard	ISO	ANSI/RESNA
Nomenclature, terms, and definitions	X	X
Determination of static stability	X	X
Determination of overall dimensions, mass, and turning space	X	x
Determination of seating and wheel dimensions		X
Static, impact, and fatigue strengths	X	X
Test dummies		X
Determination of coefficient of friction of test surfaces	X	X
Requirements for information disclosures, documentation, and labeling	X	X
Determination of flammability	X	X
Wheelchairs used as seats in motor vehicles		X
Wheeled mobility devices for use in motor vehicles	X	
Determination of performance of stand-up wheelchairs		X
Setup procedures	X	X
Maximum overall dimensions	X	X
Determination of dynamic stability of electric wheelchairs	X	X
Determination of efficiency of brakes	X	X
Energy consumption of electric wheelchairs and scooters for determination of theoretical distance range (ISO)	X	X
Determination of maximum speed, acceleration, and retardation of electric wheelchair	X	X
Climatic tests for electric wheelchairs	X	X
Determination of obstacle-climbing ability for electric wheelchairs	X	X
Testing of power and control systems for electric wheelchairs	X	X
Requirements and test methods for electromagnetic components of power wheelchairs and motorized scooters	X	X
Requirements and test methods for attendant-operated stair-climbing devices	X	
Requirements and test methods for user-operated stair-climbing devices	X	

applied these standards to manual and powered wheelchairs and seating cushions (for example, see Cooper et al., 1997a, 1999; Fass et al., 2004; Pearlman et al., 2005; Rentschler et al., 2004; Sprigle & Press, 2003).

IMPLEMENTATION AND TRAINING FOR MANUAL AND POWERED MOBILITY

As we have emphasized throughout this text, the assistive technology system includes much more than a piece of equipment. For the consumer to be satisfied and successful with an assistive device, proper implementation and training need to be part of the system. The same holds true to maximize the performance of consumers who use mobility systems.

BOX 10-4 Checklist for Wheelchair Fitting Process

Seating position
Position of control interface
Transfer method
Indoors: size, obstacles, doorways, turning circle
Outdoors: curbs, soft grass, rough ground, inclines
Distance required to travel
Maneuverability in community
Lights, horn
Care provider's training
Assembly and disassembly
Charging method
Battery life and maintenance
Transport in personal and public vehicles
Storage
Maintenance and repair

Modified from Ham R, Aldersea P, Porter D: *Wheelchair users and postural seating: A clinical approach,* New York, 1998, Churchill Livingstone, p 238.

Fitting of Mobility Systems

It is advisable that a fitting appointment be held with the consumer and caregiver. The purpose of this appointment is to make any adjustments needed to the wheelchair and to try the chair and determine whether it meets the original objectives outlined during the assessment. During the initial fitting, time should also be spent demonstrating to the user and the caregiver important features of the chair and going through instructions for maintenance. Box 10-4 shows a checklist of items to be covered during the fitting process for either a manual or powered wheelchair. Depending on the complexity of the wheelchair and whether seating components are involved, more than one fitting appointment may be necessary.

Because today's wheelchairs are often multifunctional, a number of components on the wheelchair are adjustable. Some adjustments and settings are made in the factory before shipping, but typically the provider of the wheelchair will need to make modifications to fit the chair to the user once it arrives from the factory. Adjustments to the wheelchair that can make a difference in user comfort, safety, and performance include axle position, wheel camber, and wheel alignment. Appropriate adjustment of the seat angle, back height and angle, and height and angle of leg rests and footrests is also critical to user performance. Any adjustments to the chair should be made carefully and with the user's safety in mind. After adjustments are made, the user should be cautious in trying out the wheelchair until he or she gets acclimated to the changes.

Maintenance and Repair of Personal Mobility Systems

Wheelchairs are designed to be low maintenance and there are few items on a wheelchair, particularly a manual wheelchair, that require maintenance by the user (Cooper, 1998).

BOX 10-5 Checklist for Basic Wheelchair Maintenance

On receipt	Weekly	Monthly	Periodically	
				General
X			X	Wheelchair opens and folds easily
X	X			Wheelchair rolls straight with no excess drag or pull
X			X	Footrests flip up/down easily
X			X	Legrests swing away and latch easily
X			X	Backrest folds and latches easily
X			X	Armrests easy to move and latch
X			X	All nuts and bolts are snug
				Wheels
X			X	Axle threads in easily or slides in and latches properly
X	X			No squeaking, binding, or excessive side motion while turning
X			X	All spokes and nipples are tight and not bent or nicked
X	X			Tire pressure is correct and equal on both sides
X		X		No cracks, looseness, bulges in tires
				Casters
X		X		No cracks, looseness, or bulges in caster tires
X	X			No wobbling of caster wheel
X	X			No excessive play in the caster spindle
X	X			Caster housing is aligned vertically
				Wheel locks
X		X		Do not interfere with tire when rolling
X	X			Easily activated and released by operator
X	X			Hold tires firmly in place while activated
				Electrical system
X			X	Wires show no cracks, splits, or breaks
X	X			Indictors and horn work properly
X	X			Controls work smoothly and repeatedly
X		X		Battery cases are clean and free from fluids
X			X	Motor runs smoothly and quietly
				Upholstery
X			X	No tears, rips, burn marks, or excessive fraying
X		X		No excessive stretching (e.g., hammocking)
X	X			Upholstery is clean

(From Cooper RA: *Wheelchair selection and configuration*, New York, 1998, Demos Medical Publishing.)

The user is responsible for keeping the chair clean, the tires properly inflated, the brakes properly adjusted, and seeing that the wheelchair is inspected on a regular basis. The user of a powered wheelchair needs to ensure that the correct battery for the wheelchair is used and that it is properly charged. A checklist of items that wheelchair users should monitor or have monitored regularly is shown in Box 10-5. The user manual for the wheelchair will also specify a schedule for periodic inspection and maintenance.

Developing Mobility Skills for Manual and Powered Systems

Training in mobility skills can occur before and after the delivery of the final chair to the consumer. In situations where it is undetermined which chair is most suitable for the consumer or if the consumer will be able to operate the wheelchair, a trial period takes place. During the trial period the person is loaned or leased a wheelchair, either manual or powered, which allows the consumer to test the chair and determine if it is appropriate to meet his or her needs. Often, particularly with powered mobility, this trial involves a period of training to determine if the person can develop the skills to use the wheelchair. For example, powered mobility may be identified as a goal but the individual may not yet have the skills required to control a powered wheelchair safely. If there is any question, it is best to delay making an expensive equipment purchase and risking the safety of the user and others. It is important that the potential user develop these skills through a training program before permanently acquiring the device. Implementation should not always end with the consumer's acquisition of the device. In many cases, further training sessions are necessary. When developing either manual or powered mobility skills, it is important to set specific, measurable objectives for training.

For manual mobility, basic skills include maneuvering the wheelchair indoors on a level surface, in and around tight spaces, and over surfaces such as carpet, tile, or linoleum. For the active user of a manual wheelchair, preparation in advanced wheelchair mobility skills is suggested. These skills include the ability to negotiate rough, uneven terrain; propel up and down ramps and curbs independently; and execute wheelies.

One well-researched training program is the Wheelchair Skills Program (Kirby, 2005).[6] This program was developed in conjunction with the Wheelchair Skills Test (Kirby et al., 2002, 2004). The program teaches wheelchair users basic use of the wheelchair, such as applying and releasing the brakes, removing footrests, and folding the chair. It teaches basic propulsion such as rolling forwards and backwards, turning, and maneuvering through doorways. More advanced skills include propulsion on an incline, level changes, performance of a wheelie, and various wheelie skills. Skills are classified as indoor, community, or advanced (Kirby, 2005). A version for powered mobility devices is also available, which requires users to demonstrate use of different features of the chair such as the controller, battery charger, and other functions.

Enabling development of the ability to use a powered wheelchair for mobility in young children is different than that for adults. The great majority of adults who start to use a powered wheelchair have experience with mobility and likely experience in driving a vehicle as well. Many young children do not. Rather than teaching the child how to use the chair, the goal of powered wheelchair provision is to enable the experience of movement (Kangas, 2010; Livingstone, 2010; Rosen et al., 2009). Current practice regarding use of powered mobility by young children suggests that the only prerequisite to use is motivation on the part of the child to be mobile, rather than requiring a certain level of cognitive ability. A young child who is learning to walk is not aware of dangerous situations, so it is the responsibility of the parents or caregivers to ensure that the environment is a safe one in which the child can learn. Similarly, children learning to use power mobility need to learn in a safe environment. It is the responsibility of the clinician, parents, or caregivers to shape the environment to provide a safe place for exploration of the control of a power wheelchair (Kangas, 2010; Rosen et al., 2009).

Three phases of powered wheelchair use by children have been described in the literature: (1) exploration, (2) use of the wheelchair functions, and (3) use of the wheelchair for functional activities (Kangas, 2010). Current practice guidelines recommend that children who can benefit from powered mobility be given this opportunity as soon as they show an interest in movement. The exploration stage allows the child the opportunity to explore movement and to learn about moving about the environment. Play is the primary means of facilitating this exploration. Kangas (2010) recommends providing the child with a wheelchair in his or her own environment. Wherever possible, let them move as they wish rather than directing the child to go right, left, start, or stop (which requires understanding of these concepts). She stresses that the adult is responsible for the child's safety. As the child becomes more confident with movement, the child is able to control the chair more directly, handling the joystick and appreciating the cause/effect relationship between his or her actions on the joystick and the movement of the chair. Ultimately, the control of the chair becomes a subskill (Bruner, 1973) that enables the child to complete daily activities while moving about the environment at will.

[6]Wheelchair Skills Program: www.wheelchairskillsprogram.ca.

OUTCOME EVALUATION

Outcome Evaluation Instruments

Several instruments are available to evaluate the outcome of wheeled mobility intervention. Table 10-2 provides information on several of these instruments. Some of these instruments are useful in a clinical setting, including the Assistive Technology Outcomes Profile-Mobility, the Functional Mobility Assessment, the Functioning Everyday in a Wheelchair Instrument, and the Wheelchair Outcome Measure. The Nordic outcome measure and the Wheelchair Use Confidence Measure are fairly new instruments for which ongoing research and development continues. These instruments will become more useful to clinicians in the short term.

The Participation and Activity Measurement System requires the use of sensors and a GIS system attached to the user's wheelchair. This system provides a significant amount of data about the individual's activities when using a wheelchair, as well as context for this use obtained through an interview. The technology required to collect the objective data will likely limit this system's use for research purposes, at least in the short term. Other researchers (Cooper et al., 2011; Moghaddam et al., 2011) have used data loggers and sensors to measure aspects of mobility of individuals who use wheelchairs. This quantitative data, when paired with qualitative information to provide context to the individual's movement, is facilitating a better understanding of where individuals travel with their chairs, what they are doing, and the length of time spent using their chairs during the day (Harris et al., 2010).

Outcomes of Wheeled Mobility Device Use

A significant body of research exists that evaluates different aspects of wheelchair use, such as different propulsion techniques, effect of wheelchair setup, and wheelchair training programs. This research will not be reviewed here, although some of this work is presented in earlier sections of this chapter. In this section, we consider research that explores the effect of wheelchair use on participation, in the home and in the community. Most of this research has been conducted with adults who use wheelchairs; however, we will start with the work exploring the relationship between wheelchair use and participation in children.

TABLE 10-2 Mobility Device–Specific Outcome Measures

Title	Reference	Purpose	Intended Population	Measurement Structure
Assistive Technology Outcomes Profile-Mobility	Hammel J, Southall K, Jutai J, Finlayson M, Kashindi G, Fok D: Evaluating use and outcomes of mobility technology: a multiple stakeholder analysis. *Disabil Rehabil: Assist Technol*, 8:294-304, 2013	Measures the impact of mobility devices on activity and participation	Adults who use mobility devices as primary means of mobility	68-item instrument measuring activity (physical performance and ADL) and participation (social role performance and discretionary social participaton). Computer adaptive testing methods used to administer only relevant items. Responses range from ability to perform without any difficulty to unable to do. Two scores: (1) mobility level with device and (2) capability without device
Functioning Everyday in a Wheelchair Seating-Mobility Outcomes Measure	Mills T, Holm MB, Trefler E, Schmeler M, Fitzgerald S, Bonninger M: Development and consumer validation of the Functioning Everyday in a Wheelchair (FEW) instrument. *Disabil Rehabil*, 24:38-46, 2002. Holm M, Mills T, Schmeler M, Trefler E. From www.Few.Pitt.edu	Provides a profile of function, as perceived by the user of a wheelchair or scooter	Adults with progressive or nonprogressive conditions who use a wheelchair as their primary means of mobility	Instrument consists of 10 items evaluating aspects of the wheelchair, its operation, ADL performance, transfers, mobility, and transportation while using the chair. Items are scored on a 6-point Likert scale with 1 = completely disagree and 6 = completely agree.
Functional Mobility Assessment	Kumar, A, Schmeler M, Karmarker AM, Collins DM, Cooper R, Cooper RA, Shin H, Holm MB: Test-retest reliability of the functional mobility assessment (FMA): A pilot study, *Disabil Rehabil: Assist Technol*, 8:213-219, 2-13.	Self-report measure of functional outcomes of mobility intervention, including seating and wheelchair intervention	Adults who use any form of mobility device, including manual and power wheelchairs	Instrument consists of 10 items, measuring a range of functional activities, e.g., completing daily routine, reaching and transferring objects, personal and public transportation, indoor and outdoor mobility. Scored on a 7-point Likert scale from completely disagree to completely agree.
Nordic Mobility-Related Participation Outcome Evaluation of Assistive Device Intervention	Brandt A, Iwarsson S: Development of an instrument for assessment of mobility-related participation outcomes, the NOMO 1.0, *Technol Disabil*, 24:293-301, 2012	Measure of participation outcomes related to use of mobility devices	Adult users of mobility devices; instrument available in Danish, Swedish, Icelandic, and Norwegian	Two parts: (1) difficulty and dependence in use of mobility device in different environments and (2) frequency, ease of participation, and number of activities performed.
Participation and Activity Measurement System	Harris F, Sprigle S, Sonenblum SE, Maurer CL: The participation and activity measurement system: An example application among people who use wheeled mobility devices, *Disabil Rehabil: Assist Technol*, 5:48-57, 2010.	Measure of health, activity, and participation of adults who use mobility devices	Adult users of mobility devices	Consists of two parts: (1) objective measurement, using GIS and sensors to record mobility factors such as time spent in wheelchair, use of features (tilt, recline, standing), distance traveled, destinations, time spent outside of home, and (2) prompted recall interview that provides context for the objective data acquired.
Wheelchair Use Confidence Scale	Rushton PW, Miller WC, Kirby RL, Eng JJ, Yip J: Development and evaluation of the wheelchair use confidence scale: A mixed-methods study, *Disabil Rehabil: Assist Technol*, 6:57-66, 2011.	Measures the confidence of wheelchair users when performing different activities	Adult manual wheelchair users from inpatient rehabilitation to community reintegration	Six different scales: Negotiating the physical environment, Activities performed using manual wheelchair, Knowledge and problem solving, Managing social situations, Advocacy, Managing emotions

Continued

TABLE 10-2 Mobility Device–Specific Outcome Measures—cont'd

Title	Reference	Purpose	Intended Population	Measurement Structure
Wheelchair Outcome Measures (WhOM)	Mortenson B, Miller W, Miller Polgar J: Measuring wheelchair intervention: Development of the Wheelchair Outcome Measure (WhOM). *Disabil and Rehabil: Assist Technol.* 2007; 2: 275-285. Miller WC, Garden J, Mortenson WB: Measurement properties of the wheelchair outcome measure in individuals with spinal cord injury. *Spinal Cord*, 49:995-1000, 2011.	A user-centered measure of the functional and physical outcomes of wheelchair service delivery	Adults who use a wheelchair as a primary means of mobility	Clients are asked to identify activity participation in the home and community. Activities are rated for importance (0–10 scale from not important to very important). Performance of activities is rated for satisfaction (0–10 scale from not satisfied at all to extremely satisfied). Satisfaction and importance scores are generated.

Rodby-Bousquet and Hagglund (2010) described the use of manual and/or power wheelchairs in children with cerebral palsy living in Sweden. A sample of 562 children living in south Sweden was surveyed to provide this description. The researchers found that wheelchair use increased with the age of the child and with the severity of the cerebral palsy. Children with a Gross Motor Function Classification Score of IV or V were more likely to use a power wheelchair. The researchers explored wheelchair use indoors and outdoors. Wheelchairs were used indoors by 165 children: 104 of these children were pushed by an attendant, 32 used a manual wheelchair exclusively, 12 used a power wheelchair exclusively, and 17 used both manual and power chairs. A larger number of children used wheelchairs for outdoor mobility; 228 used mobility devices for this purpose. Of this group, 66 were independent when propelling their chair (18 manual wheelchair, 36 power chair, and 12 both) (Rodby-Bousquet Hagglund, 2010). A significant proportion (162 of 228 children) were pushed when traveling outside (Rodby-Bousquet Hagglund, 2010). These numbers give some indication of the level of independence of this sample of children when using their chairs, as well as the effect of indoor versus outdoor mobility.

The RESNA position paper (Rosen et al., 2009) on provision of powered mobility for children cites numerous benefits of powered mobility use by young children. These benefits include greater likelihood of initiating movement, enhanced exploration, independence and curiosity, more interactions with peers, and greater participation in educational programs (Rosen et al., 2009).

The influence of powered mobility on function of children with motor impairments was further investigated by Bottos et al. (2001) and Jones et al. (2012). Jones et al. investigated the effect of the provision of powered mobility in a small sample of children (N = 28) with severe motor impairments, aged 14 to 30 months to determine its influence on their development and function, comparing the performance of children who received a power wheelchair with that of children who did not. Their findings suggested that receptive communication, mobility, need for caregiver assistance, and caregiver self-care change scores of the experimental group were significantly different from those of the control group. Bottos et al. (2001) found little change in gross motor function, cognition, and impact of childhood illness on parents in young children with cerebral palsy 6 months following acquisition of a powered mobility device. They did find a significant difference for the level of independence. These two studies have promising findings; however, combined with the literature included in the RESNA position paper on pediatric powered mobility (Rosen et al., 2009), they demonstrate the limited evidence base to support clinical practice in this area.

More attention has been given to adults who use wheelchairs. Here we focus on work that has investigated the influence of mobility device use on participation. The following review is not intended to be an exhaustive review of studies of the effect of wheelchair use on participation. However, the range of client populations studied and the convergence of findings across the papers enabled the identification of key themes that are reflected in our application of the HAAT model to mobility device service delivery and use. Studies were conducted with older adults (Evans et al., 2007; Lofqvist et al., 2012); adults who have sustained a stroke (Barker et al., 2006; Pettersson et al., 2006, 2007); adults with multiple sclerosis (Boss & Finlayson, 2006); and adults with spinal cord injury (Chaves et al., 2004, Cooper et al., 2011, de Groot et al., 2011; Kilkens et al., 2005).

Several themes recur in these studies. Participants experienced freedom, independence, and autonomy with acquisition of a wheelchair, either manual or powered (Barker et al., 2006; Evans et al., 2007; Pettersson et al., 2006; Rosseau-Harrison et al., 2012). Participants in several studies reported they felt less of a burden on family members (Barker et al., 2006; Boss et al., 2006).

Enhanced quality of life is another positive outcome of mobility device acquisition (Pettersson et al., 2007). In contrast to the perception of self as an independent, autonomous person, some participants reported experiencing stigma and a self-perception of greater disability, particularly following acquisition of a powered wheelchair. One study reported that participants self-limited their community mobility because of concern that they looked disabled (Evans et al., 2007). Individuals who reported greater satisfaction with their device and greater comfort when using it were more likely to have higher rates of participation (deGroot et al., 2010). Further, individuals with stronger wheelchair skills had higher levels of function (Kilkens et al., 2005).

Power mobility devices afforded greater community mobility than did manual devices, which were found to enhance occupations in the home to a greater extent than in the community (Rosseau-Harrison et al., 2012). While many studies reported that users of power mobility devices were able to do more in the community (Barker et al., 2006; Blach Rossen et al., 2012; Cooper et al., 2011; Evans et al., 2007; Lofqvist et al., 2012; Pettersson et al., 2006), barriers were also experienced that limited the choice of venues visited (Barker et al., 2006). Power mobility devices enabled individuals to travel in the community to perform necessary and desired occupations such as going for a walk or shopping and enhanced social interactions (Barker et al., 2006; Blach Rossen et al., 2012; Evans et al., 2007; Lofqvist et al., 2012; Pettersson et al., 2006), providing their destinations were accessible (Barker et al., 2006; Boss et al., 2006; Chaves et al., 2004; Evans et al., 2007; Pettersson et al., 2006). Powered mobility devices themselves hindered participation due to lack of fit with various forms of transportation (Chaves et al., 2004).

These studies demonstrate the positive benefits of mobility device use, particularly powered mobility device use, for participation of adults with mobility impairments. However, they also point out environmental accessibility issues, including transportation, that limit community participation of adults who use powered devices. The research further highlights the meaning that use of a mobility device holds for an individual, and how that influences participation. These three key findings—enhanced participation, effect on self-perception, and accessibility issues—are elements of all phases of the service delivery process and support the human-activity-context foundation that we applied in this chapter.

SUMMARY

Mobility is very important for participation in self-care, home, work, school, and leisure activities. Mobility needs for individuals with disabilities vary depending on the age and the disability status of the user. The ability to move about one's environment at will has physical, psychological, and social benefits. In this chapter we describe the general characteristics of personal mobility systems and the various types of mobility devices available to meet individual needs of the user. Personal mobility devices fall under the categories of independent manual, dependent manual, and powered mobility. Both manual and powered wheelchair options were described.

CASE STUDY 12-1

Change from Manual Wheelchair to Power

Ted is a 53-year-old man who sustained a T12 incomplete spinal cord injury in a car crash 15 years ago. Ted is a business man who commutes to work regularly using adapted public transit. His work and home are both fully accessible to support use of a manual wheelchair. Ted enjoys an active lifestyle, particularly getting out to visit friends, using his chair to travel on outdoor paths, and traveling with his wife. Ted has had increasing shoulder pain, resulting from many years of propelling his manual chair. For the past year he has found himself unable to do as much activity as he wishes because of the pain in his shoulder. He also finds that he becomes fatigued more easily when propelling his chair. Ted was recently admitted to a rehabilitation facility for a urinary tract infection. While in the facility, his wheelchair prescription is being reviewed. The seating and mobility team, with Ted, will decide if he should change to power-assist wheels or a power wheelchair. You are a clinician in the facility. Your assessment will assist with this decision.

Questions

What observations would you make during your interactions with Ted that would contribute to this decision?

What factors or observations would indicate that power-assist wheels are the best option?

What factors or observations would indicate that a powered wheelchair is the best option?

CASE STUDY 12-2

Wheelchair Safety in a Long-Term Care Facility

Maude is an 83-year-old woman who lives in a long-term care facility. She has a diagnosis of mid-stage Alzheimer's disease. Two years ago she sustained a stroke, followed immediately by a myocardial infarction. This combination of conditions resulted in the use of a powered wheelchair, following the initial recovery from the stroke. In the past 6 months, staff and residents in the long-term-care facility have expressed concerns about Maude's safe use of her powered wheelchair. She has had many collisions with doorframes and walls when traveling in the facility and several times has come close to colliding with staff or other residents. Last week Maude ran over the foot of one of the staff members. A family meeting will be held in two days to discuss these safety concerns and the plan to change to use of a manual chair. The staff members expect that the family will express concerns that this change will limit Maude's independence. You are a clinician in the long-term-care facility and will participate in the family meeting because you interact with Maude on a regular basis.

Questions

What information is important to provide in each of the following areas?

- Physical abilities
- Cognitive abilities
- Emotional state
- Environmental aspects

What is the context in which incidents of unsafe use of the chair occur?

What features of a manual wheelchair do you think will be important to include to minimize the effect this change will have on her mobility?

CASE STUDY 12-3

Pediatric Wheelchair Training

Matthew is a 4-year-old boy who just started preschool. He has severe cerebral palsy, affecting upper and lower extremities, trunk, and head control. At rest his tone is low. When excited or when completing an activity, his tone increases. His head control is fair. He is unable to sit independently. He has a slight startle reflex to loud noises. Matthew has some right hand function, as evidenced by his ability to play computer games using a four-position switch array. Matthew is nonverbal and communicates with facial expressions, gestures, sounds, yes/no signals, and a picture board. His communication is purposeful. He is able to express his needs and engage in a limited conversation with his picture board. His vocabulary is increasing rapidly now that he has some means to communicate. His functional vision appears to be intact.

Matthew's parents have used a solid based stroller for mobility. They did not want to obtain a wheelchair as they wanted Matthew to walk. However, recently they realized that Matthew wants to be able to move about his environment independently and agreed to the purchase of a powered wheelchair. He recently received his powered wheelchair, with a four-position switch array embedded into the laptray as a controller. You are the clinician who is responsible for conducting his powered wheelchair training.

Questions

Describe three stages in the training in use of a powered mobility device and give an example of an activity that you think would be beneficial at each stage.

How would you arrange the environment for Matthew in the initial stages of powered wheelchair training?

What opportunities would you use to help Matthew learn to control the chair, while at the same time ensuring his safety in the environment?

What skills do you think Matthew should demonstrate consistently before he uses his powered wheelchair in an environment with other children?

STUDY QUESTIONS

1. Describe the three broad categories of wheeled mobility systems.
2. Describe one aspect of a resident's cognitive, physical, and affective behavior or skill that a clinician may observe that provides useful information for a wheelchair assessment.
3. Describe one aspect of each of the physical, social, and institutional contexts that has the potential to affect a client's ability to use a manual wheelchair.
4. Describe three situations or behaviors that a clinician might observe that would suggest that a client should change from a manual to a power wheelchair.
5. What are the two major structures of a wheelchair?
6. Describe and contrast the advantages and disadvantages of tilt versus recline systems. What are the indications for the recommendation of each?
7. Discuss the relationship of the center of mass of the user to the center of mass of the wheelchair as it was described in this chapter. What are the implications of this relationship to function?
8. What are the ways in which pediatric wheelchairs can accommodate growth?
9. List the four types of standing systems and give an advantage and disadvantage of each. What are the major benefits of these systems?
10. Define bariatrics and discuss the implications of wheelchair configuration and use for this population.
11. Discuss the considerations of wheelchair use and configuration for elderly clients.
12. Identify the different locations of the drive wheels of an electrically powered wheelchair and describe how each affects the function of the chair.
13. What types of control interfaces are typically used for powered wheelchairs?
14. What types of batteries are used in powered wheelchairs? How do they differ from automobile batteries? What is the difference between wet-cell and gel batteries?

REFERENCES

Algood SD, et al.: Effect of a pushrim-activated power-assist wheelchair on the functional capabilities of persons with tetraplegia, *Arch Phys Med Rehabil* 86:380–386, 2005.

American National Standards Institute/Rehabilitation Engineering and Assistive Society of America: *Wheelchair standards: Additional requirements for wheelchairs (including scooters) with electrical systems*, vol. 2, New York, 1998, ANSI/RESNA.

Americans with Disabilities Act of 1990, 42, U.S.C. §§ 12101 et seq.

Aylor J, et al.: Versatile wheelchair control system, *Med Biol Eng Comput* 17:110–114, 1979.

Barker DJ, Reid D, Cott C: The experience of stroke survivors: Factors in community participation among wheelchair users, *Can J Occup Ther* 73:18–25, 2006. DOI: 10.2182/cjot.05.0022.

Blach Rossen C, et al.: Everyday life for users of electric wheelchairs: A qualitative interview study, *Dis Rehabil: Assist Technol* 7:399–407, 2012, http://dx.doi.org/10.3109/17483107.2012.665976.

Boninger M, et al.: Propulsion patterns and pushrim biomechanics in manual wheelchair propulsion, *Arch Phys Med Rehabil* 83(5):718–723, 2002.

Boninger M, et al.: Pushrim biomechanics and injury prevention in spinal cord injury: Recommendations based on CULP-SCI investigations, *J Rehabil Res Dev* 42(3):9–20, 2005.

Boss T, Finlayson M: Responses to the acquisition and use of power mobility by individuals who have multiple sclerosis and their families, *Am J Occup Ther* 60:348–358, 2006.

Bottos M, et al.: Powered wheelchairs and independence in young children with tetraplegia, *Dev Med Child Neuro* 43:769–777, 2001.

Bruner JS: Organization of early skilled action, *Child Dev* 44:1–11, 1973.

Buck S: More than 4 wheels: Applying clinical practice to seating, mobility and assistive technology, Milton, ON: Therapy Now! Inc, 2009.

Center for Disease Control: State-specific prevalence of obesity among adults—United States, 2005, *Morbidity and Mortality Weekly* 55(36):985–988, 2006.

Chaves ES, et al.: Assessing the influence of wheelchair technology on perception of participation in spinal cord injury, *Arch Phys Med Rehabil* 85:1854–1858, 2004. http://dx.doi.org/10.1016/j.apmr.2004.03003.

Cooper RA: *Wheelchair selection and configuration*, New York, 1998, Demos Medical Publishing.

Cooper RA, Boninger ML, Rentschler A: Evaluation of selected manual wheelchairs using ANSI/RESNA standards, *Arch Phys Med Rehabil* 80:462–467, 1999.

Cooper RA, et al.: The relationship between wheelchair mobility patterns and community participation among individuals with spinal cord injury, *Assist Technol* 23:177–183, 2011. http://dx.doi.org/10.1080/10400435.2011.588991.

Cooper RA, et al.: Performance of selected lightweight wheelchairs on ANSI/RESNA tests, *Arch Phys Med Rehabil* 78:1138–1144, 1997a.

Cooper RA, et al.: Methods for determining three-dimensional wheelchair pushrim forces and moment—A technical note, *J Rehabil Res Dev* 38(1):41–55, 1997b.

Cossette L: *A profile of disability in Canada, 2001*, Ottawa, ON, 2002, Ministry of Industry.

Daus C: *The right fit, Rehab Manag*, Available online. Downloaded October 31, 2006. http://www.rehabpub.com/features/892003/4.asp, 2003.

deGroot S, et al.: Is manual wheelchair satisfaction related to active lifestyle and participation in people with spinal cord injury? *Spinal Cord* 49:560–565, 2011, http://dx.doi.org/10.1038/sc.2010.150.

Deitz J, Swinth Y, White O: Power mobility and preschoolers with complex developmental delays, *Am Jl of Occup Ther* 56:86–96, 2002.

Denison I, Gayton D: *Power wheelchairs selection*. Downloaded October 28, 2006 http://www.assistive-technology.ca/newdef2.htm, 2002.

Eng JJ, Levins SM, Townson AF: Use of prolonged standing for individuals with spinal cord injury, *Phys Ther* 81:1392–1399, 2001.

Eng JJ: Getting up goals, Rehab Manag. Downloaded October 28, 2006. http://rehabpub.com/features/1022004/5.asp, 2004.

Engstrom B: *Ergonomic seating: A true challenge*, Sweden, 2002, Posturalis Books.

Evans S, et al.: Older adults' use of and satisfaction with electric powered indoor/outdoor wheelchairs, *Age Ageing* 36:431–435, 2007, http://dx.doi.org/10.1093/ageing/afm034.

Fass MV, et al.: Durability, value and reliability of selected electric powered wheelchairs, *Arch Phys Med Rehabil* 85:805–814, 2004.

Finley MA, et al.: Effect of 2-speed manual wheelchair wheel on shoulder pain in wheelchair users: Preliminary findings. In *Proc 22nd International Seating Symposium*, British Columbia, 2006, Vancouver.

Furumasu J, Guerette P, Tefft D: Relevance of the pediatric powered wheelchair screeing test for children with cerebral palsy, *Dev Med Child Neuro* 46:468–472, 2004.

Giesbrecht EM, et al.: Participation in community-based activities of daily living: Comparision of a pushrim-activated, power assist wheelchair and a power wheelchair, *Disabil & Rehabil: Assist Tec* 4(3):198–207, 2009.

Ham R, Aldersea P, Porter D: *Wheelchair users and postural seating: A clinical approach*, New York, 1998, Churchill Livingstone.

Harris F, et al.: The participation and activity measurement system: An example application among people who use wheeled mobility devices, *Dis Rehabil: Assist Technol* 5:48–57, 2010. http://dx.doi.org/10.3109/17483100903100293.

Howarth S, et al.: Use of a geared wheelchair wheel to reduce propulsive muscular demand during ramp ascent: Analysis of muscle activation and kinematics, *Clinical Biomechanic* 25:21–28, 2010.

Howarth SJ, et al.: Trunk muscle activity during wheelchair ramp ascent and the influence of a geared wheel on the demands of postural control, *Arch of Phys Med Rehabil* 91:436–442, 2010.

Jones MA, McEwen IR, Neas BR: Effects of power wheelchair on the development and function of young children with severe mobility impairments, *Pediat Phys Ther* 24:131–140, 2012. http://dx.doi.org/10.1097/PEP.0b013e31824c5fdc.

Kangas K: *Powered mobility does not require any prerequisites, except the need to be independently mobile*, Orlando, 2010, ATIA. December 13, 2010.

Kaye S, Kang T, LaPlante MP: Wheelchair use in the United States, *Disability Statistics Abstract* 23, 2002.

Kemper K: Strollers: A growing alternative, *Team Rehabil Rep* 4(2):15–19, 1993.

Kermoian R: Locomotor experience facilitates psychological functioning: Implications for assistive mobility for young children. In Gray DB, Quatrano LA, Lieberman ML, editors: *Designing and using assistive technology*, Baltimore, 1998, Paul H Brookes.

Kilkens OJE, et al.: Relationship between manual wheelchair skill performance and participation of persons with spinal cord injury 1 year after discharge from inpatient rehabilitation, *J Rehab Res Dev* 42:65–74, 2005. http://dx.doi.org/10.1682/JRRD.2004.08.0093.

Kirby RL: *Wheelchair Skills Program v. 3.2*. Available from www.wheelchairskillsprogram.ca, 2005.

Kirby RL, Swuste J, Dupuis DJ, Mcleod DA: Munro, R: The wheelchair skills test: A pilot study of a new outcome measure, *Arch Phys Med Rehabil* 83:1298–1305, 2002.

Kirby RL, Dupuis DJ, MacPhee AH, et al.: The Wheelchair Skills Test (version 2.4): Measurement properties, *Arch Phys Med Rehabil* 85:41–50, 2004.

Kreutz D: Power tilt, recline or both, *Team Rehab Rep* 29–32, March 1997.

Lange M: Tilt in space versus recline: New trends in an old debate, *Tech Spec Int Sec Quart* 10:1–3, 2000.

Lange M: Power wheelchair access: Assessment and alternative access methods, *Proc 21st Int Seat Symp*, 87–88, January, 2005.

Livingstone R: A critical review of power mobility assessment and training for young children, *Disabil and Rehabil: Assist Tech* 5(6):392–400, 2010.

Lofqvist C, Pettersson C, Iwarsson C, Brandt A: Mobility and mobility-related participation outcomes of power wheelchair and scooter interventions after 4 months and 1 year, *Dis Rehabil: Assist Tech* 7:211–218, 2012. http://dx.doi.org/10.3109/17483107.2011.6194244.

Mendoza RJ, Pittenger DJ, Savage FS, Weinstein CS: A protocol for assessment of risk in wheelchair driving within a healthcare facility, *Dis Rehabil* 25:520–526, 2003.

Ministry of Industry: *Physical Activity and Limitation Survey, 2006: Tables (Part IV)*, Statistics Canada, 2010, Ottawa. Publication No: 86-628-X. Accessed February 10, 2014.

Mitchell IM, Viswanathan P, Adhikari B, Rothfels E, Mackworth AK: Shared control policies for safe wheelchair navigation of elderly adults with cognitive and mobility impairments: Designing a Wizard of Oz study, *Am Control Conf*, 2014. pre-print.

Mogul-Rotman B, Fisher K: Stand up and function, Available online *Rehab Manag*, 2002. Downloaded October 28, 2006, http://www.rehabpub.com/features/892002/3.asp.

Moghaddam AR, Pineau, J, Frank J, Archambault P, Routhier F, Audet T, Polgar J, Michaud F, Boissey P: Mobility profile and wheelchair driving skills of powered wheelchair users: Sensor-based event recognition using a support vector machine classifier, Proceedings of the Annual International Conference IEEE Engineering in Medicine and Biology Society, EMBS, art no. 6091711, 7336–7339, 2011.

Mortenson B, et al.: Perceptions of power mobility use and safety within residential facilities, *Can J Occup Ther* 72(3):142–152, 2005.

Mortenson B, et al.: Overarching principles and salient findings for inclusion in guidelines for power mobility use within residential care facilities, *J Rehab Res Dev* 43(2):199–208, 2006.

Pearlman JL, Cooper RA, Karnawat J, Cooper R, Boninger ML: Evaluation of the safety and durability of low-cost non-programmable electric powered wheelchairs, *Arch Phys Med Rehabil* 86:2361–2370, 2005.

Pettersson I, Ahlström G, Törnquist K: The value of an outdoor powered wheelchair with regard to the quality of life of persons with stroke: A follow-up study, *Assist Tech* 19:143–153, 2007.

Pettersson I, Törnquist K, Ahlström G: The effect of outdoor power wheelchair on activity and participation in users with stroke, Dis Rehabil: *Assist Tech* 1:235–243, 2006. http://dx.doi.org/10.1080/17483100600757841.

Phillips K, Fisher K, Miller Polgar J: Thinking beyond the wheelchair. *Proc 21st Int Seat Symp*, 2005, pp 97–98.

Ragnarsson KT: Prescription considerations and a comparison of conventional and lightweight wheelchairs, *J Rehabil Res Dev Clin Suppl* (2)8–16, 1990.

Rentscher, et al.: Evaluation of select electric-powered wheelchairs using the ANSI/RESNA standards, *Arch Phys Med Rehabil* 85:611–619, 2004.

Rodby-Bousquet E, Hagglund G: Use of manual and power wheelchair in children with cerebral palsy: A cross-sectional study, *BMC Pediatr* 10:59–66, 2010. http://dx.doi.org/10.1186/1471-2431-10-59.

Robson M: 25 Choices: Manual wheelchair configuration and new technology. In *Proc 20th Can Seat Mob Conf*, 2005, p 113.

Rosen L, Ava J, Furumasu J, Harris M, Lange ML, McCarthy E, et al.: RESNA Position paper on the application of power wheelchairs for pediatric users, *Assist Tech* 21:218–225, 2009.

Rosseau-Harrison K, Rochette A, Routhier F, Dessureault D, Thibault F, Cote O: Perceived impacts of first wheelchair on social participation, *Dis Rehabil: Assist Tech* 7:37–44, 2012. http://dx.doi.org/10.3109/17483107.2011.562957.

Sawatsky BJ, Denison I, Kim WO: Rolling, rolling, rolling, *Rehab Manage*, 2005. downloaded October 29, 2006. http://www.rehabpub.com/features/892002/7.asp.

Sawatsky BJ, et al.: Prevalence of shoulder pain in adult- versus childhood-onset wheelchair users: A pilot study, *J Rehabil Res Dev* 42(3):1–8, 2005.

Scherer M: Introduction. In Scherer MJ, editor: *Assistive technology: Matching device and consumer for successful rehabilitation*, Washington, DC, 2002, American Psychological Association, pp. 3–13.

Schmeler M, Bunning MJ: *Manual wheelchairs: Set-up and propulsion biomechanics*. Downloaded September 8, 2006 http://www.wheelchairnet.org/wcn_wcu/SlideLectures/MS/5WCBiomech.pdf, 1999.

Simpson R: Smart wheelchairs: A literature review, *J Rehab Res Dev* 42:423–435, 2005.

Smith ME: *The applications of tilt and recline*. Downloaded October 28, 2006. http://www.wheelchairjunkie.com/tiltandrecline.html, 2004.

Sprigle S, Press L: Reliability of the ISO wheelchair cushion test for loaded contour depth, *Assist Tecnol* 15:145–150, 2003.

Taylor SJ, Kreutz D: Powered and manual wheelchair mobility. In Angelo J, editor: *Assistive technology for rehabilitation therapists*, Philadelphia, 1997, FA Davis.

United Nations: Convention on the rights of persons with disabilities, New York: UN, 2006. Available from: www.un.org/disabilities/convention/conventionfull.shtml.

Veeger HEJ, Roxendaal LA, van der Helm FCT: Load on the shoulder in low intensity wheelchair propulsion, *Clin Biomech* 17:211–218, 2002.

Wang Q: *Disability and American families: 2000*, Washington, 2005, US Census Bureau.

Wang RH, et al.: Power mobility with collision avoidance for older adults: User, caregiver and prescriber perspectives, *J Rehab Res Dev* 50:1287–1300, 2013. http://dx.doi.org/10.1682/JRRD. 2012.10.0181.

Warren CG: Powered mobility and its implications, *J Rehabil Res Dev Clin Suppl* (2)74–85, 1990.

Wilson K, Miller Polgar J: The effects of wheelchair seat tilt on seated pressure distribution in adults without physical disabilities. In *Proceedings of the 21st International Seating Symposium*, Orlando, FL, 2005, pp 115–116.

World Health Organization: *International classification of functioning, disability and health*, Geneva, 2001, WHO.

World Health Organization: *Guidelines on the provision of manual wheelchairs in less-resourced countries*, Geneva, 2008, WHO.

World Health Organization: *World report on disability*, Malta, 2011, WHO.

CHAPTER 11

Technologies That Aid Transportation

CHAPTER OUTLINE

LEARNING OBJECTIVES

On completing this chapter you will be able to do the following:

1. Describe the correct use of child restraint systems for passenger safety
2. Describe the correct use of child restraint systems designed for children with special needs
3. Understand the basic features of standards for crashworthiness of wheelchairs and seating systems
4. Understand the use and basic features of standards for wheelchair tie-downs and occupant restraint systems
5. Identify the major components of driver evaluation
7. Discuss major design features to consider when making a vehicle purchase
8. Discuss vehicle access issues for individuals with disabilities
9. Describe vehicle modifications to promote access for individuals with disabilities
10. Describe primary and secondary driving controls

KEY TERMS

Booster Seat
Child Vehicle Restraint System
Crashworthiness
Driving Evaluation
Forward-Facing Infant Seat
Large Accessible Transit Vehicles
Original Equipment Manufacturer
Primary Driving Controls
Rear-Facing Infant Seat
Secondary Driving Controls
Universal Docking Interface Geometry
Vehicle Seat Belt Assembly
Wheelchair Tie-Down and Occupant Restraint System
Wheelchair Tie-Down System

Robert Murphy, a social anthropologist who described his experience with a spinal tumor in the book *The Body Silent*, eloquently describes how the loss of the ability to drive deprived him of the spontaneity to go places when he wanted:

> *The inability to drive was more than a retreat from mobility, for it was one step away from spontaneity and the free exercise of will. Where as I could once act on whim and fancy, I now had to exercise planning and foresight. This was true of even the simplest of actions. (Murphy, 1990)*

Chapter 10 focused on personal mobility systems, specifically manual and powered wheelchairs, that afford individuals the ability to move within their immediate environments and for short distances between local environments. This chapter considers mobility systems that afford movement over longer distances, such as movement between home, school, work, and community sites such as shopping and leisure venues, as well as travel between communities.

Technology that is important to three key activities related to transportation, driving, vehicle accessibility, and occupant protection, is the focus of this chapter. The chapter discusses technology that enables a person with a disability to ride safely in a vehicle (private or public) using devices provided by the original equipment manufacturer

BOX 11-1 Suggested Websites for Further Information on Transportation Safety

General Information

US National Highway Traffic Safety Association: http://www.nhtsa.dot.gov/

Healthy Canadians (Health Canada): http://healthy canadians.gc.ca/index-eng.php.

University of Michigan Transportation Research Institute: www.umtri.umich.edu

Monash University Accident Research Centre: http://www.monash.edu.au/miri/research/research-areas/transport-safety/

Safe Transportation for Children

American Academy of Pediatrics: http://www.healthychildren.org/English/safety-prevention/on-the-go/Pages/Car-Safety-Seats-Information-for-Families.aspx

Australian: http://roadsafety.transport.nsw.gov.au/stayingsafe/children/childcarseats/index.html

Canadian: http://www.tc.gc.ca/eng/motorvehiclesafety/safedrivers-childsafety-car-time-stages-1083.htm

Infant and Toddler Association: http://infantandtoddlersafety.ca/child-seat-safety/

Older Driver Safety

American Automobile Association Foundation: www.seniordrivers.org

American Occupational Therapy Association: www.aota.org/olderdriver

Association of Driver Rehabilitation Specialists (ADED): www.driver-ed.org

Canadian Association of Occupational Therapists Older Driver Safety: www.olderdriversafety.ca

CanDrive: www.candrive.ca

National Older Driver Research and Training Center: *http://driving.phhp.ufl.edu/*

Rehabilitation Engineering Research Center on Wheelchair Transportation Safety: www.rercwts.org

Vehicle Safety for People Who Use Wheelchairs: www.travelsafer.org

(OEM), infant/child restraint systems, or wheelchair occupant restraint systems. The chapter also describes devices that assist individuals to transfer into and out of the vehicle, including those devices that assist the caregiver. The technology aspects of driving will be considered here, but this chapter is not intended to provide a comprehensive discussion of driving assessment and rehabilitation. Box 11-1 lists a number of useful Websites.

ACTIVITY

Transportation is a support that enables individuals to access desired community venues. The UN Convention on the Rights of Persons with Disabilities (United Nations, 2006) includes the right to transportation specifically in article 9 and implies it in articles that state that persons with disabilities have the right to live independently and engage in the community, being supported by the same services as persons without disabilities (Articles 24–27, 29,30).

The WHO's ICF includes a domain specific to "moving around using transportation" (WHO, 2001, p. 146). Use of a variety of types of transportation (public and private), and operating a vehicle, whether human powered or motorized, are included in this domain, which is part of the activities and participation classification. The environment factors of the ICF include relevant domains such as products and technology that support outdoor mobility and transportation (which are congruent with the AT component of the HAAT model) as well as infrastructure, legislation, and policies related to transportation (which are congruent with the institutional aspect of the HAAT context component).

Individuals who are not able to access non-adapted public or private modes of transportation have the right to be supported in their community mobility. The lack of accessible transportation is identified as a factor that limits the ability to perform a variety of activities in the community (Hammel, Jones, Gossett, & Morgan, 2006; Kochtitzhy, Freeland, & Yen, 2011; Rimmerman & Araten Bergman, 2009; Wheeler, Yang, & Xiang, 2009). When an individual is unable to travel to the location of a desired occupation, she is clearly unable to engage in that occupation. Lack of accessible transportation limits employment, educational, recreational, and civic occupational opportunities.

The ideas expressed in the capabilities approach are useful to understand the role that transportation plays in supporting community engagement of individuals with a disability. Capabilities are understood as "substantive freedoms" (Nussbaum, 2011; Sen, 2009), which are clusters of opportunities that support choices for action. Transportation affords the opportunity to engage in desired occupations; without transportation, an individual does not have the capability to choose to exercise the opportunities that a society offers (Nussbaum, Sen). For example, an accessible place of employment is of little use if a potential employee is unable to travel from home to work because of a lack of accessible transportation. This chapter focuses on the technology aspects of accessible transportation, although other factors such as cost, attitudes, and inadequate infrastructure (e.g., accessible vehicles, schedules, information, policy) influence community mobility (Hammel, 2006; WHO, 2007).

The WHO's World Report on Disability (WHO, 2011) implicates inaccessible transportation as contributing to the poorer living situation of persons with disabilities by restricting independent access to community venues for employment, education, health care, social, and recreational occupations (p. 170). It further describes this lack of service as a barrier to participation that is present to varying degrees in all countries. This lack of transportation contributes to the development of secondary disabilities (including mental health issues and additional physical disability related to the inability to secure health care), and social isolation of the individual and their caregiver. Further, it contributes to greater financial limitations of both the individual and their caregiver when access to educational and employment opportunities are restricted (WHO, 2011).

Three main activities related to transportation are presented in this chapter: occupant protection, vehicle ingress and egress, and driving. Occupant protection refers to the structures present in the vehicle (e.g., seatbelt and airbags) and those added to the vehicle (e.g., child restraint systems and wheelchair securement systems) that contribute to the protection of vehicle occupants during regular transportation and in the event of a crash. In the first event, the activity involves secure and safe positioning while the vehicle is moving. For example, a child with muscular dystrophy loses the ability to maintain an upright seated position and to hold his head upright. He needs external support, beyond the capacity of a seatbelt, that will keep him in an upright position, preventing his head from falling forward as the vehicle moves. In this example, the inability to maintain his head in an upright position is a significant safety risk. In the second event, restraint systems secure the individual in a crash, limiting excess movement when the vehicle rapidly decelerates following a collision.

Access to a vehicle is not useful if an individual is unable to get in (ingress) or exit (egress) it. This activity is present for both public and private transportation vehicles. It includes ingress and egress with and without another type of assistive technology (usually a mobility device). It also includes prevention of unintentional egress, for example, preventing an individual with a cognitive impairment from opening the vehicle door while the vehicle is in motion.

Driving is the final activity and one that will not be fully addressed in this book because of the breadth of the topic. The WHO defines driving as "being in control of and moving a vehicle...travelling under one's own direction or having at one's disposal any form of transportation, such as a car..." (WHO, 2001, p. 147). Here differentiation is made between primary driving activities (acceleration, deceleration, stopping, and steering the vehicle) and secondary driving activities (e.g., activation of turn signals, setting the parking/emergency brake, operating lights, entertainment systems, navigation systems, temperature control, and turning the ignition on and off).

HUMAN

Occupant protection and safe driving issues are of particular concern for persons with disabilities (including children) and older adults whose age-related motor, sensory, and cognitive abilities affect their ability to drive safely.

Motor impairments that affect the ability to be protected in the vehicle, access, or drive it include musculoskeletal and neurological disorders. Individuals who are unable to sit independently (hands dependent sitters, according to the classification system described in Chapter 9) are often unable to use the OEM seatbelt safely because it does not provide enough support to enable them to maintain an upright position. Individuals with joint contractures or who use braces or casts may not have sufficient joint mobility to be seated in a vehicle. Limitations of balance, strength, range of motion, and coordination can all affect the ability to be safe when travelling in a vehicle, to enter or exit it, or to drive it (Dobbs, 2001; Charlton et al., 2004; Marottoli, Wagner, Cooney, & Tinetti, 1994; Shaw, Miller Polgar, Vrkljan, & Jacobson, 2010; Sims, McGuin, & Pulley, 2001).

Visual impairments have significant implications for the ability to drive safely (Owsley & Ball, 1992). Relevant impairments include reduction in the visual field, with particular limitation of peripheral fields of view, age-related visual changes such as slow accommodation in reaction to changes in light, need for greater contrast between figure and ground, and conditions such as macular degeneration (Dobbs, 2001, Charlton et al., 2004, Owsley et al., 2001). Age-related and other hearing impairments pose less of a challenge for driving and, on their own, do not affect the ability to be safely seated in a vehicle or enter or exit it (Charlton et al., Dobbs). As a person ages, reaction time slows, affecting the ability to drive safely (Charlton et al., Dobbs).

Cognitive impairment can affect the ability to be safely secured in the vehicle when associated behaviors result in unsafe actions, such as unbuckling the seat belt or opening the door of a moving vehicle. Cognitive impairments, particularly mild cognitive impairment and dementias, are one of the main issues of concern for safe driving as a person changes. Memory, judgment, and other executive functions all affect the ability to drive safely (Charlton et al.; Ducheck et al., 2003; Lundberg et al., 1998; Stutts, Stewart, & Martell, 1998; Whelihan, DiCarlo, & Paul, 2005).

Young children with disabilities can often be safely secured in a vehicle in an infant or child vehicle restraint system that is available on the commercial market (American Academy of Pediatrics, 1999b). Difficulties with protecting them when riding in a vehicle arise when these commercially available devices do not fit due to size or constraints related to body position, for example, when a child uses a cast or brace that keeps his hips in abduction or when she is unable to maintain a seated position safely. A child with a neurological condition resulting in very low tone may not be able to maintain an upright head position in sitting, which makes her vulnerable to strangulation when seated in a commercially available child vehicle restraint seat that positions her in an upright position (American Academy of Pediatrics). As a child with a disability grows larger, a commercially available child restraint system no longer affords adequate protection, which requires the family to seek alternative forms of occupant protection.

Similarly, adults with disabilities who are not adequately protected by the original equipment manufacturer's (OEM) seatbelt system require other types of restraint systems when travelling in a vehicle.

Adolescents and adults with disabilities who drive may not be able to use the OEM controls (e.g., steering wheel, accelerator, brake pedal, or secondary controls such as turn indicator lever, windshield wiper lever) due to physical issues such as ROM, strength, coordination, or the absence of all or part of a limb. For example, individuals with a spinal cord injury lack movement and sensation required to use the brake and accelerator pedals. Individuals with musculoskeletal conditions that limit ROM or who have pain may not be able to exert sufficient force to use vehicle controls. Individuals with neurological disorders may also have difficulties with motor coordination that limits their ability to perform driving tasks safely (AMA, 2010; AMC/CMA, 2012).

Stroke is a common condition that affects the ability to drive safely with motor, sensory, and perceptual sequelae that affect daily activities. In some jurisdictions, the driver's license of a person who has sustained a stroke is automatically revoked until medical clearance is given.

The neurological function of persons with diabetes can result in impaired sensory perception in the lower extremities, which limits the ability to use the brake and accelerator pedals safely.

Age-related changes that affect the ability to drive safely have been well documented (AMA, 2010; AMC/CMA, 2012). Age alone is not a predictor of safe driving; however, the presence of disabling conditions that affect sensory, motor, and cognitive functions are predictors and these conditions are most prevalent in older adults. Consequently, more attention is paid to the driving abilities of older adults than any other group (CAOT, 2009).

CONTEXT

Physical Context

Vehicle Selection

For the purposes of transportation and assistive technologies, the vehicle is considered to be the physical context. A number of factors are important when selecting a vehicle for a person with a physical disability. Some of these include: whether the person will use the vehicle seat or a wheelchair, vehicle access, visual aspects, location and size of primary and secondary driving controls, and seatbelt and airbag design. Resources are available to assist with the process of selecting a vehicle. Most of these are geared to the elderly population (Box 11-2).

Seniors who participated in a study by Shaw et al. (2010) reported a number of factors that made ingress and egress easier, including whether the height of the seat roughly matched the hip, a wide door opening, and some form of handle to help them steady themselves. Seats that have less bucketing also make transfers easy. The Handybar is a small after-market device that fits into the frame of the vehicle and provides a handle that is available to assist transfers (Figure 11-1). Figure 11-2 shows an after-market modification of a passenger seat that pivots 90 degrees and then moves forward and down to come out of the vehicle to facilitate transfers. Seniors also reported that the weight of the door affected ingress and egress; a door that was too heavy was a concern because seniors felt less stable when they reached out to close it. Once in the vehicle, the driver should determine access to the steering wheel, pedals, and controls for secondary functions such as windshield wipers.

Ingress and egress considerations relevant to transferring a child into and out of a vehicle include the amount of space around the seat where the child restraint system is located to enable a parent or other sufficient room to maneuver to properly position and secure both the child and the seat into the vehicle. Sufficient room is particularly important as children grow larger or where there are physical and/or behavioral aspects that make it difficult to secure the child.

Visual aspects are another consideration when selecting a vehicle. The driver needs to determine the sightlines in the vehicle and whether there is clear visual access to the front, the side, and the mirrors. Further, the driver needs to determine whether he or she can read the information on the dashboard, both during the day and at night. A final aspect of vision relates to the location of various controls. Are controls for important features such as the temperature and wipers

BOX 11-2 Resources for Selecting a Vehicle

Canadian Association of Occupational Therapists: Choosing the Right Car—the Senior Friendly Car
CarFit: www.Car-Fit.org
UMTRI: http://www.umtri.umich.edu/our-results/publications/has-time-come-older-driver-vehicle

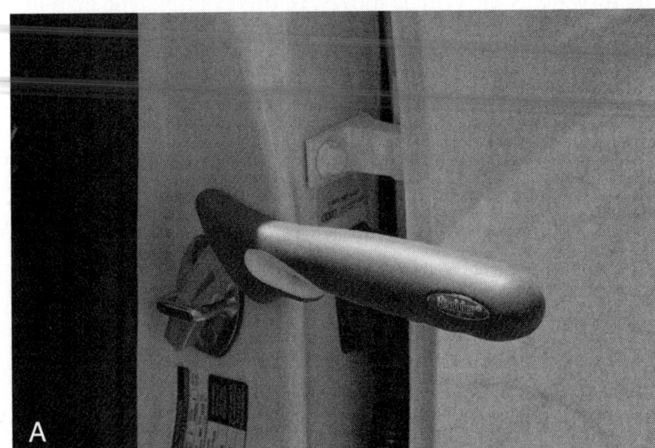

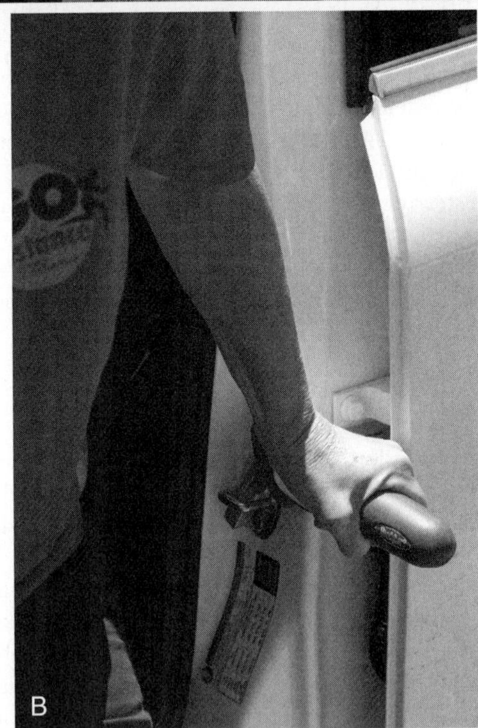

FIGURE 11-1 A, The Handybar, an after-market device that connects to the vehicle frame to assist with ingress and egress. **B,** Shows how the Handybar is used to assist the user to stand up or sit down when entering/exiting the vehicle.

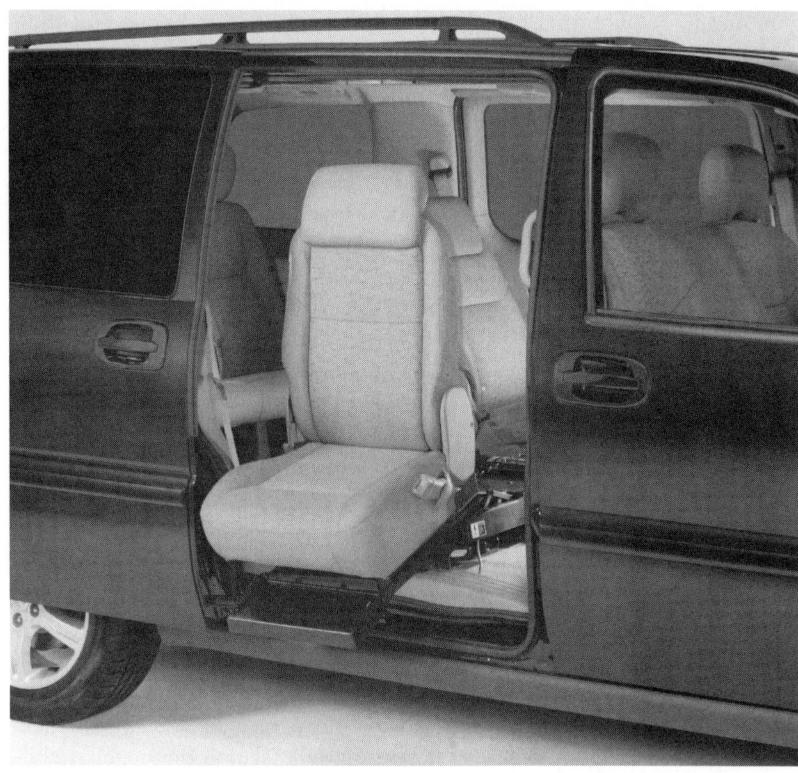

FIGURE 11-2 After-market seat modification that rotates seat 90 degrees and moves it toward outside of vehicle to facilitate transfer. (Courtesy of Braun Corporation.)

located in such a way that a quick glance away from the road is sufficient to guide a reach to use them?

The location and size of the controls have physical as well as visual implications. Consideration should be made of the range of motion required to reach vehicle controls for features such as wipers, turn indicators, temperature, and window defrost. Are they of sufficient size that the driver or passenger can target them accurately when reaching? What force is required to activate them? What action is required to activate them? Modifications to these controls are discussed in a later section.

Seniors who participated in the study by Shaw et al. (2010) overwhelmingly indicated that seatbelts were problematic. They were difficult to reach, fasten, and unfasten. Participants had difficulty seeing the coupling mechanism. In some vehicles, the location of the receiving part of the seatbelt is very difficult to see. Seatbelts did not fit properly (as described above), often sitting uncomfortably on the neck. Some after-market products are available which attempt to make the seatbelt more comfortable. These devices are not regulated, so there is the potential that they may invalidate any crash testing completed with the seatbelt and limit the potential of the seatbelt to protect the occupant in a crash. After-market devices should not alter the proper fit of the seatbelt.

Consideration should be made of the safe use of airbags. The driver should sit about 10 inches away from the steering wheel to avoid injury from an airbag that is activated at less than that distance. The height and weight of passengers is a further issue. Car manufacturers recommend that children under the age of 12 years should not occupy the front seat in a car equipped with passenger airbags because of the risk of serious injury or death. Adults who are the height or weight of a typical 12-year-old are at similar risk. Many new vehicles have sensors in the seat that vary the force with which the airbag activates or whether the airbag activates in a crash on the basis of the weight of the seat occupant.

Access to storage of a mobility device and any regularly transported equipment should be checked. If a vehicle occupant uses a wheelchair that is transported with the individual, it is important to determine whether the wheelchair will fit in the vehicle and how difficult it is to lift and position in the vehicle. This suggestion seems like a very obvious one, but it is one that can be neglected with a very frustrating outcome.

A final consideration is whether an individual who uses a wheelchair will transfer into the vehicle seat or whether he or she will be transported in the wheelchair. This discussion will focus on the driver because of access issues to driving controls, but many of the comments will be applicable to a passenger who regularly uses a wheelchair. Transfer to the vehicle seat provides the most protection for the occupant because the OEM's seat belt provides the most effective protection in a crash (Schneider & Manary, 2006). The vehicle seat back and headrest also provide better protection than that of a wheelchair seating system. The vehicle seat should put a driver in a better position to reach necessary controls. However, use of the vehicle seat does require the ability to complete a transfer relatively easily. A seating system will provide the user with a better functional position generally than a vehicle seat will do (Phillips, Fisher, & Miller Polgar, 2005). The most important limitation of using the vehicle seat concerns individuals at risk for pressure ulcers.

Vehicle seats are not designed with tissue integrity in mind and over a long trip a pressure ulcer could easily develop.

The benefits and limitations of remaining in a wheelchair during transportation are the reverse of the above with some additional factors. The wheelchair seating system is designed to give better postural control and trunk stability than a vehicle seat, which are important safety considerations for either a driver or a passenger (Phillips, Fisher, & Miller Polgar, 2005; Schneider & Manary, 2006). Any vehicle tie-down system will not be as safe a restraint as the OEM's system. A less apparent consideration is the suspension system of the wheelchair. Vehicle seats do not have suspension systems, so the seat does not move independently of the vehicle. Such is not the case with a wheelchair with a suspension system. Travel in these chairs may have the uncomfortable side effect of motion sickness (Phillips, Fisher; & Miller Polgar, 2005).

Social Context

Two aspects of the social context will be discussed: (1) the societal view of community mobility as a right for all individuals (CAOT, 2009) and (2) the perception held of older drivers by members of society (AMA, 2010). Societies that hold community mobility as a right seek ways to provide transportation options to individuals who are not able to travel in a private vehicle. Initiatives such as an age-friendly city (WHO, 2007) and inclusive designs (Sanford, 2012) have as goals transportation systems and infrastructure that are accessible to a wide range of individuals.

Central to the belief in community mobility as a right is the responsibility of the community to provide these transportation options and infrastructure. In addition to providing alternative transportation, such as large accessible transit vehicles, this responsibility extends to providing a transportation infrastructure that supports the needs of individuals who cannot access typical transit options. This infrastructure includes provision of information that is easily available to all individuals, accessible transit stops, transit operators who understand and support the needs of all transit users, and affordable options for alternative transportation (Hammel et al., 2006; WHO, 2011).

The views of society, often as influenced by the media, contribute to general perceptions held regarding older adults (AMA, 2010; CAOT, 2009). Often, older drivers are portrayed in a negative fashion, as menaces behind the wheel, whose inabilities to drive safely are threats to other members of society. When a crash involving an at-fault older driver occurs, media calls for more stringent testing of older drivers or removal or restriction of driver's licenses often follow.

Alternate views of older drivers convey paternalistic messages, suggesting that older adults must be protected; that they no longer have the capacity to make decisions regarding driving, with the result that such decisions are made for them, with the common rationale that it is *in their own best interest*. When such attitudes are prevalent, older adults find their opportunities to continue to drive restricted, with subsequent loss of independence, self-esteem, and functioning, often resulting in poor mental and physical health (Marottoli, 2000).

Social beliefs that limit transportation options for individuals with disabilities contribute to poor life circumstances. Lack of transportation may prevent an individual from employment or education, resulting in lowered income, often leading to poverty (Rimmerman et al., 2009; WHO, 2011). Similarly, it leads to poorer health when an individual is not able to travel to health care appointments and to social isolation when it is not possible to get to places where social activities with others occur (WHO).

Institutional Context

Three groups of legislation and related policies or standards affect assistive technology use related to transportation: (1) occupant protection, (2) legislation and standards related to crash-testing, and (3) legislation and policies related to licenses to drive a vehicle. Legislation concerning occupant protection includes the requirement to use seat belts and the conditions under which their use can be waived. Use of infant and child restraint systems is mandated through legislation, regulations, and policy. In most jurisdictions, conditions are established for the situations in which a child must be protected by an infant or child restraint system.

Commonly, these conditions include age, weight, and height. Most jurisdictions have legislation that requires children 40 pounds and under and/or 40 inches and under to be correctly secured in a restraint system. The recognition that children who are less than 80 (in some cases 100) pounds are still vulnerable to injury when only secured by the seatbelt has led to further legislation in some jurisdictions that require the use of booster seats that properly position the seat belt.

Standards related to crash-testing describe procedures and outcomes for restraint systems and wheelchairs when secured in a vehicle. In both cases, the system is secured in the intended manner in a rig or "sled" and then crashed into a barrier at a proscribed speed, typically in a frontal crash situation. The standards describe the tolerance levels for damage that results from the crash. These standards are context specific; a system that passes a crash test in one context may not meet the standards in another, a point that is important if the system is purchased in one jurisdiction and used in another.

Finally, legislation, regulations, and policies around vehicle licensing set out the conditions under which a person is able to control a motor vehicle. They describe the conditions under which a person can obtain and use different classifications of driver's license (for example, some types of driver's licenses require the driver to have another licensed driver in the front passenger seat).

They establish conditions such as minimum vision requirements needed to obtain a license. On- and off-road testing procedures are standardized. The consequences of certain health conditions (e.g., stroke or myocardial infarction) on retention of a driver's license are also regulated. In many contexts, a process of graduated licensing where the driver assumes greater independence in driving and ability to drive in more complex situations, such as limited access highways, is regulated. De-graduated licensing where the reverse situation occurs is less frequent, but has been posed as one way to enable older drivers to retain the ability to drive in situations that are considered to be less challenging.

ASSISTIVE TECHNOLOGY

Occupant Protection

Occupant Protection for Children

Legislation exists in most jurisdictions that requires children of a certain weight and height to travel in a **child vehicle restraint system.** The majority of jurisdictions require children weighing less than 40 pounds to be properly secured in a vehicle restraint system. An increasing number are also requiring the use of booster seats for children who weigh more than 40 pounds. Many children with mild to moderate seating needs can safely sit in vehicle restraint systems that are produced for children who have no special seating needs, so these products will be discussed first, including their proper use and installation. The array of products is vast and constantly changing. The following discussion is general and readers should review specific requirements in their own jurisdictions, particularly those related to booster seats.

Vehicle Restraint Systems for Children

There are three main types of vehicle restraint systems for children: **rear-facing infant seats, forward-facing infant seats,** and **booster seats.** A number of Websites provide access to up-to-date information on the proper use and installation of these devices for their specific jurisdictions (Box 11-3). The National Highway Traffic Safety Association (NHTSA) offers the "Seat Check" program that provides free car seat inspections and determination of whether the vehicle restraint system is properly installed.[1] NHTSA maintains current information on vehicle restraint systems.

The American Academy of Pediatrics also provides current information on vehicle restraint systems, including those specifically for children with disabilities. In addition, the University of Michigan, Transportation Research Institute (UMTRI) recently published best practice information for the use of infant and child restraint systems (Klinich et al., 2012). Federal regulations exist that govern the structure and testing of vehicle restraint systems, including those for children with disabilities. In the United States, the Federal Motor Vehicle Safety Standards (FMVSS) group produces these regulations and in Canada they are produced by the Canadian Motor Vehicle Safety Standards (CMVSS) organization. Restraint systems that meet these regulations are labeled with a sticker identifying either FMVSS or CMVSS and the specific standard that the system has met. These regulations can be found at http://www.nhtsa.dot.gov/cars/rules/rulings/ChildRestrSyst/Index.html and http://www.tc.gc.ca/eng/motorvehiclesafety/safedrivers-childsafety-car-time-stages-1083.htm for US or Canadian standards, respectively.

Rear-facing infant seats (Figure 11-3 *A*) are intended for use from the time the infant leaves the hospital after birth to the time he or she reaches 12 months and 22 pounds (10 kg). Although most vehicle restraint systems indicate a height and weight limit for the child, rear-facing infant vehicle restraint systems have an age and weight limit, which means that the child must be 12 months of age before he or she is turned to the forward-facing position. Infants younger than this age do not have sufficient head control and their bones are not sufficiently developed to withstand even a minor crash (American Academy of Pediatrics, 1996). A common error on the part of parents is to move a child to the next type of child vehicle restraint system too early (Ebell et al., 2003; Winston et al., 2000; Winston et al., 2004; Yakupcin, 2005). Many children reach the 22 pound/10 kg weight limit well before their first birthdays. In this instance, they should be moved to a vehicle restraint system that will accommodate their heavier weight but will allow them to remain in the rear-facing position. Rear-facing infant seats are typically not left in the vehicle. Rather, the child is transported in the infant seat between the vehicle and destination. The car seat belt system provides restraint for the child and the seat inside the vehicle. Some seats secure into a base that remains installed in the vehicle over the long term.

Forward-facing vehicle restraint systems (Figure 11-3 *B*) are intended to be installed in a vehicle and remain for the long term. These systems accommodate children up to 40 pounds and 40 inches. Proper installation of these systems is critical. A biomechanical study of the demands of installation of a forward-facing vehicle restraint system found that proper installation required efforts that exceeded maximal force output for many participants and postures that limited the force that could be produced, particularly in the shoulder. Further, the configuration of the vehicle interior resulted in postures that put parents at risk for low back injury (Fox, Sarno, & Potvin, 2004; Sarno, Fox, & Potvin, 2004).

Two errors are common when installing the forward-facing car seat: (1) nonuse or misuse of the tether strap and (2) improper use of the strapping system of the restraint system (Klinich et al., 2014; Kohn, Chausme, & Flood, 2000; Lane, Lui, & Newlin, 2000). These seats all fasten to the vehicle frame with a tether strap. All new vehicles are equipped with tether anchors. The tether strap must be fastened and tightened so that an excursion of the restraint system of no more than ½ inch is allowed. The strapping component of the restraint system should be snug to the seat with the chest buckle about two fingerwidths below the child's neck. Often these straps are loose, allowing the child to wiggle

[1] http://www.seatcheck.org/.

BOX 11-3 Websites of Manufacturers of Safety Systems for Children with Disabilities

Britax www.britax.ca
Besi (Securement Vests) www.BESI-INC.com
Columbia Medical www.columbiamedical.com
E-Z-On Products www.ezonpro.com
Q'Straint www.qstraint.com
Preston Medical www.prestonmedical.com
Snug Seat www.snugseat.com

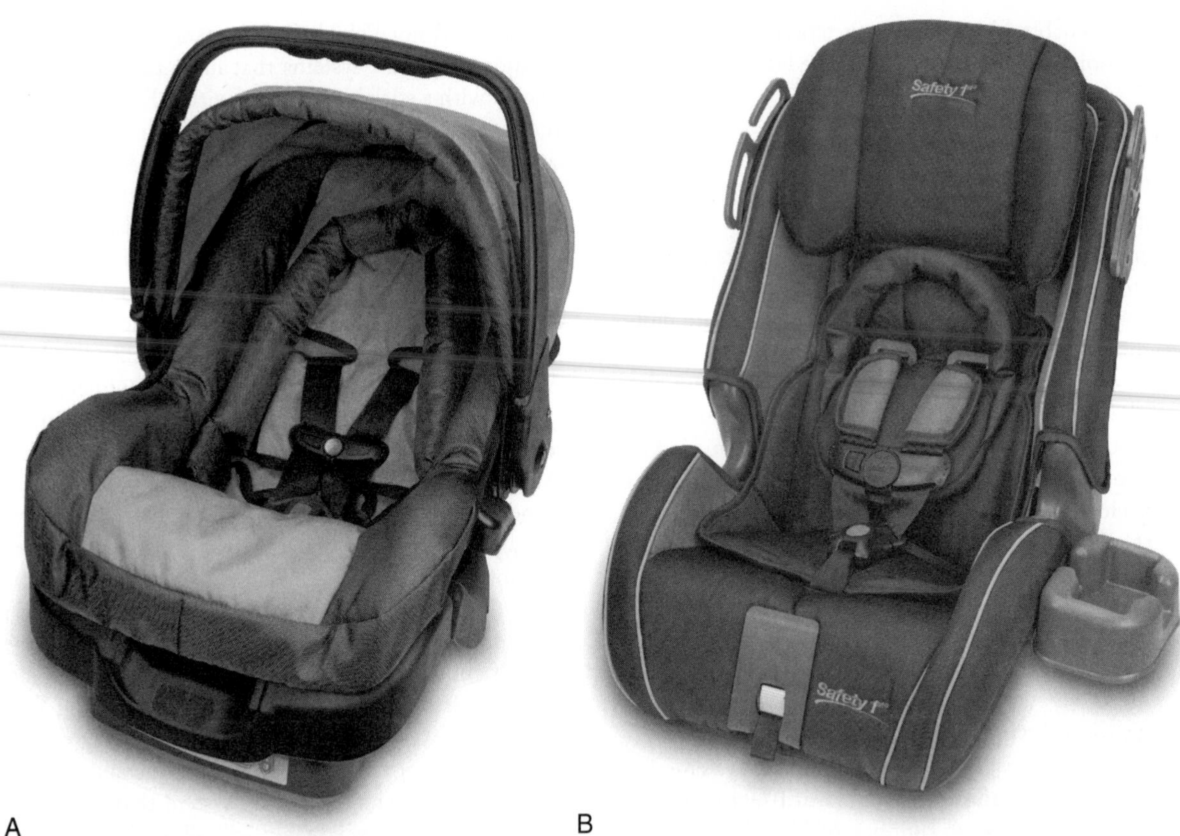

FIGURE 11-3 **A,** Rear-facing infant restraint system. **B,** Forward-facing child restraint system. (Courtesy of Dorel Juvenile Group.)

free of them. Since 2002, vehicles have been equipped with Lower Anchors and Tethers for Children (US name) and lower universal anchorage systems (Canadian name) that make installation of forward-facing car seats simpler. Clasps attached to the restraint system are attached to anchors that are fixed in the vehicle by the OEM at the level of the seat. These systems are tested to a weight of 48 pounds (21 kg).

Once a child reaches 40 pounds and 40 inches, he or she can be moved to a booster seat. These seats position the child so that the vehicle seat belts fit properly. The vehicle seat belt provides restraint when a booster seat is used. Figure 11-4 shows the proper positioning of the seat belt, coming over the shoulder, not across the neck, and across the lap, not the abdomen. Booster seat laws are relatively recent and do not necessarily have the same provisions for when the child is ready to move to use the vehicle seatbelt assembly alone. Usually, a child is ready to move to use of the vehicle seat belt only when he or she reaches 80 pounds and is at least 4 feet 9 inches in height.

Location in the Motor Vehicle

The safest location for the child in a motor vehicle is the center rear seat (American Academy of Pediatrics, 1996, 1999a; Klinich et al., 2012). When this seat is not available, the outboard seat (i.e., the seat behind the front passenger seat) is preferred because this seat is usually on the side of the lane that borders the road shoulder rather than the side that faces oncoming traffic. Booster seats require the use

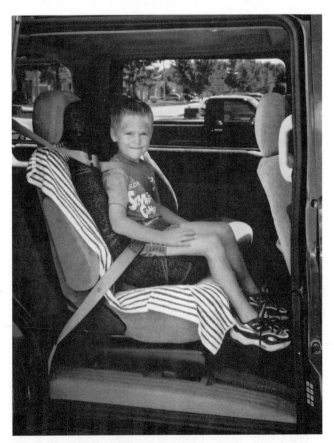

FIGURE 11-4 Proper positioning in a booster seat.

of a three-point seat belt assembly (i.e., one that has both a shoulder and a lap portion), which sometimes precludes locating the child who uses a booster seat in the rear center seat because the restraint system in this location does not always include the shoulder portion. Children under the age of 12 years should not travel in the front passenger seat of a vehicle that has passenger side airbags. The airbags can seriously injure or kill a young child when they deploy. Many auto manufacturers include "smart" airbags that sense the weight of the occupant of the front passenger seat and either adjust the force of the airbag deployment or turn it off. Many vehicles have both front and side airbags, both of which can seriously injure or kill a child travelling in the front seat.

Vehicle Restraint Systems for Children with Disabilities

As previously mentioned, some children with mild to moderate seating needs are able to use a car seat that is designed for children without disabilities. This option is preferred when possible because of the costs of vehicle restraint systems that are designed specifically for children with disabilities. In some cases, the child may be able to use the child restraint system without any modification. When modifications are required, elements of the system that are provided by the **original equipment manufacturer** (OEM) cannot be altered or removed because the system was crash tested with those elements present. Alteration or removal may limit the ability of the seat to protect the child in a crash. Similarly, nothing can be placed underneath the padding or the straps. In the case of the strapping system, placing something underneath alters the direction of the pull on the child's body and may cause him or her to be ejected from the seat in a crash.

However, rolls can be placed alongside the child's legs, trunk, or head to help maintain an upright position. A roll can also be placed under the child's knees to reduce extensor tone (American Academy of Pediatrics, 1999b).

Some children with disabilities cannot be safely transported in a child vehicle restraint system that is designed for children without disabilities, or they do not have sufficient postural control to be safely secured by the **vehicle seat belt assembly** once they become too heavy to safely use other restraint systems. Some indicators of the need for a vehicle restraint system that is specifically designed for children with disabilities are children with tracheostomies, children with either excessive high or low tone for whom the typical restraint system does not provide sufficient support, and children who have a spica cast after hip surgery.

Commercially available restraint systems accommodate children up to 130 pounds and 56 inches (142 cm). The weight limit varies on these products so the clinician needs to check to determine that the child can be accommodated safely. In addition to accommodating children who are heavier than 100 pounds, these systems provide more postural support and have the option for greater tilt of the system. Postural control may be achieved by the form of the seat shell, providing contouring of the seat and more integral fit with the child's body, or by padding that is supplied by the manufacturer. Some of these products have the option for the addition of a pommel to maintain leg abduction. Tilt in the system helps maintain postural control in a manner similar to that provided in mobility systems described in Chapter 10. These systems must meet federal safety standards and be crash tested for use as a vehicle restraint system. Systems that meet federal requirements will have the FMVSS or CMVSS sticker, or appropriate labeling from another jurisdiction.

Transportation for children who are unable to maintain a sitting position is difficult. Federal regulations exist for car beds but the companies that manufactured or distributed these devices no longer produce them. The E-Z ON Vest remains on the market as a product that will help restrain the child in the supine position. Box 11-3 lists Web sites of companies that manufacture child safety systems for children with disabilities.

SAFE TRANSPORTATION OF INDIVIDUALS IN WHEELCHAIRS

A person who routinely uses a wheelchair for mobility is safest in a motor vehicle when he or she is able to transfer into the vehicle seat and use the belt restraint systems that are supplied by the OEM. When transfers are not possible, the individual may travel in a motor vehicle while remaining seated in the wheelchair. Three factors collectively influence the increasing number of individuals who remain seated in their wheelchairs while riding in a motor vehicle: (1) legislation that promotes the rights of individuals with disabilities, (2) standards that are applied to wheelchairs and tie-down systems that relate to the design and testing of these devices for use in a motor vehicle, and (3) the increased availability of vehicle modifications that allow the wheelchair to be secured safely.

Crashworthiness of Wheelchairs and Seating Systems

Voluntary standards have been developed by the American National Standards Institute (ANSI)/Rehabilitation Engineering Society of North America (RESNA) and the International Standards Organization (ISO) that make provisions for the testing of wheelchairs and seating systems to determine their performance in a 21 g/48k m (30 mph) frontal impact crash simulation. These standards are: ISO 7176-19 *Wheeled Mobility Device for Use as Seats in Motor Vehicles* (2008), ANSI/RESNA WC4:2012-19 *Wheelchairs Used as Seats in Motor Vehicles*, ANSI/RESNA WC1:2009-1*Requirements and Test Methods for Wheelchairs (including Scooters)*, and ANSI/RESNA WC1:2009-4 *Wheelchairs and Transportation*, ISO 16480 *Seating Devices for Use in Motor Vehicles* (2004), and ANSI/RESNA WC4: 2012-20 *Wheelchair Seating Systems for Use in Motor Vehicles*. See Box 11-4 for summary of the ANSI/RESNA WC4:2012-19 standard. The first four standards identify crash test procedures and manufacturer requirements for labeling and provision of information for a wheelchair and

BOX 11-4 Summary of ANSI/RESNA WC-19 Standard

The ANSI/RESNA WC-19 standard:

- Specifies general design requirements, test procedures, and performance requirements related to frontal impact performance for manual and power wheelchairs
- Applies to passengers in paratransit, transit, school bus, over-the-road coaches, and personally licensed vehicles
- Applies to securement of wheelchairs by four-point strap-type tie-down systems that are occupied by children and adults
- Applies to a wide rage of wheelchairs, including manual, powerbase, three-wheeled scooters, tilt-in-space wheelchairs, and specialized mobile seating bases with removable seating inserts
- Specifies strength and geometric requirements for wheelchair securement points and occupant restraint anchorage points on the wheelchair
- Provides requirements and information for wheelchair accessory components, seat inserts, and postural support devices with their regard to design and use in motor vehicles
- Applies primarily to wheelchairs that are retrofitted for use as a motor vehicle seat by the addition of after-market add-on components

its dedicated seating. The use of an after-market seating system invalidates the wheelchair crash testing. Because many consumers purchase a wheelchair from one manufacturer and a seating system from another, ISO 16840 and ANSI/RESNA WC4:2012-20 make provisions for testing of a seating system independent of a specific wheeled mobility base. These standards are specific to a frontal impact; further development is required to test **crashworthiness** in side and rear impact crashes. Similar standards for wheelchair transportation exist or are being developed for Canada (Z605), Australia (AS-2942), and other parts of the world (ISO 10542, Parts 1 to 5).

More information can be found on standards for wheelchair transportation on the Web site for the Rehabilitation Transportation Safety Research Center on Wheelchair Transportation Safety (RERC WTS).[2]

In addition to describing the crash test procedure, the standards set peak excursion limits for the head, the pelvis, and the hip in the anteroposterior plane. They place restrictions on the condition of the wheelchair and seating system after the crash test and provide a rating system for the ease of use and the fit of the vehicle restraint system on the consumer's body. It is important to remember that the vehicle restraint system (i.e., the vehicle seat belt) provides restraint for the wheelchair occupant, not the straps that are fixed to the wheelchair (Bertocci, Karg, & Fuhrman, 2005; Schneider & Manary, 2006). The rating system that evaluates use of the vehicle restraint system considers the following factors: the size of the opening through which the vehicle restraint system is threaded, the contact of the system with the consumer's body and where that contact is made, the angle of the pelvic portion of the restraint system, and whether the vehicle restraint system comes into contact with any sharp surfaces (ISO 2004, 2008). As was described earlier for positioning of the vehicle restraint system for a child in a booster seat, the vehicle restraint system must sit across the pelvis, not the abdomen, and rest on the shoulder, not on the neck. Further, the vehicle restraint system must not be held away from the user's body by any part of the wheelchair or seating system.

ISO 7176-19 and the corresponding ANSI/RESNA standard require manufacture of a frame that has four securement points for a **wheelchair tie-down system**. These standards apply to manual wheelchairs and scooters. Wheelchairs that have been successfully crash tested are commonly referred to as WC-19 chairs. As noted initially, these standards are voluntary, with the result that only a small percentage of wheelchairs have been crash tested. A number of reasons for this small proportion were identified at a State of the Science Workshop on Wheelchair Transportation Safety (Karg, Schneider, & Hobson, 2005). These reasons included the concern of manufacturers to assume legal liability of marketing a wheelchair as conforming to WC-19 standards, the lack of knowledge of safe transportation requirements and issues on the part of many ATPs and consumers, the added expense to purchase a WC-19 chair, the voluntary nature of the standards, and the fact that the standards are more rigorous and conflict with federal regulations for safe transportation in a public vehicle (Schneider, Manary, & Bunning, 2005).

The requirements for manufacturers to warn users of potential hazards provide useful information regarding safe transportation for persons who travel seated in their wheelchairs. The most protected position is for individuals to be seated forward facing, yet on many public transit vehicles, the configuration for securement of a wheelchair seats the individual sideways. In addition to being unsafe in a crash, the individual feels less secure because he or she is required to adjust to the acceleration and deceleration of the vehicle. Any peripheral devices such as a communication system or a lap tray need to be removed from the chair and stored securely.

Chest harnesses are recommended only when they have a quick release mechanism. Although they may be useful in aiding proper positioning of the shoulder component of the vehicle restraint system, they do have the potential to restrict the user's airway if they become loose (Bertocci, Karg, & Fuhrman, 2005). A head restraint is also recommended (Bertocci, Karg, & Fuhrman, 2005).

Wheelchair Tie-Down and Occupant Restraint Systems

The person with a disability is best protected from injury if he or she transfers to the vehicle seat and uses the standard OEM's restraint system (see Box 11-5 for summary; J2249 Guideline, version June 9, 1999[3]). However, for many individuals with disabilities, transferring to the seat of a vehicle is not possible or practical. For these individuals, the

[2] www.rercwts.org

[3] http://www.rercwts.org/RERC_WTS2_KT/RERC_WTS2_KT_Stand/Intro_WC18.html

BOX 11-5 Principal Elements of SAE Recommend Practice J2249

1. Upper and lower torso restraint be provided
2. Restraint forces be applied to the bony regions of the body and not the soft tissues
3. Postural supports not be relied on as occupant restraints
4. The occupant faces forward in the vehicle.
5. Adequate clear space be provided around the occupants seated in wheelchairs

From: J2249 Guideline, version June 9, 1999, http://www.rercwts.pitt.edu/RERC_WTS2_KT/RERC_WTS2_KT_Stand/Standards.html.

wheelchair functions as the vehicle seat. Once the person is inside a personal or public vehicle as either a passenger or a driver, both the person and the wheelchair need to be properly secured for safety. The four-point strap tie-down system with the three-point occupant restraint system (as supplied by the vehicle OEM) is considered to be the standard means of securing a passenger who is seated in a wheelchair in a vehicle (van Roosmalen & Hobson, 2005). It is important to view **wheelchair tie-down and occupant restraint systems** (WTORS) as separate parts of a total system designed to protect the passenger or driver who uses a wheelchair (Thacker & Shaw, 1994).

The system that secures the wheelchair to the vehicle (wheelchair tie down) should be separate from the restraint that protects the occupant (i.e., the occupant restraint, which is the vehicle seat belt assembly as described above). The standards that specify the design, testing, and manufacturer labeling and information are: ISO 10542, *Parts 1-5 Wheelchair Tie-Downs and Occupant Restraint Systems* (2005). RESNA developed a recent position paper about the use of wheelchairs as seats in motor vehicles (Bunning et al., 2012). *Tie-down systems* secure the wheelchair to the vehicle floor (Figure 11-5).

There are two types of tie-downs that have been crash tested: four-point strap and docking types (ISO, 2012; Hobson, 2005). The four-belt type of tie-down, the most commonly used system in public transit vehicle, secures the wheelchair at each corner of the frame. In front the belts are attached to the frame (not the leg rests) just above the front caster pivot. WC-19 chairs have very obvious locations for the attachment of these straps. The strapping system and buckles are similar to those used in the aircraft industry for securing cargo. The major advantage of belt systems is low cost and their ability to secure most types of wheelchair frames. Their disadvantage is that use is time consuming and cumbersome and cannot be done independently by the wheelchair rider.

Docking systems have two components: a bracket that is secured to the vehicle floor and a component that is fixed to the lower portion of the wheelchair that couples with the bracket. These systems are specific to each model of wheelchair, thus limiting their use in public transit vehicles. Figure 11-6 A/B shows the E-Z Lock system. Some of these devices have an auto engage feature; all have some feedback mechanism that tells the user that the wheelchair is properly secured (Schneider & Manary, 2006). A switch control that is either activated by the wheelchair rider or by another vehicle occupant disengages the wheelchair from the docking component. The major advantages are quick and easy connection and independent use by the wheelchair rider. The disadvantage is that they require adding hardware to the wheelchair (which adds weight), and they are two to five times as expensive as belt systems.

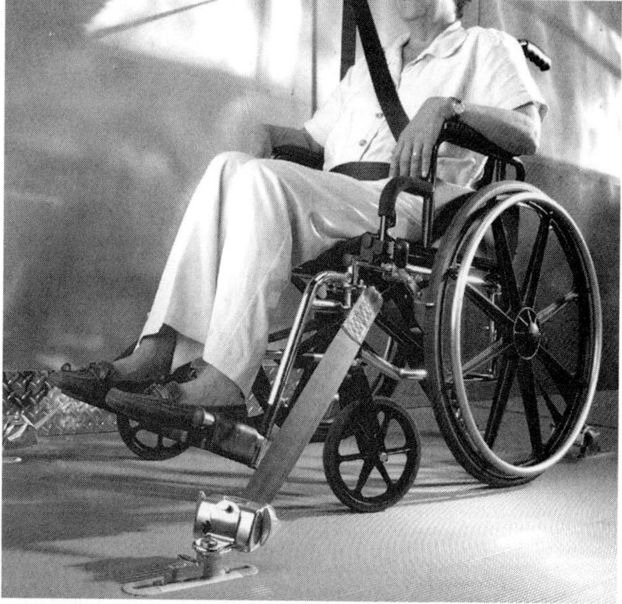

FIGURE 11-5 Wheelchair tie-down securement system for use of wheelchair in a vehicle. Q-Straint wheelchair tie-down system. (Courtesy of Q-Straint.)

For occupant restraint, variations of seat and shoulder belts used in passenger cars can be coupled with the four-belt and docking tie-downs to form a complete WTORS. The occupant restraint can be attached either directly to a van floor or to a point that is common to the tie-down attachment point. It is less likely that the wheelchair and occupant will move different distances during a collision if the occupant restraint is attached to the latter point. If they are not attached at the same point, it is likely that the wheelchair will move farther, forcing the occupant into the restraint and causing injury (Thacker & Shaw, 1994). Both the four-point strap tie-down and the docking systems described above have disadvantages. Strap systems cannot be used independently by the wheelchair rider. Current docking systems are wheelchair specific, limiting their use to private vehicles. The ISO 10542 describes specifications for a **universal docking interface geometry** (ISO, 2012). This standard specifies the dimensions and shape of the adaptor, location on the rear of the wheelchair, and dimensions of space required around the adaptor (ISO, 2012).

Another advancement in the technology for securing wheelchairs in a vehicle is a passive, rear-facing system that is being introduced in Canada, Australia, and Europe for **large accessible transit vehicles**. This technology uses a securement station based on external structures, rather than straps, to protect the passenger in the event of a crash.

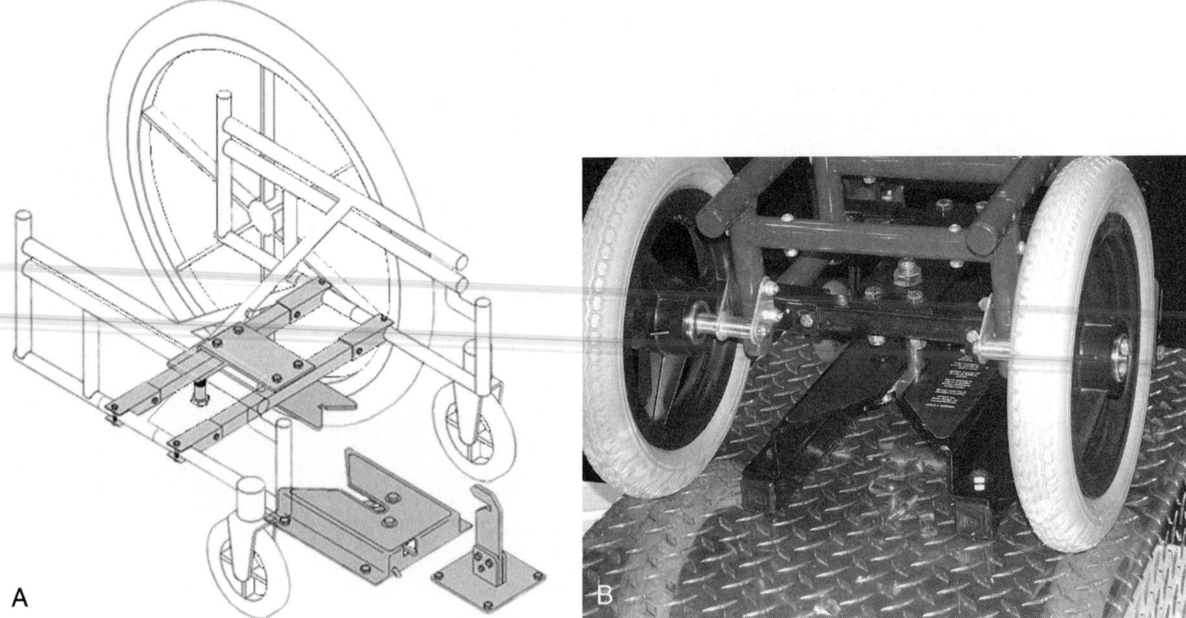

FIGURE 11-6 **A,** Schematic depicting the components of the E-Z Lock system; **B,** Wheelchair connected to E-Z Lock system in a vehicle. (Courtesy of EZ Lock: www.ezlock.net.)

A padded structure that fits closely to the person's back and head protects in forward motion, the wall of the vehicle and a bar on the opposite side limit lateral movement, and the brakes of the wheelchair and the user's ability to grasp a bar limit rearward movement (van Roosmalen & Hobson, 2005). Wheelchair riders prefer this system because they can use it independently. However, problems remain, most notably the unreliability of many manual wheelchair brakes and the great variance in the ability of individuals to grasp and hold the barrier to stabilize themselves (Hobson, 2005). No industry standards exist for these stations.

TECHNOLOGIES FOR TRANSPORTATION AND DRIVING

Driving is a valued activity, particularly in North America where people depend more on private vehicles than on public transportation. Driving affords independence and spontaneity. People are often very reluctant to give up their driver's license even when they realize that they can no longer drive safely (Vrkljan & Miller Polgar, 2007). Globally, the demographics of those who hold valid drivers licenses is changing. A recent study of these demographics in fifteen different countries showed that the percentage of older adults with valid drivers licenses is increasing in all countries studied (Sivak & Schoettle, 2012). Because the data were drawn from existing databases for each country, it is difficult to compare across countries. Of those reporting statistics for older adults 70 years and older, the US and Canada reported about 75% of the population in that age group held valid drivers licenses, Switzerland and the UK reported about 50%, while Finland and South Korea reported much smaller proportions (approximately 38% and 13%, respectively) (Sivak & Schoettle).

Vehicle Access

Ingress and egress issues for an individual who transfers into a vehicle seat were considered above. This section will discuss access issues for individuals who remain in their wheelchairs for transportation. In these instances, the vehicle will be a modified van. Also considered will be after-market devices that load and store the wheelchair once the user has transferred to a vehicle seat.

Van modifications typically involve provision of a ramp for access and a tie-down system to secure a wheelchair. The latter were discussed in an earlier section of this chapter. Ramps can be side or rear loading, manual or power operated. They provide access through the side sliding passenger door or the rear. A passenger who enters through the side can sit in either the front or the middle row of van seats. Entering through the rear of the van provides access to the rear and middle row of seats. Figure 11-7 shows a ramp that accesses the side sliding passenger door.

Newer designs store the ramp in a recessed area on the van floor so they do not interfere with access inside the vehicle. Many car manufacturers provide reimbursement for after-market modifications required to make a van accessible. The Web addresses for the main van conversion companies are listed in Box 11-6.

Integration of the wheelchair with the van modifications is critical. A mismatch between these mobility devices is a very expensive mistake. The consumer needs to know the dimensions and configuration of his wheelchair before proceeding with van modifications. The following should be considered: (1) the width of the wheelchair for movement

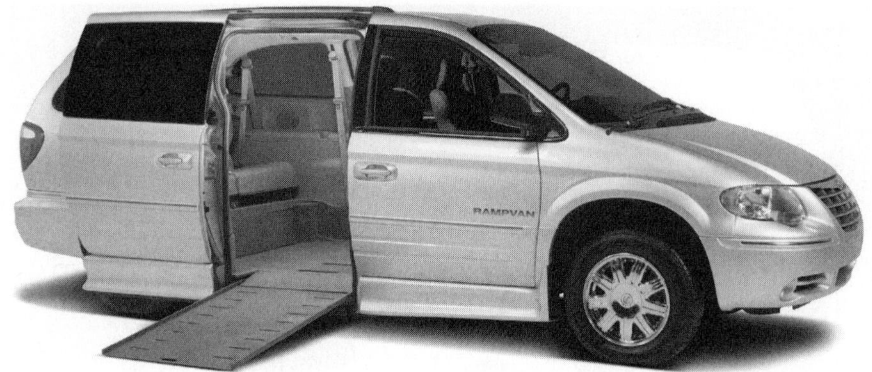

FIGURE 11-7 Side access ramp for transfer with wheelchair into and out of vehicle. (Courtesy of Braun Corporation, www.braunlift.com.)

BOX 11-6 Van Conversion Companies

Braun Corporation: www.braunlift.com
Access Mobility Systems: www.accessams.com
Ricon Corporation: www.riconcorp.com
Access Unlimited: www.accessunlimited.com

through the opening into the vehicle and maneuvering once inside the vehicle, (2) the height of the wheelchair for head clearance (remember that a tilt chair may increase the overall height, and (3) the length of the wheelchair and consequent turning radius; front rigging and the need for a reclined position will increase the length of the wheelchair. If a person remains in the wheelchair to drive, further considerations are made. He or she must be able to fit into the space allocated for the driver. The seat height must not interfere with the travel of the steering wheel. He or she must be able to reach the necessary controls and finally be able to see out of the front and side windows and access the mirrors. In some situations, if the seat height is too high, the driver will not be able to see out of the front window (Phillips, Fisher, & Miller Polgar, 2005). These are important considerations; a modified van that does not accommodate the user's wheelchair is of no benefit.

If it is not possible for the individual to load the wheelchair manually into the vehicle, there are powered wheelchair-loading devices that can assist with this function. These devices pick up and store a manual wheelchair in the back seat, in the trunk, or in a carrier attached to the roof or back of the car. Figure 11-8 shows an example of a loading device that folds and stores a conventional wheelchair inside a cover that is mounted on top of the car. The other advantage of this type of loading device is that the wheelchair does not take up room in the trunk or back seat. These devices can be operated either from outside or inside the vehicle.

Modifications for Driving

Primary Driving Controls

The **primary driving controls** are those that are used to stop (brakes), go (accelerator), and steer. Modifications are available to assist the driver to maintain a grip on the steering wheel, to access the pedals, or to control the vehicle with the hands and arms only when the driver does not have use of the legs to control the vehicle. Each of these vehicle modifications will be considered in turn.

There are a number of options to consider for steering for drivers who use one arm or use a prosthetic arm or who have impaired arm and hand function. For a driver who uses one hand to steer, a steering device allows the driver to maintain control of the wheel at all times (Lillie, 1996). Evaluation of the client's hand function determines both the type and location of the device (Bouman & Pellerito, 2006). Steering devices attach directly to the steering wheel or to a bar that stretches across the inner diameter of the wheel and attach to each side of the steering wheel. These devices are frequently removable so that another person can drive the vehicle (Bouman & Pellerito, 2006). Steering devices (shown clockwise in Figure 11-9) include palm grip, tri-pin, fork-grip or V-grip, spinner knob, and amputee ring (for use with prosthetic hooks).

Additional modifications for steering may include a reduced-effort or zero-effort steering mechanism, a steering wheel of reduced diameter, height and angle adjustments to the steering column, and reduced gain (the number of turns of the steering wheel required to pivot the wheels from fully left to fully right). Reduced- or low-effort steering systems reduce the effort required for steering a vehicle by 40%, whereas zero-effort systems are able to reduce the effort required by 70% (Peterson, 1996).

Two primary types of pedal adaptations are available: a left foot accelerator and pedal extensions (Bouman & Pellerito, 2006). The latter are available from many OEMs and are used by individuals who are not able to reach the pedals. As the name would indicate, the left foot accelerator allows the driver to control both braking and acceleration with the left foot. This device is also removable for other drivers. It requires an automatic transmission vehicle.

Hand controls for accelerator and brake consist of a mechanical linkage connected to each pedal, a control handle, and associated connecting hardware. There are four common design approaches: push-pull, push-twist,

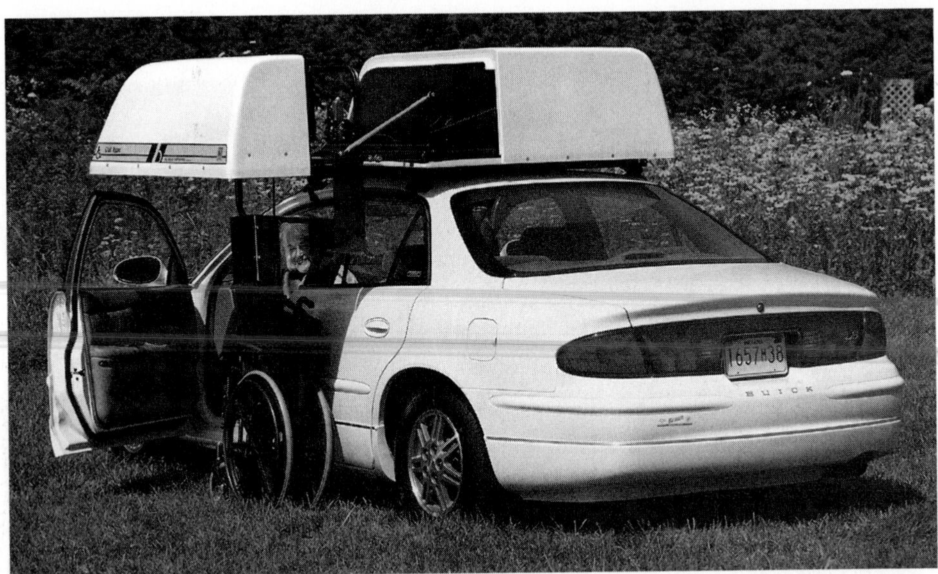

FIGURE 11-8 Wheelchair loading device for a sedan. (Courtesy of Braun Corporation, www.braunlift.com.)

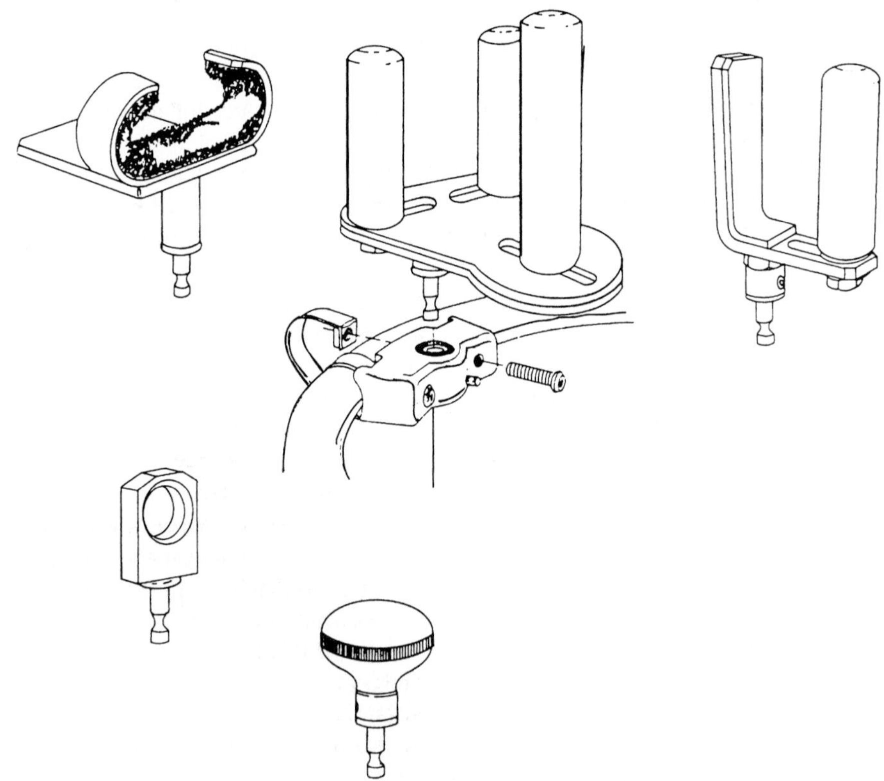

FIGURE 11-9 Different steering aids that accommodate a variety of consumer needs. (Courtesy Mobility Products and Design.)

push-right-angle-pull (Bouman & Pellerito, 2006), and push-tilt (Bouman and Pellerito). In each case the first designation (e.g., push) refers to activation of the brake and the second (e.g., pull or twist) is used for activation of the accelerator.

By using a push control (Figure 11-10, *A*), the consumer activates the brakes by pushing on a lever in a direction directly away from him or her, parallel to the steering column. Acceleration is accomplished either by pulling back on the control, rotating it, or pulling downward at a right angle to the steering column. The weight of the user's hand is sufficient to maintain a constant velocity. When the accelerator control is released, it returns to the off position. These controls are easily attached to almost any vehicle by the connecting hardware, which clamps a rod to each pedal and stabilizes them by attachment of a mounting bracket to the steering column.

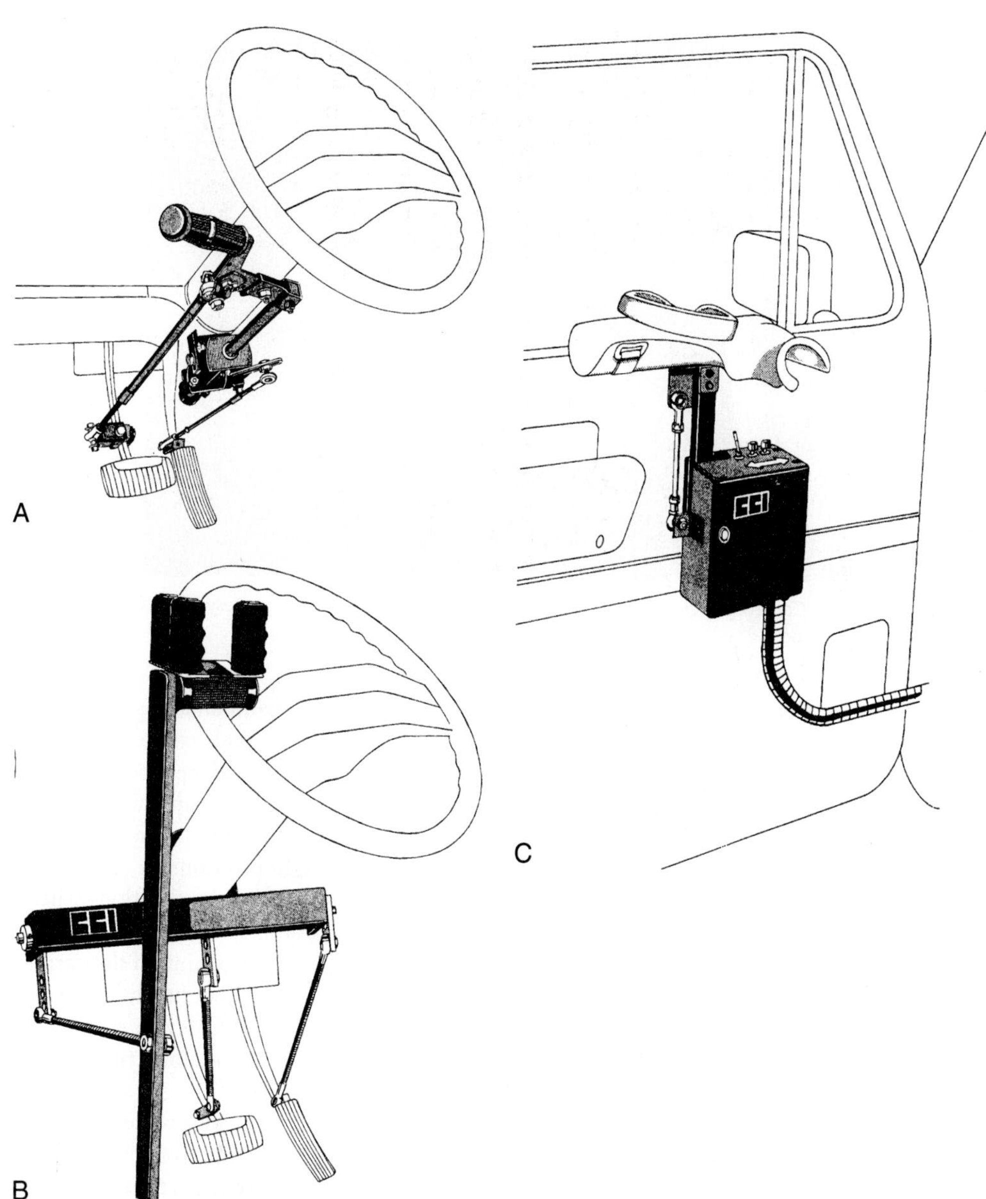

FIGURE 11-10 Hand control for braking and acceleration. **A,** A push-twist hand control. Pushing down applies the brakes, and twisting the lever to the left accelerates the vehicle. **B,** A mechanically assisted manual system. **C,** An electrically assisted controller and interface. (Courtesy Creative Controls, Inc.)

The connecting rods are adjustable in length to accommodate different vehicles. They are normally operated with the left hand, and the right hand is used for steering; however, right-hand mounting systems are also available from a variety of manufacturers (Bouman and Pellerito, 2006).

Additional assistance is required for persons with weak upper extremities (e.g., high-level spinal cord injury). There are two basic approaches: (1) mechanical assist and (2) power assist. Mechanical assist systems use one of the approaches described above, but they provide a lever arm that affords a mechanical advantage (Figure 11-10, *B*). Instead of connecting the hand control directly to the accelerator and brake pedals, there is a mechanical linkage that magnifies the force applied by the user. Typically this system consists of a long arm, attached to the floor, that is pulled back for acceleration and pushed forward for braking. The arm is also linked to the pedals through connecting hardware. Power-assisted devices use either hydraulic or pneumatic assist (similar to power brakes or steering) or electronic powered systems. Electronically powered systems add servomotors that apply force to the brake and accelerator system. An electronically assisted brake and accelerator control is shown in Figure 11-10, *C*. One of the most recent developments is the use of a joystick that the driver pushes back for acceleration and pushes forward for braking.

Secondary Driving Controls

In addition to the controls necessary to maneuver the vehicle, **secondary driving controls** are needed for safe operation of a vehicle. These include turn signals, parking brakes,

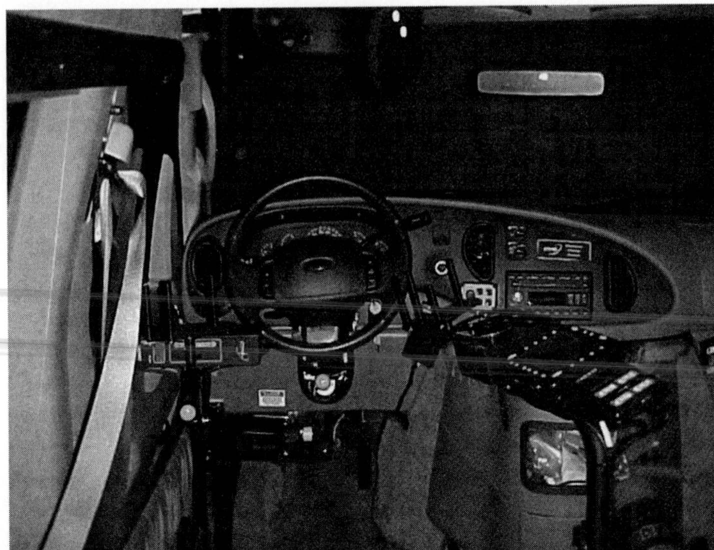

FIGURE 11-11 Control panel for primary and secondary driving control. (Courtesy of Access Mobility, www.accessams.com.)

lights, horn, ignition, temperature control (heat and air conditioning), and windshield wipers. The knobs for operating secondary controls may not be within reach of the driver or may be of such a shape that the driver cannot operate them (Bouman & Pellerito, 2006). These knobs can be adapted by adding extensions or a differently shaped control or by relocating them so the driver can use them. A control panel that contains all these functions can also replace the standard controls. This panel is a special-purpose membrane keyboard that interfaces through a microcomputer to activate the secondary functions. It is mounted to either side of the steering wheel in a location that is within reach of the driver (Figure 11-11). Drivers who have the use of only one hand have an option of a voice-activated control panel that activates the functions above through spoken commands (Bouman & Pellerito, 2006).

ASSESSMENT

A number of websites provide useful information for determining the, correct type of car seat for a child of a certain age, height and weight. Box 11-1 provides a list of some of these websites. Car seat clinics are frequently held in many communities where individuals can take their vehicle and child restraint system to a specific location where they are inspected for proper installation of the seat.

Assessment of the safest way to transport children with disabilities is not formalized, although information is available. Transport Canada produced a report: *Transporting infants and children with special needs in personal vehicles: A best practices guide for healthcare practitioners* (Transport Canada, 2008) that provides information about the most appropriate restraint options for children with special needs. The following questions guide the decision-making process:

1. Does the child meet the height and weight requirements for the infant/child restraint system being considered?
2. Can the child maintain an upright seated position safely?
   a. Consider how much support he or she needs to maintain this position. Does the system need to be tilted to allow the child to maintain an upright position?
   b. Can the child maintain an open airway for respiration in an upright position?
   c. Are there cardiac implications when seated in an upright position?
3. If the child cannot maintain an upright seated position safely, what is his or her height and weight to guide selection of an alternative device such as a transport bed or modified vest (which allows the larger child to be transported lying down)?
4. Are behavioral problems present that affect safety, such as the ability of the child to unclasp safety restraints during transportation? (Transport Canada, 2008)

Assessment for Driving

An individual may require a driving evaluation for a variety of reasons, including physical disability such as spinal cord injury, impairments resulting from a cerebral vascular accident or traumatic head injury, or age-related changes such as vision loss. A driving evaluation may be used to determine whether an individual whose license has been removed because of an illness, such as a stroke, is safe to return to driving or whether an individual who is currently driving remains safe to do so. The decision to recommend to a regulatory body that an individual is no longer safe to drive is a difficult one for two reasons: (1) the knowledge that removing a person's driver's license frequently results in withdrawal from social activities and depression (Marottoli et al., 2000) and (2) the concern that this conclusion is based on sound assessment procedures. Two consensus conferences on driving evaluation published their findings (Korner-Bitensky et al., 2005; Stephens et al., 2005). These conferences were prompted by concern that a common driving evaluation was not used. A recent publication from the National Highway and Traffic Safety Association reviews current driver assessment practices and instruments (Chardury et al., 2013). Further guidelines for evaluation of older drivers are published by the American and Association Médicale Canadienne/Canadian Medical Associations (AMA & NHTSA, 2010; AMC/CMA, 2012).

A **driving evaluation** usually has two components: an off-road assessment that is paper or computer based and an on-road component with a trained evaluator. In some situations, performance on the off-road assessment may indicate that the client is not safe to proceed with an on-road evaluation or that the on-road evaluation should be conducted in a safer environment such as a closed-circuit course.

Both consensus groups recommended that the off-road assessment should include cognitive, physical, visual, and perceptual elements, although these were not necessarily defined in the same way. The international group (Stephens et al., 2005) also included cutaneous sensation as an element, and the Canadian group (Korner-Bitensky et al., 2005) included behavior as a component. Both groups recommended that a medical history, driving history, and assessment of knowledge of rules of the road be completed. Box 11-7 provides a list of functions that are recommended for evaluation as part of a driving assessment. At this time, there is limited evidence to indicate how well performance on off-road driving assessment predict future driving abilities. However, research is currently proceeding (Classen et al., 2013; Classen et al., 2012; Marshall et al., 2013) that will provide a more evidence-based approach to driving assessment.

The Canadian group went on to make recommendations for an on-road evaluation. They recommended that the individual drive a course that includes many common driving maneuvers such as stopping at a light or stop sign, making right and left hand turns, merging and accelerating into traffic, driving in reverse, and driving on roads with a variety of speed limits. Behaviors scored during an evaluation include but are not limited to the ability to drive at a consistent, appropriate speed, stopping when appropriate and continuing when appropriate (i.e., not stopping at a green light), maintaining a safe distance from a lead car and from cars and other objects that are parked on the side of the roadway, proper lane position, and the ability to drive safely when additional cognitive tasks are present, such as when a passenger talks to the driver.

On the basis of the results of the evaluation, a recommendation for driving is made. The outcome of the evaluation can be one of the following: (1) the individual has the skills to continue to drive safely, (2) the individual does not have the skills required for safe driving, (3) the individual has the basic skills and continues with a driver training program, or (4) the individual has a specific impairment that limits the ability to drive with typical equipment so must be assessed and trained to use adapted driving controls.

The driver with a disability needs to be carefully evaluated for any modifications that are being considered. The assessment of an individual for driving modifications progresses in a logical manner, starting with an assessment of ability to operate the primary controls, followed by an assessment of the use of the secondary controls. This assessment requires specific expertise of an individual who is a driving rehabilitation specialist. Because of this expertise, the assessment is not described in detail here. Once modifications are recommended, only a reputable dealer should install them.

BOX 11-7 Common Assessment Areas for Off-Road and On-Road Driving

Cognition
- Attention (sustained, divided, alternating)
- Memory
- Orientation
- Impulse control
- Judgement
- Insight
- Planning
- Problem solving

Vision*
- Acuity
- Useful Field of View
- Contrast sensitivity
- Visual field
- Accommodation and adaptation
- Visual tracking

Motor
- Range of motion (neck, upper and lower extremities)
- Upper and lower extremity strength
- Coordination (fine and gross motor)
- Balance and postural control
- Endurance
- Reaction time

Somatosensory
- Proprioception
- Cutaneous sensation

Visual Perception
- Visual scanning
- Figure-ground
- Depth perception
- Spatial relations
- Form constancy

On-Road Evaluation
- Stop at stop sign or light
- Right and left-hand turns
- Merge into ongoing traffic
- Lane change
- Driving on roads with different speed limits
- Acceleration/deceleration
- Driving in reverse
- Driving on multiple access roadways (e.g., streets)
- Driving on limited access highways/freeways

* Many of the visual tests must or should be completed by an eye/vision care specialist (e.g., ophthalmologist or optometrist)

Sources:
AMA
CMA
Korner-Bitensky, N., et al., 2005
Stephens B.W., et al., 2005

CASE STUDY

Driving Evaluation

Sandra was 35 years old when she sustained an incomplete C5-6 spinal cord lesion. She has good control of her shoulder movement, the ability to flex and extend her elbows with gravity removed, and weak hand movements. Her muscles are stronger on her right side compared with her left. She has poor trunk control and flaccid lower extremities. Sensation is absent below the level of the lesion. She uses a mid-wheel drive power wheelchair that she controls with a joystick located on her right-hand side. She is now ready to return to driving and has been referred to you for driver evaluation and retraining and vehicle modifications. She still has the four-door sedan that she drove before her injury.

Questions

1. Describe the evaluation you would conduct for both driving and vehicle access.

Would you recommend that she drive while seated in the OEM vehicle seat or in her power wheelchair? Justify your recommendation.

2. Describe your evaluation of her vehicle. What vehicle modifications would you recommend?

Given the information you have about Sandra, what assistive technology would you recommend to enable her to drive?

OUTCOME EVALUATION

The primary outcome of the use of these technologies is incidence of crashes and crash outcome. These data are collected typically by various agencies including Ministries of Transportation, Federal Transportation Agencies, and Insurance Agencies.

Driver Training or Retraining

Driver education and training give the opportunity for the consumer to relearn driving skills or to learn driving skills in the case of an individual who is learning to drive with hand controls. This training can include classroom activities, use of a driving simulator, and on-road instruction.

Many driving schools will provide driving instruction for individuals whose basic skills are no longer safe but who have the potential to regain safe driving skills as determined by an evaluation. Classroom training is competency based and focuses on topics such as emergency driving procedures, defensive driving techniques, purchase of a vehicle, vehicle maintenance, accident responsibilities, and traffic laws. This classroom training is followed by on-road practice of basic driving maneuvers.

In addition to discussing rules of the road, programs teach safe driving strategies such as route planning, not driving at night or in bad weather, and avoiding heavily traveled freeways.

Other modules talk about cognitive and visual changes that have the potential to affect safe driving, the effect of medications on driving performance, vehicle safety features, and how to judge personal fitness to drive. Although educational programs provide excellent information, the lack of an on-road component limits the ability to ensure that participants will be safe drivers in the actual driving situation (Bédard et al., 2004).

Driving simulators allow training of specific driving skills in a safe environment (Stephens et al., 2005). There are many different types of driving simulators. The simplest form consists of one or more computers that display a preprogrammed route. A steering wheel and brake and accelerator pedals are connected to the computer. The client may sit in a regular chair, wheelchair, or a vehicle seat. More sophisticated models project a driving route onto a screen that surrounds a vehicle on three sides. A client sits in the vehicle and uses the vehicle's controls. The vehicle is usually fixed with this type of simulator. The most complex simulators use a pod that contains a vehicle with route projected onto a screen that surrounds the vehicle. This pod is mounted on a system that provides six degrees of freedom of movement in an attempt to simulate the motion of a vehicle. Although the technology is continually refined, there is concern that the simulated motion is not sufficiently coupled with the projected image, which can produce nausea in the client.

Driving simulators are useful tools for the driver education process (McCarthy, 2005). They allow the instructor to program specific driving elements into a system and vary the demands placed on the client. Routes can be simple, straightforward driving for use when an individual is learning to use hand controls, for example. The complexity increases with the addition of driving elements, interaction with other vehicles and pedestrians, and unexpected hazards. However, there are drawbacks to these systems. One drawback is the validity of these simulations with respect to actual on-road performance. The ability to predict on-road performance from performance on a simulator is not well established (McCarthy, 2005). A major drawback is simulator sickness. Many clients, particularly seniors, cannot tolerate the simulation and develop nausea and dizziness, which obviously limits the device's usefulness.

Driver assessment and rehabilitation have the primary goals of keeping safe drivers on the road and helping those who have the potential to remain safe to regain necessary skills. Evaluation and retraining are linked components of this process. Because of the increasing prevalence of senior drivers in many developed countries, many resources are available that provide information about remaining safe behind the wheel and identifying signs for when driving is no longer a safe occupation (Box 11-1).

Secondary Outcomes

Transportation supports community mobility so outcome evaluation also includes determining whether the individual and her or his family are able to use transportation to access key venues in their community. To date, little research exists that examines these outcomes of transportation technology use as most of the work in this area is focused on older drivers. Further, there is a lack of standardized instruments that evaluate the ability to be mobile in the community, using different forms of public or private transportation. The Canadian Occupational Performance Measure (Law et al., 2005) can be adapted to obtain some data on the importance of participation in and satisfaction with community engagement as supported by different forms of transportation.

SUMMARY

Access to a vehicle affords independence and the ability to participate in community activities. Technology relating to occupant protection and vehicle access, either as a driver or a passenger, needs to be considered in light of its ability to provide safety when traveling in the vehicle. This chapter considered assistive technology that aids safe transportation for individuals with disabilities. A primary concern is occupant protection, which included selection and use of proper vehicle restraint systems for children who are not able to use the vehicle seatbelt assembly and for individuals with mobility impairments who remain seated in a wheelchair while riding in an adapted vehicle. The factors that need to be considered when determining whether an individual can transfer to a vehicle seat or needs to remain in a wheelchair were discussed. Further, the voluntary standards that guide the testing and labeling of wheelchairs for use during transportation and for vehicle tie-down and occupant restraint systems were also discussed. Two further main topics were covered in this chapter: vehicle access and selection and driver evaluation and retraining, including vehicle modifications for driving.

STUDY QUESTIONS

1. What are the three main categories of child restraint systems for vehicles? What are the indications for the use of each category?
2. What modifications can be made to a child restraint system, designed for a typically developing child, that accommodate the positioning needs of a child with a disability? What types of modifications cannot be made to these systems? Why?
3. Describe the advantages and disadvantages of transferring to the OEM vehicle seat for travel in a vehicle, rather than remaining in a wheelchair. Describe the advantages and disadvantages of remaining in a wheelchair when traveling in a vehicle.
4. Name the standards that set the criteria for crash testing and labeling of wheelchairs and seating systems. What are the requirements of these standards?
5. Define a wheelchair tie-down and occupant restraint system.
6. Describe the advantages and disadvantages of each of the two types of wheelchair securement systems for vehicles.
7. What off-road components are recommended for inclusion in a driver evaluation?
8. What on-road components are recommended for inclusion in a driver evaluation?
9. Describe the major considerations for selection of a vehicle for use by an individual with a disability, as either a driver or a passenger.
10. Discuss the elements that need to be considered to ensure that an individual's wheelchair is compatible with the modified vehicle.
11. What are primary and secondary vehicle controls?
12. How are primary mechanical hand controls designed and operated? What are the major types?
13. How are secondary driving controls used?

REFERENCES

American Academy of Pediatrics, Committee on Injury and Poison Prevention: Selecting and using the most appropriate car safety seats for growing children: guidelines for counseling parents, *Pediatrics* 97:761–763, 1996.

American Academy of Pediatrics, Committee on Injury and Poison Prevention: Safe transportation of newborns at hospital discharge, *Pediatrics* 104:986–987, 1999a.

American Academy of Pediatrics, Committee on Injury and Poison Prevention: Transporting children with special needs, *Pediatrics* 104:988–992, 1999b.

American Medical Association, National Highway and Traffic Safety Association: *Physician's Guide to Assessing and Counseling Older Drivers*, 2nd ed., Chicago, 2010, AMA. Available from http://www.nhtsa.gov/people/injury/olddrive/olderdriversbook/pages/contents.html. Accessed December 15, 2013.

ANSI/RESNA: Wheelchairs 1: Section 5: *Requirements and test methods for wheelchairs (including scooters)*, 2009, ANSI/RESNA.

ANSI/RESNA: Wheelchairs 1: Section 4: *Wheelchairs and transportation*, Arlington, VA, 2009, ANSI/RESNA.

ANSI/RESNA: Wheelchairs 4: Section 18: *Wheelchair tie-downs and occupant restraint systems in motor vehicles*, Arlington, VA, 2012, ANSI/RESNA.

ANSI/RESNA: Wheelchairs 4: Section 19: *Wheelchairs used as seats in motor vehicles*, Arlington, VA, 2012, ANSI/RESNA.

ANSI/RESNA: Wheelchairs 4: Section 20: *Wheelchair seating systems for use in motor vehicles*, Arlington, VA, 2012, ANSI/RESNA.

Association Médicale Canadienne/Canadian Medical Association: *CMA Driver's Guide: Determining medical fitness to operate motor vehicles*, 8th ed., 2012. Available from https://www.cma.ca/Assets/assets-library/document/en/about-us/CMA-Drivers-Guide-8th-edition-e.pdf. Accessed December 15, 2013.

Bédard M, et al.: Evaluation of a re-training program for older drivers, *Can J Public Health* 95:295–298, 2004.

Bertocci G, Karg P, Furhman S: Wheelchair seating systems for use in transportation. In Karg P, Schneider L, Hobson D, editors: *State of the science workshop on wheelchair transportation safety: final report 2005*, Pittsburgh, PA, 2005, RERC on Wheelchair Transportation Safety, pp 35–56.

Bouman J, Pellerito JM: Preparing for the on-road evaluation. In Pellerito JM, editor: *Driver rehabilitation and community mobility*, St. Louis, MO, 2006, Elsevier Mosby, pp 239–253.

Bunning ME, Bertocci G, Schneider LW, Manary M, Karg P, Brown D, Johnson S: RESNA position paper on wheelchairs used as seats in motor vehicles, *Assistive Technology* 24:132–141, 2012.

Canadian Association of Occupational Therapists: *National blueprint for injury prevention in older drivers*, Ottawa, ON, 2009, CAOT Publications ACE.

Chardury NK, Ledingham KA, Eby DW, Molnar LJ: *Evaluating older drivers' skills.* (Report No. DOT HS 811 733), Washington, DC, 2013, NHTSA.

Charlton J, Koppel S, O'Hare M, Andrea D, Smith G, Khodr B, Langford J, Odell M, Fildes B: *Influence of chronic illness on crash involvement of motor vehicle drivers.* Monash University Accident Research Centre, *Report* 213, 2004. www.monash.edu/muarc/reports/muarc213.html.

Classen S, Wen P-S, Velozo CA, Bedard M, Winter S, Brumbach SM, Langford DN: Psychometrics of the self report behavior driving measure for older adults, *American J Occup Ther* 66: 233–241, 2012. http://dx.doi.org/10.5014/ajot.2012.001834.

Classen S, Wang Y, Winter SM, Velozo CA, Langford DN, Bedard M: Concurrent criterion validity of the safe driving behavior measure: a predictor of on-road driving outcomes, *American J Occup Ther* 67:108–116, 2013. http://dx.doi.org/10.5014/ajot.2013.005116.

Dobbs BM: *Medical conditions and driving: a review of the literature (1960-2000).* Report No. DOT HS 809 690, Washington, DC, 2001, NHTSA.

Duchek JM, Carr DB, Hunt L, Roe CM, Xiong C, Xiang K, et al.: Longitudinal driving performance in early stage dementia of the Alzheimer's type, *J Am Geriatri Soc* 51:1342–1347, 2003.

Ebell BE, et al.: Use of child booster seats in motor vehicles following a community campaign, *JAMA* 289:879–884, 2003.

Fox M, Sarno S, Potvin J: A biomechanical evaluation of child safety seat installation: forward facing. In *Proceedings of the Inaugural Ontario Biomechanics Conference*, Barrie ON, 2004, The Conference, p 53.

Hammel J, Jones R, Bossett A, Morgan E: Examining barriers and supports to community living and participation after stroke from a participatory action research approach, *Top Stroke Rehabil* 13:43–58, 2006.

Hobson D: Problem-solving the next generation of wheelchair securement for use in public transport vehicles. In Karg P, Schneider L, Hobson D, editors: *State of the science workshop on wheelchair transportation safety: final report 2005*, Pittsburgh, PA, 2005, RERC on Wheelchair Transportation Safety, pp 57–78.

ISO: ISO 16840-4: *Wheelchair seating—Part 4—seating systems for use in motor vehicles*, Geneva, Switzerland, 2004, ISO.

ISO: ISO 7176-19: *Wheelchairs: Wheeled mobility devices for use in motor vehicles*, Geneva, Switzerland, October, 2008, ISO.

ISO: ISO 10542-1: *Technical systems and aids for disabled or handicapped persons—wheelchair tiedown and occupant-restraint systems—Part 1: requirements and test methods for all systems*, Geneva, Switzerland, 2012, ISO.

Karg P, Schneider L, Hobson D: *State of the science workshop on wheelchair transportation safety: Final report 2005*, Pittsburgh, PA, 2005, RERC on Wheelchair Transportation Safety. www.rercwts.pitt.edu. Accessed November 9, 2010.

Klinich KD, Manary MA, Weber KB: Crash protection for child passengers: Rationale for best practice, *UMTRI Research Review* 43:1–15, 2012.

Klinich KD, Manary MA, Flannagan CAC, Ebert SM, Malik LA, Green PA, Reed MP: Effects of child safety restraint features on installation errors, *Applied Ergonomics* 45:270–277, 2014. http://dx.doi.org/10.1016/j.apergo.2013.04.005.

Kochtitzhy CS, Al Freeland, Yen IH: ensuring mobility supported enivornments for an aging population: critical actors and collaborations: *J Aging Res*, 2011, open access, article ID: 138931Z: http://dx.doi.org/10.4061/2011/138931.

Kohn M, Chausme K, Flood MH: Anticipatory guidance about child safety misuse: lessons from safety seat "check-ups," *Arch Pediatr Adolesc Med* 154:606–609, 2000.

Korner-Bitensky N, et al.: Recommendations of the Canadian Consensus Conference on driving evaluation in older drivers, *Phys Occup Ther Geriatr* 23:123–144, 2005.

Lane WG, Liu GC, Newlin E: The association between hands-on instruction and proper child safety seat installation, *Pediatr* 106(4 Suppl):924–929, 2000.

Law M, Baptist S, Carswell A, McColl MA, Polatajko H, Pollock N: *Canadian Occupational Performance Measure*, 4th ed., Ottawa, ON, 2005, CAOT Publications ACE.

Lillie SM: Driving with a physical dysfunction. In Pedretti LW, editor: *Occupational therapy: practice skills for physical dysfunction*, St. Louis, MO, 1996, Mosby.

Lundberg C, Hakammies-Blomqvist L, Almkvist O, Johansson K: Impariments of some cognitive functions are common in crashi-involved older drivers, *Accid Anal Prevent* 30:371–377, 1998.

Marottoli RA, Wagner DR, Coonery LM, Tinetti ME: Predictions of crashes and moving violations among older drivers, *Annal Int Med* 121:842–846, 1994.

Marottoli RA, et al.: Consequences of driving cessation: decreased out-of-home activity levels, *J Gerontol* 55:S334–S340, 2000.

Marshall S, et al.: Protocol for the CandriveII/Ozcandrive, a multicenter prospective older driver cohort study, *Accid Anal Prevent* 61:245–252, 2013. http://dx.doi.org/10.1016/j.aap.2013.02.009.

McCarthy D: Approaches to improving elders' safe driving abilities, *Phys Occup Ther Geriatr* 23:25–42, 2005.

Murphy RF: *The body silent*, New York, 1990, W.W. Norton.

Nussbaum M: *Creating capabilities: the human development approach*, Cambridge, MA, 2011, Belknap Press of the Harvard University Press.

Owsley C, Ball K: Assessing visual function in older drivers, *Clin Geriatr Med* 9:389–401, 1992.

Owsley C, Stavely B, Wells J, Sloane ME, McGwin G Jr: Visual risk factors for crash involvement in older drivers with cataract, *Arch Ophthalmol* 119:881–887, 2001.

Peterson WA: Transportation. In Galvin JC, Scherer JM, editors: *Evaluating, selecting and using appropriate assistive technology*, Gaithersburg, MD, 1996, Aspen Publishers.

Phillips K, Fisher K, Miller Polgar J: Transportation integration: thinking beyond the wheelchair. In *Proceedings of the 21st International Seating Symposium*, Orlando, FL, 2005, pp 97–98.

Rimmerman A, Araten-Bergman T: Social participation of employed and unemployed Israelis with disabilities, *J Soc Work Dis Rehabil* 8:132–145, 2009. http://dx.doi.org/10.1080/15367100903200445.

SAE Recommended Practice J2249: Wheelchair tiedown and occupant restraint systems for uses in motor vehicles, October, 1996, revised, January 1999.

Sanford JA: *Universal design as a rehabilitation strategy: design for the ages*, New York, 2012, Springer Publishing Company.

Sarno S, Fox M, Potvin J: A biomechanical evaluation of child safety seat installation: rear facing. *Proceedings of the inaugural Ontario Biomechanics Conference*, Barrie ON, 2004, The Conference, p 54.

Schneider LW, Manary MA: Wheeled mobility tiedown systems and occupant restraints for safety and crash protection. In Pellerito JM, editor: *Driver rehabilitation and community mobility*, St. Louis, MO, 2006, Elsevier Mosby, pp 357–372.

Schneider LW, Manary MA, Bunning ME: Barriers to the development, marketing, purchase and proper use of transit-safety technologies. In Karg P, Schneider L, Hobson D, editors: *State of the Science Workshop on Wheelchair Transportation Safety*, Pittsburgh, PA, 2005, final report 2005, pp 4–34. www.rercwts.pitt.edu. Accessed December 3, 2006.

Sen A: *The idea of justice*, Cambridge MA, 2009, Belknap Press of the Harvard University Press.

Shaw L, et al.: Seniors' perceptions of vehicle safety risks and needs, *Am J Occup Ther* 64:215–224, 2010.

Sims RV, McGwin G Jr, Pulley L, et al.: Mobility impairment in crash involved drivers, *J Aging Health* 12:430s, 2001.

Sivak M, Schoettle B: Recent changes in the age composition of drivers in 15 countries, *Traffic Inj Prevent* 13:126–132, 2012. http://dx.doi.org/10.1080/15389588.2011.638016.

Stephens BW, et al.: International older driver consensus conference on assessment, remediation, counseling for transportation alternatives: summary and recommendation, *Phys Occup Ther Geriatr* 23:103–112, 2005.

Stutts JC, Stewart JR, Martell C: Cognitive test performance and crash risk in an older driver population, *Accid Anal Prevent* 30:337–346, 1998.

Thacker J, Shaw G: Safe and secure, *Team Rehabil Rep* 5:26–30, 1994.

Transport Canada: Transporting infants and children with special needs in personal vehicles: a best practices guide for healthcare practitioners, *TC 14772E*, 2008.

United Nations: *Convention on the Rights of Persons with Disabilities*. New York, 2006, UN. Available from: www.UN.org/disabilities/convention/conventionfull,shtml.

van Roosmalen L, Hobson D: Looking toward future wheelchair transportation—what should be our vision and how do we realize it? In Karg P, Schneider L, Hobson D, editors: *State of the Science Workshop on Wheelchair Transportation Safety*, Pittsburgh, PA, 2005, final report 2005, pp 79–94. www.rercwts.pitt.edu. Accessed November 9, 2010.

Vrkljan B, Polgar JM: Linking occupational performance and occupational identity: an exploratory study of the transition from driving cessation in older adulthood, *J Occup Sci* 14:42–52, 2007.

Wheeler K, Yang Y, Xiang H: Transportation use patterns of US children and teenagers with disabilities, *Dis Health J* 2:158–164, 2009, http://dx.doi.org/10.1016/j.dhjo.2009.03.003.

Whelihan WM, DiCarlo MA, Paul RH: The relationship of neuropsychological functioning to driving competence in older persons with early cognitive decline, *Arch Clin Neuropsych* 20:217–228, 2005.

Winston FK, et al.: The danger of premature graduate to seat belts for young children, *Pediatrics* 105:1179–1183, 2000.

Winston FK, et al.: Recent trends in child restrain practices in the US, *Pediatrics* 113:e458–e464, 2004.

World Health Organization: *International Classification of Functioning, Disability and Health*, Geneva, 2001, WHO.

World Health Organization: *Global age-friendly cities: a guide*. Geneva, 2007, WHO Press. Available at http://www.who.int/ageing/publications/Global_age_friendly_cities_Guide_English.pdf.

World Health Organization: *World Report on Disability*, Malta, 2011, WHO.

Yakupcin JP: Child passenger safety in the school age population, *Pediatr Emerg Care* 21:286–290, 2005.

CHAPTER 12

Technologies That Aid Manipulation and Control of the Environment

CHAPTER OUTLINE

LEARNING OBJECTIVES

Upon completing this chapter you will be able to:

1. List functional manipulative tasks that can be aided by assistive technologies.
2. Describe the different ways manipulation aids are designed to enable manipulation.
3. List the features and design properties of electronic page turners.
4. List the functions carried out by electronic aids to daily living.
5. Describe the different ways that electronic aids to daily living are connected to the devices they control.
6. Describe the basic components of electronic aids to daily living and how they are implemented.
7. Discuss the uses of robotic devices in aiding manipulation by persons with disabilities.
8. Describe an assessment process to identify appropriate manipulation aids.

KEY TERMS

Alternative
Augmentative
Continuous control
Desktop Robots
Discrete control
Electrically Powered Page Turners
Electronic Aid to Daily Living
General-Purpose Manipulation Devices
Head Pointers
Infrared Light Transmission
Latched control
Mobile Assistive Robots
Momentary control
Mouth Sticks
Programmable Controllers
Radio Frequency Transmission
Reachers
Remote Control
Robotic Systems
Special-Purpose Manipulation Devices
Telephone Controllers
Trainable Controllers
Universal Remote

One of the activity outputs described in the Human Activity Assistive Technology (HAAT) model is manipulation. At the most basic level, *manipulation* refers to those activities that we normally accomplish using the upper extremities, particularly the fingers and hands. Many types of manipulation are required to use assistive devices, especially those that are electronically controlled. For example, keys must be pressed for computer entry, joysticks controlled for powered mobility, and switches activated for communication devices. We have discussed these types of manipulation in previous chapters, and

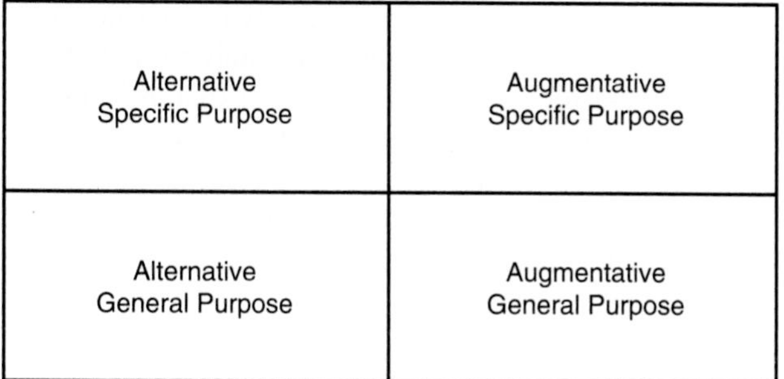

FIGURE 12-1 Assistive technologies for manipulation can be categorized in two dimensions: general purpose versus specific and alternative versus augmentative.

we exclude them from the general discussion of manipulation in this chapter. Here, we describe gross motor manipulation as reaching, grasp/release, lifting, carrying, and coordination of movements such as pushing, pulling, throwing/catching, and turning. Fine motor manipulation includes pinch, point, and dexterity of finger movements. The end goal of the integration of these manipulation components is a person's actions in daily and life activities. For example, activities such as hand writing, food preparation, eating, reaching and using controls in the environment such as door handles and elevator buttons, and appliance control depend on manipulation of physical objects. These types of activities and the technology that supports them are our focus in this chapter.

Figure 12-1 is a characterization of assistive technology devices used for manipulation. As in many other areas of assistive technology application, manipulative aids are either **alternative** (a different method of doing the same task) or **augmentative** (assistance in doing the task in the same manner as it is normally done). For manipulation, we can also distinguish devices as being either specific purpose or general purpose. **Special-purpose manipulation devices** are designed for only one task, whereas **general-purpose manipulation devices** serve two or more manipulative activities. For example, an augmentative, general-purpose approach to turning pages uses a mouth stick that is also used for other activities such as pressing a keyboard on a phone. An alternative, specific-purpose manipulation device is an electronic page turner that lifts and turns a page when a button or switch is pressed. A robotic arm is a general-purpose alternative manipulative aid. It can be used for eating, but it also has application in work site manipulation and many other areas. A hand splint that allows gripping of any utensil serves as a general-purpose augmentative aid, since it can be used to hold a fork for eating or a pen for writing. In this chapter we discuss all four categories of manipulation assistive technologies shown in Figure 12-1.

The variety and choice of technology to assist with elements of manipulation have expanded greatly over the past several years. Often a commercially available tool or appliance will work very well to assist an individual with a disability with manipulation. Many implements for activities such as cooking and gardening are commercially available with enlarged or ergonomically designed handles. Manufacturers are similarly producing implements with telescoping or long handles.

ACTIVITY COMPONENT

The definition of manipulation given at the beginning of this chapter suggested that it involves what we do with our upper extremities. Generally, it involves gross motor functions (larger and more forceful movement and function) and fine motor functions (smaller and more delicate movements). Fine motor coordination is considered to be "the smooth and harmonious action of groups of muscles working together to produce a desired motion" (Giuffrida & Rice, 2009). Let's look at the activity of dressing to illustrate gross and fine motor actions. Gross shoulder movements are needed to reach overhead, behind the back, across the midline of the body and below the waist for lower extremity dressing. Elbow range of motion is needed to assist with reaching. Grasp and release are needed to grab and hold clothes while putting them on and taking them off. Strength is needed for grasp/release as well as to pull clothing up or down, on or off. Fine motor movements are necessary to use zippers, button and unbutton, tie shoelaces, and use fasteners behind the body (e.g., buttons or hook and eye of a waistband). Gross motor functions important here include reaching, grasping/releasing an object, lifting and carrying an object, and actions such as pushing, pulling, and turning an object or control.

The WHO's *International Classification of Functioning, Disability and Health* (WHO, 2001) classifies manipulation as a mobility activity, defining it as: "carrying, moving, or manipulating objects" (WHO, p. 138). Manipulation activities are listed in the subclassification of carrying, moving, and handling objects. More specific elements are congruent with the manipulation components identified in the introduction of this chapter.

These fundamental components of manipulation support all aspects of daily life. The relevant ICF categories include self-care, domestic life (household tasks, caring for others and things), major life areas such as employment, work and community, social and civic life, which involves leisure and recreation, community activities, religious/spiritual, and political life. Like each of the other outputs of assistive technology use—communication, cognition, and mobility—manipulation enables the performance of all daily activities.

HUMAN COMPONENT

Manipulation can be affected by conditions that affect range of motion, limit strength, cause pain, or result in flexible or fixed deformities. Dexterity and fine motor coordination can be affected by tremor and imbalances of muscle tone (e.g., hyper- or hypotonus). Examples of musculoskeletal conditions that affect manipulation include rheumatoid arthritis, osteoporosis, fracture, and amputation. Neuromuscular conditions that affect manipulation include cerebral palsy, spinal cord injury, stroke, traumatic brain injury, and progressive disorders such as amyotrophic lateral sclerosis, multiple sclerosis, Parkinson's disease, and muscular dystrophy. Manipulation can also be affected by general conditions such as frailty and morbid obesity, primarily through loss of strength and endurance.

Clients with little or no manipulation skill benefit from access to and use of electronic aids to daily living or robotics, which are described in a later section on high-technology aids for manipulation. These individuals typically require the technology to replace function that they no longer have. Individuals who have sustained a high cervical spinal cord injury or traumatic head injury, or who have experienced significant decline from progressive conditions such as amyotrophic lateral sclerosis, are potential consumers of high-technology manipulation aids.

Stanger and Cawley (1996) evaluated the incidence of 12 conditions associated with reduction of upper limb function that might benefit from the use of robotic systems. These were cerebral palsy, arthrogryposis, spinal muscular atrophy, muscular dystrophies, rheumatoid arthritis, juvenile rheumatoid arthritis, multiple sclerosis, amyotrophic lateral sclerosis, poliomyelitis, spinal cord injury, head injury, and locked-in syndrome. Robotic systems also have been used with children and adults who have cognitive disabilities (Autism Spectrum Disorders ASD, intellectual disability) and elderly individuals who need assistance with daily living tasks and/or suffer from loneliness.

CONTEXT COMPONENT

Physical Context

Our discussion of the physical context relevant to manipulation aids will consider where these devices are typically used. The context is different between high- and low-tech devices. Low-tech devices such as reaching devices, utensils and tools with built-up handles, and stabilizing devices tend to be portable and useful across multiple devices. A mouth stick is a common example of a low-tech device that can be carried from one place to another and used in different locations in each setting. A mouth stick can be used to push elevator buttons or low-effort buttons for automatic doors. It can be used to dial a telephone, turn a device on/off, or type on a keyboard. When not in use, the device can be tucked away, out of sight. Low-tech devices are very commonly seen in homes, schools, work environments, and in some community and leisure settings (for example, gardening implements with built-up handles might be found in a community garden).

In contrast, high-technology devices tend to be fixed in a single location, commonly the user's residence. As will be described in a subsequent section of this chapter, these devices may be hard-wired to a building's electrical system or consist of a transmitter and receiver that are paired to each other specifically. These devices may restrict other users from controlling an appliance or entertainment unit through other means such as a television remote control, which limits their use in contexts such as an office where multiple users access the same technology (for example, a computer workstation in a commercial establishment that is used by many employees). The high cost of these devices, which is not typically funded externally, and the potential complexity of their use are additional factors that limit their use to the client's residence.

The physical context affects the ability to use some high-technology devices such as **electronic aids to daily living** (EADLs) and robots. In particular, light (natural and artificial) affects the ability to perceive visual information presented on a screen. Ambient noise can affect the function of a voice-activated device and can also interfere with the user's ability to detect information or feedback from the device that is presented auditorily.

Social/Cultural Contexts

It is difficult to separate out the social and cultural contexts in a discussion of the manipulation aids, so they are considered together in this chapter. One aspect that is clearly a social component was discussed in an earlier chapter: the influence of others in the environment. As with other types of assistive technology, the knowledge of others in the setting in which the technology is used—about both the skills of the technology user and use of the technology—affect the willingness to use a device and its integration into daily life. Some of the more complex devices that are discussed later in this chapter are difficult to set up and learn to use and often require assistance from another person for set-up—both initially and for ongoing use.

The attitudes of others in the environment also affect use of this technology. Family, friends, coworkers, teachers, and others who view technology use as simply an alternative way of completing necessary and desired activities accept and enable technology use in different settings.

It is more challenging to separate social and cognitive influences when considering how technology is integrated into our lives and how we use it. Looking first at some of the low-technology devices, such as utensils and tools with built-up handles, we see an example of how a modification that originated in a rehabilitation setting has transferred into the mainstream marketplace (refer to this discussion in Chapter 2). When you peruse the shelves of many stores, you will see many examples of devices that accommodate the needs of individuals with different abilities. In part, the "graying" of the population in many countries may be driving this expansion of ergonomically designed devices in the mainstream; as individuals age and lose function such as grip strength, they demand the availability of devices that meet their physical or sensory needs and enable them to continue with meaningful occupations such as cooking, gardening, or woodworking.

High-technology devices are fixtures in the lives of many of us, as was mentioned previously. Most of us are reliant on our smart phones for communication with others, storage of information, entertainment, and information acquisition. We accept technology that augments how we engage in our daily activities. Similarly, as will be described in the discussion of robotics, robots are commonplace in many industrial and health settings—we are more accepting of a place in our lives for robots and robotics. Consequently, culturally, we are in the midst of tremendous advancements in the types and availability of technology. We are seeing technology originally designed for individuals with disabilities move into the mainstream and devices designed for persons without disabilities being of great use to those who do have disabilities (see Chapter 2). This cultural shift bodes well for the ability of individuals with disabilities to access high-technology devices such as EADLs and robots and integrate them into their daily lives to enable occupations.

Institutional Context

Funding is the critical aspect of the institutional context related to access to EADLs and robotics (although as will be discussed, many of the robotic applications remain in the research laboratory). EADLs are expensive, and are not funded externally in most jurisdictions. Consumers have criticized the high cost of these devices (Stickel et al., 2002). In the absence of external funding, the high cost is a barrier to their acquisition. Some insurance policies provide funding for these devices and it is also possible for individuals who meet specific criteria, such as veterans, to receive some funding to obtain these high-technology devices. The increasing use of smart phone and tablet apps as EADLs has the potential to make them more economical.

LOW-TECHNOLOGY AIDS FOR MANIPULATION

In Chapter 2 we define low-technology aids as inexpensive, simple to make, and easy to obtain. Many manipulative aids fall into the low-technology category. We group these aids into general- and special-purpose devices. Within special-purpose devices, we categorize devices according to the major performance areas of the Human Activity Assistive Technology (HAAT) model: self-care, work or school, and play or leisure. The examples and other aids to daily living are available from many sources, including home health stores, online, and mail-order catalogs.[1]

General-Purpose Aids

To be classified as general purpose, a manipulation aid must serve more than one need. Three general-purpose aids are described here because they are commonly found in most environments: mouth sticks, head pointers, and reachers. The first two of these are often used as control enhancers in conjunction with control interfaces. In Chapter 7 head pointers and mouth sticks are discussed in detail, including their use as control enhancers for activating control interfaces. Both **mouth sticks** and **head pointers** are used for direct manipulation. A mouth stick is usually a wooden dowel with different attachments at one end and a molded piece at the other end that allows the person to hold the stick in his or her mouth. A head pointer is similar in design, except the dowel is fixed to a headband that is worn around the forehead. Both of these devices are controlled by head movements. Turning pages is often accomplished with a mouth stick or head pointer used in conjunction with a book or magazine mounted on a simple stand. A ballpoint pen tip or a pencil can also be attached to a mouth stick for writing. Additional attachments include a pincher that is opened or closed by tongue action and a suction cup end that can be used to grip objects (e.g., a page) by sucking on the end of the mouth stick. Many tasks require sliding objects (e.g., paper, pens) around on a desk or table. Both mouth sticks and head pointers can be used for this task. Mouth sticks or head pointers can also be used for such functions as dialing a telephone, typing, and turning lights on and off.

Many individuals need to extend their physical range. Often the need for extended range is a result of being seated in a wheelchair and wanting to reach an object on a counter or in a cabinet. In other cases it is a need to reach an object on the floor when bending is restricted or stability is poor. Reaching to the floor or in a forward direction is difficult following a hip replacement or a hip fracture when the individual has limitations in hip movements. In all these cases, **reachers** can be useful. A reacher consists of a handle grip that is used to control the jaws of the reacher in order to grasp an object. The grasp required to activate the grip may be of several types: squeeze with the whole hand, pistol grip with all the fingers, or trigger with the index finger. Overall length varies from 24 to 36 inches, and some models fold for ease of carrying. The gripper portion of the reacher may be circular for ease of gripping cans or pincher-like for picking up smaller objects. Rubber or other nonslip materials are often used for reacher grippers. Reachers can be used to manipulate many objects, including food (e.g., cans, packages), cooking utensils (e.g., pans, pots, plates, dishes), office objects (e.g., paper, books, magazines), and recreational or leisure objects (e.g., books, tapes, CDs).

Reachers are used in many ways to manipulate objects. They can act in similar ways to head pointers and sticks to push or pull objects into a space that is usable by the individual. Reaching devices can assist with activities such as dressing, hygiene and other self-care activities, and household activities—any activity that requires grasp and retention of an object that is outside of the individual's reach. It is important to note that because a reaching device extends the length of the arm, it also extends the length of the lever arm, resulting in increased force required to lift the object. As an experiment, try lifting a book and holding it close to your body. Hold it in that position for about 30 seconds. Sense its weight. Now hold the book at arm's length. Hold it in this position for 30 seconds. Notice the difference in the sensation of weight. The book feels like it weighs much more when held away from the body; more force is required to hold it. Keep this consideration in mind when encouraging a client to use a reacher.

Special-Purpose Aids

Because special-purpose low-tech aids are designed for one or two tasks only, they serve those tasks very well. However, because they are so specialized, it may be necessary to have several of these available to meet the demands of self-care, work, and leisure.

[1] Suppliers of the aids described in this section include: Maddak Ableware® (www.maddak.com), Patterson Medical (www.pattersonmedical.com). Useful websites for further information on devices described in this section include: Ability Hub (www.abilityhub.com) and Abledata (www.abledatacom).

Most special-purpose adaptations of products involve one of four modifications: (1) lengthening a handle or reducing the reach required, (2) modifying the handle of a utensil for easier grasping or manipulation, (3) converting two-handed tasks to one-handed ones (providing an alternative method of stabilizing the tools that are being used), and (4) amplifying the force that a consumer can generate with his or her hands. These include enlarged grips for easier grasping, cuffs that hold a utensil and circle the fingers, angled handles for ease of scooping (for people with limited wrist movement), swivel handles that allow the end to be oriented differently for different positions in space (e.g., on a table or near the mouth), and handles requiring limited grasp.

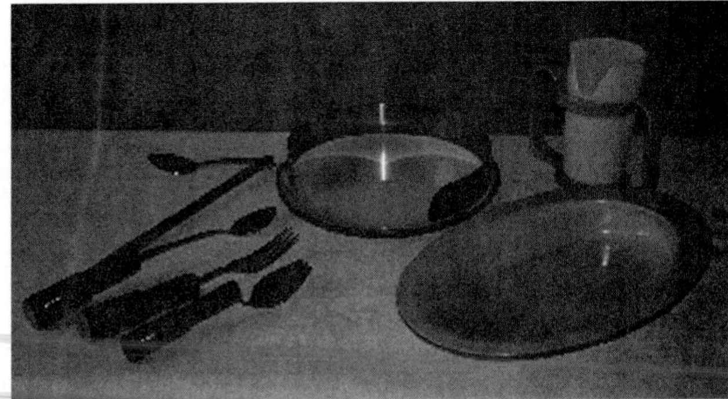

FIGURE 12-2 Low-technology aids for food consumption: Left to right: long-handled spoon with adjustable angle, utensils with built-up handles, plate guard, scoop dish, and cup holder.

Self-Care

Self-care includes aids for assistance in several areas: food consumption, food preparation, dressing, and hygiene. Food consumption aids include a variety of modifications to utensils, such as enlargement and ergonomic shapes of handles, swivel handles so the bowl of the spoon retains a level orientation, lengthening of handles, and combinations of utensils called "sporks" (i.e., a spoon and fork combination). Modifications to plates include suction cups for stability, enlarged rims that make it easier to scoop food onto a utensil (scoop dish), and removable rims that attach to any plate (plate guard). Drinking aids include cups with caps and "sipper" lids through which fluid can be sucked; nose cutouts that allow drinking to occur without tipping the head back; and double-handled cups for two-handed use. Figure 12-2 shows a number of low-tech devices to assist with food consumption.

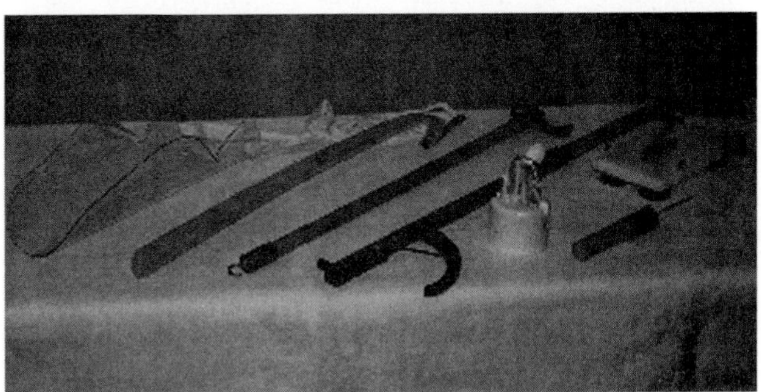

FIGURE 12-3 Low-technology aids for dressing and hygiene. Left to right: sock aid, long-handled shoehorn, dressing stick, reacher, toothpaste holder, button hook, and nail clipper on stable base for one-handed use.

Dressing aids designed to compensate for poor fine motor control include adapted button hooks for single-handed buttoning and zipper pulls. These are available with enlarged, suction, and quad grip handles. For limited reach, there are aids for pulling on socks and pantyhose, long-handled shoehorns, and trouser pulls. A variety of dressing aids and a reacher are shown in Figure 12-3.

Areas of hygiene that can be aided by special-purpose devices include: hair combing and brushing, tooth brushing, shaving, bathing, and toileting. Adapted aids are available that enlarge, change the angle of, or lengthen the handle of hairbrushes, combs, toothbrushes, bath sponges, and manual razors. Toothpaste and shaving cream containers can be adapted with a simple device that allows one-handed dispensing of the product. Devices are available that attach an implement such as nail clippers or electric shaver to a base, thus stabilizing them for one-handed use. Some of these devices are shown in Figure 12-3.

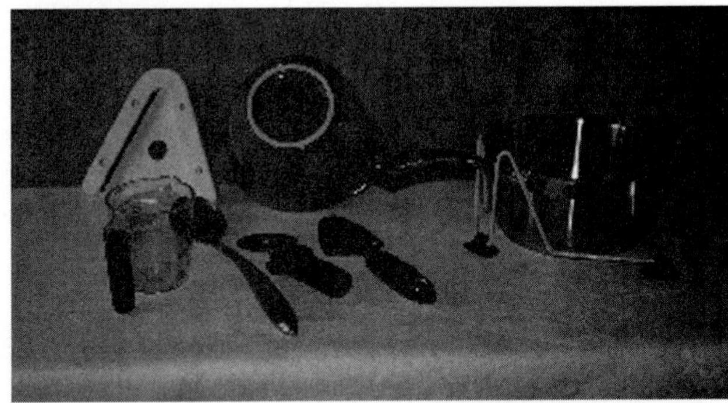

FIGURE 12-4 Low-technology aids for food preparation. Rear left to right: one-handed jar opener and bowl with non-slip base. Front left to right: measuring cup with enlarged handle, commercially available kitchen implements with enlarged, ergonomic handles, and pot holder to stabilize pot for one-handed use.

Examples of food preparation adaptations include one-handed holders for can and jar opening, brushes with suction cups for one-handed scrubbing of vegetables, bowls with suction cup bottoms for stability while stirring with one hand, bowl and pan holders (some of which tilt for pouring), and cutting boards that stabilize food during cutting. Modified handles are available for knives and serving spoons, as well as for other utensils. Many of these devices are shown in Figure 12-4, which includes both commercially available and rehabilitation products. Other self-care items intended for use in the home include cuffs that are used to grip brooms and mops, extended handles on household items such as dustpans and dusters, and key holders. Many of these products are commercially available.

Devices such as universal cuffs are available for individuals unable to grasp, for example, following a spinal cord injury. These devices function in two ways, either as a cuff that is attached to the hand or a rigid, shaped bar that can be slid onto the hand, between the thumb and forefinger.

When a universal cuff is used, implements such as a comb, toothbrush, or pen are inserted into a sleeve that crosses the palm to allow use of the implement without the need for grasp.

Work and School

Throughout this book we have described assistive technologies that aid consumers in accomplishing work- and school-related tasks (e.g., computers, augmentative communication devices). In this section we discuss low-tech aids that specifically help with work and school in the areas of writing and reading.

Handwriting for written communication is a requirement of work and school occupations. Special-purpose manipulative aids that assist handwriting focus on one of two problems: holding the pen or pencil and holding the paper. Some consumers lack the ability to grip a standard pen or pencil. Low-tech approaches to this problem include modified grippers that attach to the hand and clamp to the pen or pencil; wire, wooden, or plastic holders that support the pen or pencil off the paper and allow it to slide across the paper; weighted pens (with variable amounts of weight) that help reduce problems associated with tremor; and pens with enlarged bodies to make them easier to grasp. There are several different designs for holding paper in place for one-handed writing. Generally the paper is held to a plate using either clips or a magnet (in this case the plate is steel). Desks can also be modified with a "lazy Susan" device that rotates to bring items within reach. File folders can be modified for easier grasp by putting hooks or loops on them. The loop or hook protrudes above the folder so that it can be grasped more easily.

Low-tech reading aids are used to hold a book or turn a page. Book holders provide support for the reading material so the consumer does not have to hold it. Page turning is done either by hand or with a head pointer or mouth stick. In a following section we discuss electrically powered page turners and other electronic devices that aid reading. Figure 12-5 shows some low-tech aids that can be used in the work, school, or leisure settings.

Play and Leisure

As with other types of manipulative aids, lack of grasping ability in recreational or leisure aids is generally accommodated for by altering the type of handle. Recreation and leisure examples include cameras with modified shutter release, modified grip scissors, modified handles on garden tools, and modified grasping cuffs for pool cues, racquets, or paddles. Again, some of these modifications are readily available in commercial outlets. A person with limited manipulation strength can fly a kite by adding special wrist or hand cuffs for holding the string. Pinball machines can be adapted with larger buttons to allow control by children and adults with disabilities[2]; the paddles can be controlled by puff-and-sip or any other switches. This makes it possible for a consumer to compete in a fast-paced, interesting game. Computer access methods that were described in Chapter 8 enable an individual to play computer games in the same way they provide access to educational materials.

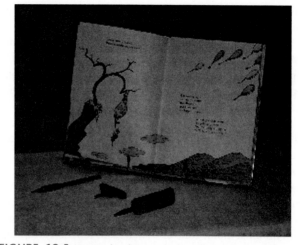

FIGURE 12-5 Low-technology aids for play, school, and work. Rear: book stand. Front left to right: pencil grip, key holder, and universal cuff holding a pen.

One example of a holder is a gooseneck arm attached at one end to a table clamp. At the other end is a bracket that holds an embroidery frame. Using this device, an individual can embroider, crochet, or mend using only one hand. Other examples of devices designed for one-handed assistance are playing card holders, knitting needle holders, and card shufflers. For individuals with limited two-hand function, there are handheld playing card holders.

Devices that aid lack of reaching ability include a mobile bridge for holding the end of a pool cue off the table (a small bracket with wheels to allow positioning of the pool cue) and ramps for use while bowling (the ball is placed at the top of the ramp and the user releases it after aiming the ramp toward the pins). Different grips are available to help a player hold a hockey stick or tennis racquet or other sports equipment to enable participation in most sports.

SPECIAL-PURPOSE ELECTROMECHANICAL AIDS FOR MANIPULATION

Electrically Powered Page Turners

Access to books, magazines, and other reading material is important for the acquisition of information for school, work, or leisure. There are many individuals with disabilities who are able to read, but who cannot physically manipulate the pages of the reading material. Several approaches can be used to assist these individuals. A book holder and mouth stick (see the section on low-tech aids in this chapter) allow independence in page turning for some persons. The major limitation of this approach is the requirement that the book be set up and properly positioned for both visual and physical access. This method also requires a high degree of head control and the ability to hold a mouth stick. A mechanical head pointer eliminates the last requirement, but there are

[2] For example: http://www.rehabilitystores.com/.

still limitations of access. Fatigue often limits the ability to use these devices for a length of time.

Audio books are readily available and provide an alternative to physically manipulating pages. These are discussed in Chapter 13. Using an EADL (described in the next section), a person with fine motor limitations can control the device that plays an audio book.

The recent advent of e-readers[3] and smart phone and tablet apps that function as e-readers has significantly enhanced access to books and other reading materials. The user can download reading material directly to the device. Most of these products have options to change font size and contrast. They can be positioned on a stand to relieve the need to hold the device. A touch screen is used to turn the pages with minimal motor control. When hand function is limited, other options for turning pages are available. For example, Airturn[4] makes a wireless hands-free device that allows the user to change pages through the use of a foot switch. We describe other switch access methods for smart phones and tablets in Chapter 8.

A final alternative is an **electrically powered page turner.** From a manipulative point of view, page turning requires two primary actions: (1) separating the page to be turned from the other pages and (2) physically moving the page from one side to the other (forward or backward). Additional useful but not essential features include scanning a number of pages, turning to a specific page, and locating a bookmark and turning to that page. Turning a single page is the most difficult for page turners, and its success for any page turner is a major indicator of the quality of the unit. Because reading materials differ widely in size, binding (e.g., uniform, spiral, loose leaf), and paper types (e.g., rough, slick, newsprint), it is important to evaluate any individual page turner with reading materials that vary in size, paper type, and binding style. Once the page to be turned is successfully isolated, the page turner must move it to the opposite side of the book or magazine.

Currently available page turners employ one of two methods to accomplish the first task of separating pages. Some devices use a vacuum pump that sucks the first page up and holds it away from the remaining pages. Other devices use a sticky roller that is placed on top of the page. When it rotates, the roller causes one page to be separated from the others. The roller may employ putty, rubber gum (like a pencil eraser), or double-sided tape.

The Gewa page turner[5] (Figure 12-6) uses a rotating roller to separate pages from each other and then moves the entire roller from one side of the book or magazine to the other after the page has been separated. The standard control for the Gewa is a four-direction joystick. Two joystick directions cause roller rotation either clockwise or counterclockwise, and the other two cause the roller to move forward or backward. Any other four-switch control interface can also be used. An additional accessory for the Gewa is a scanning selection method in which a single switch is used to select one of the four control functions as they are presented in sequence. The display of functions consists of small LED indicators, each labeled function corresponding to one joystick direction.

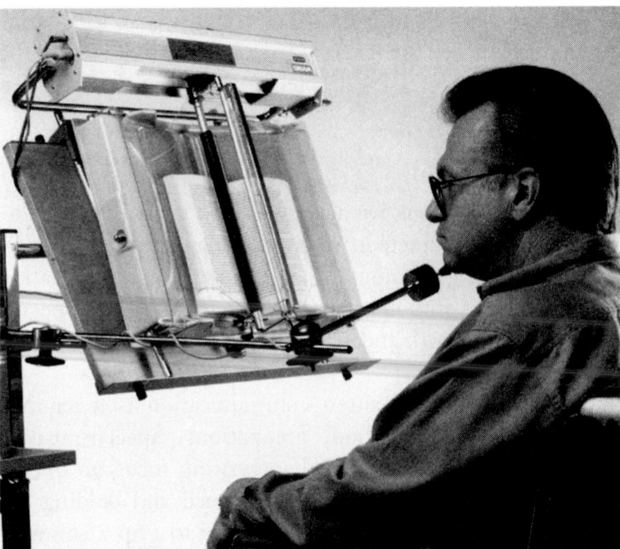

FIGURE 12-6 The Gewa page turner. (Courtesy Zygo Industries.)

Other page turners have different mechanisms. The Touch Turner[6] uses a rubber-coated wheel to separate the pages, and then a rotating semicircular disk pushes the separated page from one side to the other. As the disk rotates, the page is moved forward or backward, depending on the direction of rotation of the disk.

ELECTRONIC AIDS TO DAILY LIVING

Daily activities routinely involve manipulation of appliances, controls, electronic devices, and environmental features such as doors and window coverings. Technology is readily available that replaces the need to physically manipulate the controls of many devices and features in our environment. For example, most of us have remote control devices that allow us to turn the TV or DVD player on and off, select the channel or disk, control the volume, program events such as recording a favorite show, and adjust other settings such as color contrast on the display. Similarly, many vehicles use a remote key entry system that eliminates the need to physically manipulate the key in the lock to unlock the car door. Some of these systems also remotely open the door. Simple security features are wired into new houses that automatically turn home lights on and off at preset times or when motion is detected. In the community, many buildings have at least one entrance where the door is controlled either through a mechanical switch or a sensor that detects when someone approaches. Voice control is an emerging means of

[3] For example Kindle, Nook, and Kobo and their apps for iOS and Android operating systems.

[4] www.airturn.com.

[5] In North America, distributed by Zygo Industries, Portland, OR, http://www.zygo-usa.com/.

[6] Touch Turner Company, Everett, WA, www.touchturner.com/.

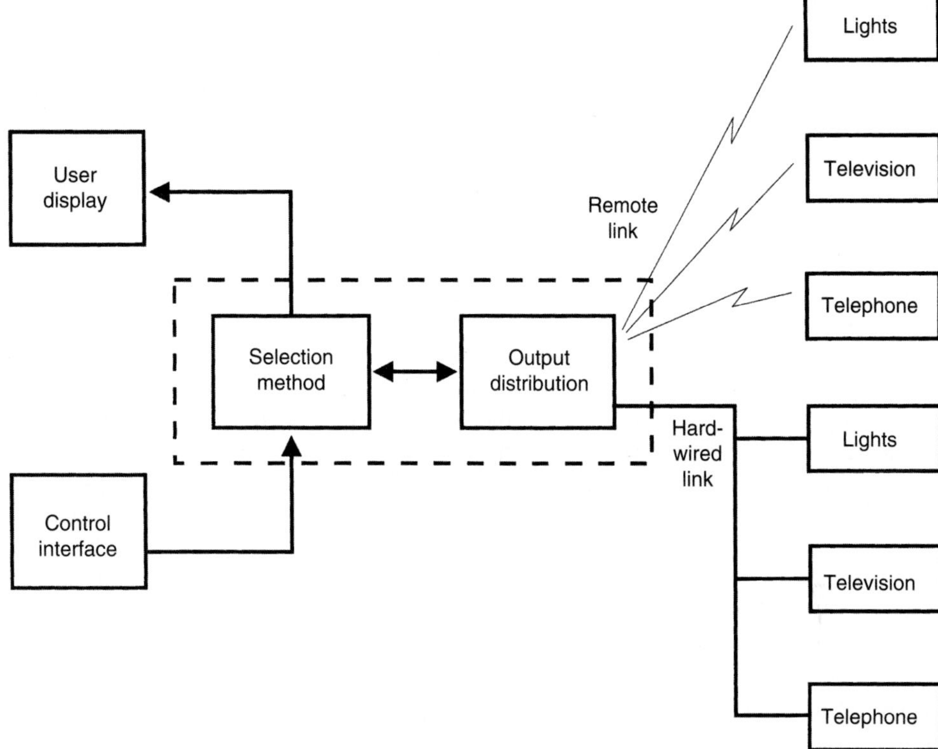

FIGURE 12-7 The major parts of an electronic aid to daily living. The *control interface* and *user display* constitute the human/technology interface. The components within the dotted box are the processor. The appliances listed on the right side of the figure are the activity output.

controlling functions of phones and vehicle controls (e.g., temperature). All of these are examples of existing commercial means to control our environment.

Many objects still require fine motor control to operate them, such as electrically powered appliances (e.g., room lights, fans, kitchen appliances such as blenders or food processors) or environmental features such as doors, windows, and security systems. Doors and windows can be modified by adding electrically powered actuators that are remotely controlled. The majority of these electrical appliances and controls are powered from standard house wiring (110-volt AC in North America, 220-volt AC in Europe and other countries). When an individual does not have sufficient motor skills to manipulate these devices directly, an electronic aid to daily living can be used. We will describe the components of an EADL, including transmission and selection methods, assessment considerations, and integration of multiple function EADLs with needs of the user.

Figure 12-7 shows the different components of an EADL. It depicts a user who wants or needs to control a device, the device to be controlled, and the processor (the selection method and the output distribution unit.) The means by which the user accesses the EADL is the control interface or input device (see Chapter 7). The control interface can include a keyboard or keypad, joystick, and single or multiple switches. The selection method refers to how users indicate their choice (e.g., direct selection or scanning; see Chapter 6). Feedback is provided to the user by some form of user display, which might be a monitor or screen, a light or sound. The control interface and user display constitute the human/technology interface. They are connected to the rest of the system and to each other by a block labeled *selection method.* The output distribution component translates the selection into some form of control of the device, which is connected to the output distribution component either directly (i.e., hard wired) or via a remote (wireless) link. Together the selection method and the output distribution component make up the processor element of the HAAT model as described in Chapter 2. Examples of the appliances to be controlled via an EADL are shown on the right-hand side of the diagram. The devices are hard wired to the home wiring and have some form of receiver (either integrated into the device as with a TV or connected to the device) that receives the signal from the output distribution unit.

In some cases the human/technology interface and the selection method are provided through an augmentative and alternative communication (AAC) device (see Chapter 16) or powered wheelchair control (see Chapter 10) or a computer (see Chapter 8). Control through another device can reduce the total number of interfaces in the user's work space and also provides an identical user interface for both functions (e.g., EADL plus wheelchair control, AAC, or computer use. Tablets and smart phones can also control EADL devices, as we discuss later in this chapter.

The EADL may simply turn the appliance on/off or open/close a door or window covering. This simple function is referred to as **discrete control.** An on/off or open/close function is referred to as binary, since there are only two responses possible. Other examples of discrete control involve selection of a single event such as selection of a TV channel or a pre-stored telephone number. Each of these events is a discrete entry, and its selection produces a unique result. The other type of control function employed in EADLs is continuous. **Continuous control** results in successively greater or smaller degrees of output. Examples of EADL continuous control are opening and closing draperies, controlling volume on a television or radio, and dimming or brightening lights.

There are two types of switch outputs available on most EADLs: (1) **momentary control** and (2) **latched control.** A momentary switch closure is active only as long as the switch is pressed. In the case of the EADL, this output remains active only as long as the control interface is activated (e.g., a switch is pressed). The momentary output mode is useful for continuous functions such as closing draperies.

The output can be sustained as long as the person desires it to be (e.g., to open drapes half way). In the latched mode, a switch closure is turned on by the first activation and off by the next activation, and it toggles between these two states with each activation. This feature can be useful when turning on an appliance such as a light or radio, or when sustained switch activation is difficult for the user. Single-switch activation of a complete control cycle is also used. An example of this type of control is that used in many remote garage door openers, which require a single press and release to start the door opener. The process then proceeds automatically until the door is open, without any further action by the user. This type of appliance control device is often used by persons with disabilities to open other doors (e.g., house or apartment), which may require either that the switch on the garage door opener be adapted or that the entire function be incorporated into the EADL.

Functions of Electronic Aids to Daily Living

Little (2010) identifies four functions of EADLs: (1) environmental regulation, (2) information acquisition, (3) safety/security, and (4) communication. Environmental regulation allows the user to adjust the temperature, lighting, and some pressure relief devices. Individuals with spinal cord injuries, multiple sclerosis, and some other conditions are more sensitive to temperature changes than individuals without disabilities. Increases in temperature can have significant negative effects on their ability to function, so having a means to control the temperature independently is of great importance. Devices in this category may also be used to open and close window coverings.

Devices that enable information acquisition are used to control audio-visual equipment, electric page turners, and other electronic devices. Perhaps the most commonly used devices in this category are those that are like the remote control that most of us use to control the TV, DVD, and similar entertainment devices. EADLs for safety and security purposes notify users that someone is at the entrance to their home or apartment, allow them to see that individual and to remotely unlock (and then relock) the door so it can be opened and closed. Other functions include systems that detect an emergency situation and/or contact a service in the case of an emergency or monitor distant areas of a home. Communication functions enabled by EADLs include use of the telephone to both place and receive a call, intercom systems, and attendant calls (Little, 2010).

Transmission Methods

All EADL systems must transmit a signal to the appliance to be controlled. There are several methods used for this transmission. We discuss four methods below: direct connection, house wiring (X10), infrared transmission, and radio frequency transmission. We use the term **remote control** to mean the absence of a physical attachment among the various components shown in Figure 12-7. Typically remote control occurs between the output unit and the appliances it controls. However, it is also possible to have remote links between the control interface and the processor.

Direct Connection

Direct wiring requires that the controlled devices be physically close together or necessitates the installation of special wiring just for the EADL. Devices wired to the EADL can include telephone lines, intercom systems, bed control, nurse call, and external speakers (Little, 2010). Benefits to this transmission method include increased reliability and control of devices not suitable for remote control methods. The primary disadvantage is that the device is tethered to what it controls (Little, 2010). Although it is theoretically possible to connect all the appliances to be controlled directly to the rest of the EADL via wires, this method is not practical.

House Wiring—X10

The industry standard for communication among devices using home automation, also called the power line control method, uses the household wiring (power line) to carry short-wave radio frequency (RF) signals to devices that need to be controlled (i.e., the devices are plugged into the home wiring system) (Little, 2010). Figure 12-8 shows how this approach works. Digital control signals are transmitted over the house wiring from the distribution control device to individual appliance modules, which are plugged into the standard electrical outlet. The distribution and control unit is also plugged into a wall outlet. This unit has a transmitter that sends out two codes over the house wiring. The first code identifies the device to be controlled, and the second selects the function to be performed (e.g., turn on or off, dim or brighten a light). Each appliance to be controlled is plugged into a module, which is then plugged into the wall. Each module contains a receiver that can interpret the codes sent out by the distribution and control unit. This type of appliance control was designed for use by the general population, and consequently, it is common and inexpensive. Devices are available at many consumer electronic stores. This type of device can be a completely adequate EADL for individuals who are able to press the buttons on the control unit.

The major advantages of house wiring transmission are that no modification is needed to the home electrical system and the technology is relatively inexpensive (Little, 2010). Disadvantages include (1) the lack of privacy, (2) possible interference

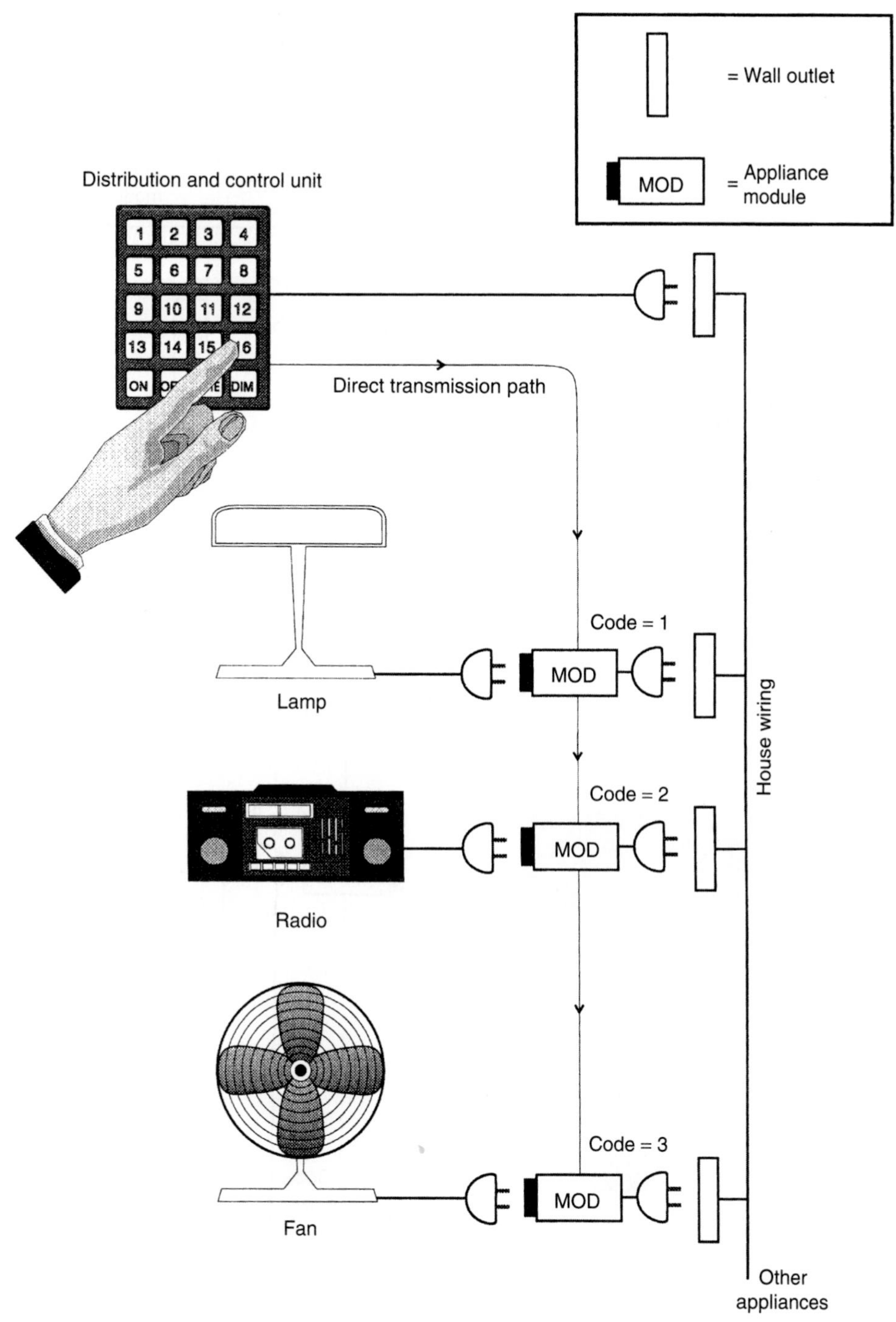

FIGURE 12-8 A direct-selection EADL. Each appliance has a numeric code, and the keypad is used to select the appropriate module. Control functions such as ON, OFF, and DIM are also activated by pressing the proper key on the keypad. This figure also illustrates the use of house wiring for distribution of the control signals to the appliance modules.

between systems on the same electrical power system (e.g., in an apartment building) resulting in unreliable performance, (3) the inability to transmit when multiple circuits are used for the wiring system, and (4) the lack of portability.

Multiple circuits are often used in house and commercial wiring. Each circuit has a separate circuit breaker, and they are physically separate from each other, which means that a module connected to one circuit does not receive the control signals from a transmitter connected to a different circuit.

Infrared Transmission

Another mode is based on the use of invisible **infrared (IR) light transmission** as the medium. This method is the most common in the control of home electronics (e.g., television set, cable television, DVD/CD player). Infrared remote controls are used for binary discrete and continuous types of control. Generally each remote device has a set of unique codes; a remote unit manufactured by one company cannot be used with a system manufactured by

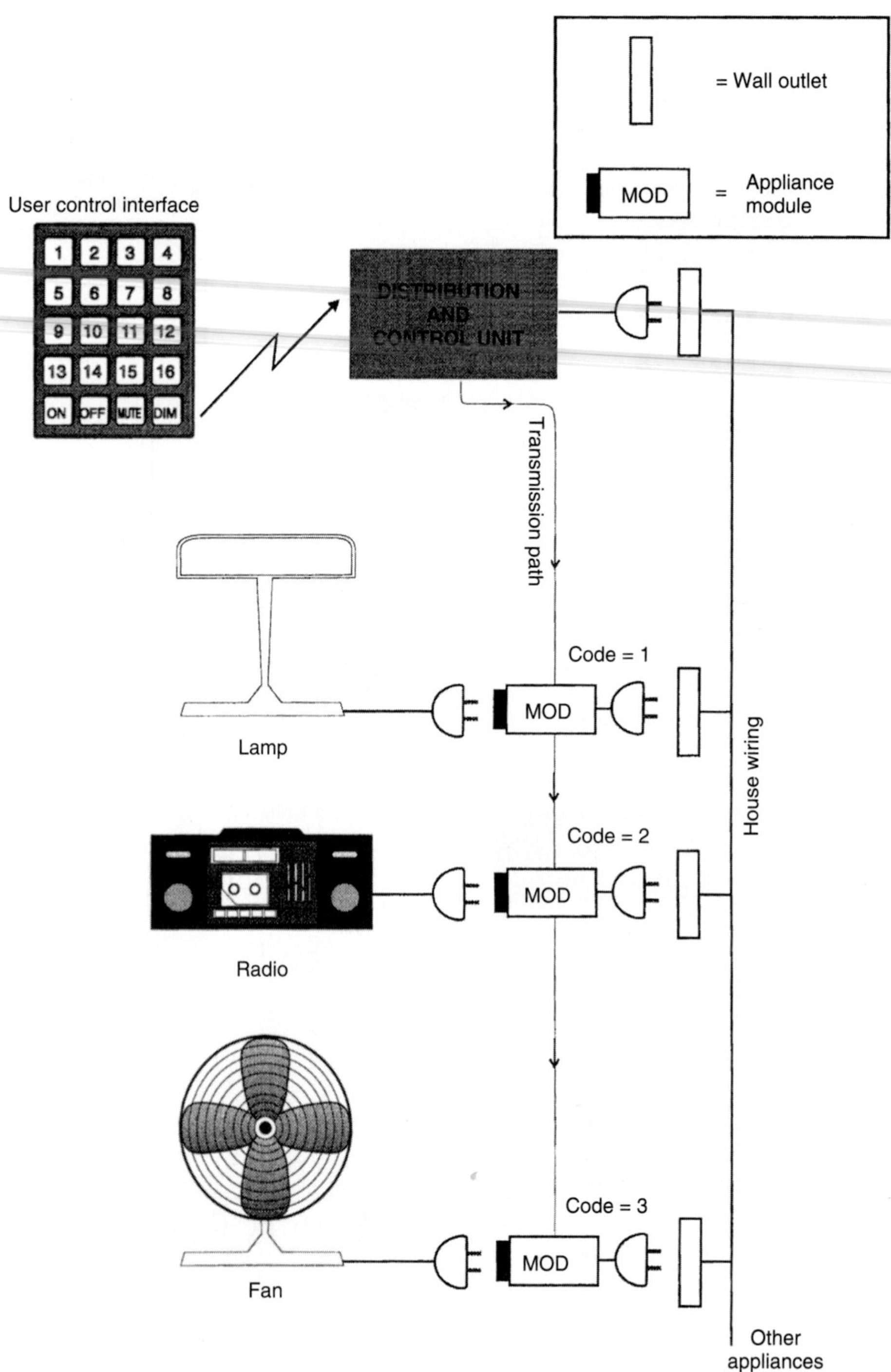

FIGURE 12-9 An EADL that employs infrared transmission from the control interface to the distribution and control unit. As in Figure 12-8, house wiring is used for transmission from the distribution and control unit to the appliance modules.

someone else, which means that several remote controllers may be necessary to manage TV, cable, and other devices, unless a "universal remote" is programmed to control all these appliances.

Infrared remote control is also used in EADLs. The remote link between the control interface and the distribution and control unit in Figure 12-9 is often implemented using IR in the same way that TV and other IR controls are used. Sometimes the link between the control and distribution unit and the remote appliances is also implemented using IR transmission.

The major advantages of IR devices are no installation costs (as compared with hard wiring) and ease of portability (Little, 2010). A major disadvantage is that the signal, because it is a light wave, can be blocked by many materials and a direct line of sight between the transmitter and receiver is generally required (Little, 2010), which means that the transmitter and receiver must be in the same room.

Because the receiver must be connected to the controlled appliances (possibly through the house wiring), the line-of-sight requirement limits the range of application (e.g., outside, inside, different rooms). Because IR devices are light sensitive, they often do not work well in bright sunlight. Recall that the HAAT model includes a consideration of the physical context (see Chapter 3, Figure 3-8) in which a given activity is taking place. In this case, the EADL is typically used in an interior location where light, heat, and sound can be controlled.

Radio Frequency Transmission

A final transmission approach is the use of radio frequency (RF) waves as the link between the distribution and control unit and the control interface, the controlled appliances, or both. The most common mainstream examples of this type of remote control are garage door openers and mobile phones. The term *RF transmission* is used because the signals are in the same range as broadcast FM radio. **Radio frequency transmission** is used as the link between the control interface and the processor.

The major advantage of RF transmission is that it is not blocked by common household materials (it can be blocked by metal that is connected to the ground), and transmission can be over a relatively long distance throughout a house and yard. Because it is less restricted, it has the major disadvantages of interference and lack of privacy. The interference problem is generally approached by reducing the distance between the transmitter and the receiver and by having several transmission channels available. The user can switch between channels (or the device will automatically scan) to find the strongest signal. Privacy is addressed by allowing the user to select a transmission code and then matching the transmitter and receiver codes—often called registering two devices.

Two of the most common RF transmission methods are Bluetooth and Wi-Fi. Bluetooth[7] is used to link phones, computers, and other network devices remotely over short distances using low-power radio transmission. There is a specification that must be followed to ensure that all Bluetooth devices can communicate with each other (IEEE Standard 802.15.1). Bluetooth communication is used in some EADLs. Originally designed for personal computers and peripheral devices as well as mobile technologies such as phones (e.g., for hands-free operation) Bluetooth has a useful range of up to 30 feet.

Another form of wireless technology similar to Bluetooth is ZigBee. In addition to providing control that has all the advantages of RF transmission, ZigBee has low power consumption (meaning longer battery life) and long range of operation (range enough to control the whole home from anywhere inside it, not just the immediate room). ZigBee is ideally suited for low data rate applications (i.e., applications in which the amount of information to be transmitted is small as in simple on/off controls) such as EADLs (Bessell et al., 2006). Specifications for ZigBee applications are made available through the ZigBee Alliance.[8] The goal of the alliance is to build wireless intelligence and capabilities into everyday devices. This cooperation will lead to companies having a standards-based wireless platform optimized for the unique needs of remote monitoring and control applications that include simplicity, reliability, low cost, and low power (Kinney, 2003).

Another common form of radio frequency transmission is Wi-Fi.[9] Wi-Fi is typically used to connect to networks. Most mainstream technologies (e.g., computers, smart phones, and tablets) have Wi-Fi capability. Wi-Fi is based on a series of evolving IEEE standards referred to as 802.11 with a letter following that have been adopted by the Wi-Fi Alliance. Networks using Wi-Fi may be local (e.g., providing a wireless connection from a computer to a printer) or they may connect devices to a Wi-Fi router that then connects to the Internet. Wi-Fi communication is employed in some EADLs.

Selection Methods

Control of EADLs is achieved through voice recognition, single or dual switch, touch screen, integrated with other controls such as for Augmentative and Alternative Communication or joystick on w/c or alternative computer access (Little, 2010). In Chapter 6 we define several selection methods used for control of assistive technology devices. These include direct selection, scanning, directed scanning, and coded access. Each of these can be used with EADLs. Direct selection occurs when the user of the system can choose any output directly. For example, an EADL for controlling a room light, a fan, or a radio on/off control may have one control interface (possibly a key on a small keyboard or speech recognition) for each of the three functions (Figure 12-9). If the same three-unit system is to be operated via scanning access, then the keyboard can be replaced by a scanning panel and each of the three items to be controlled has a corresponding light. When the light of the device to be activated comes on, the user activates a control interface to select that item. Finally, a code such as Morse code (see Chapter 6) can be used for one of the four output devices. The user enters a series of dots and dashes corresponding to the numerical code required to activate the desired appliance.

Each of these selection systems is used in current EADLs, and some EADLs have multiple options available. We discuss specific selection methods in the remainder of this section. Choice of a control interface for use with an EADL is based on the considerations presented in Chapter 7.

Trainable or Programmable Devices

Remote devices that utilize either IR or RF typically are designed for operation with only one appliance (e.g., TV, DVD player). If an individual owns several remotely controlled devices, this can lead to "controller clutter," with a separate control required for each device. To reduce this problem,

[7] http://compnetworking.about.com/cs/bluetooth/g/bldef_bluetooth.htm.

[8] http://www.zigbee.org/en/about/.

[9] http://www.techterms.com/definition/wifi.

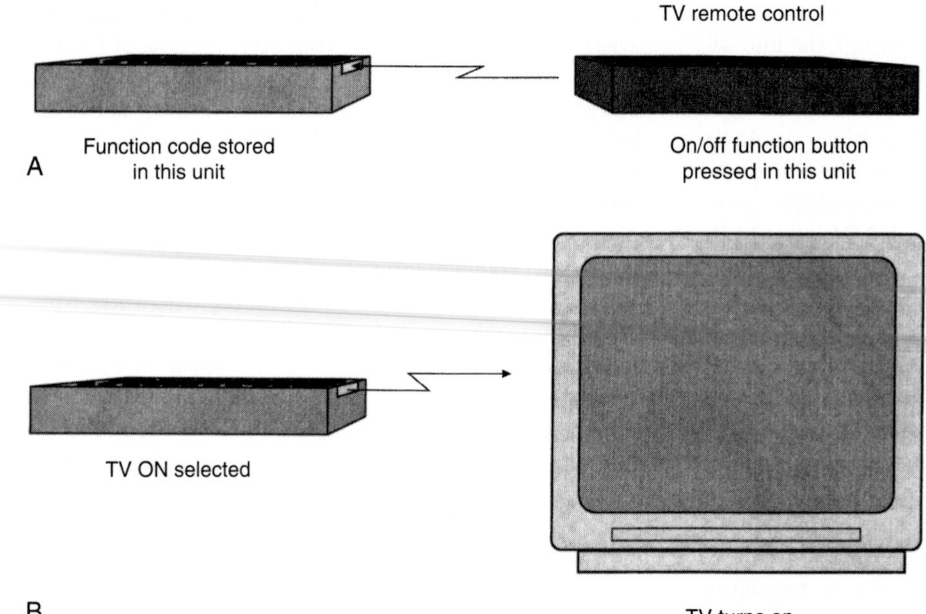

FIGURE 12-10 A trainable infrared controller. The trainable or programmable controller is shown on the left. **A,** Training is accomplished by aiming the device-specific control at the trainable controller and pressing the desired button (in this case, TV ON). **B,** The trained unit can then be used with the appliance to accomplish the desired function.

several manufacturers produce remote control units that can be adapted to work with any appliance. Some of these are called **trainable controllers.** These devices operate by storing the control code for any specific appliance function (e.g., on/off). As shown in Figure 12-10 *A*, the storage is often accomplished by pointing the trainable controller at the controller for the specific appliance and sending the specific function code (TV ON in Figure 12-10). The trainable device then stores this code for future use. When the stored code is sent to the appliance, it is received and used as if it had been sent by the appliance's own controller. This process is illustrated in Figure 12-10 *B.* In this manner, all the functions of the individual appliance controllers can be stored in one master controller and the user need only activate this one device. Most of these controllers have two modes: train and operate. Figure 12-11 shows a programmable EADL unit mounted to a wheelchair and used for controlling appliances such as the television.

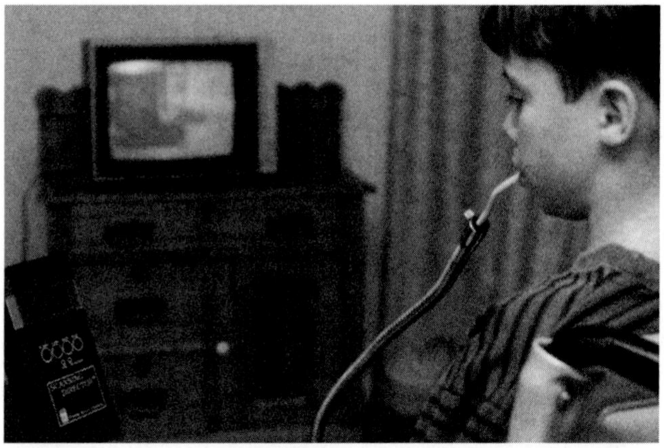

FIGURE 12-11 A trainable infrared EADL with scanning access. The EADL is shown mounted to a wheelchair. It is positioned so there is a line-of-sight link to the television for use of IR control. (Courtesy APT Technology, Inc., DU-IT CSG, Inc., Shreve, OH.)

Some controllers have codes for many appliances permanently stored in them. The user selects a code corresponding to the appliance owned (e.g., a television set made by a specific manufacturer) by looking up the correct controller code in a table. Once this code is entered into the controller, it is able to control the appliance. We refer to these as **programmable controllers.**

Trainable or programmable controllers designed for the general home electronics market can be of benefit to persons with disabilities who are able to press the small keys associated with these devices. For those persons who cannot use standard controllers, there are specially adapted trainable or programmable units that provide both direct selection and scanning selection.[10] Control interfaces include expanded keyboards or a built-in keyboard or single switches for scanning access. In the latter case, one of two methods is typically used: (1) small lights that are located next to each button are sequentially illuminated or (2) alphanumeric labels or numeric codes for each function are sequentially displayed. For each of these approaches, the user presses the switch when the desired choice is presented.

Most of the trainable or programmable EADL devices can be interfaced to other electronic devices (e.g., AAC devices, computers, powered wheelchair controllers) via a USB port. To control the EADL, a code must be sent from the communication device or computer to the controller, and all specific functions and separate appliance codes must be stored in the communication device or computer. Several manufacturers include control software for EADLs in their communication software programs (see Chapter 16). When the EADL is controlled by a computer or communication device, the software program generates the control signals and sends them through the USB port to the EADL.

[10] For an excellent description of EADLs, including a comparison chart, go to Michelle Lang's website, www.atilange.com, and choose Resources.

To facilitate the control of appliances, cell phones, and other electronic devices the concept of a **universal remote** was developed (Zimmerman et al., 2004). The universal remote standard is intended to allow users (including EADL users) to interact with networked devices and services in their environments. The universal nature of the controller specification means that all devices meeting the standard will be able to interact because they will follow predefined protocols rather than being unique to each manufacturer. The universal remote standard provides a versatile user interface description for devices and services, called a "user interface socket" to which any universal remote console (URC) can connect. Each URC can electronically "discover" remote devices or services in its range and then access and control them. Examples of services include cell phones and wireless computer networks. Devices could be any of these described for EADL control (e.g., television, CD/DVD players, standard telephones). A major advantage is that with only one user interface description, diverse URC technologies can be supported, including connection via desktop and laptop computers and mobile technologies like smart phone and tablets.

Telephone Control

Persons with physical disabilities of the upper extremities often have difficulty in carrying out the tasks associated with telephone use. These include lifting the handset, dialing, holding the handset while talking, and replacing the handset in its cradle. Telephones differ greatly in design (e.g., portable, speaker, rotary, or touch-tone dial), but all require that the listed tasks be performed. As in many other areas of assistive technology, there are a variety of ways to accomplish the same tasks. Mouth sticks or head pointers (see the section on low-tech aids earlier in this chapter) can be used to press a button to open a line on a speaker phone (equivalent to lifting the hand set), dial by pressing buttons, and hang up at the end of a conversation. There are also simple holders that position a handset for hands-free operation and mechanical switches with long handles that control the switch hook for answering a call or hanging up after a call. Finally, telephone companies provide operator-assisted calling for persons with disabilities, so it is only necessary to press 0 for an operator, who then dials the call for the consumer. Our emphasis in this section, however, is on electronic telephone access systems, which are often integrated into EADLs.

Because modern telephones are actually sophisticated electronic devices, automation via electronic **telephone controllers** is relatively easy, and there are a variety of commercial products available to accomplish telephone access for persons with disabilities.[11] Many of the general-purpose EADLs have telephone functions built in.[12] The functional components of a telephone controller are shown in Figure 12-12. Individual devices may group these components differently. Telephone controllers for a person with a disability are built around standard telephone electronics. In some cases the controller is connected into the standard telephone, whereas in others the telephone is bypassed and the controller plugs directly into the telephone line. These devices enable several of the important functions common to consumer telephones, such as automatic dialing of stored numbers and redial. Another useful feature of currently available adapted telephones is that the user can answer electronically rather than physically picking up the handset. This action is done as an additional choice on a scanning menu or a direct selection on an EADL telephone control panel.

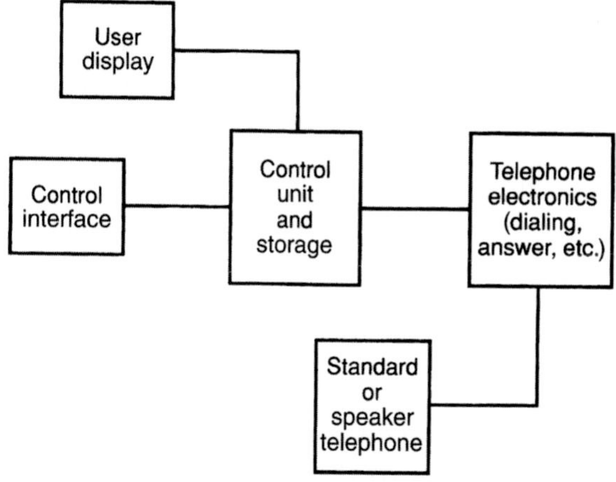

FIGURE 12-12 Functional components of an automatic telephone dialer. The *control interface* and *user display* constitute the human/technology interface, the *control unit and storage* and *telephone electronics* are the processor, and the *telephone* constitutes the activity output.

Other parts of the telephone controller shown in Figure 12-12 are necessary only for persons who require single-switch access to the system (e.g., the user display). The control interface is connected to a control unit that also interfaces with a display and with the telephone electronics. Although systems vary in their design, a typical approach is for the device to present digits sequentially on the display. When the digit to be dialed is presented, the user presses the switch to select the number and the scan begins again at zero. In this way, any phone number can be entered. Once the number is entered, it is sent to the telephone electronics for automatic dialing.

Many persons with disabilities respond slowly, and each switch press may take several seconds. If we assume that it takes 2 seconds to respond, then we must display each number for at least 3 seconds, which may require scanning through 10 numbers (30 seconds) just to get to the desired number. If all the desired numbers were large (e.g., 7, 8, 9), it could take almost 5 minutes (300 seconds) to dial one long-distance (11-digit) number. For this reason, all practical systems use stored numbers and automatic dialing. They also allow numbers to be entered and either stored or dialed using scanning. Redial also can speed things up, and this feature is normally included as well. Another unique feature in most telephone dialers designed for persons with a disability is the inclusion of a HELP (e.g., a neighbor) or EMERGENCY (911) phone number that can be dialed quickly.

[11] See comparison chart at www.atilange.com.
[12] See comparison chart at www.atilange.com.

There are several modes of operation in automatic telephone dialers that require a selection by the user. First, the user must choose among dial, answer, or hang up. If dial is chosen, then the user must decide whether to access a stored number, redial, call for help, or dial an unstored number. When single-switch devices are used as the selection method, this decision is generally made in one of two ways: (1) the system sequentially presents the choices to the user and the user waits until the desired choice is presented before pressing the switch, or (2) two switches are used: one to access the operational modes only (e.g., dial, answer, store) and the second switch to select numbers. In either method, if HELP is selected, it is automatically dialed with no further entry. Some units merely reserve the first place in the stored number directory for HELP, whereas others use a special selection scheme for it (e.g., a long switch press). The next place in the phone list is generally redial.

If redial is not chosen, then stored numbers are presented, usually by a code. Many systems allow a picture of the person to be presented with his or her number, greatly simplifying the selection process, especially for individuals who have a cognitive disability (see Chapter 15). Most systems have a capacity for multiple stored numbers. The user merely waits until the code or picture for the number of the person he or she wants to call is presented and then presses the switch. At this point, everything else is automatic. If the user wishes to dial or store a new number, he or she waits until that choice is presented and then activates the switch. Once in this mode, the method discussed above is used to enter the number, and the user then tells the controller whether to enter it into memory or to dial it.

Because the telephone controller obtains access to the telephone lines in the course of its normal operation, it is relatively easy to include other telephone-based functions in the adapted controller's operation. For example, apartment buildings often use the telephone system for the intercom and front door latch, and the adapted telephone dialer can access these by including additional codes selected by the user.

When a computer is used as part of an EADL, the telephone dialing functions can be implemented using software programs coupled with an electronic telephone interface that connects to the telephone line. These software and electronics are common for use in modems for communication between computers (e.g., for Internet access), and they have been adapted for some EADL systems. Similarly, applications (apps) available for smart phones and tablet computers can augment the dialing functions.

Configuring Electronic Aids to Daily Living

Having looked at the components that normally make up EADLs, we now move to a discussion of how EADLs are selected and configured to meet the specific needs of a person with a disability. The first step in this process is to carry out an assessment of the person's needs and skills.

Single-Device Binary Control EADLs

Electronic aids to daily living that control only one appliance can be useful in developing motor control, as well as cognitive concepts such as cause and effect.[13] In Chapter 6 we describe a motor training program that utilizes these types of EADLs. Most of these have both momentary and latched modes, and they include a timer to activate the appliance for a preset number of seconds. These devices are useful when only a single device control can be understood by the user (e.g., in the case of developmental disability) or when only one device is required (e.g., a radio or light). The cost is low (less than $200), and there can be a significant increase in independence. The use of single-function EADLs often leads to the use of multiple-function EADLs or electronic communication devices (see Chapter 16). This progression is described in Chapter 6.

TABLE 12-1 Functions Performed by EADLs

Functions	Methods of Implementation
Binary latched control of AC appliances (e.g., lights, radio, on-off only)	House wiring transmission Direct ultrasound control
Discrete or continuous appliance (e.g., TV, VCR, CD, cassette tape control)	IR remote transmission
Momentary control of appliances (e.g., door opener, drapery control)	RF remote transmission
Telephone control	Hard wired switch control
Switch control (any device requiring one or two switches)	Hard wiring IR link to switch box

Matching the Characteristics of Multiple-Function EADLs to the Needs of the User

When planning an EADL to meet specific needs, it is useful to group the tasks (determined during the assessment) into the five categories shown in Table 12-1. This grouping, based on the common ways of implementing specific functions, is the first step in specifying an EADL. The EADL functions required can be identified in the left-hand column of Table 12-1. The corresponding information in the right-hand column identifies the methods available for EADL implementation, which allows options to be considered.

The first group in Table 12-1 is binary (on/off) latched (stays on or off until the next activation) control of appliances that operate from standard household wall current. As we have described, there are two basic ways that current EADLs control such appliances: (1) by plugging them into receivers that plug into the house wiring and transmit control signals over the house wiring and (2) by direct transmission (infrared, or radio frequency) to a receiver into which the appliance is plugged. The most common commercially available components for use with house wiring transmission are the X10 modules and

[13] For example, the Power Link, Ablenet, Minneapolis, MN, www.ablenetinc.com.

controllers.[14] These modules are incorporated into many EADLs.

The second category in Table 12-1 is appliances that require discrete or continuous control, such as television channel selection or volume control. The most common EADL control method for discrete or continuous appliances is IR remote transmission; several EADLs utilize integrated trainable or programmable IR controllers. This technology allows several devices (e.g., TV, CD/DVD) to be incorporated into one package controlled by the EADL. Each of these devices must have its own IR control to be incorporated into the trainable or programmable controller. The options available to the clinician depend on what appliances the consumer has and whether they have IR remote control. If IR remote devices are available, then the choice is to use an EADL with a trainable or programmable IR device. If the consumer needs continuous or discrete control but does not have IR-controlled appliances, then the clinician should consider EADLs with built-in discrete or continuous control, which may require modification of the appliance or purchase of a stand-alone IR controller.

If the consumer wants to control items such as draperies, then momentary control (i.e., the appliance is turned on for a variable period of time and then turned off) is required. For example, a drapery motor or bed elevation control may be turned on long enough to move the curtain or the bed to the proper position, and then the motor must be turned off. A latched control generally presents problems in this scenario. Very short activation times are not possible with latched control, especially if the user has delays in muscle motor response. In some cases the range of movement for the task is always the same (e.g., when opening a door), and we can use a device that is started by the user and automatically stopped at the end of the task by the device (e.g., when the door is fully open or fully closed). This type of control is often implemented using RF transmission. Hard-wired switch control can also be used for these functions. Common examples are the enlarged switches often placed near doors for persons with disabilities or the active floor mats or light sensors used to trigger the opening of these doors.

Telephone control is listed separately in Table 12-1 because the functions performed are different from other EADL tasks. Generally telephone controllers use switches connected directly to them (hard wired). Integrating all EADL functions is often desirable. If the consumer is also going to use IR continuous or discrete control, the clinician should consider the use of an IR-controlled telephone. This option allows the consumer to control the telephone in the same way as he or she controls the TV, CD/DVD, and so on.

The final category in Table 12-1 is for devices that require one- or two-switch control. Other examples of appliances requiring switch control are call signals and drapery and door controls. The simplest method to implement this type of control is hard wiring of the switch to the EADL component. However, this approach has two major disadvantages: (1) the user is forced to go to the device to be controlled and use the switch at that location, so flexibility in movement is limited; and (2) it is difficult to integrate the switch control with other EADL functions into a total package controlled by only one control interface. If a consumer must use different switches for different devices, then independence can be reduced. If the individual does not have good motor control and requires careful positioning of the control interface for successful use, the problem is even more difficult.

One way to integrate switch control with other EADL functions is to use a component that can detect IR, or Bluetooth signals and generate a switch-type output. This type of output is sometimes referred to as *relay output.* For example, if the consumer is using a trainable or programmable IR EADL controller for TV, CD/DVD, and telephone use and needs to control a drapery motor as well, a two-output IR trainable switch box (as shown in Figure 12-13) can be used. The IR EADL can provide the equivalent of a switch output directly, and the consumer does not need to have two additional switches to control the drapes (e.g., one switch to open them and one switch to close them). Some EADLs have built-in switched or relay outputs.

Not all remote control utilizes IR transmission. Binary latched control of electrical appliances is often implemented by RF transmission, and trainable or programmable IR controllers are not usable for these functions. Two basic approaches are used to integrate binary appliance control and remote IR controllers. The first of these, shown in Figure 12-13, has a control and distribution unit that employs IR transmission. The transmitted codes are used to select an appliance (the number of appliances can vary from 4 to 256) and the function to be accomplished (on/off or dim/brighten for lights only). The trainable or programmable IR device is programmed to recognize these codes, and the remote unit treats the appliance control and dual-switch receiver as IR-controlled devices.

The second approach to integration of discrete or continuous IR control with binary latched appliance, is to incorporate RF control into the trainable or programmable device together with IR transmission. In this case there is no need for a separate IR transmission distribution and control unit, since the RF transmission is built into the trainable or programmable remote controller. This technology combines the trainability of the IR unit for TV, CD/DVD, and so on with the simplicity of RF transmission for binary control of appliances. This configuration allows more flexibility in the choice of individual environmental control components, and allows us to focus on the needs of the EADL user rather than on the devices that may be available.

ROBOTIC AIDS TO MANIPULATION

Because *robots* or **robotic systems** are intended to assist with manipulation, they are a natural alternative manipulation device for persons who have disabilities. There are, however,

[14] X-10 Powerhouse, Inc., Northvale, NJ, www.X-10.com.

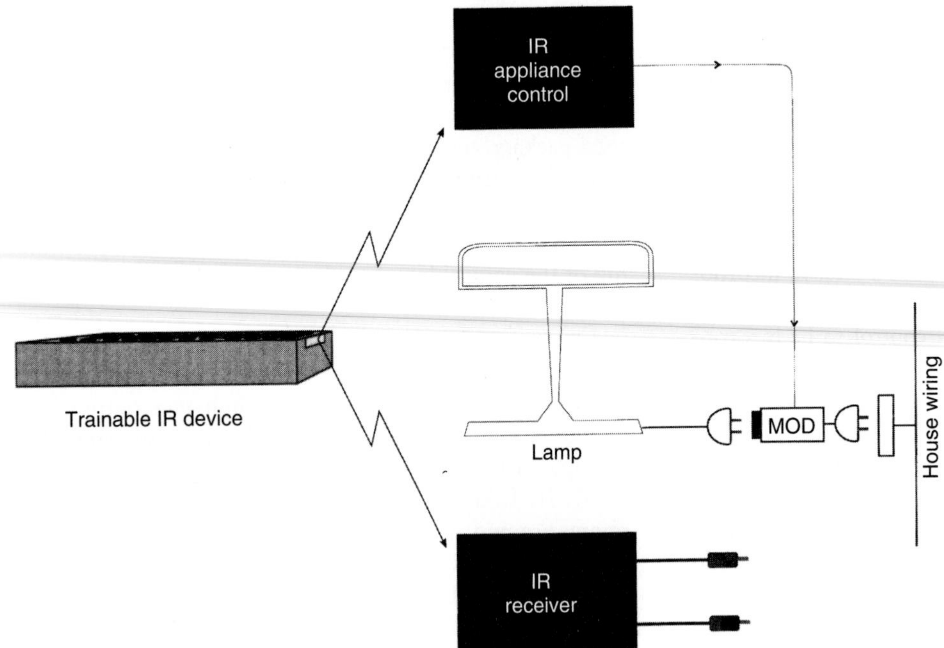

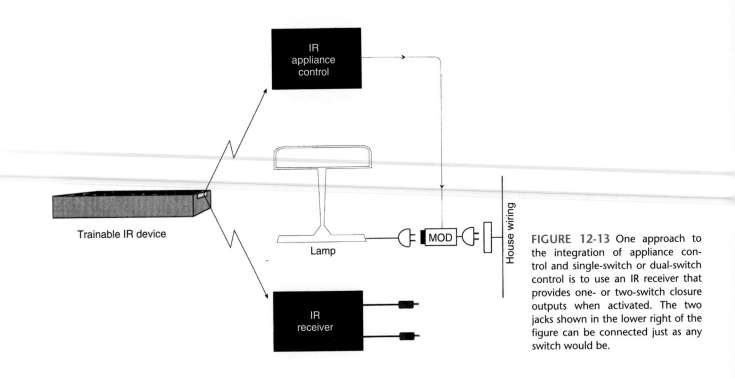

FIGURE 12-13 One approach to the integration of appliance control and single-switch or dual-switch control is to use an IR receiver that provides one- or two-switch closure outputs when activated. The two jacks shown in the lower right of the figure can be connected just as any switch would be.

some significant differences between the use of robots by persons with disabilities and their use industrially. Industrial robots often have the role of *replacing* the human operator for reasons of strength, safety, or precision. In production line environments (e.g., automobile manufacturing), it is often necessary to lift large or heavy objects and position them for attachment to other parts. Robots are stronger than humans and are not subject to fatigue after hours of service. Many work environments are hazardous (e.g., those involving radiation or very high or low temperatures). To ensure safety of the operator, handling of objects in these environments is done by a robotic manipulator controlled by the human operator. At the opposite extreme from heavy object positioning is the repeated assembly of small parts (e.g., electronics assembly). Robots can be programmed to carry out the exact same task over and over without fatigue or loss of accuracy. In each of these cases, the human is an ancillary part of the total system.

In contrast, with assistive robotics the human operator is at the center of the process. Instead of replacing the user, the goal is to enhance the user's ability to manipulate objects and to function independently, which makes issues of safety more important for assistive robots. Assistive robots perform many functions, in contrast to the relatively limited repertoire of an industrial robot. Although some tasks (e.g., feeding) are repeated, the assistive robot must be able to carry out totally unplanned movements spontaneously.

Brose et al. (2010) described advances in assistive robotics that have the potential of assisting persons with disabilities. They divided assistive robots into two broad categories: physically assistive robots (PARs) and socially assistive robots (SARs). PARs are designed to provide assistance with manipulation of objects. Feil-Seifer and Mataric (2005) defined SARs as robotic devices with the goal "to create close and effective interaction with a human user for the purpose of giving assistance and achieving measurable progress in convalescence, rehabilitation, and learning" (Feil-Seifer & Mataric, 2005, p. 465).

Principles of Assistive Robots

A robot is defined as "an automatically controlled, reprogrammable, multipurpose manipulator programmable in three or more axes, which may be either fixed in place or mobile for use in industrial automation applications" (International Standard ISO 8373). This definition applies to applications other than industrial applications, including assistive robots used for the amelioration of physical sensory and cognitive limitations in children and adults with disabilities (Cook et al., 2010).

Degrees of Freedom

The number of degrees of freedom (DOF) is how many variables are required to determine the position of a mechanism in space. In a robotic arm, each joint (base, shoulder, elbow, wrist (may have multiple joints)) represents a degree of freedom. The human wrist has pronation/supination, flexion/extension, and left/right lateral movement (ulnar/radial deviation). Thus, it requires three degrees of freedom to determine its position in space. If each degree of freedom associated with a joint were to be controlled by a bidirectional switch, it would be very difficult to carry out complex movements. To understand this complexity, place a pencil or pen on the table. Now reach for it and pick it up, but only move in one of the degrees of freedom (i.e., one joint) listed above at a time. This type of movement takes great concentration. Now, reach for the pen or pencil as you normally would. This is called end-point positioning, and it is much easier to accomplish, but it makes the control system and robot much more complicated.

If an assistive robot is on a mobile stand, it will have additional degrees of freedom that must be controlled by the user to position the robot for a specific task. This action is similar to the task of driving a remote-controlled car. In some cases, assistive robotic arms are mounted to wheelchairs. In that case, some degrees of freedom necessary to position the arm in space are controlled by the position of the wheelchair. For example, turning the wheelchair may be used to move the robot hand left to right.

Coordinate Systems

The type of control (joint, end-positioning, etc.) is related to the coordinate system in which the robot operates. The user has to develop a new coordinate system for controlling the robot, one related to the workspace of the robot rather than to the user's own body. This change in frame of reference can be difficult, and mastering control of the robot requires practice.

Several coordinate systems can be used. Joint positioning, as described above, is one approach, but it is difficult and tiring to use for extended operations. It might be used to train a robot arm movement, store it, and then replay it later. Operating in a tool coordinate system is more common. Here the user must control the robot arm to move relative to the object to be manipulated. The disadvantage of this mode is that it requires that one control interface for each degree of freedom must be available. For individuals who have limited motor control, this approach can be limiting. One approach to dealing with the need for many control signals is to use indirect selection methods (e.g., scanning; see Chapter 6).

Levels of Autonomy

Robots can operate at different levels of autonomy with respect to the control exerted by the user. At one extreme, the robot can accept high-level commands that define a task to be completed (e.g., take a glass from the shelf, fill it with water, and bring it to the user). The robot will perform whatever subtasks are necessary and make necessary decisions (e.g., determining the glass is full) without requesting any human intervention. This is referred to as being *fully autonomous.*

Alternatively, the user has direct control over the robot movements throughout the task. This is referred to as *teleoperated.* Multiple controls are then necessary to each robot degree of freedom, as described above.

Between these two extremes of autonomy (autonomous and teleoperated robot), several levels of autonomy, shown in Box 12-1, can be defined (Parasuraman et al., 2000). Assistive robots are often employed at a midrange of autonomy, in which the user merely needs to hit or press and hold a switch to replay a prestored movement.

Configuration

Stand-alone assistive robots are table-mounted, attached to wheelchair frames, mounted on mobile bases, or attached to overhead tracks (Figure 12-14). Some commercial robots are flexible in terms of the ways they are configured. Others are designed for a specific application (e.g. mounted to a wheelchair).

BOX 12-1 Sheridan's Levels of Robotic Autonomy (Parasuraman, et al., 2000)

1. Computer offers no assistance; human does it all.
2. Computer offers a complete set of action alternatives.
3. Computer narrows the selection down to a few choices.
4. Computer suggests a single action.
5. Computer executes that action if human approves.
6. Computer allows the human limited time to veto before automatic execution.
7. Computer executes automatically then necessarily informs the human.
8. Computer informs human after automatic execution only if human asks.
9. Computer informs human after automatic execution only if it decides to.
10. Computer decides everything and acts autonomously, ignoring the human.

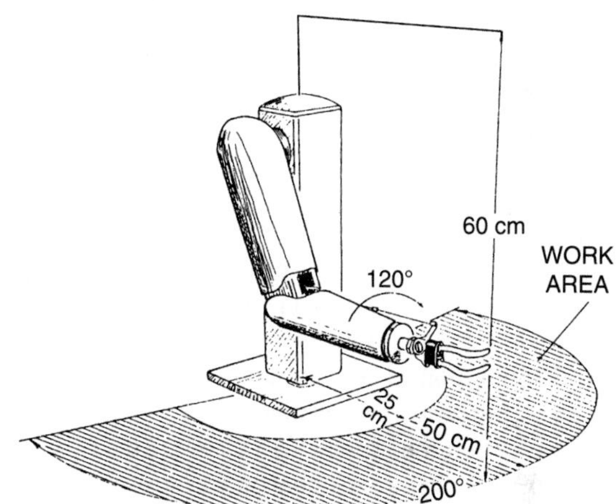

FIGURE 12-14 The coordinate system and working envelope of the APL RAWT system. (From Seamone W, Schmeisser G: Early clinical evaluation of a robot arm/worktable system for spinal-cord-injured persons, *J Rehabil Res Dev* 22:38-57, 1985.)

Robots as Personal Assistants

In this section we discuss the basic principles underlying development and application of assistive robots. In contrast to technologies discussed in other sections of this chapter, assistive robots are still largely in the research and development stage, and application of these systems is not yet widespread although many clinical and community-based evaluations have been reported (Brose et al., 2010).

Robots are often employed as personal assistants, in which the goal is to provide manipulation aids to people with motor impairments and/or intellectual disabilities. Typical tasks that are assisted include everyday functions such as eating or personal hygiene. Personal assistants may be stand-alone robotic arms, often called robotic workstations, integrated into a wheelchair or autonomous mobile robotic platforms.

Robotic Workstations

A workstation can be defined as an area dedicated to the performance of a specific job or activity. Examples of activities are design (e.g., a computer workstation for engineering students), reading (e.g., a library-based workstation), and clerical tasks (e.g., a workstation for word processing, telephone answering, and manipulation of files). These workstations involve manipulation of papers, books, and other devices. When the user of the workstation has difficulty with upper extremity function and manipulation, **desktop robots** can play a major role in creating full access to the workstation. Because the workstation is fixed in one location, the design of the robotic system can focus on manipulation of objects only, rather than movement to the object and then manipulation of it.

Birch et al. (1996) carried out a study to determine actual costs if using a robotic assistant as compared with using a personal assistant for office-related tasks. They used a simulated office environment and standardized tasks. They found that, although the robotic assistant did reduce assistant time and therefore cost, it also resulted in decreased productivity by the user. They attributed this reduction in productivity to waiting times necessitated by robotic movements, which were slower than the corresponding human attendant actions.

Mobile Assistive Robots

Because we rarely do all our manipulation from a fixed location, **mobile assistive robots** have been developed. These fall into one of two general classes: (1) wheelchair mounted and (2) mounted on a mobile base that is controllable by the user. The major limitation of the first approach is that the most functional robot arms are relatively large. This large size, coupled with the other apparatus that must be attached to the wheelchair, makes attachment of the arm to the wheelchair impractical in many cases. Recent miniaturization of these arms has solved this problem. The separate mobile base approach solves these problems, and it is practical in the home or at the work site. However, this approach also has disadvantages. The mobile robot requires that the user add "steering" to the required control commands. Because the user of a robot most likely has a restricted set of control signals available, the addition of these steering commands may be impossible. It is also difficult to transport the mobile base from one location to another. It is like having two powered wheelchairs to transport. Thus the most practical application of mobile robots is within one location. This location can, of course, include all rooms in a house or any location within a school, factory, or office.

Wheelchair-Mounted Robotic Arms

The Manus manipulator (currently known as the Intelligent Assistive Robotic Manipulator, iARM),[15] pictured in Figure 12-15, is a robotic arm mounted to a wheelchair (Verburg et al., 1996; Driessen et al., 2001). It is designed to serve as a general-purpose manipulative aid for people who have severe upper extremity limitations. The robotic arm has eight degrees of freedom, can lift a 1.5-kg weight when the arm is fully extended, and can exert a gripping force of 20 N. The iARM weighs 9 kg. The iARM can be customized with specific functions prestored for replay from a menu. The iARM can be controlled by a keypad, a joystick, or single-button control. The iARM allows use in different coordinate system frameworks. For example, what is called Cartesian, or straight line, control provides movement along straight lines by automatically adjusting each joint to keep a cup or plate level during movement. The iARM also stores particular positions that are frequently used. They can be recalled with one selection from a menu. Several research groups have made adaptations to the iARM to increase its clinical functionality. Brose et al (2010) describe some of these.

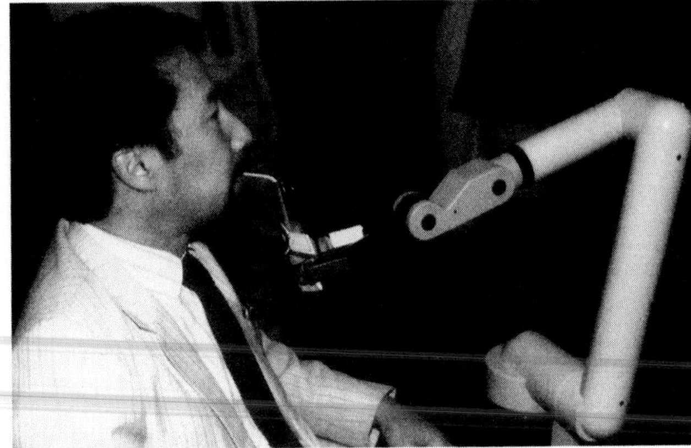

FIGURE 12-15 The Manus wheelchair-mounted robotic arm. (Courtesy CW Heckathorne, Northwestern University Rehabilitation Engineering Research Center, Chicago, IL.)

Use of the Manus system was evaluated by 14 individuals in six European countries (the Netherlands, Germany, Norway, France, Italy, and Switzerland) (Oderud, 1997). These community-based evaluations demonstrated that the Manus manipulator was frequently used at home for activities of daily living (e.g., fetching objects, eating and drinking, preparing food in a microwave oven). Limitations in this home environment included the added size and weight of the wheelchair when the Manus was mounted to it and the need for training of the user and significant others. In these studies the Manus was not frequently used for vocational tasks because it could not be preprogrammed for repetitive tasks. The iARM functionality has overcome this limitation.

Another robotic arm developed for rehabilitation application is the JACO manufactured by Kinova[16] (Maheu et al, 2011). The JACO arm system (Figure 12-16) is a lightweight (6 kg) robotic manipulator that is typically mounted on a wheelchair. The Jaco arm can also be attached to a table, a bed or a workstation. The hand is 12 cm and has three fingers, that can each move independently. The arm can lift 1.5 kg (3.3 pounds) and can reach up to 90 cm (36 inches). The seven degrees of freedom allow it to reach anywhere within its workspace and to approach objects from any direction or orientation. The JACO arm can move in three-dimensional space (up, down, left, right, back and forth—3 DOF). There are 6 movements of JACO's wrist (abduction, adduction,

[15] Exact Dynamics, http://www.exactdynamics.nl/site/.

[16] http://kinovarobotics.com/products/jaco-rehab-edition/.

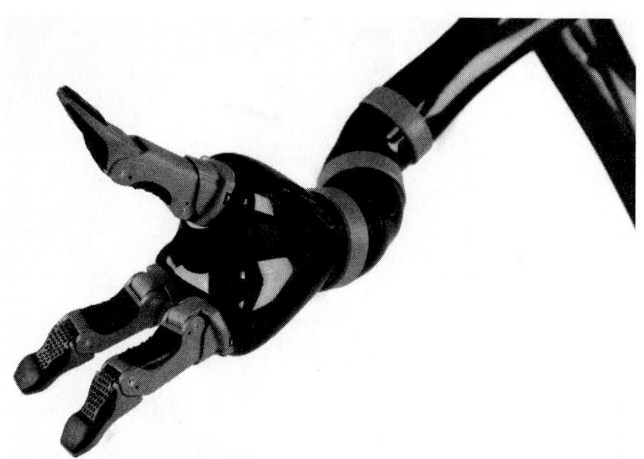

FIGURE 12-16 JACO arm system.

flexion, extension, pronation, supination (6 DOF) and opening and closing of the 3 fingers (1 DOF).

The JACO arm is controlled with a three-axis joystick that can be mounted on the wheelchair armrest or positioned for access when the arm is mounted on a table, bed or workstation (Maheu et al, 2011). The three axes are: (1) shaft forward or backward; (2) shaft right or left; (3) handle turned clockwise and counter-clockwise. There are three control modes that are accessed by two pushbuttons. In the first control mode, the user can move the robot's hand in three-dimensional space with the orientation of the hand fixed. In the second control mode, the user can modify the orientation of the hand, but the hand is kept centered at the same point in space. A third control mode allows the user to grasp and release the hand, using either two or three fingers.

The JACO arm was evaluated by 34 participants between 18 and 64 years old who were users of power wheelchairs controlled by a standard joystick and who were able to press the control buttons on the joystick (Maheu et al, 2011). The arm was fixed on a table. The participants were asked to perform JACO's 16 basic movements twice, which include all possible actions of the robotic device: These actions were touching targets located left, right, up and down; rotating the hand; pushing objects; activating the grasp function; placing the arm in its retracted position. The participants also had to accomplish a series of six tasks shown in Box 12-2. The perceived ease of completing the tasks was assessed as well as the satisfaction and estimated importance of performing each task.

Maheu et al found that the majority of the participants were able to accomplish the testing tasks on their first attempt. A majority of the participants thought that the JACO arm was very easy to use, and the majority were able to perform all of the 16 basic movements and the 6 ADL-related tasks.

In order to assess the degree to which the participants thought the JACO arm would assist with ADLs, they were asked what the average time spent by a caregiver was for several ADLs. They then asked the participants to indicate whether they would be "fully able" or "very able" to perform these same tasks using the JACO arm. "Fully able" responses varied from 26% to 47% of the participants, and "very able" from 48% to 79%. They also determined that caregivers supply an average of 3.2 ± 2.1 hours daily to the participants for the selected ADLs. To assess the paid caregiver weighted time savings, the results for the mean of the "fully able" and "very able" results were used to calculate an "average of time saving." The result was a mean potential time reduction of 1.31 hours per day leading, Maheau et al to conclude that the use of the JACO arm system could potentially reduce caregiving time by 41%.

BOX 12-2 Six Tasks Participants Performed with the JACO Arm

Grasping a bottle located on the left side of the table
Grasping a bottle located on the right side, on a surface near the ground and placing the bottle on the table
Pushing the buttons of a calculator
Taking a tissue from a box on the table
Taking a straw from a glass located on the table
Pouring water from a bottle into a glass.

Robots for Social Integration

The development of artificial intelligence led to socially assistive robots (SAR) that show aspects of human style intelligence. SARs are characterized by their physical form (in general, anthropomorphic), personality traits, and emotional expression (Seelye et al, 2012). A SAR provides assistance to human users through nonphysical social interaction. Through the use of a variety of sensors, these socially interactive robots are able to perceive and interact with their environment. These features have led to their use in promoting social integration. Two major target populations are identified for social assistive robots: children with autism spectrum disorder and elderly individuals who require companionship. Tele-operated robotics include video-monitoring by a caregiver or health care provider while the senior is living independently (Seelye et al, 2012).

These robots allow users to stay connected with family members or friends. Tele-operated robots are controlled remotely, and they generally do not provide the same level of human–robot social interaction as SARs.

Social Assistive Robots for Individuals with Autism Spectrum Disorder

Studies have been conducted to establish the effectiveness of robots in ameliorating the impacts of autism. Individuals with autism spectrum disorder have impaired social interaction, social communication, and social imagination (Dautenhahn and Werry, 2004). Robots could be helpful when human intervention is a barrier to learning, as might be the case with children with autism spectrum disorder (Dautenhahn and Werry, 2004). It is also hypothesized that the "social" relationship the child with autism spectrum disorder might develop with the robot can then be transferred to humans. Developments in this area include both stationary robots that imitate human facial expressions and gestures, and mobile robots that interact with children through movement (Michaud et al, 2007).

Fong, Nourbakhsh and Dautenhahn (2003) surveyed socially interactive robots for children with autism.

Robots Supporting Older Adults

Assistive robots that promote older adults' interaction with others have gained recent interest. There are two main categories of such SAR and tele-operated (remote control) robotics (Seelye et al, 2012). We describe evaluations of examples from each of these categories. An increasing trend is to consider the use of robots as helpmates for elderly individuals who require significant amounts of assistance for tasks of daily living (Brose et al, 2010).

Robots have also been proposed as companions for individuals (mostly senior) who are isolated and lonely (Seelye et al, 2012). These applications of robots raise major ethical questions which we discuss in Chapter 4.

Socially Assistive Robots for Seniors

The developments in socially assistive robots have led to the suggestion that they can serve as companions for seniors who are living alone. Often these robots are developed to resemble animals. Shibata et al (2012) describe a user evaluation of Paro, a socially assistive robot designed to resemble a baby harbor seal. To create more realistic facial expressions each eyelid moves independently to allow expression of both happy and sad emotions. The use of this animal representation was intentional to avoid preconceptions associated with common pets like a cat or dog. However, developers took care to make the robot resemble a human baby in size and shape with a warm body temperature like a real animal. It has also been called a "mental commitment robot" designed to coexist with people and provide them with joy and relaxation through physical interaction. All of these features contribute to some of the ethical concerns regarding the misleading perception by the human that the robot actually feels and responds to emotions as pet animals or other persons do (see Chapter 4). In this study people accepted the unfamiliar animal easily. Paro was first sold commercially in Japan; over 1000 units have been sold.

Shibata et al (2012) examined people living with Paro during the period March 28, 2005 to July 24, 2007. The results showed that interaction with Paro improved the mood of elderly people and patients, making them more active and communicative with each other and their caregivers. Subjective evaluation varied depending on the robot's movement, appearance, generated sounds, and sense of touch. Data were analyzed by gender with about 72% of Paro owners who participated in the study being female. The most important characteristics for males were: "eye blink" 16 (72%), "face" 11 (50%), "cry" 11 (50%), "body shape" 13 (59%), with the main reason for acquiring the robot being "Healing effect is expected" 16 (73%). For females the characteristics of importance were: "tactile texture" 46 (75%), "blink" 42 (69%), "face" 36 (59%), "cry" 35 (57%), and their major reason for acquiring the robot was also "Healing effect is expected" 37 (61%). These design features of Paro are typical of those of socially assistive robots designed for seniors living at home.

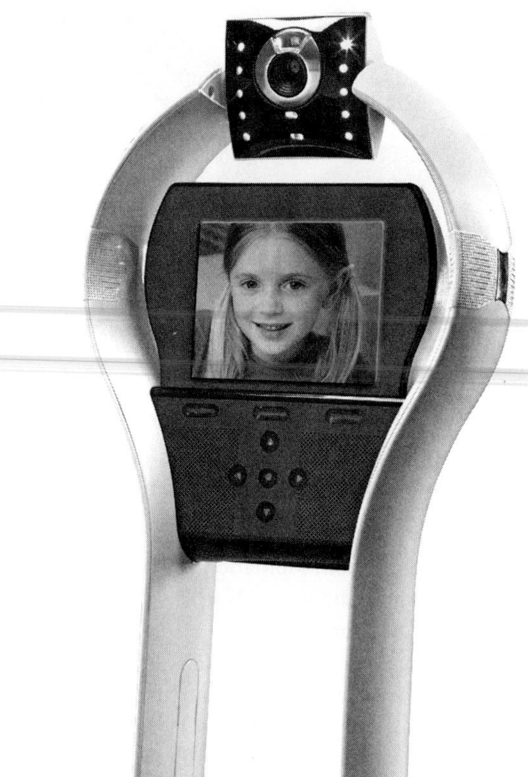

FIGURE 12-17 The VGo robot system is intended to provide both monitoring and some social interaction in the home.

Tele-Operated Robots for Assisting Seniors in Their homes

Mobile autonomous platforms with and without robotic arms have been developed to assist elderly people and people with disabilities in their homes (Dario et al, 1999; Michaud et al, 2008). In this section we explore one such application in more detail.

Seelye et al (2012) studied the feasibility of use and acceptance of a remotely controlled robot with video that included monitoring and communication features. The VGo robot system (VGo Communications[17]) (see Figure 12-17) was used in this study. This robot system includes a remotely controlled robot with a handheld local controller, and a remote driving controller. In-home use requires an 802.11 broadband wireless local Wi-Fi network with high speed Internet access. It is equipped with a screen, camera microphone, and speakers for two-way remote communication.

Attitudes and preferences of eight cognitively intact older adults living independently and their families and care providers, collectively referred to as *collaterals* (the term used to describe family members, care providers, and others involved with the senior) were evaluated. The participants were drawn from a longitudinal cohort established to understand how various methods of pervasive home computing and other technologies may support or improve the health and independence of people as they age. They generally appreciated

[17] www.vgocom.com/.

the potential of this technology to enhance their physical health and well-being, and to connect them with family and friends. Collaterals found it easy to install and set up the robot system and they particularly liked having the ability to move the robot around during calls. They also appreciated the potential to increase their loved one's safety and social connectedness. Challenges in operation of the system would most likely be increased if the individuals had cognitive impairments.

Robot Use by Children for Play and Learning

The pioneering work of Seymour Papert (1980) demonstrated that robots can enhance motivation and provide a test bed for "learning by doing." Robots can provide a means for children who have disabilities to engage in play and academic activities, especially those that involve exploration and manipulation of the environment (Cook et al., 2005).

Most rehabilitative robotic systems have been designed for adults (e.g., those with high-level spinal cord injuries), and their control requires relatively high-level cognitive skills that exceed the developmental level of younger children (Van Vliet & Wing, 1991). Severe physical disabilities may also limit the access to standard rehabilitation robots (Eberhardt et al., 2000). The educational setting places additional constraints on the robot system. First, the user may be very young, which necessitates simplified, age-appropriate control schemes and user interfaces. Second, a robot that is intended for use by young children has added safety demands since school children cannot be expected to exercise the same caution as adults.

Robots as Aids to Learning for Children with Disabilities

Kwee et al (1999, 2002) adapted the Manus arm for various pick and place academic activities with six participants, 7 to 29 years old, all of whom had cerebral palsy. The required adaptations focused on two areas: the physical control of the robot and the cognitive understanding of the required tasks. Difficulties in directly controlling the robot were generally addressed by using scanning rather than direct selection. Single-switch scanning was used to select the direction of movement, and activation of the arm. However, scanning requires greater cognitive skill and these adaptations for physical performance resulted in control schemes that required significant amounts of training and practice in order to understand the cognitive aspects involved (Van Vliet and Wing, 1991).

Open-ended tasks such as drawing have also been carried out using single-switch scanning with the Handy 1 Robot (Smith and Topping, 1996). In this case, selection of the color of a pen, the position of the pen, up (move) or down (draw), and the pen's movement are accomplished using single-switch scanning. Tasks such as these are cognitively demanding, and widely varying levels of success were reported for the three subjects included in the study.

A specially designed robot for access to science lab activities was trialed with seven students aged 9 to 11 years who had physical disabilities (Howell & Hay, 1989). The Aryln Arm robotic workstation was developed specifically for educational applications (Eberhardt et al, 2000). It has a portable base and a six degree-of-freedom arm. A two-joystick control system is used to position the arm, control the end effector (a "pseudo hand"), and direct the moveable base. There is also a built-in vacuum system. Eberhardt et al (2000) used the arm with five subjects who had disabilities preventing participation in science and the arts. Using the arm system these subjects completed projects in these two subject areas. Robots have also been used as tools in therapeutic play activities (Latham et al, 2001). In this approach, a series of sensors are attached to a child to detect arm, finger or head movement. Those signals are then used to control a robot. A storytelling robot was employed to address cognitive, language, and emotional rehabilitation needs in children with disabilities.

Another system for classroom use was developed in Great Britain (Harwin et al, 1988). This system differed from other educational applications in the inclusion of a vision system based on a television camera and image recognition software, which allowed the system to be used for more sophisticated tasks such as finding and stacking blocks. Three tasks were used with this system: (1) stacking and knocking down blocks with two switches (yes/no), (2) sorting articles by shape or color with four switches (one for each feature) or two switches (yes/no), and (3) a stacking game with five switches (left, middle, right, pick up, release). Children with motor disabilities who used this system enjoyed it and were able to successfully complete the tasks described. By using the robotic arm, they could accomplish otherwise impossible tasks.

PlayROB is a dedicated robot system to help children with severe physical impairments use Lego bricks (Kronreif et al, 2005). Trials were conducted with three able-bodied children (between 5 and 7 years old) and three disabled children (between 9 and 11 years old; child 1 – multiple disabilities; child 2 – tetra paresis; child 3 – transverse spinal cord syndrome). Kronrief et al reported that the majority of the children enjoyed playing with the robot and that it was able to provide the necessary support for manipulating the Lego bricks. To investigate possible and estimated learning effects, a multicenter study was conducted with an upgraded version of the robot system in which children with and without disabilities participated (Kronreif al, 2007).

Mathematics instruction is most effective when young students both participate interactively with hands-on activities and reflect on what they have learned verbally (Van De Walle et al, 2010). Students with severe physical disabilities combined with complex communication needs may not be able to manipulate the materials used in mathematics instruction. To address the problem of physical access to instructional materials in mathematics, Adams and Cook (2013) used a robot controlled via a speech generating device (SGD) (see Chapter 16) to enable students with physical and communication limitations to demonstrate their knowledge in math measurement activities. An integrated communication and robotic manipulation system allowed students with disabilities to engage in math instruction and work with objects to "construct ideas of number, devise your own problems, think about what you are doing and express what you have learned" (Ginsberg et al, 1998, p. 440).

Three students participated in a study to use robots as manipulative aids in mathematics instruction: a 14-year-old girl, a 10-year-old boy, and a 12-year-old girl. All had severe physical disabilities and complex communication needs (CCN) and each used the IR output of an SGD to control a Lego MindStorms robot. The SGD was mounted to their wheelchair. Selections were via scanning head movements detected by two switches. A standard mathematical curriculum was used for the study. Students manipulated objects by controlling the Lego robot and at the same time expressed themselves using their SGD. They performed the manipulative mathematics tasks using the robot enabled, which allowed the teacher to assess the procedural knowledge of each student. A procedural gap in the knowledge of the participants was not recognizing that they had to " line up ends of items" to compare objects. This action had always been done by their teacher or educational assistant before asking which object was longer. Without the direct manipulation this gap would not have been detected.

The combination of the robot and SGD gave participants multiple means of demonstrating their understanding of concepts. They could use whatever method was most effective for demonstrating or explaining, and, since both modes were always available, they could augment one with the other.

All of the participants demonstrated and explained their understanding of math concepts, and some gaps in their knowledge were revealed that might have been missed without the combination of manipulation and communication. The EAs felt these gaps were caused by lack of experience in doing the activities independently.

Robots to Enable Play for Children with Disabilities

The most common traits of play are: (1) intrinsic motivation, (2) process rather than product oriented, (3) enjoyment and pleasure, (4) active engagement and internal control, and (5) suspension of reality (Bundy, 1993). As the most prevalent activity in childhood, play has an instrumental role in a child's development (Ferland, 2005). Playing provides the opportunity to discover and test capabilities, try-out objects, make decisions, comprehend cause and effect relationships, and understand consequences (Missiuna & Pollock, 1991). Free play provides children the opportunity to learn through creative problem solving and interaction with objects and people. They also experience a sense of internal control and mastery (Bundy, 1993).

Due to their disabilities, children with motor impairments may suffer from play deprivation (Missiuna & Pollock, 1991). The consequences of play deprivation include anxiety, frustration, and passivity in children, which often leads to secondary disabilities. Secondary disabilities include a decrease in the child's sense of self-efficacy, self-confidence, satisfaction, and well-being (Blanche, 2008). Based on these considerations, several groups are addressing the more general problem of developing robots that can be children's partners or playmates (e.g., Howard et al, 2008; Besio, 2008).

Besio (2008) framed the development of robots that enable play in educational and therapeutic settings for children with physical and/or cognitive impairments in terms of the Children and Youth version of the *International Classification of Functioning and Disability* (WHO, 2001). The ICF-CY was chosen for many of the same reasons that we have used the primary ICF as a framework in this text: it takes into account all aspects related to the individuals and their life environments and examines technology as an important tool for enabling activity and participation. The ICF-CY directly addresses specific issues related to child and youth development.

Besio identified five main clusters as detailed in the ICF-CY that are related to robot-mediated play of children with disabilities:

- Factors related to the *individual*
- Factors related to the *context*
- Factors related to *technology and robotics*
- Factors related to *methodology*
- Factors related to *play*

Based on this framework, play scenarios were developed based on children's functional impairments, as described by the ICF-CY (Besio, 2008). Since the robots are intended to be used in educational inclusive settings, environmental factors in the ICF-CY also have been taken into account (Besio, 2008). This framework contemplates possible play activities from simple sensory play to more complex games with rules that require a range of body functions (e.g., voice and speech, mental, musculoskeletal, and sensory functions). Activity and participation components such as general tasks and demands, communication, and mobility are also included in the play framework. As we have described, technology is included in the environmental components of the ICF. The products and technologies (adapted or not) for communication and play constitute the tools that enable play for children with disabilities.

ASSESSMENT FOR USE OF MANIPULATION AIDS

This section primarily addresses an assessment process that will result in the recommendation for an EADL, smart technology, and in the future, robotics. As we discuss in Chapter 5, the initial assessment step is to determine the consumer's needs carefully, especially in the context of daily living demands (e.g., home, employment). The client, clinician, and family (as appropriate) collaboratively frame the needs of the client that have the potential to be addressed by this type of technology. Use of the ICF categories can assist the clinician to identify activities that are necessary and desired. Manipulation aids can assist the client to reach, grasp, and retrieve objects; to open/shut a door; and to control various appliances, home features, and devices. Smart technology can support the client with many communication and cognitive activities. Robots have the potential to perform many activities for the client. A measure such as the *Canadian Occupational Performance Measure* (COPM; Law et al, 2005) can be used to identify key occupations in which the client wants/needs to engage.

Consistent with the previous discussion of the application of the HAAT model (Chapters 3 and 5), consideration of the human factors follows the identification of target activities. Assessment of client manipulation, both fine and gross motor, provides information on the client's performance in this area and the degree of support required by a device. The clinician identifies one or more movements (e.g., finger movement, inhalation/expiration, eye blinks) that can be used reliably to control an EADL or robot. Cognitive function is evaluated since the initial learning process and ongoing use can require high-level cognitive abilities, particularly if the device has multiple functions or requires several steps in the selection process. Sensory function—in particular vision, audition, and touch perception—are also evaluated for their role in the human/technology interface (HTI).

As with other technology, the clinician should determine the meaning that technology use has for the client, the readiness of the client to use it, and their previous experience with it. At this point, having identified the target activities and assessed the client's functional abilities and readiness for technology, the client and clinician can now set goals for use of high-tech devices.

Consideration of the context(s) in which the technology will be used is the next step. Context is most important when considering high-tech devices. Previously, we identified physical aspects of light and sound that affect technology use. The physical dimensions of the client's residence and features to be controlled are determined. For example, if an EADL is installed to open/close an entrance door, consideration of the physical dimensions of the door, whether it opens into the residence or out of it (or perhaps is a sliding door) is necessary to select the appropriate device. When the device will be connected to the home's wiring, such details are also necessary. Funding possibilities are explored as part of the assessment.

The outcomes of an EADL assessment include: (1) identification of control sites and control interfaces, (2) determination of cognitive abilities related to understanding EADL operation, (3) listing of EADL functions desired (in priority order), (4) evaluation of the consumer's motivation to use electronic environmental control, (5) a listing of other electronic devices that the consumer uses, and (6) identification of the environments in which the EADLS will be used. The listing of functions may include such things as lighting, TV, and drapery control. The listing of other electronic devices should include both consumer electronic devices (such as TV, CD/DVD player, computer, and speaker telephone) and assistive technologies (such as communication devices and powered wheelchairs). Armed with this information, it is then possible to work with the consumer to select an EADL that meets his or her needs.

Holme et al (1997) conducted a survey of occupational therapists (OTs) working in spinal cord injury and disease centers. Although this study is fairly old, a more recent study is not in the literature and the results of this work remain informative. The purpose of the survey was to determine the use of EADLs by persons who have had spinal cord injuries, reasons for recommendations for EADLs (or not) by OTs, and the skills required to assess consumers for use of EADLs and recommend appropriate devices. They found that 84% of the OTs working in these centers used EADLs with their clients as part of the in-patient rehabilitation process. Consumers who had injuries at the C4 or higher level were generally viewed as able to benefit from EADLs. The top four reasons for recommending an EADL were: (1) empowerment of the client, (2) improvement in the client's quality of life, (3) increased access to call systems, and (4) decreased need for attendant care. Holme et al (1997) also found that more than 50% of the EADLs recommended and purchased for clients were still in use. They identified the major reasons for *not* recommending an EADL as: (1) lack of funding (64% of respondents), (2) high cost of EADLs (47%), (3) unavailability of EADLs for trial, and (4) lack of EADL knowledge by the OT responsible for the client's rehabilitation. The major reason that clients did not use EADLs recommended for them was a preference for having another person provide the necessary assistance. Holme et al (1997) concluded that more frequent recommendation of EADLs by OTs is dependent on two factors: (1) outcome studies that identify the effectiveness of EADLs and their cost effectiveness and (2) inclusion of knowledge and skills related to EADLs in OT training.

Acute Care and Rehabilitation Contextual Implications

In the acute care setting, the client has experienced a sudden change in the ability to engage in daily activities, for example loss of motor skills and sensation following a spinal cord injury, changes in motor control and cognitive function following a traumatic brain injury, or change in the underlying condition of a progressive disease such as amyotrophic lateral sclerosis. The client has limited physical abilities and in the case of a spinal cord injury, no longer knows what his body can do or how she can control her environment. The client's world is limited to a bed and hospital room for extended lengths of time. Necessary activities in this context include use of the call bell for nursing assistance and perhaps controlling a TV. At this point, provision of a simple EADL that offers control of these two devices can demonstrate to the client that he or she can still engage in some activities and control the environment with a degree of independence. The acute care setting may be able to provide professionals with expertise in EADLs to support the client's use of the technology.

When a client moves to a rehabilitation context, he or she typically is learning how to engage in many more activities and may have regained some motor function. This setting is more likely to employ professionals with EADL expertise who will be involved in assessment, recommendation, set-up, and training of the technology. The client will have greater mobility and will be learning to use a powered wheelchair that enables more independence and the ability to move about the facility and its grounds. During the rehabilitation period, the client also has the opportunity to go out to the community. The rehabilitation period affords the client the opportunity to learn how to use EADLs that support more complex functions, such as the use of a telephone or controlling different appliances.

Community Context

Once clients return to the community, either to their own homes or to some form of supported living, they need to engage in many more activities. The focus of EADL use in the home is to enable engagement in daily activities.

For example, a client returning to his or her own home needs to be able to identify someone at the door, unlock/open the door to admit the person as appropriate, and then close the door. This activity is an example of something that was not required in either of the other previous two settings. Similarly, the client needs to control different aspects of the environment such as temperature and lighting, using a phone in an emergency or controlling window coverings that were not required in the previous two settings. The support and training of a caregiver or support personnel in the home is less than what is available in the rehabilitation setting, particularly in the initial period following the return home. The home environment does provide the opportunity to determine the requirements for EADLs in a stable environment and how this technology needs to be integrated into the user's daily life.

Little (2010) describes several issues that affect the introduction of EADLs. In the acute phase, post-trauma, the response to the EADL will vary and the devices may be rejected because the client needs time to adjust to his or her altered function and to recognize how technology can enhance that function. Arguments for introduction of the EADL during the acute hospital phase of rehabilitation include developing a sense of control and possible independence in the client and providing the system while there is significant support available for set-up and training (Ability Research Centre, 1999). Early introduction of a device to someone with a progressive disease allows the opportunity to concentrate on becoming proficient with the use of the device rather than attempting to both learn how to use the device and adapt to loss of function at the same time. Little (2010) suggests the introduction of a device early in rehabilitation but waiting to obtain a device until the client has returned to the community so there is a better sense of what the client can do and needs to do as well as the environmental support for the use of the device.

OUTCOMES OF EADL USE

Little research has been conducted that provides evidence for the outcomes of implementation of EADL technology. What work has been done, though, investigates its use in the client's residence. Two reasons are behind the lack of this research. The technology is complex and changing rapidly, which makes it difficult to conduct research that provides generalizable results across client populations and which evaluates current technology. This research is also hampered by the lack of any outcome measure that is specific to EADL (or other high-technology) use (Boman et al, 2007). Existing studies use measures described in Chapter 5: PIADS and QUEST, which provide a general understanding of psychosocial impact of device use (PIADS) and satisfaction with (QUEST) device use.

Box 12-3 summarizes research on factors that influence EADL use and non-use, as well as clinicians' reasons for recommending or not recommending such devices. Some of the themes that describe reasons for device use and non-use are echoed in research exploring outcomes of the use of these devices. A small number of studies in the literature explore

BOX 12-3 What the Research Says: Consumers' Use of Electronic Aids to Daily Living and Clinicians' Reasons for Recommending Them

Factors that Influence Use of EADLs

Training and ongoing support are available for the user, caregivers, and staff (Ability Centre, 1999, Boman et al, 2007)
The device is reliable, consistently doing what it is intended to do with few errors or malfunction (Ability Centre, 1999)
The user has the opportunity to try the device for a period of time (e.g., 2 weeks) before purchase (Boman et al, 2007)
The device affords the user an enhanced sense of security and comfort, allowing them to spend longer periods of time alone (Verdonck et al, 2011)
User identifies applications of the device for communication, safety/security, household, employment, and educational tasks (Boman et al, 2007)

Factors that Influence the Discontinuation or Lack of Use of EADLs

When the situations described above are not present, the device is more likely to be abandoned in the short or long term
User may prefer to have another person (caregiver, personal attendant) provide assistance for the tasks that could be completed with the use of an EADL (Palmer & Seale, 2007)

Primary Reasons for Recommendation of EADLs (Holme, 1997)

Empowerment of the client
Improvement of the client's quality of life
Reduce the need for attendant care
Provide access to attendant call systems and other devices in the environment

Primary Reasons Why EADLs Are not Recommended (Holme et al, 1997)

Lack of external funding, paired with the high cost of the devices
Limited availability of different types of devices due to the infrequency with which many providers make recommendations for these devices
When service providers do not regularly recommend these devices, their knowledge may be limited to only a narrow range of devices
The expense of the equipment and the complexity of set-up restricts opportunities users have to trial the devices

the influence of EADL acquisition and use. These studies investigate EADL use only by adults, primarily adults living in the community. Client populations include individuals with high cervical spinal cord injuries, multiple sclerosis, traumatic brain injury, muscular dystrophy, and stroke.

Users' perceptions of the benefits of EADLs were evaluated throughout the assessment and acquisition process using the PIADS (Ripat & Strock, 2004). In the pre-acquisition phase, potential EADL users predicted that there would be positive impact on feelings of competence and confidence and that an EADL would enable them in a positive way. One month after obtaining an EADL the perceptions were still positive but less so than in the pre-acquisition phase. After 3 to 6 months the level of positive perception had returned to the pre-acquisition level, indicating that the original predictions were actually met. The most likely reason for the reduced positive impact perception in the middle phase is that the users were learning the new device and were adjusting to carrying out activities of daily living in a new way with the EADL.

Ripat (2006) reported results of a follow-up study. This study found that the positive benefits were sustained over time, as measured by the COPM and PIADS (see Chapter 5 for a description of both measures). New and more experienced users both perceived an overall positive impact of EADLs (Ripat, 2006). Both the COPM, which measures an individual's perception of performance and satisfaction with performance in activities of daily living, and the PIADS which measures the impact of assistive technology on an individual, yielded positive results that were highly correlated with each other. Stickel et al (2002) reported similar results, concluding that satisfaction with EADL use was prevalent and stable over time.

Studies of EADL use have concluded that these devices are useful and easy to use (following a training and skill development period) (Boman et al, 2007). The finding that EADL that fits into the client's routine and existing habits rather than disrupting their patterns is interesting, although perhaps not surprising (Boman et al. 2007; Erikson et al, 2004). Clients who use EADLs report higher quality of life over those who do not (Boman et al, 2007; Rigby et al, 2011). Palmer and Seale (2007), Rigby et al (2011), and Verdonck et al (2011, 2014) offer some explanation for the findings that demonstrate satisfaction with device use and greater quality of life.

Palmer and Seale (2007) used a grounded theory methodology to explore attitudes toward electronic control systems (ECS) by individuals with physical disabilities. They describe utility of the device, in which the device is seen as a tool, as the primary theme. Individuals who described utility of these systems in a positive manner expressed the opinion that it was more than a tool; that use of an ECS changed their life. In contrast, participants with a more negative view of ECS use reported dissatisfaction with the outcome of the device use. The participants in the Palmer and Seale study varied on their upper extremity function, which was proposed as the distinguishing factor in whether ECS use was a satisfactory or unsatisfactory experience. Participants with greater upper extremity function had more options for ways to engage in an activity and were more likely to view ECS use negatively (Palmer & Seale, 2007).

Rigby and colleagues (2011) explored quality-of-life issues with individuals with tetraplegia who used EADLs, in comparison with those who did not. They used the Quality of Life Profile—Physical Disabilities (Renwick et al, 2003) to compare quality of life across these two groups. Their participants all had a spinal cord injury at the C5/6 level or higher. The Functional Independence Measure was used to measure disability; no difference was found between the two groups (Rigby et al, 2011). The quality-of-life measure consists of three domains: being, belonging, and becoming. Being consists of physical, psychological, and spiritual being; belonging involves physical, social, and community belonging; and becoming involves practical, leisure, and growth (personal development) domains (Renwick et al.). Respondents rate the importance of and their satisfaction with each of these domains. No significant differences were found between the groups. Satisfaction with all three of the becoming scales, the total quality of life score and physical being were significantly higher in the group of EADL users than in the non-users (Rigby et al, 2005).

Verdonck and colleagues (2011, 2014) conducted a phenomenological study of the experience of EADL use among individuals with high cervical spinal cord injuries. Autonomy was identified as the overarching theme, described as being able to do what you want (Verdonck et al, 2011). Two sub-themes were related to autonomy: time alone and changed relationships. The respondents indicated that use of EADLs enabled them to be alone, giving them privacy and their own space.

They were also able to get away from their home with these devices. The theme of changed relationships described the experience of feeling less of a burden, not having to apologize, and experiencing less annoyance (on the part of the individual and others) (Verdonck et al, 2011). In a recent publication, Verdonck and colleagues describe the interplay between hassle and engagement in the use of EADLs (Verdonck et al, 2014). Six individuals with a high cervical spinal cord injury were provided with a "trial pack" of ECS devices and then interviewed after a period of use of these devices. They described a tension between the hassle with use of the technology, including the need to break habits in order to use the devices, and engagement in occupations facilitated by their use. Engagement was described as having fun, feeling good, and being surprised by the impact of the ECS on their lives (Verdonck, 2014).

Collectively, these studies provide some evidence for the positive influence of EADLs on the user's quality of life and the enabling influence of these devices on function. Verdonck's work (2011, 2014) provides interesting insight into the experience of using these devices. Rigby's work (2011) provides preliminary evidence of specific areas of quality of life in which EADL use has an influence. These studies all have small sample sizes, in part due to the small number of individuals who use these devices. They are also limited by the availability of measurement tools specific to this type of device use. These issues aside, the small body of literature available in this area has promising results that demand more research to enhance the evidence base supporting use of these devices.

SUMMARY

Assistive technologies designed to aid manipulation help consumers in accomplishing tasks for which they normally use their upper extremities. Some manipulative aids are general purpose, meaning they serve multiple functions, and some are special purpose, designed for one task. In some cases the manipulative aid assists with normal hand function (e.g., hand-writing aids); we refer to these as *augmentative.* In other cases an *alternative* method is used (e.g., a robotic arm for moving items on a desk). In addition, special-purpose and general-purpose devices may be either high or low tech.

Low-tech general-purpose manipulation aids include mouth sticks, head pointers, and reachers. Special-purpose devices are available to meet needs in the general performance areas of self-care, work or school, and recreation or leisure.

There are two types of general-purpose electrically powered devices: EADLs and robotic systems. Electronic aids to daily living include appliance control; telephone access; TV and CD/DVD control; and remote access to doors, drapes, and windows. Robots are used to meet manipulative needs in the home, at work, and in the classroom. Both EADLs and assistive robots are controlled by computers, and each may be accessed by a variety of control interfaces and selection methods.

CASE STUDY 12-1

EADLs for Increased Independence

Joyce is 39. She has cerebral palsy, and she has just moved into an apartment with an attendant. She is unable to speak, and she uses a communication device based on a laptop computer. Joyce controls her scanning communication device with a tread switch mounted near her knee. The communication device consists of a software program running on a laptop computer. The communication and environmental control aspects of Joyce's system were integrated by using an IR trainable or programmable remote device interfaced to the serial port of the laptop computer. The remote device is activated by the scanning communication software computer program, and it controls a TV and DVD directly.

A two-channel IR receiver with switch output is used to control an automatic telephone dialer. The telephone controller also allows control of four ultrasound receivers that Joyce has connected to two lamps and to a drapery control to open her curtains automatically. All the EADL functions are controlled by selecting the device from a menu and then sending a command through the IR remote unit to activate it (turn on the switch to the telephone dialer, change TV channels, and so on).

*Scanning WSKE, Words Plus, Lancaster, CA., www.words-plus.com
†Relax II, TASH Inc, Ajax, ON Canada, www.tashinc.com
‡E.A.S.I. Dialer, TASH, Ajax, ON, Canada, www.tashinc.com

CASE STUDY 12-2

EADLs Following a Stroke

Eileen, who is 62 years old, suffered a brainstem stroke and requires maximal assistance for daily living. She sits in a reclining chair at home for the majority of the day. Eileen is able to use head movement to make communication selections using a built-in Madentec Tracker light pointer mounted on a headband to control a communication device.

Eileen also needs a simple EADL that can control the TV (turn it on, select channels, and control volume), a lamp, and a call signal to use when her husband is out of the room. She controls a scanning trainable IR remote† using a single switch mounted next to her head. This directly accesses the required TV functions. For the call system, an IR-sensitive switch is used to control an X-10 module. The module can be plugged in anywhere in the house, and her husband carries it with him when he goes outside or into a remote part of the house. In this way Eileen can summon him at any time if necessary. She can activate the switch using her head movement, without having to have the light pointer taken off. This makes her communication function independent of her EADL function, and it offers a contrast to Joyce's preference of having them integrated.

*Edmonton AB, Canada, www.madentic.com
†Vantage, Prentke Romich, Wooster, Ohio, www.prentrom.com/
‡Relax II, TASH Inc., Ajax, ON, Canada, www.tashinc.com

CASE STUDY 12-3

EADL and a progressive condition

Dorothy, a 45-year-old woman who has amyotrophic lateral sclerosis, lives with her son, daughter, and husband and receives attendant care daily. Dorothy uses a computer for written communication and an EADL for telephone, door, and electrical bed and appliance control. For writing, she uses a trackball with a virtual keyboard software program for text entry (see Chapter 7).

Appliance and telephone control were implemented using a stand-alone EADL accessed using a single-touch switch. This approach was taken, instead of combining the communication and environmental control functions, because Dorothy generally does not need access to the EADL functions while she is writing. Automatic telephone dialing is accomplished by the scanning approach described above. Dorothy's needs for controlling AC appliances are met by using X-10 modules plugged in to the house wiring. The EADL also plugs in to the house wiring to communicate with the modules. These can control lights, appliances, or a call signal. The electric door opener is controlled by a switch output on the EADL.

*Conrol 1, formerly available from Prentke Romich, Wooster, Ohio

STUDY QUESTIONS

1. List and describe the four categories of aided manipulation.
2. Identify the four kinds of product modifications of low-tech special-purpose aids to manipulation. Give an example of each.
3. What are the primary types of self-care activities supported by low-tech manipulation aids?
4. What are the two major approaches used in electrically powered page turners?
5. What are the functions provided by electrically powered page turners?
6. What are the four control functions implemented in EADLs? Describe the differences between them and give an EADL example of each.
7. Discuss the relative advantages and disadvantages of the two modes of binary latched AC appliance control.
8. What are the four major transmission modes used in EADL systems?
9. How does a trainable or programmable IR controller work, and what are the major advantages of these types of device?
10. What is the difference between a trainable and a programmable IR controller?
11. Describe the functions of an automatic telephone dialer.
12. List the major assessment areas to be considered when determining the best EADL for a specific user.
13. What are the key factors that contribute to use or non-use of EADLs by persons with spinal cord injuries?
14. Describe the key design features of the Manus mobile robotic arm.
15. How do the Manus design features contribute to or detract from its effectiveness and consumer satisfaction?
16. What are the key factors considered when determining if a Manus robotic arm is suitable for a consumer's needs and goals? Do you agree with these? Why or why not?
17. Describe the major differences between desktop and mobile robots from the point of view of both the required design and the user interaction with the robot.
18. How do educational applications of robotic systems differ from vocational or daily living applications?
19. How can robotic systems be used to evaluate and perhaps enhance cognitive and language functioning in young children?

REFERENCES

Ability Research Centre: *Environmental control systems for people with spinal cord injuries.* Retrieved from http://www.ability.org.au/images/stories/ftp/research/environmental_controls_systems_report.pdf, 1999.

Adams K, Cook A: Access to hands-on mathematics measurement activities using robots controlled via speech generating devices: Three case studies, *Disabil Rehabil: Assist Technol*, 2013 (Online August).

Besio S, editor: *Analysis of critical factors involved in using interactive robots for education and therapy of children with disabilities*, Italy, 2008, Editrice UNI Service.

Bessell T, Randell M, Knowles G, et al.: Connecting people with the environment—a new accessible wireless remote control, *Proceedings 2004 ARATA Conference*, November 17, 2006. Retrieved from.

Birch GE, et al.: An assessment methodology and its application to a robotic vocational assistive device, *Tech Disabil* 5:151–165, 1996.

Blanche EI: Play in children with cerebral palsy: doing with—not doing to. In Parham L, Fazio L, editors: *Play in Occupational Therapy for Children*, St Louis, 2008, Mosby Elsevier, pp 375–393.

Boman I-L, Than K, Granqvisst A, et al.: Using electronic aids to daily living after acquired brain injury: a study of the learning process and the usability, *Disabil Rehabil: Assist Technol* 2:23–33, 2007, DOI: 10.1080/17483100069856213.

Brose SW, Weber DJ, Salatin BA, et al.: The role of assistive robotics in the lives of persons with disability, *Am J Phys Med Rehabil* 89(6):509–521, 2010.

Bundy A: Assessment of play and leisure: delineation of the problem, *Am J Occup Ther* 47(3):217–222, 1993.

Cook AM, Bentz B, Harbottle N, et al.: School-based use of a robotic arm system by children with disabilities, *IEEE Trans on Neural Systems and Rehabilitation Engineering* 13:452–460, 2005.

Cook A, Encarnação P, Adams K, Robots: assistive technologies for play, learning and cognitive development, *Technology and Disability* 22(3):127–146, 2010.

Dario P, Guglielmelli P, Laschi C, et al.: MOVAID: a personal robot in everyday life of disabled and elderly people, *Technol Disabil* 10:77–93, 1999.

Dautenhahn K, Werry I: towards interactive robots in autism therapy: background, motivation and challenges, *Pragmat Cognition* 12(1):135, 2004.

Driessen BJ, Evers HG, van Woerden JA: MANUS—A wheelchair-mounted rehabilitation robot, *Proc Inst Mech Eng [H]* 215: 285–290, 2001.

Eberhardt SP, Osborne J, Rahman T: Classroom evaluation of the arlyn arm robotic workstation, *Assist Technol* 12(2):132–143, 2000.

Erikson A, Karlsson G, Soderstrom M, Tham K: A training apartment with electronic aids to daily living: lived experiences of persons with brain damage, *Am J Occup Ther* 58:261–271, 2004.

Feil-Seifer D, Mataric MJ: *Defining socially assistive robotics*, Presented at the International Conferenceon Rehabilitation Robotics (ICORR'05), Chicago, IL, 465–468, 2005.

Ferland F: *The Ludic Model*, ed 2, Ottawa, 2005, CAOT Publications ACE.

Fong T, Nourbakhsh I, Dautenhahn K: A survey of socially interactive robots, *Robotics and Autonomous Systems* 42:143–166, 2003.

Ginsburg HP, Klein A, Starkey P: The development of children's mathematical thinking: connecting research with practice. In Siegel IE, Renninger KA, editors: *Handbook of child psychology, Volume 4: Child psychology in practice*, ed 5, New York, 1998, John Wiley and Sons, pp 401–476.

Giuffrida G, Rice MS: Motor skills and occupational performance: assessments and interventions. In Blesedell Crepeau E, Cohn ES, Boyt Schell BA, editors: *Willard and Spackman's occupational therapy*, ed 11, Philadelphia, 2009, Lippincott, Williams & Wilkins, pp 681–714.

Harwin WS, Ginige A, Jackson RD: A robot workstation for use in education of the physically handicapped, *IEEE Trans Biomed Eng* 35:127–131, 1988.

Holme AS, et al.: The use of environmental control units by occupational therapists in spinal cord injury and disease, *Am J Occup Ther* 51:42–48, 1997.

Howard AM, Park H, Kemp CC: Extracting play primitives for a robot playmate by sequencing low level motion behaviors. In *Proceedings of the 17th IEEE International Symposium on Robot and Human Interactive Communication*, Munich, Germany, August 13, 2008, Technische Universitat Munchen.

Howell R, Hay K: Software based access and control of robotic manipulators for severely physically disabled students, *J Art Intell Educ* 1(1):53–72, 1989.

Kinney P: *ZigBee Technology: Wireless control that simply works*, Communications Design Conference, October 2003 July 10, 2014. Retrieved from http://www.zigbee.org/en/resources/#WhitePapers.

Kronreif G, Prazak B, Mina S et al: PlayROB—robot assisted playing for children with severe physical disabilities, *Proceedings of the 9th IEEE International Conference on Rehabilitation Robotics*, June 28–July 1, 2005, Chicago, IL.

Kronreif G, Kornfeld M, Prazak B et al: Robot assistance in playful environment—user trials and results, *Proceedings of IEEE International Conference on Robotics and Automation*, April 10-14, 2007, Rome, Italy.

Kwee H, Quaedackers J: POCUS project adapting the control of the Manus manipulator for persons with cerebral palsy, *Proceedings ICORR: International Conference on Rehabilitation Robotics*, Stanford, CA, pp. 106–114, 1999.

Kwee H, Quaedackers J, van de Bool E, et al.: Adapting the dontrol of the MANUS manipulator for persons with cerebral palsy: an exploratory study, *Technol Disabil* 14(1):31–42, 2002.

Latham C, Vice JM, Tracey M, et al.: Therapeutic play with a storytelling robot, *Proc. Conf. Human Factors in Computing Systems*, 27–28, 2001.

Law M, et al.: *Canadian Occupational Performance Measure*, ed 3, Toronto, 2005, CAOT/ACE Publications.

Little R: EADL, *Phys Med Rehabil Clin N Am* 21:33–42, 2010, http://dx.doi.org/10.1016/j.pmr.2009.07.008.

Maheu V, Archambault PS, Frappier J, et al.: Evaluation of the JACO robotic arm: clinico-economic study for powered wheelchair users with upper-extremity disabilities. *2011 IEEE International Conference on Rehabilitation Robotics*, ETH Zurich Science City, Switzerland, June 29-July 1, 2011, Rehab Week Zurich.

Michaud F, Boissy P, Labonte D, et al.: A Telementoring robot for home care, technology and aging, selected papers from the, *2007 International Conference on Technology and Aging* 21, 2008.

Michaud F, Salter T, Duquette A, et al.: Perspectives on mobile robots used as tools for pediatric rehabilitation: assistive technologies, *Special Issue on Intell Syst Ped Rehabil* 19(1):21–36, 2007.

Missiuna C, Pollock N: Play deprivation in children with physical disabilities: the role of the occupational therapist in preventing secondary disabilities, *Am J Occup Ther* 45:882–888, 1991.

Oderud T: Experiences from the evaluation of a Manus wheelchair-mounted manipulator. In Anogianakis G, Bühler C, Soede M, editors: *Advancement in assistive technology*, , Amsterdam, 1997, IOS Press.

Palmer P, Seale J: Exploring the attitudes to environmental control systems of people with physical disabilities: a grounded theory approach, *Technol Disabil* 19:17–27, 2007.

Papert S: *Mindstorms: children, computers, and powerful ideas*, New York, 1980, Basic Books.

Parasuraman R, Sheridan TB, Wicke CD: A model for types and levels of human interaction with automation, *IEEE Transactions on Systems, Man, and Cybernetics—Part A: Systems and Humans* Vol. 30(No. 3):286–297, May 2000.

Renwick R, Nourhaghighi N, Manns PJ, et al.: Quality of life for people with physical disabilities: a new instrument, *Int J Rehabil Res* 26:279–287, 2003.

Rigby P, Ryan S, Joos S, et al.: Impact of electronic aids to daily living on the lives of persons with cervical spinal cord injuries, *Assist Technol* 17(2):89–97, 2005.

Rigby P, Ryan S, Campbell K: Electronic aids to daily living and quality of life for persons with tetraplegia, *Disabil Rehabil: Assist Technol* 6:260–267, 2011, http://dx.doi.org/10.3109/17483107.2010.522678.

Ripat J: Function and impact of electronic aids to daily living for experienced users, *Technol Disabil* 18:79–97, 2006.

Ripat J, Strock A: User's perceptions of the impact of electronc aids to daily living throughout the acquisition process, *Assist Technol* 16:63–72, 2004.

Seelye AM, Wild KV, Larimer N, et al.: Reactions to a remote-controlled video-communication robot in seniors' homes: a pilot study of feasibility and acceptance, *Telemed E-Health* 18(10):755–759, 2012.

Shibata T, Kawaguchi Y, Wada K: Investigation on people living with seal robot at home: analysis of owners' gender differences and pet ownership experience, *Int J Soc Robot* 4:53–63, 2012.

Smith J, Topping M: The introduction of a robotic aid to drawing into a school for physically handicapped children: a case study, *Brit J Occ Ther* 59(12):565–569, 1996.

Stanger CA, Cawley MF: Demographics of rehabilitation robotics users, *Technol Disabil* 5:125–137, 1996.

Stickel MS, Ryan S, Rigby P, Jutai J: Toward a comprehensive evaluation of the impact of electronic aids to daily living: evaluation of consumer satisfaction, *Disabil Rehabil* 24:115–125, 2002, DOI: 10.1080/0963828011006679 4.

Van De Walle JA, Karp KS, Bay-Williams JM: *Elementary and middle school mathematics: teaching developmentally*, , Boston, 2010, Allyn and Bacon.

Van Vliet P, Wing AM: A new challenge—robotics in the rehabilitation of the neurologically motor impaired, *Phys Ther* 71(1):39–47, 1991.

Verburg G, et al.: Manus: the evolution of an assistive technology, *Technol Disabil* 5:217–228, 1996.

Verdonck M, Chard G, Nolan M: Electronic aids to daily living: being able to do what you want, *Assist Technol* 6:268–281, 2011. http://dx.doi.org/10.3109/17483107.2010.525291.

Verdonck M, Steggles E, Nolan M, Chard G: Experiences of using an electronic control system for persons with high cervical spinal cord injury: the interplay between hassle and engagement, *Disabil Rehabil: Assist Technol* 9:70–78, 2014. http://dx.doi.org/10.3109/17483107.2013.823572.

World Health Organization: *International classification of functioning, disability and health*, Geneva, 2001, WHO.

Zimmermann G, Vanderheiden G, Gandy M: Universal remote console standard—toward natural user interaction in ambient intelligence. *Extended Abstracts for the 2004 Conference on Human Factors in Computing Systems*, pp. 1608-1609, New York: ACM Press, 2004. Retrieved from. http://myurc.org/publications/2004-CHI-URC.php Novermber 28, 2006.

CHAPTER 13

Sensory Aids for Persons with Visual Impairments

CHAPTER OUTLINE

LEARNING OBJECTIVES

On completing this chapter, you will be able to do the following:

1. Describe the major approaches to sensory substitution for visual function, including the advantages and disadvantages of each
2. Describe the major causes of vision loss that can be aided by assistive technologies
3. Describe device use for reading and mobility by persons who have visual impairment
4. Describe how computer outputs are adapted for individuals with visual limitations
5. Describe the major approaches to creating visual access for mobile technologies
6. Describe the major approaches to Internet access for persons with visual impairments
7. Describe the contextual factors that affect assistive technologies for visual impairment
8. Describe the major assessments of visual function that are relevant to assistive technology use

KEY TERMS

Accessibility
Alternative Mobility Device
Braille
Closed-Circuit Television
Digital Talking Books
Electronic Travel Aid
Graphical User Interface
Internet
Magnification Aids
Optical Aids
Optical Character Recognition
Orientation and Mobility
Privacy
Quality
Reading Aid
Refreshable Braille Display
Screen Readers
Scripts
Spatial Display
Universal Access
User Agent
User Display
Video Magnifiers

When an individual has a visual sensory impairment, assistive technologies can provide assistance in the input of information. This chapter emphasizes approaches that are used to either aid or replace seeing. This includes sensory aids that are intended for *general use* in aiding reading or mobility and assistive technologies (AT) that are used specifically for providing visual access to computers and mobile technologies such as phones and tablets.

ACTIVITY COMPONENT

Visual function is important (but not essential) for the effective use of assistive technology systems, especially regarding access systems. For example, in using augmentative communication systems (Chapter 16), individual items must be found in arrays of vocabulary elements, scanning cursors must be tracked, and visual feedback is often used to signify successful message generation. Likewise, to use a powered wheelchair (Chapter 10), visual scanning of the environment must be present, and there must be adequate acuity and visual field to guide the chair around obstacles effectively, safely, and efficiently. For individuals who have visual impairments, reading print material or computer displays can be difficult or impossible, and assistive technologies can be of help. We discuss AT for visual impairment in this chapter.

Impact of Vision Loss on Activity

Patients with low vision were surveyed to determine their major needs for assistive devices (Stelmack et al., 2003). Sixty-three activities in the categories of travel, food and shopping, communications, household tasks, self-care, recreation and socialization, and contrast were included in the survey. The informants were 149 individuals in the age range of 51 to 96 years (mean 76 years). Two thirds were male. The survey consisted of asking participants whether they could perform the activity independently or if they used a low-vision device or whether they thought it was important to use a device to perform the activity independently. The highest-ranked items involved travel (find a clear path, identify landmarks, recognize traffic signals, step off a curb), self-care (apply makeup, shave), reading (large print, sign checks, find food in kitchen), and recreation (see television, recognize persons close up); Stelmack et al. (2003) provide detailed results. Assistive devices designed to meet the needs identified in the Stelmack survey are discussed in this chapter.

Studies of Computer Use by Adults with Visual Impairments

It is not surprising that computer use by individuals who are blind or who have low vision is less than by nondisabled individuals. Individuals with visual disabilities have less access to the Internet, are online less often, and are more likely to be online from work than are individuals without disabilities (Gerber & Kirchner, 2001). Severity of impairment and existence of multiple impairments each reduce the access and use further. Individuals under 65 years of age have greater use and access than do those older than 65 years (Gerber & Kirchner, 2001). This finding is important given the high prevalence of visual impairment in the population over 65 years old. People who are employed are more likely to use computers and the Internet, regardless of whether they are disabled, and the percentage of people using computers is almost identical for the two groups.

Activities of daily living (ADLs) are supported by mainstream appliances, entertainment products, and productivity tools for work. These technologies are continually improved with many electronically sophisticated new features. People with visual impairments worry that they will be left behind if these electronic advancements are not visually accessible. Universal design (see Chapter 2) principles become very important in this context.

HUMAN COMPONENT

The term *low vision* indicates that the individual is able to use the visual system for reading but that the standard size, contrast, or spacing are inadequate. The term *blind* refers to individuals for whom the visual system does not provide a useful input channel for computer output displays or printers. For individuals who are blind, alternative sensory pathways of either audition (hearing) or touch (feeling) must be used to provide input. Because low vision and blindness needs are so different from each other, they are discussed separately.

Common Visual Disorders

There are many diseases of the eye that lead to low vision or blindness (Galloway et al., 2006). The low vision that results from some types of diseases can be aided by assistive technologies. In this chapter we focus on the most common of these: age-related macular degeneration (ARMD), glaucoma, cataracts, and diabetes-related vision loss.

Congenital Blindness

Globally, the major causes of blindness in children vary widely by region (Gilbert & Foster, 2001). Major determining factors are socioeconomic development and the availability of primary health care and eye care services. Lesions of the optic nerve and higher visual pathways are the major cause of congenital blindness in high-income countries. In low-income countries additional causes include corneal scarring from measles, vitamin A deficiency, the use of harmful traditional eye remedies, and ophthalmia neonatorum.[1] Retinopathy of prematurity is an important cause in middle-income countries. Cataract, congenital abnormalities, and hereditary retinal dystrophies are significant causes in all countries. "It is estimated that, in almost half of the children who are blind today, the underlying cause could have been prevented, or the eye condition treated to preserve vision or restore sight" (Gilbert & Foster, 2001).

Age-Related Macular Degeneration

Age-related macular degeneration is the most common cause of blindness in seniors in western countries (Galloway et al., 2006). It occurs most frequently in individuals over 65, beginning in one eye and progressing gradually to both eyes. There are two types of ARMD: "dry" or atrophic and "wet" or endovascular. The dry form is much more common, but the wet form accounts for 80% to 90% of the cases of ARMD-related blindness. ARMD primarily affects the central vision with the peripheral vision being preserved. As it progresses, the size of the impaired central field gradually increases. A useful resource about ARMD, its treatment, and information for patients and families is the AMD alliance (http://www.amdalliance.org/en/home.html).

[1] Ophthalmia neonatorum is conjunctivitis that occurs in a newborn. Conjunctivitis is an inflammation of the surface or covering of the eye. Any eye infection that occurs in the first month of a baby's life can be classified as ophthalmia neonatorum (http://pediatrics.med.nyu.edu/conditions-we-treat/conditions/ophthalmia-neonatorum).

Additional information and resources are available from the US National Institutes of Health.[2]

Glaucoma

Glaucoma is a group of eye diseases caused by increased intraocular pressure that damages the optic nerve (Galloway et al., 2006). It is most common in individuals over 60 years old. In contrast to ARMD, the effect on vision of glaucoma is loss of the peripheral visual field, with the central visual field retained. In early stages there are treatments that can prevent further vision loss.[3] As the disease progresses, assistive technologies for low vision such as those discussed in this chapter can be helpful.

Cataracts

A cataract is a clouding of the lens of the eye that results in blurred vision (Galloway et al., 2006). The most common treatment is surgical replacement of the lens with an artificial lens. In some cases assistive technologies for low vision are useful if there is vision loss from cataracts or cataract surgery.[4]

Diabetic Eye Disease

Individuals who have diabetes are also more likely to have eye diseases that can cause severe vision loss (Galloway et al., 2006). Diabetic-related eye disease may include diabetic retinopathy, cataract, and glaucoma. Cataracts develop earlier in people who have diabetes, and a person with diabetes is nearly twice as likely to get glaucoma. Diabetic retinopathy is the most common type of eye disease that accompanies diabetes and is a leading cause of blindness.[5] It is caused by changes in the blood vessels of the eye that affect the blood supply to the retina. The result is loss of parts of the visual field seen as black areas at random points.

ASSISTIVE TECHNOLOGIES FOR VISION

Chapters 1 and 3 describe the human component of the human activity assistive technology (HAAT) model in some detail. Two primary intrinsic enablers of the human in this model are sensing and perception. If there are impairments in either of these functions, it is necessary to use sensory aids. When sensory aids are designed or applied, the level of impairment becomes a critical issue. If there is sufficient residual function in the primary sensory system being aided, the input is augmented to make it useful to the person. For example, eyeglasses magnify (augment) the level of visual information. On the other hand, if there is insufficient residual sensory capability, then the sensory aid must use an alternative sensory pathway. For example, braille (tactile pathway) can be used for reading when vision is not functional. We describe both augmentation and replacement for visual information in this section.

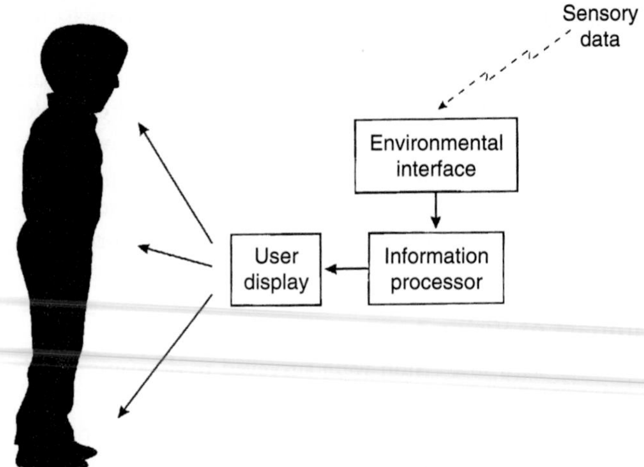

FIGURE 13-1 The major components of all sensory aids.

Fundamental Approaches to Sensory Aids

Figure 13-1 shows the major components of a sensory aid based on the parts of the assistive technology component of the HAAT model. The *environmental interface* detects the sensory data that the human cannot obtain through his or her own sensory system. This is typically a camera for visual data, a microphone for auditory data, and pressure sensors for tactile data. The environmental interface signal is fed to an information processor, the function of which depends on the type of aid. For sensory aids that use the same sensory pathway, the information processor primarily amplifies the signal. Examples include closed-circuit television (CCTV) for visual input and hearing aids for auditory input. In other cases, the information processor may be more complicated. For example, in an auditory substitution reading device, the information processor may take visual information from the sensor, convert it to speech, and then send it to the user as auditory information. In the case of the sensory aid, the human/technology interface is a **user display**, which portrays the sensory information for the human user. The processed information is presented to the user so that the alternative pathway can process it. For the visual pathway this is a visible display (e.g., a video monitor), for the auditory pathway it is an audio display (e.g., a speaker), and for the tactile pathway it is a vibrating pin or electrode array through which pressure or touch data are provided to the user.

Augmentation of an Existing Pathway

For someone who has low vision, the primary pathway (i.e., the one normally used for input) is still available; it is just limited. The limitation may be one of several types. The most common type of limitation is one of *intensity*. For visual information, this limitation means that the size of the input signal is too small to be seen. Eyeglasses are the most common type of aid used for this problem, but other ways can be

[2] http://www.nei.nih.gov/health/maculardegen/armd_facts.asp#1a.
[3] http://www.nei.nih.gov/health/glaucoma/glaucoma_facts.asp.
[4] http://www.nei.nih.gov/health/cataract/cataract_facts.asp.
[5] http://www.nei.nih.gov/health/diabetic/retinopathy.asp..

used to magnify the signal. The second type of impairment is referred to as a *frequency* or *wavelength* limitation. For visual input, this is manifest in inadequacy in discerning colors or the contrast between foreground and background, and this problem can be addressed with filters or by varying contrast (e.g., black on white rather than white on black). Finally, there are *field* limitations. The most common approach to problems of this type is to use lenses that are designed to widen the field.

Use of an Alternative Sensory Pathway

When a sensory input modality is so impaired that there can be no useful input of information through that channel, we must substitute an **alternative sensory system**. The use of braille for reading by persons who are blind is an example of tactile substitution for visual input. Tactile and auditory systems replace the visual system, and visual and tactile systems substitute for auditory input of information. Visual and tactile substitutions for auditory information are discussed in Chapter 14. When this type of substitution is made, the assistive technology practitioner (ATP) must be aware of fundamental differences among the tactile, visual, and auditory systems.

Tactile Substitution

The tactile system has been used as the basis for many visual substitution systems. Visual information is spatially organized (Nye & Bliss, 1970). This means that visual information is represented in the central nervous system by the relationship of objects to each other in space; that is, the left, right, up, down, far, and near features of objects are preserved. In contrast, the auditory system is temporally organized (Kirman, 1973). This means that it is the time relationships in auditory signals that provide information. For example, it is the temporal sequence of sounds in speech that the auditory system uses to form words and derive meaning. Finally, tactile information is both temporally and spatially organized (Kirman, 1973), and sensory input from the tactile system requires both spatial and temporal cues. For example, the fingers are capable of distinguishing fine features such as those found on coins. However, to distinguish one denomination of coin from another, it is necessary to manipulate them in the hand. This movement of the coins provides temporal (time sequence) information that helps clarify the spatial information, and it is very difficult to distinguish two denominations of coins merely by placing a hand on top of them without movement. This combination of movement and texture is referred to as *spatiotemporal information*. The combination of tactile and kinesthetic or proprioceptive information is called the *haptic sensory system*.

Kirman (1973) presents an example that illustrates the differences between visual and tactile information for reading. Print on a page is organized spatially. People read by using saccadic eye movements, which jump from one group of letters to another. With each new point of focus, new information is taken in. This allows the visual system (including the eyes, peripheral pathways, and central nervous system components) to use its spatial feature extraction to recognize shapes as letters, to assemble them into words, and to associate meaning with them. In contrast, a person reading with braille moves his or her hand across the line of raised dots, obtaining both spatial (the organization of the six braille cells) and temporal (the moving pattern under the finger) information. If the sighted person were to use the method used with braille, the text would constantly move before the eyes, and this would result in a blurred image because the spatial information would be constantly changing. Thus we can say that the movement (temporal aspect) interferes with the visual input of information. On the other hand, if the braille user were to use the approach used by the sighted reader he or she would place a finger on a character, input the information, and then jump to the next character. This would severely limit the input of braille information because the movement required by the tactile system would be absent. Thus the visual and tactile methods of sensory input are very different, which must be taken into account when one system is substituted for the other.

When vision is used for mobility rather than reading, there are some differences. In this case the visual image is constantly changing as the individual walks. The eyes scan the environment, and information is derived from the spatial arrangement of objects and people and from changes in the person's position relative to these objects as he or she moves. The visual system (including oculomotor components) functions to stabilize images on the retina for input of data, even during movement. This maximizes input of changing spatial information. Ways in which persons with visual impairments use other senses and assistive devices for mobility are discussed in the section on mobility later in this chapter.

Auditory Substitution

The auditory system has been used to substitute for visual information in several ways. Some of these have been more successful than others, and the reasons for success or failure illustrate the challenges of substituting one sense for another. The least successful approaches have been those that converted a visual image of letters into a set of tones. One such device was the Stereotoner (Smith, 1972). The environmental interface for this device was a camera consisting of a set of horizontal slits. As the camera passed over a letter, a black area (i.e., a part of a letter) resulted in a tone being produced and a white area (no letter) resulted in silence. As the camera moved over a letter, a series of tones was heard as changing musical chords. Although some individuals were able to use this information at a reading rate of 40 words per minute, the device was generally unsuccessful. Cook (1982) cites several reasons for this. First, the device required the user to recognize a chord pattern, then assemble that into a letter, and then to put the letters together into a word that was meaningful in the context of the whole sentence. This is a difficult and unnatural process for the auditory system. Second, the necessity to read letter by letter using this approach resulted in a slow input speed and placed additional memory requirements on the user. Finally, the Stereotoner was tiring to the user because of the intense concentration required. The major lesson to be learned from this example is that the auditory system is ideally suited to the receipt of language information in certain forms (e.g., speech), but it is poorly suited to complex signals that represent spatial patterns, as in the case of the Stereotoner. This is the primary reason that reading devices using auditory substitution all use speech as the mode of presentation of information.

Devices for visual mobility have used auditory substitution with greater success. This is because mobility depends much more on gross cues than on precise spatial information as in reading. In mobility, the problem becomes one of identifying large objects as potential hazards.

Reading Aids for Persons with Visual Impairments

The major problems faced by persons with visual impairments are (1) access to printed reading material, (2) orientation and mobility (i.e., moving about safely and easily), and (3) access to computers, mobile phones, and tablets, including the **Internet.** This section first describes reading aids for people with low vision who still obtain information through the visual system. Then tactile and auditory alternatives for people who are blind are discussed. The term *reading* is used here to include access to text, mathematics, and graphical representations (e.g., maps, pictures, drawings, and handwriting). As discussed later, some types of reading have very specialized alternatives (e.g., talking compasses in lieu of maps, talking bar code readers for medicines and food cans).

Magnification Aids

There are three factors related to visual system performance for reading: size, spacing, and contrast. This section discusses the principles of low-vision aids for reading print material. These devices are generally referred to as **magnification aids.** Magnification may be vertical (size) or horizontal (spacing) or both. *Magnification* also includes assistive technologies that enhance contrast. There are three categories of magnification aids: (1) optical aids, (2) nonoptical aids, and (3) electronic aids (Servais, 1985). Examples of these are listed in Box 13-1.

BOX 13-1 Categories and Examples of Low-Vision Aids

Optical Aids
Handheld magnifiers
Stand magnifiers
Field expanders
Telescopes

Nonoptical Aids
Enlarged print
High-intensity lamps
Daily living aids
High-contrast objects

Electronic Aids
CCTVs
Portable CCTVs
Slide projectors
Opaque projectors
Microfiche readers

Data from Servais SP: Visual aids. In Webster JG et al, editors: *Electronic devices for rehabilitation,* New York: John Wiley, 1985.

Assistive technologies can also be used to enhance visual cues for children who have low vision (Griffin et al., 2002). Color and contrast can be enhanced by using hues (the named color, red, blue, etc.), lightness (perceived intensity), and saturation (perceived differences in color). Deficits in color vision may be difficult to detect in children. Griffin et al. provide the following guidelines for use in visual magnifiers, software, or Website design for children with low vision: (1) use colors that differ as little as possible in lightness, (2) avoid colors from the ends of the spectrum, (3) avoid white or gray with any color of the same lightness, (4) avoid colors adjacent to each other in the color spectrum, and (5) avoid use of pastel colors. Spatial considerations are another issue in enhancing visual access for children with low vision (Griffin et al., 2002). Space includes size, patterns, outlines, and clarity of text and pictures. Optical magnifiers, software programs, and Websites can address these features.

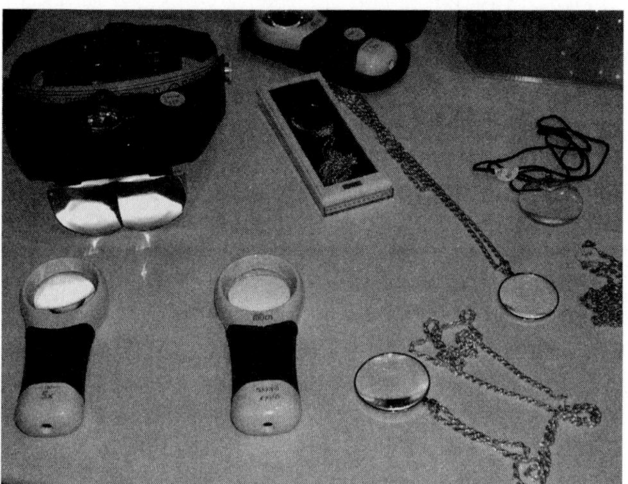

FIGURE 13-2 A selection of optical aids for low vision.

Optical Aids

More than 90% of all individuals who have visual impairments have some usable vision (Doherty, 1993). Thus it is important to carefully choose low-vision devices to meet their needs. With the use of **optical aids,** individuals with low vision may be able to see print, do work requiring fine detail, or increase the range of their visual fields. Optical aids directly affect the image that is presented to the eye.

The simplest of optical aids is the handheld magnifier. Among the advantages of these devices is that they require little training, they are lightweight and small (can fit in a pocket or purse), and they are inexpensive. Some also have a built-in light to increase contrast, and others have several lenses, which can be used alone or in combination, depending on the application. A selection of optical aids is shown in Figure 13-2. Sometimes it is difficult to hold a lens and carry out a task (e.g., a two-handed task such as embroidery).

In other cases it may be difficult to hold a magnifier steady (e.g., for someone who is elderly or in poor health). In these situations, stand magnifiers, some of which have a built-in light, are useful. Some magnifiers are mounted on eyeglass frames to free both hands.

One approach to limitations of visual field is the use of field expanders. These are generally prisms or special lenses built in to eyeglass frames. When magnifying lenses are used, the expansion of the field reduces the size of the image and a tradeoff occurs. This effect can be seen on some automotive side mirrors that give an expanded field, but reduce the size of objects in that field. It is also the same effect observed when viewing a map on the computer screen. As you zoom out the field is expanded, but the image has less detail. The image is not reduced in size when prism lenses are used to expand the field.

Telescopes assist with distance vision. These may be either worn on the head or held in the hand, and they may be monocular or binocular (Mellor, 1981). They may be used, for example, by students who need to see a chalkboard or an adult who needs to monitor children playing outdoors. Telescopic aids provide an enlarged but narrowed visual field. Head-mounted units may be attached to eyeglass frames or have a separate frame. Head-mounted devices are particularly useful when long periods of wear are necessary, such as when watching television.

CASE STUDY 8-1

Living with Glaucoma

Karen is a 68-year-old woman with glaucoma. Her central vision is intact, but she is losing her peripheral vision. She has spent most of her time lately playing bridge, quilting, and reading. She would like to continue these activities as long as possible. What types of optical aids might help her continue with her recreational activities?

Nonoptical Aids

This approach to magnification is based on changes in the actual material that is to be read (Servais, 1985). Common examples are large-print books or other materials such as menus, programs, and newspapers. High-intensity lamps can significantly increase contrast of reading materials, and high-contrast objects in the environment can aid in localization. For example, brightly colored furniture or dishes can help with visualization. A glass that stands out from a countertop is easier to find and fill with liquid. As Servais (1985) points out, nonoptical aids can be very useful under the right circumstances, but they are limited in application because they are specialized to one or a few tasks.

Electronic Aids

Optical approaches to magnification use fixed lenses and this limits the amount of magnification and contrast enhancement that can be obtained. Electronic low-vision aids are called **video magnifiers.** These devices were originally based on **closed-circuit television** (CCTV) systems and this terminology is still used by some manufacturers. There are two primary advantages of CCTV devices: (1) the amount of magnification can be much more than for optical aids, and (2) the image can be manipulated and controlled. This is the principle used in the zoom feature on digital cameras. For example, contrast can be dramatically affected by the use of color or reversed images (e.g., white type on black background). Most current video magnifiers are based on computers, so many of the common features of word processors such as searching a document or other text manipulation can be incorporated into the video magnifier. Image contrast can be dramatically affected by the use of color or reversed images (e.g., white type on black background).

The major components of a video magnifier are a camera (environmental interface), a video display (user display), and a unit that controls the presentation of the image (information processor). Commercial devices are available with flat panel video displays. The material to be read is placed on a scanning table that easily moves both left to right and forward and back to image different portions of the page or other objects being viewed (e.g., a prescription bottle, recipe, photo of a grandchild). The scanning table can also be locked once the desired portion of the image is magnified. There may be mechanical notches that help align the material, and some devices have adjustable margins.

When the text is enlarged, the relative position of the material on the page is lost, and a spotlight of high intensity is sometimes used to show the user which part of the page is being imaged. With use of a split video screen, video magnifiers can be operated in conjunction with enlarged computer displays to allow magnification of both computer data and the video image of standard print material. Other contexts in which video magnifiers are used are to complete job-related tasks, to access educational materials at all levels, and for recreational reading or hobbies such as sewing or painting.

CASE STUDY 8-2

Managing ARMD

Marco is 65 and recently retired. He has ARMD and is loosing his central vision. He wants to be as independent as possible in his daily life. This includes taking care of his own finances (including reading bills, writing checks, managing the family budget) and doing minor maintenance on the family car (his wife now does the driving, but he still wants to check the oil level, measure the tire air pressure, etc.) as he has always done. He has asked you for suggestions of assistive devices that might be helpful for him. What would you tell him? Consider all of the low-vision aids discussed in this chapter.

An example of a video magnifier in use is shown in Figure 13-3. There is, however, a relatively wide range of features available in specific devices. The two broad categories of video magnifiers are desktop and portable. Size and spacing are controlled primarily by two factors in desktop units: (1) size of the video monitor and (2) amount of enlargement provided by the electronics. Typical video monitors range in size from 17 to 25 inches, and maximal electronic magnification ranges from 45 to more than 80 times. There is a major tradeoff between monitor size and overall space

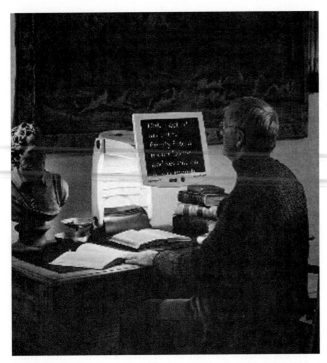

FIGURE 13-3 A video magnifier in use. (Courtesy NanoPac, Tulsa, Okla.)

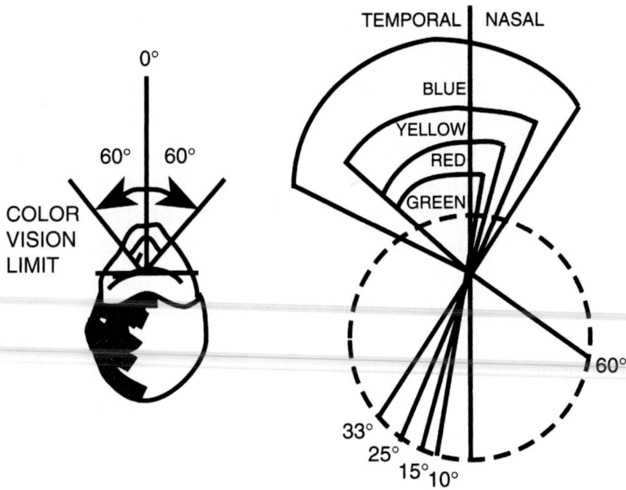

FIGURE 13-4 Color response of the eye differs with visual angle. (Modified from Woodson W and Conover D: *Human engineering guide for equipment designers*, Berkely, Ca.: University of California Press, 1964.)

required for the unit. Space requirements are often a significant limitation if a computer terminal, printer, and other office equipment must share space with the video magnifier. A split-screen system that allows access not only to printed material but also to the computer video screen overcomes this space problem to a large degree. One such product is Topaz,[6] which allows the screen to be split into two. One half is used for video magnifier display of printed material and the other is used for enlarged computer output. This system also functions as either a computer screen magnifier only or video magnifier only. Other manufacturers have similar products. Most video magnifiers have simple controls for magnification (generally a rotating dial), contrast, and brightness. The controls are located directly under the video display for convenient access.

A major challenge for people using video magnifiers is navigation around the text because it is often so enlarged that only a portion of a line or two of text is visible. This situation can result in missed words or difficulty in finding the beginning of the next line. One approach is to create a digital image of the page and then let the computer-based magnifier automatically scroll through the text.[7] Automatic reading can be one long row that scrolls across the screen, a column of text wide enough that it all appears on the screen at once or one word at a time with the user controlling the rate at which each word is displayed. Scrolling rate, magnification, and cursor movement around the text field are all adjustable and controllable by the user.

Contrast enhancement is provided either by gray scale or color. In the former approach, the foreground and background contrast is adjustable and may be reversed (e.g., black letters on white or white letters on black). Color adds significant contrast enhancement because the user can choose alternative background and foreground colors. Not all persons with visual impairments have the same color vision, and color vision varies with visual field (see Figure 13-4). Having some control over the foreground-background color combination allows the display to be customized to the needs of an individual user. Some commercial video magnifiers include selection of contrast from a group of 20 or more preset foreground/background color combinations. Another advantage of color displays is that the original color of the print material can be retained. Maps with colored areas can be imaged; a preprinted form that calls for a signature "on the red line" shows the line as red, and so on. The major tradeoff with color monitors is that the image may not be as sharp as the black and white image, especially at large magnifications. Most video magnifiers also have a black and white mode when a sharper image is required.

Fully portable magnifiers are designed to be carried with the user. The most significant differences between these portable units and desktop CCTVs are size, weight, and battery power. Portable units weigh as little as 1.2 pounds and measure only about 9 by 3 inches for the display and 4 by 2 inches for the camera.[8] Some portable units have a handheld camera that is moved over the page and others have folding stands that can be set up to image a page, a whiteboard in a classroom, or other objects such as a medicine bottle.

Portable magnifying devices called *portable readers* include storage of text in digital form.[9] These devices have

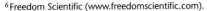

[6] Freedom Scientific (www.freedomscientific.com).

[7] myReader, Human Ware, Concord, Calif (http://www.humanware.com/en-international/home).

[8] For example, Smartview, HumanWare, Inc., Concord, Calif. (www.humanware.com); Magnilink, Vision Cue (http://www.visioncue.com).

[9] For example, Intel Reader (www.intel.com/healthcare/reader/about.htm); KNFB Reader (http://www.knfbreader.com/products-mobile.php).

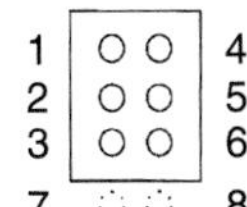

Standard braille cell

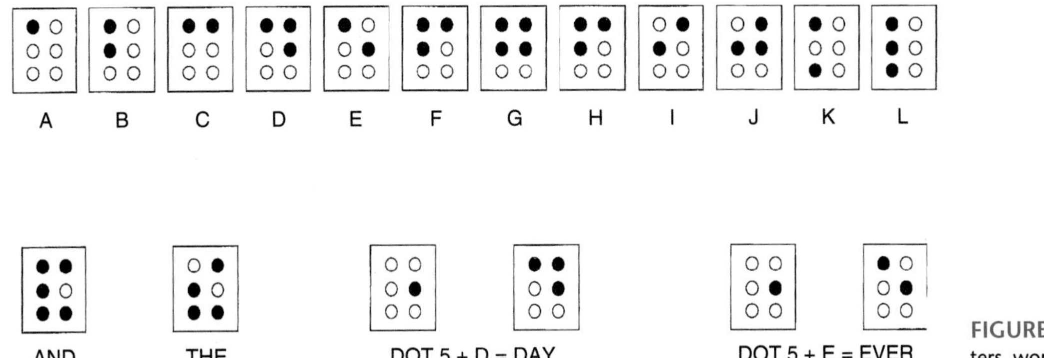

FIGURE 13-5 Examples of braille letters, word signs, and contractions.

a built-in high-resolution camera. The displayed image can be enlarged. Some portable devices are based on cell phone technology and others have a custom-designed computer and packaging. Using the built-in camera, these portable readers take a picture of text and magnify it for display on the built-in screen like other portable magnifiers (much like taking a picture with a digital camera). The image is then enlarged or converted to speech. The user can zoom in on a portion for greater magnification. Some devices also include a translation to auditory form via speech synthesis for users who are blind. Earphones provide privacy and avoid disturbing others. Stored data can be uploaded to a computer for further processing or conversion into MP3 or DAISY format.

Several portable video magnifiers connect to laptop computers for the image display.[10] Portable units consist of a camera and software to allow control over the video magnification. Maximal magnification varies from 3 to 64 times. Some units also allow the camera to be connected to a desktop video monitor or standard television set to display the video magnifier output, which allows it to be used in a portable or stationary mode, depending on the needs of the user. These cameras are extremely small (e.g., 2 inches × 2 inches × 4 inches, weighing 6 ounces). This flexibility is useful when greater magnification is needed for certain material (e.g., fine print) or at certain times (e.g., at the end of the day, when fatigue is greater), and when the user must travel to different settings during the day. Portable video magnifiers are useful for students and in business applications where travel to various locations is important.

[10] For example, Smart View Graduate, Human Ware (www.humanware.com); Pearl, Freedom Scientific (www.freedomscientific.com).

Braille as a Tactile Reading Substitute

The most widely used tactile substitution device for persons with visual impairments is **braille**, although only 10 to 15% of individuals who are blind can access it. Each braille character consists of a cell of either six or eight dots. Standard six-dot braille is shown in Figure 13-5. The seventh and eighth dots are used for computer access to show cursor movement or to provide single-cell presentation of features such as upper and lower case alphabet, numbers, special symbols, and control characters like ENTER. Figure 13-5 shows examples of letters and numbers. When text is directly translated into braille letter by letter, it is referred to as *Grade 1.* Also shown in Figure 13-5 are some braille codes for words (called *wordsigns*) and word endings. The use of these contractions significantly speeds up the rate of reading, and this type of braille is called *Grade 2* or *Grade 3,* depending on the number of contractions used. Reading rates with Grade 2 braille are about 104 words per minute (wpm) (Sardegna et al., 2002). Grade 1 reading rates are about 75% of Grade 2 rates (Legge et al., 1999). Grade 3 has more contractions and eliminates some vowels, and it is used primarily for taking notes (Sardegna et al., 2002). Traditionally, braille has been produced by embossing on heavy paper, and this method is still widely used. For persons who develop skill with it, braille can be a fast and efficient method for accessing print materials.

Limitations of Printed Braille

Embossed braille material is heavy and bulky, and each braille page has significantly less information than a printed page of the same size. For example, a braille version of a book would be about two and a half times bigger than a printed version (Lazzario, 2001). A second disadvantage is that the cost of producing braille in an embossed form is high compared

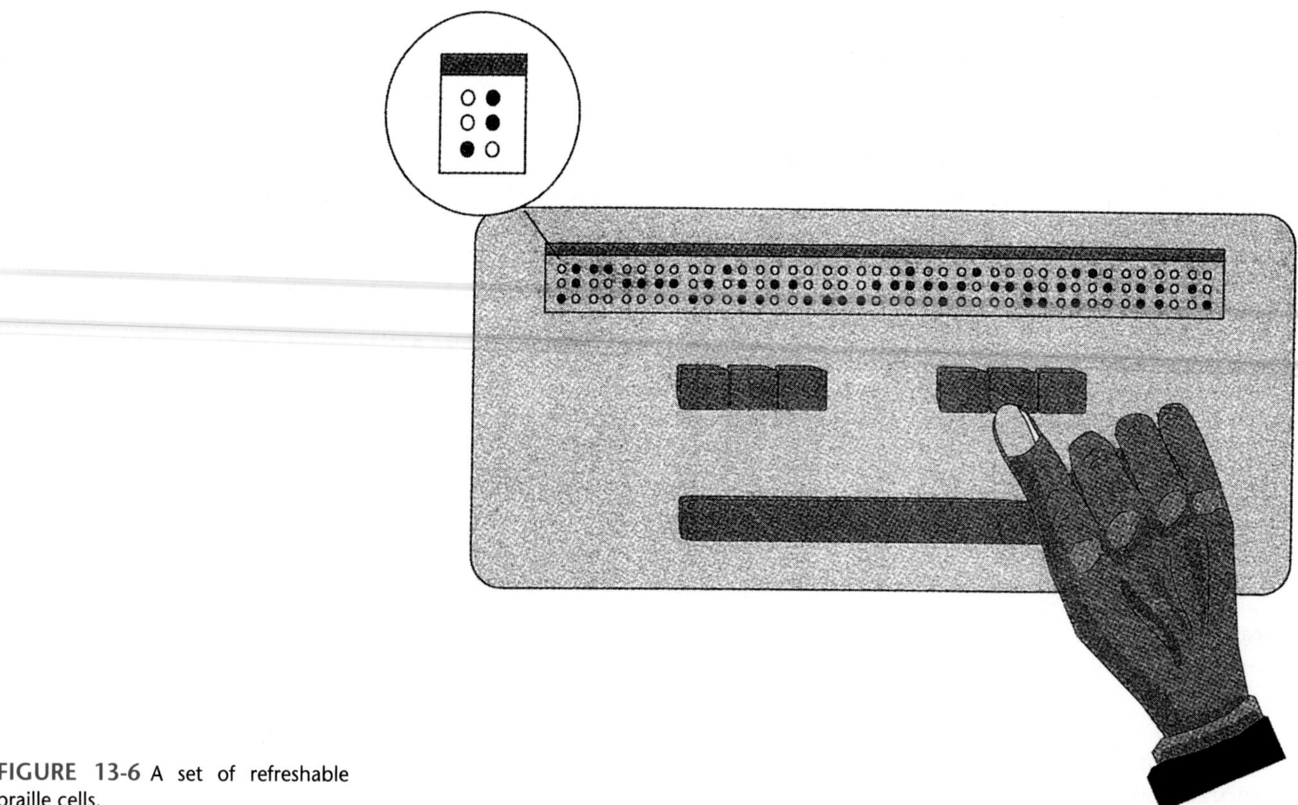

FIGURE 13-6 A set of refreshable braille cells.

with print materials. For this reason, only a fraction of the total print literature is available in embossed braille form. It is difficult to scan a braille document to find the particular piece of text as is typically done with print material. Finally, braille embossers do not allow corrections to be made.

Braille itself, regardless of format, has limitations as well. The most significant is that very few persons with severe visual impairment learn to use it. This is partially because the majority of all persons who become blind do so after age 65 years, and many of these cases are the result of diabetes, which also affects the tactile sense, making braille less desirable than other alternatives such as talking books. Despite all these disadvantages, braille is the modality of choice for many persons with severe visual impairment, and the use of a format other than embossed paper significantly enhances the effectiveness of this modality. One of the most widely used of these alternative formats is refreshable braille cells consisting of raised pins. Computer output systems use either a refreshable braille display or hard copy generated by use of braille printers.

Refreshable Braille Displays

Because braille is represented by a series of dots, raised pins can be substituted for the traditional embossed paper format. This approach, called **refreshable braille display**, is shown in Figure 13-6. There are several advantages to this format. The most significant of these is that the refreshable display is controlled by an electronic circuit that can be interfaced to computer displays or braille keyboards. This allows information to be stored electronically and greatly reduces the bulk compared with embossed braille. Second, because the text material is in electronic form, it can be edited, searches can be made, and copies of braille material can be easily produced in electronic form and saved or shared via storage media. The refreshable braille cell (or cell array) can also be used as the output mode for an automatic reading machine. Some portable reading and note taking aids, discussed later in this chapter, also use refreshable braille cells.

Each refreshable braille cell has a set of small pins arranged in the shape of a standard braille cell. The pins that correspond to the dot pattern for a letter or word sign are raised. Both Grade 1 and Grade 2 braille can be presented on refreshable displays by use of software that converts text from ASCII format to braille. Arrays of from 1 to 80 cells are available. Some braille displays also include a braille keyboard.[11]

Stationary refreshable braille displays have arrays with multiple braille cells that are connected to a computer through a USB interface. Typically the array sizes are 20, 40, or 80 cells.[12] These refreshable braille arrays can be used as an alternative to the computer video display. Many refreshable braille displays also have a wireless Bluetooth link to increase flexibility of use.

[11] For example, BrailleNote or Braille Displays Humanware, Concord, CA (www.humanware.com), Focus 40, Freedom Scientific, St. Petersburg, Fla. (http://www.freedomscientific.com/), ALVA BC640, Vision Cue, Portland, OR (http://www.visioncue.com).

[12] For example: Brailliant BI 40, Brailliant B 80 and Brailliant BI 32, Humanware, Concord, CA (www.humanware.com); Focus 40, Freedom Scientific, St. Petersburg, Fla. (http://www.freedomscientific.com/); ALVA BC640 or ALVA BC680, Vision Cue, Portland, OR (http://www.visioncue.com).

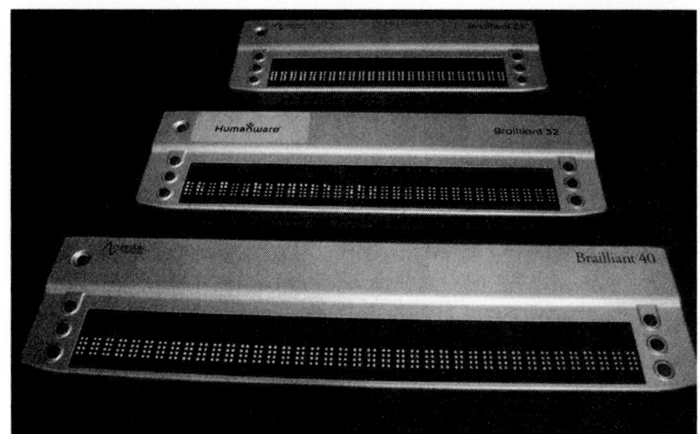

FIGURE 13-7 Refreshable braille cells are available with a variable number of cells.

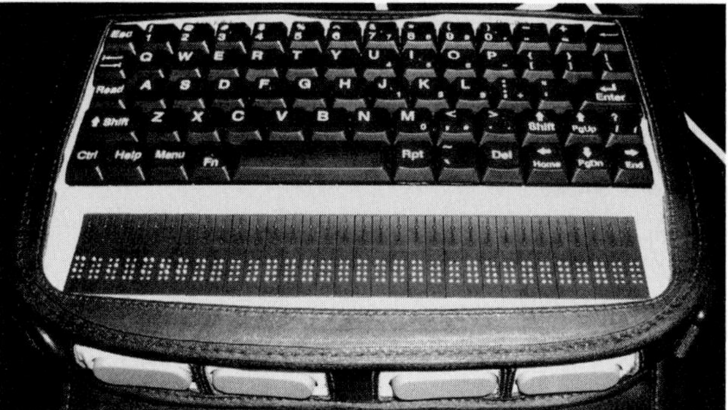

FIGURE 13-8 A personal organizer with braille display and synthesized speech output.

The ALVA[13] braille terminals provide 44-, 70-, and 80-cell refreshable displays for desktop use and 23- and 44-cell displays for portable applications (battery operated). All versions have eight-dot braille cells. All ALVA models also provide extra status cells that display the location of the system cursor, which line of text is displayed in braille, which attributes are active, and the relationship of those attributes to the characters on the screen. This information can be monitored with the left hand while the right hand reads the text on the braille display. USB and serial ports are available for data transfer. Text is provided in both Grade 1 and Grade 2 braille.

Freedom Scientific[14] makes 40- and 80-cell braille displays. The 40-cell unit includes a braille keyboard. Both the 40- and 80-cell versions have navigation features accessible through a series of buttons on the display. Combinations of buttons are used to enter commands. Another product, the PAC Mate Omni™ portable braille display, is a 20- or 40-cell refreshable braille display that functions as a portable computer. It can be connected to any computer through a USB port to synchronize email, calendars, or transfer files. This unit uses a seamless design between braille cells that makes the display feel like paper. It works with most Windows-based software packages.

Human Ware[15] makes a series of refreshable braille displays, shown in Figure 13-7. The 40-cell and 24-cell Brailliant refreshable braille displays are designed for use with a laptop or desktop computer. The Brailliant 32, 64 and 80 are eight-dot braille displays for desktop computers. All these models are configured for split-window display or as programmable status cells and all include Bluetooth and USB connectivity. The latter are accessed by clicking a sensor located above one of the braille cells to instantly move the mouse pointer or cursor to a new location for editing. Grade 2 braille translation is included on all models.

For computer users who are familiar with braille, refreshable braille cells can be more effective than screen readers. However, a combination of approaches may be most effective with braille and speech combined. If done thoughtfully and carefully, the hardware and software designed for braille can be used together with that developed for screen reading with speech synthesis. Supernova (Dolphin Computer Systems, San Mateo, Calif., www.dolphincomputeraccess.com) provides screen magnification (2 to 32 times) and speech and braille output in one package for Windows applications. There are six viewing modes: full screen, split screen, window, lens, autolens, and line view (for smooth scrolling). Speech output is available letter by letter during typing or word by word. A variety of languages and speech synthesizers can be used with Voyager. "Hooked access" allows parts of the screen, such as the current line of a word processor, to be permanently displayed. Supernova also supports graphic object labeling and provides speech output and a braille layout mode.

Portable Braille Note Takers and Personal Organizers

Many individuals who are blind use digital recording for note taking at meetings or in class. Others use portable braille note takers as stand-alone data managers or personal organizers. These units vary in size from a compact 4.5 inches square and about 1.5 inches thick to the size of a laptop computer (approximately 9 × 12 inches).[16] A typical model is pictured in Figure 13-8. Some models use a braille keyboard for input and others use a standard QWERTY keyboard. The braille keyboard has one key for each of the eight dots in a braille cell. Additional keys are used for control, editing, and data management. Synthesized speech is available in all units with either a speaker or earphone output for the synthesized speech. Some models include a refreshable Grade 2 braille display (from 8 to 32 braille cells) either alone or paired with synthetic speech. The speech synthesizer and refreshable braille display can also be used as outputs (replacing the output from the video monitor) on the unit or

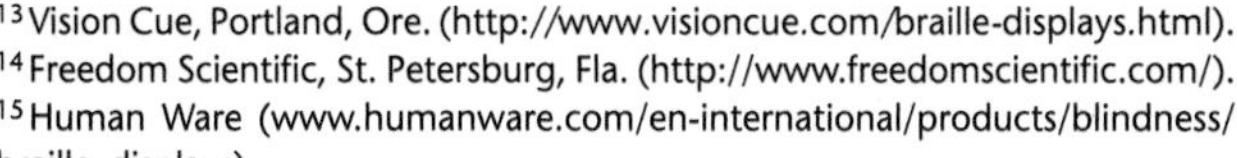

[13] Vision Cue, Portland, Ore. (http://www.visioncue.com/braille-displays.html).
[14] Freedom Scientific, St. Petersburg, Fla. (http://www.freedomscientific.com/).
[15] Human Ware (www.humanware.com/en-international/products/blindness/braille_displays).

[16] For example, the Braille Desk 2000, Braillino, Handy Tech Elektronik GmbH, Germany (www.handytech.de); Braille Note, HumanWare, Concord, Calif. (www.humanware.com); Aria, Sensory Tools, Robotron Proprietary Limited, St. Kilda, Australia (www.sensorytools.com/products.htm); PacMate, Freedom Scientific, St. Petersburg, Fla. (http://www.freedomscientific.com/).

TABLE 13-1 Audiobook Formats

Features and Functionality	Downloadable DAISY (AudioPlus)	DAISY CDs (AudioPlus)	WMA Downloadable (AudioAccess)
Requires separate purchase of specialized DAISY hardware and/or software	Yes	Yes	No
Compatible with MP3* players and Windows Media Player**	No	No	Yes
Download chapters or sections of a book	No	No	Yes
Enhanced (DAISY) navigation, bookmarking, and variable speed control	Yes	Yes	No
Requires online access	Yes	No	Yes
Compatible with iOS devices	Yes	No	No

Downloadable DAISY Books provide instant access with enhanced navigation, bookmarking, and variable speed control. Play from Microsoft® Windows® compatible computer with RFB&D enabled software or specialized DAISY players.
DAISY CDs offer enhanced navigation and play on RFB&D enabled specialized DAISY players.
Downloadable books in WMA (Windows Media Audio) play on Microsoft Windows-based computers using Windows Media Player version 10 or higher. These books can be synched to commercial MP3 players with DRM capabilities.
Courtesy Recording for the Blind and Dyslexic (www.rfbd.org).
*MP3 players must have DRM (Digital Rights Management) capabilities to play encrypted content.
**Windows Media Player 10 or higher.

in conjunction with screen reader software on a PC. Additional outputs available on selected models include computer file transfer, Internet and email access, and print. Some models also dial a telephone automatically from the data in the built-in address book.

Built-in programs vary somewhat among various note taker models. All include word processing for writing away from a computer (e.g., while sitting by the pool or riding a bus to work), editing documents developed on a PC word processor, and taking notes in class or at meetings. Other programs built into specific models, in various combinations, include a calendar, address book, calculator, timer or watch, email access, and Internet browser, all with full access through speech or braille. Storage of data is in both computer memory and flash memory cards. Direct transfer of data from a PC to a portable reader or vice versa is available using a USB port. MP3 music players and Web access via Bluetooth or Wi-Fi protocols is also available on many units. Some note takers can also be used as computer keyboards through the built-in USB port or function as cell phones. Storage and manipulation of information may be in the form of braille or print or both. Control features may be via additional keys with specific functions or via a speech output menu of choices.

CASE STUDY 13-3

Braille Note Taking in School

Jenny is an eighth-grade student. She uses many pieces of technology to assist her in being successful at school. She has been using a Braille 'n Speak since the fifth grade to take class notes, complete assignments, take tests, keep an assignment notebook, and maintain a personal phone and address book. Review the features of this device (http://www.freedomscientific.com/) and list those that are likely to benefit Jenny in each of these applications.

Speech as an Auditory Reading Substitute

Because reading is based on visual language, it is logical that auditory substitution for reading also uses language—that is, speech. Audio technology is the primary method for information storage and retrieval used by individuals who are blind (Scadden, 1997). All the approaches discussed in this section have speech as the output mode. Synthetic speech for reading systems designed for the blind is available in a variety of languages using the approaches described in Chapter 6.

Recorded Audio Material

The oldest and still the most prevalent use of auditory substitution for persons with visual impairment is recorded material. Current technology used in recorded audio material is CDs and digital recording (e.g., MP3 device format and downloadable files).[17] There are still sites that provide books on cassette tapes, for those who do not have access to digital media. Special machines are needed for high-speed cassette playback. These are available from some libraries, including the National Library Service for the Blind (NLS).[18] The variable speed allows the listener to review material more quickly than it was originally spoken. With practice, it is possible to understand speech up to four times as fast as normal speaking rates. Some people use digital recording and playback to record lectures and then review the material in lieu of note taking. The common current digital formats are shown in Table 13-1 (Courtesy Recording for the Blind and Dyslexic).

The use of CDs allows a great deal of information to be placed on a single disk. One CD-ROM can store a large amount of data, and reproduction costs are low. The major advantages of CDs are greatly increased fidelity resulting from greater frequency response and indexing, which can be used to find a particular track. The use of digitized

[17] For example, Recording for the Blind and Dyslexic (www.rfbd.org); National Library Service for the Blind and Physically Handicapped, Library of Congress (http://www.loc.gov/nls/index.html). Recording and Playback Devices at National Federation of the Blind (https://nfb.org//).
[18] http://www.loc.gov/nls/index.

audio information allows voice recordings to be mixed with headings that allow easier searching of the text. Multimedia presentations are also commonplace with digitized audio information, allowing both visual and auditory presentation of information and thereby increasing the potential market and reducing price.

Audio displays are also being used for the presentation of mathematical information by computers and speech synthesizers and as a substitute for data presentation (e.g., tables, charts) (Scadden, 1997). In this form a book can be loaded into a PC word processor (either Windows or Apple OS based) and displayed on the screen. Because the CD-ROM is basically a storage medium for the computer, sophisticated search strategies can be used to find a particular item or place in the text. For persons with low vision or blindness, the availability of CD-ROM–based reading materials opens up many options for obtaining access to print materials. For example, with an enlarged screen output, reading material on a CD-ROM can be accessed and presented to a person with low vision by use of a computer. More significant, however, is the use of either braille or speech output from the computer to allow individuals who are blind to read from the CD-ROM.

One of the challenges in any electronic format is standardization. Different countries have different recording formats for talking books on tape, and there are many formats for word processors in digital form. For this reason an international group, the DAISY Consortium (www.daisy.org) has developed an international standard for **digital talking books** (Kerscher & Hansson, 1998). This standard includes production, exchange, and use of digital talking books. The goal of the DAISY Consortium is to promote the use of digital books that comply with an international standard. The members of the consortium are associations and organizations across the world that are involved in the provision of reading materials for individuals who are blind. The DAISY standard is hardware platform and operating system independent, and it makes use of the Web accessibility standards developed by the World Wide Web Consortium (W3C). There are several online sources for books in the Daisy format.[19] Many of the books are available in both Daisy and BRF Grade-II braille format for printing books or using refreshable braille displays. These sites have thousands of titles, including books for children and adults, textbooks, and newspapers. Many of the books are available in both DAISY and Braille Reading Foundation Grade II braille format for printing books or using refreshable braille displays. Players for Daisy format CDs are available from several manufacturers.[20] A typical DAISY format reader is shown in Figure 13-9.

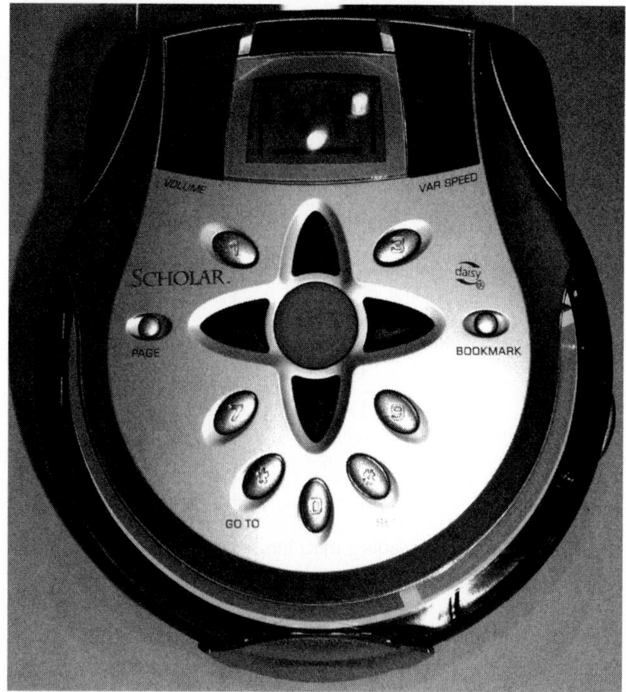

FIGURE 13-9 Typical DAISY reader.

Devices That Provide Automatic Reading of Text

Automatic reading of text requires the three components shown in Figure 13-1: an environmental interface, an information processor, and a user display. The environmental interface is a camera that provides an image of the printed page, and the user display can be either tactile (braille) or speech synthesis. A block diagram showing the major components of an automatic reading machine is presented in Figure 13-10.[21] Device operation involves scanning, **optical character recognition** (OCR), and the translation of recognized characters and either text-to-braille or text-to-speech conversion Most reading machines provide speech output, and some provide braille or both braille and speech. Synthetic speech for automatic reading systems is available in a variety of languages. Some automatic reading devices utilize standard computers with special software for information processing and output to a refreshable braille display or speech synthesis program.[22]

Stand-alone automatic reading machines include scanners in the basic system and offer simple one-button operation to scan a document and have it read. These units also provide manual access to features such as cursor keys to move around in the text, storing and retrieving files, and transferring the text to a computer or a disk. Automatic reading systems can also be used in conjunction with screen readers and web browsers.

[19] For example, Benetech (www.bookshare.org), National Library Service for the Blind and Physically Handicapped, US Library of Congress (www.loc.gov/nls), Recording for the Blind and Dyslexic is now LearningAlly (https://www.learningally.org/); Dolphin Audio Publishing http://www.yourdolphin.com/.

[20] For example, FSReader, Freedom Scientific, St. Petersburg, Fla. (http://www.freedomscientific.com/); EasyReader, Dolphin Computer Access (http://www.yourdolphin.com/index.asp); Victor Reader, Human Ware, Concord, Calif. (http://www.humanware.com/en-international/products/blindness/dtb_players).

[21] For example ScannaR Compact, Humanware (www.humanware.com/).

[22] For example Open Book, Freedom Scientific (www.freedomscientific.com/).

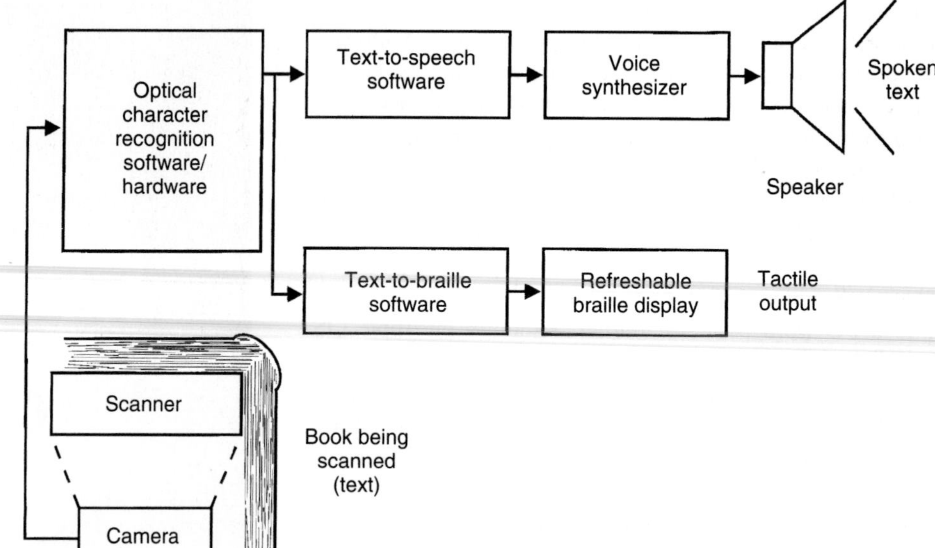

FIGURE 13-10 The major components of an automatic reading machine for persons with total visual impairment.

Some desktop reading systems have scanners built into them.[23] These systems include a flatbed scanner, built-in computer, voice output, and hard drive with room for up to 500,000 pages of text. In some cases DAISY reading capability for digital books (see above) is included. Scanned documents can be saved in MPS, WAV, DAISY, or plain text format. Many of these systems require only a single button to be pressed to scan and read a document. Some units also provide multiple languages for spoken output.[24] Other reading systems are software products that include optical character recognition and text-to-speech synthesis and are designed to use external commercial scanners and computers.[25] Some systems are fully portable, such as the ReadDesk[26] scanning, reading, and magnifying device that weighs just 1.5 lb and folds into a laptop bag.

Camera and Scanner Characteristics for Automatic Reading

To input the information into the machine, reading devices may use a flatbed scanner, a handheld scanner, or a combination of the two. Flatbed scanners have a glass plate 18 to 24 inches long and 10 to 14 inches wide. Scanners are usually defined as letter or legal size depending on the dimensions of the flat bed. This type of scanner, also called a *desktop scanner*, resembles a photocopy machine; however, the thickness is only about 3 to 4 inches. The material to be read is placed on the surface of the glass, and one advantage of this type of unit is that it can scan almost any kind of document, from a single sheet to a bound magazine or book. An automatic document feeder attachment can also be added to many flatbed scanners. This allows multiple sheets to be loaded and scanned. Scanners are widely used for home or business applications such as scanning photographs for use on Webpages or scanning documents for editing when an electronic copy is not available. For this reason, the technology is improving and the prices are falling as a result of the general market demand (Grotta & Grotta, 1998). This has resulted in advances that benefit blind users of automatic reading systems. For scanners narrower than the page, the camera must be moved across a line of text and then moved down to the next line, and so on all the way down the page. This can be difficult for a person who is blind because there is no frame of reference to keep the scanner on one line or to move just one line down. Flatbed scanners overcome this problem. The handheld scanner can image most types of material, including single sheets and bound documents. An additional advantage is that it can be used with a laptop computer to create a portable reading machine.

Optical Character Recognition

The camera and scanner provide an image, consisting of an array of dots (called pixels) in black and white or color dots. Optical character recognition software is used to translate the image into speech or braille. The primary function of the OCR is to analyze the raw pixel data and assemble it into letters, spaces (to delineate words), and punctuation. Graphics (pictures or drawings and the elaborate characters sometimes used to begin chapters in books) must be

---

[23] For example, Ovation, Telesensory, Sunnyvale Calif. (http://www.telesensory.com/product.aspx?category=4&id=6); Sara, Freedom Scientific, St. Petersburg, Fla. (http://www.freedomscientific.com/); PlusTech Book Reader V100 (www.plustek.com); POET-Compact 2, Baum (www.baum.de/index-e.php); ScannaR Compact 2, HumanWare, Concord, Calif. (www.humanware.com); Sophie, Handy Tech Elektronik GmbH (https://www.handytech.de/downloads/pdfs/29_pdf_en_SOB_ENG_V24.pdf).

[26] Read Desk, Issist, Georgetown, Canada (http://pediatrics.med.nyu.edu/conditions-we-treat/conditions/ophthalmia-neonatorum).

[24] For example, Open Book, Freedom Scientific (www.freedomscientific.com/), SARA CE (http://www.freedomscientific.com/products/lv/SARACE-product-page.asp); CleaReader (http://uk.optelec.com/); Poet BE (http://pamtrad.co.uk/); ExtremeReader (http://www.guerillatechnologies.com/index.html).

[25] For example, Open Book, Freedom Scientific, St. Petersburg, Fla. (http://www.freedomscientific.com/products/fs/openbook-product-page.asp); Cicero, Dolphin Products (www.dolphincomputeraccess.com).

[26] Read Desk, Issist, Georgetown, Canada (http://pediatrics.med.nyu.edu/conditions-we-treat/conditions/ophthalmia-neonatorum).

removed from the text. There are a number of problems that OCR software must solve. The most significant of these is that letter recognition must occur with different print fonts. OCRs that accomplish this are called *omni-font OCRs*. Most scanners have an OCR product bundled with the scanner. These OCRs provide basic OCR capabilities, but they do not match stand-alone OCR products. Automatic reading systems use the professional stand-alone OCR products to achieve the best possible results. Some companies that provide automatic reading systems have their own proprietary OCR software, and others use professional-quality OCR software developed for business applications. The majority of the commercial software incorporated into automatic reading systems uses either the Xerox or Caere OCR software. Most current scanners use OmniPage LE (Nuance Corp., Burlington, Mass., www.nuance.com), TextBridge (Nuance Corp.) Classic, or proprietary OCR software. All OCR software available separately is compatible with the Windows operating system, and several automatic reading systems use standard PCs, OCR software, and an external scanner.

Making Mainstream Technologies Accessible for Individuals Who Have Low Vision or Are Blind

Access to computers is essential for business, home, education, and recreation. Desktop and notebook computers have built-in accessibility features that enhance access for individuals who have visual impairments. Third-party products expand the options for computer use. Increases in the power of mobile technologies (phones and tablets) provide significant opportunities for people with disabilities, especially those with low vision or blindness. It is possible for a user to store customized programs on the network (e.g., in cloud servers) and download them as needed from any remote location.

Principles of Mainstream Adaptations for Visual Impairments

ICT (Information and communication technology, e.g., computer, smart phone, and tablet) interaction is bidirectional, and it is important to understand how ICT outputs can be adapted for persons with sensory impairments. ICT user output is generally provided by a visual display, and the input choices (keyboard or icons) are presented visually as well. This type of display is also referred to as *soft copy*. Output from a printer is referred to as *hard* copy. ICTs also provide auditory outputs of sound, music, or synthetic speech. These outputs are important to individuals who have visual impairments. Standard visual ICT outputs are often not suitable for use by persons who have vision impairments.

Graphical User Interface

The most commonly used method for inputting information into a computer and many other mainstream technologies such as smart phones and tablets is through a **graphical user interface** (GUI). The GUI has three distinguishing features: (1) a mouse pointer, which is moved around the screen, (2) a graphical menu bar, which appears on the screen, and (3) one or more windows, which provide a menu of choices (Hayes, 1990). Movement of the mouse or a mouse equivalent (e.g., keystrokes, trackball, head pointer, or joystick, touch screen) causes the pointer to move around the screen. Two primary characteristics of GUIs are particularly important in assistive technology applications: (1) the use of graphical menus and icons to which the user can point and click or tap for input instead of using the keyboard and (2) multitasking capabilities, which allow more than one program to be loaded and run simultaneously. The creation of a graphical environment can save typing, reduce effort, and increase accuracy. Since they depend on recognition memory rather than recall, icons generally aid users with memory problems. The GUI allows the use of windows, which partition the screen into smaller screens, each showing a particular application. When an application or function is opened or run by clicking or tapping, a feature (e.g., a calculator) or application (e.g., a word processor) is displayed in a window. Several windows may be open at the same time. Figure 13-11 shows multiple windows open and examples of menus and dialog boxes used for manipulating data and information. Specific implementations of GUIs have slightly different modes of operation, but the basic principles are similar to those described here.

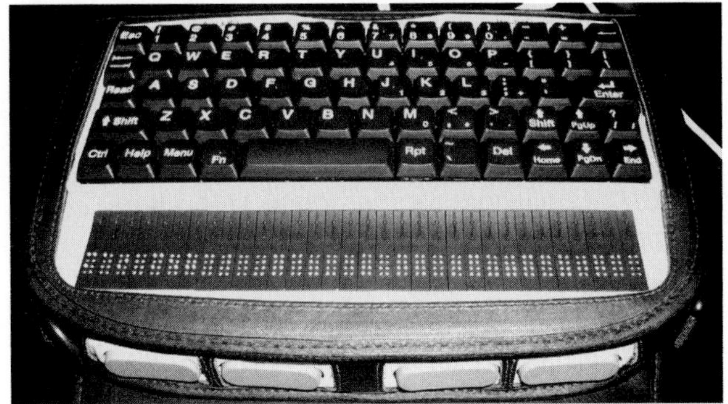

FIGURE 13-11 An example of a graphical user interface with several windows open for different applications. (Courtesy of Microsoft).

The GUI has both positive and negative implications for persons with disabilities. The positive features are those that apply to nondisabled users. The major limitation of GUI use in assistive technology is that the user may not have the necessary physical (eye–hand coordination) and visual skills. In addition, adaptation for alternative input or output devices is often difficult, and adaptations must be redone when changes are made to the basic operating system. The GUI is the standard user interface because of its ease of operation for novices and its consistency of operation for experts. The latter ensures that every application behaves in basically the same way (e.g., screen icons for the same task look the same, operations such as opening and closing files are always the same). Another feature of the GUI is that it provides a specific, consistent layout of controls on the screen. This aids the user (especially a novice) in accessing programs because everything is consistent from one application program to another and within an application.

The GUI: Challenges for Individuals with Visual Impairments

The GUI presents unique and difficult problems to the blind user because of an approach to video display that creates many more options for the portrayal of graphical information than just text. Many different graphical symbols can be created. These symbols are useful to sighted computer users because they can rely on "visual metaphors" (e.g., a trash can to represent deleted files) (Boyd, Boyd, & Vanderheiden, 1990). The graphical labels used to portray these functions are referred to as *icons*. The GUI presents several problems to the blind user. First, the graphical characters are not easily portrayed in alternative modes. Text-to-speech programs and speech synthesizers are designed to convert text to speech output (see Chapter 6). However, they are not well suited to the representation of graphics, including the icons used in GUIs. Most icons used in GUIs have text labels with them, and one approach to adaptation is to intercept the label and send it to a text-to-speech voice synthesizer system. The label is then spoken when the icon is selected.

Another major problem presented to blind users by GUIs is that screen location, important in using a GUI, is not easily conveyed by alternative means. Visual information is spatially organized, and auditory information (including speech) is temporal (time based). It is difficult to convey the screen location of a pointer by speech alone. It is difficult to portray two-dimensional spatial attributes with speech. An exception to this is a screen location that never changes. For example, some screen readers use speech to indicate the edges of the screen (e.g., right border, top of screen). One approach that is used frequently is to step through the icons one at a time speaking the name of each.

For mouse use, a significant problem is that the mouse pointer location on the screen is relative, rather than referenced to an absolute standard location. This means that the only information available to the computer is how far the mouse has moved and the direction of the movement. If there is no visual information available to the user, it is difficult to know where the mouse is pointing.

Other challenges presented to the visually impaired user of a GUI include the organization of the screen with elements spatially clustered visually; multitasking in which several windows are open simultaneously, with one possibly occluding another (i.e., visually displayed "on top" although both windows are active); spatial semantics (information presented through position in tables, groupings etc.); and graphical semantics (information portrayed through visual elements such as font size, colors, style) (Ratanasit & Moore, 2005).

Another obstacle faced by individuals who are visually impaired is the use of graphical information in tables and graphs. Three primary issues are the size of the table (i.e., providing information about the boundaries), overloading with speech information, and knowledge of current location within the table. Various methods have been developed to represent this information auditorally (Ratanasit & Moore, 2005). Nonspeech sounds are used to provide spatial relationships (e.g., a plucked violin string earcon might be used to represent the lines in a table or graph) and the text-based information contained in the table or graph is provided by synthesized speech. Another technique used is to associate higher pitches with larger numbers and lower pitches with smaller numbers in portraying trends and similar graphical data. Evaluation with visually impaired participants indicated greater success in using tables when nonspeech cues were combined with speech-based information. Another graphical approach is to represent numerical values by pitch, as above, but use a different timbre (instrument sound) for each axis. Box 13-2 describes research in nonspeech auditory representation of icons.

BOX 13-2 Research in Nonspeech Sounds

Ratanasit and Moore (2005) reviewed three primary types of nonspeech sound cues used for representing visual icons used in GUIs: (1) auditory icons, (2) earcons, and (3) hearcons. Auditory icons are everyday sounds used to represent graphical objects. For example, a window might be represented by the sound of tapping on a glass window or a text box by the sound of a typewriter. The Screen Access Model and Windows™ sound libraries are used in some applications. Earcons are abstract auditory labels that do not necessarily have a semantic relationship to the object they represent. Motives are components of earcons such as rhythm (e.g., the length of a musical note, a latin beat), pitch (e.g., a musical C vs A), timbre (e.g., sound of a type of instrument), and register (e.g., octaves on the musical scale). An example of an earcon is a musical note or string of notes played when a file, window or program is opened or closed. Different musical instruments may be used to represent different actions, such as a trumpet representing opening a file and a drum representing closing. In evaluations by blind users, earcons associated with musical characteristics were more effective than those using unstructured sounds (i.e., lacking rhythm, pitch, and other cues). Hearcons are either nature sounds or musical works or instruments. Hearcons are completed musical sounds such as those produced by a running river or birds or a musical work whereas earcons are separate audio components. In an evaluation by visually impaired participants, hearcons did not sufficiently portray semantic relationships to be effective. Font types have been represented by male versus female synthesized voices for normal and hyperlink text or softer and louder sounds for normal versus bold font.

Various methods have been developed to represent spatial information auditorally (Ratanasit & Moore, 2005). Nonspeech sounds are used to provide spatial relationships (e.g., a plucked violin string might be used to represent the lines in a table or graph) and the text-based information contained in the table or graph is provided by synthesized speech. Another technique used is to associate higher pitches with larger numbers and lower pitches with smaller numbers in portraying trends and similar graphical data. Evaluation with visually impaired participants indicated greater success in using tables when nonspeech cues were combined with speech-based information. Another graphical approach is to represent numerical values by pitch, but use a different timbre (instrument sound) for each axis.

TABLE 13-2 Proposed Revision of Categories of Visual Impairment (From WHO)

	Presenting distance visual acuity	
Category	**Worse than:**	**Equal to better than:**
Mild or no visual impairment 0		6/18 3/10 (0.3) 20/70
Moderate visual impairment 1	6/18 3/10 (0.3) 20/70	6/60 1/10 (0.1) 20/200
Severe visual impairment 2	6/60 1/10 (0.1) 20/200	3/60 1/20 (0.05) 20/400
Blindness 3	3/60 1/20 (0.05) 20/400	1/60* 1/50 (0.02) 5/300 (20/1200)
Blindness 4	1/60* 1/50 (0.02) 5/300 (20/1200)	Light perception
Blindness 5	No light perception	
9	Undetermined or unspecified	

*Or counts fingers (CF) at 1 meter

Computer Adaptations for Visual Impairments

Computer users generally receive output from a computer by looking at a visual display. In order to assist individuals who have visual limitations, it is necessary to understand how computer outputs can be adapted. Video displays are found in computers, personal digital assistants (PDAs), cell phones, and many other devices. Printed output is also commonly used in computer applications. Computers also provide auditory outputs of sound, music, or synthetic speech. These outputs are important to individuals who have visual impairments.

Standard visual computer outputs are often not usable by persons who have vision impairments. The degree of vision loss (as in Table 13-2) determines the amount and type of adaptation necessary for successful computer access. For individuals who are blind, we must use tactile or auditory pathways to provide input. Because low-vision and blindness needs are so different from each other, we discuss them separately. Box 13-3 describes research related to computer use by individuals who have a visual impairment.

BOX 13-3 What the Research Tells Us: Computer Use by Visually Impaired Adults

Computer use by individuals who are blind or have low vision is less compared to nondisabled individuals (Gerber & Kirchner, 2001)
- Less access to the Internet
- Are online less
- More likely to be online from work than at home

- Effect of severity of impairment and existence of multiple impairments

  Individuals under 65 have greater use and access than those over 65

  Important given the high prevalence of visual impairment in the population over 65

  People who are employed are more likely to use computers, and the Internet, with same percentage as nondisabled population
- Computer usage patterns of individuals who have visual impairments (Gerber, 2003)
  - Focus groups at national conferences of subscribers to a technology and visual impairment publication*
  - This sample represents the group of visually impaired individuals who use computers and the Internet, but it is not representative of the broader visually impaired community
  - 50% had no useable vision, and the other 50% had variable amounts of vision
  - 50% had been blind since birth, 85% had some university education, and 73% were employed
  - Computer allows access to employment and the creation of flexibility in finding work, including telecommuting
  - Computer also allowed employed individuals to create a cultural identity by being successfully employed
  - Computer use created access to information including newspapers and magazines as well as Web-based sources of information
  - Respondents reported that it was rewarding to read for themselves using technology rather than have someone read to them
  - Improvement in writing skill also occurred
  - Major benefit of computer use is social connections made through the Internet that reduced feelings of isolation and loneliness: independently sending and receiving email, participating in online discussions
  - Concerns

  Lack of training in use of adapted computers

  Training material in accessible form

  Being shut out of advances due to accessibility lags
- Training availability (US focused) (Wolfe, 2003)
  - Group training more common than individual training
  - More demand than available opportunities
  - Training for all major technology types
  - Major challenge is keeping trainers up to date as technologies change
- Quality of training (Wolfe, Candela & Johnson, 2003).
  - Positive comments: good overall quality of the training, greater self-confidence of the trainees following training, and (to a lesser extent) the quality of the trainers
  - Negative comments: training was too short or too infrequent, too few computers were available for hands-on practice, training was not relevant to technology available on the job, the pace of training was too slow or too fast, material was presented at too basic a level, and there was too much variability in trainee experience which limited content that could be covered
  - There is a need to stay abreast of technology changes
- The amount and type (e.g., social networks, email, shopping, banking, etc.) of use of the Internet were not statistically related to either the perception of social support received or a sense of well-being among individuals with visual impairments (Smedema & McKenzie, 2010)

**Access World: Technology and People with Visual Impairments*, American Foundation for the Blind, New York, http://www.afb.org.

TABLE 13-3 Simple Adaptations for Visual Impairment*

Need Addressed	Software Approach**
User cannot see standard size text or graphics	Magnifier (M), Zoom (A)
User cannot see status of open windows, dialog boxes, etc.	Audio Description (M), ToggleKeys (M), Talking Alerts (A)
User requires greater contrast between foreground and background or greater size of characters on the screen	Magnifier or High Contrast color scheme (M) Zoom or High Contrast color scheme (A)
User requires speech output rather than visual output	Narrator (M), VoiceOver (A)

*Software modifications developed at the Trace Center, University of Wisconsin, Madison. These are included as before-market modifications to Microsoft Windows and Apple OS X and iOS X operating systems, as well as some smart phones.
**M = Microsoft Windows, A = Apple OS X or iOS X.

Access to Visual Computer Displays for Individuals with Low Vision

Screen-magnifying software that enlarges a portion of the screen is the most common adaptation for people who have low vision. The unmagnified screen is referred to as the *physical screen*. There are three basic modes of operation for screen magnifiers: lens magnification, part-screen magnification, and full-screen magnification (Blenkhorn et al., 2002). At any one time the user has access to only the portion of the physical screen that appears in this magnified viewing window. Lens magnification is analogous to holding a handheld magnifying lens over a part of the screen. The screen magnification program takes one section of the physical screen and enlarges it. This means that the magnification window must move to show the portion of the physical screen in which the changes are occurring. Part-screen magnification is similar to lens magnification, except that the magnified portion is displayed in a separate window, usually at the top or bottom of the screen.

The enlarged portion of the screen is called the *magnification window*, and the size of text in this window is the *magnification*. The magnification varies from 2 to 36 times or more in current magnifier programs. The magnification program will follow a particular part of the screen referred to as the *focus* of the screen (Blenkhorn et al., 2002). Typical foci are the location of the mouse pointer, the location of the text-entry cursor, a highlighted item (e.g., an item in a pull-down menu) or a currently active dialog box. Screen magnifiers automatically track the focus and enlarge the relevant portion of the screen and the magnification window tracks any changes that occur on the physical screen. For example, if a navigation or control box is active, then the viewing window can highlight that box. If mouse movement occurs, then the magnification window can track the mouse cursor movement. If text is being entered, then the magnification window can follow the text entry cursor and highlight that portion of the physical screen.

Adaptations that allow persons with low vision to access the computer screen are available in several commercial forms. Lazzaro (1999) describes several potential methods of achieving computer access. The simplest and least costly are built-in screen enlargement software programs provided by the computer manufacturer (see Table 13-3). One system for the Macintosh OS X operating system is *Zoom*. This program allows for magnification from 2 to 40 times and has fast and easy text handling and graphics capabilities. There are options for the focus of the magnification, for contrast colors, for cursor size, and for the way in which the user can enable the magnification. More information is available on the Apple accessibility website.[27] *Magnifier* (see Table 13-3) is a minimal function screen magnification program included in Windows.[28] It displays an enlarged portion of the screen (from 2 to 9 times magnification). Other *Magnifier* options include inverted (e.g., black background, white letters), changing the location of the magnification pane, and high-contrast modes. For individuals who need only the *High Contrast* option (available in the control panel Accessibility icon) there are many color combination options for text, background, windows, and other GUI features. None of these built-in options are intended to replace third-party full-function screen magnifiers. The mouse pointer settings under the Windows "Mouse" control panel provide for changing the size, style, and color combination of all the pointers used during GUI interaction.

There are many screen magnification programs available for use with Windows (see www.microsoft.com/enable/ click "Products" tab) or Macintosh (see www.apple.com/accessibility/macosx/ select "Mac OS X solutions from third parties") operating systems.[29] These software programs offer wider ranges of magnification and have more features than built-in screen magnifiers. These programs generally offer access to Windows™ applications including spreadsheet and word processing, email, and Internet browsers. Many can also run with a screen reader (speech output utility). In some cases the screen reader is bundled with the magnification software, and in other cases the screen magnifier speech output runs in conjunction with a separate screen reader. Magnification of up to 36 times or more is available. The various screen modes described above are available in most screen magnification software. These programs also allow

[27] www.apple.com/accessibility/macosx/.
[28] www.microsoft.com/enable/.
[29] For example, SuperNova from Dolphin, Computer Access, San Mateo, Calif. (http://www.yourdolphin.com/); MAGic, Freedom Scientific, St. Petersburg, Fla. (http://www.freedomscientific.com/); Zoom Text, Zoom Text Mac, Zoom Text Large-Print Keyboard, Zoom Text ImageReader, Zoom Text USB, Zoom Text Camera and Zoom Text from AI Squared, Manchester Center, Vt. (www.aisquared.com).

tracking of the mouse pointer, location of keyboard entry, and text editing. The magnification window can be coupled with one or more of these to facilitate navigation for the user. All screen images (including windows, control buttons, and other windows objects) are magnified. Automatic scrolling of the screen (left, right, up, down) is also available to make it easier to read long documents when they are magnified.

For individuals who have low vision, hard copy (printer) output is also a challenge. If the output is to be read by a person with normal vision, the text can be edited on the screen using the methods described earlier and then printed in a standard printer font size. If, however, the user with visual impairment needs to access the hard copy output, then an enlarged printout is desirable using a laser printer coupled with a special software program to create larger characters.

CASE STUDY 13-4

Computer Access for Low Vision

Cheryl is a college student. Her visual limitations prevent her from using the standard computer display. She has asked the ATP to help her find a way to use the computer. The constraints on her situation are that she must use several different computers during the day: her own home computer, a laptop that she carries to class for note taking, and the computers in the student laboratory. What approach would the ATP recommend for her? Would the ATP recommend that she buy special hardware or software to meet her needs, or can she make use of features built into Windows? How would the ATP evaluate the success of your solution for Cheryl?

Access to Visual Computer Displays for Individuals Who Are Blind

Individuals who are blind and want to access a computer will need to have an alternative to the video screen that provides the screen information in either tactile or auditory form. The two primary options are to present text or graphical information as either speech or braille. Systems that provide speech or braille output for blind users are called **screen readers.** A computer user who is blind should be able to access all the same graphics and text as a person who is sighted. Windows™ includes a basic function screen reader utility called *Narrator*[30] (see Table 13-3) that reads text that is displayed on the screen. Audio description provides a speech description of videos played in Windows. *Toggle Keys* (Table 13-3) generates a sound when the CAPS LOCK, NUM LOCK, or SCROLL LOCK key is pressed. The Apple Macintosh OS X operating system includes VoiceOver.[31] This utility provides voice description of the screen as well as reading text. It also includes plug-and-play capability for many braille displays. Talking Alerts automatically speak the contents of dialogs and alerts similarly to Toggle Keys.

A sighted computer user will often scan a screen for a specific piece of information or to obtain a sense of the continuity and flow of the written material, which includes looking for specific screen attributes (such as highlighted or underlined material and features of the GUI). For the user who is blind, duplicating this capability requires that the adapted output system provide reading of text and descriptions of graphics. Finally, screen reader programs provide on-screen messages or prompts for the user input during program operation. Graphic characters should have text labels attached to them. These can be read to the consumer by use of speech synthesis software.

Currently available screen reader programs provide navigation assistance by keyboard commands. Examples of typical functions are movement to a particular point in the text, finding the mouse cursor position, providing a spoken description of an on-screen graphic or a special function key, and accessing help information.[32]

Screen readers also monitor the screen and take action when a particular block of text or a menu appears (Lazzaro, 1999). This feature automatically reads pop-up windows and dialog boxes to the user. Screen readers can typically be set to speak by line, sentence, or paragraph. Other features are also available; for example, Jaws for Windows[33] allows the user to read the prior, current, or next sentence or paragraph in all applications by using specified keystrokes (e.g., read prior sentence = ALT + UP ARROW; read next sentence = ALT + DOWN ARROW; read current sentence = ALT + NUM PAD). The user may use the standard Windows method of switching between applications (ALT + TAB). There are many other key combinations used in Jaws for navigating through text, tables, Webpages, and other documents. There are also special functions for individual programs like those in Microsoft Office,[34] Web browsers, and others.

All screen readers provide navigation; however, their specific keys and ways of organizing the functions vary. Some screen readers also provide a "window list" in which applications that are running appear in alphabetical order. This allows the user to switch between, close, or see the state of any active application. This is a faster way to switch between applications when a user has many windows open, rather than moving the cursor to a pull-down menu or "close" box. SuperNoval[35] is a screen reader designed to operate with the visible information on the screen. SuperNova recognizes objects by looking for distinct attributes, shapes, borders, highlights, and so on. This is in contrast to using the standard labels of Windows, and it means that SuperNova is independent of whether an application has obeyed the rules of Windows programming. SuperNova recognizes objects by their final shape on the screen, rather than their Windows attributes. The advantage of this approach is that once set

[30] www.microsoft.com/enable/.

[31] www.apple.com/accessibility.

[32] For example, Jaws for Windows from Freedom Scientific, St. Petersburg, Fla. (http://www.freedomscientific.com/); Zoom Text Magnifier/Reader from AI Squared, Manchester Center, Vt. (www.aisquared.com); Supernova ScreenReader from Dolphin Computer Access, San Mateo, Calif. (www.yourdolphin.com); Magnum and Magnum Deluxe from Artic Technologies, Troy, Mich.; Protalk32 for Windows; Window Eyes from GW Microsystems, Fort Wayne, Ind. (www.gwmicro.com).

[33] Freedom Scientific, St. Petersburg, Fla. (http://www.freedomscientific.com/).

[34] Microsoft Corporation, Seattle, Wash. (www.microsoft.com/).

[35] Dolphin Computer Access, San Mateo, Calif. (http://www.yourdolphin.com/).

up for one application, all similar-looking applications will talk correctly without any adjustment to the settings. Most screen readers include a braille output mode that interfaces to many different refreshable braille displays via a USB port. These are only examples of product features; as is true for any computer application, rapid advances are common.

Many screen readers have applications for specific types of programs, procedures or applications. Examples include SuperNova,[36] JAWS for Windows,[37] and Window Eyes.[38] These applications, called **scripts,** are small computer programs that contain sequences of individual steps used to activate and control a wide variety of computer applications. Scripts are used to make screen readers and screen magnifiers work well with specific programs. The script runs when a user loads a document and provides a way for an application to be customized for a particular user. Each script or function contains commands that tell the screen reader how to navigate and what to read under different conditions. These features are automatically loaded anytime the application program is loaded. Scripts are used for software applications like email, Web browsing, word processing, and other applications. Screen readers generally allow modification of scripts and provide development tools for scripts used to make any application accessible with the screen reader. By analyzing what actions are taking place in a given application, the script can optimize the screen reader for the use. Scripts require access to a proprietary scripting language that varies by the screen reader/magnifier manufacturer.

Window-Eyes[39] uses the Microsoft Excel DOM (document object model) to communicate directly with Microsoft Word and Microsoft Excel and includes the ability to save specific settings (i.e., headers and totals and monitor cells) for specific documents. VIRGO 4[40] uses Microsoft Visual Basic as a scripting language to customize the screen reader for specific applications. Users who have computer programming skills can write their own scripts to automate tasks or to optimize their readers for specific applications.

These applications all require that the special script or application file be developed individually for a particular application. An alternative approach is to develop software that automatically develops a script based on what the user is doing at the time by observing his or her actions (Ma et al., 2004). The software also informs the user when a script exists that is relevant to the application being used. Examples of scripts that might be developed are finding a weather forecast or a stock price. The Intelligent Screen Reader (Ma et al., 2004) works with the built-in macro recorder of JAWS and a script generation interface to automatically generate a script with *plan recognition networks* (PRNs). PRNs are probabilistic models of procedures produced by an automated synthesis of plan recognition networks (Huber & Simpson, 2004).

[36] Dolphin Computer Access, San Mateo, Calif. (www.yourdolphin.com/).
[37] For example: JAWS, Freedom Scientific, St. Petersburg, Fla. (http://www.freedomscientific.com/).
[38] GW Microsystems, Fort Wayne, Ind. (www.gwmicro.com).
[39] GW Microsystems, Fort Wayne, Ind. (www.gwmicro.com/gwie).
[40] Baum, Germany (www.baum.de).

The key to this software approach is the ability to identify the user's intentions as the task is being performed. The advantage of this approach is that the user does not need to learn the script programming method and also does not need to depend on the prestored scripts developed by the manufacturer.

For computer users who are familiar with braille, refreshable braille displays can be more effective than screen readers. However, a combination of approaches may be most effective with braille and speech combined. The hardware and software designed for braille can be used together with that developed for screen reading using speech synthesis.

Printed braille output is produced by *embossers.* Embossers are available in both single- and double-sided formats. They include both portable and stationary systems with a variety of printing speeds from 30 to 60 characters per second and with line widths of 32 to 40 characters (single-sided) and 55 characters per second with 56-character line widths (double-sided).[41] The Viewplus Braille Embosser Series[42] are embossers that print in different paper weights at high speeds for use in production. The Mountbatten Brailler[43] is a braille writer with a braille keyboard, built-in memory, autocorrection features, and extensive formatting controls. The Mountbatten can be used as an embosser for a computer or as a braille translation device. It can translate from print into braille or braille into print and is available in both AC and battery-operated models. All these embossers include internal software that accepts standard printer output from the host computer and converts it to either six- or eight-cell braille embossed on heavy paper. American Thermoform Corporation[44] makes a variety of braille embossers. These cover applications from mass production to systems for individual users.

Braille translation programs are available from Duxbury Systems.[45] These programs convert computer data (word processor text files, spreadsheets, database files) to Grade 2 braille in hard copy form for either Macintosh OS X or Windows operating systems. Duxbury Braille Translation provides translation and formatting capabilities to automate the process of conversion from regular print to braille (and vice versa) and also provides word processing functions for working directly in braille or print format. Braille characters can be displayed on the screen for proofreading before printing. This software is typically used both by individuals who do not know braille and those who do. The Duxbury Braille Translator allows the user to create braille for schoolbooks and teaching materials, office memos, bus schedules, personal letters, and signs. The software allows importing of files from popular word processors and other sources.

[41] Enabling Technologies, Jenson Beach, Fla. (http://www.Brailler.com/index.htm); Pulse Data Human Ware, Concord, Calif. (http://www.pulsedata.com); GW Microsystems, Fort Wayne, In. (https://www.gwmicro.com/); View Plus, Corvallis, Ore. (http://www.viewplus.com).
[42] Human Ware, Concord, Calif. (http://www.humanware.com/en-international/home).
[43] Quantum Technology, Sydney, AU (http://www.mountbattenbrailler.com/).
[44] La Verne, Calif. (http://www.americanthermoform.com/index.html).
[45] Westbury, Mass. (http://www.duxburysystems.com/).

Access to Mobile Phones and Tablets for Individuals with Low Vision or Blindness

Cellular telephones and tablets have become more powerful, with capabilities similar to personal computers. Fruchterman (2003) describes four significant factors to assist people with disabilities, especially those with low vision or blindness: (1) standard cell phones have sufficient processing power for almost all the requirements of persons with visual impairments,[46] (2) software apps can be downloaded into these phones easily, (3) wireless connection to a worldwide network (including the cloud) provides a wide range of information and services in a highly mobile way, (4) many of these features are built into standard cell phones, making the cost low and accessible by persons with disabilities. Much of the cell phone industry (the iPhone is an exception) has moved away from proprietary software to an open source approach, much like personal computers. This has led to a greater diversity of software for tasks such as text-to-speech output, voice recognition, and OCR in a variety of languages. Many applications for people with disabilities can be downloaded from the Internet. For example, downloading a DAISY reading program into a cell phone can provide access to digital libraries, and outputs in speech or enlarged visual displays allow access to standard text messaging.

Accessible mobile phones and tablets with the capability of adding software apps for specific functions open up a range of options for people who have a visual impairment. These options include calendar/appointments, personal contact databases, note taking, multimedia messaging, and Web browsing. Many other possibilities exist as well; for example, with a built-in camera and network access a blind person could obtain a verbal description of a scene by linking to online volunteers who provide descriptions of images. Advances of this type will occur rapidly.

One reason for the optimism surrounding these types of advancements is the increasing application of universal design in information technology products (Tobias, 2003). Universal design principles (see Chapter 2) call for mainstream technologies to be accessible to a wide range of individuals with and without disabilities. Tobias (2003) describes government regulations that underlie access in many countries and the challenges in implementing them. When mainstream technologies employ open source operating systems, network-based accommodations can be accessed by users without specially designed equipment. This can reduce cost and thereby increase availability. These applications include ATMs, cell phones, vending machines, and other systems that are encountered on a daily basis (Tobias, 2003).

The Royal National Institute of Blind People (RNIB) in Britain has information regarding mobile phone and tablet accessibility (http://www.rnib.org.uk/Pages/Home.aspx). The RNIB provides many useful resources for persons with visual impairments who want to access computers, cell phones or tablets. Another useful Website for cell phone accessibility is www.accessible-devices.com. This site has both product information and user case studies that provide lots of practical advice for people with low vision in selecting and using a cell phone.

Another useful source of information for individuals with visual impairments who want to access tablets and mobile phones is Code Factory (http://www.codefactory.es/en). Code Factory develops accessible software applications for mobile phones. Their Website includes a selection wizard to help individuals find specific products that will meet their needs based on the tablet or mobile phone that they intend to use. Products described include screen readers, screen magnifiers, GPS navigation aids, and a mobile DAISY player.

Code Factory has three types of products for mobile phones: (1) screen readers[47] for mobile phones using text-to-speech software and the speaker or a headset on the phone, (2) screen magnifiers[48] for mobile phones, and (3) mobile tools for navigation (Mobile Geo GPS aid), mobile DAISY Player, and a color identification app.

Accessibility features of the Apple iPad, iPhone, and iTouch are described on the Apple Website (www.apple.com/accessibility). The standard or built-in features are a screen reader (VoiceOver), screen magnifier (Zoom), and reverse (white on black) contrast. All of these features take advantage of the touch screen and the use of gestures (e.g., swipe or tap) to make a choice or to navigate around Webpages. There are also a number of third-party hardware and software products that adapt the iPhone for people with disabilities. These are listed on the Apple accessibility website.

Accessibility for individuals with visual impairments who want to use Android phones and tablets is available at: http://eyes-free.googlecode.com/svn/trunk/documentation/android_access/index.html. Built-in features as well as third-party apps are described for both low vision and blindness. Voice output is built in to Android devices as well as accessibility features that can change font size and contrast. Because it is an open source system there is also extensive information for developers on making their apps accessible.

There are many apps for iOS (at iTunes) (www.apple.com/accessibility/third-party/) and Android (https://play.google.com/store/search?q=accesibility&c=apps) devices (at Google Play Store). Apps include screen readers, self-care such as reading bar codes using voice output, navigation aids, and recreation (e.g., visually adapted games).

The built-in approaches and apps based on the standard hardware are sometimes not sufficient to provide access for individuals who are blind and want to use mobile technologies. Other approaches based on combinations of speech and tactile displays have been developed. Oliveira et al. (2011) evaluated four approaches for touch screen text-entry with 13 blind people as participants. All text-entry methods were implemented as Android applications on a Samsung Galaxy S

[46] Popular applications-oriented operating systems include Android (http://market.android.com/); Apple's iOS (http://www.apple.com/accessibility/third-party/); and BlackBerry OS (http://us.blackberry.com/apps-software/blackberry6/).

[47] Mobile Speak (Symbian, Windows Mobile), Mobile Accessibility (Android), Oratio (BlackBerry).

[48] Mobile Magnifier (Symbian, Windows Mobile).

touch screen device. Two of the applications were similar to the Apple iOS VoiceOver feature. The *QWERTY* text-entry method used the traditional computer keyboard and the *MultiTap* approach used a layout similar to keypad-based devices. In both approaches, the user can enter the letter by split-tapping or double tapping anywhere on the screen. A third approach, NavTouch, is a gesture-based approach with an adaptive rather than fixed layout. Text entry is accomplished via a navigational approach: with speech feedback in which gestures to left and right navigate through the alphabet horizontally and gestures up and down navigate vertically (i.e., between vowels). To select the current letter users can perform a split or double tap. The final system evaluated, BrailleType, requires that the user know braille. Six large targets, corresponding to the six braille cells, are mapped to the corners and edges of the screen for easy access. To mark/clear a dot, a long press is required and auditory feedback is provided. The user double taps anywhere on the screen for entry after selecting the six dots for a braille character (in any order).

Guerreiro et al. (2008) identified three determining characteristics of individual users that impacted the effectiveness of touch interfaces: (1) spatial ability, (2) pressure sensitivity, and (3) verbal IQ. Identifying these characteristics is important because most approaches neglect the individual differences among blind people and their impact on users' performance. Results of testing indicated that participants felt that NavTouch was easier to use than MultiTap, and BrailleType was easier to understand than both the MultiTap and QWERTY methods. BrailleType and NavTouch had the fewest user mistakes and were also the slowest in terms of WPM; this result was reflected in the questionnaire as lower user preference for these methods. NavTouch and BrailleType were slower but also easier and more accurate systems. Errors with MultiTap were due to difficulty in multitapping,

Oliveira et al. (2011) found that spatial ability, pressure sensitivity, and verbal IQ played important roles in the blind user's ability to use and perform accurately with a touch screen. Younger users always performed faster than older users, independently of the text-entry method used. Participants with better pressure sensitivity performed significantly better on the MultiTap method. For the two methods where exploration of the screen is vital, QWERTY and MultiTap, participant performance was significantly related to spatial ability. Different levels of computer experience did not lead to statistically significant differences on the QWERTY method, in terms of speed and accuracy. Participants who were faster at reading braille were fastest with BrailleType. NavTouch and MultiTap were more demanding in terms of memory and attention. This study is important in that it demonstrates that one size does not fill all when it comes to touch screen access for individuals who are blind.

Visual Access to the Internet

As the Internet becomes more and more dependent on multimedia representations involving complex graphics, animation, and audible sources of information, the challenges for people who have disabilities increase. The most obvious barriers are for those who are blind. People who have learning disabilities and dyslexia also find it increasingly difficult to access complicated Websites that may include flashing pictures, complicated charts, and large amounts of audio and video data. The challenges faced by these populations are discussed in Chapter 15. It is estimated that as many as 40 million persons in the United States have physical, cognitive, or sensory disabilities (Lazzaro, 1999). Thus, the importance of making the Internet accessible to all is great.

Many of the approaches to computer input and output discussed in this chapter are important to the provision of access to this information for persons who have disabilities. Emiliani, Stephanidis, and Vanderheiden (2011) provide a comprehensive review of the issues related to Internet access by persons with disabilities. Two useful sources of information regarding Internet access for people with disabilities are the World Wide Web Consortium Web Accessibility Initiative (W3C WAI; www.w3.org) and the Trace Center (www.trace.wisc.edu/world/web). The W3C consortium has provided guidelines for web content accessibility at www.w3.org/WAI/WCAG20/quickref/.

User Agents for Access to the Internet

Access to the Internet must be independent of individual devices. This device independence means that users must be able to interact with a *user agent* (and the document it renders) using the input and output devices of their choice on the basis of their specific needs. A **user agent** is defined as software that is used to access Web content (www.w3.org/wai). This includes desktop graphical browsers, text and voice browsers, mobile phones, multimedia players, and software assistive technologies (e.g., screen readers, magnifiers, keyboard and mouse emulators) that are used with browsers. Input devices that are used for Internet access include many of those described earlier in this chapter and in Chapter 9. Mouse and mouse-alternative pointing devices, head wands, keyboards and keyboard alternatives such as on-screen keyboards, braille input keyboards, switches and switch arrays, and microphones can all serve as input devices for user agents. Output devices for Internet access are also those described in this chapter (e.g., screen readers, screen magnifiers, braille displays, and speech synthesizers).

The W3C WAI project provides practical solutions for the development of accessible user agents based on existing and emerging technologies. The most useful commercial products maximize compatibility between graphical desktop browsers and dependent assistive technologies (e.g., screen readers, screen magnifiers, braille displays, and voice input software). These developments will also benefit those who access the Internet through palmtop computers, telephones, and tablets. Users may also have difficulty reading or comprehending text. Users who have low vision or blindness will require adaptations for computer access and user agents need to be accessible.

The W3C WAI has developed guidelines to inform user agent developers of design approaches required to make their products more accessible to people with disabilities. The W3C WAI project also provides practical solutions for the development of accessible user agents on the basis of existing and emerging technologies. These resources will also increase usability for all users. The W3C initiative emphasizes the use of designs that facilitate compatibility between graphical desktop browsers and independent assistive technologies (e.g., screen readers, screen magnifiers, braille displays, and voice input software). These developments will also benefit those who do not use the standard keyboard and mouse to access the Internet (e.g., those who are mobile and access the Web through smart phones, tablets, and auto terminals).

The W3C WAI user agent guidelines are based on several principles.[49] The first is to ensure that the user interface is accessible to a consumer using an adapted input system in the same way that it is accessible to a nondisabled person using standard keyboard, mouse, and video display. Second, the user must be able to control the style (e.g., colors, fonts, speech rate, and speech volume) and format of a document. Many of the screen magnifier approaches described earlier in this chapter (e.g., easy scrolling, and viewing windows that follow changes) help make access to content easier. When using a screen reader or magnifier a challenge for the user is to know where they are on a Website or a linked Website if that is needed. We typically have this information visually, but when using speech or braille or a magnified screen it is often hard to keep track of links on a Website or follow links to similar Websites. Thus, a third principle for user agents is to help orient the user to where he or she is in the document or series of documents. This function can be accomplished by showing how many links the document contains and the number of the current link or other numerical position information that allows the user to jump to a specific link.

Web Browsers

Web browsers incorporate accessibility features to varying degrees. The W3C initiative describes standards for browsers at www.w3.org/standards/agents/browsers. There are many features of browsers that are independent of the operating system, and the accessibility of browsers varies. Cascading style sheets (CSS) allow a Webpage to be viewed in any layout chosen by the user (Lazzaro, 1999). Style sheet layouts that are compatible with screen magnifiers, screen readers, and braille are available. One example of an HTML accessibility standard is the alt-"text" HTML attribute. This function associates text with each graphic object. By pressing the ALT key on the keyboard, a description of the object is displayed. This can also be linked to a screen reader or braille output device.

Microsoft Internet Explorer[50] contains a range of features for people with disabilities. These include keyboard navigation (among links, frames, and client-side image maps), optional display of text descriptions with images, multiple font sizes and styles, and an optional disabling of style sheets so that the user's font, color, and size settings (their personal style sheet) will be used. This allows turning sounds, videos, pictures, and backgrounds off or on. Toolbar button size and icon size, text color, font, and size are all adjustable. Automatic fill in of user names, passwords, web addresses, and routine forums is also included. Internet Explorer also uses the High Contrast function to increase legibility and incorporates Microsoft Active Accessibility to provide information about the document. Internet Explorer is compatible with most screen readers and magnifiers.

Safari[51] is a browser included with the Macintosh OS X operating system. It is also available for Windows and the mobile iPod Touch, iPhone, and iPad. Safari has features for accessible Web browsing. For example, the user can click on a box to prevent text from being displayed in a size smaller than the setting for the screen. There are also special features that aid in navigation of a Webpage. Additional special accessibility features can be added using cascading style sheets accessed through a pop-up menu. CCS-based adjustments to a Webpage include color, font size, number of columns, and other ways of modifying the way Webpages are displayed.

The auditory interfaces of screen readers do not filter the content, so everything is spoken and there can be significant information overload. Mahmud, Borodin, and Ramakrishnan (2008) developed a simple approach to doing Web transactions using nonvisual modalities. They used the context and keywords to identify various concepts surrounding links to other pages presented on a Webpage (e.g., "add to cart," "item description"). This helps users to reduce the information overload and improve the browsing experience. Most concepts can be divided into three broad categories: (1) those that can be detected using keywords (e.g., "Add To Cart"), (2) those that can be captured by simple patterns or rules, and (3) those that have a variation of content and presentation styles across different Websites. The third type cannot be detected with keywords and patterns alone (e.g., "Item Detail"). The approach was evaluated with 12 typical adults. Overall, 11 out of 12 of the evaluators felt that the system was adequate to perform transactions.

Chrome and Android operating systems share many of the same accessibility features.[52] These include screen layout such as font size, contrast, and screen zoom. ChromeVox is a screen reader add-on to Chrome that provides text-to-speech output. Other accessibility features for both users and developers are shown on the Google Accessibility Website (https://play.google.com/store/search?q=accesibility%26c=apps). Firefox[53] has similar features regarding font size, contrast, zoom, and other accessibility features for individuals with visual impairments. The Fangs Screen Reader Emulator renders a text version of a Webpage similar to how a screen reader would read it to illustrate to developers how a screen reader would access their Web content.

[49] W3C WAI Webpage (www.w3.org/wai).

[50] Microsoft: Seattle, Wash. (www.microsoft.com/enable/).

[51] www.apple.com/safari.

[52] http://www.google.ca/accessibility/products/#blind-low-vision.

[53] https://play.google.com/store/search?q=accesibility%26c=apps.

BOX 13-4 Quick Tips to Make Accessible Websites

Images and animations. Use the "ALT" attribute to describe the function of all visuals.
Image maps. Use client-side map and text for hot spots.
Multimedia. Provide captioning and transcripts of audio, and descriptions of video.
Hypertext links. Use text that makes sense when read out of context. For example, avoid "click here."
Page organization. Use headings, lists, and consistent structure. Use cascading style sheets for layout and style where possible.
Graphs and charts. Summarize or use the "longdesc" attribute.
Scripts, applets, and plug-ins. Provide alternative content in case active features are inaccessible or unsupported.
Frames. Use "no frames" element and meaningful titles.
Tables. Make line-by-line reading sensible. Summarize.
Check your work. Validate. Use tools, checklist, and guidelines at www.w3.org/tr/wai-webcontent.
For complete guidelines and checklist, see www.w3.org/wai.

Special Considerations for Seniors

Many individuals who have low vision or blindness are also seniors. They may not have had experience with computers and they may not be comfortable with the many features available on many screen readers/screen magnifiers. To meet the need for this population to have access to computer programs like email or Web browsing, Dolphin has developed the Dolphin Guide.[54] This program is based on a simple menu-driven user interface that makes it easier for a partially sighted person to access the computer. All commands and screen elements are available in both speech and enlarged text formats. Automatic speech recognition (see Chapter 8) can also be used for input, creating a completely hands-free environment.

Making Web Sites Accessible

The W3C WAI has also developed guidelines for creating accessible Websites. Their Quick Tips are shown in Box 13-4. These guidelines particularly address the way in which Websites are laid out and the programming that is done to create the Website. The guidelines facilitate access to the Webpage by people using alternative input or output methods and give designers guidelines for making their content accessible to individuals who have visual, auditory, or manipulation disabilities. The technical terms that appear in the guidelines (e.g., cascading style sheets, HTML, scripts, applets) are defined on the W3C WAI home page.

Evaluating Web Sites for Accessibility

There are a number of approaches to the evaluation of a Website to determine how accessible it is. The W3C initiative is a good source of information regarding how to determine if a Website is accessible, where to find tools to aid in the determination of accessibility, an outline of a general procedure for evaluation, and tips for making accessible Websites (http://www.w3.org/standards/webdesign/). Evaluation of accessibility varies for different disabilities and for different situations, such as development of a Website versus on-going use. The W3C Website also describes the pros and cons of using Web evaluation tools (www.w3.org/WAI/eval/). The main advantage of evaluation tools is the saving in time and effort. However, these tools do not replace human judgment, which may require manual testing of the Website. Finally, the Website also lists considerations that are important to the selection of a web evaluation tool.

MOBILITY AND ORIENTATION AIDS FOR PERSONS WITH VISUAL IMPAIRMENTS

Orientation refers to the "knowledge of one's location in relation to the environment" (Scadden, 1997, p. 141). There are five approaches used to aid blind travel: a sighted guide, dog guides, the long cane, electronic aids, and alternative mobility devices. The last three are discussed in this section.

For individuals who have low vision or blindness, mobility and orientation are major challenges. The blind traveler uses many methods to orient himself or herself to the environment and move safely (American Foundation for the Blind, http://www.afb.org). Attention to sensory inputs of smell, sound, air currents, and surface texture alert the blind person to the terrain and environment, and a blind person can learn to pick up cues regarding objects. Sound cues are derived from reflections, sound shadows, and echo location. Temperature changes are also important. For example, passing a window on a cold day or passing under a canopy on a warm day provides information that is used in orientation. Odors from restaurants and crowds and other strong smells also provide information. Input regarding the texture of a sidewalk or grass is provided by the kinesthetic sense. Finally, persons with visual impairments also use travel aids, some of which are discussed in this section.

Canes

The most common mobility aid for persons with visual impairments is the long cane (Farmer, 1978). The standard cane consists of three parts: the grip, the shaft, and the tip. The entire cane is designed to maximize tactile and auditory input from the environment. The grip (which forms the handle) is made of leather, plastic, rubber, or other materials that easily transmit the tactile information to the user's hand. The shaft and tip work together to sense and then relay the tactile information to the grip. The tip (especially a metal tip used on a hard surface such as concrete) is a major source of high-frequency auditory input used by pedestrians who are blind to detect obstacles and landmarks by echolocation. A careful balance is obtained between sufficient rigidity to resist wind and bending and adequate flexibility to transmit the tactile and auditory sense of the surface texture. The advantages and limitations of the long cane are shown in Table 13-4. It takes between 6 and 12 weeks to develop proficiency in using a long cane (Ramsey et al., 1999).

Many blind travelers use folding or telescoping canes, which offer the advantage of easy storage when not in

[54] www.yourdolphin.com/productdetail.asp?pg=1&id=30.

TABLE 13-4 Pros and Cons of the Long Cane

Advantages	Limitations
Low cost	Only detects obstacles one step in front of the user
Simplicity of use	Doesn't sense objects above waist level (e.g., the cane may pass between table legs, under the tabletop)
Well developed training programs	Doesn't sense head-height obstacles such as tree branches

use. Typically these are made of composite materials such as carbon fiber. When collapsed, they can be placed in a pocket or purse.

The primary advantages of canes are the low cost and the simplicity of use. They have significant limitations, however. One of these relates to the range over which sensory information is obtained. In use, the cane is moved in an arc approximately one step in front of the user. Any obstacles outside this range are not detected, and in some cases it is difficult for the blind traveler to adjust and avoid an obstacle within the space of only one step. A second limitation is that the cane only senses obstacles that are below waist level. In many cases, objects above knee level are not sensed until it is too late. For example, if there is a table in the path of the user, the cane may pass between the table legs, under the tabletop. The user will be unaware of the table's existence until he or she runs into it. Obstacles that are above waist height are also not sensed. Those of most concern are head-height obstacles such as tree branches.

Alternative Mobility Devices

Roentgen et al. (2008) identified 12 devices designed specifically for obstacle detection and orientation. The term **alternative mobility device** is used to describe a variety of methods used to aid mobility for individuals who are blind, particularly young children (Skellenger, 1999). Many of these devices are custom made from items such as hula hoops, toy shopping carts, PVC attached to an arm, and similar objects. Skellenger (1999) defines alternative mobility devices as "travel propelled devices other than the long cane that are held relatively statically in front of the traveler and are used primarily to detect obstacles and changes in depth" (p. 517). Skellenger found that these devices are widely used with children under the age of 5 years by orientation and mobility trainers, but they are rarely used with adults. The alternative devices are used primarily for training and are generally replaced by one of the other means of mobility assistance.

Electronic Travel Aids for Obstacle Detection, Orientation, and Mobility

Electronic travel aids (ETAs) have been developed to overcome some of the limitations of the long cane. These aids supplement rather than replace the long cane and guide dog. They are designed to provide additional environmental information over that sensed with a cane and to detect those obstacles typically missed by the long cane. ETAs also provide information that can assist with orientation for pedestrians who are blind (Scadden, 1997). We discuss both these applications in this section.

ETAs have the three components, as shown in Figure 13-1: an environmental interface, an information processor, and a user display. The environmental interface is typically both an invisible light source and a receiver (usually in the infrared range) or an ultrasonic transmitter and receiver. Both these technologies are similar to those used in television remote controls. The information processor may be a special-purpose electronic circuit or a microcomputer-based device. The user display may be either an auditory tone of varying frequency (e.g., higher as an object gets closer) or a haptic interface. Haptic interfaces are those that provide tactile input by use of vibrating pins or motors that vibrate faster as an object is closer. Zelek et al. (2003) developed and tested a haptic glove with three separate motors providing vibration to the thumb, middle finger, or little finger, depending on whether an obstacle was to the right, center, or middle of the user. The vibration of the motors was updated two to three times per second. The evaluation of the glove indicated that blind subjects navigated an unknown space efficiently (measured by the length of the path) and accurately (measured by avoidance of obstacles). Zelek et al. (2003) also described the concept of visual-tactile mapping.

Electronically Augmented Canes

Over the years several alternatives have been developed to extend the range of the standard cane and add the capability of detecting overhangs and/or sensing of drop-offs. Figure 13-12 *A* illustrates the principle of operation of electronically augmented canes. From one to three narrow beams of laser light or high-frequency sound (ultrasound) are projected from the cane. Commercial products have one, two, or three beams. One beam is directed upward, and it detects obstacles at head height. If an object is encountered in this beam, the reflected signal causes the vibration of pins or an auditory tone of rising pitch as objects are detected closer and closer. The pins and speaker for tones are located in the handle of the cane, where the fingers can comfortably rest on them (Figure 13-12 *B*). The final beam is aimed downward, and it is intended to detect drop-offs. If the reflected beam is interrupted (because the drop-off does not reflect light in the same way as a level surface), then a low-frequency tone is emitted. In some cases the auditory and tactile signals from the laser cane are misleading to the user (Mellor, 1981). For example, the laser beams could travel through a plate-glass door or window without being reflected, and the glass would not be detected. Nonglass portions of the door (e.g., frame or handle) were generally detected, but they had to be recognized as part of a door on the basis of laser cane signals. Highly reflective shiny surfaces also provided confusing reflections to the cane user.

A current ETA based on the cane is the UltraCane,[55] which uses ultrasound. The UltraCane, shown in Figure 13-13 *A*, provides all the information normally obtained

[55] Sound Foresight LTD, Barnsley, UK (www.ultracane.com).

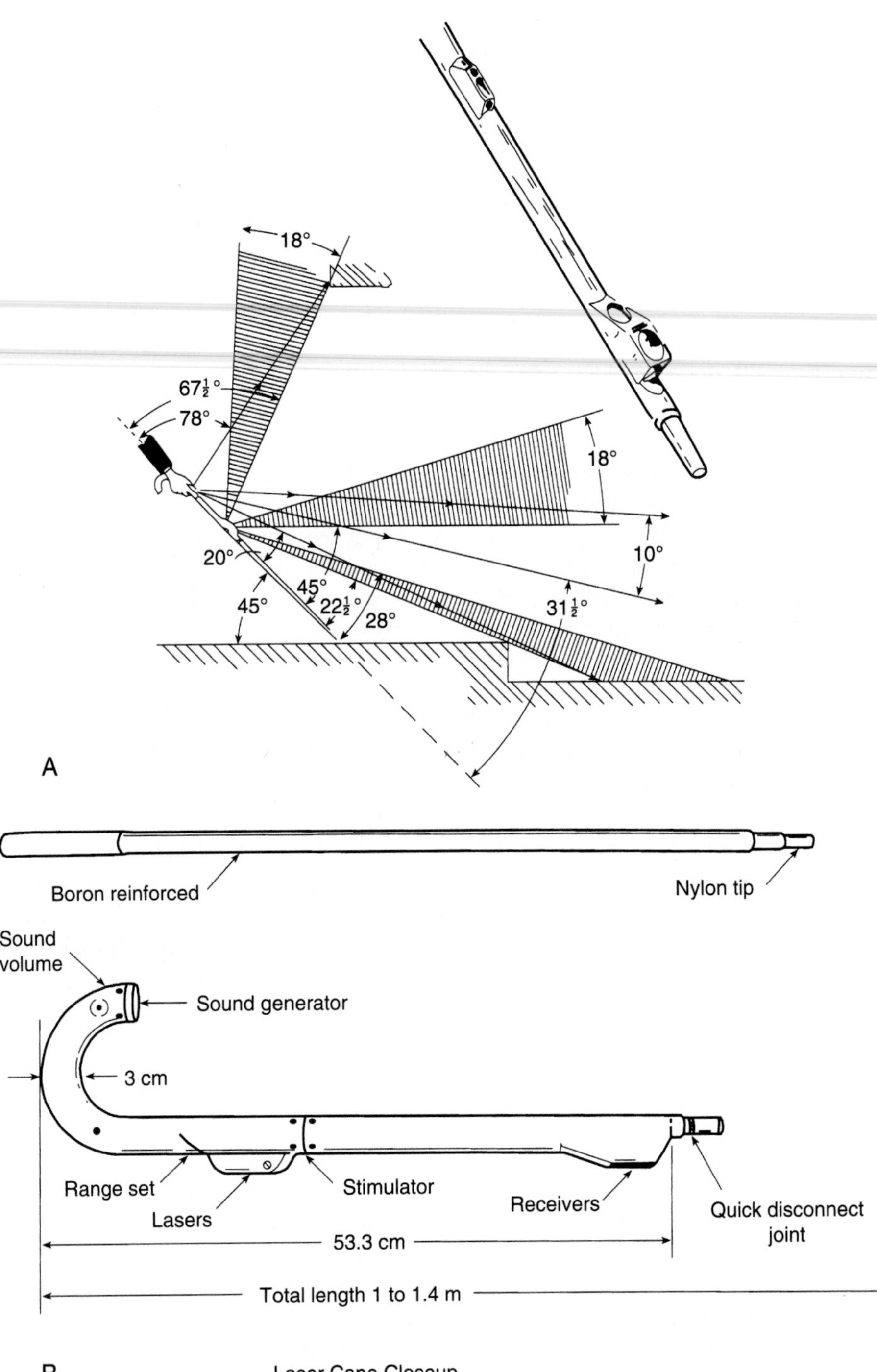

FIGURE 13-12 The laser cane. **A,** The triangulation method used. **B,** The major components. (From Nye PW, Bliss JC: Sensory aids for the blind: A challenging problem with lessons for the future, *Proc IEEE* 58:1878–1879, 1970.)

from the long cane and adds two ultrasound beams and sensors. One detects objects directly in front and one detects objects at head height. It comes in seven lengths from 105 cm (41 inches) to 150 cm (59 inches). The ultrasound beam avoids the problems of transparent glass encountered by the laser cane because the ultrasound beam is reflected from glass or shiny surfaces without distortion. The user display (Figure 13-13 *B*) provides tactile feedback with three vibrating pins located on each side and in the middle to indicate where the detected object is located. The intensity of the vibration indicates how close the object is. In contrast to the earlier laser cane, the UltraCane is collapsible and lightweight. It is used in the same way as the standard long cane. The user sweeps the cane in an arc in front as he or she walks. Although it is not quite as responsive as a standard long cane, primarily because of the added electronics in the handle, the laser cane can also provide conventional tactile and auditory information. One major advantage of the UltraCane is that it is fail safe; if the batteries run down or an electronic failure occurs, the cane can be used like a standard long cane. The laser cane was also used during mobility training, helping the trainee understand how to hold the cane correctly and move it in

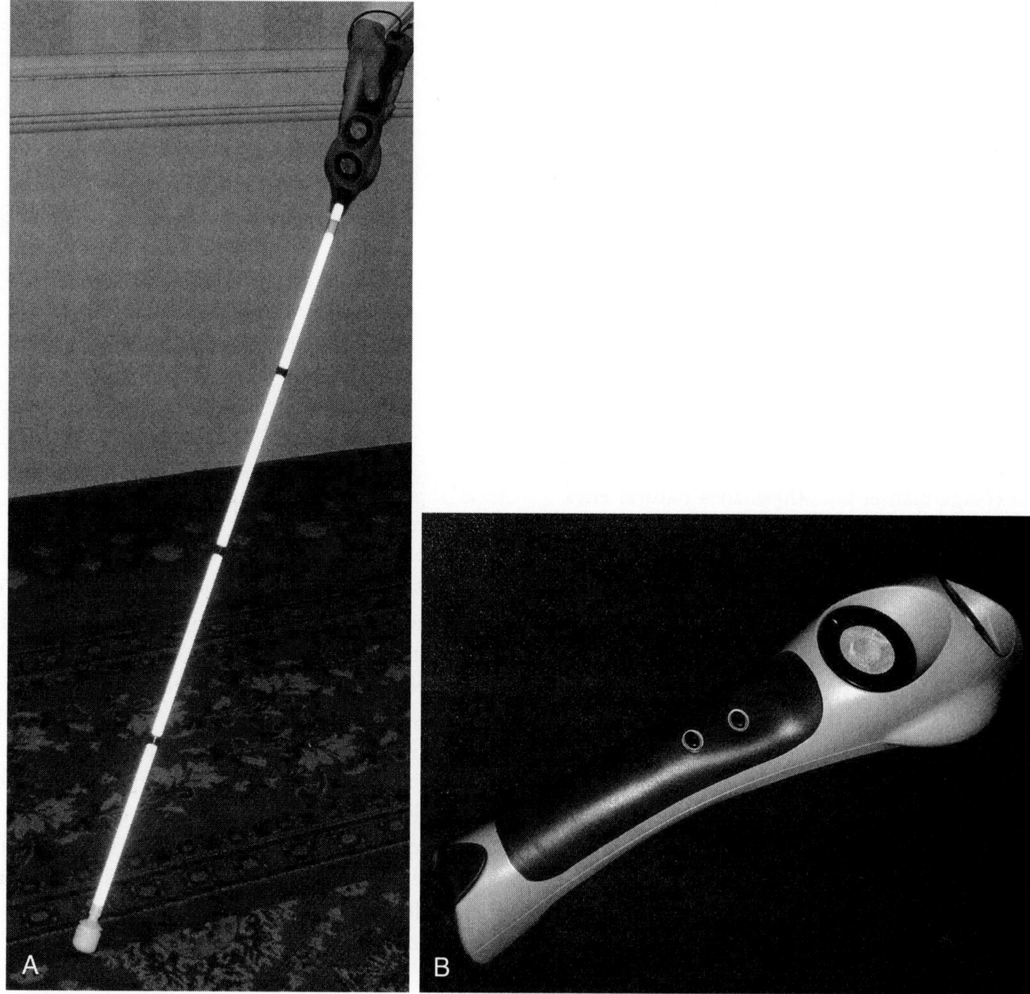

FIGURE 13-13 **A,** The UltraCane provides all the information normally obtained from the long cane. **B,** Two ultrasound beams and sensors are built into the handle.

the correct arc (Mellor, 1981). The UltraCane can be used in a similar fashion. After the training is complete, the trainee can choose either to use the standard cane or to continue with the UltraCane. The UltraCane can also provide important information for a congenitally blind child regarding the size of objects and their location in space.

Another ETA based on the long cane is the EasyGo[56] ultrasound transmitter/sensor that can be attached to a standard long cane. The sensor is aimed forward. When an obstacle is detected by the ultrasound beam, the handle provides tactile feedback to the user through a ring, which is integrated into the handle. During use, the user's finger rests on the ring, which rotates around the grip when an object is detected. The user can use the cane like a standard long cane while walking. Two ranges are available from the ultrasound sensor by turning the ring to the right (2.5 meters) or left (4 meters).

The most significant disadvantage to augmented canes is the cost/benefit ratio. These devices are up to 8 times more expensive than the long cane, and each individual user must decide how important the additional information received from an augmented cane is to his or her work, lifestyle, or safety. There are a variety of other augmented canes of both the specially designed type and devices that attach to the standard long cane (Roentgen et al., 2008).

Navigation Aids for the Blind

The electronic travel aids for obstacle avoidance do not address orientation that keeps an individual apprised of location and heading. To be effective, a navigation system should (1) keep track of the user's current location and heading as he or she moves through the environment, (2) find the way around and through a variety of environments, (3) successfully find and follow an optimally safe walking path to the destination, and (4) provide information about the salient features of the environment (Walker & Jeffery, 2005). To develop navigation aids, it is necessary to decide what environmental elements are important and then to develop technological approaches to detecting those elements, and finally to provide a nonvisual means by which the information can be provided to the user.

As described, the most effective auditory method for presenting information is speech, which has been the major

[56] Q-tec B.V., The Netherlands (www.q-tec.nl/uk/easygo.htm).

approach for descriptive information in navigation aids. Synthetic or recorded speech cues and environmental descriptions are typically used in navigation aids. Other auditory cues are used as well to identify way points along a path (e.g., beacon signals that break down a long path into short segments with an auditory signal toward which the user walks), specific objects (e.g., furniture), locations (e.g., office, laboratory, or shop), or transitions (e.g., carpet to tile, curb cuts). It is important that the presentation of auditory information not interfere with natural environmental cues (e.g., sounds of traffic, water, etc.).

A major difficulty in electronic travel aids is the identification of obstacles against a busy or cluttered background. Sonification is the process by which environmental data are transformed into auditory signals to allow interpretation or communication (Nagarajan et al., 2004). In a natural environment, background objects can dominate the sonification "image." To overcome this problem, Nagarajan, Yaacob, and Sainarayanan used signal processing that mimics the natural human eye. Because the system is used in a real-time mode, the processing time for each signal is short (about 0.7 to 1 second). Two primary types of processing are used: edge detection and background suppression. Edge detection highlights the boundaries of key objects in the environment, making them stand out. This is similar to emphasizing borders of objects in a visual image. Because some background objects may be important (e.g., a large tree), the background is suppressed, not eliminated. The end result is that objects that are important for navigation are enhanced and those that are less important are reduced in intensity.

In normal vision, turning the head is used to scan the environment. In the auditory substitution system this technique is also applied, keeping the object of interest in the center of the digital camera used to sense the environment. Stereo signification uses a number of acoustic attributes to add richness to the user display. These attributes include pitch, loudness, timbre (the waveform of the sound that gives a trumpet a different sound than a violin), and location. Localization of objects is aided by the stereo presentation and enhanced by rotating the head and listening to the change in the signals presented to each ear. Nagarajan, Yaacob, and Sainarayanan (2004) describe the signal processing algorithms used in their system.

The simplest devices for assisting with orientation are adapted compasses. The braille compass has the major north, south, east, and west directions labeled in braille and the intermediate points labeled with raised dots. The face opens, much like a braille watch, so that the direction can be felt. The C2 Talking Compass[57] Figure 13-14 uses spoken output to help orient the user. The user points the compass in one direction and presses a button. The compass then speaks the direction as north, east, south, west, or intermediate directions (e.g., north-west). The compass can be purchased with two languages installed, and 20 languages are currently available.

[57] Sensory Tools division of Robotron Group (www.sensorytools.com/c2.htm).

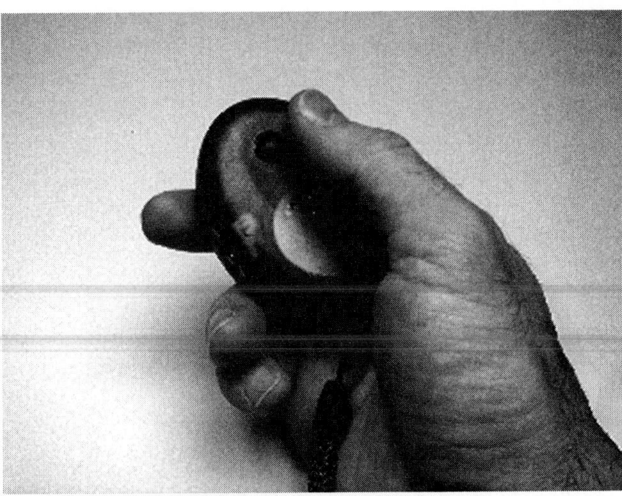

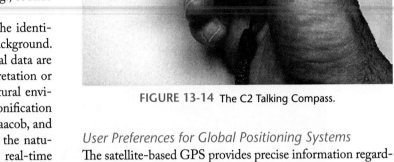

FIGURE 13-14 The C2 Talking Compass.

User Preferences for Global Positioning Systems

The satellite-based GPS provides precise information regarding features, terrain, vehicles, or buildings. It was initially developed for military applications. The GPS technology is ideally suited to use in navigation systems for persons who are blind. Golledge et al. (2004) conducted a survey of blind individuals to determine their preferences for the development of GPS-based navigation aids. The most common problems reported were dealing with street crossings, avoiding unknown obstacle hazards, learning new routes, and taking shortcuts. Difficulty in gaining access to navigational information was identified in several areas, including knowing and keeping track of the direction to walk to a destination, knowing which way the person was facing, knowing that they were at a street corner, where to turn, and the location of specific landmarks such as stores and bus stops. The type of needed navigational information identified (in priority order) was information about landmarks, streets, routes, destinations, buildings, and transit. All participants identified automatic speech recognition (see Chapter 8) as the most desirable form of input to the device. Other highly rated input choices were a QWERTY keyboard, braille keyboard, and telephone keyboard. The most acceptable output device for providing navigational information to the user was a collar- or shoulder-mounted speech or sound device. On the basis of the loss of ambient auditory information when headphones were used, this mode was the least acceptable. The Wayfinding Group is collaborating on the development of GPS-based devices (http://www.senderogroup.com/wayfinding/).

Global Positioning System Displays

To determine the most effective user display for a GPS system, Loomis et al. (2005) evaluated five spatial displays. A **spatial display** is one that provides direct spatial information about the directions and distances to environmental locations relative to the user. The five displays evaluated were (1) virtual speech, (2) virtual tone, (3) haptic pointer interface (HPI), and tone, (4) HPI and speech, and (5) body pointing. The HPI is like the talking sign technology (see below) that can receive an identifying signal that is produced by an environmental object. Virtual speech and tone provide description information that is localized to the direction from which the signal is received by using a stereophonic user display. The HPI used by Loomis et al. consisted of a handheld pointer with a compass attached. Their HPI-based displays provided auditory information (tone or speech) that corresponded to the direction in which the pointer was aimed. The body pointing display was identical to the HPI-tone device except that the compass was mounted on the waist rather than held in the hand. Results indicated that the virtual speech was judged to be the best display; body pointing was preferred to the other HPI options and virtual tone displays. One negative feature of the speech was the use of headphones, which limited ambient input. Alternative auditory displays are mandatory.

GPS-Based Mobility Aids

There are three approaches used for GPS-based systems for the blind traveler: (1) stored digital maps or databases of locations, street names, postal codes; (2) the use of databases only; and (3) systems that have no maps or databases and rely on the user generating the route (Roentgen et al., 2008). If using the first type of device, routes can be planned and information about the user's current location and points of interest in the environment are included. The second type uses only a database with checkpoints along a route to guide the blind traveler. For the third type of device, the user must store a series of announcements (e.g., street names, waypoints, individual points of interest with voice descriptions) that are used as landmarks during travel. All of the GPS-based systems are intended to be used in conjunction with other mobility aids such as a guide dog, cane, or ETA. Examples of each of these categories of navigation aids are described in this section.

One approach uses the PAC Mate Omni (running Windows Mobile 6.0 operating system) as a platform for the StreetTalk VIP software[58] combined with a GPS receiver resulting in a navigation aid with either braille or speech output for the user. The database contains millions of points of interest such as restaurants, banks, and parks. Maps can be purchased for specific regions on flash cards that are inserted into the PAC Mate Omni. Routes that are repeated can be saved to aid in travel. The routes can be printed on embossed paper, uploaded, and saved or emailed to other users.

GPS LookAround[59] is a talking map that can be loaded as an app for both iOS and Android-based products. In operation, a shake of the phone will display the current heading, street, city, cross street, and nearest point of interest (POI). The POI information is based on the selection of a category from a database consisting of points of interest including street names and other points of interest such as bus stops, favorite restaurants, frequently visited shops, friends' houses, public buildings, landmarks, and museums. At the press of a button a "where am I feature" is activated and the LookAround tells the user the current location. Another feature tells the user what points of interest are in the immediate vicinity.

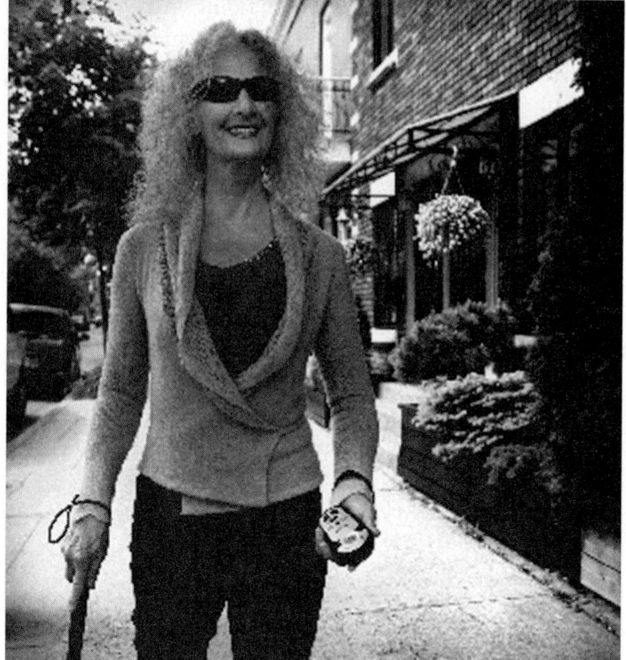

FIGURE 13-15 The Trekker Breeze is a handheld GPS system.

The Trekker Breeze[60] (Figure 13-15) is a palm-sized GPS device that can be controlled by one hand and includes digital maps and a point of interest database. Trekker Breeze verbally announces names of streets, intersections, and landmarks during travel. When a single button is pressed, Breeze speaks the current location. When used in a vehicle, Trekker Breeze speaks the names of intersections. Breeze also provides locations and points of interest in the immediate vicinity of the user. It also records the path for a journey and slows it to be played back to repeat the path. Recording the path can be used to record a path while guided by a sighted person and then play it back for independent travel at a later time. Information can be entered via speech or written text. A wide variety of maps are available covering most Western countries. Maps can be downloaded from the Internet. Trekker Breeze can record landmarks along a route, such as the user's home or favorite restaurant, and they will be announced when the user passes by

The BrailleNote GPS[61] is an accessory to portable braille or voice note takers consisting of software and a cell phone–size GPS receiver. It relays information from GPS satellites that can be used by the portable note taker to calculate where the user is and to plot a route to a destination of choice. The BrailleNote GPS includes GPS software with maps and hundreds of points of interest. The user can calculate the distance and direction to a street address or intersection, find out the relative location of points of interest, automatically

[58] Freedom Scientific (http://www.freedomscientific.com/).

[59] Sendros, Davis, Calif. (www.senderogroup.com/index.htm).

[60] Humanware, Concord, Calif. (http://www.humanware.ca/).

[61] Humanware, Concord, Calif. (http://www.humanware.ca/).

create routes for either walking or riding in a vehicle, and provide detailed information about speed and the direction of travel.

iWalk is a navigation app for people with visual impairments that runs on iPhone, Blackberry, and Android smart phones (Stent et al., 2010). It does not rely on special-purpose hardware. iWalk provides navigation services using real-time turn-by-turn walking directions in speech and text. It includes GPS-enabled navigation services in addition to street names so that users are not forced to read street signs. iWalk accesses various servers in the cloud as needed for functions including: automatic speech recognition, local business search, geocoding and reverse geocoding, and routing. Here is how iWalk would provide navigation to a pizza restaurant (Stent et al., 2010):

During query the user provides information about a location (e.g., a pizza restaurant), giving the name, or address if known.

iWalk collects the user's current location from the GPS.

iWalk uses the input query and user location to retrieve up to ten listings from a business listing database comprising tens of millions of listings.

The user can move through the listings using the left and right soft keys, or the Next and Back buttons.

iWalk then presents these listings to the user one-by-one in increasing order of distance from the user's current location.

iWalk might say to the user "Destination: PizzaGrille, 3HeadquartersPlaza, 0.23miles (about 3 minutes)."

When the desired destination is presented, the user can click either on the listing summary or on the Directions button.

iWalk then gives directions using distance and estimated time information as well as street names

Indoor Navigation

The main problem with GPS-only based systems is that they cannot provide guidance when the GPS signal is lost (e.g., indoors and at urban locations with tall buildings). Because GPS signals are not available indoors, some other positioning technology is needed. Wi-Fi tracking has been proposed, but it is accurate only at the room level and could only be used for tasks such as going to a specific seat in a specific room. If maps of indoor spaces are available (and some companies are developing them) then a cloud-based approach for indoor navigation would be possible. The addition of image processing to detect people in the surroundings or optical character recognition to detect signs in the building would further enhance indoor navigation. A database of places previously visited could be stored in the cloud and retrieved when the user revisits.

When indoor navigation is required, the environment is constrained and the technology can be simplified. Ross and Henderson (2005) developed an indoor navigation system called Cyber Crumbs. The concept is to load directions for navigation within a building into a central database. When an individual with a visual disability enters the building, he or she will use an information kiosk to select a desired destination in the building. The kiosk will then compute the most direct route for the person to take and download the route into the user's badge in the form of an ordered list of cyber crumb addresses. The stored speech instructions are provided to the user though a bone conduction headset that does not block the input of natural auditory information. As the individual traverses the course toward the destination, the badge detects each strategically located cyber crumb and updates the instructions accordingly. The cyber crumbs are located at key locations such as elevators, hallway intersections, exits, and entrances. The user's badge has a repeat button. Instructions are repeated only when this button is pressed. In a pilot trial of the cyber crumbs system, visually impaired users improved their performance. In baseline trials without the technology, visually impaired people were 35% as fast as sighted users. With the cyber crumb technology they were 80% as fast as the sighted control group (Ross & Kelly, 2009).

Indoor navigation systems like Cyber Crumbs rely on a particular infrastructure. These systems do not take full advantage of resources made available by cloud computing providers or location-specific resources on the Internet. Angin and Bhargava (2011) describe an alternative approach that takes advantage of currently available infrastructure as well as cloud computing to create a context-rich and extensible navigation system. The primary components of their system design are shown in Figure 13-16. The camera is built into sunglasses to ensure that the image being processed is based on the user's line of gaze. The visual data are combined with an integrated compass and positioning module and computation in the cloud. This proposed system leverages GPS, Wi-Fi access points, and cell tower triangulation to increase the information available to blind travelers. Context-relevant local data, such as crossing guidance at urban intersections, detection of moving/stationary obstacles, and identification of bus stops, are also included. Speech output is used to provide context-relevant feedback to the user and speech recognition is used for the user to query the system. Angin and Bhargava choose the Android mobile platform for development because of its open architecture.

Provision of guidance for crossing at urban intersections is an important aspect of outdoor navigation in busy urban areas. In their conceptual model, Angin and Bhargava (2011) developed a pedestrian signal detector using an Android mobile phone and a cloud -based crossing guidance program running on a cloud server. Their proposed system, shown in Figure 13-17, illustrates some of the issues to be solved and the possibilities provided by combining existing resources locally and in the cloud to achieve enhanced navigation information for the traveler who has a visual impairment. The operation of the system has several steps detailed by Angin and Bhargva (2011, p. 5):

The Android application captures the GPS signal and communicates with the Google Maps Server to detect the current location of the blind user.

Once the application detects that the blind user is at an urban intersection, it triggers the native camera to take a picture (or multiple consecutive pictures) and sends the picture to the server running on the Amazon EC2 Cloud.

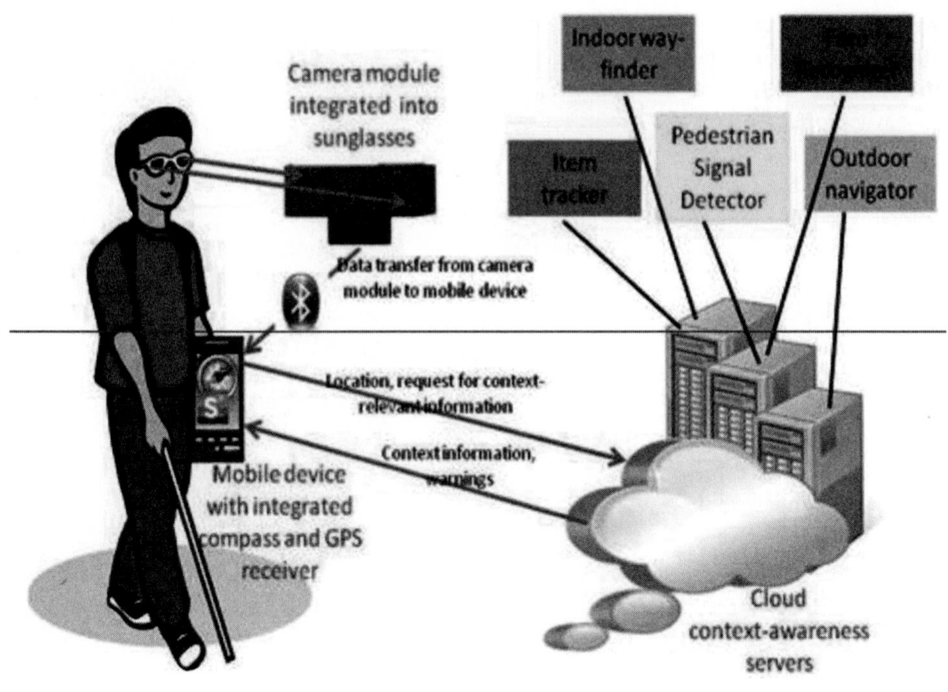

FIGURE 13-16 Proposed enhanced navigation system for blind mobility (system architecture). (Angin and Bhargava, 2011, p. 3.)

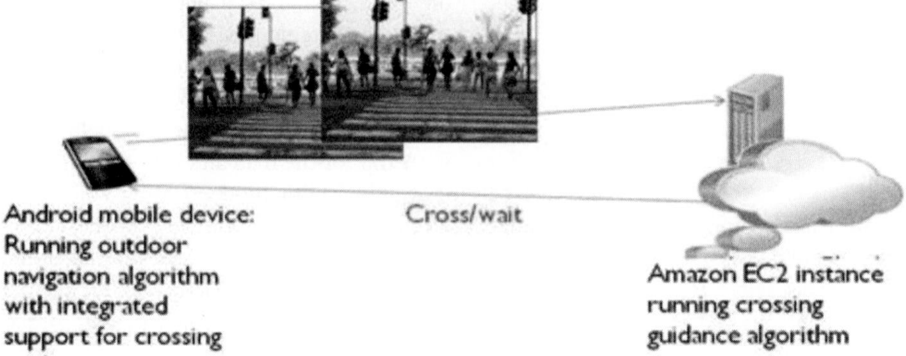

FIGURE 13-17 System architecture for pedestrian signal detector. (Angin and Bhargava, 2011, p.3.)

The server does the image processing, applying the Pedestrian Signal Detection algorithm, and returns the result as to whether it is safe for the user to cross.

The system uses contextual clues, including other pedestrians crossing in the same direction, a crosswalk, and the status of traffic lights in the same direction. This example, which is further detailed by Angin and Bhargva, shows how a mix of local (camera, phone) and cloud-based resources can enhance the information available to the user.

Navigation Aids Based on Environmental Data

Street signs and building signs provide a significant amount of our orientation as sighted travelers. Individuals who are blind or who have trouble reading require that same information in order to maintain their orientation as they travel. The Talking Signs[62] voice message originates at the sign and is transmitted by infrared light to a handheld receiver at a distance. Because of the nature of infrared transmission, the transmission is directionally selective. When the user aims the receiver directly at the sign, the intensity and clarity of the message increases. This change allows the user to focus the Talking Signs system and orient himself or herself to his or her actual location. In order to operate, Talking Signs transmitters must be installed as adjuncts to all signs. This is a large task, but many signs have been installed. Talking Sign can also be used to label objects such as building entrances, drinking fountains, phone booths, or restrooms (Scadden, 1997).

Cloud-Based Navigation Aids for Persons Who Are Blind

One aspect of wayfinding technology is the concept of "smart environments" (Baldwin, 2003). These environments are conceived of as having a series of embedded transmitters (e.g., form signs, intersections, store logos, etc.) that are linked to GPS-based networks and stored maps.

[62] Talking Signs, Inc., Baton Rouge, La. (www.talkingsigns.com).

The location-based technology has two components: a wireless system for labeling, and latitude and longitude geographical databases. These smart environments will be of benefit to the general public (e.g., in navigational aids for traveling) and can be considered part of universal design for the environment (see Chapter 2). If sensors for these networks are built into "wearable computers," the sensing and user display functions will be both unobtrusive and effective in facilitating independent mobility for blind travelers on the basis of existing wayfinding technologies developed for the general public. Baldwin (2003) describes how these mainstream technologies will benefit blind travelers.

Special-Purpose Visual Aids

In developing the HAAT model in Chapter 3, we defined three categories as part of the activity: self-care, work and school, and play and leisure. Persons with blindness or low vision may have needs in each of these areas, and there are special-purpose devices that can provide assistance. These devices are in addition to those serving needs for reading and orientation/mobility, which are used in all three performance areas. In this section we describe some of the special-purpose devices that serve these needs. The American Foundation for the Blind[63] (AFB), Sensory Access Foundation,[64] Smith-Kettlewell Eye Research Institute, Rehabilitation Engineering Center,[65] and New York Lighthouse, Inc.[66] are good sources of information regarding specific needs. Several companies sell large numbers of products for all three performance areas.[67]

Devices for Self-Care

Auditory or tactile substitutes can be used for many household tasks. The American Foundation for the Blind[68] Website lists almost 200 devices for use in household tasks, self-care, and independent living. For example, braille tape (similar to the tape used for labeling, with raised letters) can be used to label canned foods and appliance controls. Another approach to identification of household objects is the use of bar codes and recorded speech (Crabb, 1998). Bar codes are typically used in supermarkets for checkout scanning. However, the codes used are stored in the grocery store computer, so they can't be read at home. Crabb developed a device called the I.D. Mate Quest[69] that allows a sighted individual to sweep a reader over the bar code and then record a short spoken message describing the contents (e.g., "Campbell's tomato soup"). This information is then played back to the user who is blind when he or she scans a similar can at the grocery store. Over 1 million items are contained in the I.D. Mate Quest database. Other household items can also be scanned.

[63] New York City (www.afb.org).
[64] Palo Alto, Calif.
[65] San Francisco, Calif.
[66] New York (www.lighthouse.org).
[67] LS&S Group, Northbrook, Ill. (www.Lssgroup.com); Maxi Aids, Farmingdale, N.Y. (www.maxiaids.com); Independent Living Aids, Inc, Plainsview, N.Y. (www.independentliving.com).
[68] www.afb.org/ProdBrowseCatResults.asp?CatID=3.
[69] En-Vision America, Normal, Ill. (www.envisionamerica.com).

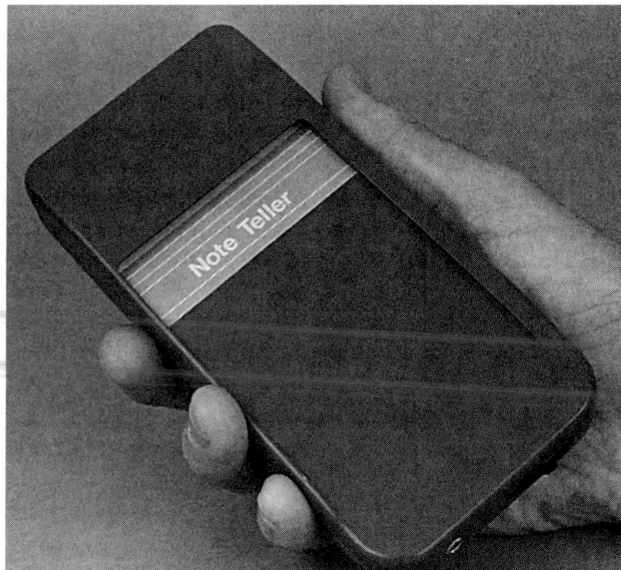

FIGURE 13-18 The Note Teller paper money reading device. (Courtesy Brytech, Nepean, Canada.)

Approximately 90% of the items sold in the United States have bar codes on them, including playing cards, cassette tapes, CDs, and many other items. The I.D. Mate Quest can also be personalized by entering a bar code and recording a corresponding message. This method can be useful for labeling household objects, clothing, and similar personal items.

Digit-Eyes[70] is an app for the iPad and iPhone that reads bar code labels for over 34 million products using VoiceOver. Individualized QR code labels can be made on the Digit-Eyes Website and printed on address labels. The label can be attached to a a calendar or a box of leftovers. Preprinted washable labels can be sewn into clothing with a recorded message about the item (e.g., color, fabric care, or what it should be worn with). Digit-Eyes is available in English, Danish, French, German, Italian, Polish, Portuguese, Norwegian, Spanish, and Swedish.

Voice output is also available on some appliances, such as microwave ovens. Kitchen timers, thermometers, and alarm clocks are available in both enlarged and auditory or tactile forms. Talking wristwatches are used by individuals who are blind. Electrical appliances often have controls marked with tactile labels to allow a blind person to adjust the control. Raised or enlarged print telephone dials can also be obtained from local telephone companies. There are also devices that read paper money and speak the denomination of the bill. These are similar to change machines or those used for automatic purchase of public transportation tickets in many cities. A portable paper money reader is shown in Figure 13-18.[71] When a paper monetary note of $1 to $100 value is inserted into the device, it automatically turns on and speaks the denomination of the note. Both English and Spanish voice outputs are available, and a headphone may be

[70] www.Digit-Eyes.com.
[71] Note Teller2, Brytech, Ottawa, Canada (www.brytech.com).

used for privacy. When the note is removed, the unit automatically turns itself off. Versions specifically for US and Canadian currencies and a universal model are available.

The use of tactile labels (e.g., braille) and speech output have made automatic teller machines (ATMs) usable by both sighted persons and persons with visual impairments. Banking over the Internet is also available for persons who are blind or have low vision. Regulations concerning ATMs are contained in the Americans with Disabilities Act Access Guidelines (ADAAG).[72] In Ontario, Canada, similar legislation is contained in the Accessibility for Ontarians with Disabilities Act (Legislative Assembly of Ontario, 2005). These guidelines provide performance standards for people with vision impairments. To provide nonvisual information from the ATM, braille instructions and control labels are used. For user feedback during use, audible devices and handsets are recommended to provide access while maintaining privacy. Braille output is not required. Touch screens with appropriate software and hardware can also be made accessible to persons who are blind. The major provisions of the standards are[73]: differentiation of each control or operating mechanism by sound or touch, provision of opportunity for input and output privacy, marking of function keys with tactile characters, provision of both visual and audible instructions for operation, dispensing of paper currency (if available) in descending order with the lowest denomination on top, and options to receive a receipt in printed or audible form or both.

Because a leading cause of blindness is diabetes, there are insulin injection devices that provide independence for blind users. Specially adapted syringes and holders for bottles are available. The holder guides the syringe into the bottle, and the syringe can be set to allow only the amount necessary for one dose to be drawn out of the bottle. Other home health care devices include thermometers with speech output and sphygmomanometers (for blood pressure measurement) that use either raised dots on the pressure meter face or synthesized speech output.

Devices for Work and School

The major needs within vocational and educational applications are for access to reading, mobility, and computers. The approaches and devices in the sections on reading and mobility, and computer access in this chapter often meet these needs. To be operated as they were designed, many tools require the use of vision. It is possible to use either tactile or auditory adaptations to make these tools available to individuals who have visual impairments. A carpenter's level with a large steel ball and center tab has an adjustment screw on one end. The screw is calibrated with half a degree of tilt corresponding to one turn. To level the device, the carpenter adjusts the screw until the ball is at the center. The user then knows how many degrees of tilt there are and can correct for the tilt. There is also a tactile tape measure with one raised dot at each quarter-inch mark, two at half-inch increments, and one large dot at each inch mark. Calipers, protractors, and micrometers use a similar labeling scheme. An audible device is used by machinists to determine depth of cut when using a lathe. There are also talking tape measures, calculators, scales, and thermometers. Many of these also have tactile versions.

Many electronic test instruments use digital (numerical) displays, which are easily interfaced to speech synthesizers. The output of the meter (e.g., a voltage measurement by a technician) is heard instead of read. Oscilloscopes are also available in both auditory and tactile forms. Electronic calculators that have speech output provide an alternative to visual display–based devices. It is possible for a person with total visual impairment to perform virtually all the tasks required for electronic or mechanical design, fabrication, and testing by using adapted tools and instruments. The Color Teller (Brytech, Ottawa, Canada, www.brytech.com/) is a handheld device that detects colors, tints, and shades like pink, pale blue-green, dark brown, and vivid yellow. The color is spoken in English, French, or Spanish with adjustable volume. It can also be used to determine whether the lights in a room are on or off.

Devices for Play and Leisure

Almost any common board game can be obtained in enlarged form. There are also enlarged and tactually labeled playing cards, and braille or other versions exist for common board games and dice. Computer games that emphasize text rather than graphics can be used with computer screen reading software.

More active games include "beeper ball," in which auditory signals replace visual cues. In this softball-like game, the ball contains an electronic oscillator that emits a beeping sound. The batter can aim for the sound. Bases are also labeled with sounds. Similar approaches are available for playing Frisbee, soccer, and football. In each case the object to be thrown or kicked emits a beep and goals are labeled with auditory markers. Individuals who are blind can snow ski with the assistance of both sighted guides and auditory signals from barriers such as slalom poles and fences.

CASE STUDY 13-5

Changing Needs for Visual Aids

Ken has enrolled this fall semester as a student at the state college. He has retinitis pigmentosa. Retinitis pigmentosa is a midperipheral ring scotoma that gradually widens with time so that central vision is frequently reduced by middle age. Night blindness occurs much earlier, and total blindness may eventually ensue. Ken has recently noticed that his vision seems to have deteriorated significantly. He would like to study to become a journalist. Ken lives alone in an apartment close to campus so he can walk to school or, when it is raining, take the bus. As Ken's retinitis pigmentosa advances, what types of assistive technology for sensory impairments might be useful to enable him to continue with his activities in the following areas: (1) school, (2) home/self-care, and (3) recreation/leisure?

[72] http://www.access-board.gov/ada-aba/adaag/about/guide.htm#Automated.
[73] Trace Center, University of Wisconsin (trace.wisc.edu).

CONTEXT COMPONENT

There are several important differences between sensory input for reading and for mobility. Inaccuracies in reading result in loss of information, but errors in **orientation and mobility** can result in injury or embarrassment. In a **reading aid** the input is constrained. This means that the information to be sensed is always in a text or graphics form. Although there are differences in text fonts and reading needs, the differences across all reading materials are relatively small.

In mobility, however, the range of possible inputs is large. The blind traveler needs to avoid obstacles as varied as a roller skate and a tree. The environment changes frequently (e.g., a chair is moved to a new location), and the blind person must be able to sense these differences. The obstacles of most concern to blind travelers are bicycles, streets, posts, toys, ladders, scaffolding, overhanging branches, and awnings. We define the environmental input required for mobility as being unconstrained because these changes are not predictable and cover a wide range of inputs. To be successful, the design and specification of mobility aids for blind persons must take into account these factors.

Individuals who have low vision or blindness describe several types of problems in accessing and using cell phones (Kane et al., 2009). Environmental lighting dramatically affects readability for people with low vision, and this is made worse by fatigue. The most common assistive devices used are portable braille note takers with phone capabilities. The relatively high cost of specialized assistive technologies lead many participants to opt for standard devices even if the devices were less effective in meeting their needs. Some also mentioned that there was an inherent stigma in using an assistive device because it identified them as disabled whereas using a standard commercial device did not (Kane et al., 2009).

The embedded environment and the cloud (see Chapter 2) provide an important environment for navigation aids and applications requiring large amounts of content. Mobile technologies linked to this environment provide intelligent personal assistants that are invisible, and enhanced functionality can be provided without having an impact on the physical size and weight of the mobile technologies used.

The use of the ambient environment and cloud servers for storage of personal data and profiles also presents challenges in terms of **privacy** (Angin & Bhargava, 2011). For example, if a blind user submits location information to the cloud there are concerns that this information could be used to locate the user and harm or exploit him or her. If the blind user submits information about personal contacts to the cloud for later use in making phone calls or navigating to their location it creates the possibility of security concerns for both the user of the service and all those who are identified as contacts. "The data submitted could include pictures (of the people in the immediate environment of the user), phone number (which could be of use in cell-phone based tracking) and address (to deduce the likelihood of a person's being at a specific place at a specific time) of a contact, which are all part of personally identifiable information" (Angin & Bhargava, 2011, p. 9). Older adults may reject the use of canes because they believe canes make them look vulnerable—which is an element of the social environment.

ASSESSMENT

Visual Function

Visual function is measured by several parameters. Those most important for assistive technology applications are discussed in this section.

Visual Acuity

Visual acuity is measured by determining the refractive index of the eye, and is usually reported in terms of the Snellen chart in which letters are read from a fixed distance. The results are reported as the relative distance at which a normal person would be able to read the letters that the person being tested is reading at 20 feet (6 meters). Three methods are used to report this score. In the United States and some other countries, the score is reported as a fraction. A value of 20/20 means that the person's vision is normal. The metric equivalent is 6/6. In some countries a decimal is used in which 1.0 is normal. Better than normal would be 20/10, 6/3, and 2.0. The World Health Organization definitions for levels of visual impairment based on visual acuity are shown in Table 13-2.

A visual impairment does not mean the individual has no ability to see. Frequently, persons with a visual impairment have some vision, but the level of impairment interferes with function. The Participation and Activity Limitation Survey (PALS) (Statistics Canada, 2006) defines low vision as difficulty seeing someone from a distance of 12 feet or reading a newspaper despite the use of corrective lenses. In other words, even with vision correction devices such as glasses, visual abilities are still limited, although the individual is able to see some things.

Visual Accommodation

In the normal eye at rest, distant objects are focused on the retina. As the object is brought closer, the image falls in front of the retina unless the curvature of the lens is changed. Visual accommodation is the process by which the ciliary muscles change the curvature of the lens and hence the focal point of the eye. For a person less than 20 years of age with normal visual accommodation, the eye is able to accommodate for an object located at about 10 cm. Ability to accommodate decreases as an individual ages. For example, at age 50 years the eyes cannot accommodate to objects closer than approximately 30 cm. This situation leads to the prescription of reading glasses. Many types of disabilities affect accommodation; limitations in accommodation are referred to as *accommodative insufficiency*, which can be a significant factor when assistive technologies are used. For example, if a person is using a keyboard device with a visual display, the separation of these two system components may require constant accommodation as visual gaze is directed at

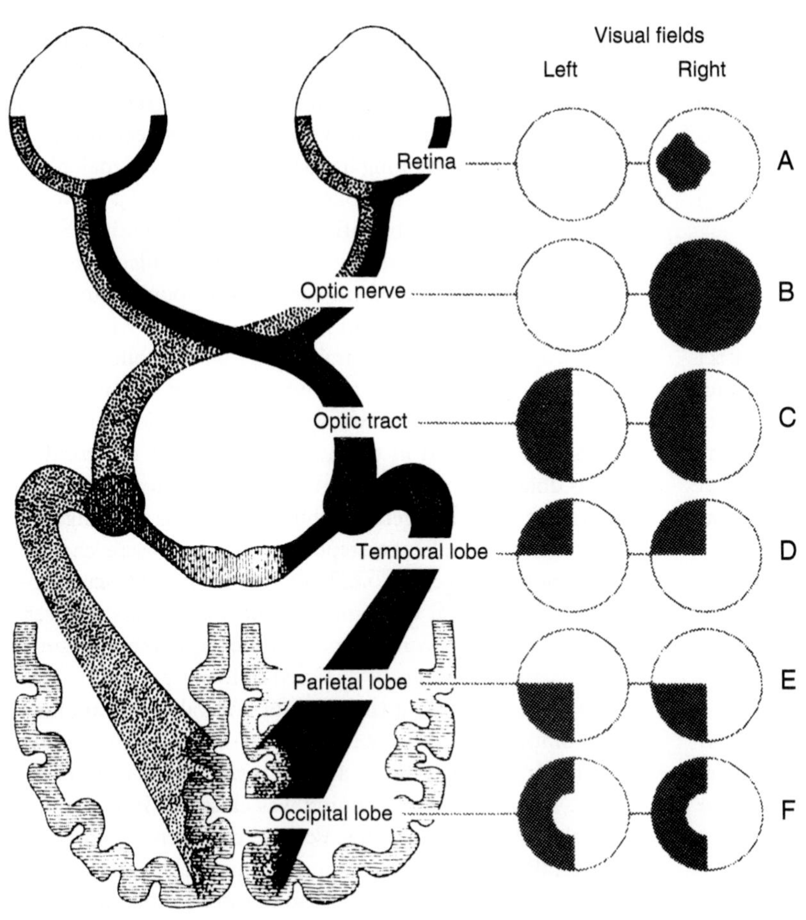

FIGURE 13-19 Types of visual field deficits. **A,** Retinal lesion: blind spot in the affected eye. **B,** Optic nerve lesion: partial or complete blindness in that eye. **C,** Optic tract or lateral geniculate lesion: blindness in the opposite half of both visual fields. **D,** Temporal lobe lesion: blindness in the upper quadrants of both visual fields on the side opposite the lesion. **E,** Parietal lobe lesion: contralateral blindness in the corresponding lower quadrants of both eyes. **F,** Occipital lobe lesion: contralateral blindness in the corresponding half of each visual field, but with macular sparing.

the keyboard and then at the display and back to the keyboard. Appropriate placement of the keyboard and visual display can reduce the amount of accommodation that is required and can result in significantly improved overall system performance.

Visual Field

Another measure of visual function is visual field. With the head and eyes fixed on a central point, the normal range of peripheral vision in the right eye is 70 degrees to the left and 104 degrees to the right (Bailey, 1989). If the eyes are allowed to rotate but the head remains fixed, the range is 166 degrees to each side of the central point. The WHO standard states that "If the extent of the visual field is taken into account, patients with a visual field of the better eye no greater than 10° in radius around central fixation should be placed under category 3" [in Table 13-2 (World Health Organization, 2010, p. 51)].

This typical visual field may be altered in several ways by disease or injury to the eyes, visual pathways, or brain. The most common types of visual field deficits are shown in Figure 13-19. Visual loss may occur in one or more of the quadrants of the left or right field. Dunn (1991) discusses the major causes of these losses. These types of losses are common in persons with disabilities such as cerebral palsy, traumatic brain injury, and diseases affecting the eyes and visual system. When assistive technology systems are specified and designed, the size and nature of the individual's visual field must be taken into account.

Orientation and Mobility Assessment

Because of the large number of options for display and sensing and the unconstrained environmental data when developing auditory navigation systems, Walker and Jeffrey (2005) used a virtual environment as a developmental tool. This approach allows the control of environmental obstacles, the evaluation of alternative user display technologies and formats, and alternative environmental sensing methods. They used this virtual environment to develop the System for the Wearable Audio Navigation (SWAN) and evaluated it with both blind and sighted subjects. Three different sound beacon maps were evaluated. A broadband noise beacon provided the best performance because it was easy to localize. Their study also showed that practice significantly improved performance, even over a short number of trials. Walker and Jeffrey also concluded that the virtual environment training carried over to natural environmental navigation. They also found few differences in performance by blind and sighted individuals.

Mobility performance can be quantified using an indoor mobility course, with various obstacles that must be avoided (Leat & Lovie-Kitchin, 2006). Measurements include the time taken to complete the course and the number of errors (mobility incidents or collisions with objects). Parameters typically measured include: mobility errors, walking speed, preferred walking speed (PWS—no obstacles), D: percentage preferred walking speed (PPWS—with obstacles), visual object detection distance (VDD), and visual object identification distance (VID).

OUTCOMES

Throughout this chapter we have discussed outcome studies relating to specific devices. There are also measures related to more global outcomes such as computer use and the effect of user training. Assistive technologies that support reading are effective both for individuals who have low vision and those who are blind. Screen readers provide access to computers. Carefully designed Websites enable access by blind and partially sighted individuals. There are also studies that have looked at more global issues.

To obtain more detailed information about the computer usage patterns of individuals who have visual impairments, Gerber (2003) conducted a series of focus groups. Four focus groups were used, three at national conferences and one based on subscribers to a technology and visual impairment publication (*Access World: Technology and People With Visual Impairments*, American Foundation for the Blind, New York, http://www.afb.org/). Half the participants reported no usable vision, and the other half had variable amounts of vision. Half the respondents had been blind since birth, 85% had some university education, and 73% were employed. This sample represents the group of visually impaired individuals who use computers and the Internet, but it is not representative of the broader visually impaired community. The leading reason why technology was important and helpful was access to employment and the creation of flexibility in finding work. For some individuals, computer access allowed telecommuting and access to employment from home. The computer also allowed employed individuals to create a cultural identity by being successfully employed.

The second major benefit of computer use identified was access to information, including newspapers and magazines as well as Web-based sources. This benefit is only recently available because more and more information is available digitally through the Internet. Independence in obtaining this information was a major benefit identified. Respondents talked about how rewarding it was to read for themselves using technology rather than have someone read to them. Improvement in writing skill was identified as a benefit of computer use.

A final benefit identified by the focus group participants was the social connections made through the Internet, such as independently sending and receiving email using adapted computers. Participation in online discussion groups related to their disability or to other topics of interest helped remove feelings of isolation and loneliness. Lack of training and not having accessible training materials were identified as a major barrier to computer use. Getting help in an accessible form was identified as a major difference between users who had visual impairments and those who did not. Being shut out of advances because of lack of accessibility, especially as computers and software change, was a major fear for many of the participants. For example, if a new version of Windows is developed, it may not be compatible with the accessible screen reader or braille display the person has been using.

Because lack of training has been identified as a major barrier to computer access, Wolfe (2003) conducted a survey of public and private rehabilitation agencies in the United States to determine the availability of training specifically related to individuals with visual impairments. Group technology-related training (general and job related) was provided more frequently than individual training by both public and private agencies. A variety of products including screen readers, screen magnifiers, web browsers, CCTVs, and electronic note takers were included in the training. These are all described in this chapter. The demand for training was reported to be far greater than the agencies' ability to provide training. The major training challenges reported by Wolfe were changes in technology requiring staff upgrading, lag between new advances in general consumer products and accessible versions, availability of computers and other equipment to use in training, and a shortage of qualified trainers.

To learn more about the need for and value of training, a series of focus groups were held with visually impaired adults who had received training and with trainers (Wolfe et al., 2003). The adequacy of training was clustered into positive, neutral, and negative groups. Positive comments focused on the overall quality of the training, greater self-confidence of the trainees after training and (to a lesser extent) the quality of the trainers. Neutral comments reflected adequacy of the training in general rather than specific areas of training. Negative comments fell into six areas, including (1) training was too short or too infrequent, (2) too few computers were available for hands-on practice, (3) training was not relevant to technology available on the job, (4) the pace of training was too slow or too fast, (5) material was presented at too basic a level, and (6) there was too much variability in trainee experience that limited content that could be covered. The trainers focused on issues of curricular content and trainee preparation for training, but there was no consistency in either of these areas. The need to stay abreast of technology changes was also a challenge listed by this group.

SUMMARY

For persons who have low vision, it is possible to improve performance by increasing size, contrast, and spacing of the text material. Low-cost magnification aids and filters can help in this regard, but electronic aids provide much greater flexibility. Reading aids for persons who are blind rely on either tactile or auditory substitution. The most effective of these are language based (e.g., speech or braille). Fully automated reading devices are capable of imaging print documents and converting them to speech by use of voice synthesis.

ETAs for persons who are blind serve a useful but limited purpose in aiding mobility and orientation for blind travelers. Just as reading aids use alternative sensory pathways of auditory and tactile input, so do ETAs. The basic structure of a sensory aid shown in Figure 13-1 applies to ETAs as well as to reading aids. The environmental interface is either a light (laser or infrared emitter and sensor) or sound (ultrasound), and the user display is either an auditory tone or series of tones of varying frequency and amplitude or tactile vibration. The information processor converts the reflected light or ultrasound information to the audible or tactile display information presented to the user. Current technology provides only limited substitution or augmentation for the long cane. By concentrating on achieving input that is more informative regarding obstacles and the orientation and location of objects in the environment, the utility of these devices will be greatly enhanced. Electronic aids that assist blind travelers with orientation are also available; some make use of GPS information.

Mobile technologies are being exploited increasingly for both reading and mobility/navigation applications. Apps for Android, iOS, and Blackberry platforms are available.

STUDY QUESTIONS

1. What are the two basic approaches to sensory aids in terms of the sensory pathway used?
2. List the three basic parts of a sensory aid and describe the function of each part.
3. What is visual accommodation, and how can it affect assistive technology use?
4. What are the three major characteristics that can be changed to increase visual input?
5. If you knew that a person with whom you were working had a severe peripheral visual loss, what color of stimulus would you use to try to maximize visibility (refer to Figure 13-4)?
6. Compare the visual, auditory, and tactile systems in terms of their basic function and as substitutes for each other.
7. What is a GUI? What advantages does it provide for persons with disabilities?
8. What special problems does the GUI present for persons who are blind?
9. What are the features included in mainstream accessibility options that assist individuals who have low vision or blindness?
10. What are the three factors that must be considered when accommodating for low vision? How are they normally dealt with in access software?
11. What are optical and nonoptical aids for low vision?
12. What are the three modes used in screen magnification software?
13. What are the primary assistive technology approaches to assisting individuals who have visual field problems?
14. What is the primary tactile method used for computer output?
15. What special adaptations are made to a braille cell specifically for computer output use?
16. What does the term *navigation* mean in describing a screen magnification or screen reading program?
17. Describe the major benefits of computer use reported by individuals who are blind or who have low vision.
18. What are the major barriers to computer use reported by individuals who are blind or who have low vision?
19. What is a Web browser? What features are necessary in a Web browser to ensure that people who have disabilities can use it?
20. List the major features of accessible Websites. What tools are typically used to test accessibility of Websites?
21. What are the major challenges for people with low vision or blindness in using mobile technologies, including smart phones and tablets?
22. What are the major differences in the effects of errors in low vision and blindness devices for devices for reading and those developed for mobility?
23. What are the major limitations of the long cane for use as a mobility aid by persons who are blind?
24. What is an electronic travel aid?
25. What are the major assistive technologies applied to orientation for people who are blind?
26. How are GPS systems used to aid people who are blind?
27. Pick a tool or measurement instrument and figure out how to adapt it for both a person with low vision and one who is blind. Repeat for a task of daily living such as food preparation and for a recreational activity.

REFERENCES

Angin P, Bhargava BK: Real-time mobile-cloud computing for context-aware blind navigation, *Proceedings of the Federated Conference on Computer Science and Information Systems*, pp. 985–989, 2011.

Bailey RW: *Human performance engineering*, ed 2, Englewood Cliffs, NJ, 1989, Prentice Hall.

Baldwin D: Wayfinding technology: A roadmap to the future, *J Vis Impair Blindness* 97:612–620, 2003.

Blenkhorn P, Gareth D, Baude A: Full-screen magnification for Windows using directx overlays, *IEEE Trans Neural Syst Rehabil Eng* 10:225–231, 2002.

Boyd LH, Boyd WL, Vanderheiden GC: The graphical user interface: Crisis, danger, and opportunity, *J Vis Impair Blindness* 84:496–502, 1990.

Cook AM: Sensory and communication aids. In Cook AM, Webster JG, editors: *Therapeutic medical devices*, Englewood Cliffs, NJ, 1982, Prentice-Hall.

Crabb N: Mastering the code to independence, *Braille Forum* June:24–27, 1998.

Doherty JE: *Protocols for choosing low vision devices*, Washington, DC, 1993, National Institute on Disability and Rehabilitation Research.

Dunn Winnie: Sensory Dimensions of Performance. In Christiansen C, Baum C, editors: *Occupational Therapy: Overcoming Human Performance Deficits*, Thorofare, NJ, 1991, Slack.

Emiliani P, Stephanidis C, Vanderheiden G: Technology and inclusion—Past, present and foreseeable future, *Technol Disabil* 23(3):101–114, 2011.

Farmer LW: Mobility devices, *Bull Prosthet Res* 30:41–118, 1978.

Fruchterman JR: In the palm of your hand: A vision of the future of technology for people with visual impairments, *J Vis Impair Blindness* 97:585–591, 2003.

Galloway NR, Amoaku WMK, Galloway PH, et al.: *Common diseases of the eye*, ed 3, London, 2006, Springer-Verlag.

Gerber E: The benefits of and barriers to computer use for individuals who are visually impaired, *J Vis Impair Blindness* 97:536–550, 2003.

Gerber E, Kirchner C: Who's surfing? Internet access and computer use by visually impaired youth and adults, *J Vis Impair Blindness* 95:176–181, 2001.

Gilbert C, Foster A: Childhood blindness in the context of VISION 2020: the right to sight. *Bulletin of the World Health Organization*, 79(3), 227–232, 2001. Retrieved September 19, 2014, from http://www.scielosp.org/scielo.php?script=sci_arttext&pid=S0042-96862001000300011&lng=en&tlng=en. 10.1590/S0042-96862001000300011.

Golledge RG, et al.: Stated preference for components of a personal guidance system for nonvisual navigations, *J Vis Impair Blindness* 98:135–147, 2004.

Griffin HG, et al.: Using technology to enhance cues for children with low vision, *Teaching Except Child* 35:36–42, 2002.

Grotta D, Grotta SW: Desktop scanners: What's now…what's next, *PC Mag* 17:147–188, 1998.

Guerreiro T, Lagoa P, Nicolau H, et al.: From tapping to touching: Making touch screens accessible to blind users, *Accessibility and Assistive Technologies*, pg 48–50, IEEE, 1070-986X/08/, 2008.

Hayes F: From TTY to VDT, *Byte* 15:205–211, 1990.

Huber MJ, Simpson R: Recognizing the plans of screen reader users: Proceedings of the *AAMA*S 2004 *workshop on modeling and other agents from observation* (MOO 2004), New York, NY: www.marcush.net/irs_papers.html. Accessed March 8, 2006.

Kane SK, Jayant C, Wobbrock JO et al: Freedom to roam: a study of mobile device adoption and accessibility for people with visual and motor disabilities, *ASSSETS '09, Pittsburgh, PA, USA*, pp. 115–122, 2009.

Kerscher G, Hansson K: Consortium—Developing the next generation of digital talking books (DTB): *Proceedings of the CSUN conference*, 1998. http://www.dinf.org/csun_98_065.htm.

Kirman JH: Tactile communication of speech: A review and analysis, *Psychol Bull* 80:54–74, 1973.

Lazzaro JL: Helping the web help the disabled, *IEEE Spectrum* 36:54–59, 1999.

Lazzaro JL: *Adaptive technology for learning and work environments*, ed 2, Chicago, 2001, American Library Association.

Leat SJ, Lovie-Kitchin E: Measuring mobility performance: Experience gained in designing a mobility course, *Clin Exper Optom* 89(4):215–228, 2006.

Legge GE, Madison CM, Mansfield JS: Measuring braille reading speed with the MNREAD test, *Vis Impair Res* 1(3):131–145, 1999.

Loomis JM, et al.: Personal guidance system for people with visual impairment: A comparison of spatial displays for route guidance, *J Vis Impair Blindness* 99:219–232, 2005.

Ma L et al.: Effective computer access using an intelligent screen reader, *Proc 26th RESNA Conf*, Atlanta, 2004, Rehabilitation Engineering and Assistive Technology Society of North America.

Mahmud JU, Borodin Y, Ramakrishnan I: Assistive browser for conducting web transactions. In *IUI '08*: *Proceedings of the International Conference on Intelligent User Interface*, Canary Islands, Spain, January 13–16, 2008, pp 365–368.

Mellor CM: *Aids for the '80's*, New York, 1981, American Foundation for the Blind.

Nagarajan R, Yaacob S, Sainarayanan G: Computer aided vision assistance for human blind, *Integrated Computer-aided Eng* 11:15–24, 2004.

Nye PW, Bliss JC: Sensory aids for the blind: A challenging problem with lessons for the future, *Proc IEEE* 58:1878–1879, 1970.

Oliveira J, Guerreiro T, Nicolau H, et-al: Blind people and mobile touch-based text-entry: acknowledging the need for different flavors, *Proceedings of ASSETS'11*, October 24–26 2011 Dundee, UK 2011

Ontarians with Disabilities Act, Bill 118, Chapter 11 of Statutes of Ontario, Legislative Assembly of Ontario, 2005.

Ramsey VK, Blasch BB, Kita A, et al.: A biomechanical evaluation of visually impaired persons' gait and long-cane mechanics, *J Rehab Research Dev* 36(4):323–332, 1999.

Ratanasit D, Moore M: Representing graphical user interfaces with sound: A review of approaches, *J Vis Impair Blindness* 99:69–93, 2005.

Roentgen UR, Gelderblom GJ, Soede M, et al.: Inventory of electronic mobility aids for persons with visual impairments: A literature review, *J Vis Impair Blindness* 102:702–724, 2008.

Ross DA, Henderson VL: Cyber crumbs: an indoor orientation and wayfinding infrastructure: *Proceedings of the 28th Annual RESNA Conference*, June 2005, http://www.resna.org/ProfResources/Publications/Proceedings/2005/Research/TCS/Ross.php. Accessed November 26, 2005.

Ross DA, Kelly GW: Filling the gaps for indoor wayfinding, *J Vis Impair Blindness* April:229–234, 2009.

Sardegna J, Shelly S, Rutzen AR, et al.: *The encyclopedia of blindness and vision impairment*, Facts on File, 2002. New York, NY.

Scadden LA: Technology for people with visual impairments: a 1997 update, *Technol Dis* 6:137–145, 1997.

Servais SP et al.: Visual aids. In Webster JG, editor: *Electronic devices for rehabilitation*, New York, 1985, John Wiley.

Skellenger A: Trends in the use of alternative mobility devices, *J Vis Impair Blindness* 93:516–521, 1999.

Smedema SM, McKenzie AR: The relationship among frequency and type of Internet use, perceived social support, and sense of well-being in individuals with visual impairments, *Disabil Rehabil* 32(4):317–325, 2010.

Smith GC: The Stereotoner—A new sensory aid for the blind, *Proc Annu Conf Eng Med Biol* 14:147, 1972.

Stelmack JA, et al.: Patient's perceptions of the need for low vision devices, *J Vis Impair Blindness* 97:521–535, 2003.

Statistics Canada: The 2006 Participation and Activity Limitation Survey: Disability in Canada, 2006, http://www5.statcan.gc.ca/bsolc/olc-cel/olc-cel?lang=eng&catno=89-628-X. Accessed January 20, 2014.

Stent A, Azenko S, Stern B, (2010) iWalk:ALightweight NavigationSystemforLow-VisionUser, *ASSETS' 10.* October 25–27, 2010. Orlando, Florida, USA, 2010, ACM978-1-60558-881-0/10/10.

Tobias J: Information technology and universal design: An agenda for accessible technology, *J Vis Impair Blindness* 97:592–601, 2003.

Walker BN, Jeffery J: Using virtual environments to prototype auditory navigation displays, *Assist Technol* 17:72–81, 2005.

Wolfe KE: Wired to work: An analysis of access technology training for people with visual impairments, *J Vis Impair Blindness* 97:633–645, 2003.

Wolfe KE, Candela T, Johnson G: Wired to work: A qualitative analysis of assistive technology training for people with visual impairments, *J Vis Impair Blindness* 97:677–694, 2003.

World Health Organization, Cumulative Official Updates to the ICD-10 (pp. 51–52), 2010, http://www.who.int/classifications/icd/Official_WHO_updates_combined_1996_2009VOL1.pdf, accessed January 20, 2014.

Zelek JS, et al.: A haptic glove as a tactile-vision sensory substitution for wayfinding, *J Vis Impair Blindness* 97:621–632, 2003.

CHAPTER 14

Sensory Aids for Persons with Auditory Impairment

CHAPTER OUTLINE

LEARNING OBJECTIVES

On completing this chapter, you will be able to do the following:

1. Describe the major types of hearing loss and their cause.
2. Describe the types of hearing aids and their features.
3. List ways that people who are hard of hearing or deaf can use telephones.
4. Describe how common devices can be adapted for use by a person who is hard of hearing or deaf.
5. Discuss the major approaches used to support communication for individuals who are deaf and blind.
6. Describe how computer outputs are adapted for individuals with auditory limitations.

KEY TERMS

Accessibility Options
Alerting Devices
Alternative Sensory Pathway
Assistive Listening Devices
Captioning
Closed Captioning
Cochlear Implants
Environmental Sensor
Hearing Aids
Hearing Carry-Over
Short Message Service
User Display
Voice Carry-Over

When an individual has a sensory impairment, access to information via vision or hearing is restricted. Assistive technologies can provide assistance with the input of information via sensory systems. In this chapter we focus on assistive technologies designed to meet the needs of persons with auditory limitations. This includes sensory aids that are intended for *general use* as well as assistive technologies that are used specifically for providing auditory access to computers.

ACTIVITY COMPONENT

Impairment of auditory function has two major effects: loss of input information and inability to monitor speech output. The latter can result in significant difficulties in oral communication. There are several assistive technology approaches to providing oral communication assistance to persons who have an auditory impairment. One approach is to provide feedback, either visual or tactile, that represents the person's speech patterns and relates them to typical speech. A second approach is to provide alternatives to oral communication, such as visual displays that are read by the listener. These and other approaches are discussed in this chapter. Assistive technologies can provide great improvement in the lives of persons who have either partial or total auditory impairments.

HUMAN COMPONENT

Auditory Function

Auditory function can be measured in several ways. *Auditory thresholds* include both the *amplitude* and *frequency* of audible sounds. The amplitude of sound is measured in decibels (dB). The minimal threshold for normal hearing is 25 dB in adults and 15 dB in children. The different cutoff levels for each reflect the fact that children are still acquiring speech and language skills and therefore the demands for hearing are even greater. For perspective, Figure 14-1 shows sound pressure levels for a variety of typical sounds (Bailey, 1989). The typical range of frequencies that can be heard by the human ear is 20 to 20,000 hertz (Hz), but the ear does not respond equally to all frequencies in this range (Martin and Clark, 2012). The ear is most sensitive to sounds that cover the speech frequencies (250 to 8000 Hz). There are several types of tests that audiologists use in assessing hearing. Pure tone audiometry presents pure (one-frequency) tones to each ear and determines the threshold of hearing for that person.

CASE STUDY 14-1

Carolyn

Carolyn frequently goes shopping at a large mall (70 dB background noise) and goes out to dinner often. For dinner, her choice of restaurant may be a noisy fast-food place (70 to 80 dB) or a quiet, elegant restaurant (50 to 60 dB). Because normal conversational levels are approximately 60 dB (see Figure 14-1), the quiet restaurant is more amenable to this activity. With these data, different voice output communication devices can be evaluated to see whether they will meet Carolyn's needs. For example, assume that the specification for system one is a maximum of 50 dB and for system two it is 75 dB; the greater output of system two generally results in a heavier and larger device because the speaker and the batteries must both be larger to allow greater volume output. If some other things are known about Carolyn, such as whether she is able to walk or uses a wheelchair and how stable she is when walking, the extra size and weight can be traded off against the greater output amplitude capability.

Hearing Loss

On the basis of these and other tests, the audiologist determines both the degree of hearing loss and the type of loss. Four types of hearing loss are typically defined (Martin and Clark, 2012). These are (1) conductive loss associated with pathological defects of the outer and/or middle ear, (2) sensorineural loss associated with defects in the cochlea and/or auditory nerve, (3) centrally induced damage to the auditory cortex of the brain, and (4) functional deafness resulting from perceptual deficits rather than physiological conditions. Some patients may have a mixed hearing loss, which is a combination of impairments such as conductive and sensorineural. Auditory impairment is considered slight if the loss is between 20 and 30 dB, mild if from 30 to 45 dB, moderate if from 60 to 75 dB, profound if from 75 to 90 dB, and extreme if from 90 to 110 dB (Martin and Clark, 2012). Causes of hearing loss include congenital loss, physical damage, disease, aging, and effects of medications (Martin and Clark, 2012). These conditions can affect the outer, middle, or inner ear.

FUNDAMENTAL APPROACHES TO AUDITORY SENSORY AIDS

Chapter 13 describes the fundamental approaches to sensory aids. Figure 13-1 applies to auditory as well as visual sensory aids. Augmentation of an existing pathway and use of an alternative pathway are the two basic approaches to sensory assistive technologies. When applied to the auditory system, the alternative pathways are tactile and visual. Each of these approaches is discussed in this chapter.

Augmentation of an Existing Pathway

When someone is hard of hearing, the primary pathway (i.e., the one normally used for input) is still available; it is just limited. Insufficient intensity means that the signals are too weak to be heard, and an amplifier is required. Certain frequencies may be more limited than others for people who are hard of hearing, and the hearing aid must be designed or specified to take this into account. For example, in aging there is usually a greater hearing loss in high rather than low frequencies. Augmentation of the auditory pathway is by use of hearing aids, cochlear implants, bone anchored hearing aids (BAHA), or assistive listening devices (ALDs).

Use of an Alternative Sensory Pathway

There are two alternate sensory pathways available to someone who is deaf. The most common example is the use of manual sign language (visual substitution for auditory). Chapter 14 discusses the fundamental differences among the tactile, visual, and auditory systems.

Tactile Substitution

Substitution of tactile input for auditory information differs from the substitution of tactile input for visual information (i.e., braille). One major difference is that the rate at which the auditory information changes is relatively high compared with the time required for the tactile system to input information. Engineers refer to this as the relative *bandwidths* of the two systems. The auditory system has a broader bandwidth (more information can be handled in a given amount of time) than the tactile system. Because auditory information is a sequence of sounds, these must be translated into tactile information for presentation to the user. These tactile signals are then detected and assembled into meaningful units by the central nervous system. Because the tactile system requires spatial and temporal information, its rate of input is slower than for the auditory system. Another major limitation of the tactile system for auditory input is that it lacks a means of converting sound (mechanical vibrations) into neural signals. This is the function normally carried out by the cochlea.

The only tactile method for input of auditory information that has been successful is the *Tadoma method* used by individuals who are both deaf and blind. In this method, which was used by Helen Keller, the person receives information by placing his or her hands on the speaker's face, with the thumbs on the lips, index fingers on the sides of the nose,

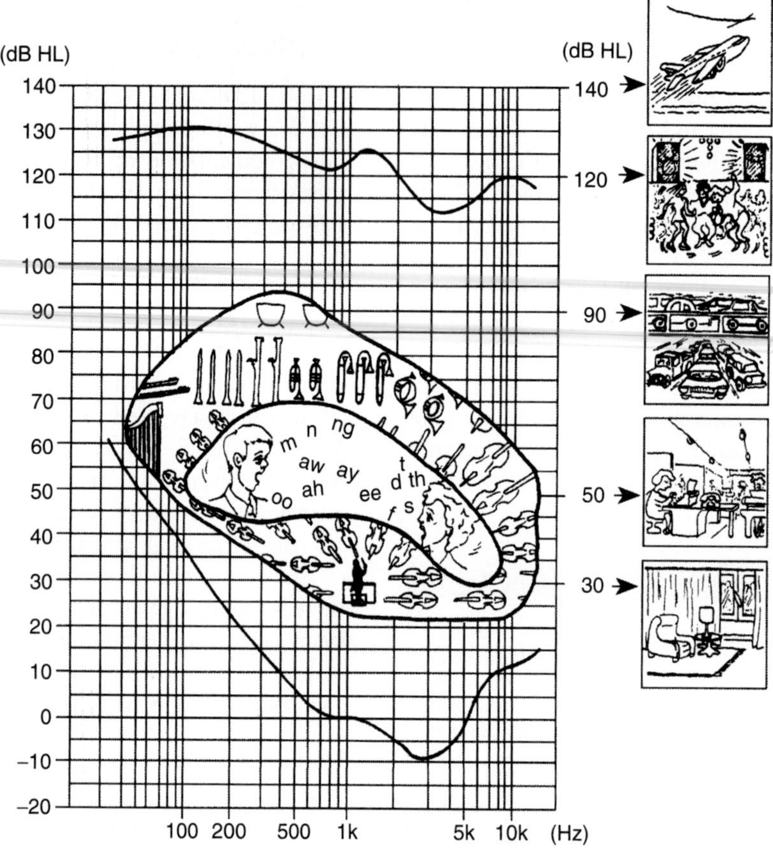

FIGURE 14-1 The sensitivity of the human ear to frequency is shown on the plot. This curve is normalized to zero dB at 1000 Hz. The reference pressure is 0.0002 dynes/cm2. Along each side and in the center of the plot are shown frequencies and intensities of common sounds and speech.

little fingers on the throat, and other fingers on the cheeks. During speech, the fingers detect movements of the lips, nose, and cheeks and feel the vibration of the larynx in the throat. Through practice, kinesthetic input obtained from these sources is interpreted as speech patterns. One reason for the success of this method is that there is a fundamental relationship between the articulators (reflected in the movements of the lips, nose, and cheeks) and the perceived speech signal, and this relationship is at least as important as the acoustic information (pitch and loudness) in the speech signal for individuals using the Tadoma method (Lieberman, 1967).

Visual Substitution

Visual displays of auditory information can take several forms. One example, sometimes used in speech therapy or as an aid to deaf individuals who are learning to speak, is to display a picture of the speech signal on an oscilloscope-like screen. Often a model pattern portraying the ideal is placed on the top half of the screen, and the pattern from the person learning to speak is placed on the bottom half of the screen. The learner attempts to match the model through practice. Some current devices also use computer graphics to make the process more interesting and motivating. This type of sensory substitution of visual for auditory information is a rehabilitative technology that is not practical for assistive technologies. The reasons for this parallel those presented for the Stereotoner in relation to auditory substitution for vision (see Chapter 13).

Visual substitution for auditory information has been successful in several areas. These include visual alarms (e.g., flashing lights when a telephone or doorbell rings) and the use of text labels for computer-generated synthetic speech. Speech is the most natural auditory form of language. Likewise, written text is the most natural way of presenting visual language. Thus, a major design goal for assistive devices that use visual substitution for auditory communication is to provide speech-to-text conversion. In this type of device, speech is received and converted by computer to text and displayed so that the person with an auditory impairment can read it.

AIDS FOR PERSONS WITH AUDITORY IMPAIRMENTS

Hearing Aids

Hearing aids are often conceived of as simple devices that amplify sound, primarily speech. Although hearing aids do contain amplifiers, hearing loss is rarely consistent across the entire speech frequency range, and hearing loss is generally greater at some frequencies than at others. This relationship is taken into account in the design of digital hearing aids. If all frequencies were amplified the same amount, the sound would be unnatural to the user. Subsequently, the hearing aid frequency response is programmed using the measured thresholds or audiogram of the user. The hearing aid response for each ear is matched separately since loss can be different in left and right ears. An additional difficulty encountered in providing hearing aids of high fidelity is that the components are small, and this miniaturization can limit the frequency response of the microphone and speaker, further reducing the quality of the aided speech.

Approximately 60% of the *acoustic energy* of the speech signal is contained in frequencies below 500 Hz (Martin and Clark, 2012). However, the speech signal contains not only specific frequencies of sound but also the organization of these sounds into meaningful units of auditory language (e.g., phonemes), and more than 95% of the *intelligibility* of the speech signal is associated with frequencies above 500 Hz. For this reason, speech intelligibility rather than sound level is often used as the criterion for successful fittings of hearing aids.

Electroacoustical Parameters of Hearing Aids

Hearing aid output is typically specified in decibels (dB) referred to as a standard of 20 micropascals. Sound pressure level (SPL) is used to designate this parameter. Standards for hearing aid specification have been developed by the American National Standards Institute (S3.46, 1997; http://web.ansi.org/) and the *International Electrotechnical Commission* (60 118-0-10; http://www.iec.ch/). These standards allow for the comparison of hearing aids from different manufacturers, and they specify parameters that are used in this comparison.

When hearing aids are fitted, it is important to know the output levels that are delivered from the hearing aid to the listener. Average conversational speech can range from 40 to 80 dB SPL depending on both how far away the talker is from the listener and the talker's vocal effort (Olsen, 1988). Therefore, the hearing aid output is assessed in response to a variety of input types and levels (e.g., pure tones and speech or speech-like signals). Powerful hearing aids are capable of producing output SPLs of 130 to 140 dB. These levels can damage the hearing mechanism even if the duration of the input is short. Therefore, the maximum power output of a hearing aid also needs to be specified to ensure that the level of the hearing aid output will not cause further discomfort or further hearing loss. Dillon (2001) provides a thorough review of the electroacoustical performance and measurement of hearing aids.

Types of Hearing Aids

Conventional hearing aids can be divided into two types: air conduction and bone conduction. All air conduction hearing aids deliver the hearing aid output into the listener's ear canal. However, some people are unable to wear air conduction hearing aids as a result of chronic ear infections or malformed ear canals. For these individuals, a bone conduction hearing aid is most appropriate. The most common type of bone conduction hearing aid is a bone-anchored hearing aid (BAHA) (Figure 14-2). An abutment is surgically attached to the skull, and osseointegration during healing covers the abutment with bone tissue (D'Eredità et al, 2012). Implant stability increases rapidly over the first 2 weeks and becomes stable 3 weeks after surgery. Through a similar process in children, the transcutaneous BAHA implant is screwed into the skull behind the ear a where a snap coupling attaches the sound processor to the implant (Miculek, 2009). Inputs to this type of hearing aid are converted to mechanical waves that vibrate the skull through the implanted abutment. BAHAs take advantage of the fact that, at a sensory level, it does not matter whether sounds come from an air conducted hearing aid or a bone conducted hearing aid (Snik et al, 2005). User evaluations of BAHA performance have shown general satisfaction, including an 18-year retrospective study of adults who received implants (Rasmussen et al, 2012), patients with unilteral conductive hearing loss (Hol et al, 2005), and children (Hickson et al, 2006; Mulla et al, 2013). Specifically, users reported benefits in daily living, sound localization, and speech recognition (when speech and nosie were spatially separated). Challenges reported included localization (for some users), phone use, and lack of availability of ongoing support. The BAHA is also used to address single-side deafness (Kerckhof et al., 2008). FM transmission is provided to link the BAHA to personal FM systems, personal listening devices, and some mobile phones.

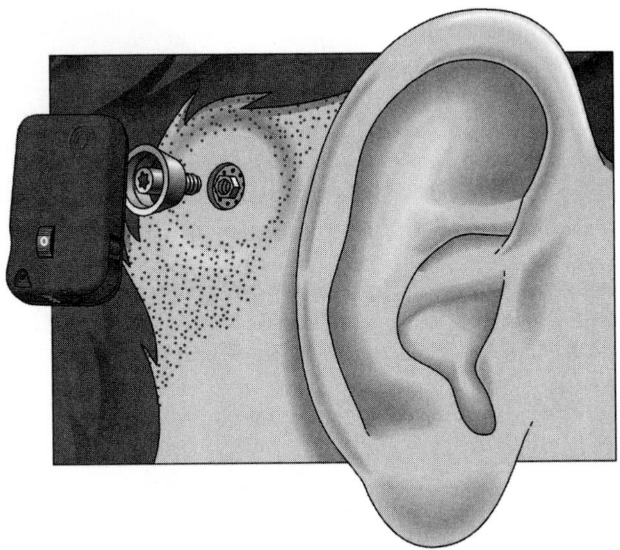

FIGURE 14-2 Bone-anchored hearing aid. (Courtesy Entific Scientific.)

Air conduction hearing aids are available in several different configurations (Palmer, 2009). Figure 14-3 illustrates several commonly used types of aids. The major types of ear-level aids are behind-the-ear (BTE), in-the-ear (ITE), in-the-canal (ITC), and completely-in-the-canal (CIC) aids. Body-level aids are used in cases of profound hearing loss. The processor is larger to accommodate more signal processing options and greater amplification and is mounted at belt level. The body-level aid is usually used only when other types of aids cannot be used.

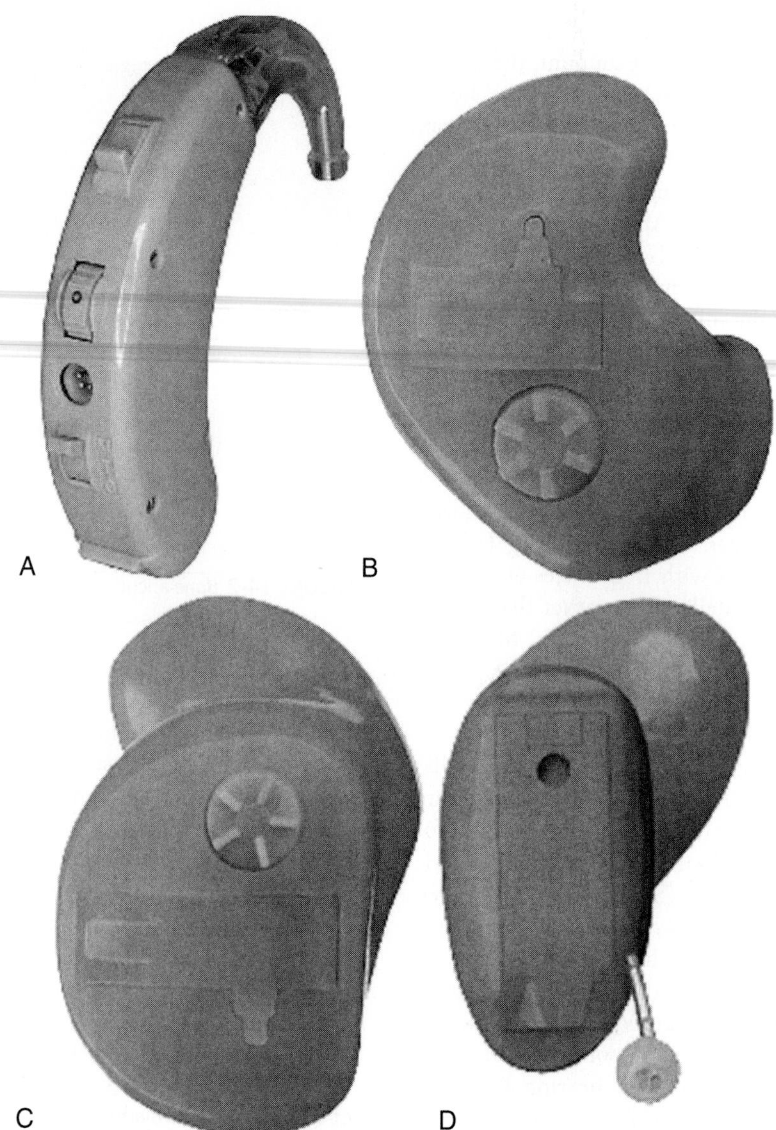

FIGURE 14-3 Types of hearing aids. **A,** Behind the ear (BTE). **B,** In-the-ear (ITE). **C,** In-the-canal (ITC). **D,** Completely in-the-canal (CIC). (Courtesy Siemans Hearing Instruments, Inc.)

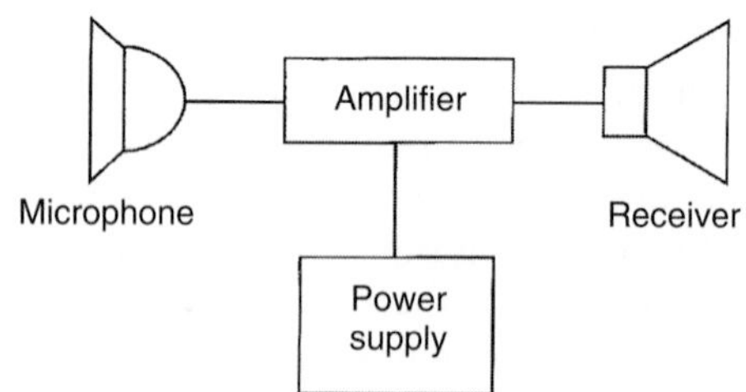

FIGURE 14-4 The major components of a hearing aid.

BTE hearing aids, which fit behind the ear, contain all the components shown in Figure 14-4. The amplified acoustical signal is fed into the ear canal through a small ear hook that extends over the top of the auricle and holds the hearing aid in place. A small tube directs the sound into the ear through an ear mold that serves as an acoustical coupler. This ear mold is made from an impression of the individual's ear to ensure comfort to the user, maximize the amount of acoustical energy coupled into the ear, and prevent squealing caused by acoustic feedback. When the mold is made, a 2-ml space is included between the ear mold and the eardrum. A vent is added to molds (all types) in part to prevent occlusion, improving sound quality for the user, but it can introduce feedback and distortion if the aid is not fit or programmed correctly. Individual anatomy is a great limitation in fitting air conduction hearing aids. An external switch allows selection of the microphone (M), a telecoil (T) for direct telephone reception, or off (O). The MTO switch and a volume control are located on the back of the case for BTE aids.

Some types of hearing loss affect only a portion of the frequency range (usually higher frequencies) with other parts (typically lower frequencies) within the normal range. Hearing aids used for this situation are called *open fit* because they do not use an ear mold. They have a wire that runs to a speaker that fits into the ear canal but does not block out the sounds that are still heard normally. This type is one

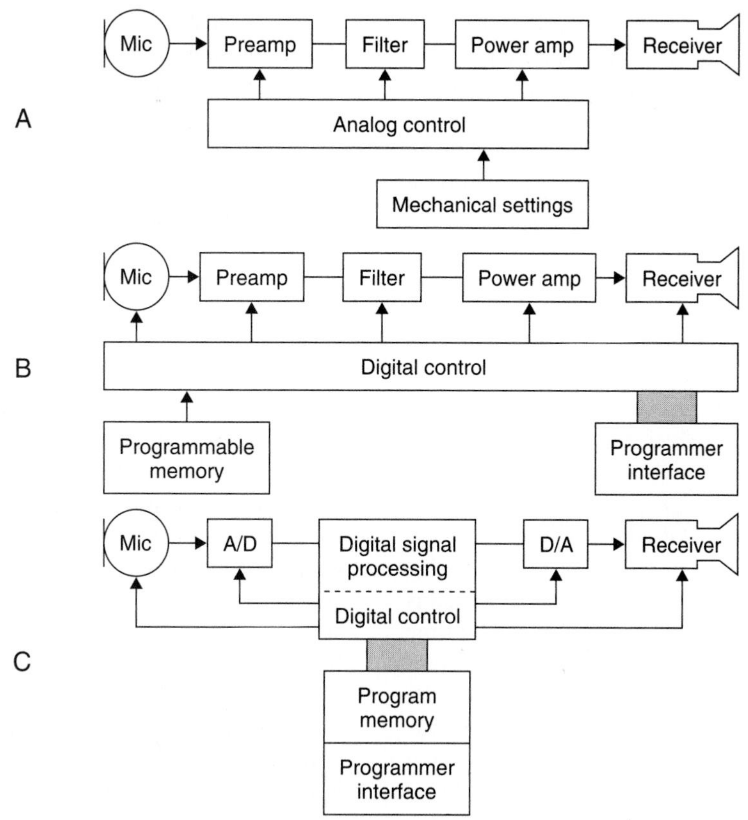

FIGURE 14-5 Three approaches to the electronic design of hearing aids. **A,** An analog hearing aid. **B,** A digitally controlled analog hearing aid. **C,** A digital signal processing hearing aid. (Modified from Stach BA: *Clinical audiology,* San Diego: Singular Publishing Group, 1998.)

form of a receiver-in-the-canal (RIC) model. The receiver (speaker) is connected to the body of the BTE hearing aid case via a wire running down a thin tube. The RIC has a smaller case for the BTE hearing aid while still providing the same amplification power. Open fit aids are often used for individuals whose hearing loss is due to aging. RIC aids can be either open fit or closed (ear mold) fit (Palmer, 2009). Open fit allows for frequencies in the normal range (usually low) to be heard naturally by the person, helping to limit complaints of occlusion. This is possible through advancements in feedback management technology. RICs may also provide more gain because of the increased distance between the microphone and receiver.

The ITE aid makes use of electronic miniaturization to place the amplifier and speaker in a small casing that fits into the ear canal. The faceplate of the ITE aid is located in the opening to the ear canal. The microphone is located in the faceplate. This provides a more "natural" location for the microphone because it receives sound that would normally be directed into the ear (Palmer, 2009). External controls on the ITE include an MTO switch and volume control. The ITC is a smaller version of the ITE. The CIC type of hearing aid is the smallest, and it is inserted 1 to 2 mm into the canal with the speaker close to the tympanic membrane. Because this type does not protrude outside the ear canal, it is barely visible. Any controls for the aid are fit onto the faceplate of the ITE, ITC, and CIC types of aids or connected via remote controls.

Basic Structure of Hearing Aids

Figure 14-5, *A* through *C,* illustrates the basic components of analog and digital hearing aids. The microphone is the **environmental sensor** (see Figure 13-1); it is the component that receives the speech or other sound signal. Overall fidelity of the hearing aid is directly related to the quality of this component. Several types of microphones are used in hearing aids (see Palmer, 2009). The function of the microphone is to convert the sound signal into an electrical signal, which is sent to the amplifier. Microphones may be omnidirectional (amplify sound from any direction) or directional. Directional microphones have a significant benefit in listening in noisy environments (Palmer, 2009). In contrast to an omnidirectional microphone that has equal sensitivity in all directions, a directional microphone is maximally sensitive in the direction the individual is facing and has reduced sensitivity in the back and/or to the sides. By digitally adjusting the response of the microphone, the hearing aid circuitry allows the user to adjust the hearing aid to focus on sounds from the front, left, right, or back (Palmer, 2009).

The information processor (see Figure 2-3) in a hearing aid is the amplifier. It performs several functions. The first and most basic of these is amplification of the input signal with a frequency response (amplifier gain between the input and output, which is different at different frequencies) that is matched to speech signals. Second, the information processor limits loud input signals to prevent distortion and discomfort and to protect the user from damage to the peripheral auditory system. Finally, signal processing is provided to minimize noise and maximize the speech signal.

Digital signal processing allows the hearing aid response to be matched to the acoustic properties of the auditory system of an individual user. Digital hearing aids also have lower distortion, less acoustical feedback, more precise compression of loud signals, and greater fidelity and intelligibility in the speech signal supplied to the ear. Dynamic and comfortable sound level ranges are acquired through proper fitting, including measured discomfort levels. The majority of hearing aids currently in use are digital (Palmer, 2009).

Digital processing allows much greater sophistication in signal processing. One area in which this has been particularly useful is in the differential amplification of speech and reduction in the amplification of noise. The way this is done is to assume that the noise signal is constant and the speech signal is varying over time (Palmer, 2009). The incoming signal is constantly evaluated in terms of whether the signal is varying in intensity over time (noise) or steady state over time (speech). If the signal processing algorithm detects constant signal, it is assumed that the signal is mostly noise and the signal-to-noise ratio is improved by decreasing the microphone sensitivity in the direction of the noise by adjusting the directional microphone. Despite these advances, hearing in background noise remains one of the most challenging tasks for an individual with hearing loss. This is partly because what they often don't want to hear (noise) is actually surrounding speech. Kerckhof, Listenberger, and Valente (2008) describe noise reduction techniques in detail.

The user display (see Figure 2-3) for a hearing aid is the *speaker.* This component is often referred to as the *receiver,* and it converts the electrically amplified signal to an acoustical waveform that is coupled to the ear. The small size of these devices severely limits the frequency response of the hearing aid for signals above the range of speech. As mentioned previously, most receivers are air conduction types, which acoustically couple the speech signal to the ear canal. However, when the middle or outer ear precludes the use of an ear mold (e.g., chronic draining in ears, atresia, absence of the pinna), bone conduction receivers may be required.

Hearing Aid Signal Processing

Digital hearing aids are based on low-power, small, digital signal processing circuits (Palmer, 2009). One of the advantages provided by digital circuitry is the capability of shaping the frequency response of the hearing aid. This provides the possibility of canceling acoustical feedback and increasing the signal-to-noise ratio of the hearing aid (Palmer, 2009). For example, there are programs that amplify speech selectively in a noisy environment. Directional microphones can be adjusted to have an improved signal-to-noise ratio in certain directions (e.g., the side, front or back of the user). Volume levels can be adjusted for each ear independently. These and other features are often controlled through a handheld remote control. Many hearing aids also have a Bluetooth link that can be used with a mobile phone or entertainment appliance (TV, DVD, music player) (Palmer, 2009). The Bluetooth linkage makes it possible for the person using the hearing aid to selectively adjust volume and perform other features (e.g., answering a mobile phone). Since Bluetooth receivers cannot currently be included in the hearing aid body due to power restrictions, some hearing aids include an accessory pendant that hangs around the individual's neck and receives the Bluetooth signal. This signal is then coupled to the hearing aid. Kerckhof, Listenberger, and Valente (2008) describe Bluetooth options for hearing aids in detail.

Cochlear Implants

If there is damage to the cochlea of the inner ear, an auditory prosthesis can provide some sound perception. The first reported use of electrical stimulation of the inner ear was made by the Italian physicist Alessandro Volta (for whom the volt is named) more than 200 years ago. He inserted wires into his ear and connected them to a 50-volt battery, and he experienced an "auditory sensation" when the voltage was applied. More recently, engineers and physiologists have developed sophisticated aids that accommodate for lost cochlear function.

These devices, termed **cochlear implants,** have the components shown in Figure 14-6 (Feigenbaum, 1987). As long as the eighth cranial nerve is intact, it is possible to provide stimulation by use of implanted electrodes. Cochlear implants have been shown to be of benefit to adults and young persons who have adventitious hearing loss (i.e., hearing loss after acquiring speech and language) (Sarant, 2012). Significant benefits also have been reported for cochlear implants in young prelingual children (Balkany et al, 2002; Waltzman et al, 2002). Children as young as 18 months old are developing speech largely through auditory input. In recent years, younger and younger children have received cochlear implants to take advantage of their neural plasticity (Ramsden, 2002). There are two major parts of most cochlear implants (Ramsden, 2002). External to the body are a microphone (environmental interface), electronic processing circuits that extract key parameters from the speech signal, and a transmitter that couples the information to the skull. The implanted portion consists of an electrode array (1 to 22 electrodes), a receiver that couples the external data and power to the skull, and electronic circuits that provide proper synchronization and stimulation parameters for the electrode array. Ten-year failure rates are reported to be less than 3% for the internal and external elements combined (Ramsden, 2002).

Candidates for cochlear implants must meet certain audiological and age criteria. Severe or profound (>90 dB) bilateral pure tone hearing loss, sentence recognition scores of less than 30%, and age 2 years or more with >90 dB loss in children are the primary criteria for cochlear implants (Loizou, 1998). Age at implant for children and duration of deafness for adults are important factors in obtaining success (Ramsden, 2002). Better results occur for children at younger implant ages and for adults who have had shorter periods of deafness.

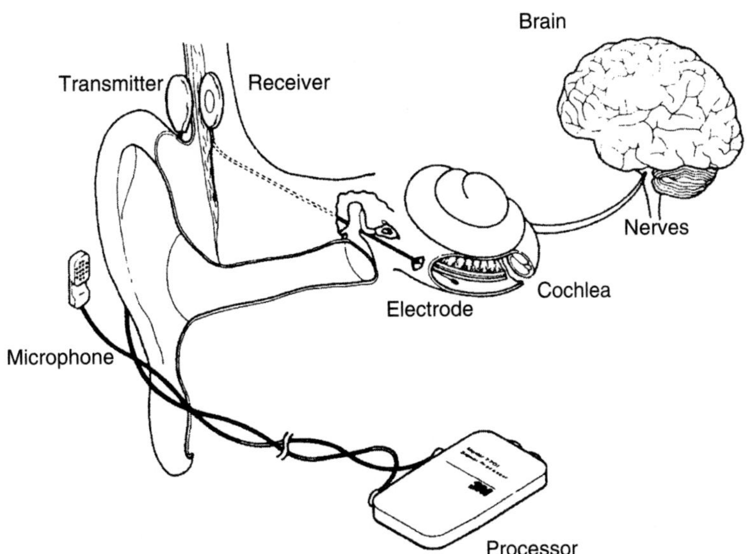

FIGURE 14-6 The components of a cochlear implant. (From Radcliffe D: How cochlear implants work, *Hearing J* November:53, 1984.)

Surgical procedures consist of insertion of the electrode array into the cochlea and implantation of the internal components and linking antenna for transcranial transmission of data and power. Ramsden (2002) describes the surgical procedures and possible surgical complications. After the implant is inserted, a period of 1 month or so is allowed for healing, and then a process of "switch-on and tuning" is carried out. Two thresholds are measured: minimal perception of sound and the level at which the sound just ceases to be comfortable. Then the electrode array is tested and signal processing is applied.

The operation of a four-channel cochlear implant system is shown schematically in Figure 14-7 (Loizou, 1998). Sound received by an external microphone is sent to a speech processor. The processed signal is coupled through the skin by a radio frequency transmitter-receiver pair. The internal signal is then fed to the electrode array implanted in the cochlea. One type of process is also illustrated in Figure 14-7; a bank of filters processes the speech information and then converts it into pulses that are sent to the electrodes. Signal processing is discussed in more detail later in this section. The resulting electrical signals at each point in the system are illustrated at the bottom of Figure 14-7. Current approaches to cochlear implants differ in several important respects. The main distinguishing characteristics, shown in Box 14-1, are discussed in depth by Loizou (1998) and summarized in this section.

Electrodes

The three major considerations in design of electrodes are: (1) biocompatibility of materials, (2) placement of electrodes, and (3) the number of electrodes in the array (Shallop and Mecklenberg, 1988). The stimulating portion of most electrodes in current devices is made of platinum-iridium because it is electrically stable and does not react with biological tissue. The "leads," wires that connect the stimulator to the platinum-tipped electrode, need to be flexible enough to curve around the cochlea, but they also must be rigid enough not to bend as they are inserted. The electrode array and the lead wires are coated with polytetrafluoroethylene (Teflon) or silicone to insulate them from each other and from the tissue. If there are small holes or breaks in the insulation, the tissue near the break will be exposed to electrical current. This can damage both the wire and the tissue. The insulation material must also be impervious to leakage of ionic fluids in the body.

Electrode placement is intracochlear (inside the cochlea), and the size of the electrode is dictated by the microanatomy of the cochlea. The average cochlea is about 32 mm long, and electrode arrays can be up to 25 mm long for insertion into this cavity (usually the scala tympani). Stimulation is either monopolar or bipolar. Monopolar stimulation places one reference electrode outside the cochlea and an array of single electrodes inside the cochlea along the basilar membrane. This arrangement requires less power for stimulation but results in less specific and less focused stimulation in the cochlea. Bipolar stimulation places electrode pairs along the membrane. This results in much more localized and specific stimulation, but it requires more power. Greater power means larger size, and this dictates the type of external packaging. The external package may be in either a BTE or body-level type. The majority of cochlear implants to date have been body-level types. As miniaturized technologies have been enhanced, BTE types have become more prevalent. The minimal spacing between electrode tips, on the basis of electrical stimulation parameters, is 0.5 to 4 mm (Loizou, 1998; White, 1987). This sets a practical limit of 22 electrodes in an array. Several different numbers of electrodes have been used in cochlear implants. Initially all devices used only one electrode. Currently available types of cochlear implants[1] have 12, 16, or 22 electrodes (Loizou, 2006).

[1]Clarion, Advanced Bionics Corp., Sylmar, Calif., www.cochlearimplant.com/; Nucleus 24, Cochlear Inc., Lane Cove, Australia, www.cochlear.com/; PUL SARCI, Med El, www.medel.com/.

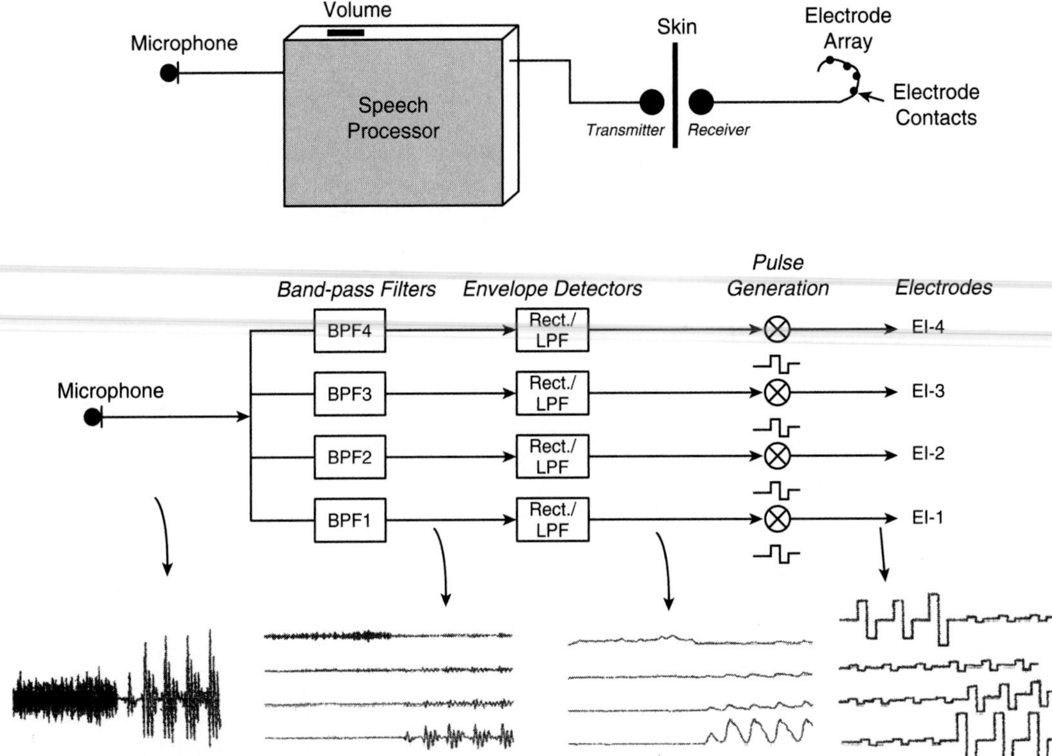

FIGURE 14-7 Diagram showing the operation of a four-channel cochlear implant. Sound is picked up by a microphone and sent to a speech processor box worn by the patient. The sound is then processed, and electrical stimuli are delivered to the electrodes through a radio-frequency link. The bottom figure shows a simplified implementation of the CIS signal processing strategy using the syllable *sa* as an input signal. The signal first goes through a set of four band-pass filters that divide the acoustic waveform into four channels. The envelopes of the band-passed waveforms are then detected by rectification and low-pass filtering. Current pulses are generated with amplitudes proportional to the envelopes of each channel and transmitted to the four electrodes through a radio-frequency link. Note that in the actual implementation the envelopes are compressed to fit the patient's electrical dynamic range. (From Loizou P: Mimicking the human ear, *IEEE Signal Process Mag* 15:101-130, 1998.)

Transmission of Power and Data

Because the microphone and speech processing components of cochlear implants need to be adjusted and because of their size and weight, they are placed outside the skull. The electrode array must be inside the cochlea, and there must be a connection through the skull. Initially this was done with wires that passed through the skull and a percutaneous plug that was used when the wires were removed. This type of percutaneous connection is subject to infection, and it has been replaced by a transmitter-receiver approach (Ramsden, 2002). A small induction coil on the external skin surface is connected to the transmitter. This coil transmits through the skin to the receiving coil located directly opposite, under the skin. The receiving coil is connected to the internal electronics and the electrode array. Power for the internal electronics is also coupled through the skin. In some cases the internal circuitry is totally passive and merely passes the stimulation signal to the electrodes. In other cases (such as that shown in Figure 14-6) the internal circuitry processes the incoming signal and distributes it to the different electrodes in the array. This consumes power, which is normally coupled through the skin just as the data are.

BOX 14-1 Varying Characteristics of Cochlear Implant Systems

Electrode design: Number of electrodes, electrode configuration
Type of stimulation: Analog or pulsatile
Transmission link: Transcutaneous or percutaneous
Signal processing: Waveform representation or feature extraction

From Loizou P: Mimicking the human ear, *IEEE Signal Process Mag* 15:101-130, 1998.

Speech Processing

The purpose of the cochlear implant is to provide an electrically triggered physiological signal that can be related to speech and environmental sounds. The process by which the cochlea, auditory nerve, and higher centers process speech is complex, and it is difficult to design an electronic speech processor that provides physiologically meaningful data to the electrode array.

The area of speech processing or coding of the signals to be sent to the electrode is one in which differences exist among different cochlear implants. Digital processing of the speech signal is aimed at extracting the relevant speech data from the microphone and converting it to a form that provides the most possible information to the user by stimulation of the auditory nerve. To recognize speech, it is necessary to encode frequency, intensity, and temporal patterns (Loizou, 1998, 2006). One approach, shown in Figure 14-7, uses a "vocoder" approach in which the incoming signal is broken down into a set of signals of different frequency through a filter bank. Frequency is encoded in the normal cochlea by location along the basilar membrane (referred to as *tonotopic organization*). A multiple electrode array can provide different frequencies at different locations along the basilar membrane, but the normal cochlea uses other, more sophisticated methods to further encode frequency (Loizou, 1998). Intensity or amplitude (what we subjectively perceive as loudness) can be encoded by the magnitude of the stimulus at any electrode location. However, the normal cochlea also uses "recruitment" of adjacent hair cells to reflect increased intensity. Recruitment or interaction between the electrode channels can also happen with electrical stimulation of neural tissue as the intensity of the stimulus increases.

Continuous interleaved sampling (CIS) signal processing was developed to avoid some of the problems of channel interactions by delivering temporally offset trains of pulses to each electrode (Loizou, 1998; Wilson et al, 1993). CIS is based on the use of nonsimultaneous interleaved stimulation. In interleaved stimulation, electrodes at different parts of the cochlea are stimulated in sequence rather than those adjacent to each other being stimulated in sequence, and only one electrode is stimulated at one time, helping to eliminate interaction between channels. A key feature is a relatively high rate (greater than 800 pulses per second) of stimulation on each channel, which provides the basis for tracking rapid variations in speech by use of pulse amplitude variations presented to the electrodes. The tradeoff for use of high stimulation rates is more cross-channel interaction. The amplitude of the incoming speech signal must be compressed to avoid damage resulting from overstimulation. As in hearing aids, this process is called compression. Because of the nature of the auditory system, a nonlinear (logarithmic) compression is typically used in cochlear implants (Loizou, 1998, 2006). Intensity of the electrical signal in microamps is analogous to the intensity of the acoustical stimulus in dB. A refinement on the CIS processing approach detects the peaks of the speech signal in several bands. The number of frequency bands is greater than the number of electrodes, and the signals sent to the electrodes are based on the bands with the highest output at any given time. This approach is called ACE (previously called SPEAK) and is implanted on the Nucelus-24 devices (Cochlear Inc., Lane Cove, Australia, www.cochlear.com/). Sentence recognition tests with the CIS, SPEAK, and ACE signal processing approaches demonstrated that significantly higher scores were obtained with the ACE than with the SPEAK or CIS strategies (Loizou, 2006). Loizou (1998, 2006) discusses speech processing for cochlear implants in depth and describes current commercial approaches.

Major cochlear implant manufacturers also provide software that is used to program the signal processing characteristics of the implant to match the needs of the user. These are used after the surgery has been completed and healing has taken place. Signals are supplied to the implant and psychophysical measurements are made to determine the optimal type of signal (pulse or analog) and electrode combinations. This uses pure tone responses. Then speech input is evaluated and adjustments are made to maximize speech intelligibility.

User Evaluation Results

Almost all postlingually deaf individuals can obtain some degree of open set (the test words or sentences are not known) speech perception without lip reading by use of cochlear implants (Ramsden, 2002). Some users can also communicate over the telephone. The degree of improvement depends on many factors, including the characteristics of the cochlear implant technology used. In general, more channels or electrodes result in greater speech perception (Loizou, 1998). Increasing the number of electrodes or channels will not be effective if there is a smaller number of surviving auditory neurons. The type of signal processing also affects cochlear implant outcomes. For example, the spectral processing method yields greater than 90% correct speech recognition even with a small number of channels, whereas the CIS processing method required up to 8 channels to achieve similar results (Loizou, 2006). An area of continued research is aimed at increasing music perception and enjoyment.

In the case of prelingual children, the need for effective auditory perception is critical in the development of spoken language. For deaf children, the cochlear implant has been shown to facilitate development of language at a rate comparable to that of typical hearing children (Balkany et al, 2002). These results are dependent on a number of factors, including age at implantation, length of deafness, and length of use (habituation to the cochlear implant) (Waltzman et al, 2002). Children who receive an implant at an age younger than 5 years perform much better on speech perception tests than do children who are older at the time of implantation. Children who receive an implant before the age of 2 years perform equally well with children who are between 2 and 5 years old when they receive their implant. The minimum age is now 12 months (Balkany et al, 2002). Children who use the cochlear implant full time perform significantly better than those who do not. In general, as the duration of use increases, the performance improves (Balkany et al, 2002; Waltzman et al, 2002). In one study, word recognition scores increased from less than 1% before implantation to 8.9% at 1 year, to 30% at 3 years, and eventually reached 65%, and sentence recognition scores increased from 18% (1 year) to 42% (3 years) to 80% (Waltzman et al, 2002). These average scores were affected by age at implantation (higher scores for those implanted at younger ages). Waltzman et al (2002) describe the recommended criteria for selecting candidates for implantation and for choosing the ear to be used. Cochlear implants are typically implanted in only one ear. This makes auditory localization more difficult and can result in uneven auditory input.

Use of unilateral cochlear implants can cause difficulties in the location and discrimination of sounds in noisy environments, and they can require effort to track a conversation. Bilateral cochlear implants overcome some of these problems (Kimura and Hyppolito, 2013). In binaural stimulation, the auditory input is provided to both ears and integrated into the auditory sensory pathway. This process can lead to greater spatial localization of sounds.

When an individual uses a unilateral cochlear implant, one of the limitations is the ability to perceive multiple entries with segregated independent sources. This reflects the difficulty in understanding speech in the presence of competitive signals and identifying the location of the sound in the environment. Bilateral hearing has three primary advantages when compared to unilateral hearing: reducing the head shadow effect, reducing the squelch effect, and binaural summation. Head shadow refers to the blockage of the arrival of sounds at the two ears by the head. For example, if only the left ear has a cochlear implant, sounds arriving at the right ear may be blocked by the head. The squelch effect is the ability of the auditory system to use the sounds received at the two ears to separate speech and competing sounds. Binaural summation describes the ability of the auditory system to make use of signals from two ears to process auditory signals.

Kimura and Hyppolito (2013) describe indicators for bilateral cochlear implants in adults and children. In general, for children the indicators are severe to profound bilateral sensorioneural hearing with no cognitive impairment. Users with bilateral cochlear implants placed between 5 and 18 months of age showed auditory and language development equal to hearing children with the same chronological age. Adults with bilateral cochlear implants have shown great spatial localization and increased listening comfort. It is also claimed that early bilateral cochlear implantation results in the preservation of the central auditory system.

An alternative approach when there is some residual hearing in one ear is to use a hearing aid in one ear and a cochlear implant in the other (Ching et al, 2001). Clear benefits have been demonstrated from having the combination of a hearing aid and cochlear implant, but there are several important factors to consider. The use of the cochlear implant may lessen the desire for using the hearing aid because the hearing aid is less attractive or is perceived to interfere with the speech perception from the cochlear implant. If the child is used to the hearing aid, the cochlear implant may not be used as often as is necessary for habituation. Ching et al (2001) present four case studies of children fitted with both a hearing aid and a cochlear implant; they describe success factors and strategies for optimizing effectiveness of this combination of devices.

Sarant (2012) reviewed cochlear implants in children. Speech perception results in children implanted with cochlear implants have been comparable to postlingually deafened adults using cochlear implants, and to those achieved by children with moderate hearing loss using hearing aids. As children receive implants at younger ages and have access to constantly improving technology, even better speech perception abilities are demonstrated.

Cochlear implants provide children with an environmental awareness because they hear sound like water running, birds singing, the kettle whistling, the car turn signal clicking, and the phone ringing. Awareness of these sounds makes children feel more connected to the rest of the world and also provides a degree of safety. Localization of sound sources is rarely obtained with a unilateral cochlear implant. Much of the improvement in speech perception scores is due to advancements in technology, and particularly to the development of more effective speech processing strategies. There is great variation in all of the results with children. However, some children who are implanted at younger ages acquire spoken language comparable to children with mild to moderate hearing loss, and children who receive the implants at very young ages with improved technology achieve spoken language development at similar rates to children with normal hearing. "There is also no evidence that children with cochlear implants in mainstream educational settings, where speech is used exclusively for communication, have an increased incidence of social or emotional difficulties compared to children in special educational settings" (Sarant, 2012, p. 345). Speech perception performance with bilateral cochlear implants exceeds that of those with unilateral implants. No clear benefit for sound localization has been demonstrated for bilateral cochlear implantation in children.

Gaylor et al (2013) carried out a systematic review of cochlear implantation in adults. A review of 42 studies showed that unilateral implants showed a statistically significant improvement in mean speech scores as measured by open-set sentence or multisyllable word tests. A meta-analysis revealed a significant improvement in quality of life after unilateral implantation. Studies of bilateral implantation showed greater improvement in communication related outcomes than for unilateral implants. Sound localization was also shown to be improved with bilateral implants. Quality of life results varied across studies, but only a few studies addressed this issue.

Telephone Access for Persons Who Are Deaf

The isolation imposed on deaf persons by the telephone is ironic given that Alexander Graham Bell was working with the deaf when he invented it. For some individuals, additional amplification is sufficient to make the telephone accessible. This may be built into the person's telephone or it may be an add-on unit that can be placed over the earpiece of any telephone. Both types of devices are available from local telephone companies. As discussed in the previous section, many hearing aids have a magnetic induction feature (telecoil) that allows the output of the telephone to be coupled to the hearing aid electromagnetically, and other hearing aids link to mobile technologies via Bluetooth. There are also devices that link to external Bluetooth devices for people who wear hearing aids or cochlear implants with a telecoil.[2] As in other Bluetooth links for hearing aids, the user wears a pendant around the neck with the loop supporting the pendant serving as an antenna to the hearing aid telecoil.

For many individuals with severe hearing loss, even increased amplification does not make the telephone signal audible. For these persons to obtain access to telephone conversations, a device that can visually send and receive telephone information is used. These individuals also often use master ring indicators, which either amplify the ringing of the telephone or connect the ringer to a table lamp that flashes when the telephone rings. These adaptations are also available from local telephone companies.

Telephone Devices for the Deaf

Originally, deaf individuals used teletype (TTY) devices designed for sending weather and news information over telephone lines to provide a "visual telephone." Many of these TTYs were donated by IBM and other companies to help deaf people talk to each other. The original TTY, now obsolete, consisted of a typewriter and electronic circuitry for converting the typed letters to pulses that could be sent over the telephone line to another TTY. The second TTY converted the pulses back into text that was typed on paper on the remote TTY. Because of their low cost, especially for surplus units, TTYs were very popular with deaf individuals, and some are still in use. A good source of information is the Gallaudet University Technology Assessment Program (http://tap.gallaudet.edu).

Electronic versions of earlier TTYs are still referred to as TTYs. Several models of current TTYs are lightweight, battery-powered devices for portable use.[3] They use a keypad, a visual display, and a modulator-demodulator (modem) to convert the electronic signal to pulses. Connection to the telephone service is by one of three methods: (1) an acoustical coupler that couples the pulses directly to the telephone handset, (2) direct connection to the telephone line by a cable, and (3) cable connection to a cell phone. Some TTYs also function as telephones with additional amplification for users who are hard of hearing. Some of these units are compatible with cell phones, further increasing access for users who are deaf.

Other TTY features include use with an answering machine, remote retrieval of messages, message notification via paging, and a printer. The printer function gives both a permanent record of the conversation and a chance to review messages before responding to them. Some TTYs also include the "Sticky keys" feature (see Chapter 8, Table 8-2) that supports one-handed typing for modifier keys such as shift and control. Many TTYs plug directly into cellular and cordless telephones to allow mobile use. Some are designed for battery powered portable use. An example of a TTY is shown in Figure 14-8. An acoustic coupler is required when calling from a pay telephone.

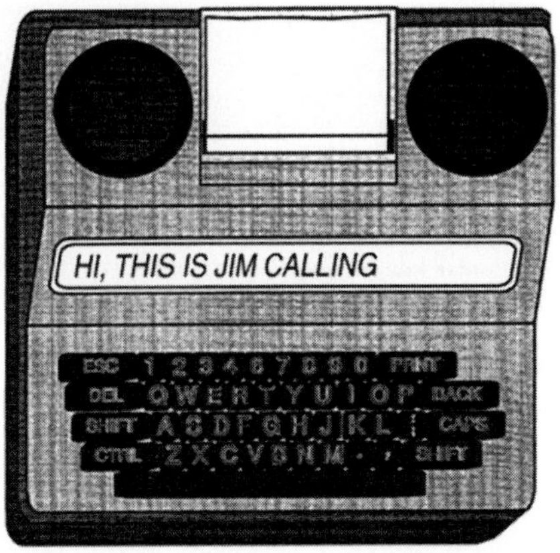

FIGURE 14-8 A typical TTY has an electronic display and a keyboard for typing messages.

There are two primary ways to use the TTY with the telephone. If both parties have a TTY, then each simply types their message, sends a "go ahead" (the letters *GA*) command to indicate that he or she is finished, and then waits for an answer. Some TTYs include a button that sends GA with one key press. If the deaf person needs to talk to someone who does not have a TTY, then a relay operator is provided by the telephone company. The operator has a TTY and reads the message sent by the deaf person to the hearing person. The response is then spoken to the operator who types the message to the deaf person's TTY. For people who can speak but not hear, **Voice Carry-Over** (VCO)[4] phones allow communication by both voice and text. These individuals can use the relay service by speaking naturally and reading the responses on the screen. For those who can hear but not speak, **Hearing Carry-Over** (HCO) allows individuals to type their message and listen to the response. The HCO user types a message for the Relay Operator to read aloud to the other party. TTYs also support **Short Message Service** (SMS),[5] the text communication protocol that enables text messaging using cell phones.

Advanced TTY features include use with an answering machine, remote retrieval of messages, message notification via paging, and a printer. The printer function gives both a permanent record of the conversation and a chance to review messages before responding to them. Some TTYs plug directly into cellular and cordless telephones to allow mobile use.

There are a large number of deaf persons who have and use TTYs (Baudot protocol), and there are also many individuals who have personal computers with modems that use the ASCII protocol. Therefore, current TTYs often include both ASCII and Baudot, and computer programs that convert from one code to another are available. To use a

---

[2]For example: Linear Blue SLC, http://www.independentliving.com/prodinfo.asp?number=617400.

[3]For example: Clarity, http://shop.clarityproducts.com/products/ameriphone/; Compu-TTY, http://www.computty.com/; Ultratec,. http://www.ultratec.com/products.php.

[4]For example: Clarity, http://shop.clarityproducts.com/products/ameriphone/; Compu-TTY, http://www.computty.com/; Ultratec, http://www.ultratec.com/products.php.

[5]SMS is based on the original short messaging used in TTYs.

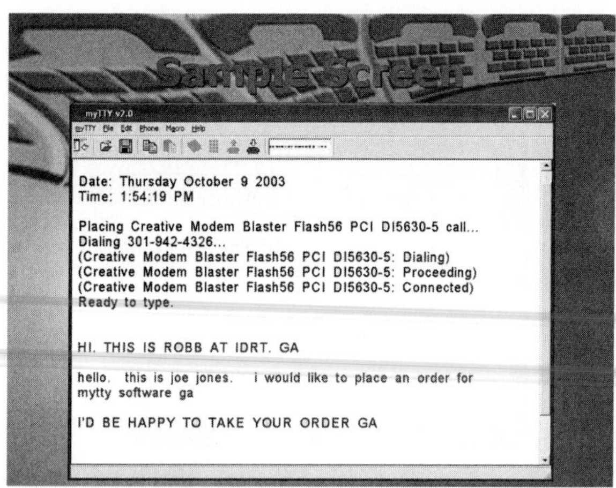

FIGURE 14-9 A screenshot of a software-based TTY system. (Courtesy of SoftTTY, Inc.)

computer for TTY communication, the user must have both TTY software and a modem that can emulate a TTY (Baudot at 300 baud).[6] The TTY software generates the Baudot codes and sends information to the TTY modem (hardware plugged into the computer). The modem then communicates with a stand-alone TTY at 300 baud. The modem must meet all the transmission protocols (e.g., frequency, 5-bit code, half-duplex communication) of the Baudot TTY in order for the communication to be successful. These protocols are not available on standard computer modems, and that is the reason a special TTY modem (with a setting of 300 baud to communicate in Baudot code with other TTYs) is required for successful communication with a TTY. A typical screenshot of a software-based TTY program in use is shown in Figure 14-9. Several windows are used including incoming and outgoing messages, a phone book, and a log of past messages.

If the deaf person needs to talk to someone who does not have a TTY, then the telephone company provides a relay operator. The operator, who has a TTY, reads the message sent by the deaf person to the hearing person. The response is then spoken to the operator who types the message to the deaf person's TTY. Under the provisions of Title IV (telecommunications) of the Americans with Disabilities Act (ADA), all telephone services offered to the general public must include both interstate and intrastate relay services for persons who use TTYs. The Federal Communications Commission (FCC) issued the rules for Title IV, and this agency monitors compliance. These rules also require that both ASCII and Baudot capabilities be provided by the relay services. Approximately 95% of the calls through a relay operator use Baudot data format. Title IV regulations also specify the conduct of relay operators. The most important features of these rules are complete confidentiality and verbatim transmission of messages.

[6]For example: Next TalNXi Communications, Inc., http://www.nextalk.net/nextalk62/nextalk.pl?rm=homepage; Phone-TTY, Inc., www.phone-tty.com; Ultratec, Inc., www.ultratec.com.

AT&T uses an interesting combination of the technologies described in this chapter in its relay services (Halliday, 1993). A blind operator serves as a relay communications assistant. Incoming voice messages are relayed by typing on a computer terminal that sends the message to the deaf person's TTY. Incoming TTY messages are converted to braille by use of a refreshable braille display and are then relayed by voice to the hearing person. This is a unique combination of technologies for persons who are deaf and who are blind, and it takes advantage of the skills of each individual.

One of the major advantages of the Baudot-based TTYs is simplicity because all have the same transmission protocol. Use of ASCII offers a variety of protocols that differ in significant ways, and a successful transmission depends on both the transmitting and the receiving parties having the same setup. This requires that the sender know the protocol of the receiver. A hearing person can obtain this information by voice, an option not available to the deaf caller.

CASE STUDY 14-2

Selecting a TTY Program

The educational audiologist at a local school approached the assistive technology practitioner (ATP) for advice regarding a young child who is profoundly deaf. The family does not have a stand-alone TTY, but they do have a computer. They are interested in using it as a TTY. The computer has the advantage of being a full-screen, full-keyboard computer that may be easier for the child to use and to read than one-line, cramped-keyboard traditional models. However, the computer is not as portable. Also, if the phone rings with a TTY call while the computer is off, the call will be missed. The price of each approach is about the same. What approach should the ATP take to help the family make this choice? Special attention should be paid to helping them (1) decide whether their computer and modem will work with TTY software and (2) determine the tradeoffs between the stand-alone TTY and a computer-based TTY with TTY software.

Visual Telephones for the Deaf

Because it requires typing of each utterance, TTY telephone transmission is slow, typically one third to one fourth the rate of human speech (Galuska and Foulds, 1990). Visual sign language, on the other hand, results in communication rates comparable to human speech, and it is the primary form of communication used by individuals who are deaf. It does, of course, require that both the speaker and the listener understand sign language or that an interpreter be available. There are many situations in which this option is unavailable or impractical. For example, in a work setting it is not always practical to have an interpreter available for casual or unscheduled conversations. If standard telephone lines could be used to send visual images of manual signs, it would significantly increase communication rates over those obtained with use of TTYs.

In a work environment there is an alternative to the visual telephone that can provide many of the same benefits: the use of personal computers (PCs) and local area networks (LANs). A LAN can be used to provide interpretive services

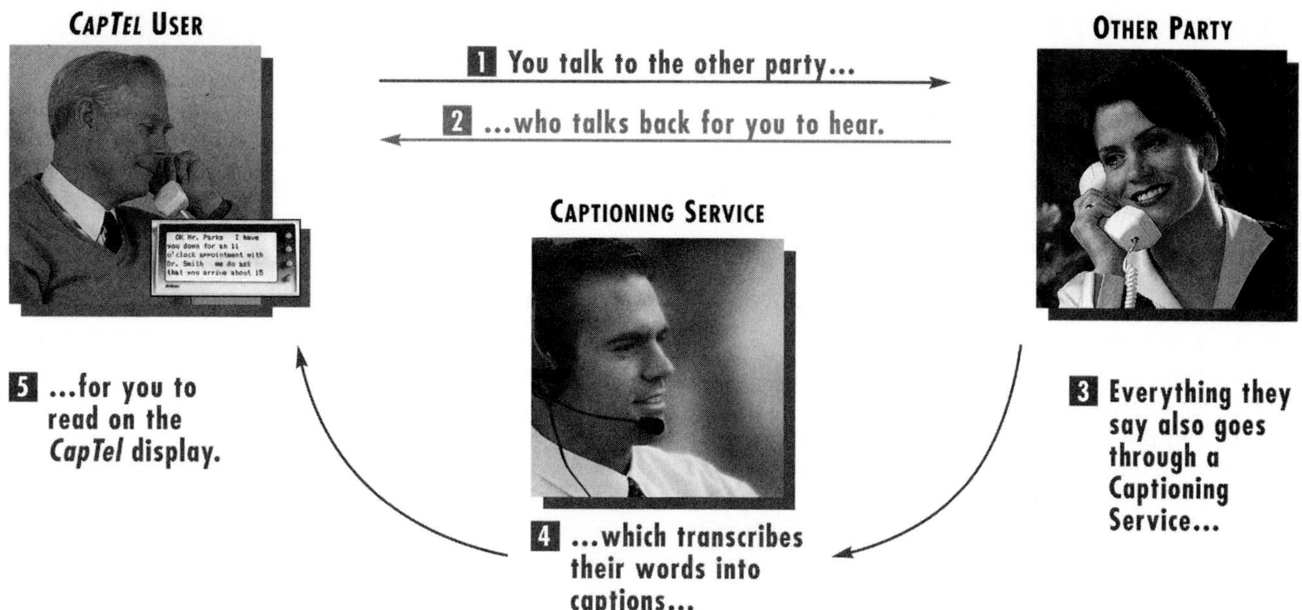
CAPTEL USER
1 You talk to the other party...
2 ...who talks back for you to hear.
OTHER PARTY
CAPTIONING SERVICE
5 ...for you to read on the CapTel display.
3 Everything they say also goes through a Captioning Service...
4 ...which transcribes their words into captions...

FIGURE 14-10 The CapTel private phone captioning system is built on the same concept as a telephone relay operator. (Courtesy of CapTel.)

to a deaf employee or customer. The interpreter can be connected by video on the network to the employee. A speakerphone provides audio connection from the meeting to the interpreter and from the hearing impaired person (by the interpreter) to others at the meeting. The network video provides signed interpretation to the individual with a hearing impairment from the interpreter and from the hearing impaired individual to the interpreter for voice relay to the meeting. Applications that support relay calling are also available for mobile phones.[7]

Another approach is to take advantage of the Internet and to use an interpreter located at a remote location who hears the conversation and then signs it over video for the individual who is deaf. This approach is enabled by a broadband videophone appliance specifically designed for deaf and hard-of-hearing individuals (Sorenson VP-100).[8] Sorenson Video Relay Service is a free service to conduct video relay calls with family, friends, and business associates through a certified sign language interpreter, Sorenson videophone, television, and a high-speed Internet connection. The deaf user sees an interpreter on their television and signs to the interpreter who then contacts the hearing user by a standard phone line and relays the conversation between the two parties. There are also apps available for mobile phones that support interpreter services.[9]

The use of an intermediary relay operator has been extended by one company to include a person who listens to the call as it comes in and captions the auditory information onto a small display built into the telephone. Figure 14-10 shows how the system works. With this system, the user dials a call as on any other telephone. As the call is dialed, it is also connected to a captioning service. In addition, the user captioning service transcribes everything the other party says into written text by use of voice-recognition technology. The written text appears almost simultaneously with the spoken word on a visual display on the captioning phone. The cost of the captioning service is covered by Telecommunications Relay Service funds as part of Title IV of the ADA. This approach requires both a special phone and the availability of the CapTel captioning service as part of the relay service provided by the state.[10] This system also works with external voice answering machine messages. There are also apps available for mobile phones that support interpreter services.[11]

Voice Over Internet Protocol

Most telephone calls are made over the public switched telephone network, or PSTN. Increasingly, hearing users are moving to Internet-based telephone service, referred to as voice over Internet Protocol (VoIP). There are many advantages to this change, including lower cost, inclusion of multimedia, and the features commonly available with cell phones or land-based networks, such as voicemail, caller ID, three-way calling, and other features included in the basic price of VoIP software or a VoIP service subscription. Originally Internet phone calls stayed within the Internet (PC to PC), but VoIP now bridges to the PSTN.

Although there are many reasons that both hearing and deaf users are attracted to VoIP, there are some issues of accessibility for VoIP (Harkins, 2004). One disadvantage is relay

[7]For example: Android, https://play.google.com/store/apps/details?id=us.purple.purplevri&hl=en.

[8]Sorensen Communications, Inc. Salt Lake City, Utah, www.sorenson.com/.

[9]For example: Android, https://play.google.com/store/apps/details?id=us.purple.purplevri&hl=en.

[10]CapTel, Ultratec Madison, Wis., http://www.captel.com/.

[11]For example: Android, https://play.google.com/store/apps/details?id=us.purple.purplevri&hl=en, iOS: http://support.apple.com/kb/HT4526.

operator service, which is mandated by the PSTN regulator (FCC) under the ADA and into which PSTN companies pay a fee from each user. VoIP companies do not participate in this program and do not typically provide relay service. A second accessibility issue is that VoIP will often garble TTY messages, especially with heavy traffic on the network. TTY messages can also be garbled if lower-quality speech coding is used for the call to save bandwidth. Many TTYs cannot connect to VoIP phones and some VoIP phones cannot connect to any TTY except by acoustical coupling. This reduces access below that of the hearing user. There is technology (NexTalk VM, NXI, www.nxicom.com/products-biz/nextalk_vm.html) that allows Internet protocol (IP)-to-IP text inside an organization's IP network and allows outside communication with TTYs that are on the public switched telephone network. This is a limited solution relevant only to the organizations that have this technology, not the entire network. Voice quality can also vary over VoIP, which can affect individuals who are hard of hearing. The multimedia aspect of VoIP can lead to more effective use of video and its application to the use of sign language interpreters or lip reading. Advances will undoubtedly be made rapidly in VoIP as it becomes more popular, and this will include TTY compatibility.

Access to Mobile Phones for People Who Are Deaf

Mobile phones are used by people who are deaf to meet needs in six broad categories: social, safety, communication, transportation, consumption, and entertainment (Chiu et al, 2010). These are interrelated, with social linkages being the most important. There are mobile phone features that are useful in order to meet these needs. Many people who are deaf rely on short message service (SMS) (generally referred to as "texting") for their mobile phone communication (Power et al, 2007). Deaf users of mobile phones indicated that touch screen keyboards, handwriting recognition, and QWERTY keyboard layouts support SMS capability (Chiu et al, 2010). As we have described, visual telephones are used to support sign language conversations. Deaf users would like this capability to be included in mobile phones (Chiu et al, 2010). Specific features that support signing are cameras located on the same side as the display and large screens. A number of needs are met through smart phone access to the Internet. For those functions people who are deaf desire Wi-Fi and wireless network linkages. Other desirable features are text-to-speech for monitoring of speech input to the device and improving communication with others, and speech-to-text for presenting received auditory content in readable form (Chiu et al, 2010).

Some people who are deaf want to use their mobile phone as a TTY. This usually requires an adapter of some sort (often just a cable) and an application that provides TTY functionality. Mobile phone apps that support TTY functions are available.[12]

There are many apps for mobile phones that are aimed at meeting the needs of people who are deaf or hard of hearing.[13] These include TTY functions, sign language communication, alternatives to auditory ring (flashing or vibration) with unique patterns for caller ID, and social communication apps to link deaf users with each other and with hearing friends.

Technology for Face-to-Face Communication Between Hearing and Deaf Individuals

The Sorenson method can be effective for face-to face conversations, but it requires time for setup and must be planned in advance for work meetings or casual conversations. For these purposes, assistive technologies that allow communication without speech or sign language interpretation can be very effective. One product, the Interpretype,[14] is designed specifically for this application. This system consists of a preprogrammed laptop-style computer that is able to send typed messages to other TTY units or a computer (Gan, 2005). A built-in display shows the text that is received from the communication partner and displays messages typed into its keyboard. The major advantage of this approach is its simplicity; however, these stand-alone devices are expensive relative to TTYs. For this reason some companies have developed simple modifications to TTYs to allow them to be used as face-to-face communication devices.[15] In this case the TTYs are interconnected, rather than being connected to a telephone line. Once connected, they function like the TTY device: one person types and the text shows up on the other person's screen. The primary advantage of using simple technology for face-to-face communication is that it is simple to set up, lightweight to carry, and intuitive to use. Because many deaf individuals have portable TTYs, the modification for face-to-face use is more cost-effective. They still need to buy a second unit, but the total cost for both units can be less than $600 and the total weight can be less than 3 pounds (1.5 kg).

Alerting Devices for Persons with Auditory Impairments

There are many environmental sounds other than speech about which a person who is deaf needs to know.[16] Examples are telephones, doorbells, smoke alarms, and a child's cry. There are **alerting devices** available that detect these sounds and then cause a vibration, a flashing light signal, or both to call attention to the sound. Some devices are very specific. For example, one device is tuned to the frequency of a smoke alarm and it responds only to that sound. When the smoke

[12]For example: Android, https://play.google.com/store/apps/details?id=us.purple.purplevri&hl=en.

[13]http://code-idea.org/index.php/accessibility-tools/applications.

[14] ITY, Interpretype, Rochester, NY, www.interpretype.com/index.php.

[15]Modern Deaf Communication, Inc., Danbury, Conn., http://www.moderndeafcommunication.org; Independent Living aids, http://www.independentliving.com/default.asp?division=sb&amsutm_medium=email&utm_source=Independent+Living+Aids%2c+LLC&utm_campaign=1509312_FriJuly27reminder&utm_content=LowHearing&dm_t=0,0,0,0,0&dm_i=ZQ7,WCLC,6Y5OJQ,2ODVA,1.

[16]For example, see: http://www.hearmore.com/store/default.asphttp://www.lssproducts.com/category/alerting-devices, and similar sites.

alarm auditory signal is detected, the visible smoke detector transmits a flasher, which can be connected to a standard lamp. The lamp flashes as long as the smoke detector is active.

Telephone alerting devices include amplified ringers that plug into a standard telephone jack and provide up to 95 dB of ringing sound (McFadden, 1996). Another approach is to use a flashing light that is connected to the telephone line. This can alert the person who is deaf that there is an incoming TTY call. Some systems have a strobe light connected to them; others use a table lamp plugged into the alerting device. The only modification required for these adaptations is a two-plug telephone adapter to allow plugging in of both the adapted alerting device and the telephone.

Doorbells can be both directly wired into a flashing light and detected by a microphone and then converted into a visible (typically a flashing light) or tactile (vibration) signal. For more general sound detection, there are silent alarms that can detect any signal and then transmit to a wrist-worn receiver. This both vibrates and flashes a light to indicate that the sound has occurred. Some devices can accommodate 16 or more channels, and different lights flash for each sound. A microphone and transmitter can be placed in each of the locations where an important sound may occur. For example, one can be near the front door, another near the telephone, another in the baby's room, and a final one near the back door. When a sound is detected at any of these locations, the wrist unit vibrates and one light is illuminated to indicate which sound has been detected.

Alarm clocks for persons who are deaf generally are either visible (flashing light on a bedside table) or tactile (vibration under the pillow). They may either be built into an alarm clock (e.g., the entire face of the clock flashes) or they may detect the clock's alarm and then cause the vibration or flashing light (or both).

One of the major difficulties faced by persons who are deaf is the lack of awareness of sounds associated with traffic. Sirens, horns, and ambient traffic noise all contribute to our ability to drive. Traffic horns of different types (air horn on a truck versus a car horn), sirens, railroad crossing gate, or train each have a unique sound and may require a different response.

> **CASE STUDY 14-4**
>
> ***Living with Hearing Loss***
>
> Sandra Robinson lives alone in the home that she and her deceased husband Russell bought 40 years ago. She is very attached to the house and wants to continue to stay there. Unfortunately, her hearing loss has been steadily increasing and she is unable to hear the telephone, doorbell, kitchen timer, and microwave beeper and alarms (smoke, home security system). Her daughter, Ann, is concerned about her mother's increasing isolation. You have been asked to recommend things that might help her become more connected to her family (some of whom live several hundred miles away) and to feel safer in her home surroundings. What would you recommend?

Assistive Listening Devices

All the devices discussed in this chapter have been designed for use by hearing impaired individuals. There is also a class of assistive devices that are intended to be used in noisy environments for individual face-to-face conversation or in group settings, such as lecture halls, churches, business meetings, courtrooms, and broadcast television. These are called **assistive listening devices.**

Individual Assistive Listening Devices

For many individuals who have auditory impairments, hearing aids are only effective for one-on-one conversations at close range (and possibly for telephone use). These individuals may also have difficulty if the environment has reverberations, such as a "live" room with echoes. Because of the abnormalities in the auditory system, the speech signal becomes buried in the background noise. A hearing aid amplifies both the desired signal (e.g., speech) and the background noise to the same degree (unless it has signal processing to separate noise and speech signals as discussed earlier). The person with a hearing loss will have increased difficulty hearing when there is noise present. In order for the person using a hearing aid to be able to distinguish speech from background noise, the speech must be 5 to 10 times louder than the noise. Wireless technology can preserve speech in the presence of background noise. Sometimes these systems are referred to as small-group or personal listening devices.

The wireless technology is called an FM system, and it consists of a microphone and a battery-powered radio transmitter that are worn by the person speaking and a receiver that is carried by the person with an auditory impairment. The output of the receiver can either be fed into earphones (personal FM system) or coupled directly to the hearing aid via telecoil loop or Bluetooth. If the person does not normally use a hearing aid or the hearing aids used do not accommodate direct coupling of the signal, earphones are used. The speaker uses a microphone and whatever she says is then transmitted to the listener with a high signal-to-noise ratio. There are also hearing aids with built-in FM receivers that facilitate these listening devices (Palmer, 2010). FM systems are useful in a variety of situations (see http://www.hearingli nk.org/fmsystems for a detailed description).

Several manufacturers produce devices that combine a conventional BTE hearing aid with an FM system. Some manufacturers use a "boot" that fits over the bottom of the BTE device and directly couples the amplified sound to the hearing aid. Other manufacturers have built the FM receiver directly into the case of the BTE. In either case, a transmitter sends the radio signal from the person who is speaking to the wireless receiver attached to or built into the BTE device. The hearing aid user can switch between hearing aid only, hearing aid plus FM, and FM only modes. In FM only mode, the user would hear only the speech of the person wearing the transmitter. However, if the user wanted to monitor his/her own voice or hear another child's answer to a question in class, the hearing aid plus FM mode might be more appropriate.

The functions of a personal listening device can also be accomplished using a smart phone with some accessories. One case study was described using the iPhone with a directional microphone and noise canceling headphones

(Eisenberg, 2012). When in a noisy environment, hearing aids may not be effective. By removing the hearing aids, attaching a directional microphone to the iPhone, and launching an app[17] all the functions of an FM listening device can be obtained.

When there are sound sources other than speech that need to be amplified (e.g., television, DVD player) there are systems called hearing loop systems that connect to the sound source and then transmit throughout a room via a coil.[18] The coil can either run around the edges of the room or be placed inside a mat that sits beneath a chair, or in a pad under a cushion.

Small-Group Devices

For many individuals who have auditory impairments, hearing aids are only effective for one-on-one conversations at close range (and possibly for telephone use). When these individuals are in a group, even a small group of five or fewer persons, it is very difficult for them to understand what is being said; *small-group* or *personal listening devices* are helpful in this situation.[19] For small-group meetings with several participants, the speaker and microphone can be placed in the middle of the conference table to pick up all the voices. Small-group devices can have multiple receivers for one transmitter if there is more than one person requiring amplification or they can have multiple receivers for one transmitter if there is more than one person requiring amplification. Digital FM systems pair the transmitter and receiver so that multiple users can each receive private messages from different speakers. The specificity of digital transmission makes it possible to have an increased level of security over previous analog systems. Each transmitter and receiver is paired by the transmitter sending a coded key to the receiver.

Classroom Applications

Several acoustical parameters affect speech perception in a classroom environment (Crandell and Smaldino, 2000). These are signal-to-noise ratio (SNR), reverberation time (RT), and distance from the speaker.

Classroom noise can be external to the classroom (outside the building such as street noise or inside the building such as other classes, hallway noise, etc.) or inside the classroom (other students talking, heating and air conditioning, moving of furniture). The SNR is the relationship between the speech amplitude from the teacher and the background noise. As the noise level increases, the perception of speech by children with and without hearing impairment falls. The decrement in speech perception is greater for children with sensorineural hearing loss. The greatest effect is on consonant perception. Because noise tends to mask frequencies above it in frequency, the effect is greater with low-frequency noise. Crandell and Smaldino (2000) recommend a SNR of at least +15dB.

RT is the prolongation or persistence of sound as it reflects off hard surfaces, specified as a time delay. Shorter RTs are better for speech perception. RT is longer with lower frequencies because sound is absorbed more readily at high frequencies. Like SNR, RT has a greater effect on children with hearing loss than on typically hearing children. Recommended RT values for classroom are lower than 0.6 seconds (Crandell and Smaldino, 2000).

The final factor is distance from the speaker. As this distance increases, the sound level decreases up to a critical value determined by the volume of the room, directionality of the speech signal relative to the listener, and the RT. Beyond the critical distance, reverberated signals arrive from sources closer than the speaker (e.g., walls, ceiling) and mask the original signal to a greater extent. Positioning a child in the front of the room near the teacher does not solve the problem because reverberated signals and other speech (e.g., a child participating in a discussion) come from throughout the room. These factors indicate that a room that is acoustically well designed (low noise sources, short RT) and has a uniform speaker-to-listener distance will be most effective for children with and without hearing limitations. Classrooms designed within these guidelines have been shown to positively affect academic performance in reading, spelling, concentration, and attention (Crandell and Smaldino, 2000).

One approach to achieving uniform sound throughout the room and avoiding the problems of distance from the speaker is the use of sound field systems (Ross and Levitt, 2002). As shown in Figure 14-11, the teacher's voice is transmitted to speakers located around the room, so the teacher's voice is presented uniformly throughout the classroom. The original systems used FM radio transmission. Recently, infrared (IR) transmission systems have come into use. The primary advantage of the IR systems is that the signal is contained within the classroom and there is no interference between classrooms or from outside radio sources. Sound from a teacher is typically at a level only about 6 dB above

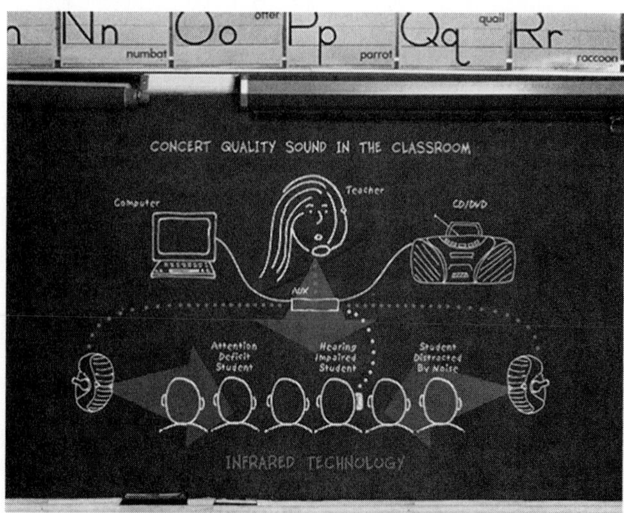

FIGURE 14-11 A typical sound field system setup. (Courtesy of Telex.)

[17]soundAMP R, https://itunes.apple.com/ca/app/soundamp-r/id318126109?amp;mt=8.

[18]For example: Contacta, http://www.contactainc.com.

[19]For example: http://www.williamssound.com/catalog/pkt-c1.

background noise in a typical classroom. Sound field systems can boost this to 8 to 10 dB, which is a much more suitable SNR (Ross and Levitt, 2002). The effectiveness of these systems depends on sound acoustical room design to maximize SNR and minimize RT. The maximum benefit of sound field systems is to children with mild hearing loss and those with attention deficit and learning disabilities. For children with more profound hearing loss, sound field systems also allow direct transmission to an individual student through earphones by coupling to a personal FM system. Sound field systems have been shown to increase speech perception, improve academic skills (reading, spelling), and address learning disabilities (e.g., attention). Typically hearing students have also been shown to benefit from sound field systems and teachers benefit from greater student attention and less vocal strain. One additional benefit of some sound field systems is the use of ambient noise compensation (ANC) (Ross and Levitt, 2002). ANC uses digital signal processing to automatically increase amplification if the noise level rises temporarily because of factors such as a transient noise (e.g., air conditioning starting up) or a decrease in the teacher's speaking volume. Adjustment for these changes in the ANC allows the sound field system to maintain a constant SNR for the student.

Large-Group Devices

The problems addressed by small-group devices also exist in large meeting rooms such as concert halls, lecture auditoriums, and churches. Under the provisions of the ADA in the United States and similar legislation in other countries, these areas must be equipped with assistive listening devices. There are several approaches possible, all of which are directly coupled to the public address system of the facility being equipped. These are (1) hard-wired jacks for plugging in earphones, (2) FM transmitter-receiver setups similar to small-group devices, and (3) audio induction loops for transmission to hearing aids equipped with telecoils. Hard-wired systems have the advantage of privacy (there is no transmission over the air) and simplicity of technology. There are two primary limitations of this approach, however. First, rewiring a facility has a high cost and, unless the wiring is done during construction, it is usually not feasible. Second, persons requiring the use of the assisted listening device are forced to sit in a few predetermined locations (where there are earphone jacks).

Audio induction loop devices have their roots in Europe. They require that the user's hearing aid have an induction coil (*telecoil*). The major limitations of the induction coil approach are the large amount of power required to drive the induction coil transmitter and susceptibility to interference. FM transmission coil systems are similar to the home-based coil but with much more powerful amplification. They have a lower level of interference and a large transmission range. FM systems have the advantage that the listener can sit anywhere within range, and they can easily be wired into the normal public address system. Limitations of this approach include varying degrees of strength in the signals being received by the receivers in different hearing aids and a nonuniform transmission pattern resulting in unequal signal strength.

Other assistive listening devices have been developed for television viewing and for use as personal amplifiers (Stach, 1998). Personal amplifiers are hard-wired microphones connected to an amplifier and to earphones worn by the person who is hard of hearing. They are used in hospitals and similar situations for temporary amplification when hearing aids are not available or not worn. Television listeners are assistive listening devices that connect directly to the audio of the television set and transmit the signal to a receiver by FM or ultrasound. The user has earphones connected to the receiver.

Captioning As an Auditory Substitute

Captioning is a process whereby the audio portion of a television program is converted to written words, which appear in a window on the screen. Captioning substitutes visual (text) information for auditory information (dialogue, narration, and sound effects). Originally focused on broadcast television and films, captioning has been expanded to include cable television, webcasting, home video and DVD, and government and corporate video programming. Captioning is also used as an alternative to sign language interpreters in classrooms, meetings, and for face-to-face conversations.

The National Captioning Institute[20] (NCI) in the United States is a leading provider of closed captioning and other media access services. NCI provides subtitling and language translation services in over 50 languages and dialects. The NCI can also caption live programs such as news broadcasts, presidential speeches, and coverage of the Olympics. Captions can aid those learning English as a second language and provide assistance in efforts to eradicate illiteracy. The European Captioning Institute (ECI) provides similar services throughout Europe. Similar organizations exist in most countries.

Closed Captioned Television and Movies

When captioning is used in public media (television, movie theaters), it is **closed captioning.** It is called *closed* because the words are not visible unless the viewer has a closed caption decoder. In the United States the Telecommunications Act of 1996 resulted in FCC regulations requiring television broadcasters to provide closed captioning. New programming released after January 1, 1998, must be "fully accessible." *Fully accessible* means that 95% of the nonexempt programming must be closed captioned. All television sets currently being produced have a built-in closed caption converter. It takes between 20 and 30 hours to close caption a 1-hour television program. The individual broadcasters make decisions regarding which programs are captioned consistent with the regulations described above. Some programs, such as live newscasts, are captioned on the fly, whereas others are captioned in postproduction.

---

[20]www.ncicap.org.

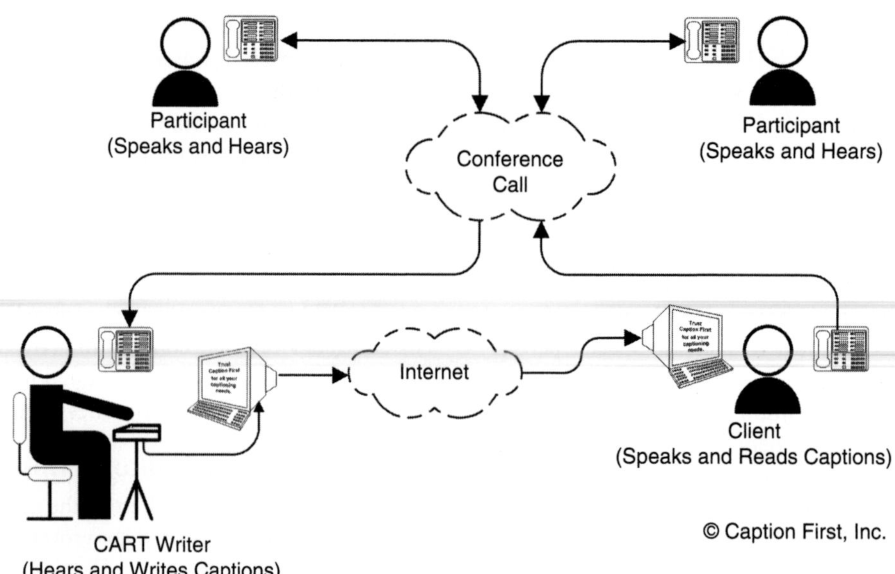

FIGURE 14-12 Schematic representation of computer-assisted real-time (or remote) transcription (CART). (Courtesy of Caption First, http://www.captionfirst.com/.)

More than 3000 titles of home videos and nearly 500 hours of network, cable, and independent programming a week are now available in closed caption form. Closed captioning includes movies, network news, comedies, sporting events, dramas, and educational, religious, and children's programming. In excess of 550 national advertisers have closed captioned more than 13,000 commercials.

Real-Time Captioning for Education and Business Applications

Computer-assisted real-time (or remote) transcription (CART) has been applied in several different ways (Figure 14-12). For lectures or meetings where there is one deaf participant, CART can be provided one-on-one where a stenographer translates speech into text in real time and it is displayed on a monitor for the individual who is deaf. For meetings in which there is more than one deaf participant, the text output is projected on a screen, generally from a computer. The Internet can also be used to assist deaf individuals with spoken language interpretation. The stenographer has voice connection through the Internet to the meeting or classroom and enters text with a stenotype machine. The text is translated through computer software to text, transmitted over the Internet back to the classroom or meeting, and then read by the deaf individual. Several vendors provide CART services.[21]

Another example is computer-assisted note-taking (CAN) (Youdelman and Messerly, 1996). A fast typist enters text with a standard computer keyboard and with use of abbreviations (see Chapter 6) to maximize speed of data entry. As in the CART method, text is displayed on a screen. The rate of entry is too slow for the speech to be converted directly to text, so a summary is used. The accuracy of the summary is estimated to be in the 90% to 95% range. In an evaluation study, Youdelman and Messerly (1996) found that notetakers found this approach to be superior to pencil and paper methods because speed could be increased without sacrificing legibility, text could be easily edited, printed copies could be made available to students immediately, and emphasis of important points could be enhanced by bold, italic, or underline formats. The teachers felt that the CAN approach helped students obtain more information than they had with previous methods and that the printed method improved spelling skills. Because CAN was applied to uncaptioned videotapes and other media, it had an additional benefit. The teachers also noted a positive impact on the entire class, not just on the hearing impaired students, because it helped the entire class focus on the material covered and helped them develop good note taking skills. The hearing impaired students stated that CAN helped them understand the material and keep up with the teacher. The children without hearing impairments observed that it was helpful to glance at the display as the teacher was talking to gain information missed orally. They also benefited from the printed notes.

Basic Principles of Computer Adaptations for Auditory Impairments

Increasingly, there is auditory information that is included with software application programs or webpages. For persons who are deaf, this information may be inaccessible. If an individual is hard of hearing, the system volume can generally be increased. It is also possible to use headphones and link more directly to the user's auditory system. Computer interaction is bidirectional, and the clinician must understand how computer outputs can be adapted for persons with sensory impairments. Persons who are deaf or hard of

[21]For example: Hear Ink, www.hearink.com/; Caption First, www.captionfirst.com/.

TABLE 14-1 Built-in Adaptations for Auditory Impairment

Need Addressed	Software Approach
User cannot hear speech and sounds produced by programs, webpages, or change of operation or error during program operation	Screen Flash (OS X), Visible and Vibrating Alerts (iOS and Blackberry), Visual Notifications (Windows)*
User wants to use sign language for communicating through the device	FaceTime (OS X and iOS)
User has limited hearing in one ear only	Mono Audio (OS X and iOS); also available on Android and Blackberry phones
User who is deaf wants to view multimedia programming (movies, TV shows, and podcasts)	Closed caption (OS X, iOS, Windows, Blackberry)

Software modifications developed at the Trace Center, University of Wisconsin, Madison. These are included as before-market modifications in most personal computers.
*Visual Notifications: Windows Microsoft, Seattle, Wash., www.microsoft.com/enable/; Screen Flash (OS X): Apple Computer, Cupertino, Calif., http://www.apple.com/accessibility/.

hearing also may have difficulties in recognizing auditory computer outputs, such as sounds or speech.

Built-in options can increase usability by persons who are deaf. Adaptations that facilitate some of these functions and that are included in the accessibility options in Windows, OSX, iOS, and Android devices are shown in Table 14-1. Major functions that are changed are the use of visual or vibrating alerts in place of auditory tones. Captioning or multimedia (movies, TV shows, and podcasts) is also available. For those who are deaf in only one ear and want the full stereo experience presented at one ear, conversion of stereo to monaural sounds can be used. Text captions can be displayed in place of sounds to indicate that an activity is happening (for example, when a document starts or finishes printing).

There are also apps for iOS, Android, and Blackberry devices that support people with hearing impairment. Examples are support for sign language transmission (high-fidelity video), alerts such as vibrating patterns that distinguish specific callers, alternatives to auditory alarms (vibrating or flashing alerts), and TTY-type functions.

Access to the Internet When Auditory Information Is Difficult for the User

Because webpages are a mixture of text, graphics, and sound, they can present challenges to individuals who are deaf or hard of hearing. As the amount of auditory web content increases, people who are deaf are also prevented from accessing information. Chapter 13 describes general issues of access and how webpages are developed, including the use of programming languages such as hypertext markup language. The World Wide Web Consortium (W3C) (see Chapter 13) recommendations include accessibility for deaf and hard of hearing users. By using the Microsoft Synchronized Accessible Media Interchange, authors of webpages and multimedia software can add closed captioning for users who are deaf or hard of hearing. This standard simplifies captioning for developers, educators, and multimedia producers and designers and is available to the public as an open (no licensing fees) standard. This approach is similar to the use of closed captioning for television viewers. The W3C Web Accessibility Initiative synchronized multimedia integration language is designed to facilitate multimedia presentations in which an author can describe the behavior of a multimedia presentation, associate hyperlinks with media objects, and describe the layout of the presentation on a screen. These features allow integration of timing of multimedia presentations into hypertext markup language programs.

Aids for Persons with Both Visual and Auditory Impairments

Individuals who are both deaf and blind must use tactile input to obtain information about the environment and to communicate. There are two basic methods used by this group of people. The Tadoma method (described earlier in this chapter) is used to understand speech; finger spelling, with the deaf-blind individual sensing the signs in his or her hand, is used when both persons in the conversation know signing or one person acts as an interpreter.

Devices for Face-to-Face Communication with Individuals Who Are Deaf and Blind

A common approach to communication between a nondisabled person and and individual who is both deaf and blind is to use a standard keyboard and visual display for the nondisabled person and a braille keyboard and display for the person who is deaf/blind.[22] This configuration enables direct face-to-face communication with individuals who have no knowledge of sign language or braille to communicate with a person who is both deaf and blind. It does require knowledge of braille by the person with a disability.

FaceToFace[23] uses a portable note-taking device (PACMate) with built-in braille keyboard and refreshable display (see Chapter 13) together with a software application on a PDA or portable computer. The two devices communicate via Bluetooth. The deaf/blind person types a message on the braille keyboard and it is displayed as text on the PDA or computer screen. The communication partner types on the PDA or computer and it is shown on the braille display. A similar approach is available in the Deafblind Communicator[24] from Humanware.

[22]For example: ITY, Intertype, Rochester, NY, http://www.interpretype.com/pricing-ordering-dbcs-2.php; FSTTY and FSCommunicator, Freedom Scientific, St Petersburg, Fla., www.freedomscientific.com/fs_products/FlyerPDFs/FSTTYFlyer.pdf; Telle-touch, Perkins, Watertown, Mass., http://support.perkins.org/site/PageServer?pagename=Webcasts_Communication_Technology.
[23]Freedom Scientific, St Petersburg, Fla., http://www.freedomscientific.com/products/fs/facetoface-product-page.asp.
[24]http://www.humanware.com/usa/products/deafblind_communication_solutions.

The TTY function provides the capability for the deaf/blind person to talk to other people who have a TTY or, through a relay operator, to anyone with a telephone. The keyboards (braille and QWERTY) and displays (braille and visual) allow face-to face communication.

Finally, another approach uses two separate devices connected by cable or wireless transmission.[25] Both the hearing and deaf/blind user have a keyboard and display, which may be QWERTY or braille keyboard and visual or braille display. The advantage of this approach is that the two people communicating can have a more comfortable physical spacing as they communicate because they each have their own device. The device can either be a stand-alone system designed for this purpose or a computer running special software.

Many of the same functions as the devices described can be accomplished using a portable braille notebook (see Chapter 13) with a link to a Bluetooth enabled smart phone. With a software app that converts braille to text and vice versa, the smart phone can provide visual text and typing in standard text and the portable braille reader can provide both input and output in braille. It is possible for persons who are deaf/blind and have this combination of technologies to carry them with them; when they encounter someone who wishes to converse, they simply hand the smart phone to the other person and begin a conversation by typing on the braille keyboard.

CONTEXT COMPONENT

Helen Keller, who was both deaf and blind, is reported to have been asked whether she would prefer to have her vision or her hearing if she could have one or the other. She responded that she would prefer to have her hearing because she felt that people who are blind are cut off from things, whereas those who are deaf are cut off from people. It is important to keep this concept in mind when considering aids for persons who are deaf or hard of hearing. Auditory impairment is often not as obvious as visual impairment, and society does not view it as having the same degree of significance as visual impairment. It is natural for a person to wear glasses as a part of the inherent process of aging. However, many people are embarrassed to admit hearing loss sufficient to require a hearing aid. Despite these considerations, hearing loss is significant, and it can be socially isolating.

There is a stigma associated with the use of hearing aids that does not apply to glasses for vision. We work hard to make hearing aids nonvisible while treating eye glasses as fashion statements (Pullin, 2009). Hearing loss is often associated with aging and is therefore further stigmatized as a symbol of "age-related decay." Hearing aid manufacturers advertise aids "that no one else can see." Designer hearing aids that make fashion statements similar to glasses have also been developed (for example, see: http://www.audicus.com/blogs/hearing-aids-blog/6071796-putting-the-cool-in-hearing-aid-design).

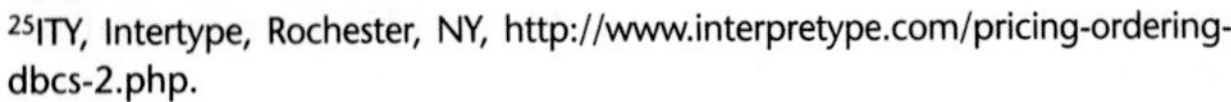

[25]ITY, Intertype, Rochester, NY, http://www.interpretype.com/pricing-ordering-dbcs-2.php.

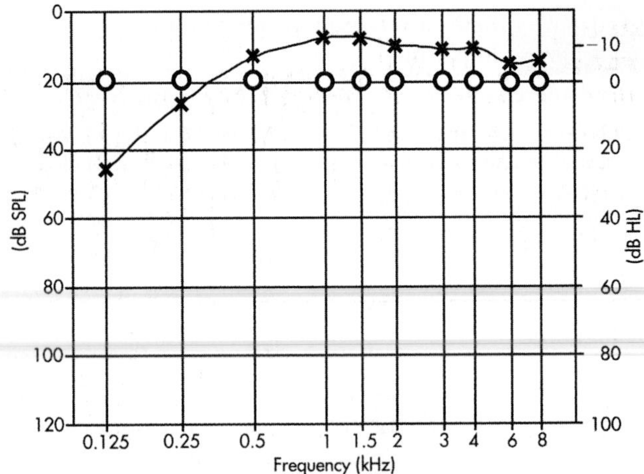

FIGURE 14-13 Typical audiogram test results for pure tone testing. SPL, Sound pressure level. (From Ballantyne D: *Handbook of audiological techniques*, London: Butterworth-Heinemann, 1990.)

Pullin (2009) describes the concept of "hear wear" design for hearing, paralleling "eye wear" for seeing. This approach is intended to reduce the stigma of hearing loss by making it fashionable to have attractive hearing aids.

ASSESSMENT

Auditory Thresholds

The typical range of frequencies that can be heard by the human ear is 20 to 20,000 hertz (Hz) (Martin and Clark, 2012). The ear does not respond equally to all frequencies in this range, however, and Figure 14-3 shows the response curve of a normal ear. The vertical axis of Figure 14-3 is the sound pressure measured in decibels. The horizontal axis shows the frequencies of sound applied. The curve in this figure is the minimal threshold for detecting the sound for each frequency. The tone presented at 1000 Hz requires an intensity of 6.5 dB to sound as loud as a tone presented at 250 Hz with an intensity of 24.5 dB. This curve illustrates why alarms and other audible indicators usually have a frequency near 1000 Hz.

There are several types of tests that audiologists use in assessing hearing. Pure tone audiometry presents pure (one-frequency) tones to each ear and determines the threshold of hearing for that person. The intensity of the tone is raised in 5-dB increments until it is heard; then it is lowered in 5-dB increments until it is no longer heard. The threshold is the intensity at which the person indicates that he or she hears the tone 50% of the time. A typical audiogram is shown in Figure 14-13. On the curve shown in Figure 14-13, all values are displayed as hearing loss, and the "normal" level is shown as 0-dB loss. The curve of Figure 14-3 is incorporated into the plot of Figure 14-13. Thus for 125 Hz, a tone of 90.5 dB was heard 50% of the time in the right ear (45.5-dB threshold from Figure 14-3 added to 45-dB loss from Figure 14-13). At 1000 Hz the threshold presented was 36.5 dB. This test gives the audiologist information regarding the range of frequencies over which the person can hear and hearing losses at specific frequencies.

Speech Recognition Threshold

Although the frequencies presented in the pure tone test are in the range of speech (125 to 8000 Hz), this test alone does not indicate the person's ability to understand speech. To evaluate this function, the audiologist uses a speech recognition threshold test. In this evaluation, speech is presented, either live or recorded, at varying intensity levels, and the person's ability to understand it is determined. The person is asked to repeat either words or sentences presented at these varying intensities.

The concept of sound pressure level and the values shown in Figure 14-3 are particularly important in consideration of the context for assistive technology use. One example of the application of these principles is Carolyn's use of an augmentative communication device that has voice synthesis output (Case Study 14-1).

SUMMARY

Hearing aids provide assistance for persons whose hearing is inadequate for conversation. Recent trends in hearing aid design have focused on improved fidelity and digital speech processing. An individual who has damage to the cochlea may benefit from the use of cochlear implants. Emphasis on speech processing algorithms will continue to provide better understanding of how stimulation by cochlear implants can aid speech recognition.

Aids for persons who are deaf use either visual or tactile systems as alternatives. Speech-to-text (sound-to-visual display) devices are not as well developed as text-to-speech aids, and visual information is most commonly used for alarms rather than for communication. Exceptions to this are telephone communication using telephone devices for the deaf (TTYs).

Mobile technology apps are available both for individuals who are hard of hearing and those who are deaf. Some adaptations for these populations are also built into computers and mobile devices.

Aids for persons who are both deaf and blind must use tactile substitution. The major approach is braille output with a text-based keyboard for communication between a sighted and a deaf-blind individual. The availability of portable systems that provide braille for the person who is deaf/blind and visual text for the communication partner has been helpful for face-to-face communication.

STUDY QUESTIONS

1. What are the two basic approaches to auditory sensory aids in terms of the sensory pathway used?
2. List the three basic parts of an auditory sensory aid and describe the function of each part.
3. Discuss the major differences between blindness and deafness in terms of the effect on the individual's social, work or school, and private life.
4. What are the major parts of a hearing aid, and what is the function of each?
5. What are the types of hearing aids?
6. What is acoustic coupling, and how does it affect hearing aid performance?
7. How does a bone-anchored hearing aid function, and when is it used?
8. List the major functions that a cochlear implant must accomplish.
9. What are the major advantages provided by digital hearing aids?
10. How are data and power coupled to cochlear implants?
11. What is the relationship between the number of electrodes and the functional performance of a cochlear implant?
12. What are the major differences between a channel and an electrode in cochlear implants?
13. Describe the major approaches to signal processing used in cochlear implants. What are the advantages and disadvantages of each?
14. What are the advantages of binaural cochlear implants?
15. What is required to make a computer communicate with a TTY?
16. What is required to make a mobile phone communicate with a TTY?
17. List the major ways that mobile phones are used by individuals who are deaf.
18. What is a TTY, and why is the Baudot code used?
19. What is CapTel and how does it work?
20. Compare a stand-alone TTY with a computer TTY modem using Baudot coding. What advantages does each offer to a deaf user?
21. Why can't a standard computer modem be used to communicate with a TTY without special software?
22. What are the major limitations to the use of standard telephone lines for visual information transmission (such as for manual signing)?
23. What is computer-assisted real-time transmission and how does it apply to education, business, and personal use?
24. What are alerting devices? For what purposes are they normally used?
25. What are FM transmission systems for group listening, and how are they typically used?
26. What are the three major assistive technology approaches used for deaf/blind individuals to obtain communication input? What are the relative advantages of each approach?
27. Discuss the major differences between blindness and deafness in terms of the effect on the individual's social, work or school, and private life?

REFERENCES

Bailey RW: *Human performance engineering*, ed 2, Englewood Cliffs, NJ, 1989, Prentice Hall.

Balkany TJ, et al.: Cochlear implants in children—a review, *Acta Otolaryngol* 122:356–362, 2002.

Ching TYC, et al.: Management of children using cochlear implants and hearing aids, *Volta Rev* 103:39–57, 2001.

Crandell CC, Smaldino JJ: Classroom acoustics for children with normal hearing and with hearing impairment, *Lang Speech Hearing Serv Schools* 31:362–370, 2000.

Chiu H-P, Liu C-H, Hsieh C-L: Essential needs and requirements of mobile phones for the deaf, *Assist Technol* 22(3): 172–185, 2010.

D'Eredità R, Caroncini M, Saetti R: The New Baha Implant: A Prospective Osseointegration Study, *Otolaryngol Head Neck Surg* 146(6):979–983, 2012.

Dillon H: *Hearing aids*, New York, 2001, Thieme.

Eisenberg A: *For hard of hearing, clarity out of the din. NY Times*, May 5, 2012. Downloaded October 5, 3013, from http://www.nytimes.com/2012/05/06/technology/audio-devices-give-new-options-to-those-hard-of-hearing.html?_r=0.

Feigenbaum E: Cochlear implant devices for the profoundly hearing impaired, *IEEE Eng Med Biol Mag* 6:10–21, 1987.

Galuska S, Foulds R: A real-time visual telephone for the deaf. In *Proceedings of the 13th Annual RESNA Conference*, Washington, DC, 1990, RESNA, pp 267–268.

Galuska S, Grove T, Gray J: A visual "talk" utility: using sign language over a local area computer network. In *Proceedings of the 15th Annual RESNA Conference*, Washington, DC, 1992, RESNA, pp 134–135.

Gan K: *Interpretype—assistive technology for face-to-face communication. Proceedings of the CSUN Conference.* Accessed April, 2007 http://www.csun.edu/cod/conf/2005/proceedings/2168.htm, 2005.

Gaylor JM, Raman G, Chung M, et al.: Cochlear implantation in adults: a systematic review and meta-analysis, *JAMA Otolaryngol Head Neck Surg* 139(3):265–272, 2013.

Halliday J: How can braille help people who are deaf, *Hum Awareness Newsl Autumn*, 1993.

Harkins J: Voice over IP: some accessibility issues. In *The blue book: 2005 TDI national directory and resource guide*, Silver Spring, Md, 2004, TDI, pp 21–23.

Hickson, Louise, Mackenzie, Deborah, Gordon, Juliet, Neall, Vanessa, Wu, Desmond Wu, Janice. The outcomes of bone anchored hearing Aid (BAHA) fitting in a paediatric cohort. *Australian and New Zealand Journal of Audiology*, 28, 75–89, 2006. doi:10.1375/audi.28.2.75

Hol, Myrthe KS, Snik, Ad FM, Mylanus, Emmanuel AM Cremers, Cor W. R. J. Does the bone-anchored hearing aid have a complementary effect on audiological and subjective outcomes in patients with unilateral conductive hearing loss? *Audiology & Neurotology*, 10, 159–168, 2005. doi:10.1159/000084026

Kerckhoff J, Listenberger J, Valente M: Advances in hearing aid technology, *Contemp Issues Communic Sci Disorders* 35:102–112, 2008.

Kimura MYT, Hyppolito MA: Reflections on bilateral cochlear implants, *Int J Clin Med* 4:171–177, 2013.

Lieberman P: *Intonation, perception and language*, Cambridge, MA, 1967, MIT Press.

Loizou P: Mimicking the human ear, *IEEE Signal Processing Mag* 15:101–130, 1998.

Loizou P: Speech processing in vocoder-centric cochlear implants, *Adv Otorhinolaryngol* 64:109–143, 2006.

McFadden GM: Aids for hearing impairments and deafness. In Galvin JC, Scherer MJ, editors: *Evaluating, selecting and using appropriate assistive technology*, Rockville, MD, 1996, Aspen Publishers.

Martin FN, Clark JG: *Introduction to audiology*, ed 11, Upper Saddle River, NJ: PearsonEducaton, 2012.

Miculek, A: Placement of the Baha osseointegrated implant in children, *Operative Techniques in Otolaryngology-Head and Neck Surgery* 20(3):197–201, 2009.

Miyazaki S, Ishida A: Traffic-alarm sound monitor for aurally handicapped drivers, *Med Biol Eng Comput* 25:68–74, 1987.

Mulla, Imran, Wright, Nicola Archbold, Sue. The views and experiences of families on bone anchored hearing aid use with children: A study by interviews. *Deafness & Education International*, 15(2), 70-90, 2013

Olsen W: Average speech levels and spectra in various speaking/listening conditions: a summary of the Pearson, Bennett and Fidell (1977) report, *Am J Audiol* 7:21–25, 1988.

Palmer CV: A contemporary review of hearing aids, *Laryngoscope* 119:2195–2204, 2009.

Power D, Power MR, Rehling B: German deaf people using text communication: Short Message Service, TTY, relay services, fax, and e-mail, *Amer Ann Deaf* 152(3):291–301, 2007.

Pullin G: *Design meets disability*, , Cambridge, MA, 2009, MIT Press.

Ramsden RT: Cochlear implants and brain stem implants, *Br Med Bull* 63:183–193, 2002.

Rasmussen, Jacob, Olsen, Steen Ostergaard Nielsen, Lars Holme. Evaluation of long-term patient satisfaction and experience with the Baha bone conduction implant. International Journal of Audiology, 51, 194-199, 2012. doi:10.3109/14992027.2011.635315

Ross M, Levitt H: Classroom sound-field systems, *Volta Voices* 9-2:7–8, 2002.

Sarant J: Cochlear implants in children: a review. In Naz S, editor: *Hearing loss. InTech Open*, 2012, pp 331–382.

Shallop JK, Mecklenberg DJ: Technical aspects of cochlear implants. In Sandlin RE, editor: *Handbook of hearing aid amplification*, vol. 1. Boston, 1988, Little, Brown.

Snik AFM, et al.: Consensus statements on the BAHA system: where do we stand at present? *Ann Otol Rhinol Laryngol* 114(Suppl 195):1–12, 2005.

Stach BA: *Clinical audiology*, San Diego, 1998, Singular Publishing Group.

Waltzman S, et al.: Long-term effects of cochlear implants in children, *Otolaryngol Head Neck Surg* 126:505–511, 2002.

Whit RL: System design of a cochlear implant, *IEEE Eng Med Biol Mag* 6:10–21, 1987.

Wilson BS, et al.: Design and evaluation of a continuous interleaved sampling (CIS) processing strategy for multichannel cochlear implants, *J Rehabil Res* 30:110–116, 1993.

Youdelman K, Messerly C: Computer-assisted note taking for mainstreamed hearing-impaired students, *Volta Rev* 98: 191–200, 1996.

CHAPTER 15

Assistive Technologies for Cognitive Augmentation[1]

CHAPTER OUTLINE

LEARNING OBJECTIVES

On completing this chapter, you will be able to do the following:

1. Apply the human activity assistive technology model to help identify appropriate assistive technologies for individuals with cognitive disabilities.
2. Identify cognitive skills that underlie functional performance for persons with cognitive disabilities.
3. Understand what cognitive faculties are commonly compromised in specific disorders.
4. Understand the role of assistive technologies in aiding cognitive function.
5. Identify and describe some of the technologies, both mainstream and assistive, that are currently available to assist individuals with cognitive impairments.

KEY TERMS

Alternative Input
Alternative Output
Attention
Attention Deficit Hyperactivity Disorder
Autism Spectrum Disorder
Cerebral Vascular Accident
Cognitive Assistive Technologies
Cognitive Prosthesis
Dementia
Developmental Disabilities
Generalization
Information Processing
Intellectual Disability
Knowledge Representation
Learning Disabilities
Media Presentation
Memory
Mild Cognitive Disabilities
Problem Solving
Prompting
Smart Home
Stimuli Control
Tracking and Identification
Traumatic Brain Injury
Vigilance

The majority of currently available assistive technologies are designed to meet the needs of individuals who have motor or sensory limitations. Those assistive devices are the subject of most of this book. Recently, designers of assistive technologies have turned their attention to the needs of individuals whose limitations are primarily cognitive. An example of this type of technology is shown in Figure 15-1. This chapter explores applications of cognitive assistive technologies (CATs).

Interventions for cognitive impairment to avoid risky behaviors are generally carried out through physical restriction

[1] In the previous edition of this book this chapter was co-written by Kim Adams, Roger Calixto, Lui Shi Gan, Andrew Ganton, Andrew Rees, Tyler Simpson, and Rebecca Watchorn.

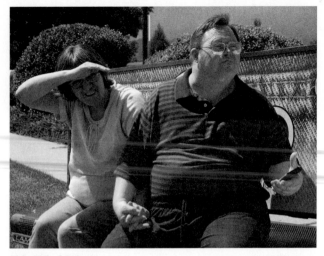

FIGURE 15-1 A specially programmed mobile technology can help an individual with a cognitive disability to achieve a greater level of independence. (Courtesy of AbleLink Technologies, http://www.ablelinktech.com/.)

of behavior (e.g., removal of individual from situation), medications, or behavior modification, all of which seek to limit risky behavior (Gillespie et al, 2012). In contrast, the use of CATs seeks to extend or augment cognitive function.

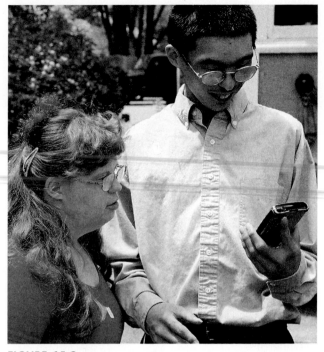

FIGURE 15-2 Mobile technologies can be used by persons with intellectual disabilities for a variety of tasks. (Courtesy of AbleLink Technologies, http://www.ablelinktech.com/.)

ACTIVITY COMPONENT

Gillespie et al (2012) examined the relationship between cognitive assistive technologies (CATs) and cognitive function using a systematic review. Using the definition of CATs as "any technology which compensates for cognitive deficit during task performance" (p. 2), they identified 89 publications that included 91 studies. The WHO *International Classification of Functioning, Disability and Health* (ICF) (see Chapter 1) was used to categorize the cognitive domains that were being assisted and the tasks being performed. ICF classification of "activities and participation" (d110-d999) includes learning and applying knowledge, general tasks and demands, communication, mobility, self-care, domestic life, interpersonal interactions, major life areas, and community, social, and civic life.

The HAAT model (see Chapters 1, 2, and 3) consists of four elements: Human, Activity, Context, and Assistive Technology (Figure 1-1). In this chapter we focus on human cognitive skills and activities that require those skills. As shown in Figure 15-2, the context might be the community. We can look for assistive technologies that can aid or replace the required cognitive skill. The expected skills and limitations presented in this chapter are general and every individual is unique.

To apply the HAAT model, a desired activity is identified. For example, the activity might be carrying out a sequence of steps such as for making a bed. The context would also be identified, and in this example it is the home. Given the activity and the context, the required set of skills to accomplish the activity can be determined. If there is a gap between the skills required to complete the task and the skills that the individual brings to the task, the use of assistive technologies to aid or replace the required skill should be considered. In this case, if the person has an **intellectual disability** that affects her ability to remember the required sequence of steps to make the bed, then a **prompting** device might be helpful. For any particular disability a skill set and possible limitations can be identified. The process of identifying and applying assistive technologies for cognitive assistance is illustrated in the following case study.

CASE STUDY 15-1

Intellectual Disability and Tasks of Daily Living

William is a 38-year-old man with an intellectual disability. He lives in a group home with five other men. He is expected to carry out duties to contribute to the program at the home. His task is to set the table for dinner. Currently, he is only successful in completing this task if he has continuous prompting from a member of the staff. This is limiting both to William, because he is not independent, and to the home because the staff is occupied making dinner during the time William is to carry out this task. Fortunately, there are assistive technologies available to assist William in this task. List the characteristics you think such a technology should have and then look at the descriptions later in this chapter of approaches that have been taken. Did you come up with better ideas than what is available?

HUMAN COMPONENT

"Cognition is the mental process of knowing, including aspects such as awareness, perception, reasoning, and judgment."[2]

[2]The free dictionary: http://www.thefreedictionary.com/cognition.

Cognitive is the adjective referring to cognition. Cognitive disabilities may be present at birth or result from injury or disease. Of those present at birth, some are genetically transmitted, others result from prenatal or perinatal conditions, and for many cases there is no identifiable cause. Acquired cognitive disabilities are the result of injury or disease. Impairments that result from cognitive disabilities include memory loss, **dementia**, language disorders, the ability to make decisions, and the capability to function independently.

There are over 20 million individuals with a cognitive disability in the United States (Braddock et al, 2004). This number can be broken down into categories: mental illness: 27%; Alzheimer's disease: 20%; brain injury: 27%; mental retardation/**developmental disabilities**: 22%; and stroke: 4%.

Cognitive Skills

Cognitive functions that have typically been aided by assistive technologies include attention, calculation, emotion, experience of self, higher level cognitive functions (planning and time management), and memory (Gillespie et al, 2012). Understanding the cognitive demands of various tasks can help us understand why an individual may find a seemingly simple task to be very difficult, while a seemingly difficult task may be carried out virtually effortlessly.

Some cognitive skills such as **memory**, **attention**, **information processing**, and **problem solving** are better understood than others (Sternberg, 2003). The definitions of some of the cognitive skills for which assistive technologies have been developed are listed in Box 15-1. Each skill listed will be described briefly in this section; for more detailed descriptions refer to a cognitive psychology textbook (e.g., Sternberg, 2003).

Perception

Perception is the interpretation of sensory information received through our eyes, ears, and skin—that is, what we see, hear, and feel (Anderson, 2000). Perception is a very basic cognitive skill that is integrated with higher order cognition to achieve various skills, such as sequencing the steps required to make a bed. Impairments that affect perception limit an individual's ability to use information from the environment to assist with daily activities. For example, someone with reduced visual acuity may have difficulty perceiving text that is presented on a computer screen. In this case, enlarged letters and auditory feedback may aid the person when using a computer for word processing.

Attention

Attention is the ability to focus on a particular task (Willingham, 2001). For example, selective attention refers to the ability to shift attention between competing tasks, which requires selectively attending to one stimulus while ignoring another (Golisz and Toglia, 2003). The characterization of different types of attention provides insight into different areas in which people may have strengths and weaknesses and for which assistive technologies may be of help.

Attention has been characterized by different levels. Any task can involve more than one type of attention. The first of these is the detection or observation of a particular stimulus or signal (e.g., an object or event occurring in the environment). Signal detection is a process by which an individual must detect the appearance of a particular stimulus. We can detect a signal in two ways. **Vigilance** refers to paying close and continuous attention over a prolonged period in order to detect a signal. *Sustained attention* is similar to vigilance, but there isn't necessarily a competing stimulus present. *Search* is the active scanning of the environment to find a particular stimulus or particular features. Vigilance and sustained attention require the person to wait for the signal to appear, and search requires the person to actively seek out a target signal. For example, after an earthquake a person might be vigilant in watching for smoke, and if smoke were detected, he or she might then actively search for the source of the smoke (Sternberg, 2003).

Using *selective attention* is how we filter out distractions and focus on the event we have chosen (Ashcraft, 1998). Variability in our selective attention skills is common, especially when there are distractions. For some individuals the influence of distractions is such that they are unable to focus on a task when another stimulus (e.g., a conversation) is occurring in the background. For example, individuals with attention deficit disorder have difficulty focusing on the teacher in class. There are other situations in which we are required to devote attention to two or more tasks at the same time using *divided attention*. One example is listening to a lecture and taking notes. Students need auditory attention and processing skills to understand what the teacher is saying, and additionally, require visual and tactile skills to take notes. While the activities of listening to a lecture and taking notes appear to be concurrent, in fact attention is moving quickly between the two tasks.

In contrast to selecting only one stimulus to attend to, at times it is necessary to allocate attention to multiple stimuli at one time. This is referred to as *divided attention*, such as listening to a lecture and taking notes. Research in this area has shown there are serious limits to the number of things people can do at one time. Often, rather than attending to multiple stimuli simultaneously, people actually switch their attention back and forth between tasks so rapidly that they are unaware of the switching. As the individual tasks become more and more cognitively demanding, the switching becomes harder to do and they are less likely to be able to truly perform the tasks concurrently (Galotti, 2004).

Memory

Short-term memory refers to storage of information for up to about 20 seconds. Various strategies, such as rehearing the information to be remembered, can be used to maintain information in the short-term store. To remember something for a longer period of time it is necessary for it to be transferred to *long-term memory*. In order for memory to be useful, the input must be perceived, recognized as something that is important to retain, encoded, stored, and then

BOX 15-1 Definitions of Cognitive Skills

Perception
Interpretation of the sensations received from environmental stimuli (through the sense organs)

Attention
Link between the limited amount of information that is actually manipulated mentally and the enormous amount of information available through the senses, stored memories, and other cognitive processes

Signal detection: Detecting the appearance of a particular stimulus
Vigilance: Paying close and continuous attention
Search: Active scanning of the environment for particular stimuli or features
Selective: Tracking one stimulus or one type of stimulus and ignoring another
Divided: Allocating available resources to coordinate performance of more than one task at a time

Memory
Drawing on past knowledge to use it in the present

Encoding: Physical and sensory input is transformed into a representation that can be stored in memory
Storage: The movement of encoded information into memory and the maintenance of information in storage
Sensory: The smallest capacity for storing information (i.e., for only a fleeting sensory image) and the shortest duration for memory storage (i.e., for only fractions of a second)
Short-term: A modest capacity (i.e., for about seven items) and a duration of a number of seconds unless strategies (e.g., rehearsal) are used for keeping the information in the short-term store for longer periods of time
Long-term: A greater capacity than both the sensory store and the short-term store, and it can store information for very long periods of time, even indefinitely
Retrieval: Recovery of stored information from memory, by moving the information into consciousness for use in active cognitive processing
Implicit: Enhanced performance on a task, as a result of prior experience, despite having no conscious awareness of recollecting the prior experience
Explicit: Consciously recalling or recognizing particular information
Recall: Retrieving memories with no hints
Recognition: Retrieving memories with hints

Orientation
Knowing and ascertaining one's relation to self, to others, to time, and to one's surroundings

Person: Awareness of one's own identity and of individuals in the immediate environment
Place: Awareness of one's location, such as one's immediate surroundings, one's town or country
Time: Awareness of day, date, month, and year. Also, time management: ordering events in chronological sequence, allocating amounts of time to events and activities
Quantity: Activity involving numbers (counting) and other incremental problems

Knowledge Representation
The mental representation of facts, objects, and skills

Mental Representation
Declarative: Recognition and understanding of factual information about objects, ideas, and events in the environment ("knowing that")
Procedural: Understanding and awareness of how to perform particular tasks or procedures ("knowing how")
Grouping
Categorization: The characterization of the relationship among objects, concepts, or thoughts
Sorting: Organizing objects, concepts, and thoughts into defined categories
Sequencing: Ordering objects or activities according to a set of rules

Problem Solving
A process for which the goal is to overcome obstacles obstructing a path to a solution.

Problem identification: Awareness of and definition of the problem
Judgment: Ability to make sound decisions, recognizing the consequences of decisions taken or actions performed
Decision making: Selecting a course of action from defined alternatives
Reasoning
Deductive: To draw a specific conclusion from a set of general propositions
Inductive: To reach a probable general conclusion on the basis of specific facts or observations
Planning: Anticipating events so as to formulate a course of action to achieve a desired outcome
Evaluation and iteration: Monitoring the status of the problem, evaluating if the goal has been achieved, and if not, making another iteration of the problem-solving cycle
Transfer: The carryover of knowledge or skills from one context to another

Language
A system of communicating objects, concepts, emotions, and thoughts through the systematic use of sounds, graphics, gestures, or other symbols

Data from Sternberg RJ: *Cognitive psychology*, ed 3, Belmont, CA: Wadsworth, 2003.

retrieved. Memory impairment can occur at any one of these parts of the process.

Two common ways of retrieving information from memory are *recall* and *recognition*. Free recall tasks provide virtually no hints at all, while cued recall tasks add in a small amount of information about the material the participant is supposed to recall (Willingham, 2001). *Recognition* tasks provide the target (material to be remembered) along with other material meant to distract the person; for example, a multiple choice question often involves recognition.

Stored memory is accessed through a *retrieval* process, by which stored information is moved into consciousness for use in active cognitive processing. Often people are aware of their memory retrieval and are able to accurately report that they are using information they have previously stored. This is referred to as *explicit* memory. A second type of memory, *implicit* memory, is demonstrated when an individual shows enhanced performance on a task as a result of prior experience, despite having no conscious awareness of the prior experience.

Orientation

A simple walk down the street during lunch hour provides an abundance of information about the noisy construction site, the smell of the flowers, or the number of cars waiting at a stoplight. These things, as well as all the other information that we attend to on a constant basis, help us to orient ourselves. Orientation can be interpreted in different ways, depending on the perspective. To someone who works with an individual with a visual impairment, orientation means moving about the environment. For an individual with a cognitive impairment, the link to movement is not required, but it is often an important part of orientation. There are three types of orientation that are important: person, place, and situation or time.

Our awareness of our own identity and that of others in our environment is called *orientation to person* (WHO, 2001). Orientation to person is commonly affected in disorders such as dementia and **traumatic brain injury** (TBI), where people forget not only who others are, but also who they are. A simple assistive technology that can aid orientation to person is a card listing the person's address and phone number that can be presented to a passerby if they become lost.

We must constantly be aware of where we are and where we are going by paying attention to clues such as streets and landmarks or by knowing that home lies east. But more importantly, we require the ability to guide ourselves from point A to point B using these clues, which is called *orientation to place* (WHO, 2001). Assistive technology wayfinding devices can aid people who have orientation to place limitations.

Orientation to time is what permits us to know it is lunch time and that we can go on our daily walk (WHO, 2001). For individuals who have difficulty reading standard clocks, there are assistive technologies that provide a sense of when events are to occur and the amount of time that must elapse before the event occurs. Orientation to time is broader than time of day. Often the question is what day is it? It also involves orientation to things like time of year, such as certain holidays, which are cues for behaviors and activities.

Knowledge Representations

Knowledge representations help us relate to things, ideas, and events. The mental representation of facts (e.g., gravity makes things fall), objects (e.g., our house or car), and skills (e.g., how to wash our hands) is also related to memory. *Declarative memory* is what allows us to know what an object is (e.g. a ball.) *Procedural memory* allows us to correctly remember a sequence of operations necessary for performance of a task or procedure (e.g., tying a shoe). Both of these can be important in the application of assistive devices to aid cognitive function.

Grouping similar items together is important in representing knowledge. *Categorization* is the basis for ordering and organizing objects based on their characteristics and how they relate to each other. Categorization of clothes could identify the type of clothing (e.g., socks, pants, skirts) or the color or the style or many other features. Once we have decided on a set of categories, the objects, concepts, or thoughts can be organized into defined categories by *sorting*, the second step of organizing. If the objects, concepts, or thoughts to be organized have a numerical relationship, then the sorting task is called *sequencing* (e.g., items to be placed in the correct numerical order). Sequencing could refer to the step required to set the table, make a bed, or take a bus to work. Assistive technologies exist that can help individuals who have difficulty sequencing.

Problem Solving

There are different terms used for cognitive skills. We have chosen the term problem solving as a key skill area. The ICF classification that includes problem solving is *applying knowledge*. In the hierarchy of Box 15-1, the first step in problem solving is *identification of the problem*. If a person has difficulty identifying problems, various devices such as ones that prompt or cue may help.[3] *Judgment* is the ability to make sound decisions, recognizing the consequences of decisions taken or actions performed. *Decision making* is the cognitive process of selecting a course of action from defined alternatives. Two types of *reasoning* are deductive and inductive. *Deductive* reasoning is a process by which an individual tries to draw a logically certain and specific conclusion from a set of general propositions. For example, when using an assistive device that requires touching a screen location (a button) to create an action, the statements, "All buttons make something happen when you push them" and "This is a button" leads to the conclusion, "Something will happen if this button is pushed." *Inductive* reasoning is a process by which an individual tries to reach a probable general conclusion, based on a set of specific facts or observations. This conclusion is likely to be true based on past experience, but there is no guarantee that it will absolutely be true (Hunt and Ellis, 1999).

In assistive technology design the existence of various types of reasoning implies that steps required for operation of a device must be logical and intuitive from the user's point of view, not just from the designer's point of view. For example, a navigational aid designed for someone with intellectual disabilities needs to present information via voice in simple direct commands (e.g., "go to the white building") rather than in more abstract general terms (e.g., "turn right 45 degrees and walk 20 meters, then turn right 30 degrees").

Planning is the process of anticipating future events so as to formulate a course of action to achieve a desired outcome. A person's ability to perform these tasks may be impacted by congenital conditions affecting brain development or by injury or disease. For these individuals, the best approach is often to reduce the number of alternative solutions, make the options clear, and reduce the reliance on anticipation of future consequences of decisions. Once a problem solution has been derived, the next step in problem solving involves confirming the successful conclusion of the task. The problem solver must *evaluate* the outcome of his or her actions and determine if the task has ended successfully, or if it

[3] For example: The Independent Living Suite, Ablelink Technologies, Colorado Springs, Co. www.ablelinktech.com.

requires continuation or repetition (called *iteration)*. **Generalization** is the carryover of knowledge or skills from one kind of task or one particular context to another kind of task or another context. Knowledge is most likely to be generalized when the conditions under which the knowledge is to be used are very similar to those under which the knowledge was acquired (Hunt and Ellis, 1999).

Language and Learning

Language is fundamental to cognitive task representation. Through language and the process of exchanging information, we can express our thoughts, needs, and ideas. *Language* is a method of communication and is composed of the rules (grammar) and symbols expressed by gestures, sounds, or writing. When teaching a skill or task, language is used to portray the desired outcome.

Learning is the process by which knowledge, skills, or attitudes are acquired and it can be attained through study, experience, or teaching. In Box 15-1 we placed learning at the end of the hierarchy because we believe it builds upon the previously mentioned skills, like building blocks. *General learning* refers to the basic ability to acquire knowledge, skills, or attitudes used as a necessity for the more specific types of learning: mathematics, reading, and writing. The ability of someone to learn and comprehend in each of these categories helps define both the features the technology must have and the skills the person needs in order to use it.

DISORDERS THAT MAY BENEFIT FROM COGNITIVE ASSISTIVE TECHNOLOGIES

Cognitive skills may be compromised as a consequence of a number of disorders. Congenital disorders (those present at birth), include intellectual or developmental disabilities (DD), **learning disabilities** (LD), **attention deficit hyperactivity disorder** (ADHD), and **autism spectrum disorder.** (ASD). Acquired disorders that can lead to cognitive limitations include dementia, traumatic brain injury (TBI), and **cerebral vascular accidents** (CVA). The characteristics of these disorders are summarized in Table 15-1.

There are other conditions that are typically thought of in terms of their motor limitations that also may have some cognitive involvement. Cerebral palsy (CP) is primarily a motor congenital disorder that may have a concurrent intellectual disability. In addition to the progressive motor limitations, multiple sclerosis (MS) may result in cognitive involvement and include behavior changes as the disease progresses. Aging is a physical process that limits motor function and also affects cognitive skills, such as memory.

Congenital Disabilities

Intellectual Disabilities

Intellectual disability is typically defined as a disability where the person has a below average score on an intelligence or mental ability test and a limitation in functional

TABLE 15-1 Disorders That May Benefit from Cognitive Assistive Technologies

Disorder	Incidence	Characteristics
Intellectual Disability	8 individuals per 1000 (http://www.cdc.gov/mmwrhtml/00040023.htm)	Limitations in functional skills, impairments in memory, language use, and communication, abstract conceptualization, generalization, and problem identification/problem solving (Wehmeyer, Smith, and Davies, 2005)
Learning Disability	2% of children	Significant difficulties in understanding or in using either spoken or written language; evident in problems with reading, writing, mathematical manipulation, listening, spelling, or speaking (Edyburn, 2005)
ADHD	4% (Daley, 2006) and 5%-7% (www.adhd.com)	Typical capacity to learn and to use their skills confounded by factors that make it difficult to fully realize that potential; easily frustrated, have trouble paying attention, prone to daydreaming and moodiness; fidgety, disorganized, impulsive, disruptive, or aggressive (Schuck and Crinella, 2005) (www.adhdcanada.com)
ASD	1 child per 165, 25% exhibit intellectual disability, 4 times more prevalent in boys than girls (Chakrabarti and Fombonne, 2001)	Varying degrees of impairment in communication and social interaction skills or presence of restricted, repetitive, and stereotyped patterns of behavior
Dementia	0.5%-1% (<65 years), 7%-10% (65-75 years), 18%-20% (75-85 years), 35%-40% (85+ years)	(1) Decline of cognitive capacity with some effect on day-to-day functioning, (2) impairment in multiple areas of cognition (global), and (3) normal level of consciousness (Rabins, Lyketsos, and Steele, 2006)
TBI	Mild: 131 per 100,000 Moderate: 15 per 100,000 Severe: 14 per 100,000 people (21 per 100,000 if prehospital deaths included) (Dawodu, 2006)	See Table 15-6
CVA	160/100,000 (overall), 1000/100,000 (age 50-65 years), 3000/100,000 (>80 years) (Demaerschalk and Hachinski, 2006)	Visual neglect, apraxia, aphasia; dysphagia; perceptual deficits, impaired alertness, attention disorders, memory disorders, impaired executive function, impaired judgment, impaired activities of daily living (O'Sullivan and Schmitz, 1994)

skills (Wehmeyer, Smith, and Davies, 2005). These functional skills include but are not limited to communication, self-care, and social interaction. The terms *developmental disability, cognitive disability,* and *mental retardation* are often used to describe individuals with intellectual disabilities. Intellectual disability can range in severity from mild to severe.

Learning Disabilities

Learning disabilities are disorders in which the person has near-normal mental abilities in general but a deficit in the comprehension or use of spoken or written language. These disabilities may be manifested as a significant difficulty with reading, writing, reasoning, or mathematical ability. Because students with LDs tend to perform poorly on standardized tests, it was long thought that LDs were a mild form of intellectual disability. This assumption is untrue; LDs can be thought of as a deficit in the processing and integration of information in an area (e.g., reading) as opposed to limitations in the basic ability in that specific area of learning. People with LDs have typical age-related capacity in all areas. Table 15-2 lists abilities associated with learning disabilities. However, processing deficits lead to the hallmark difficulties that are commonly experienced (Johnson et al, 2005).

Attention Deficit Hyperactivity Disorder

Attention deficit hyperactivity disorder (ADHD) is defined as a pattern of inattention, hyperactivity, and/or impulsivity that is more frequent or severe than for typical people of a given age (http://www.nimh.nih.gov/health/topics/attention-deficit-hyperactivity-disorder-adhd/index.shtml). The delay aversion hypothesis of ADHD posits that the ADHD child distracts himself or herself from the passing of time when he or she is not in control, explaining daydreaming, inattention, and fidgeting (Daley, 2006). Children (and adults) with ADHD have a normal capacity to learn and to utilize their skills, but suffer from confounding factors that make it difficult to fully realize that potential (Schuck and Crinella, 2005).

TABLE 15-2 Categorization of Abilities Associated with Learning Disabilities

Explicit Abilities	Implicit Abilities
Reading skills (dyslexia)	Visual or auditory discrimination
Mathematical skills (dyscalculia)	Visual or auditory closure
Writing skills (dyslexia, dysgraphia)	Visual or auditory figure-ground discrimination
Language skills (dysphagia)	Visual or auditory memory
Motor-learning skills (dyspraxia)	Visual or auditory sequencing
Social skills	Auditory association and comprehension
	Spatial perception
	Temporal perception

Particularly, those with ADHD can be easily frustrated, have trouble paying attention, are prone to daydreaming and moodiness, and are fidgety, disorganized, impulsive, disruptive, and/or aggressive (http://www.caddra.ca/).

Autism Spectrum Disorder

ASD is a developmental disorder characterized by varying degrees of impairment in communication and social interaction skills or the presence of restricted, repetitive, and stereotyped patterns of behavior. A commonly used definition for autism is that of the *Diagnostic and Statistical Manual of Mental Disorders–Fourth Edition* (DSM-IV) (American Psychiatric Association [APA], 2000), which classifies autism as a *pervasive development disorder* (PDD). As the term implies, this disorder covers a wide spectrum of conditions, with individual differences in number and kinds of symptoms, levels of severity, age of onset, and limitations with social interaction. Major subtypes of ASD include *autistic disorder, Asperger's syndrome, Rett syndrome, childhood disintegrative disorders,* and PDD *not otherwise specified* (NOS). Individuals with ASD typically demonstrate deficits in communication skills including delay in or total lack of spoken language and *spontaneous speech*; unusual speaking patterns (e.g., echolalia or idiosyncratic language); and underdeveloped social interaction skills (including problems interpreting facial expressions, gestures, and intonation while interacting with other people) (Maenner et al, 2013). They might also seem evasive, avoid eye contact, and appear to lack initiation and desire to share joy or interest. Children with ASD also have inflexible adherence to specific routines and demonstrate unusual persistence and intense focus on a specific subject or activity. Many children with ASD have unusual (hypersensitive or hyposensitive) responses to sensory information, which could lead to the lack of or aversive response to sensory input.

Individuals with ASD also have strengths and unique abilities. For example, some individuals with ASD have unusually good spatial perception and visual recall or accurate and detailed memory for information and facts, are able to concentrate for long periods of time on particular task or subjects, and are more attentive to details than most people. These abilities may allow them to excel in areas of music, science, math, physics, and other specialized areas.

Acquired Disabilities

Dementia

The word *dementia* comes from the Latin *de mens,* which means "from the mind." Dementia is best defined as a syndrome, or a pattern of clinical symptoms and signs, that can be defined by the following three points: (1) decline of cognitive capacity with some effect on day-to-day functioning, (2) impairment in multiple areas of cognition (global), and (3) normal level of consciousness (Rabins et al, 2006). Dementia is distinguished from congenital cognitive disorders (such as intellectual disability, LDs, etc.) by its age of onset and its degenerative component. It is also important to note that, although it must affect multiple areas of cognition, not all areas are affected.

Traumatic Brain Injury

People who experience a traumatic brain injury (TBI) often lose significant cognitive function. A TBI may occur when the head or brain is struck by an external force, such as from a fall, gunshot wound, or motor vehicle accident. The causes of TBI are described in Table 15-3. The extent of the trauma to the brain is the determining factor in diagnosing TBI, not the injury itself. For instance, it is possible to incur TBI as a result of both open-head injuries (the brain is exposed to air) and closed-head injuries (no brain exposure). The effect of a TBI on an individual's cognitive ability varies from case to case, in terms of both severity and the set of skills affected.

Not all head injuries give rise to TBI, and there is an accepted protocol for diagnosing such an injury. One tool available to assist with diagnosis is the Glasgow Coma Scale (GCS), a rating system used for describing the severity of a coma (Dawodu, 2006). The GCS ranks comas on a scale of 3 (most severe) to 15 (mildest) according to eye response, verbal response, and motor response categories. A score on the GCS of 12 or lower is a mild brain injury and below 8 is considered a severe injury.

If the GCS does not indicate TBI, one of the following two criteria must be satisfied for a TBI diagnosis: either the client has amnesia for the traumatic event or the individual has a documented loss of consciousness. It is common to have a *recovery period* after the injury. This recovery usually plateaus within 12 months after injury, and the extent of recovery is both variable and unpredictable (Cicerone et al, 2005). A good measure of the extent of an individual's recovery from a TBI is his or her return to preinjury activities of daily living. Two main recovery indicators are the return to work and the return to driving, both important tasks for independent living. Data on the return to work are summarized in Table 15-4, and similar data for the return to driving are shown in Table 15-5 (Novack, 1999). In both cases, very little improvement was observed beyond 12 months after injury. Typical cognitive and behavioral difficulties that a person with TBI may encounter are listed in Table 15-6 (Novack, 1999; Rehabilitation Engineering Society of North America [RESNA], 1998). Two areas of importance are memory and language skills because these may benefit from intervention with assistive technology.

TABLE 15-3 Data on Causes of TBI (Injury Control Research Center [ICRC])

Cause	Percentage of Total
Motor vehicle crashes	64%
Gunshot wounds	13%
Falls	11%
Assault	8%
Pedestrian	3%
Sports	1%

Data from TBI Inform, June, 2000. Published by the UAB-TBIMS, Birmingham, AL. © 2000 Board of Trustees, University of Alabama, http://www.uab.edu/medicine/tbi/.

Stroke

A *stroke*, or cardiovascular accident (CVA), is an incidence of irregular blood flow within the brain causing an interruption in brain function. A stroke may arise from a lack of blood flow to the brain (known as an *ischemic stroke*) or

TABLE 15-4 Return to Work

	Student	Employed	Home	Retired	Unemployed
Onset	11%	57%	1%	11%	21%
6 months	7%	17%	None	10%	67%
12 months	7%	26%	None	8%	57%

Data from ICRC Study, 1999, http://neuroskills.com/whattoexpect.shtml.

TABLE 15-5 Return to Driving

	Percent Return to Driving		
	No	Partially	Yes
6 months	69%	13%	19%
12 months	60%	10%	30%

Data from ICRC Study, 1999, http://www.Neuroskills.Com/Whattoexpect.Shtml.

TABLE 15-6 List of Typical Cognitive and Behavioral Difficulties after TBI

Type of Difficulty	Examples
Cognitive	Processing of visual or auditory information
	Disrupted attention and concentration
	Language problems (i.e., aphasia)
	Difficulty storing and retrieving new memories
	Poor reasoning, judgment, and problem-solving skills
	Difficulty learning new information
Behavioral	Restlessness and agitation
	Emotional lability and irritability
	Confabulation
	Diminished insight
	Socially inappropriate behavior
	Poor initiation
	Lack of emotional response
	Projecting blame on others
	Depression
	Anxiety

from ruptured blood vessels in the brain (a *hemorrhagic stroke*). The neurological damage incurred as the result of a stroke produces symptoms that directly correspond to the injured area within the brain (O'Sullivan and Schmitz, 1994). A CVA causes acute damage to the brain; there are no degenerative effects after the onset of injury. As with TBI, persons who have sustained a stroke often have a recovery period when portions of the brain learn to compensate for damaged areas. Typical cognitive and behavioral difficulties associated with stroke are shown in Table 15-7. Most recovery (as observed by the return to activities of daily living) occurs within 6 months after onset (Bruno, 2005). The majority of persons with CVA are able to return home after the initial hospitalization period. A summary of discharge locations after hospitalization for stroke is shown in Table 15-8. These data suggest that the number of people returning home after a CVA is increasing, which might be attributed to improvements to hospital care at the onset of stroke. Children may have a more pronounced recovery than adults because their brains have a greater degree of plasticity. Also, women may display greater recovery of lost language skills than men because the language centers of the brain are larger in women than in men.

TABLE 15-7 List of Typical Cognitive and Behavioral Difficulties after Stroke

Type of Difficulty	Examples
Cognitive	Visual neglect, hemianopsia
	Apraxia
	Language problems (i.e., aphasia, dysarthria)
	Perceptual deficits (i.e., figure-ground impairment, disorientation)
	Impaired alertness, attention disorders
	Memory problems, both short-term and long-term
	Perseveration
	Decreased executive function
Behavioral	Impaired judgment
	Impulsiveness
	Emotional lability
	Confabulation
	Poor initiation
	Mood alterations
	Depression

TABLE 15-8 Discharge Data for CVA from the Canadian Heart and Stroke Foundation

Discharge Destination	1993	1999
Home	33%	56%
Inpatient rehabilitation	41%	32%
Nursing home or long-term care	26%	11%

Data from Heart and Stroke Foundation of Canada. Stroke statistics: www.heartandstroke.com.

Cognitive Skills Related to Specific Disorders

Figure 15-3 relates the disorders described in Table 15-1 to the cognitive skills described in Box 15-1. The listed cognitive skills are judged to be those that may be aided or replaced through the use of assistive technologies. Cognitive skills are listed along the top row and disabilities and disorders along the vertical axis. Items marked with an X are the skills that may be limited or absent in the corresponding disorder. This table can be used to identify assistive technologies (rows) that aid or replace skills (columns) to enable a person to carry out functional tasks. It can be used to identify both compensatory and enhancement approaches to the use of assistive technologies for individuals who have cognitive disabilities.

The cognitive skills are roughly arranged such that, moving from left to right in Figure 15-3, the skills build on each other. This figure illustrates *possible* skills that may be affected for a person with a specific disorder, but each case must be considered to determine specific impacts for a given individual. Most of the disorders and disabilities that have cognitive implications are quite variable from individual to individual, and not all of the possible limitations included in Figure 15-3 will necessarily exist for any specific person.

Figure 15-4 relates cognitive skills and disorders to possible assistive technology characteristics that can address needs. Entries in Figure 15-4 are marked with X, A, or R, where X indicates that the skill is required by the technology, A indicates that the technology aids that skill, and R indicates that the technology replaces that skill. Figure 15-4 is based on clinical experience and published literature regarding assistive technologies frequently used by people with cognitive limitations. Specific needs served by the type of assistive technology and examples of specific devices are also shown in Figure 15-4 for each category.

For each entry in this table, the frame of reference is the person with a disability (i.e., the skill is restricted or absent in the person). Figure 15-4 can serve as a checklist to ensure that all of the skills that might be affected and aided by assistive technologies are identified. If there is a gap between the skills required to complete a task and the skills that the individual brings to the task, the use of assistive technologies to aid or replace the required skill should be considered.

ASSISTIVE TECHNOLOGIES THAT ADDRESS COGNITIVE NEEDS

General Concepts

Assistive technologies are applied to the amelioration of a wide range of cognitive problems. These applications vary by the type and severity of the cognitive limitations faced by the individual. In this section we first discuss aspects of AT application specific to three broad categories of cognitive need: congenital disabilities further categorized as mild and moderate to severe, and acquired cognitive disabilities. Both the

Domain	Skill	Subskill	CVA	TBI	DEMENTA	ASD	ADHD	LD	ID
Perception			X	X		X		X	
Attention	Signal Detection	Vigilance	X	X			X		
		Search	X	X		X	X		
	Selective		X	X	X		X		
	Divided		X	X	X	X	X		
Memory	Encoding		X	X	X				
	Storage	Short-Term	X	X	X		X	X	
		Long-Term	X	X	X				
	Retrieval	Recognition	X	X	X				
		Recall	X	X	X				
Orientation	Place		X	X		X		X	
	TIme		X	X	X	X		X	
	Person		X	X	X			X	
	Quantitative		X	X		X		X	
Knowledge Representation and Organization	Mental Representations	Declarative/know what	X	X	X	X			
		Procedural/know how	X	X	X	X			
	Grouping	Categorization	X	X		X			
		Sorting	X	X		X			
		Sequencing	X	X		X			
Problem Solving	Identify Problem		X	X		X			
	Judgment		X	X	X	X	X	X	
	Decision Making		X	X		X	X	X	
	Reasoning	Deductive	X	X	X	X			
		Inductive	X	X	X	X			
	Planning		X	X		X			
	Evaluation and Iteration		X	X	X	X			
	Transfer/Generalization		X	X		X			
Language			X	X		X			
Learning	General		X	X		X		X	
	Mathematics		X	X		X		X	
	Reading		X	X		X		X	
	Writing		X	X		X		X	

FIGURE 15-3 Skills versus disorder matrix.

Skill			Memory Aids: Recorders	Memory Aids: Word completion/prediction	Memory Aids: Information retrieval	Time Management	Prompting/Cueing	Stimuli Control: Auditory (noise reduction)	Stimuli Control: Visual field	Stimuli Control: Media presentation	Concept Organization	Language Tools	Alternative Input	Alternative Output	Tracking	ID
Attention	Signal Detection	Vigilance	X	X			A	A		A	A	X		X		
Attention	Signal Detection	Search		X	X	X		A	A	A	X	X	X			
Attention	Selective					X		A	A	A	A			X		
Attention	Divided			X	X		X			A	A	X				
Perception			X	X	X	X	X	A	R	A	X	X	X	R		
Memory	Storage	Short-Term	R			R	R				A				R	R
Memory	Storage	Long-Term	R	X	X	R	R				A	X				R
Memory	Encoding										A					
Memory	Retrieval	Recognition		X	X	X	R				A	X				R
Memory	Retrieval	Recall	R	A	A	R	R				X	R			R	R
Information Processing/ Orientation	Quantitative						A								A	
Information Processing/ Orientation	Visuospatial								A		A				R	A
Information Processing/ Orientation	Temporal		A			R	R									
Information Processing/ Orientation	Personal															R
Knowledge Representation and Organization	Categorization				X						A	X				
Knowledge Representation and Organization	Sorting										A					
Knowledge Representation and Organization	Sequencing				X						A	X				
Knowledge Representation and Organization	Mental Representations	Declarative/know what	R	A	A		R				X	A			R	R
Knowledge Representation and Organization	Mental Representations	Procedural/know how	X	X	X	X	R				X	X	X			X
Problem Solving	Identify Problem						A								R	
Problem Solving	Judgment						R									
Problem Solving	Decision Making			X	X	X	R				A	X				
Problem Solving	Reasoning	Deductive					R				X					
Problem Solving	Reasoning	Inductive					R				X					
Problem Solving	Planning						R				A					
Problem Solving	Evaluation and Iteration			X	X		R				X	X	X		R	
Problem Solving	Generalization						A				A					
Language			X	X	A	X	X			X	X	A	A	A		
Learning	General		X	A	A	X	R	A	A	A	A	A	X	A		
Learning	Mathematics						R							A		
Learning	Reading			X			R		A	A	X	A		A		
Learning	Writing			A	A		R				X	A		A		

FIGURE 15-4 Skills versus assistive technology matrix. An "X" indicates that the cognitive skill is required to use that type of assistive technology. An "A" indicates that the type of assistive technology might aid the cognitive skill in an activity. An "R" indicates that the type of assistive technology might replace the requirement for that cognitive skill in an activity. Note that these entries are with respect to the assistive technology.

general characteristics of cognitive assistive technologies and technologies designed to meet specific needs are described.

Considerations for Individuals with Mild Cognitive Disabilities

Individuals with **mild cognitive disabilities** have needs that are more subtle and harder to define than in the case of physical disabilities or more severe cognitive disabilities. For example, learning disabilities typically involve significant difficulties in understanding or in using either spoken or written language, and these difficulties may be evident in problems with reading, writing, mathematical manipulation, listening, spelling, or speaking (Edyburn, 2005). Although there are assistive technologies that are specifically designed to address these areas (discussed later in this chapter), many of the technological tools are useful for all students and are part of instructional technology (Ashton, 2005). Even the identified assistive technologies have features (e.g., multimedia, synthetic speech output, voice recognition input) that are useful to all learners.

Chapter 1 distinguishes between educational technologies (or instructional technologies) and assistive technologies. This distinction works well for sensory and motor assistive technologies. The distinction is much more blurred for cognitive assistive technologies (Ashton, 2005; Edyburn, 2005). For example, some spell checkers, word prediction, and talking word processors have been specifically designed for individuals with learning disabilities.[4] These programs are discussed later in this chapter. As Ashton (2005) points out, each of these technologies is potentially useful to all students, not just those with learning disabilities. In that sense they are educational or instructional technologies. The issues surrounding assistive technologies and competency are described in Box 15-2.

Edyburn (2005) points out that many other productivity tools can function as assistive technologies for individuals with mild disabilities. He cites the example of the *Ask* web search engine,[5] which could provide assistance to a child who has difficulty retrieving information. Edyburn poses the following question: if the student knows that he or she can find the names of all the US presidents using this or another search engine, then isn't that as useful an educational outcome as having memorized the names for a test? The question of information retrieval using the Internet is part of the larger issue of compensation versus remediation in cognitive assistive technologies (Edyburn, 2002).

Throughout this text a four-part approach to assistive technology applications has been emphasized: human, activity, context, and assistive technology (the HAAT model of Chapters 1, 2, and 3). When a clinician is dealing with motor disabilities, the starting point is a careful description of the activity to be performed. An evaluation of the individual's skills relevant to the activity leads to a clear picture of what assistive technology needs the individual has. The context (physical, social, and cultural milieu and institutional environment) then moderates the choices of assistive technologies. The assistive technology includes both soft technologies (training, strategies) and hard technologies (devices) or, in Edyburn's (2002, 2005) terminology, remediation (soft technology) and compensation (hard technology).

For sensory or motor disabilities, we don't much care how the function is accomplished as long as the activity can be satisfactorily completed. Other issues, such as how much energy it takes to walk versus using a power wheelchair for someone with severe cerebral palsy, are matters of personal choice. The situation changes dramatically, however, in dealing with cognitive assistive technologies. Should the child in our example be required to learn the presidents' names (remediation) or be allowed to use an assistive technology (e.g., *Ask*) as a compensatory tool, and why is its use

BOX 15-2 Compensation vs. Remediation

What constitutes independence?

Do we care how the function is accomplished as long as the activity can be satisfactorily completed?

Sensory or motor disabilities: how much energy it takes to walk vs. use a powered wheelchair for someone with severe cerebral palsy are matters of personal choice.

Cognitive disabilities: Should a child in our example be required to learn the presidents' names (remediation) or be allowed to use an assistive technology (e.g., *Ask*) as a compensatory tool, and why is its use considered "cheating" by some educators and parents?[20]

The role of time:

- In community settings time is not as critical (e.g., allowing additional time for an individual who is blind to cross the street using a long cane is an accepted part of human performance).
- In vocational settings, completion time for a task also varies from individual to individual and is acceptable within wide limits.
- Why, then, in educational contexts is time fixed (e.g., for an exam) and accomplishment variable?[20]
- Restricting time, learning activities, instructional approaches, and other classroom variables to a "one-size-fits-all" constraint in educational settings means that high standards of performance cannot be achieved.[20]
- While many students with special needs are given extra time to complete an exam, the level of competence they achieve is still variable and time (even expanded time) is fixed.
- If achievement were to be fixed, then each student would be allowed as much time as necessary to complete the task.
- If uniformly high performance and preparation for later vocational success are the goals, then compensation, using both hard and soft assistive technologies, must be an alternative for individuals with mild cognitive disabilities as it is for their counterparts with motor, sensory, or communication disabilities.
- Time considerations can also apply in other rehabilitation settings. For example, if caregivers/teachers/CNAs intervene to speed up a task (like dressing or feeding) due to time limitations it can decrease the individual's independence, confidence, and self-esteem and increase the learned helplessness cycle.

[4] For example: Co-Writer and Read-Outloud, Don Johnston, Inc, Volo, IL, http://donjohnston.com/.

[5] www.ask.com.

considered "cheating" by some educators and parents (Edyburn, 2005)?

A related concern is the concept of time in educational contexts. Time is fixed and accomplishment varies (Edyburn, 2005). This is not true in the case of sensory or motor disabilities where additional time (e.g., for an individual who is blind to cross the street using a long cane) is an accepted part of human performance. In vocational settings, completion time for a task also varies from individual to individual and is acceptable within wide limits. Why, then, is this not the case in an educational context? Restricting time, learning activities, instructional approaches, and other classroom variables to a "one-size-fits-all" constraint in educational settings means that high standards of performance cannot be achieved (Edyburn, 2005).

Although many students with special needs are given extra time to complete an examination, the level of competence they achieve is still variable and time (even expanded time) is fixed. If achievement were to be fixed, then each student would be allowed as much time as necessary to complete the task. If uniformly high performance and preparation for later vocational success are the goals, then compensation, using both hard and soft assistive technologies, must be an alternative for individuals with mild cognitive disabilities as it is for their counterparts with motor and sensory disabilities.

Considerations for Individuals with Moderate to Severe Intellectual Disabilities

Several ways of characterizing cognitive needs have been used in consideration of assistive technology applications for individuals who have intellectual disabilities. One method considers the cognitive impairment exhibited, such as impairments in memory, language use and communication, abstract conceptualization, generalization, and problem identification/problem solving (Wehmeyer et al, 2005). Assistive technology characteristics that address these impairments include simplicity of operation, capacity of the technology to support repetition, consistency in presentation, use, and inclusion of multiple modalities (e.g., speech, sounds, and graphical representations). Wehmeyer et al (2005) discuss assistive technology characteristics and approaches for each of these impairments. Many of these technologies are covered in the subsequent sections of this chapter.

Granlund et al (1995) take a different approach and define five content areas for technological assistance to individuals who have moderate to severe intellectual disabilities. The content areas, on the basis of cognitive structures, are the following:

- Quality (What is this?)
- Causal patterns (Why? And if so?)
- Space (Where?)
- Quantity (How much? How big?)
- Time (When? Duration?)

Within these content areas, individuals with intellectual disabilities typically have difficulties in organization and reorganization, performing operations with cognitive structures, and symbolic representation.

Wehmeyer et al (2005) described eight primary factors of cognitive ability: (1) language, (2) reasoning, (3) memory and learning, (4) visual perception, (5) auditory perception, (6) idea production, (7) cognitive speed, and (8) knowledge and achievement. They argue that the promise of technology for aiding individuals with intellectual disabilities lies in enhancing human capacity in these areas rather than compensating for deficits. An important element in this approach is the application of the principles of universal design (see Chapter 2) to ensure that mainstream technologies are designed in such a way that individuals with a range of intellectual abilities can access them.

As an example of the impact of universal design principles on access for individuals with cognitive disabilities Stock et al (2008) evaluated a multimedia cell phone interface prototype and compared it to a typical mainstream cell phone. The custom interface was implanted using a Pocket PC/PDA phone edition operating system. To place a call, the user taps the picture of the person to be called, and a recorded audio message is played stating: "To call the person you see on the screen, tap the picture again." If the user selects the wrong person's picture, a Stop button (e.g., a typical Stop sign) is displayed. When the stop sign is tapped the software returns the person to the original address book. For an incoming call the phone rings loudly, the picture of the calling person is displayed, and an audio prompt to "Press the picture to answer this person's call" plays. This sequence continues until the user taps the caller's picture and talks as with a typical cell phone. The Stop button is tapped to end the phone conversation. Participants required significantly less help and made significantly fewer errors when making and receiving calls using the specialized multimedia phone system as compared with a mainstream Nokia cell phone. This study demonstrated that people with ID can benefit from the use of cell phone technology that includes universal design features to enable cognitive access.

The design of the human/technology interface (HTI) (see Chapter 6) in the HAAT model is an example of the difference between a compensation approach and the concept of enhancement of the technology characteristics to make it more accessible. If an individual with an intellectual disability has difficulty accessing a screen because of language problems (e.g., reading), one approach is to use a compensatory approach and provide auditory output instead of text, avoiding the necessity for reading. If the problem is too much clutter on the display, then the best approach may be to simplify the display (i.e., enhance it) so that the information is more accessible. The following sections of this chapter describe technology approaches that use both enhancement and compensation strategies. For individuals with intellectual disabilities, Wehmeyer et al (2004) present a thorough literature review of approaches that have been taken to enhance performance in each of the eight cognitive factors.

Palmer et al (2002) surveyed families of persons with intellectual disabilities to determine their use of computers and other technologies. They compared their results to the earlier study by Wehmeyer (1998). The 2002 study showed that although the use of computers was more prevalent, other technology use frequency was much the same as in the 1998 survey. The 2002 survey and other studies have shown that access to technologies is limited for people with intellectual disabilities and when it is available it is underutilized. There were more families who indicated that their family member with an intellectual disability could benefit from technology but did not have access than families that indicated that the family member had access. The technologies that had the highest reported effectiveness were palmtop computers or personal data assistants (PDAs), a technology replaced by smart phone apps, followed by auditory prompting devices, electronic and information technologies, video devices, and augmentative communication devices. Reported use of communication devices by family members with an intellectual disability was 13%. Independent living devices were used by 5% of the families and consisted of eating aids, cell phones with preprogrammed numbers, environmental controls, alert buttons, door openers, various remote controls, and a scheduler for someone who cannot tell time. Almost half (49.7%) of the survey sample used computers in some way. Computers were used for writing, budgeting money, doing work-related tasks, Internet access, email, and recreation (e.g., computer games). Comparison of Palmer et al's result with earlier surveys indicated that the percentage of technology use over time has been essentially constant or increased slightly. Use of common electronic information technologies for emailing, using a digital camera, and using a mobile phone was at lower rates than the general population. Full and equal access to mainstream technologies is still elusive for individuals who have intellectual disabilities. The increasing availability of smart phones and tablets has increased opportunities for societal participation by individuals with intellectual disabilities (Kagohara et al, 2013). There are still major challenges in obtaining access due to both physical and cognitive skills and family support (Gillespie et al, 2012).

Considerations for Individuals with Acquired Disabilities

Individuals with acquired cognitive disabilities resulting from injury (e.g., TBI) or disease (e.g., CVA or dementia) retain a wide variety of cognitive skills. The majority of assistive technologies and strategies that have been used to aid persons with acquired cognitive disabilities are designed to compensate for deficits by building on remaining strengths (LoPresti et al, 2004). Collective technologies and strategies that help a person with cognitive deficits function more independently in certain tasks have been called assistive technology for cognition (ATC) (LoPresti et al, 2004), **cognitive prosthesis** (Cole and Mathews, 1999), or **cognitive assistive technologies** (CATs) (LoPresti et al, 2008). We will use CAT. A CAT is an entire system of hardware, software, and personal assistance that is individualized to meet specific needs. As the HAAT model (see Chapter 1) implies, a cognitive prosthesis includes a custom-designed computer-based compensatory strategy that directly assists in performing daily activities.[6] It may also include additional technologies such as a cell phone, pager, digital camera, or low-tech approaches.

To be effective CATs that assist dementia care must address the so-called "three pillars of dementia care" (Rabins et al, 2006). First is to treat the disease, which helps identify current needs and future necessities as the disorder progresses. Second is treatment of the symptoms. By treating the symptoms, the quality of life of the client will improve in the cognitive, functional, and behavioral domains. Medications and technology are the two main ways to accomplish this task. Third, client support is important and leads to ensuring that the client's needs are met and quality of life is improved as much as possible.

De Joode et al (2012) surveyed 147 professionals in cognitive rehabilitation and interviewed fifteen patients with acquired brain injury (ABI) TBI, and stroke and 14 caregivers regarding perceptions and use of CATs, particularly the application of PDAs, in treatment of ABI. When asked about use of technology, all patients and caregivers reported use of personal computers, but only two patients and three caregivers used PDAs. Four patients used cell phones as cognitive aids. Portability and having all functions present in one device (PDA) were viewed as important reasons to use it. Patients mentioned cost as a barrier more often than caregivers.

However, more caregivers than patients considered AT unsuitable. Learning time to become proficient with the CAT was not considered a barrier to adoption. Although most professionals were willing to use AT in the future, only 27% currently used CATs in the clinical setting. The amount of experience was a factor in the attitude of the professionals toward CATs. Those with CAT experience were more positive about the potential effectiveness than those without experience. Lack of insurance funding for CATs was perceived as an important barrier for more widespread use.

A treatment model for adults with ADHD that involved a combination of CATs and OT support was evaluated by Lindstedt and Umb-Carlsson (2013). The Quebec User Evaluation with Assistive Technology (QUEST 2.0) (see Chapter 5) was used to measure the participants' satisfaction with the CATs. Seventeen participants evaluated 674 CAT products over a one-year period. At the conclusion of the study 45 CAT products were retained and 29 returned. Reasons for returning devices include malfunctions and devices being no longer needed. The three most highly rated devices were weekly schedules (paper, metal plates with magnetic tags, plastic laminated paper, and/or regular calendars), watches/alarm clocks, and weighted blankets. More of the participants were employed at the end of the study than at the beginning. The four most frequent supports in terms of the ICF domain of "Activity and Participation" were carrying out daily routines (code d230) (27.3%), economic self-sufficiency (code d870) (9.0%), undertaking a single task (code d210) (8.3%), and looking after one's health (code d570)

[6] Institute for Cognitive Prosthetics, http://www.brain-rehab.com/.

TABLE 15-9 Categories of Assistive Technologies to Aid Cognitive Function

AT Category	Needs Served	Examples
Memory Aids	Augment or replace the primary memory functions	Recording/playback, word completion/prediction, information retrieval
Time Management	Planning, prioritizing, and execution of daily and time-dependent tasks	Alternative formats, reminders, schedulers; some prompt visually or auditorally as well as alarm for reminder
Prompting/Cueing	Guidance for procedural or navigational sequencing tasks	Auditory (verbal and sounds), visual (pictures or drawings), or word-based; can be customized for individual tasks; may use other data such as GPS location
Stimuli Control	Address attention or perception problems by limiting or manipulating the information presented to the user	Noise reduction techniques, visual field manipulation, and media presentation techniques
Language Tools	Assist with writing	Word completion/prediction, spell checking, concept mapping
Alternative Input	Assist with reading	Voice recognition software, simplified user interface and desktop
Alternative Output	Assist with reading and writing	Synthesized or digitized speech output, graphic alternative to text, e-books, variation in font size, background/foreground color combinations, contrast, spacing between words, letters, and paragraphs
Tracking and Identification	Safety for users who might not have the cognitive skills required to work their way out of problematic situations	Wearable electronic monitoring device, home monitoring systems

(8.3%) (WHO, 2001). The ICF domain "Environmental Factors" (where assistive technologies are located in the ICF classification) was also identified. An interesting finding was that participants expressed less satisfaction with domestic chores, organized leisure activities, and family relations at the end of the intervention than at the beginning. Lindstedt and Umb-Carlsson (2013) offered two explanations: (1) the intervention had a negative effect on these aspects of family life and (2) "the intervention contributed to increased aspirations but also to increased awareness of limitations in performance of the activities in question and satisfaction of family relations" (p. 5). They viewed the second option as more likely.

Cognitive Assistive Technologies

Characteristics of Cognitive Assistive Technologies[7]

Categories of assistive technologies for cognitive assistance are listed in Table 15-9. This categorization is similar to that used by others (e.g., Cole and Mathews, 1999; Edyburn, 2005; Granlund et al, 1995; LoPresti et al, 2004; LoPresti et al, 2008; Braddock et al, 2004; Wehmeyer et al, 2004; Wehmeyer et al, 2005; Gillespie et al, 2012). Specific needs served by the type of assistive technology and examples of specific devices are also shown in Table 15-9 for each category. Some devices fit in more than one category. For example, time management requires memory and prompting can have a temporal element if sequencing of tasks is required. Many mainstream technologies, including computers and smart phones, support more than one cognitive function and this complicates the mapping of devices to functional categories.

[7]Dan Davies of AbleLink Technologies, Inc., provided significant insight to this section.

Gillespie et al (2012) identified the following five classifications of CATs based on the cognitive function being supported:

1. Alerting: Devices that draw attention to a stimulus present in the external or internal environment
2. Reminding: Devices providing a one-way, usually one-off, time-dependent reminder about something not in the immediate environment which is intended to be an impetus to action (e.g., reminder about an appointment)
3. Micro-prompting: Devices using feedback to provide detailed step-by-step prompts guiding the user through an immediately present task
4. Storing and displaying: Devices that store and present episodic memories, without being a time-dependent impetus
5. Distracting: Devices that distract users from anxiety provoking stimuli such as hallucinations

These classifications are similar to those shown in Table 15-9.

Many of the functions included in mainstream technologies such as mobile phones and computers are as useful to individuals with cognitive disabilities as to those without cognitive disabilities. For someone who has a cognitive disability these features may be even more important because the individual depends on them to carry out independent daily activities. The features included in mobile phones and other similar technologies can help compensate for certain abilities that are limited due to the cognitive disability. Specific functions of mainstream technologies that are important to all users, including those who have cognitive disabilities, support activities of productivity, leisure, and self-care (e.g., communicate, remember schedules, learn new information, listen to music, access online information and services, etc.). Mobile technologies can be programmed, and many people have developed applications for them. Many of these applications are specifically developed for people who have cognitive needs and many others developed for the general population are useful to them.

Mainstream technologies can be complex to use, and there are also specially designed cognitive support technologies that have been developed to compensate for cognitive limitations or provide access to the same basic functionality that exists in everyday technologies when the mainstream options that are available are too complex to operate. Different applications for the same person could use the same technology device, and there could be further confusion for the person with a cognitive disability.

For example, notebook computers, mobile phones, and tablets have been programmed to function as both augmentative communication devices (see Chapter 16) and as cognitive assists (Stock et al, 2008). Many applications (apps) for these two functions utilize an input method of a touch screen or small keyboard, and they have an output of either speech or visual characters and text. These input/output features may be operated in many different ways. The surface features of the two applications may appear to be identical, and indeed the same device could be used for both applications with a change in software. However, the function will be very different because of the characteristics of the application's software loaded into the device. If the user attends only to the existence of the input and output features and the size, color, and shape of the device, then some of the operational parameters of the device may not be understood. If he or she has previous experiences with one type of application (for example, a prompting app) that uses the smart phone, then he or she may not recognize that a new application (for example, an augmentative communication app) is functionally different since the hardware (the phone) is the same.

To be useful to people who have cognitive disabilities, technologies must be accessible. Accessibility in this case means that complexity is reduced, multiple modes of presentation of choices are available, and operation is consistent with the cognitive skills of the potential user. To achieve this level of accessibility commercial developers of technology must incorporate cognitive accessibility into their products utilizing universal design principles (see Chapter 2).

Support tools and services must also be developed to ensure they can be used by as wide a range of users with cognitive disabilities as possible. Currently, this level of cognitive accessibility is rarely achieved for mainstream technologies, and individuals who have cognitive disabilities must rely on specially designed assistive technologies to meet their needs.

For individuals who have cognitive disability to effectively use the technology (either mainstream technology or specialized AT) the technology must have been made cognitively accessible. Accessible technology is only the starting point. Successful use of CATs is also dependent on the availability of soft technologies (see Chapters 1 and 2) that include effective selection, training, and implementation of technology solutions. Support can come from a wide variety of individuals (and usually multiple individuals) who are part of the life of those with cognitive disabilities, including rehabilitation professionals, living skills counselors, home health care providers, friends, and other family members.

Individuals who support people in the use of CATs typically represent a wide range of knowledge and experience in the use of technology by individuals with disabilities. However, unlike some categories of assistive technology that have been around for several decades (AAC, vision products, wheelchairs, etc.), most of the technology that is considered "cognitively" accessible is less than a decade old. Therefore, there is often a lot of new learning necessary on the part of all individuals, regardless of their knowledge of other areas of assistive technology. Tips for supporting people who use cognitive assistive technologies are listed in Box 15-3 (Courtesy of Dan Davies, AbleLink Technologies).

For example, people with intellectual disabilities have the ability to learn basic ICT skills given the right environment and training tools. Evaluation of an e-mentoring program for young people with disabilities found that those who had been mentored learned a lot about how to use the Internet while also gaining social benefits (Chadwick et al, 2013).

Devices to Aid Memory

Memory aids are those devices or software apps that augment or replace memory by providing a means to store commonly used information or to retrieve information. These devices can be subdivided into three categories on the basis of their primary tasks: recording, word completion/prediction, and information retrieval.

Recorders are devices that store information that can be replayed at a later time to aid in the recall of facts or appointments. The most common devices in this category are those that record voice information as short memos. This feature is often built into small Dictaphones, PDAs, mobile phones, and tablets. Word completion and prediction solutions are software packages that aid memory during a written communication task by giving a user a series of contextually significant words/phrases that he or she may wish to use. This technology is also discussed in Chapter 6, where its use was to reduce time required to input text or to reduce the number of required keystrokes.

Reminding people to take their medication is one of the main uses of memory assistance technologies. Low-tech medication reminders (e.g., boxes with seven or more compartments labeled by the day and/or type of medication) have been in widespread use for many years. However, these devices do not alert the person that it is time for the medication. If an alert is needed, then electronic medication reminders are required (Mann, 2005). A watch-based medication reminder, such as the Cadex Medication Reminder Watch,[8] provides up to 12 daily reminders that have an audible alarm and a display of the required medication. While this format is convenient due to its small size, it has a small

[8] Cadex Medication Reminder Watch, http//:www.cadexproducts.com.

BOX 15-3 Tips for Supporting Individuals Who Have Cognitive Needs

Dan Davies, President of AbleLink Technologies, a developer of cognitive technologies, provided these tips that address some of the issues that are particularly important for individuals such as caregivers, siblings, parents, or spouses who are responsible for supporting assistive technology application.

- Start small. Individuals with cognitive disabilities, as well as caregivers, can easily become overwhelmed by technology. It is best to identify the most important needs an individual has for the technology, and begin with meeting one of those needs. When the individual becomes comfortable with the use of the technology and experiences success with using it, then addressing another need with the technology can be added.
- Understand the different user settings that can be changed to simplify the program to meet a particular individual's needs. Then start the individual with the interface that best meets his or her current need for support. Well-designed cognitive support technology will provide the ability to modify the user interface for different individuals to ensure the interface is not cluttered with buttons and other program options that the individual will not be using.
- Talk with others who have used cognitive support technology. The nature of cognitive technology is that it can be used many different ways to help people with cognitive disabilities, even ways not envisioned by the developer of the technology. It is good to learn from others, such as through online communities, and contribute as well so others can learn from your experiences.
- Cognitive technologies are usually not designed as "out of the box" solutions that are one-size-fits-all. Good cognitive technologies are usually best applied by adding content that is appropriate for the individual. For example, the best task prompting systems come with authoring tools to allow the caregiver to create a task that meets the specific needs of the individual they are serving, such as specific instructions for how to do his or her laundry. Generic instructions for performing activities of daily living are rarely useful for individuals with cognitive disabilities, other than for a general orientation to the task. Actually performing the task independently will often require customized steps with pictures of the individual's own washer and dryer (for example), and audio instructions designed for the cognitive level of the individual. Sometimes task libraries may be available (e.g., www.aimsxml.com) where previously created tasks can be downloaded and then customized with new pictures and audio files to make the downloaded task meet the needs of the particular individual. To get the most benefit out of cognitive technologies, it is very important to make full use of the ability to customize the relevant content to meet the unique needs of the individual with the cognitive disability. The time spent in creating custom content is well worth it given that the individual will then be able to do many things that he or she has been dependent on others for in the past.
- Use cognitive technology to help learn how to use cognitive technology. One of the unique benefits of cognitive support technology is that it can be used to provide very easy to follow instructions for using the technology itself.[38]

(Courtesy of Dan Davies, AbleLink Technologies.)

display and limited memory. Pagers and cell phones are also used as medication reminders with dosage, type of medication, and instruction provided via text messaging from a central service. Software apps for mobile technologies[9] provide medication alerts with detailed information regarding pill type and dosage, a medication log, refill reminder, and emergency information (Mann, 2005).

More sophisticated medication reminders make use of the Internet and the concept of ambient environments (see Chapter 2). These devices attempt to ensure that the person takes his or her medications by reporting to a care provider if they don't.[10] Each medication bin (for a single day or a single medication on a single day) is programmed by the provider on the web and is automatically downloaded to the device on the next phone connection. The care provider selects the optimal times to take the medication, indicates how many to take, and chooses optional warnings or instructions applicable to the drug. For example, auditory, text, or graphic alerts can be provided to the individual who is to take the medication and these alerts can be repeated until the user takes the medication or until disabled by the carer remotely. When the lid of a bin is opened the time is recorded in memory. Pill-taking histories are sent daily by telephone line or Internet upload. The caregiver who needs to check charts can view them via the Internet. These systems allow online remote programming of prescription or regimen changes. These systems have both an initial equipment charge and a monthly fee for the monitoring function.

There are also other specialized memory aids. Reminder messages can be used for prompting; for example, a voice prompt may remind a person to pick up her keys or lock the front door when leaving home or reminding the person of daily appointments. Safety reminders are often helpful for people with dementia (e.g., to tell them not to go out at night or not to trust bogus callers at the door or on the phone). Locator devices can be attached to items that are often mislaid.

Pressing a color-coded button on a transmitter causes the object with the same color code to beep. Fastening the transmitter to the wall will help to ensure that the transmitter itself will not be mislaid. Reminders of time and day are discussed in the next section of this chapter. The WatchMinder2: Training and Reminder System, which is described in the time management section, can also serve as a memory aid.

Information retrieval systems are devices or software packages that categorize and organize words/phrases so that they may be retrieved through associations. A number of information retrieval aids have been designed that use PDAs, smart phones, or tablets. Features of these devices

[9] For example: On-Time-Rx for iOS, Android, Blackberry, or Windows, www.ontimerx.com.

[10] For example: MedSignals, https://www.medsignals.com/MEDMinding.aspx; Philips Medication Dispensing Service: http://www.managemypills.com/.

[38] For example: the Learning Library (http://trainer.aimsxml.com/) from AbleLink Technologies, a cognitively accessible web-based training system using step-by-step prompting technology to provide picture-, audio-, and video-based instructions for how to use cognitive support technologies. See text for more information.

that are particularly useful include small size for portability, flexibility in programming for customization, large storage capacity, a variety of input and output modalities, and interfacing to other technologies (e.g., desktop or notebook computers, cell phones) (Szymkowiak et al, 2005). When PDAs or smart phones are used by individuals who have disabilities, two usability issues arise: changes in sensory processing and the small size of the keyboards and screens. Individuals with cognitive limitations from aging, injury (TBI or CVA), or dementia often have accompanying visual problems (declining acuity and contrast sensitivity, including color discrimination). The interconnectivity of mobile technologies provides the opportunity for interfacing with the Internet to retrieve a much wider range of information. Personalized profiles, possibly with features downloaded from the cloud as needed (Lewis and Ward, 2011) and integrated with sensors such as cameras and GPS receivers and internal features such as phone and calendar (Lewis et al, 2009), can be used to support reminders of activities on specific days or specific times or provide navigation assistance via GPS location with spoken data presentation.

Daily schedulers and reminder alarm devices based on mobile technologies (both of which are produced in a wide variety of formats) (Figure 15-5) are technologies that tend to provide the most immediate benefit to people with TBI (Kim et al, 1999; Van Hulle and Hux, 2005), CVA, aging (Szymkowiak et al, 2005), and intellectual disabilities (Davies et al, 2002). Software packages for these devices have also been designed to include prompting cues to aid memory (Bergman, 2002). These specially designed systems can be customized to meet the needs of a specific user and they have user-friendly interfaces and are easy to carry (Gorman et al, 2003). The mobile technology–based information retrieval aids require the user to display some degree of sensory perception, language use, memory, or learning skill to be of practical benefit. Because the software can be customized, the complexity of these functions can be adjusted to fit the skills of a wide variety of users. Case study 15-2 illustrates the application of mobile technologies as memory and organization aids.

CASE STUDY 15-2

Memory Challenges After Traumatic Brain Injury

Darrell is a 30-year-old man who sustained a TBI 3 years ago. His ability to read and write was severely affected, but he is able to communicate well through speech. Darrell also has trouble with time management and often forgets to complete daily tasks. He acknowledges his weaknesses and has been actively seeking out technologies that could help him to live more independently. One of Darrell's main concerns is addressing his forgetfulness. Ever since returning to work, he has had to rely on constant reminders from his supervisor to complete tasks. He found that his inability to read or write was not affecting his job performance, but it was limiting his ability to use written reminders to help with his memory difficulties. In addition to seeking help completing his work duties more independently, Darrell was also hoping to find something that would help him remember to take his medication at the right times throughout the day.

Essentially, what Darrell requires is both a "things-to-do" checklist and an alarm capable of signaling reminders at preset times throughout the day. One major restriction is that he must be able to interact with the device in some way that does not require reading or writing. Aside from that, Darrell has said he would prefer that the device be portable, and that it should have at least enough battery life to last an entire 8-hour work shift.

A smart phone app with voice recognition software was recommended for Darrell. After a brief training period, he was able to dictate a list of things he needed to do, store them in the phone's memory, and then play them back for future reference using the device's text-to-voice synthesizer. In this manner, Darrell was able to set up a schedule in the mornings and complete his work duties without constant reminders from his supervisor. He was also able to program a spoken reminder that indicated when it was time to take his medication. Darrell enjoyed the flexibility of this system because, after some training with the device, he was able to program new checklists and alarms as needed. Overall, he was very satisfied with the independence he gained from using the device.

What other alternatives to voice input/output would be appropriate for Darrell's needs? If Darrell was able to read and write, would this affect the choice of technology? Could the same functionality be obtained with a less costly device or combination of devices? Is there a low-tech solution?

Devices for Time Management

Time management technologies are those devices that aid in the planning, prioritizing, and execution of daily and time-dependent tasks. One class of devices uses an alternative format for representing time to make it more accessible to individuals with intellectual disabilities. One example is the Quarter Hour Watch[11] (Figure 15-6), which offers an alternative and potentially more intuitive representation of the passage of time (Granulund et al, 1995). The Quarter Hour Watch uses an entirely different concept of time by presenting a 2-hour time frame in 8 one-quarter-hour steps. Rather than clock hands or numbers, the watch display has eight circles, one for each quarter hour. The user of the watch must understand elapsed time rather than absolute time based on standard clocks. Events are represented by pictures on plastic chips (about 2 inches square) that are placed into the Quarter Hour Watch. A care provider sets the time of the event on the back of the plastic chip, which is read by the watch. When the chip is inserted into the watch, the display indicates how much time remains until the event should occur. If the time to the event is greater than 2 hours, then all eight circles are dark. After each quarter hour, a circle turns from dark to light until they are all light. At that time a signal sounds and the circles flash. The individual using the watch chooses the chip (e.g., time for favorite TV program, time to go to work) and then is able to tell when that time has arrived.

The WatchMinder[12] (Figure 15-7) is a device that reminds a user when a given preprogrammed task or event is scheduled

[11] Made by Handitek AB, Sweden: available from http://www.abilia.org.uk/produkter/produkt.aspx?productgroup=266921&product=261468.

[12] Irvine, CA, http://watchminder.com/.

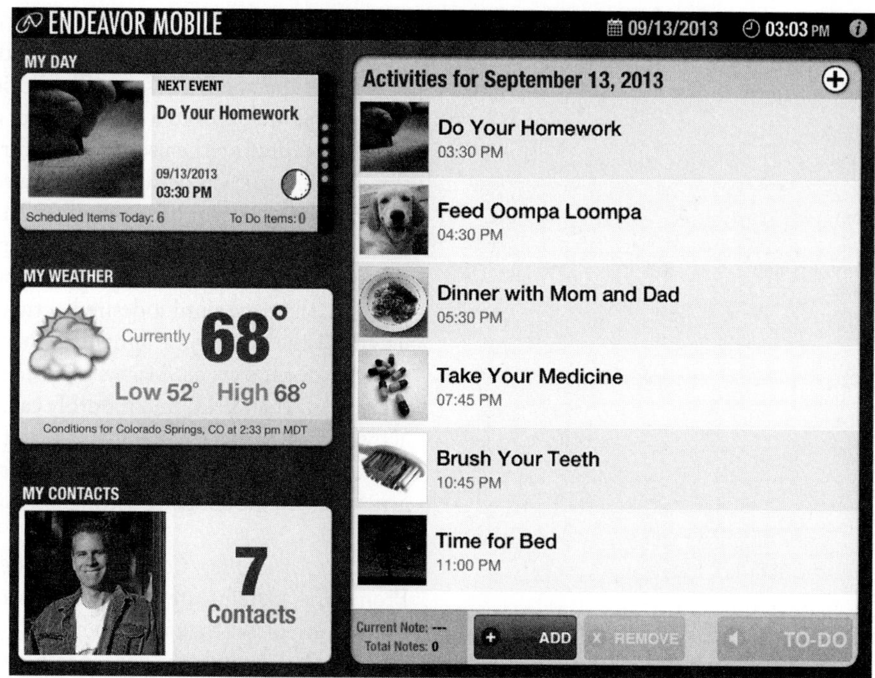

FIGURE 15-5 Devices based on smart phones and tablets can assist with scheduling and reminders for individuals with cognitive impairments.

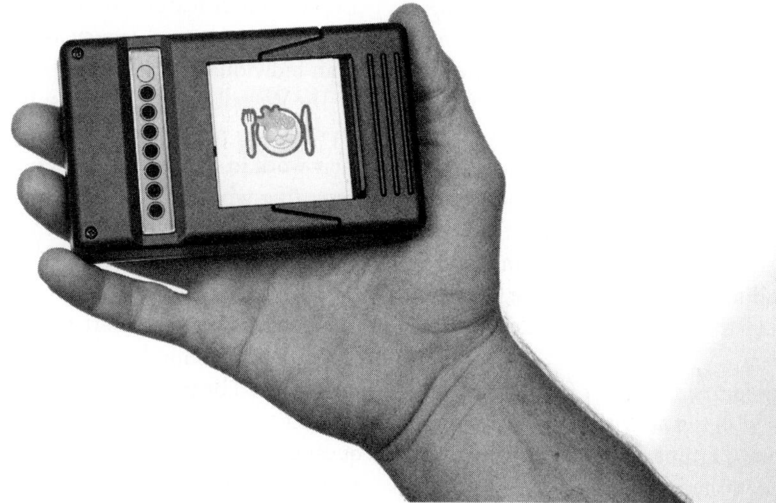

FIGURE 15-6 The Quarter Hour Watch. (Courtesy Abilia AB www.abilia.org.uk.)

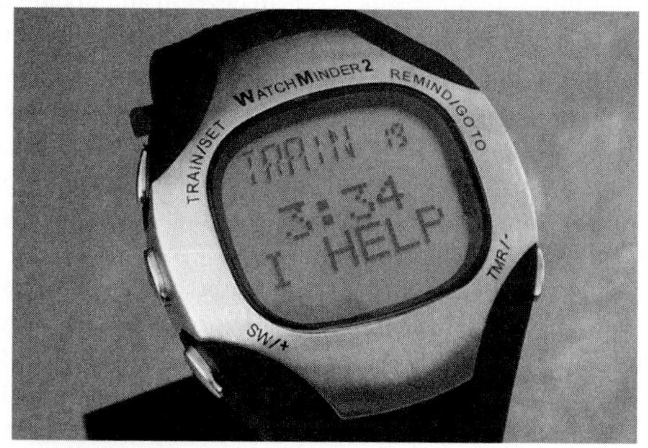

FIGURE 15-7 WatchMinder. (Courtesy WatchMinder, Irvine, CA, Watchminder.com.)

to occur. This device was designed for people with ADD, ADHD, LD, chronic diseases, stroke, or brain injury. A silent vibrating reminder system or beeping alert with 30 programmable alarms is included with both a training and reminder mode. The reminder mode is for remembering specific tasks such as taking medication and doing homework or chores. The training mode is for behavior change and self-monitoring. Box 15-4 shows preset messages for the WatchMinder2. This device also can be programmed with three personalized messages. The WatchMinder2 has two possible schedule modes: *fixed* (every 2, 3, 5, 10, 15, 20, 30, 45, or 60 minutes) or *random* (CPU randomly chooses from 2, 3, 5, 10, 15, 30, and 60 minutes). The person programming the device chooses one of these modes and the daily start (S) time and end (E) time.

BOX 15-4 Examples of WatchMinder2 Preset Messages[39]

BATHRM (bathroom)
BE POS (be positive)
BREATH (breathe)
COUGH
FOLDIR (follow directions)
FOLRUL (follow rules)
GIVPOS (give positive reinforcement)
GOODJB (good job)
HANDUP (raise hand)
IGNORE
POSIMG (positive image)
POSTUR (posture)
PRAY
PYATTN (pay attention)
RELAX
REST
SIT
STOP
STRTCH (stretch)

The MEMOplanner[13] (Figure 15-8) is a planning board or day planner that facilitates the sequencing and organization of an individual's tasks and events for a given period of time. This panel helps teach concepts such as understanding units of time (e.g., "How long is an hour?") and elapsed time (e.g., "Why can't I have lunch now?"). This device also helps individuals to independently answer daily life questions (e.g., "Do I have time to eat before the bus comes?" or "How long until we go swimming?"). Like the Quarter Hour Watch, the MEMOplanner displays time with four lighted elements per hour, each signifying 15 minutes. The total period of time is adjustable with preset division of the day into morning, midday, afternoon, evening, and night and day, week, or month. Changing these can be hidden from the user if they would cause confusion.

Activities can be displayed in either a list (with the time in text) or timeline format with the activities shown next to the row of lighted elements. Current activities are outlined in red. Activities can be identified by graphic information (digital photos or scanned drawings) or descriptive text. Activities can be "signed off" when completed by touching a square in the activity window where the following is displayed: date, starting and stopping time, activity icon (picture, drawing), activity name, sign-off box (if sign-off is selected), description (if entered), activity tasks (if entered), speaker icon for audio message concerning start and stop times, speaker icon for speech synthesis (if selected), delete button, make a copy button, edit button, and OK button. These can all be edited and customized for an individual user via the built-in touch screen or from another computer over the Internet. Remote control allows the user or family member to make settings or adjustments in the device from a distance.

The activity tasks provide a prompting structure for the user. The start of activities is prompted by audio alarms or as recorded personal messages. The device can be set to send text (SMS) messages to a care provider or family member or someone expecting the user to arrive for an activity. The time slot adjacent to each light can be labeled with an activity by using text, pictures, or other symbols. The current time is represented either by a column of lights starting with the current time and proceeding in 15-minute intervals or by a single dot of light. The time until a desired activity is indicated by the length of the column of lights from the present time to the start time of the event. Alarms can be set for each 15-minute increment. The weekly and monthly calendars provide similar activity display in a smaller format. Past activities are crossed out. The MEMOplanner can be used in an individual living arrangement, group living setting, or a classroom.

Prompting/Cueing/Coaching Devices

Prompting systems are those devices or software packages that inform a user that an action should be taken and provide visual, verbal, or auditory cues as to how to accomplish a task. In most cases the systems allow a care provider to enter the relevant information regarding events, times, and frequency. Some devices also allow collection of data regarding ease of use, and others feature communication with a central station for data logging, emergency assistance requests, or tracking of an individual's actions and location.

The Wearable Coach[14] is a suite of smart phone/computer apps to help people who have cognitive disabilities perform their work in the proper sequence and stay on task without forgetting what they are doing. The system is also designed to allow managers to check the progress of workers during the day or update a worker's schedule during the day as conditions change via a phone signal or Wi-Fi connection. The worker wears a smart phone equipped with the daily schedule and reminders on his or her shoulder. Reminders are triggered by timers and schedules along with the worker's interaction via gesture. Many of the reminders are framed as questions to help to keep the worker's mind engaged in the task. The supervisor and/or coach use a computer and phone or tablet interface and connect to the worker's phone via the Internet.

This link allows the supervisor to develop and update the schedule and monitor the worker's progress throughout the day. Other interactions include updating the schedule at whatever completion or interim points the supervisor designates and texting the supervisor or someone else when an unexpected event happens (such as a task taking too long or the GPS sensing that the worker is not where he or she should be).

Individuals who have cognitive disabilities also need navigation assistance that can be provided by a smart phone with GPS and speech output capability. Boulis et al (2011) describe how GPS systems that are included within mainstream mobile technologies can serve as a platform for the

[13] Abilia, http://www.abilia.org.uk/index.aspx.
[39] Irvine, CA, Watchminder.com.

[14] Source America, http://www.sourceamerica.org/.

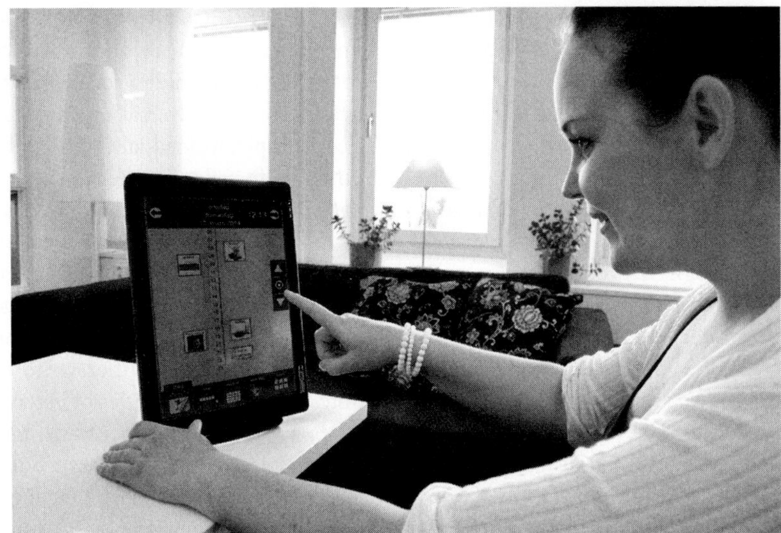

FIGURE 15-8 The MEMOplanner provides reminders of activities throughout the day. (Courtesy of Abilia, www.abilia.org.uk.)

development of devices to aid navigation and emergency calling for people with cognitive disabilities, including the elderly. The built-in GPS can locate the individual and the phone can transmit messages such as instructions for finding a location. If the individual encounters an emergency situation he or she can send a message via 911 or a text message to a familiar contact. The contact or 911 service will know where the individual is and can respond. Boulos et al (2011) describe several products and development projects that are designed for monitoring the location and status of vulnerable persons utilizing the GPS function of mainstream mobile phone systems.

A navigational device based on a GPS cell phone, called Opportunity Knocks, was designed specifically for people with cognitive limitations (Kautz H et al, 2004). This device learns the patterns of the user, and uses that pattern to help the user find the most familiar (not necessarily the shortest) route, recover from mistakes, and receive prompts when needed. If an error occurs (e.g., a user misses a bus stop that is routinely taken) the device verbally prompts the user with prompts such as "I think you made a mistake" or "May I guide you to [location]." The user can indicate which location by touching a picture of it on the display of the cell phone. Then a mode of transportation (e.g., walk or bus) is chosen in the same way. Using the stored patterns, the system then directs the user to that location. Using stored information, the system can also determine if the user is on the wrong bus, and direct him or her to get off at the next stop. Instruction can then be provided to get the person back on track to the correct destination. These concepts have been realized in a number of smart phone and iPhone apps.[15] Voice output for navigation helps individuals who cannot read.

WayFinder[16] is a smart phone–based application designed to enable people with intellectual and other cognitive disabilities to travel via bus or light rail more independently using audio and visual cues generated based on their GPS location. WayFinder includes an optional tracking feature that allows a family member or caregiver to track the location of a user using instant messaging and Google Maps.

For individuals who have difficulty understanding text and who need assistance with sequential activities, the Visual Assistant[17] provides task prompting using digital pictures and custom recorded audio or video messages. Step-by-step instructional supports are provided by allowing caregivers to set up instructional tasks. To provide multimodal cues for task completion, each step has recorded instructions and corresponding pictures. The most useful pictures are of the user performing the step in the actual environment. Visual Assistant can be used for more complex or detailed tasks where the addition of a picture or video clip can increase accuracy. Instructions can branch to different alternative sequences based on the choices made by the end user. Any step can be time based to advance automatically or provide periodic reminders to complete the current step.

An example of a prompting app designed for the iPhone and iPad is CanPlan developed at the University of Victoria in Canada. Activities are broken into a sequence of easy-to-follow steps labeled with both audio and graphic (e.g., photos) identifiers. The user goes through the activity under the direction of a support person or family member. Photos are taken of each step in the task and text or audio is added as needed. The task is categorized for storage and recall. Typical categories include areas such as food preparation, household chores, shopping, transportation, exercise, and workplace tasks. Scheduling and reminders are included for each task. CanPlan was developed to aid people who have difficulty

[15] For example: Google Maps Navigation, http://www.google.com/mobile/maps/; iNav, http://www.inavcorp.com/?gclid=CKSmhcPQ2qMCFVjW5wodkVDR9g.

[16] AbleLink Technologies, http://www.ablelinktech.com/.

[17] http://www.ablelinktech.com/index.php?id=33.

with activities consisting of sequences of steps, including those with TBI, dementia, ASD, dyslexia, and developmental disabilities.

The ISAAC™ Cognitive Prosthesis[18] System is a wearable and highly customizable device that provides procedural information and personal information storage (Cole and Dehdashti, 1998). This system is a fully individualized cognitive prosthetic system that assists the user to live and work more independently through the organization and delivery of individualized prompts and procedural and personal information. A care provider enters the content with the use of an authoring system. The content is then delivered to the individual with a cognitive disability in English or Spanish as synthesized speech audio, text, checklists, or graphics. Prompts can be delivered on the basis of specified conditions, such as the time of day, to prompt for an action by the user. User input is through a pressure-sensitive touch screen.

Mihailidis, Fernie, and Barbenel (2001) developed a prompting system for hand washing to assist individuals who have dementia. The system, called COACH, uses a video camera, personal computer, and artificial intelligence software. The system monitors progress of the person and provides auditory prompts when steps are skipped or mistakes are made. The system also learns the patterns of the individual users and adapts its settings and cues to match them. In a single subject design study with 10 elder participants, the COACH system led to significant improvement in completion of hand-washing tasks without caregiver assistance (Mihailidis, 2004).

Low-tech devices can also aid a user in performing a task by providing concrete feedback as to the proper course of action to undertake. For example, a microwave button shield only lets a user see/use those buttons that are needed for a specific task or raised lines on paper give a user an idea of where symbols should be placed to enhance readability. Task-specific jigs enable people to perform tasks that they may not otherwise be able to perform. For example, weighing and counting tasks in manufacturing and assembly can be difficult for workers who have cognitive disabilities. One approach to modifying, weighing, and counting is to use a talking scale connected to a controller that provides prompting and feedback as necessary (Erlandson and Stant, 1998). For counting tasks, a bin with a specified number of locations is weighed. If the bin is properly filled, the weight is correct and the user is prompted to proceed with the next step. If the weight is too low, the user is told to check all the bins, and if it is too high the user is prompted to be sure only one element is in each bin. For weighing, objects placed on the scale are compared with stored weight limit values, and the user is prompted if the weight is above or below the weight range. Visual and auditory prompts are included. Erlandson and Stant (1998) describe the successful use of this system in a nail-counting task for a construction supply company by a woman with mild intellectual disability.

[18] www.cosys.us/.

Devices That Can Help Control Extraneous Stimuli

For some individuals the influence of distractions is such that they are unable to focus on a task when another stimulus, such as a conversation, is occurring in the background. For example, individuals with attention deficit disorder have difficulty focusing on the teacher in class. There are other situations in which we are required to devote attention to two or more tasks at the same time using *divided attention.* One example is listening to a lecture and taking notes. Students need auditory attention and processing skills to understand what the professor is saying, and additionally, require visual and tactile skills to either write or keyboard as they take notes. While the activities of listening to a lecture and taking notes appear to be concurrent, in fact attention is moving quickly between the two tasks. Sustained attention is similar to vigilance, but differs in that there isn't necessarily a competing stimulus present.

The family of **stimuli control** devices includes technologies that address attention or perception problems by limiting or manipulating the information presented to the user. They can be subdivided into three categories that best capture their intended application: noise reduction techniques, visual field manipulation, and **media presentation** techniques. Auditory (noise reduction) systems are those devices that filter out extraneous noise so the user may focus on one specific source. An example of such a system is a transmitter/headphone receiver link between a student and teacher in a classroom setting similar to those used for students who are hard of hearing (see FM systems in Chapter 14). Visual stimuli can be altered in a similar fashion, through the use of prism glasses or special lenses that correct for double vision or neglect (e.g., in TBI) (see Chapter 13).

Media presentation is an important design consideration for many visual display applications. Websites, computer monitors, and other visual displays need to be carefully designed to avoid extraneous information that might be distracting to a person with an attention disorder. By reducing clutter, increasing clarity, and simplifying visual displays, information can be presented in a way that is best perceived and understood by a broad target audience. Key concepts in web design for individuals with cognitive disabilities are shown in Table 15-10. The WebAim project[19] has many useful resources for making websites accessible to individuals who have cognitive disabilities. These include evaluation packages to check websites for accessibility, guidelines for developing accessible websites, and tools for making websites more accessible to this population.

Internet access for individuals with intellectual disabilities can provide benefits in self-esteem and self-confidence, independence in vocational and living contexts, opportunities for training, self-directed activities, and use of their time for pursuits that are stimulating and informative (Davies et al, 2001). Unfortunately, access to the Internet for this population is often limited by standard web browsers that require high-level cognitive skills, particularly in reading and

[19] Center for Persons with Disabilities, Utah State University, www.webaim.org.

TABLE 15-10 Key Concepts in Web Design for Individuals with Cognitive Disabilities

Challenges	Solutions
Users may become confused at complex layouts or inconsistent navigational schemes.	Simplify the layout as much as possible.
	Keep the navigation schemes as consistent as possible.
Users may have difficulty focusing on or comprehending lengthy sections of text.	Where appropriate, group textual information under logical headings.
	Organize information into manageable "chunks."
One method of input may not be sufficient.	Where appropriate, supplement text with illustrations or other media, and vice versa.

(From WebAIM, http://www.webaim.org/techniques/cognitive/.)

writing. A pilot project was designed to compare a specially designed web browser (Web Trek) with a standard browser (Internet Explorer) (Davies et al, 2001).

Web Trek used graphics, reduced screen clutter, audio prompts, and personalization and customization to maximize accessibility to individuals with intellectual disabilities. Twelve participants evaluated the two browsers in three tasks: searching for a website, saving websites to a favorites list, and retrieving sites from the favorites. Three measures of performance were used: independence (fewer prompts), accuracy (errors made), and task completion (completed with three or fewer prompts). All three measures showed statistically significant differences favoring the Web Trek browser, indicating that Internet access for persons with intellectual disabilities is feasible. Web Trek is also a part of the AbleLink technologies Endeavor Desktop Environment.[20]

Tools for Concept Organization and Decision Making

Concept mapping is a process of conceptualizing information using graphics and text. Inspiration® concept mapping software[21] is designed to help students in sixth through twelfth grade to plan, organize, and write research papers. As shown in Figure 15-9, its alternative format for representing ideas with both text and graphics, ability to import concepts from the Internet and other sources, and the provision of a large number of templates make Inspiration useful to students who have learning disabilities (Ashton, 2005; LoPresti et al, 2004). Inspiration also allows the students to toggle between text and concept map as they develop their report. Using Inspiration, eighth-grade students who had learning disabilities produced essays that were significantly above their pretest levels in number of words, concepts included, and holistic writing scores (Sturm and Rankin-Ericson, 2002).

An application that helps create access to portable electronic systems for people who have intellectual disabilities, autism, Down syndrome, traumatic brain injury, and Alzheimer's disease is the Pocket Ace. This software application creates a simplified interface for cell phone use. Pocket ACE uses audio messages and images to navigate the phone structure to make and receive phone calls. A central element is a picture-based address book that allows a user to merely tap on the picture of the person he or she wants to talk to in order to place the call.

Likewise, pictures of incoming callers who are in the address book are displayed and the user can recognize the caller and answer by tapping the picture. The Pocket Ace software runs on the Pocket Ace phone and allows individuals to make personal, business, and emergency phone calls without assistance.

The Schedule Assistant is a PDA and smart phone app intended for use by individuals who are unable to use mainstream text-based scheduling because of literacy limitations. It uses a multimedia approach that presents information in visual (picture, symbol) or auditory form. Appointments or events are entered into the system by recording an audio message and selecting a relevant digital picture or icon to be displayed when the message is activated. The day(s) and time for the message to activate are also selected. The Schedule Assistant can be used for meeting bus schedules, medication reminders, taking work breaks, and maintaining classroom schedules or morning routines. Schedule Assistant, Pocket Ace, and Visual Assistant are available as part of the Community Integration Suite or Pocket Endeavor products from AbleLink Technologies.[22]

Individuals with intellectual disabilities have a very high unemployment rate. The increasing complexity of the work environment is one of the major reasons for this (Davies et al, 2003). People with intellectual disabilities are often not able to learn complex decision-making skills that are essential for work.

The Pocket Compass[23] is a PDA-based device specifically designed to assist in decision making. The Pocket Compass uses graphic and audio prompts to guide a user through a decision-making process when participating in complex tasks. The decision-making process contains a branching sequence of cued steps with decision points based on a task analysis of the desired job activity. In the setup mode the work supervisor or care provider creates cueing sequences described by pictures and recorded audio instructions. Decision points in a decision-making process can be identified with these pictures and audio labels. Once a setup has been entered into the device, the user can move through the sequence of instructions and decision points by using the graphic and auditory prompts and making entries (beginning with START and then NEXT after each choice is presented) through a touch screen on the PDA. Up to four pictures can be presented at decision points.

[20] http://www.ablelinktech.com/index.php?id=18.

[21] Inspiration software, Inc, Beaverton OR, http://www.inspiration.com/.

[22] http://www.ablelinktech.com/index.php?id=37.

[23] Replaced by the Visual assistant for Android devices, http://www.ablelinktech.com/index.php?id=33.

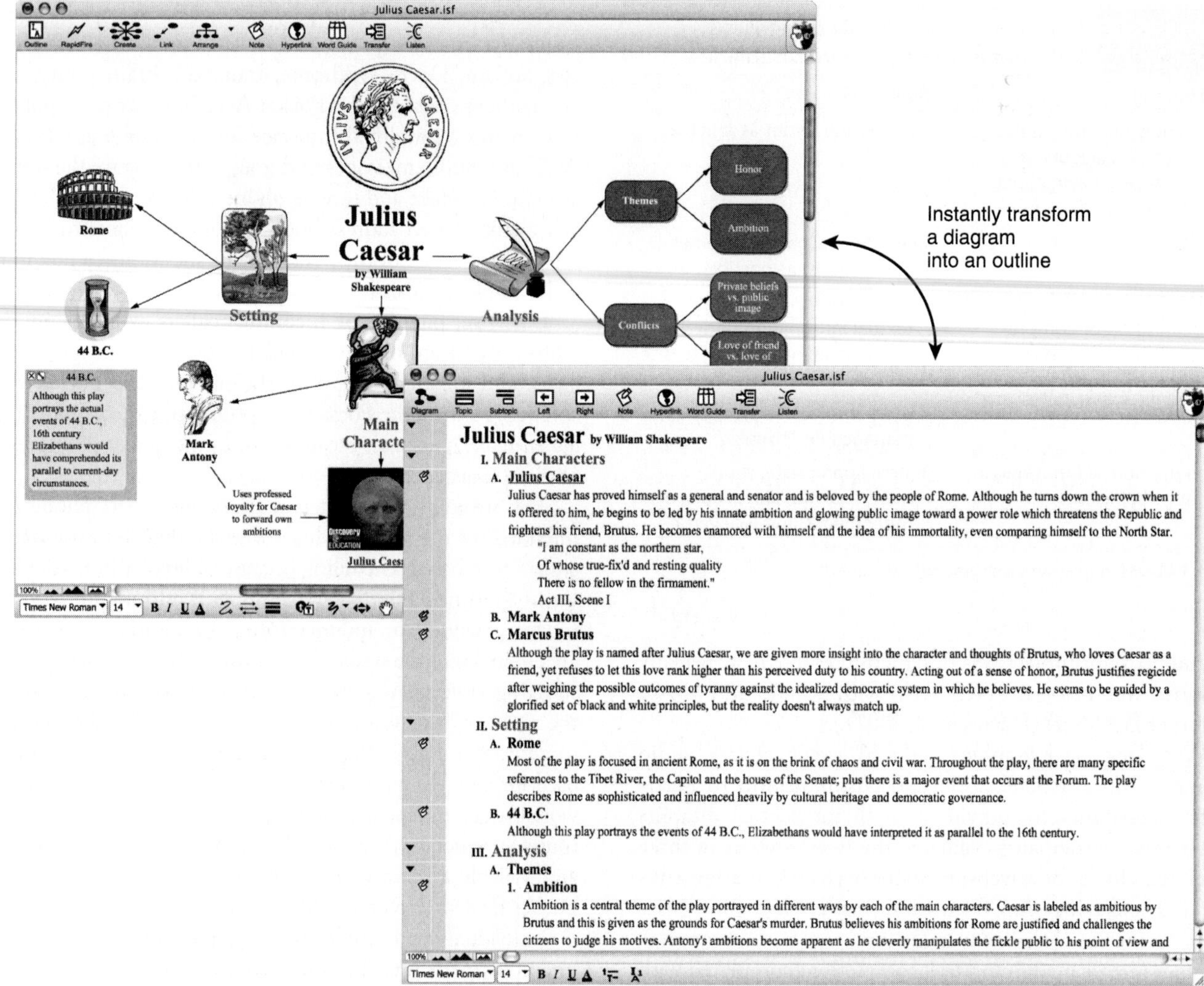

FIGURE 15-9 Inspiration software allows the development of ideas in a graphical format and automatic conversion to text. (Courtesy Inspiration Software, Inc, Beaverton, OR, http://www.inspiration.com/.)

The Planning and Execution Assistant and Trainer™ (PEAT)[24] is an Android™ smart phone or tablet application designed to assist individuals with cognitive disorders resulting from brain injury, stroke, Alzheimer's disease, and similar conditions (Levinson, 1997). PEAT uses artificial intelligence to automatically generate plans and also to revise those plans when unexpected events occur. PEAT uses a combination of manually entered schedules and a library of stored scripts describing activities of daily living (e.g., morning routine or shopping). Scripts can be used for both planning and for execution. Planning involves a simulation of the activity with key decision points presented and necessary prompts (auditory and visual) supplied to aid the individual through the planning process. The plan to be executed can be either the stored script or a modified script based on the simulation. The PEAT artificial intelligence software generates the best strategy to execute the required steps in the plan (LoPresti et al, 2004). PEAT also automatically monitors performance and corrects schedule problems when necessary.

[24] Attention Control Systems, Mountain View, Calif., www.brainaid.com/.

Language Tools

Many forms of assistive technology are *language tools* that assist with reading or writing. Many devices focus on the memory requirements of language. For example, word completion programs (see Chapter 6) are useful for people who are poor at spelling. They predict whole words on the basis of the first few letters typed by the user. A list of possible word choices is presented, and the user need only recognize the intended word from that list. Dictionaries and thesauruses are low-tech alternatives to word completion programs because they also operate on the basis of using word recognition to rectify deficiencies in word retrieval. For TBI, word prediction software programs have all been shown to be useful in clinical trials (Kim et al, 1999; Van Hulle and Hux, 2005).

Word prediction has been shown to be a promising strategy for improving text entry speed of students with learning disabilities as they move from hand writing to computer writing by using a word processor (Lewis, 2005). Word prediction programs written specifically for students with learning disabilities[25] include features that make them more effective. In addition to simple word prediction, these programs often include dictionaries to suggest alternatives that increase the richness and interest of the writing on the basis of the topic being discussed, and they can be personalized for an individual student. Another program, WordQ,[26] takes into account phonetic spelling mistakes.

Spell checking programs are helpful to students with learning disabilities as editing tools, but grammar checkers are not (Lewis, 2005). Spell checking programs are designed to primarily detect typographical errors, not misspellings resulting from phonetic errors (Ashton, 2006). Thus, the target word for a student with a learning disability who is spelling phonetically is often not the first word listed by the spell checking program. Despite this limitation, students with learning disabilities were able to detect their target word 95% of the time, even if it was not the first word listed (Ashton, 2006). The reason for the lack of success with grammar checkers is that they often rely on text to have correct spelling (Lewis, 2005). When evaluated on the basis of types of spelling errors made by students with learning disabilities, spell checkers vary widely in effectiveness (Sitko et al, 2005). Spell checking programs are most effective when they are integrated into a word processing program.

Providing Alternative Input

Alternative input technologies offer the user different modalities for providing input commands or information to a device. One example is the use of voice recognition software instead of text-based or icon-based pointing or tapping (see Chapter 8). Voice recognition can be useful for generation of text input by individuals with cognitive disabilities that limit their ability to write (LoPresti et al, 2004). Users are able to enter information or commands to a computer through voice dictation instead of the GUI screen. For TBI, speech recognition programs have all shown to be useful in clinical trials (Kim et al, 1999; Van Hulle and Hux, 2005). Voice recognition can be very effective in improving writing for students with LDs (Sitko et al, 2005). A person with an LD may be able to verbally articulate thoughts very well but, because of visual processing problems, may have trouble getting words down on paper: "the words jump all over the page." Automatic speech recognition provides an alternative for this type of individual.

Voice memo recorders are used in a similar manner, replacing pen-and-paper or keyboard entry as a means of storing messages for future reference. For those who are unable to make the fine motor movements required for handwriting, a portable notebook computer with abbreviation expansion or word completion/prediction (see Chapter 6) may be more efficient. Buttons with descriptive pictures and text may make the function of input controls more obvious.

An advantage of smart phones and tablets is that the user interface can be customized via software, and the complexity of input operating functions can be adjusted to fit the skills of a wide variety of users. One example of customization of the user interface is AbleLink's Pocket Discovery Desktop.[27] This software tool is helpful for people who have difficulty using smart phones because of their complexity. The Pocket Discovery Desktop software interfaces to the operating system desktop and provides a simplified interface for accessing programs. Picture- or audio-based messages can be programmed into on-screen buttons for any application on the phone. The picture and audio labels help users identify different programs. Pocket Desktop can avoid accidental activation of the physical buttons by deactivating or causing them to have specific functions on the phone. Discovery Desktop Pocket is available as part of the Community Integration Suite from AbleLink Technologies.

Endeavor Desktop Environment (EDE)[28] is designed for people who need a simplified Windows desktop. The program provides a picture-based log-in screen and allows the creation of custom, single-click picture buttons for everyday technologies, such as social networking, online access and communication, and productivity. EDE incorporates the Web Trek accessible browser to enable web browsing, Endeavor email, a picture-based address book, a visual media player, and access to news via an accessible RSS reader. Within each user's custom desktop, personalized content is available using dynamic buttons configured with descriptive images and audio to facilitate access. Because multiple users can each have their own unique desktop on a single computer, Endeavor Desktop Environment is useful in classrooms or group living settings. The desktop also identifies the user so that any programs customized for that user will be loaded, if available. EDE is available as part of the Computer & Web Access Suite or as part of the Smart Living Suite from AbleLink technologies.

A software application for Internet access that addresses impairments in language and communication ability is SymbolChat (Keskinen et al, 2012). This software is customizable by end users and their support personnel. The picture-based instant messaging system uses input via a touch screen and output via speech synthesis. Nine adult users evaluated the SymbolChat prototype and demonstrated that users can express themselves in spontaneous communication even without prior training in the use of symbols. These results indicate that it is possible to provide alternative means for individuals with cognitive disabilities to access computers and the Internet.

Options for Alternative Output

Alternative output technologies offer users a nontraditional means of acquiring feedback or information from a device. Some individuals are more visually oriented and print or

[25] For example: Co-Writer, Don Johnston, Inc, Volo, Ill., http://donjohnston.com/.
[26] http://www.synapseadaptive.com/quillsoft/WQ/wordq_description.htm.
[27] Part of the Community Integration Suite, http://www.ablelinktech.com/index.php?id=36.
[28] http://www.ablelinktech.com/.

screen displays work well for them. For others, information is easiest to access in auditory form. Synthesized or digitized speech output is often used for auditory information. The principles of electronically generated speech and its application in augmentative communication systems are discussed in Chapter 16. Many devices that were originally developed for individuals who have limited vision make use of synthesized speech to enhance or replace a typically visual output. Examples of these devices include text-to-speech screen readers for computer applications, talking calculators, a tape measure with speech output, and bar code scanners (see Chapter 13).

Synthesized speech and digitized speech (see Chapter 7) are both used to provide auditory information to children and adults with intellectual disabilities (see prompting/cueing section in this chapter). Synthesized speech associated with a word processor[29] for students with LDs can provide an additional modality that is helpful in writing and editing. The greatest benefit may be in reducing the most common misspellings (i.e., those that are "nonreal" words such as "thar" for "there" as opposed to word substitutions such as "to" for "two") (Lewis, 2005). Synthetic speech output also was useful when the spell checker could not suggest any words because of gross misspelling. The impact of speech output is more significant for younger learners than for secondary students because it may be a distraction for older students, drawing attention away from the writing task. In some cases, the impact of speech synthesizers in providing writing assistance to students with LDs is less significant than the effective use of spell checkers and word prediction (Lewis, 2005). However, as illustrated by the following case study, auditory output by speech synthesis is an effective tool for students with reading or writing difficulties associated with LDs (Sitko et al, 2005). Students can often detect errors in their writing more easily if they hear the words as opposed to reading them in written form. Adding speech synthesis to the presentation of screen-based text provides a multimodal output that also assists in reading and writing.

CASE STUDY 15-3

Learning Disability and Alternative Input for Reading

Daniel is a student in a regular educational program. He has an LD that makes it difficult for him to read printed material. The system provided for Daniel allows him to have an alternative input modality for his reading. He completes the printed lesson that requires him to fill in blanks on a worksheet by using a scanner that digitizes his lesson and puts it into a word processor. He listens to the text using earphones so as not to disturb the other students. With this system he is able to mark and copy the text using a reading program like those described in this section. He also makes use of word prediction, spell checking, and grammar checking in completing his assignments.

Because many individuals with LDs have greater comprehension of auditory than written information, synthesized speech output in "talking books" or "e-books" has been shown to be effective in improving reading abilities

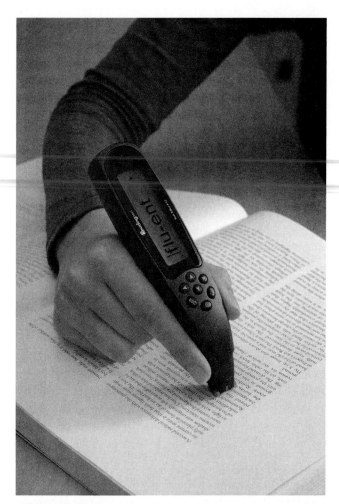

FIGURE 15-10 The Quicktionary Text-to-Speech Reading Aid. Text is scanned into the pen's memory. (Courtesy WizCom technologies, Ashton, MA, www.wizcomtech.com/.)

(Ashton, 2005). E-books have a number of features that are useful for students who have LDs. For example, words can be highlighted in the text as they are spoken or the document can be presented in an enlarged font. For students who need spelling practice, a spelling activity can be selected that uses the words from the story. Using software and online tools, teachers can create their own e-books (Ashton, 2005).

The Readingpen,[30] an assistive reading device (Figure 15-10), is a handheld scanner designed specifically for school-age reading levels. As the pen is moved across a word or full line of text, the text is spoken aloud. Using a children's dictionary and thesaurus, the device also provides information to the student about word meaning and alternative words through a three-line built-in display. The pen provides a portable way for people with reading difficulties, LDs, or dyslexia to get immediate word support when they are reading. The scanned text may be spoken word by word or line by line. An earphone connection is available for privacy.

Altering the visual appearance of the computer screen can also aid individuals with disorders such as dyslexia (LoPresti et al, 2004). Changing features such as font size,

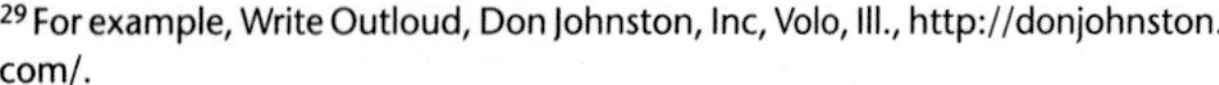

[29] For example, Write Outloud, Don Johnston, Inc, Volo, Ill., http://donjohnston.com/.

[30] WizCom Technologies, Ashton, Mass., www.wizcomtech.com/

background/foreground color combinations, contrast, spacing between words, letters, and paragraphs, and use of graphics can all improve access to screen-based information.

The World Wide Web Consortium (W3CWeb Content Accessibility Guidelines) (see Chapter 13) has developed strategies for web designers that support online access for individuals with cognitive disabilities. These include (Chadwick et al, 2013):

- Text alternatives for nontext content;
- Captions and other alternatives for multimedia;
- Content can be presented in different ways;
- Content is easier to see and hear;
- Users have enough time to read and use the content;
- Content does not cause seizures;
- Users can easily navigate, find content, and determine where they are;
- Content is readable and understandable;
- Content appears and operates in predictable ways;
- Users are helped to avoid and correct mistakes;
- Content is compatible with current and future user tools.

Tracking and Identification

This final category consists of technologies that involve the **tracking and identification** of people or items. Such devices often provide an extra degree of safety for users who might not have the cognitive skills required to work their way out of problematic situations. For instance, individuals with Alzheimer's disease often have periods of forgetfulness and disorientation. The disorientation can lead to wandering behavior that is unsafe to the person and very worrisome to the caregivers and family. Global positioning systems (GPS) have been used to assist these individuals by providing their location to the caregiver (Mann, 2005). The GPS Locator Watch[31] is designed to track children, but its features apply well to persons with dementia. The watch has a wireless transmitter/receiver that transmits the location of the person and allows transmission of information to the watch. For individuals whose disability makes it difficult to understand the purpose of the watch and who try to remove it, the watch has an electronically activated lock to keep it in place. The lock can be remotely released for removal. The device also has a built-in pager, clock, and emergency call function.

Individuals who have cognitive disabilities also need navigation assistance that can be provided by a smart phone with GPS and speech output capability. Boulis et al, 2011 describe how GPS systems that are included within mainstream mobile technologies can serve as a platform for the development of devices to aid navigation and emergency calling for people with cognitive disabilities, including the elderly. The built-in GPS can locate the individual and the phone can transmit messages such as instructions for finding a location. If the individual encounters an emergency situation they can send a message via 911 or a text message to a familiar contact. The contact or 911 service will know where the individual is and can respond. Boulis et al (2011) describe several products and development projects that are designed for monitoring the location and status of vulnerable persons utilizing the GPS function of mainstream mobile phone systems. They also point out the dangers inherent in GPS systems if the technology fails to provide accurate information or if there is over-reliance on the technology. The ethical implications of the use of monitoring technologies in these ways are discussed in Chapter 4.

WayFinder[32] is a smart phone–based application designed to enable people with intellectual and other cognitive disabilities to travel via bus or light rail more independently using audio and visual cues generated based on their GPS location. WayFinder includes an optional tracking feature that allows a family member or caregiver to track the location of a user using instant messaging and Google Maps.

Because these individuals often try to remove unfamiliar objects like bracelets and leg bands that are often used for attaching GPS-based monitoring devices, the effectiveness of GPS systems can be limited. Procedural memory is often preserved in patients with dementia and individuals typically get dressed as part of their daily routine. The GPS shoe[33] takes advantage of these characteristics by installing a GPS receiver and transmitter in the patient's shoes. The GPS signal can be monitored from a smart phone or from the Internet. The patient's travel is superimposed on a map for display to family or other care providers.

An iPhone application called Community Sidekick[34] sends automated email messages containing Google Map links that show the user's location. This allows the care provider or family to track the person's travels in the community. When the user starts a trip and launches the program, automated location information is sent via emails every few minutes. The user can also send simple stored messages by pressing one key. Sample messages include "I am OK," or "Please contact me," if the person has a question, needs assistance, or wants to speak with someone directly. Sidekick is intended to support parents of children with autism, spouses of people with traumatic brain injuries or other cognitive injuries, and support staff for people with intellectual and developmental disabilities.

CASE STUDY 15-4

Dementia and Wandering

Tito is 70 years old and has recently been diagnosed with Alzheimer's dementia. He lives with his wife Betsy in the small house in which he raised his family. His son comes by and checks up on his parents three to four times a week and is readily available should necessity arise. Because of Tito's condition he is forgetful about turning things off, which require vigilance, and has been found taking "walks" late at night. Unfortunately, Tito has had problems finding his way home during his outings and his son has received calls from the local police on two occasions regarding this problem. Betsy helps him remember to take his medicine and makes sure he doesn't forget the time of his weekly bingo game, and he still has no problem remembering old friends' names or solving his morning crossword puzzles. Given this profile, what types of assistive technologies might benefit Tito?

[31] Wherify, www.childlocator.com/.

[32] AbleLink Technologies, http://www.ablelinktech.com/.

[33] http://www.gpsshoe.com.

[34] http://itunes.apple.com/us/app/community-sidekick/id413107872?mt=8.

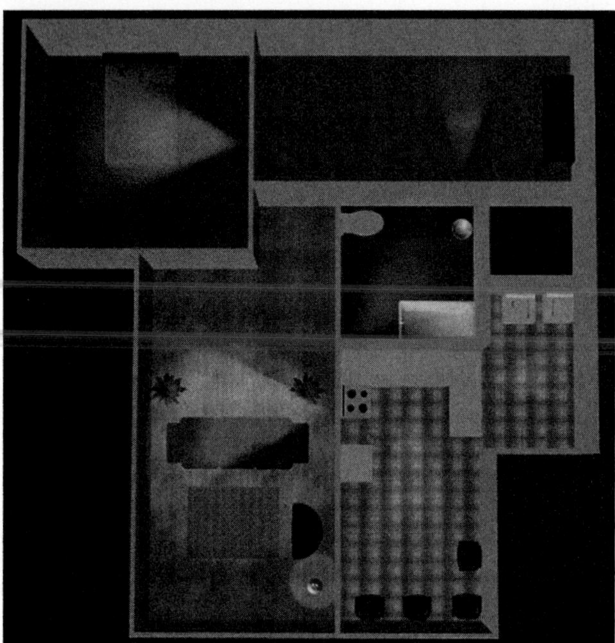

FIGURE 15-11 SmartHouse conceptualization. 1. Insulation and weatherization. 2. Heating and cooling. 3. Water heating. 4. Windows. 5. Lighting. 6. Appliances. 7. Water conservation.

Another method of tracking is home monitoring systems that can keep track of the status of a person with cognitive disabilities. The concept of a **smart home** (Figure 15-11) has been used to denote living environments in which automation is used to provide automatic functions including monitoring, communication, household functions (lights, air conditioning/heating, door locks), physiological measurements, and medication alerts (Mann, 2005). These systems include monitoring of the environment within a house (e.g., gas or smoke detectors), cardiac parameters (heart rate, arrhythmias), objects, and people (e.g., sensors that determine whether a person has left his or her bed by monitoring the weight applied to a pressure sensor placed under the bed frame), and emergency call (a button that is pushed and automatically dials a central station). The suppliers of these systems describe many case examples on their websites[35] that illustrate how these systems can make it possible for persons with memory loss, wandering, and other cognitive limitation continue to live at home (see case study 15-4).

Smart homes have the potential to allow greater independence to individuals with cognitive limitations, and in the case of elderly individuals, a chance to stay in their homes rather than move to group living facilities. Mann (2005) describes levels of a smart home from basic communications (Internet, phone) through complex monitoring and tracking of the resident's health, behavior, and needs. The core of the smart home is a processing and communication system linked to a sensory array. One example of a monitoring application is described in the following case study. The system aids a user in performing common tasks of daily living by assessing the person's current physiological state and the state of various utilities throughout the home and providing the user with feedback should he or she become disoriented or confused on a given task (Haigh et al, 2006). Mann (2005) describes several smart home projects.

A smart home includes heating systems, cooking, white appliances (dishwasher, washing machine, freezer etc.), home entertainment devices (radio, TV, video recorders, etc.), telecommunications devices (telephone, video telephone, fax), safety alarm systems, health monitoring systems, home safety monitors and sensors (water, smoke, fire, stoves, movement, etc.), special furniture (electrically adjustable beds, cupboards, and washbasins), and environmental control systems (door intercoms, doors, curtains, windows, lights, etc.) (Emiliani et al, 2011). These appliances and other equipment are becoming "intelligent"—that is, they have computing power and can be networked together for data sharing and control. Their software also allows decision making based on what they sense. For example, a washing machine could send a message when the cycle is over or a refrigerator could notify the owner that the egg tray is almost empty and add eggs to the shopping list on his or her phone.

Aldrich (2003) proposed five hierarchical classes of smart homes: (1) environments that contain intelligent objects—environments contain single, stand-alone applications and objects that function in an intelligent manner; (2) environments that contain intelligent, communicating objects—environments contain appliances and objects that function intelligently in their own right and also exchange information between one another to increase functionality; (3) connected environments—environments with internal and external networks, allowing interactive and remote control of systems, as well as access to services and information, both within and beyond the environment; (4) learning environments—patterns of activity in the environments are recorded and the accumulated data are used to anticipate users' needs and to control the technology accordingly; and (5) attentive environments—the activity and location of people and objects within the environments are constantly registered, and this information is used to control technology in anticipation of the occupants' needs (cited by Emiliani et al, 2011, p. 111). The interaction of these elements in the smart home depends on communication and control between objects and services. Because of the complexity of the smart home environment and the possible number of choices required for control, the user interface is important and should act as an intelligent intermediary between the complex system and the user. Emiliani et al (2011) provide a detailed analysis of the "intelligent kitchen" that includes the concept of ambient intelligent environments.

[35] For example, in Canada, www.lifeline.ca/; in the United Kingdom, http://www.tunstall.co.uk/home.asp; and in the United States, http://www.lifestation.com/?ASK=Medical-Alert.

CASE STUDY 15-5

Dementia: Assistive Technology to Allow Staying at Home

Eighty-six-year-old Emily has lived in her own home for many years. She and her husband (deceased) raised their family in this home, and her daughter still lives nearby. Emily now lives alone in the home. She has had difficulty remembering things and occasionally gets confused since she sustained a series of ministrokes a few years ago. Although her daughter helps out as much as she can, her own family and full-time job limit her availability. Emily's confusion and memory loss have resulted in her leaving the gas stove in her house turned on but not lit. Several possible solutions were proposed by the local assistive technology clinic. Because Emily still enjoyed cooking her own meals, turning off the gas permanently was ruled out. An electric stove was suggested, but Emily had spent her life cooking on a gas stove and didn't want to "learn how to cook all over again." A microwave oven was ruled out for the same reason. The solution that was implemented involved using a gas sensor connected to a shut-off valve. The sensor was originally connected to an audible alarm, and its use to control the shut-off valve required modification. The system was also set up to notify a central home monitoring system that a gas leak had been detected. The home monitoring center then notified Emily's daughter, who was able to go to the home and turn the gas back on. This approach allowed Emily to remain at home and to continue preparing her own meals. In the past year or so, her daughter has only had to reconnect the gas about four times in total.

Adapted from the Safe Home Project.

The COACH and the smart home are examples of *context-aware cognitive orthoses* (LoPresti et al, 2004). Each of these systems provides cueing and prompting on the basis of a combination of prestored information and data obtained from sensors in the environment. The use of context-based information can relieve anxiety, reduce the cognitive load, and overcome a lack of initiation by the individual using the device. In terms of the HAAT model, this functionality provides important information about one of the four elements of the model: the context. LoPresti et al (2004) also describe other examples of context-aware cognitive orthoses.

Ideally, technologies intended to support the smart home concept should be adapted to the user's needs. This requires a manual setup and adjustment for each user by themselves or (more likely) a care provider. To make that process more intuitive and easier to use for the care provider, mathematical models based on the probability that certain behaviors will occur are used. Hwang et al (2013) describe how these models are developed and how they function to translate user needs into a "caregiver interface" that will allow more sophisticated customization of cognitive technologies to meet user needs.

CONTEXT COMPONENT

There are four contexts to consider for assistive technology applications: physical, social, cultural, and institutional (see Chapters 1 and 3). There are implications for CATs in each of these.

The physical context for cognitive assistive technologies includes the concept of cloud computing (Lewis and Ward, 2011). Using networked computers (the cloud) to manage information and programs offers opportunities for improved services for people with cognitive disabilities. As discussed earlier in this chapter, there are web features that enhance cognitive access, such as access to definitions of unfamiliar words and audio presentation of web information. Unfortunately, these are not always incorporated into webpages. It is possible to have these and other accessibility features managed by software that resides in the cloud. Users could create information presentation preference profiles, stored in the cloud, and download them when they are needed for access to any site, from any device. Cloud services can make it possible for any text on any website to be read at the user's request.[36] These tools work by sending content from a webpage to a text-to-speech service running on a computer accessed via the web.

Individuals with cognitive disabilities often have trouble reading and when they are able to read they may frequently encounter words they do not understand. Having a dictionary of common words in the cloud would have the advantage of being available for any website and any device from which the cloud is accessed. The BrowseAloud tool provides this capability. Because a generic dictionary cannot contain all of the needed words or definitions, terms with special uses will have to be provided by site designers.

Another use for the cloud is to store user preferences in a user profile that can be downloaded to different devices. For example, things like font size, audio presentation of information, and links to cloud services can be included in a user profile. If a user has difficulty remembering and typing an email address it can also be stored in his or her profile. Because sensitive private information is included in the cloud profile, security is a prime concern. Automatic configuration of a range of devices such as a new smart phone is also possible using a stored user profile. Some individuals with intellectual disabilities have instruction books that include easily accessible information that they use to operate ICT devices. Rather than having to carry such a book with them, it could also be stored in the cloud and made available whenever and wherever they are.

A major part of the social context is the stigma associated with the use of CATs. The degree of stigma differs according to the type of assistive technology (Parette & Scherer, 2004); for example, hearing aids have more stigma than glasses. Individuals with intellectual disabilities and their families may view the use of assistive technologies as generating heightened attention and scrutiny and therefore reducing their comfort level in community settings. The reduced level of comfort may be due to actual perceived danger or due to vulnerability portrayed by the type of AT or it can be embarrassment due to having to depend on AT for function. Some technologies (e.g., those that have auditory output) can also call attention to the user. This added attention is often undesired.

[36] For example, BrowseAloud (http://www.browsealoud.com), or WebAnywhere (http://webanywhere.cs.washington.edu/).

The stove timer is installed in the homes of many older adults to compensate for cognitive impairment. Although these devices may be used as a standard safety precaution in any home, they can also be viewed as assistive technologies when they are procured to meet a cognitive weakness (Nygård, 2009). The way they are viewed has a large impact on how the client and his or her family, the home service aide, and the professional involved view both the client and the device. "A stove timer was thus often perceived by clients as a stigmatizing sign of old age, confirming a hidden disability of being 'old and forgetful.' It was even suggested that for older women, questioning their ability to manage the stove by suggesting a stove timer could be equivalent to withdrawing the driving licence for older men" (Nygård, 2009, p. 61).

The use of surveillance technologies is an increasingly dangerous special situation that can result in stigma. Social acceptability of surveillance technologies has a large influence on the acceptance and use of a particular technology by persons with developmental disabilities and its acceptance by their family (Niemeijer et al, 2010). Surveillance and monitoring AT may be particularly stigmatizing because the individual may feel that they have been "tagged." However, some types of tags are more acceptable than others. For example, a GPS-based surveillance transmitter mounted unobtrusively in a shoe may be more acceptable than a wrist or ankle bracelet to a person with dementia. Likewise, a monitoring app loaded into an iPod carried by a teenager with developmental disabilities may be more acceptable than a more conspicuous monitoring device while providing the same surveillance. In any case, the need to be monitored or tracked may be taken to reflect the social value attributed to that group, an aspect of the cultural context (Niemeijer et al, 2010). There is the danger that surveillance technologies marginalize individuals with dementia by overtly identifying them as incapable of managing their own lives.

In considering monitoring and surveillance systems, stigma is only one of the issues. These technologies are highly invasive and reduce the user's choice and control. We discuss the impact of this situation from an ethical point of view in Chapter 4.

It is also possible for assistive technologies to impact stigma in a positive way. For people with intellectual disability (ID), the disability is so visible and strong that it often is the primary identity a person has (Chadwick et al, 2013). The ID label can result in life-long stigma and societal discrimination. Social exclusion, increased vulnerability, and reduced life opportunities are also facts of life for individuals with ID, and the magnitude of the problems increases with the severity of the disability. When the person with an ID utilizes assistive technologies, especially those based on mainstream technologies, there is a perception of competence and skill resulting from device use that can positively impact social interaction and self-image.

The Internet in general and social media in particular have the potential to significantly reduce the impact of many of the negative aspects of ID (Chadwick et al, 2013). The Internet provides an opportunity for individuals with ID to "present themselves outside of their disability" when interacting online through social media (Chadwick et al, 2013, p. 385). When interacting online, individuals with ID have the option of whether or not to disclose their disability. People with ID often experience discrimination based on physical appearance, mannerisms, or behaviors, so the interaction without disclosing the disability can overcome some of the challenges inherent in developing meaningful relationships. Young people with mild to moderate ID reported that "the online medium rendered their disabilities invisible and made them feel like 'typical teenagers'" (Chadwick et al, 2013, p. 386).

Participating in social media also provides the potential to reduce feelings of loneliness and significantly improve frequency and quality of social interactions. Young people with mild intellectual disabilities used the Internet for social and romantic purposes and preferred to visit sites that were not restricted to those with disabilities (Chadwick et al, 2013). Having support to go online may help people with ID to cope with negative stereotypes, attitudinal biases, and social and physical exclusion.

An aspect of the institutional context is the policies and practices that accompany CAT use by individuals with ID. For example, people with intellectual and developmental disabilities are much less likely to have access to and use the Internet than are their nondisabled peers. Family and caregiver concern for safety often leads to blockage of Internet access by parents and caregivers. Some would argue that this overprotection denies the individual "the right to risk." There are, however, real risks of bullying and invasion of privacy that may be difficult for an individual with ID to recognize and then to resist or avoid. Lee (2012) gives a number of useful tips and strategies to support people with ID in accessing the Internet.

Family and caregivers may also believe that the Internet is beyond the skills of people with ID, creates a barrier to social inclusion and interpersonal interaction, and is inappropriate for older people with ID and those with more significant cognitive impairments (Chadwick et al, 2013). Computers can also be "cognitively inaccessible" for many individuals with ID. As we discussed earlier, attention to design features that enhance accessibility can dramatically improve this situation.

Chadwick et al (2013) summarize the situation as follows: "Despite claims that the Internet will bestow benefits, empirical verification of the actual social benefits and development opportunities provided by the Internet for people with ID is lacking.... Our understanding of how to enable people with ID to participate more fully in the online aspects of our society remains limited. The evidence base that does exist points to simplified Universal Design for the Internet, improved training and time for carers to facilitate access, building ICT into organisational cultures and addressing carer and societal attitudes to people with ID and to such people accessing the Internet" (p. 391).

Reluctance to be stigmatized can also have institutional context implications. For example, this factor also influenced the clients' motivation or lack of motivation to apply for a stove timer (Nygård, 2009). Clients were reluctant to get a stove timer because of the infringement on their independence. When the counterargument was made that it was a free service provided by the government, some responded that they "did not want to apply for funding from the city as they did not want to be a burden to society" (p. 58). This response is common when working with seniors and assistive technologies.

Nygård's (2009) study also showed that "when many different types of professionals take part in a process without sharing a model or structured frame of reference, it is likely that they act from different incentives and motives" (p. 6) and the client is not well served. The installer and manufacturer only delivered and set up the device. The OTs felt they were finished when the recommendation for funding was submitted. The home service aides realized that their initial impression of the stove timer as being very simple was in error and they did not really understand how it worked; this in turn led them to doubt whether the client was capable of learning to use the timer. The end result is often frustration with the technology, even if it is appropriate for the need and does support the desired activity.

ASSESSMENT

Measures such as the Canadian Occupational Performance measure (see Chapter 5) can be used to gain an understanding of the activities that the person (or family) wants to achieve through the use of CAT. Having identified activities, it is then possible to identify the skills required to utilize CATs for accomplishing those activities (see Box 15-1 and Figure 15-1). Many of the cognitive skills that are aided by CATs as well as those skills required to operate the CATs are assessed though typical psychological testing. Some assessments specially designed for CATs also have been developed. One of these is discussed in this section.

For the content areas defined by Granlund et al (1995) (Table 15-11), adults with cognitive disabilities may encounter problems in activities such as choosing a leisure activity, using public transportation, being on time for work, and preparing meals. Typical assessment questions and assistive technology examples for each content area are listed in Table 15-11.

One systematic approach developed for assessing ICT skills for people with cognitive disabilities is the EasyICT framework (Dekelver et al, 2010). The EasyICT was developed to assess and train children with cognitive disabilities between the ages of 6 and 18. For assessment of ICT, skill items were categorized in four main groups: (1) managing the computer (identifying parts, handling mouse), (2) browsing the Internet, (3) using email, and (4) using ICT to communicate in a safe, sensible, and appropriate way. For each category subtasks are identified such as mouse entry via clicking. Test questions were developed for each task. The test sessions were kept to an hour or less to avoid loss of concentration by the participants and provisions were made to stop and restart tasks if the participant did lose concentration.

Some exercises (e.g., clicking and dragging) were developed in a simulated environment in a game format. Others (e.g., opening a browser) were performed on the participant's familiar desktop. Observations were also recorded (e.g., appropriately handling the hardware). Based on these measurements and observations a client profile is generated that includes the acquired skills as well as the ones not yet acquired. The report also includes a list of steps in the prescription process adapted to people with ADHD:

Stage 1 Assess the need for CAT.

Stage 2 Test, adapt, and select an appropriate product.

Stage 3 Customize the product where necessary. A diversity of solutions was attempted; sometimes several products were required to support a single function.

Stage 4 Instruct, train, and inform. The participants were given generous time and resources to work out routines on how to apply the CAT.

Stage 5 Follow-up and assess the function and benefit of CAT.

One issue that is characteristic of virtually all assistive technology applications is who the user is because AT use often involves people other than the actual user (Nygård, 2009).

TABLE 15-11 Assessment Questions and Assistive Technology Examples

Content Area	Typical Assessment Questions	Examples of Applicable Assistive Technology
Quality	How does the person classify objects? Are one, two, or more dimensions used?	Sorting jigs, graphic symbol labels for categories
Causal Patterns	How many steps in a process or chain can be understood? Can outcomes of accomplishing a task in different ways be compared?	Sequencing jigs, PDA-based prompting and cueing
Space	Can the person find his or her way with a map? Does he or she use shortcuts? Can he or she ask directions?	Paper maps, dynamic display in GPS on PDA with speech output
Quantity	How is money handled? Is conservation of volume present?	Money-sorting jigs, matching task rather than counting, parts-counting jigs
Time	Can a watch be used? Is the duration of an activity or waiting period understood?	Quarter Hour Watch, electronic pocket calendars with reminders, PDA with reminder and voice output

From Granlund M et al: Assistive technology for cognitive disability, *Technol Disabil* 4:205-214, 1995.

In the case of the simple stove timer that automatically turns of the stove if it is not attended to in a preset period of time, some home service aides perceived the stove timer to be a device for both the client and themselves since they could use the stove for cooking, and the client could safely maintain the perception of independence in cooking. Other home service aides believed that they were the users of the stove and the stove timer since the timer only existed because the client could not safely manage the stove alone. A third group of home service aides believed that the user was the client exclusively since the device had been obtained to meet their needs. The OTs and nurses concluded that each client, with his or her family, is responsible for the stove timer and how to use it since procurement is individualized.

Another issue that frequently arises is determining the perceived purpose of a CAT. An example is provided by the stove timer (Nygård, 2009). All groups (client, family, homecare workers, and professional OTs and nurses) agreed on the primary purpose of the device being to ensure safety, and on the importance of timing and clients' motivation. The importance of safety without changing everyday life was also a goal. But other meanings also were attributed to the stove timer. One of the most important was the role of the timer as delaying a move to sheltered living where the client might be better served. Some informants felt that the stove timer hindered their clients with dementia by postponing them from getting needed care.

OUTCOMES

The use of mainstream technologies by individuals with intellectual disabilities requires a carefully developed training program. Taber et al (2003) developed a training paradigm based on a least to most prompting system to teach students with intellectual disabilities how to answer a cell phone and describe their location through landmarks or use a speed dial function to call for assistance. One aspect of the training was establishing the concept of being "lost" since this is not intuitive. They used a cell phone that did not have a screen-based interface or features such as those described by Stock et al (2008). Training took place in school (known settings) first, and then in unfamiliar community-based settings. After training, students were able to complete the phone answering–description task with 70% or greater accuracy and the speed dialing task with nearly 100% accuracy. This reinforces the value of single key (speed dial–like) function keys for phones intended for people with intellectual disabilities.

Kagohara et al (2013) reviewed the use of iPads and iPods with individuals who have developmental disabilities. The 15 papers reviewed included applications in five areas: (1) academic, (2) communication, (3) employment, (4) leisure, and (5) transitioning from school settings. The participants in these studies had a diagnosis of either autism spectrum disorder or intellectual disability. The focus of the studies was either to deliver instructional prompts (see descriptions of example apps in this chapter) or to teach the operation of the iPod or iPad. Detailed descriptions are provided for each of the 15 studies. The conclusion was that "iPods, iPod touch, iPads and related devices are viable technological aids for individuals with developmental disabilities" (Kagohara et al, 2013, p. 147).

Studies of the impact of apps on the writing abilities of students with learning disabilities have led to mixed results (Sitko et al, 2005). In small sample studies, word prediction programs have been shown to improve writing by addressing word finding problems. When coupled with speech synthesis, the results are improved further. Results vary for word completion versus word prediction (see Chapter 6), with word prediction being more effective because it includes the context of the sentence as well as that of the word.

The Gillespie et al (2012) systematic review of the use of CATs included studies that investigated electronic technologies as compensations for cognitive impairment to enable or enhance task performance. Participants had cognitive impairments affecting functions in attention, memory, psychomotor, emotional areas, perceptual, thought, higher-level cognitive tasks, calculation, mental sequencing of complex movements, and experience of self and time. They evaluated the effectives of devices based on the clinical evidence presented in reviewed papers.

The review revealed 12 clinical trials that have used CATs to shift attention and found that the evidence for the effectiveness of these devices is good. The most common ICF mental function for which CATs have been used is time management. Gillespie et al (2012) found good evidence for effectiveness in improving task performance for devices that provided content-free cueing. The CAT that supports the ICF area of self and time related to the awareness of one's identity, one's body, one's position in the reality of one's environment, and of time are those dealing with navigation. Gillespie et al found the effectiveness of navigation devices to be promising. Several CATs provide time management via visual or auditory reminders to assist in task performance.

The evidence for the effectiveness of time management CATs is strong. Some CATs assist higher level organization and planning by providing step-by-step support during task performance. Studies of these devices shows moderate support for their effectiveness. CATs often support daily routines (personal hygiene, food preparation, and movement within and outside of the home). Prompting devices are the most frequent type of CAT used in this area. Gillespie et al reported substantial evidence for the efficacy of reminding devices and strong evidence for alerting, distracting, and prompting devices.

Prompting systems have been used with autistic individuals for initiation, maintenance, or termination of an activity (Goldsmith and LeBlanc, 2004). Coyle and Cole (2004) reported a decrease of off-task behavior in three autistic students when an auditory timer was used to prompt self-monitoring of on-task behavior in classroom settings. Taber et al (1999) similarly reported a decrease in teacher-delivered prompts and in off-task and inappropriate behavior in a

12-year-old student when a self-operated auditory prompting system was used. Tactile systems were investigated in a few studies to increase verbal initiation (Shabani et al, 2002; Taylor and Levin, 1998) and to seek assistance when lost (Taylor et al, 2004).

Forty participants who had intellectual disabilities participated in a pilot study of Pocket Compass in an activity developed from a task in which different pieces of software were packaged for shipping (Davies et al, 2003). Participants using the device made fewer errors performing the task and fewer errors in decision points, and less assistance was required using the technology than when they had only a job coach. Davies, Stock, and Wehmeyer (2002) concluded that technology can significantly assist persons with intellectual disabilities in accomplishing relatively complicated work-related tasks independently.

The Discovery Desktop and Visual smart phone apps were evaluated by a 19-year-old man with moderate intellectual disability due to Down syndrome (Lachapelle et al, 2011). The participant was asked to choose the sequence of travels he wanted to do and four new destinations were identified. The step-by-step procedures required to achieve specific targeted tasks were entered into the app configured with audio and picture prompting. The participant was very excited, enthusiastic, and effective at using the technology from the very first trip. Both caregiver and participant comment input using the QUEST (see Chapter 5) indicated a high level of satisfaction with the device. The father commented: "I am convinced of the effectiveness of this assistant for independent travel. I sincerely believe that the task assistant can significantly promote the development of self-determined behavior of people with disabilities. In addition, it can help increase self-esteem for the person who finds it can quickly and easily perform a task without assistance or supervision of a teacher or parent. Thanks to his electronic personal assistant, the participant is able to move autonomously!" (p. 376). One challenge to the participant was that the screen saver was displayed following a long period of inactivity. This situation was confusing to the participant because he had only used the screens that were part of the app. Having the device revert to the basic operations rather than a specialized app is a major concern when using mainstream technologies as assistive technologies.

Davies, Stock, and Wehmeyer (2002) evaluated a palmtop-based time management and scheduling system designed for individuals who have intellectual disabilities. The Schedule Assistant was evaluated in a pilot study with 12 participants who had intellectual disabilities. Each participant was asked to complete an eight-item schedule using the Schedule Assistant and using a traditional written schedule. A care provider entered a schedule of daily events into the Schedule Assistant and the device provided visual and auditory (speaker or earphone) prompts that corresponded to those events at the appropriate time. A typical use of this type of device is shown in Figure 15-2. The reminders can be replayed automatically until acknowledged or by a request from the user. Results showed that participants required significantly less assistance when using the Schedule Assistant than with the written instructions, leading to the conclusion that electronic scheduling and prompting systems have value for individuals who have intellectual disabilities.

Studies conducted to determine the effectiveness of CATs have generally resulted in identified benefits. The results have varied by the type of disability and the specific characteristics of the CATs. The use of mainstream technologies offers promise for individuals with cognitive disabilities.

SUMMARY

Individuals who have cognitive disabilities of various types and severity can benefit from the use of cognitive assistive technologies. The implementation of these assistive technologies and strategies is based on the augmentation of or substitution for cognitive skills that are required for the completion of specific functional tasks. Cognitive disabilities represent a wide variety of skill levels and severity, and an equally wide range of types of assistive technologies are available to ameliorate these conditions. Increasingly, mainstream mobile technology apps are being developed to meet the needs of individuals who have cognitive disabilities.

STUDY QUESTIONS

1. Pick a specific cognitive disability, an activity, and a context and describe how the HAAT model as described in Chapter 1 would be applied to determine the best assistive technology approach (hard and soft technologies) for that individual.
2. How do assistive technology approaches differ for congenital and acquired cognitive disabilities?
3. What are the main challenges in applying mainstream mobile technologies to meet the needs of people who have cognitive disabilities?
4. List three benefits of making mainstream mobile technologies accessible for people with cognitive disabilities.
5. Pick a specific disorder and describe both the cognitive skills that are likely to be available for use of an assistive device and those that may need to be replaced or augmented by such a device.
6. List the major characteristics of mild cognitive disabilities as they relate to the use of assistive technologies.
7. List the major characteristics of intellectual disabilities as they relate to the use of assistive technologies.
8. List the major characteristics of dementia that may be aided by cognitive assistive technologies.
9. In terms of recommendations of assistive technologies, how do CVA and TBI differ from other acquired cognitive disabilities and from each other?

10. How do the considerations for mild cognitive disability, intellectual disability, and acquired disability differ? What are the implications of these differences for the application of assistive technologies?
11. Why is ADHD not considered an LD?
12. What interventions are commonly applied to the treatment of LDs?
13. Describe the differences between remediation and compensation as they apply to cognitive disabilities.
14. How do the terms remediation and compensation differ when applied to sensory (Chapters 13 and 14) or motor (Chapters 6 through 12) disabilities as opposed to cognitive disabilities?
15. What are the currently available assistive technologies that are beneficial to children with ASD? What are the efficacies and feasibilities of these technologies in replacing or augmenting skill deficits?
16. What are the characteristics of PDA-based time management systems for persons with intellectual disabilities?
17. Describe the general characteristics of memory aids.
18. Contrast the use of memory aids in intellectual disabilities, dementia, and TBI.
19. Describe how systems designed to provide prompting, cueing, or coaching are applied to assist persons with intellectual disabilities.
20. How do applications of prompting, cueing, or coaching systems differ between applications for individuals with intellectual disabilities and those with dementia?
21. What is meant by the term *stimuli control*, and how is this concept applied to webpage design?
22. What are the major challenges in using assistive technologies to address the problems faced by individuals with dementia?
23. How can word completion and word prediction benefit students who have LDs? What are the limitations in this application?
24. What are the most commonly used alternatives to printed text output?
25. What should be considered when recommending a time management device for a stroke patient?
26. What is a cognitive prosthesis? Describe how these devices are applied to assist individuals with TBI.
27 How do cognitive assistive technologies contribute to stigma for people with disabilities and the elderly?
28. How can technologies help to overcome stigma and discrimination for people with intellectual disabilities?
29. What advantages does the cloud have in addressing the needs of individuals who have cognitive disabilities?

REFERENCES

Aldrich FK: Smart homes: past, present, and future. In Harper R, editor: *Inside the smart home*, London, 2003, Springer-Verlag.

American Psychiatric Association: *Diagnostic and statistical manual of mental disorders, DSM-IV. Washington DC*, ed 4, American Psychiatric Association, 2000.

Anderson JR: *Cognitive psychology and its implications*, New York, 2000, Worth Publishers.

Ashcraft MH: *Fundamentals of cognition*, New York, 1998, Addison-Wesley.

Ashton TM: Students with learning disabilities using assistive technology in the inclusive classroom. In Edyburn D, Higgins K, Boone R, editors: *Handbook of special education technology research and practice*, Whitefish Bay, 2005, Wis.: Knowledge by Design, Inc, pp 229–238.

Bergman MM: The benefits of a cognitive orthotic in brain injury rehabilitation, *J Head Trauma Rehabil* 17:431–445, 2002.

Braddock D, Rizzolo MC, Thompson M, et al.: Emerging technologies and cognitive disability, *J Spec Educ Technol* 19(4):49–56, 2004.

Boulis MNK, Anastasiou A, Bekiaris E, et al.: Geo-enabled technologies for independent living: examples from four European projects, *Technol Disabil* 23(1):7–17, 2011.

Bruno AA: Motor recovery in stroke. Available from http://www.emedicine.com/pmr/topic234.htm. Accessed April 6, 2005.

Chadwick D, Wesson C, Fullwood C: Internet access by people with intellectual disabilities: inequalities and opportunities, *Future Internet*, vol. 5:376–397, 2013.

Chakrabarti S, Fombonne E: Pervasive developmental disorders in preschool children, *JAMA* 285:3093–3099, 2001.

Cicerone KD, et al.: Evidence-based cognitive rehabilitation: updated review of the literature from 1998 through 2002, *Arch Phys Med Rehabil* 86:1681–1692, 2005.

Cole E, Dehdashti P: Cognitive prosthetics and telerehabilitation: approaches for the rehabilitation of mild brain injuries, computer-based cognitive prosthetics: assistive technology for the treatment of cognitive disabilities. In *Proceedings of the Third International ACM Conference on Assistive Technologies*, ACM SIGCAPH, Marina del Rey, CA, 1998. The Conference.

Cole E, Matthews MK: *Proceedings of Basil Therapy Congress, Basel, Switzerland, pp 111–120*. Accessed July 27, 2006 http://www.brain-rehab.com/pdf/cpt1999.pdf (June 1999).

Coyle C, Cole P: A videotaped self-modeling and self-monitoring treatment program to decrease off-task behavior in children with autism, *J Intellect Dev Dis* 29:3–15, 2004.

Daley D: Attention deficit hyperactivity disorder: a review of the essential facts, *Child Care Health Dev* 32:193–204, 2006.

Davies DK, Stock SE, Wehmeyer ML: Enhancing Internet access for individuals with mental retardation through use of a specialized web browser: a pilot study, *Educ Train Ment Retard Dev Disabil* 36:107–113, 2001.

Davies DK, Stock SE, Wehmeyer ML: Enhancing independent time-management skills of individuals with mental retardation using a palmtop personal computer, *Ment Retard* 40:358–365, 2002.

Davies DK, Stock SE, Wehmeyer ML: A Palmtop computer-based intelligent aids for individuals with intellectual disabilities to increase independent decision making, *Res Pract Persons Severe Disabil* 4:182–193, 2003.

Dawodu SY: Traumatic brain injury: Definition, epidemiology, pathophysiology, WebMD: e-medicine: http://www.emedicine.com/pmr/topic212.htm#top. Accessed August 27, 2006.

Dekelver J, Vannuffelen T, De Boeck J: EasyICT: A framework for measuring ICT-skills of people with cognitive disabilities. In Miesenberger K, et al. editors: *ICCHP 2010, Part II, LNCS*, 6180, pp 21–24, 2010.

De Joode EA, Van Boxtel MPJ, Verhey FR, et al.: Use of assistive technology in cognitive rehabilitation: exploratory studies of the opinions and expectations of healthcare professionals and potential users, *Brain Injury* 26(10):1257–1266, 2012.

Edyburn DL: Assistive technology and students with mild disabilities: from consideration to outcome measurement. In Edyburn D, Higgins K, Boone R, editors: *Handbook of special education technology research and practice*, Whitefish Bay, WI, 2005, Knowledge by Design, Inc., pp 239–270.

Edyburn DL: Remediation vs. compensation: a critical decision point in assistive technology consideration. 2002. Edyburn, D.L. (2004). Rethinking assistive technology. Special Education Technology Practice, 5(4), 16-23. Accessed August 3, 2006.

Emiliani P, Stephanidis C, Vanderheiden G: Technology and inclusion: past, present and foreseeable future, *Technol Disabil* 23(3):101–114, 2011.

Erlandson RF, Stant D: Polka-yoke process controller: designed for individuals with cognitive impairments, *Assist Technol* 10:102–112, 1998.

Galotti KM: *Cognitive psychology: in and out of the laboratory*, Belmont, Calif, 2004, Wadsworth.

Gillespie A, Best C, O'Neill B: Cognitive function and assistive technology for cognition: a systematic review, *J Int Neuropsych Soc* 18:1–19, 2012.

Goldsmith T, LeBlanc L: Use of technology in interventions for children with autism, *J Early Intens Behav Intervent* 1:166–178, 2004.

Golisz KM, Toglia JP: Perception and cognition. In Blesedell Crepeau E, et al. editors: *Willard and Spackman's occupational therapy*, ed 10, Philadelphia, 2003, Lippincott Williams & Wilkins, pp 395–416.

Gorman P, et al.: Effectiveness of the ISAAC cognitive prosthetic system for improving rehabilitation outcomes with neurofunctional impairment, *Neurorehabilitation* 18:57–67, 2003.

Granlund M, et al.: Assistive technology for cognitive disability, *Technol Disabil* 4:205–214, 1995.

Haigh KZ, Kiff LM, Ho G: The independent lifestyle assistant: lessons learned, *Assist Technol* 18:87–106, 2006.

Hunt RR, Ellis HC: *Fundamentals of cognitive psychology*, ed 6, Boston, 1999, McGraw-Hill College.

Hwang A, Liu M, Hoey J, et al.: DIY smart home: narrowing the gap between users and technology [Extended abstract]. Interactive Machine Learning Workshop, *International Conference Intelligent User Interfaces*, March 19, 2013 at Santa Monica, California.

Johnson E, Mellard DF, Byrd SE: Alternative models of learning disabilities identification, *J Learn Disabil* 38:569–572, 2005.

Kagohara DM, Meer L, Ramdoss S, et al.: Using iPods and iPads in teaching programs for individuals with developmental disabilities: a systematic review, *Res Develop Disabil* 34:147–156, 2013.

Kautz H, et al.: Opportunity knocks: a community navigation aid, University of Washington. 2004 http://www.cs.washington.edu/homes/kautz/talks/access-symposium-2004.ppt. Accessed July 27, 2006.

Keskinen T, Heimonen T, Turunen M, et al.: Symbolchat: A flexible picture-based communication platform for users with intellectual disabilities, *Interacting with Computers* 24:374–386, 2012, http://dx.doi.org/10.1016/j.intcom.2012.06.003.

Kim HJ, et al.: Utility of a microcomputer as an external memory aid for a memory-impaired head injury patient during in-patient rehabilitation, *Brain Injury* 13:147–150, 1999.

Lachapelle Y, Lussier-Desrochers D, Caouette M et al: Using a Visual Assistant to travel alone within the city. In Stephanidis C, editor: *Universal access in HCI, Part III, HCII 2011, LNCS* 6767, New York, 2011, Springer, 372–377.

Lee D: Keeping the ME in media: thoughts, ideas and tips for supporting people with intellectual disabilities to use social media. service, support and success, *Direct Support Workers Newsletter* 2(4):1–6, 2012.

Levinson RL: The planning and execution assistant and trainer, *J Head Trauma Rehabil* 12:769–775, 1997.

Lewis C, Sullivan, Hoehl J: Mobile technology for people with cognitive disabilities and their caregivers: HCI issues, *Lecture Notes in Computer Science* (including subseries Lecture Notes in Artificial Intelligence and Lecture Notes in Bioinformatics) 5614, *LNCS* Part 1:385–394, 2009.

Lewis C, Ward N: Opportunities in cloud computing for people with cognitive disabilities: designer and user perspective. In Stephanidis C, editor: *Universal Access in HCI, Part II, HCII 2011, LNCS*, 6766. 2011, pp 326–331.

Lewis RB: Classroom technology for students with learning disabilities. In Edyburn D, Higgins K, Boone R, editors: *Handbook of special education technology research and practice*, Whitefish Bay, WI, 2005, Knowledge by Design, Inc, pp 325–334.

Lindstedt H, Umb-Carlsson O: Cognitive assistive technology and professional support in everyday life for adults with ADHD, *Disabil Rehabil Assist Technol*, 8(5):402–408, 2013.

LoPresti EF, Bodine C, Lewis C: Assistive technology for cognition, *IEEE Engineer Med Biol Mag* 5:29–39, 2008.

LoPresti EF, Mihailidis A, Kirsch N: Assistive technology for cognitive rehabilitation: state of the art, *Neuropsycholl Rehabil* 14:5–39, 2004.

Maenner MJ, Schieve LA, Rice CE, et al.: Frequency and pattern of documented diagnostic features and the age of autism identification clinical guidance, *J Am Acad Child & Adolesc Psych* 52(4):401–413, 2013.

Mann WC: *Smart technology for aging, disability and independence*, New York, 2005, John Wiley.

Mihailidis A: The efficiency of an intelligent cognitive orthosis to facilitate hand washing by persons with moderate to severe dementia., *Neuropsychol Rehabil* 14:135–171, 2004.

Mihailidis A, Fernie GR, Barbenel JC: The use of artificial intelligence in the design of an intelligent cognitive orthosis for people with dementia, *Assist Technol* 13:3–29, 2001.

Niemeijer AR, Frederiks BJM, Riphagen II: Ethical and practical concerns of surveillance technologies in residential care for people with dementia or intellectual disabilities: an overview of the literature, *International Psychogeriatrics* 22(7):11291142, 2010.

Novack T: What to expect after TBI, *Presented at the Recovery after TBI Conference*. (September 1999): http://images.main.uab.edu/spinalcord/pdffiles/tbi3pdf.pdf. Accessed October 31, 2006.

Nygård L: The stove timer as a device for older adults with cognitive impairment or dementia: different professionals' reasoning and actions, *Technol Disabil* 21:5366, 2009.

O'Sullivan SB, Schmitz TJ: *Physical rehabilitation: assessment and treatment*, , Philadelphia, 1994, FA Davis.

Palmer SB, Wehmeyer ML, Davies DK, et al.: Family members' reports of the technology use of family members with intellectual and developmental disabilities, *J Intellect Disabil Res* 56(4):402–414, 2002.

Parette P, Scherer M: Assistive technology use and stigma, *Educ Train Develop Disabil* 39(3):217–226, 2004.

Rabins PV, Lyketsos CG, Steele CD: *Practical dementia care*, ed 2, Oxford, 2006, Oxford Press.

RESNA: Clinical application of assistive technology (1998): http://www.rehabtool.com/forum/discussions/94.html. Accessed April 6, 2005

Schuck SEB, Crinella FM: Why children with ADHD do not have low IQs, *J Learning Disabil* 38:262–280, 2005.

Shabani DB, et al.: Increasing social initiations in children with autism: effects of a tactile prompt, *J Applied Behavior Analysis* 35:79–83, 2002.

Sitko MC, Laine CJ, Sitko CJ: Writing tools: technology and strategies for the struggling writer. In Edyburn D, Higgins K, Boone R, editors: *Handbook of special education technology research and practice*, Whitefish Bay, WI, 2005, Knowledge by Design, Inc., pp 571–598.

Sternberg RJ: *Cognitive psychology*, ed 3, Belmont, CA, 2003, Wadsworth.

Stock SE, Davies DK, Wehmeyer ML, et al.: Evaluation of cognitively accessible software to increase independent access to cellphone technology for people with intellectual disability, *J Intellect Disabil Res* 52(12):1155–1164, 2008.

Sturm JM, Rankin-Erickson JL: Effects of hand-drawn and computer-generated concept mapping on the expository writing of middle school students with learning disabilities, *Learn Disabil Res Pract* 17:124–139, 2002.

Szymkowiak A, et al.: A memory aid with remote communication: preliminary findings, *Technol Disabil* 17:217–225, 2005.

Taber TA, et al.: Use of self-operated auditory prompts to decrease off-task behavior for a student with autism and moderate mental retardation, *Focus Autism Other Dev Disabil* 14:159–166, 1999.

Taber A, Alberto PA, Seltzer A: Obtaining assistance when lost in the community using cell phones, *Res Pract Persons Severe Disabil* 28(2):105–116, 2003.

Taylor BA, Levin L: Teaching a student with autism to make verbal initiations: effects of a tactile prompt, *J App Behav Anal* 31:651–654, 1998.

Taylor BA, et al.: Teaching teenagers with autism to seek assistance when lost, *J Appl Behav Anal* 37:79–82, 2004.

Van Hulle A, Hux K: Improvement patterns among survivors of brain injury: three case examples documenting the effectiveness of memory compensation strategies, *Brain Inj* 20:101–109, 2005.

Wehmeyer ML: National survey of the use of assistive technology by adults with mental retardation, *Mental Retardation* 36:44–51, 1998.

Wehmeyer ML, Smith SJ, Davies DK: Technology use and students with intellectual disability: universal design for all students. In Edyburn D, Higgins K, Boone R, editors: *Handbook of special education technology research and practice*, Whitefish Bay, WI, 2005, Knowledge by Design, Inc., pp 309–323.

Wehmeyer ML, et al.: Technology use and people with mental retardation, *Int Rev Res Ment Retard* 29:291–337, 2004.

Willingham DB: *Cognition: the thinking animal*, Princeton, NJ, 2001, Prentice-Hall.

WHO World Health Organization: *International classification of functioning, disability and health (ICF)*, Geneva, Switzerland, 2001, World Health Organization.

World Wide Web Consortium (W3C). Web Content Accessibility Guidelines (WCAG) Overview. Available online: http://www.w3.org/WAI/intro/wcag.php#components (accessed on November 3 2013).

CHAPTER 16

Augmentative and Alternative Communication Systems

CHAPTER OUTLINE

LEARNING OBJECTIVES

On completing this chapter, you will be able to do the following:

1. Describe the different communicative needs of persons with disabilities
2. Discuss the basic approaches to meeting these differing needs
3. Recognize the needs that individuals have for conversation and for graphical output such as writing, mathematics, and drawing
4. Describe the ways that mainstream technologies are used to meet AAC needs
5. Describe the major characteristics of alternative and augmentative communication devices
6. Describe current approaches to speech output in assistive technologies
7. List and describe the major approaches to rate enhancement and vocabulary expansion
8. Describe the major assessment questions that must be asked and answered in determining the most appropriate alternative and augmentative communication device for an individual user
9. Discuss the major goals for and the significance of training in augmentative and alternative communication device use and communicative competence
10. Delineate the steps and procedures involved in implementing an augmentative and alternative communication device for an individual consumer

KEY TERMS

Access Barriers
Amyotrophic Lateral Sclerosis
Aphasia
Apraxia
Augmentative and Alternative Communication
Autism Spectrum Disorder
Cerebral Palsy
Complex Communication Needs
Context-Dependent Communicators
Dynamic Communication Displays
Dysarthria

KEY TERMS—cont'd

Emergent Communicators
Icon Prediction
Independent Communicators
Language
Opportunity Barriers
Selection Set
Skilled Nursing Facility
Speech
Speech-Generating Devices
Traditional Orthography
Traumatic Brain Injury
Visual Scene Displays
Vocalization

Augmentative and alternative communication (AAC) is an area of clinical practice that deals with communication problems of people who have **complex communication needs** (CCN). These problems may occur at any point across the life span. Communication is the very essence of being human, and when someone is not developing **speech** and **language** skills or has lost the ability to speak and/or understand spoken or written language, then AAC intervention approaches are required to meet their CCN. People communicate differently with different partners, under different conditions, and by using a variety of tools, techniques, and strategies. AAC involves a wide range of techniques, strategies, and technologies to support the communication needs of individuals with CCN (Figure 16-1). The focus of AAC must be on augmenting communication in ways the person values. As Daniel Webster said in 1822, *"If all my possessions were taken from me with one exception, I would choose to keep the power of communication, for by it I would soon regain all the rest."*

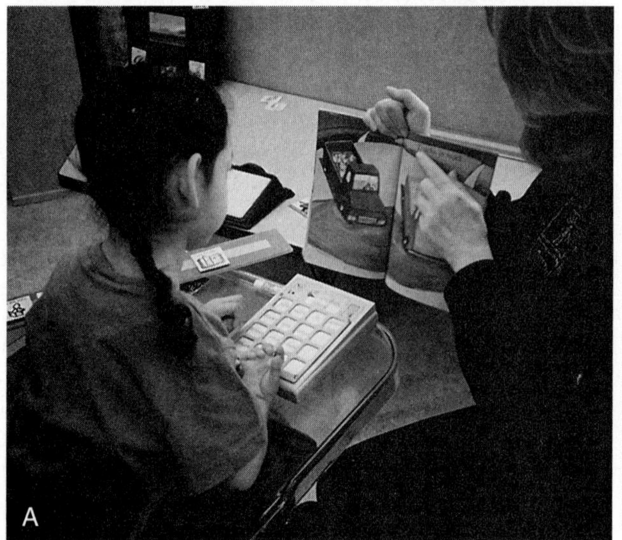

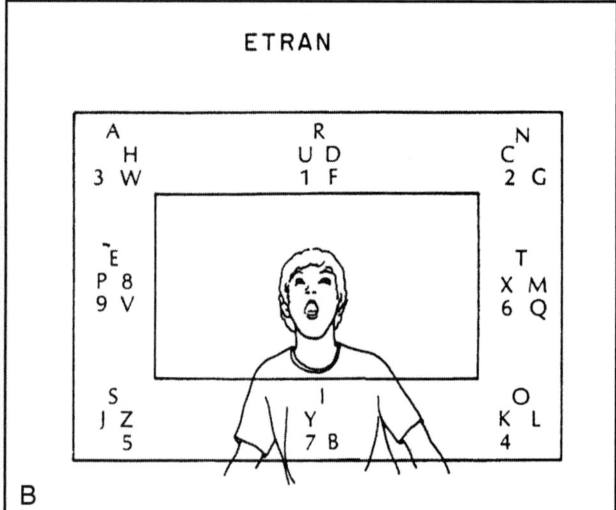

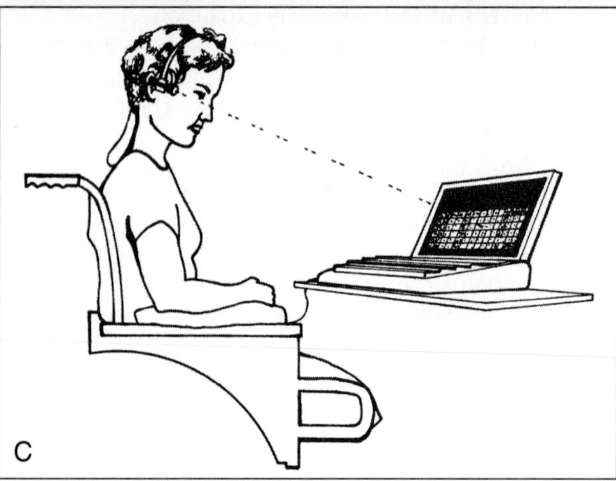

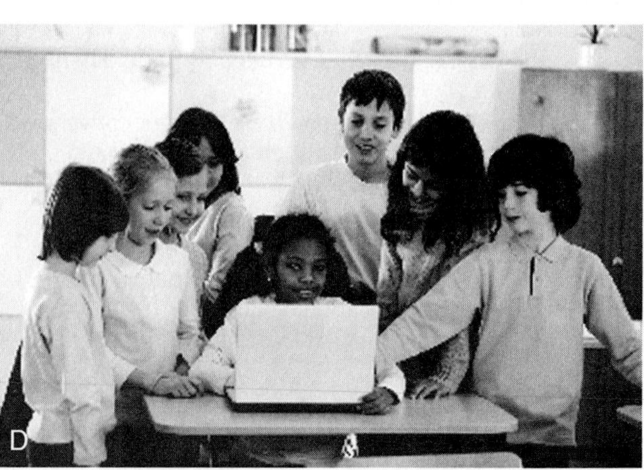

FIGURE 16-1 There are a variety of approaches and needs for augmentative and alternative communication systems. A, Conversations about a story, B, An eye transfer communication device (ETRAN). Eye gaze is used to indicate the choice. C, Head pointing is often used to make choices from a communication device. D, AAC systems with focused vocabulary are used in classrooms. (From Blackstone S: *Augmentative communication,* Rockville, Md, 1986, American Speech Language Hearing Association.)

Speech-generating devices (SGDs) produce digitally recorded or synthesized speech output. They are AAC tools that can significantly improve communication for individuals with CCN. SGDs and their accessories are commercially available and currently funded by governments and third-party payer programs in many countries. SGDs have a variety of features that have changed over time to meet the needs of individuals with CCN. An SGD may be a specially designed device, a computer program running on a portable computer, or an app for a mobile device.

This chapter is devoted to a discussion of the major aspects of AAC that are important in enabling individuals with CCN to communicate across the life span, while recognizing that each individual has unique needs, goals, preferences, skills, and abilities. The material presented in earlier chapters is applied to AAC here.

ACTIVITY COMPONENT

People with CCN are using AAC to attend schools and universities, work, carry on chats, participate in computer social networks, shop, order in restaurants, talk on the phone, and generally participate fully in society. People with CCN who have severe disabilities and who are able to obtain SGDs are living independently, getting married, and are active members of their communities. Individuals with CCN who do not gain access to AAC interventions may have limited social networks, have difficulty in reporting abuse, and be limited in their access to employment (Bryen, Cohen, & Carey, 2004; Collier, 2005).

Communication is foundational for many activities and participation classifications in the WHO *International Classification of Functioning, Disability, and Health* (WHO, 2001). Chapter 3 describes the activity categories that are specific to communication. These categories include:

1. Receiving communication
   - Via spoken means
   - Via nonverbal means, such as gestures, signs and symbols (e.g., stop sign, musical notations), drawings, and photographs
   - Via formal sign language
   - Through written messages
2. Production of communication
   - Speaking
   - Using nonverbal messaging, such as body language, signs and symbols, drawings, and photographs
   - Use of formal sign language
   - Writing messages
3. Conversation and use of communication devices and techniques
   - Conversation, including starting, sustaining, and ending a conversation, conversing with one person or many people
   - Discussion, with one person or many people
   - Use of communication devices, including telephones and similar devices, writing machines (typewriters, computers, braille writers), use of communication techniques that involve actions and tasks involved in communication such as lip reading (WHO, 2001, pg. 133-137).

What Is Augmentative and Alternative Communication?

There are many ways of looking at AAC systems. *Unaided communication or body-based modes* describe communication behaviors that require only the person's own body, such as pointing and other gestures, pantomime, facial expressions, eye-gaze and manual signing, or finger spelling. These modes are often used concurrently with each other and with speech. Even unaided modes of communication are typically culturally bound. Thus, when individuals have significant sensorimotor impairments, communication partners frequently misinterpret their nonverbal behaviors because eye gaze, facial expression, body movements, posture, traditional head nods, and pointing or reaching may be inaccurate, leading to communication misunderstandings (Kraat, 1986). Rush (1986) gives an example when he describes the difficulty his cerebral palsy causes him in delivering his line (a yell) in a play: "When a person with cerebral palsy wants to do something, he can't and when he wants not to do something, he involuntarily does it. So getting my vocal cords to cooperate with the cue was as hard as memorizing a Shakespearean play [for a nondisabled person]" (p. 21).

Aided AAC components may include a pen or pencil, a letter or picture communication board, a computer, a cell phone, and an SGD. Aided AAC may be either electronic or nonelectronic. Although a paper letter board (nonelectronic) differs from a computer-based SGD (electronic), both nonelectronic and electronic devices require that the person use a symbol system and have a way to select messages. All forms of AAC require consideration of how communication partners will participate in the communication process.

Communication Activities That Can Be Aided by Augmentative and Alternative Communication

When someone is unable to speak or write so that all current and potential communication partners can understand him or her, then an AAC system is required. As humans, we communicate in a myriad of ways depending on the circumstances. We rely most heavily on speaking and writing, but when these modes are unavailable we search for (and find) other ways of communicating. People with CCN often are unable to speak and write so others can understand them. Thus, they need AAC approaches to help them communicate face to face, on the phone, and across the Internet. Written communication includes all the things that are normally done with a pencil and paper, computer, calculator, and other similar tools. Composition of text, drawing, graphing, and mathematics are included.

Light (1988) describes four purposes of communicative interaction: (1) expression of needs and wants, (2) information transfer, (3) social closeness, and (4) social etiquette.

Expression of needs and wants allows people to make requests for objects or actions. Information transfer allows expression of ideas, discussion, and meaningful dialog. Social closeness serves to connect individuals to each other, regardless of the content of the conversation. Social etiquette is used to describe those cultural formalities that are inherent in communication. For example, students will speak differently to their peers than to their teachers.

HUMAN COMPONENT

Infants, toddlers, and preschoolers with CCN require AAC interventions that support the development of language, communication, and emerging literacy (reading and writing) skills. School-aged children with CCN need AAC interventions that enhance participation in their education, enable them to make friends, develop literacy and other academic skills, and engage with family members and people in their communities. For all children and adolescents, AAC can assist in meeting age-appropriate psychological and social development milestones. Individuals who acquire disabilities later in life need AAC to help them sustain employment and maintain their relationships and social networks, independence, and dignity.

The Importance of Augmentative Communication in the Lives of People With Complex Communication Needs

Christopher Nolan (1981), a man with cerebral palsy, wrote in the third person (as Joseph) about the importance of attentive and responsive communication partners. "Such were Joseph's teachers and such was their imagination that the mute boy became constantly amazed at the almost telepathic degree of certainty with which they read his facial expression, eye movements, and body language. Many a good laugh was had by teacher and pupil as they deciphered his code. It was in moments such as these that Joseph recognized the face of God in human form. It glimmered in their kindness to him, it glowed in their keenness, it hinted in their caring, indeed it caressed in their gaze" (p. 11).

AAC systems can enhance interaction, but they can also become the center of attention, as Rush (1986) noted:

> *My new friend (Wendy) was good looking. She was just over five feet tall and had brown eyes that matched the color of her shoulder length hair. Her skin showed a summer tan and she had a dynamite smile. "Did he show ya all his electronic stuff?" one of my dorm mates asked her. "Go on, Bill, show her." So I demonstrated the controls for my lights and clock radio. I showed off my door opener, which I could control via a radio transmitter attached to the Plexiglas tray on my wheelchair. She was impressed with the space-age technology. "Hey, show her your wheelchair and how it works. I'll never understand how it works. It baffles me," another dorm-mate said. So, wondering if I should sell tickets, I wheeled about the room. I demonstrated how I went straight, reverse, and turned left and right. I was angry at my dorm-mates because I was a man, not a side show freak. My wheelchair was a tool for my mobility, not a novelty. Why couldn't they see that? And why couldn't they see that I was trying to get to know Wendy? Why didn't they understand I had a right to my privacy just as they did? As I was wheeling around the room, I noticed that Wendy was typing something. I was disappointed in her. I thought she knew that I could hear and that she didn't have to write things to me. Apparently I was wrong. When I was done showing my electric marvels to her and the guys, I rolled back to my typewriter to read, "I wish they would go, so we could talk by ourselves." They finally left and we finally got to talk. Our friendship had started. (p. 137)*

The loss of speech can also occur later in life. Doreen Joseph (1986) lost her speech after an accident. Here's what she said, "I woke up one morning and I wasn't me. There was somebody else in my bed. And all I had left was my head. Speech is the most important thing we have. It makes us a person and not a thing. No one should ever have to be a 'thing'" (p. 8). Sue Simpson (1988) lost her speech after a stroke at age 36 years. She wrote: "So you can't talk, and it's boring and frustrating and nobody quite understands how bad it really is. If you sit around and think about all the things you used to be able to do, that you can't do now, you'll be a miserable wreck and no one will want to hang around you long" (Simpson, 1988, p. 11).

Dowden and Cook (2002) defined three types of AAC communicators. **Emergent communicators** have no reliable method of symbolic expression, and they are restricted to communicating about here-and-now concepts. **Context-dependent communicators** have reliable symbolic communication, but they are limited to specific contexts because they are either only intelligible to familiar partners, have insufficient vocabulary, or both. **Independent communicators** are able to communicate with unfamiliar and familiar partners on any topic. Each of these communicators has different needs and goals.

Self-determination is difficult for people who rely on AAC (Collier, 2005). They must know what they want, know how to get it, and have a sense of self-worth. In order to achieve these goals they need the "language of negotiation" and negotiation skills that require transactional language to supplement requesting, information exchange, and conversational control vocabulary and skill. Without these skills, individuals who rely on AAC are dependent on others for the determination of their life goals, direction, and things like medical decisions. They also need these skills to avoid abuse and harassment by caregivers and others or to report these incidents if they do occur. "Too many individuals who use AAC have been left without a way to communicate effectively and appropriately in adult situations; to refuse to be victimized, for example, and report the inappropriate behaviors of others, as needed, in a precise and confidential manner" (Williams, Krezman, & McNaughton, 2008, p 201).

Disabilities Affecting Speech, Language, and Communication

In considering communication needs, three perspectives are addressed: (1) individuals with developmental disorders, (2) individuals with acquired conditions, and (3) individuals with degenerative conditions. Although the focus of AAC interventions may vary across these groups, there is also substantial overlap in the issues faced when communication is severely limited, no matter what the causes may be.

There are many disabilities that can affect an individual's communication skills and abilities. Communication disorders can be categorized into those that affect the production of sounds and intelligible speech and those that affect cognitive and language abilities. Some individuals cannot produce speech because of conditions present at birth or acquired later in life. For some, the problem is in making sounds, although many individuals can produce sounds without being able to produce speech. The production of sounds is called **vocalization** and it can be an effective way of communicating some things like yes and no, anger (screaming), happiness (laughing), sadness (crying), and getting attention. Even if sounds can be produced, an individual may have limitations that interfere with the ability to make sounds or control the muscles of the chest, diaphragm, mouth, tongue, and throat to produce intelligible speech. **Dysarthria** is a disorder of motor speech control resulting from central or peripheral nervous system damage that causes weakness, slowness, and a lack of coordination of the muscles necessary for speech production (Anderson & Shames, 2006). Verbal **apraxia** is a disorder affecting the coordination of motor movements involved in producing speech caused by a central nervous system dysfunction (Anderson & Shames, 2006). Written communication is also important and limb apraxia may impair the ability to write. When speech and/or writing are severely impaired, AAC approaches are indicated.

Cognitive and language abilities are necessary in order to understand the speech of others and to express thoughts. There is a difference between speech disorders and language disorders A language is a set of symbols and the rules for organizing them. Each symbol represents a concept or concepts with expressive meaning. The symbols may be the familiar alphabetic written language (referred to as **traditional orthography**) or it may be a set of pictographic symbols conveying meaning (such as hieroglyphics or other special symbols) or a set of hand movements (sign language) or gestures. *Speech* is the oral expression of language.

AAC interventions for children with severe language delays or disorders are designed to support the development of receptive and expressive language and literacy (reading and writing) skills. **Aphasia** is a type of language disorder that often occurs as a result of a cerebral vascular accident or traumatic brain injury (TBI). Aphasia can affect both expression and reception of spoken and written language. For example, some people may lose the ability to recall vocabulary (e.g., names, places, events), and others may lose the ability to understand spoken language, organize language into meaningful utterances, and speak and write meaningful utterances. The degree to which various language functions are impaired is variable. AAC interventions for severe aphasia often focus on strategies that help individuals compensate for a severe loss of *language* function in ways that support functional communication.

Among the disabilities affecting communication that are ameliorated by AAC interventions are developmental conditions such as cerebral palsy (CP) and autism; acquired conditions such as TBI, stroke/cerebral vascular accident (CVA), and high-level spinal cord injury; and degenerative diseases such as **amyotrophic lateral sclerosis** (ALS), progressive aphasia, and multiple sclerosis. Estimates indicate that approximately 2 million people in the United States and from 0.3% to 1.0% of the total world population of school-aged children have a need for AAC (Beukelman and Mirenda, 2013). Not all the people in this population are served equally. Various populations are served differently. Children with CP, individuals with good cognitive skills, and adults with some degenerative diseases (i.e., ALS) receive more attention from AAC practitioners than individuals with intellectual disabilities and children and adults with autism, dual sensory impairment, TBI, and the elderly (Blackstone, Williams, & Joyce, 2002).

Approaches to AAC interventions differ depending on the severity, type, and onset of an individual's disability. There are significant differences, for example, between meeting the needs of children who have never spoken or used written language (congenital disabilities) and adults who have developed language, speech, and writing and then lost these skills because of a disease or injury. For example, young children with severe motor impairments and CCN are learning language at the same time they are learning to "talk" and "write" by using AAC approaches.

Thus, conventional means of communication (i.e., speaking and using a pencil) are unavailable to them. In addition, they have few, if any, opportunities to interact with competent AAC users who might serve as models and help them learn how to communicate using AAC. On the other hand, someone in whom ALS develops at age 46 years typically has years of experience using multiple forms of communication and intact language skills; thus, AAC interventions likely focus on providing AAC technologies and strategies so they can continue to communicate effectively with preferred partners.

AAC for Individuals With Developmental Disabilities

Because the development of speech, language, and communication begins at birth, early intervention is important. Effective AAC interventions for children with developmental disabilities requires that AAC be integrated into the child's daily experiences and interactions and that it take into account what we know about child development (Light & Drager, 2002). For example, many young children do not have the physical or cognitive skills to learn to use current AAC selection techniques (e.g., scanning or encoding) and thus are unable to access AAC systems. Also, the design of current AAC technologies often requires a child to stop playing to use a communication device. A more desirable approach is to design AAC technologies and strategies that incorporate the use of AAC into the child's play activities so the child can talk about his or her play or interact with peers while engaged in the activity. In short, to be effective, the design, type, and layout of AAC system components should match the desires, preferences, abilities, and skills of children.

A major concern for parents is whether the use of AAC will impede their child's development of speech. Research data puts all such fears to rest (see Blackstone, 2006). The use of AAC does not interfere with speech development and may in fact enhance the development or return of speech. There are a number of possible explanations for this, including increased acoustic feedback (from voice output SGD), increased experience with conversational turns and other communicative functions, reduced pressure to speak that releases motor stress, and the development of an internal phonology as a result of AAC systems use (Blishcak, Lombardino, & Dyson, 2003).

Research shows that children with a broad range of developmental disabilities can benefit from AAC interventions. This includes children with **cerebral palsy** (CP), intellectual disability, Down's syndrome, other genetic disorders, and **autism spectrum disorder** (ASD). Intellectual disabilities and more mild disorders such as learning disabilities are discussed in Chapter 15.

Cerebral Palsy

Cerebral palsy is a nonprogressive motor impairment due to a lesion or anomalies of the brain arising in the early stages of its development (Winter, 2007). Cerebral palsy syndromes describe motor disorders characterized by impaired voluntary movement resulting from prenatal developmental abnormalities or perinatal or postnatal central nervous system (CNS) damage. It is primarily a disorder of muscle tone and postural control. Individuals who have cerebral palsy will often exhibit apraxia, which is the inability to perform motor activities although sensory motor function is intact and the individual understands the requirements of the task (Crepeau, Cohn, & Schell, 2009).

Primitive reflexes, characterized by immediate and automatic movement performed at a subconscious level, also accompany cerebral palsy (Hopkins & Smith, 1993). Typically these reflexes are inhibited or (more often) integrated into volitional movements in order to control posture and perform basic movement patterns as the infant develops. Cerebral palsy may affect the degree to which these reflexes are integrated and some reflex patterns persist into adulthood for those with CP. The primitive reflexes that most commonly influence AT use are the asymmetrical tonic neck reflex (ATNR) and the symmetrical tonic neck reflex (STNR). The impact of these on AAC use is shown in Figure 16-2 (Beukelman and Mirenda, 2013).

CP is also characterized by variation in muscle tone ranging from increased tone referred to as hypertonicity or spasticity to low tone referred to as hypotonicity. In an individual child, the tone may be mixed, may vary over the course of the day, or may vary depending on the child's position (Winter, 2007). This altered muscle tone has an impact on motor control required for the use of AAC devices. Oculomotor function (problems with eye movements) is also abnormal in many children with CP. The variety of visual problems in CP is very broad, including peripheral problems such as strabismus, refraction disorders, and retinopathies as well as cerebral visual impairment (CVI) (Fazzi et al., 2012). Between 60% and 70% of children with CP exhibit CVI, defined as "... a deficit of visual function caused by damage to, or malfunctioning of, the retrogeniculate visual pathways (optic radiations, occipital cortex, visual associative areas) in the absence of any major ocular disease" (Fazzi et al., 2012, p. 730). This finding has a direct bearing on tasks that require frequent redirection of gaze such as looking at a keyboard to find the desired character and then looking at a display or screen to monitor the selections.

As Scherer (1998) points out, the person who is born with cerebral palsy is likely to have adjusted to the disability and developed strategies that help accommodate for the lack of coordinated motor control. For example, some individuals are able to use a primitive reflex to initiate a movement. Others have learned to position equipment and materials to maximize the motor control they have. These individuals are inclined to view assistive technology as opening up new opportunities for them and they often apply their developed strategies to the control of these devices (see Case Study 16-1).

CASE STUDY 16-1

Meeting a Congenital Need for Augmentative and Alternative Communication

Joyce is 39 years old. She has cerebral palsy, and she currently lives with her parents. Her speech is dysarthric, and she is unable to use a pen or pencil for writing. Her communication systems are listed in Table 16-1. Unaided communication modes include head nods and eye gaze. Joyce currently uses a tread switch (see Chapter 7) mounted near her knee to control her scanning communication device, which has synthesized speech output and a small word processing program for writing. To meet Joyce's need to activate a call device for emergency help over the telephone, she uses an alarm tied into a 24-hour surveillance company and activated by a wobble switch (see Chapter 7) using her left arm. She uses her arm for the emergency call device because this movement is less limited by being supine in bed than is knee movement. Also, when she is seated in her wheelchair, arm use does not interfere with either her powered mobility or her communication because they use other control sites.

Autism Spectrum Disorder

ASD is characterized by significant social communication challenges throughout life that reflect impairments in social interaction, verbal and nonverbal communication, and restricted, repetitive, stereotypical patterns of behavior, interests, and activities (Blackstone, 2003b). Early intervention (starting as young as age 2) improves outcomes for children with ASD. These children often have difficulty

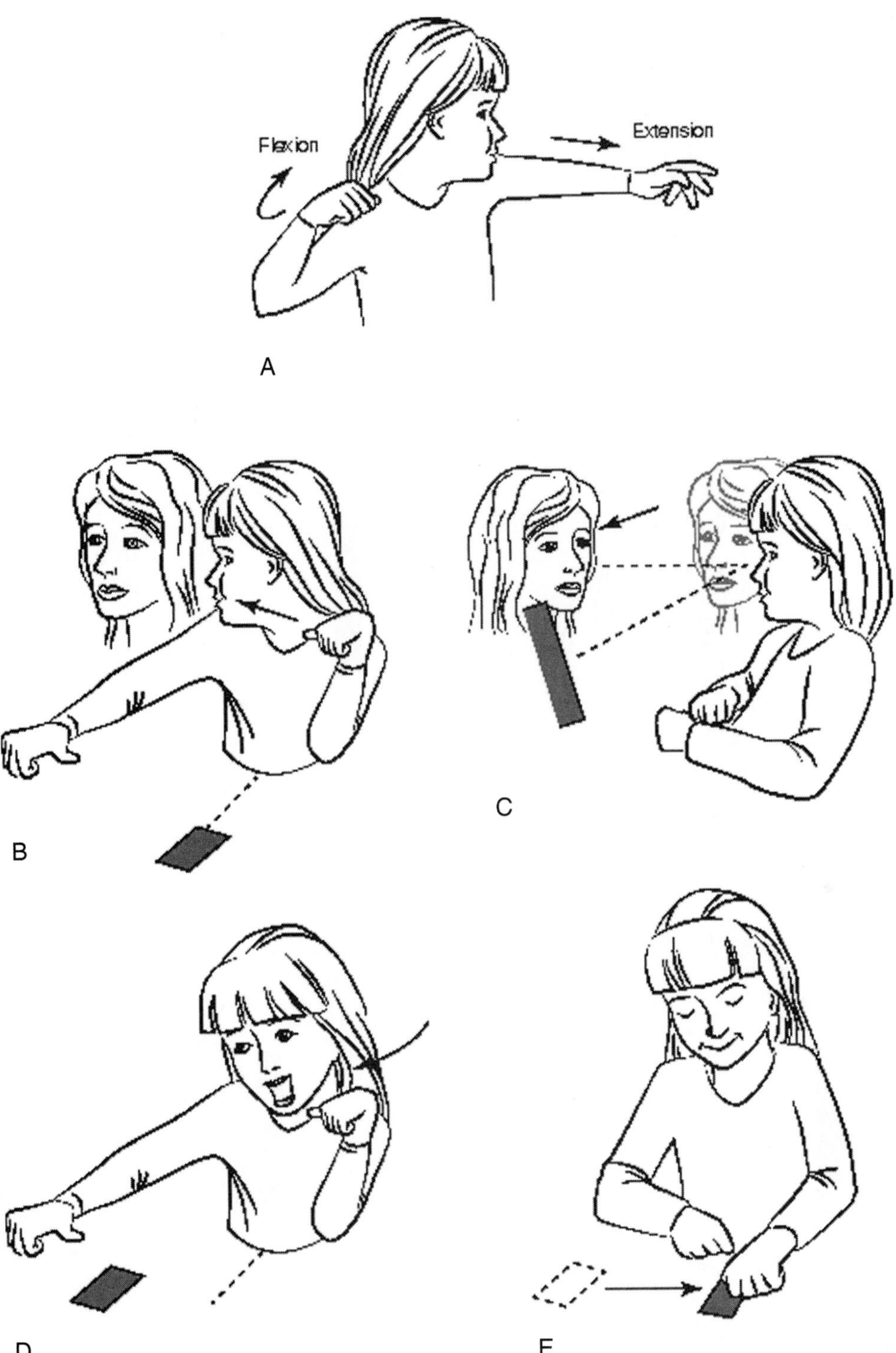

FIGURE 16-2 The asymmetric tonic neck reflex (ATNR) (left) and symmetric tonic neck reflex (STNR) (right) can impact AAC system use. (From Beukelman DR, Mirenda P: *Augmentative and alternative communication: management of severe communication disorders in children and adults*, ed 3, Baltimore: Paul H Brookes, 2005.)

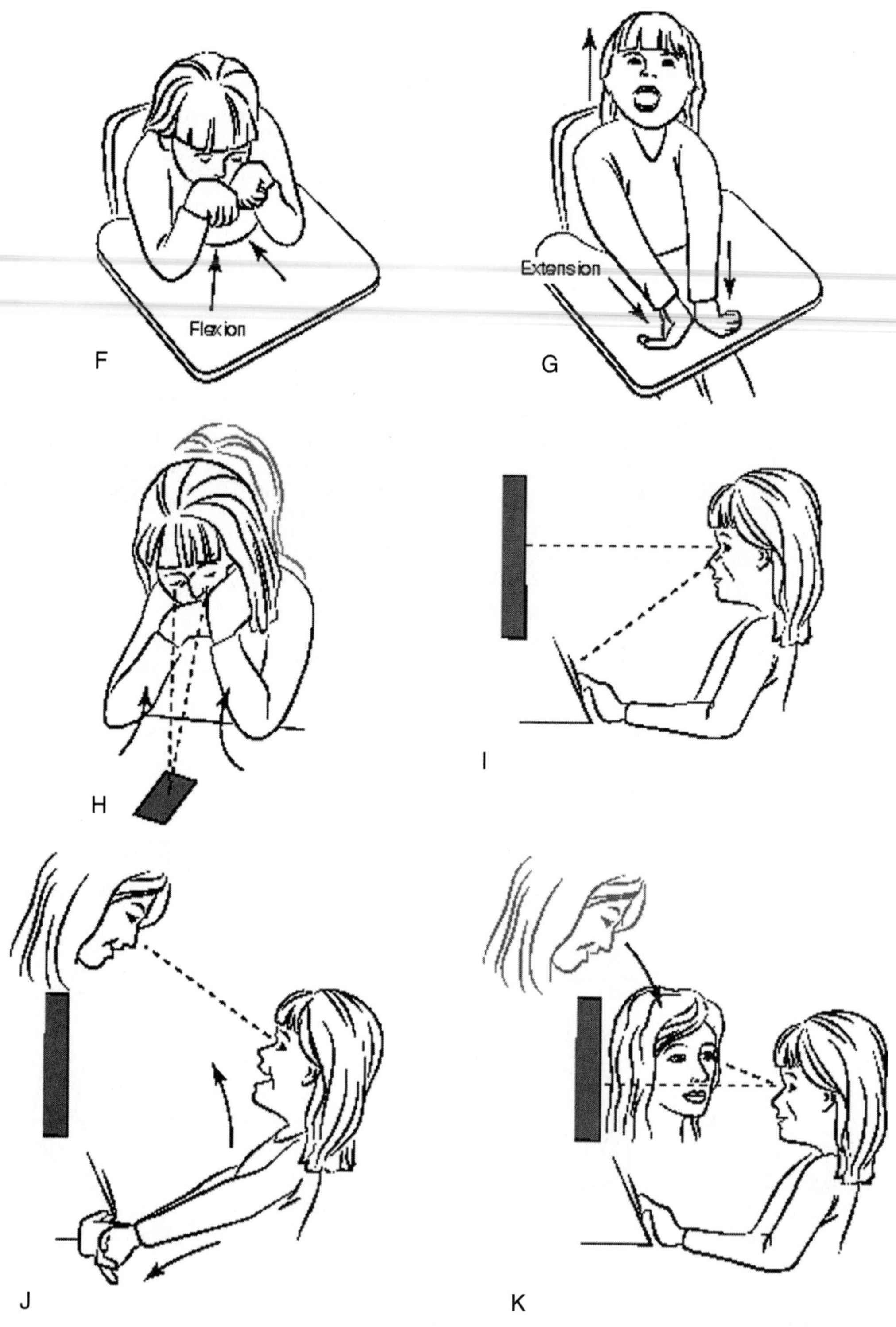

FIGURE 16-2, cont'd

with joint attention (i.e., coordinating attention between people and objects) and understanding and using symbols. Approximately one third to one half of children with ASD do not use speech functionally (Blackstone, 2003b). The learning styles of children with ASD show a strong preference for static information and, as a result, they often benefit from the use of "visual supports." Because speech and other elements of conversations are transient, AAC devices and communication displays that use static visual symbols provide possible advantages for the child with ASD. Also, because of their dependence on rote or episodic memory, children with ASD often benefit from contextual clues and prompts, and this can lead to them becoming prompt or context dependent. Thus, AAC interventions that extend the use of language and appropriate communication behaviors across different contexts and partners are needed.

TABLE 16-1 Augmentative and Alternative Communication Case Study Examples

Subject	Communication Needed	Modality	Activation/ Control
Joyce	Conversation/ Writing	Unaided	Eye gaze or head nod
		Electronic AAC device	Knee/tread switch
	Emergency call	24-hour service	Hand/wobble switch
Eileen	Conversation	Unaided	Vocalizations, head nods, facial expression
		Letter board	Eye gaze
		Electronic AAC device	Optical pointer/ head movement

BOX 16-1 Picture Exchange Communication System

The Picture Exchange Communication System (PECS) (Pyramid Educational Products, Newark, Del.) is a commercially available program developed for people with ASD that uses graphical symbols (often the Mayer-Johnson Picture Communication Symbols©) and a specific instructional method. The objective of PECS is that children or adults who are not yet initiating requests, comments, and so forth, learn to spontaneously initiate communicative exchanges. The person is initially encouraged to give something (picture/symbol) to a communication partner to complete a communication exchange. Thus, by using PECS, learners gain the attention of the communication partner to make a request. By advancing through the six phases of PECS, the student progresses from a simple exchange through increasing levels of spontaneity to sequencing words and creating sentences. No prompting is used throughout the learning process. In a study conducted by Bondy and Frost (2001) in 85 children (aged 5 years or younger), more than 95% of the children were able to exchange at least two pictures, whereas 76% began using speech with or without PECS. In other studies with smaller numbers of participants, positive outcomes in speech improvement, rapid mastery of the system, and decrease in destructive behavior or tantrums were reported anecdotally (Helsinger, 2001; Schwartz, 2001). Recent empirical studies on PECS have reported positive effects regarding rate of mastery of the system and improvement in general communication skills (Magiati & Howlin, 2003).

Blackstone (2003b) argues that AAC can be effective for children with ASD because it addresses both their unique learning styles and their communication needs.

Children with ASD can use no-technology (e.g., manual signs) and high- and low-technology approaches to AAC (Mirenda, 2003). At this time, there is no clear evidence that one approach is superior to any other. The use of total communication (speech and manual signing) provides advantages because there is no device to worry about and because it promotes more natural forms of communication. However, not all children (or their partners) do equally well with this approach. Some children develop more functional communication using low-tech aided systems. PECS (Box 16-1) is one widely used example. Voice output communication aids can also support interactions. For example, Schlosser & Blischak (2001) suggested that electronically generated speech might be beneficial for children with ASD who have difficulty processing natural speech. Also, computer aided instruction may help children with ASD attend to instructions and prompts when provided by electronic speech output. There are many considerations in choosing among the many available AAC approaches, including an individual's preferences, ease of learning, effect on the development of speech and language, ability to use the approach functionally across partners and contexts, and the communication tasks the person needs to accomplish. Finally, the degree of partner support and responsiveness is considered. Currently, best practice relies on clinician judgment as much as evidence because current research on the use of AAC approaches for individuals with ASD is promising but inconclusive in each of these areas.

AAC for Individuals With Acquired Disabilities

Adults with acquired disabilities such as **traumatic brain injury** (TBI), aphasia, and other static conditions may require the use of AAC interventions as part of the rehabilitation process (Beukelman & Ball, 2002). Persons with recovering conditions often have changing levels of motor, sensory, or cognitive/linguistic capability that benefit from the use of human/technology interfaces, including AAC, to help them accommodate. Although many people may be unable to speak or write directly after a severe head injury or brainstem or cortical stroke, most will recover these abilities. However, over the long term, some individuals continue to benefit from the use of AAC. In this section TBI and aphasia are discussed as examples of individuals with acquired AAC needs.

Traumatic Brain Injury

TBI can result in the loss of speech and often causes physical, cognitive, and language impairments (Beukelman et al., 2007). The motor impairment is often severe in TBI and the sequelae include problems with cognition (thinking, memory, and reasoning), sensory processing (sight, hearing, touch, taste, and smell), communication (expression and understanding), behavior or mental health (depression, anxiety, personality changes, aggression, acting out, and social inappropriateness). These factors frequently hamper function and often are long-term outcomes that affect communication and other function in very subtle ways, limiting the ability to access AAC (Carlisle Ladtkow & Culp, 1992). While the long-term recovery of speech is variable, immediately following the injury many individuals benefit from the AAC interventions to support functional communication.

Frager, Hux, & Beukelman (2005) found that a group of communication partners and the continuing support of an AAC facilitator contribute to success, that high-tech devices were favored over low-tech systems, and that low-tech systems were apt to be used temporarily by people with TBI who regained speech. Beukelman et al. (2007) carried out a study of AAC use by individuals who had sustained a TBI. The

BOX 16-2 AAC and TBI

What the Research Tells Us: TBI and AAC

- 68% of this sample was advised to utilize high-technology AAC devices
- 94% of these individuals and their decision makers accepted the recommendations
- After 3 years, 81% continued to use their AAC technology, 6% had not received the technology because of funding problems, and 12% had discontinued AAC device use because they did not have appropriate AAC facilitator support
- 87% used letter-by-letter spelling, while the remaining 13% relied on symbols and drawings
- Low-technology AAC options were recommended for 32% of the total group
- 100% accepted the recommendation
- After 3 years, 63% continued to use their low-technology AAC strategies at least part time
- 37% discontinued use because they regained sufficient natural speech to meet their communication needs

individuals with TBI in this study generally accepted AAC recommendations, and none of the participants rejected AAC after receiving a low-tech or high-tech AAC option. When it did occur, AAC technology abandonment usually reflected the loss of a facilitator (soft technology loss; see Chapter 1), not rejection of the technology (Box 16-2). Participants in this study relied predominantly on letter-by-letter spelling strategies, primarily due to the interference of cognitive limitations with the ability to encode messages or utilize other message formulation strategies. Beukelman et al. (2005) attempted to teach the use of encoding and/or word retrieval to several individuals with TBI who spelled their messages using AAC technology. Some were able to learn the encoding or prediction strategy in the intervention setting, but none used the strategy in their everyday communication, reporting that it was "too much work" (see Case Study 16-2).

CASE STUDY 16-2

Augmentative and Alternative Communication After a Brainstem Stroke

Eileen is a 62-year-old woman who has sustained a brainstem stroke and now requires maximal assistance for daily living. Eileen's unaided communication modalities, shown in Table 16-1, include isolated words, facial expressions, yes/no responses, and inflectional vocalizations. She also has two AAC devices. The first of these is a letter board, accessed by her eye gaze, that she uses to indicate her needs and choices (Figure 16-1, *B*). All of these systems have limitations. The unaided systems require significant amounts of interpretation by the partner, and the manual eye gaze device is slow because it relies on spelling and interpretation by her partner. These limitations are partially overcome by Eileen's electronic AAC device, which she accesses by using head movement to make selections with a light pointer mounted on a headband on the side of her head (Figure 16-1, *C*). This device includes vocabulary storage, so she can use whole words and phrases, and it provides synthesized speech output. These features allow Eileen to converse with more people, and they make it easier on the communication partner. Each of these devices contributes to the quantity and quality of her communication interactions.

Aphasia

Persons who sustain **cerebrovascular accidents (CVAs)** often have language difficulties that we collectively call *aphasia.* One lasting problem these individuals have is vocabulary retrieval or word-finding difficulties. There are several AAC-related approaches with potential for aphasia rehabilitation (Jacobs et al., 2004). For example, individuals who can recall first letters and recognize a desired word from a list may use word prediction devices/software. The individual begins typing a letter and then the device predicts several words from which to choose (see Figure 6-11). Colby et al. (1981) developed a microcomputer-driven device that used a specially designed database containing words, their frequency of use, and features of each word, which was specifically designed for persons with aphasia. Features included words that "go with" the desired word. This can be a sound-alike relationship; a semantic (meaning) relationship; a categorization (e.g., a piece of furniture or a fruit); and initial, middle, and ending letters. Each was shown to be effective for persons with certain types of aphasia. Many factors must be considered when AAC is applied in aphasia rehabilitation. Some people with severe aphasia learn to augment their speech and communication efforts by relying on gestures and an alternative symbol system (Jacobs et al., 2004). However, although persons with aphasia may be able to use graphic symbols, many find it difficult to apply them socially or to generalize their use.

One commercial device designed specifically for persons with aphasia is the Lingraphica™, which organizes symbols by semantic categories (e.g., places, foods, and clothing) and includes synthetic speech output and animation of verbs (e.g., walk, give).[1] Lingraphica provides graphic building blocks which are called icons (small pictures, sometimes animated). The icons can be manipulated to generate messages using a cursor. Lingraphica also has applications that allow favorite icons, phrases, and videos selected on the Lingraphica to be transferred to the iPhone and iPod touch. The mobile accessory can be used as an AAC device for communication or for self-cueing and scaffolding (i.e., helping to generate expressive language by providing prompts).

Other technological interventions for aphasia are focused on supporting specific communication tasks such as answering the phone, calling for help, ordering in restaurants or stores, giving speeches, saying prayers, or engaging in scripted conversations. These may be either paper-based systems or electronic devices.

Portraits (static pictures or other symbols) contain limited, usually decontextualized information (e.g., a picture of a person with a plain background), and additional information about the person(s) or object in a portrait must be generated by the individual with aphasia or speculated on by the communication partner (Beukelman et al., 2007). This spontaneous generation of additional specific and detailed information is difficult for individuals with severe chronic

[1] http://www.aphasia.com/.

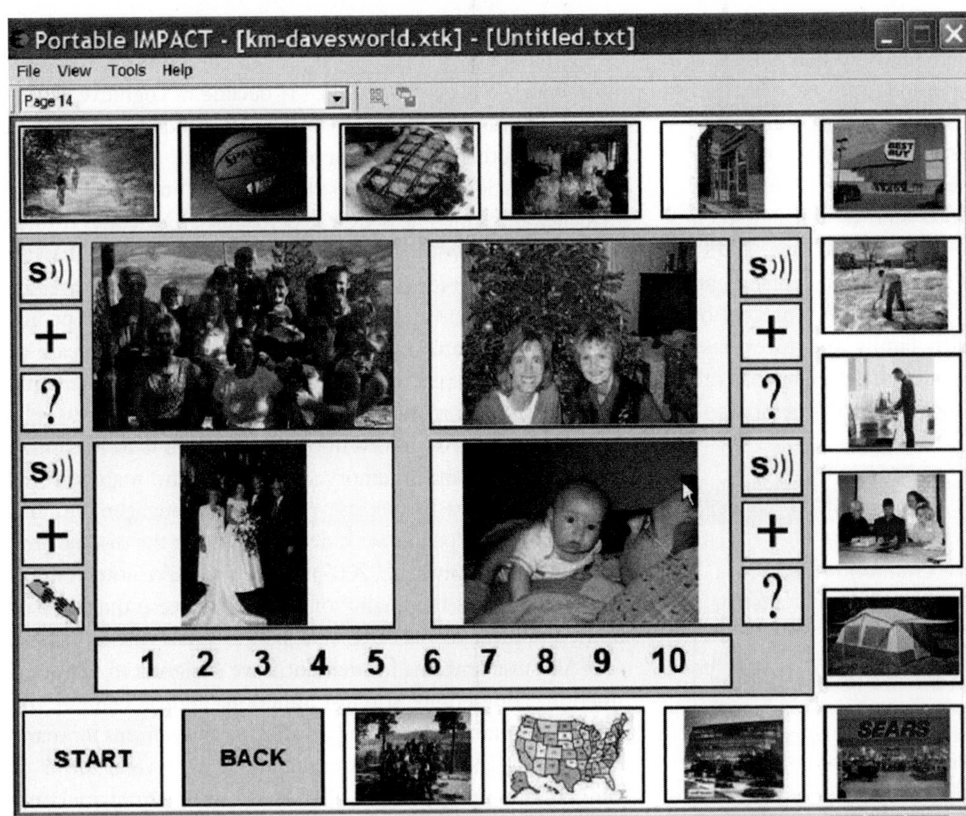

FIGURE 16-3 VSD layout for family outing or wedding (personalized). (From Blackstone S: Visual scene displays, *Augment Commun News* 16(2):1-5, 2004.)

aphasia. An alternative is **visual scene displays** (VSDs) (see Figure 16-3 and discussion later in this chapter) that use personalized digital photos of scenes and arrange these on a dynamic display device (these devices are described later in this chapter). Each element in a visual scene is pictured in its natural relationship and position to all other elements in the scene (McKelvey et al., 2007). The meaning of all elements and semantic associations are integrally tied together, creating a holistic context.

VSDs enable individuals with severe aphasia to use familiar photographs to engage partners in interactions about multiple topics. In addition, the design of the technology makes it relatively easy for partners to provide conversational supports such as prompting with familiar reminders. The individual with aphasia and the communication partner co-construct "the gist" of the visual scene. Contextualized pictures are paired with text and voice output to communicate specific messages, ask questions, and/or provide support for the communication partner. Because of the dynamic nature of the display, the user is continually prompted regarding the available choices, reducing the individual's need to rely on recall memory. It is also possible to use the same approach with paper-based displays. There is a template provided by the University of Nebraska at http://aac.unl.edu/intervention.html.

AAC for Individuals With Degenerative Conditions

A degenerative condition in which speech or language functions are gradually lost presents a different set of challenges for the person with CCN and for AAC interventions. For many conditions, multiple AAC modes are necessary as the disease worsens. Persons with degenerative conditions often have changing levels of motor, sensory, or cognitive/linguistic capability that require the adaptation of the human/technology interfaces to accommodate their changing motor and cognitive skills.

ALS

Amyotrophic lateral sclerosis, one of the motor neuron diseases, is a rapidly progressing neuromuscular disease that affects speech in the majority of cases (see the following case study of Mr. Webster). There are two types of ALS: bulbar or brainstem ALS and spinal ALS (Beukelman & Mirenda, 2013). The bulbar form affects speech and swallowing before it affects other motor control, and individuals are initially able to control AAC devices with hand and finger movement. They lose this motor control over time and need to shift to head control or eye tracking. Individuals with spinal ALS initially have progressive muscle weakness in the extremities stage before the loss of speech, requiring assistance with writing tasks. Dependence on AAC for conversation comes at a later stage.

Although persons with ALS use the same AAC systems as others, there are unique factors considered during the intervention process. For example, it is not uncommon for someone to begin using a direct-selection AAC system and later on require scanning to continue communicating. If this type of transition is not planned for initially, it can be very hard for the person to maintain effective interactions. Families differ in their desire and ability to deal with the longer term

(Blackstone, 1998). Some families prefer to "plan ahead" and consider future needs, whereas others prefer to take things as they come. Some SGDs can accommodate direct selection and a variety of indirect selection modes, so these are often recommended. But they are often heavy and hard to carry and thus may be less useful at the outset when the person is still ambulatory. Patients with ALS tend to use high-tech aids with strangers and for conversation (Blackstone, 1998). No-tech approaches, including 20 questions (the person can answer yes or no by head nod, eye blink, or other means) or gestures may be most effective with family and to express basic needs. Low-tech approaches such as letter boards are more often used with strangers than with family members.

CASE STUDY 16-3

Augmentative and Alternative Communication and Amyotrophic Lateral Sclerosis: Changing Needs

Mr. Webster was assessed for an AAC device shortly after he began to lose the ability to speak as a result of ALS. He received a direct-selection spelling device, which he accessed with his right index finger. This device was highly effective for him, and he was fond of making lists of tasks to be done around the house, planning menus, and creating shopping lists for his wife and son, which allowed him to maintain his role as head of the household. Unfortunately, Mr. Webster eventually lost the ability to use his finger to type and was again referred for an AAC assessment.

A new device was recommended and purchased for him. This device used single-switch scanning accessed through eyebrow movement. This system was not effective for Mr. Webster. Several factors led to the difference in results between the two systems. First, there was an 11-month period between when he was unable to use the first system and the delivery of the second system. This time without a functional communication system probably contributed to a much more dependent role in the family for Mr. Webster, and he told us that he had "nothing to say" when we asked about his nonuse of the new system. His dependent role in communication also changed his role as head of the household. The new system was also more complicated to set up and to operate. It required his wife and attendant to learn more about the system, and he had to wait for one of them to set it up for him. The effort involved on everybody's part may have been overwhelming.

Acceptance of AAC by persons who have ALS is reported by several authors. In one 4-year study, more than 96% of those given the choice of AAC accepted that choice (Ball, Beukelman, & Patee, 2004). There are several factors leading to acceptance and successful use of AAC by persons with ALS. First, it is important that clinicians provide information regarding the speech-language characteristics of ALS at the outset of intervention. There is a relationship between speaking rate and intelligibility, with 80% intelligibility occurring at about 130 words per minute (Ball, Beukelman, & Patee, 2004). Speech rate is used to determine the timing of AAC interventions. The rate continually drops as ALS progresses, and evaluation is initiated when the rate is at 90%. The second success factor is maintaining continuous contact to monitor speech rate and intelligibility along with other routinely measured motor system parameters. Finally, it is important that the family remain aware of AAC service intervention opportunities. Flexible AAC devices and strategies that will accommodate for changes over the course of the disease are important. A key reason for acceptance of AAC by persons with ALS is their desire to continue interacting with communication partners in a variety of contexts. The literature strongly supports the use of AAC as a key component of evidence-based practice in the treatment of ALS.

Dementia

Dementia is a syndrome, or pattern of clinical symptoms and signs, which can be defined by: (1) decline of cognitive capacity with some effect on day-to-day functioning; (2) impairment in multiple areas of cognition (global); and (3) normal level of consciousness (Rabins, Lyketsos, & Steele, 2006). The incidence of dementia is expected to grow. Currently 10% of people aged 65 years and 47% of people 85 years and older have been diagnosed with Alzheimer's disease (McKelvey et al., 2007). This percentage translates into about 4 million people in the United States, a number that is expected to increase to 14 million by the year 2050. A major characteristic of dementia is difficulty in communicating, both receptively and expressively.

The aim of AAC intervention in dementia is to maximize communicative and memory functioning to maintain (or increase) activities to increase participation/engagement, and quality of life for people with dementia across the disease progression (McKelvey et al., 2007). Successful AAC intervention may also increase the quality of life and decrease the stress of family and professional caregivers of individuals with dementia.

AAC interventions for dementia are designed to maintain function, compensate for lost function, and/or counsel the individual or family regarding conditions and options for managing the symptoms of dementia. There are several forms of compensatory support typically used. Low-technology communication cards and books, pictures, drawings, and printed reminders can be designed to support those with dementia to remind them of temporal or semantic information. High-technology support such as computerized memory aids for visual or auditory information is also available (see Chapter 15). AAC in dementia intervention is typically designed to support the individual, rather than to support his or her communication interactions, per se (McKelvey et al., 2007).

AAC interventions for dementia are relatively new, but there is mounting evidence of their effectiveness. Investigation of the use of AAC and cognitive support technology by persons with dementia is encouraging. Most approaches involve low-technology memory and communication books and high-technology displays that are positioned within the individual's living space. Additional techniques include modifications of the communication partner's behavior during communicative interactions by: reduction of distractions, using short simple sentences, reducing questions to yes/no format, allowing time for the individual with dementia to respond, and assisting with word finding strategies such as word description if a word cannot be retrieved.

Other AT interventions for dementia are discussed in Chapter 15. Case Study 16-4 illustrates the application of AAC for each of these major disorders.

CONTEXT COMPONENT

Partners of People With Complex Communication Needs Who Rely on Augmentative and Alternative Communication

Communication almost always involves a partner who may be in the room, on the phone, or a continent away on email.

CASE STUDY 16-4

AAC in an Adult Care Center

You work as a member of the transdisciplinary rehabilitation team in an adult day health program. The program has participants with a variety of disabilities and needs, and some have difficulty speaking. The center offers nursing, social work, physical therapy, speech-language pathology, occupational therapy, a variety of activities, and meals. There is an Individual Program Plan (IPP) in place for each participant. Some participate in the program's art activities in small groups with an instructor or aide; others are in supported employment for half days and in the center for the other days. Other participants are in the center all day and they have occasional community outings with care staff to recreational sites, stores, and physical activity venues (e.g. swimming). You have been asked to help address the communication needs of four of these participants:

- A 25-year-old man with TBI living in an apartment with supported living services and a roommate
- A 40-year-old man with severe intellectual disability, ambulatory, good fine motor control, living in an group home with other adults functioning at about the same level
- A 19 year-old-woman with cerebral palsy that limits her fine and gross motor abilities in all four limbs, who lives with her sister, her primary caregiver
- A 67-year-old woman with aphasia secondary to a CVA living at a board and care home

None of these individuals have functional speech that is consistently understood by strangers or even their caregivers who know them well.

What things are important to know as you prepare to consult with the interdisciplinary rehab team and the participant's family members and/or care giving staff attend the interdisciplinary team meeting to discuss these participants' augmentative communication assessment needs?

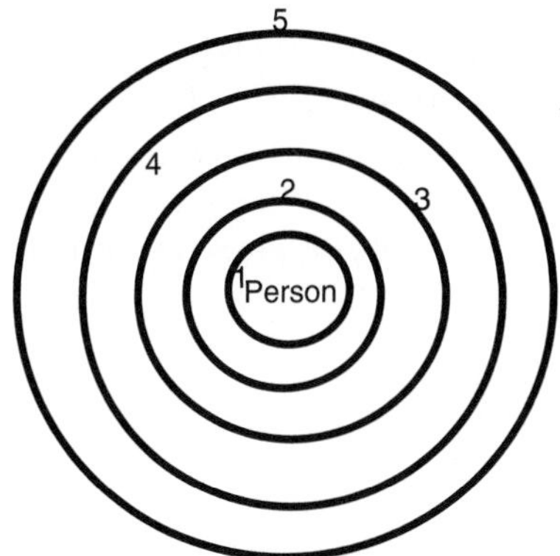

FIGURE 16-4 The circle of communicative partners. First circle—The person's life-long communication partners. Second Circle—Close friends/relatives. Third circle—Acquaintances (neighbors, schoolmates, bus driver, shop keeper). Fourth circle—Paid workers (SLP, PT, OT, teachers, teacher assistant, babysitter). Fifth circle—Unfamiliar partners ("everyone else" who doesn't fit in the first four circles).

Some "partners" may be merely imagined, as when someone writes a story. The Circle of Communication Partners (Figure 16-4) is helpful in defining the range of partners that a person with CCN who relies on AAC might encounter (Blackstone, 2003a). The first circle represents the person's life-long communication partners. This is primarily immediate family members. The second circle includes close friends (i.e., people who you tell your secrets to). These are often not family members. Acquaintances such as neighbors, schoolmates, coworkers, distant relatives (such as aunts and cousins), the bus driver, and shopkeepers are included in the third circle. The fourth circle is used to represent paid workers such as a speech-language pathologist (SLP) or a PT, OT, teacher, teacher assistant, or babysitter. Finally, the fifth circle is used to represent those unfamiliar partners with whom the person has occasional interactions. This includes everyone who does not fit in the first four circles.

The familiarity with partners decreases as we move from circle 1 to 5 and the modes of communication required to communicate with people in each circle will vary. Table 16-2 shows that as we move from circle 1 to 5 the modes of communication required to communicate with people in each circle also varies (Blackstone & Hunt Berg, 2003). For example, gestures and speech (even if it IS difficult to understand) are often preferred modes in circles 1 and 2. Circle 2 also includes some nonelectronic communication boards as well as telephone and email. Circle 4 reflects the school, work, and professional provider partners and therefore a wide range of modes are used. Circle 5 relies primarily on nonelectronic communication boards and books and SGDs of various types.

Although the experience of the clinician with individuals who have CCN may be limited to a brief encounter, the family has a long-term relationship with the individual and is a key member of the AAC assessment and decision-making team (Parette, Botherson, & Huer, 2000). In fact, when one family member relies on AAC, it always has an impact on the entire family (Goldbart & Marshall, 2004). Parents, spouses, and siblings need clear, jargon-free information that is presented objectively and honestly. Information about options, funding, timelines, and training in the use of the recommended AAC device or strategy is particularly important (Parette, Botherson, & Huer, 2000). There is great diversity among families, of course, and this will affect the way they respond to their family member's communication needs and to AAC itself (Goldbart & Marshall, 2004). For example, parents report feeling additional pressure to use AAC in communicating with their child and to help others to do so (Angelo, 2000). Researchers also report that the goals of mothers and fathers may differ for their children (Angelo, Kokoska, & Jones, 1996). Mothers ranked social opportunities with both nondisabled children and other AAC users, integrating AAC into the community, and planning for future needs as their highest priorities. Fathers focused on planning for future needs, knowing how to program, repair, and maintain the SGD; integration of AAC into educational settings; and obtaining computer access with the SGD. Parents also indicated that they have to become strong advocates for their child to receive necessary services (Goldbart & Marshall, 2004).

Raghavendra et al. (2012) investigated the current patterns and frequency of Internet use by young people with disabilities who had a mean age of 14.6. They found that

TABLE 16-2 Partners and Modes of Communication in the Circles in Figure 16-4

Circle	Partners	Commonly Used AAC Modes and Techniques[19]
1	Life-long communication partners, immediate family members	Facial expressions, gestures, vocalizations, speech, manual signs
2	Close friends, i.e., people who you tell your secrets to, often not family members.	Facial expressions, gestures, vocalizations, nonelectronic communication boards and books, telephone, email
3	Acquaintances such as neighbors, schoolmates, coworkers, distant relatives, such as aunts and cousins, regular shopkeeper or bus driver	Facial expressions, gestures, vocalizations, low-tech and high-tech dedicated SGDs, telephone, email
4	Paid workers such as a speech-language pathologist (SLP) or a PT, OT, OTA, PTA, speech assistant, teacher, teacher assistant, or babysitter	Facial expressions, gestures, vocalizations, manual signs, nonelectronic communication boards and books, writing, low-tech and high-tech dedicated SGDs, mainstream-based SGDs
5	Unfamiliar partners with whom the person has occasional interactions, e.g., the bus driver and seldom visited or new shopkeepers	Facial expressions, gestures, nonelectronic communication boards and books, low-tech and high-tech dedicated SGDs, mainstream-based SGDs

[19]Blackstone SW, Hunt Berg M: *Social networks: A communication inventory for individuals with complex communication needs and their communication partners: Inventory booklet*, Monterey, CA: Augmentative Communication, Inc, 2003.

their participants used the Internet for a variety of purposes. Some found that the Internet was an extension of offline connections providing additional connections that helped to strengthen friendships. The role of friends was particularly important in learning how to use social media and access the Internet. Participants tended to connect only with friends and others known through school or clubs. Having family resources sufficient to purchase computers and Internet service provider services and literacy skills of parents were significant factors influencing usage.

Attitudes About and Acceptance of Augmentative and Alternative Communication

McCarthy and Light (2005) reviewed 13 research studies on attitudes toward individuals who rely on SGDs. They identified several factors affecting attitudes: characteristics of typically developing individuals, characteristics of the person using AAC, and characteristics of the AAC system. These are elements of the social context of the human activity assistive technology (HAAT) model. Attitudes toward individuals who use AAC vary across the parameters of gender, type of disability, age, experience of the user of AAC, experience and familiarity with disability and AAC by the partner, and social context. Attitudes appear to be formed by the interaction of many of these factors.

The attitudes of children who do not have disabilities toward children who do and who use AAC is influenced by their familiarity with children who have disabilities (i.e., whether the nondisabled students had a classmate with a disability) and by age (older children are less positive than are younger children) (Beck et al., 2002). In general, girls are more positive toward disabled peers than boys are (Beck & Dennis, 1996). Although the number of conversational turns (one exchange between the speaker and partner) was almost identical in both groups, children who use AAC communicate mostly through responses and their typically developing peers initiate almost all of the requests (Clarke & Kirton, 2003). Beck et al. (2002) reported that the longer the messages produced (two- vs. four-word utterances), the more positive were the peers' attitudes toward the child using AAC. Consistent with the second-circle relationship, much of the interaction among peers involves expressions of humor and intimacy (e.g., laughing, joking, teasing, tickling, etc.). In general, the attitudes of peers toward an AAC user do not appear to be affected by the type of AAC system used (Beck & Dennis, 1996). However, in one study the use of voice output led to more positive peer attitudes than when the output was only visual (letters on a display) (Lilienfeld & Alant, 2002).

Many students who use AAC are enrolled in inclusive classroom settings. Thus, the attitudes of general education teachers (circle 4) toward AAC are important to their success (Kent-Walsh & Light, 2003). Both the students who use AAC and their typically developing classmates in general education classes can develop skills and positive interactions during classroom activities. However, unequal status with classmates and dissimilar interests lead to social exclusion for students who rely on AAC. Often peers speak to the teacher or teacher's assistant rather than directly to the student. Teachers are also concerned about lack of academic gain. Some device features (e.g., speech synthesis) are perceived as disruptive to other students. School-related barriers to successful inclusion include large class sizes, the physical layout of the classroom, and the tendency of the schools to apply inclusion guidelines very liberally without a focus on educational needs. Teachers require time to adjust to the idea of having students with disabilities in class, full access to school resources for the AAC students, and availability of specialists for consultation and training.

Employers and coworkers are also influenced by workers who use AAC (McNaughton, Light, & Gulla, 2003). Benefits for the worker using AAC are social interaction, personal enjoyment, and financial gain. Benefits to the employer include positive impacts on other employees, high quality of work performance by the employee using AAC, loyalty of the employee, and the ability to fill "hard-to-fill positions." Employment challenges fall into several themes: finding a good job match to individual skills, communication challenges (e.g., noisy AAC device, speaker phone use), difficulty with typical office tasks (e.g., manipulation of paper, telephone use), education or vocational skill level too low, lack of knowledge of work culture, and physical challenges necessitating assistance from other workers and financial (e.g., insurance costs to company).

ASSISTIVE TECHNOLOGIES FOR ALTERNATIVE AND AUGMENTATIVE COMMUNICATION

We all use a variety of communication modes (e.g., phones, email, computers) to interact with others and accomplish our activities of daily living. In order to meet all of their needs, people with complex communication needs require multiple communication methods and devices.

Many communicators use "no-technology" or body-centered methods such as speech, gestures, facial expressions, and vocalizations (nonspeech sounds). They also use "low-technology" systems such as paper communication boards and books, where their choices are indicated by pointing or paper and pencil for writing messages. Some individuals who have CCN use "high-technology" electronic devices including talking picture frames, smart phones, computers that have speech outputs, and devices specially designed for AAC use called speech-generating devices. AAC systems can take on many forms. Not everyone uses all of these approaches, but many people do.

In a paper written from the point of view of accomplished augmentative communicators, five principles were identified as essential to the next 25 years of AAC (Williams, Krezman, & McNaughton, 2008). One of the principles is "One is never enough." Individuals with CCN need more than one device, have more than one communication partner, develop multiple communication strategies, and communicate in a range of environments. These factors dictate that multiple communication modes, devices, and strategies must be available. "AAC should not be thought of as an attempt to create some minimal approximation of speech—it is a collection of techniques and strategies meant to support participation in a wide range of communication activities in a wide range of social and physical environments, each with its own unique challenges and demands" (Williams, Krezman, & McNaughton, 2008, pp. 196-197). There should at least be a low-tech back-up to the high-tech system.

Funding agencies generally dictate that only one speech-generating device be provided for an individual. Some agencies (such as Medicare in the United States) also restrict the range of communication activities (e.g., no access to the Internet, mobile phone, or computer via the SGD).

In general, only minimal training for the individuals and communication partners is funded. The restrictions work against the principle of "one is not enough" and, most important, prevent the full range of communication options for individual with CCN that are available to the rest of society. Williams et al. (2008) summarize the benefits of communication options:

> *The development of a rich and dynamic collection of AAC strategies and technologies has many benefits. First, access to a variety of communication techniques helps to ensure that an individual can have access to an appropriate tool for a desired goal: We need AAC techniques to support delivering a lecture in a high school social studies class and to communicate raucous joy at a sporting event; to send an emergency message when a bus is delayed; and to share the good news when a job is obtained. (p. 197)*

Another principle proposed by Williams et al. is "My AAC must fit my life: AAC systems must be highly individualized and appropriate to individual needs" (p. 195). This is a recognition that AAC needs of children, adolescents, and adults vary and that each has unique needs in both their AAC systems and the strategies for their use. Vocabulary needs vary as do situations in which communication occurs. Adolescents want to communicate at a noisy rock concert, adults have many communication partners, children are developing language abilities. Each of these unique situations places equally unique demand on the AAC methods and systems required.

Ways of Representing Language in AAC

AAC systems can use a variety of symbol systems that are understood by an individual and used to communicate. The most flexible symbols are letters and words (called traditional orthography). However, the use of traditional orthography depends on spelling ability and literacy (reading and writing) skills. Spontaneous spelling requires the person to spell the requested word letter-by-letter like the typical spelling test for children in school. This is the most flexible and versatile capability, and it allows traditional orthography to portray any concept about which the user wishes to communicate. Sixth-grade spelling is generally recognized as the minimal level for general communication. Even if spontaneous spelling is weak, the individual may be able to choose the first letter of the desired word and recognize the completed word from a list presented by the SGD word completion function (see Chapter 6). Even without first letter spelling, *recognition spelling* that requires the individual to pick the correct entry from a list of options can be used with a paper communication board or SGD that presents word lists or other stored vocabulary choices and relies on recognition memory. If the person has a large word recognition vocabulary, the AAC system vocabulary choices for the user should be based on words with possible "carrier phrases" that are filled in with limited spelling (e.g., "I would like a drink of ____").

When spelling or word recognition is not possible, alternative symbol systems are used. A variety of symbol types are shown in Figure 16-5. Perhaps the most concrete type of symbol is the use of real objects (full size or miniature). However, to a person with cognitive disabilities, a miniature object may not appear to represent the full-sized version, and

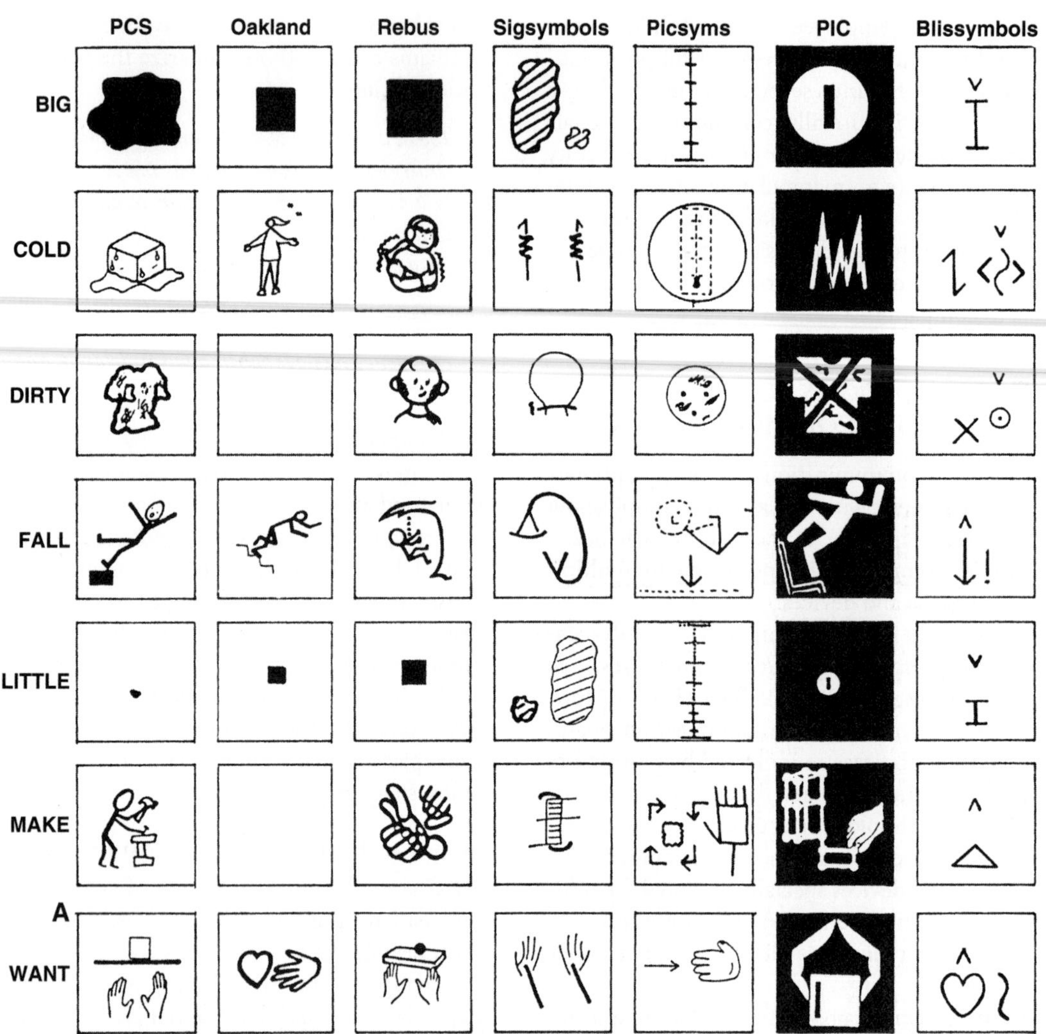

FIGURE 16-5 Examples of the variety of symbol systems that have been developed for AAC use. (From Blackstone S: *Augmentative communication,* Rockville, MD: American Speech Language Hearing Association, 1986.)

care must be taken to ensure that the concrete association is made between the two different sized objects by the user (Lloyd, Fuller, & Arvidson, 1997). Real objects and photographs have the disadvantage that many communicative concepts (e.g., good, more, go, hurt) are difficult to portray using these symbols.

Pictographic symbols include provisions for more abstract concepts and allow much greater flexibility in developing vocabulary usage. A more flexible symbol type is the use of a symbol system possessing grammar and syntax (e.g., Blissymbols). The nature of this symbol system allows the inclusion of more linguistic functions, such as categorization by parts of language.

Figure 16-6 illustrates the use of line drawings, words, and photographs to portray similar concepts. As can be seen, photographs can sometimes be less clear than line drawings.

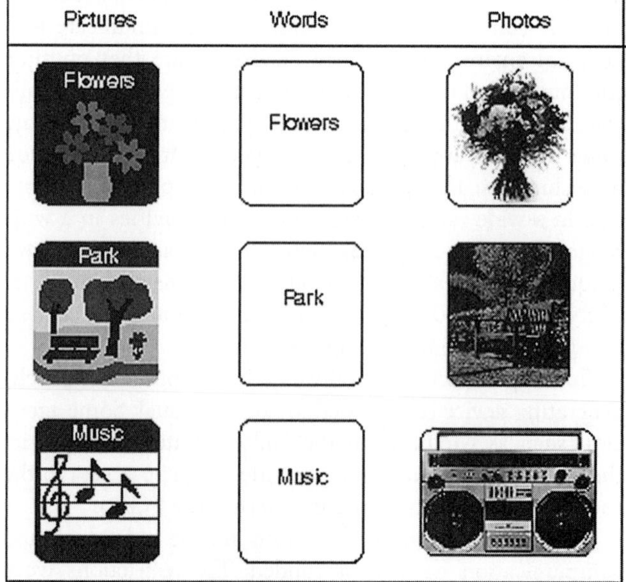

FIGURE 16-6 A comparison of drawings, words, and photographs to describe the same topic.

No-Tech AAC Systems

Gestures, facial expressions, and body movements help display emotional states, regulate and maintain a conversation, and support information exchange. Formal gestural codes

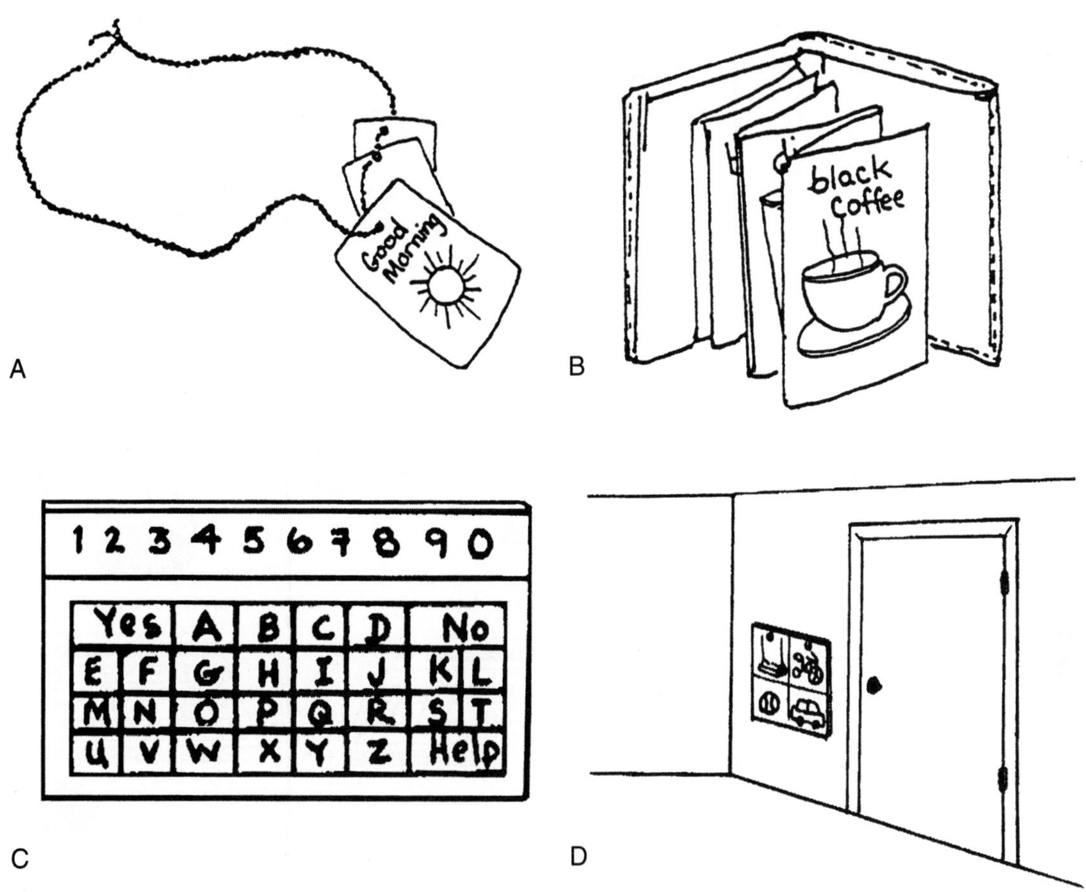

FIGURE 16-7 Low-tech communication aids.

(American Indian, Tadoma) and formal manual sign systems (e.g., ASL, SEE) are examples of more formal approaches (Beukelman and Mirenda, 2013).

Low-Tech AAC Systems

Low-technology refers to inexpensive devices that are simple to make and easy to obtain. Many types of AAC approaches fit into this category. Examples of low-technology approaches are shown in Figure 16-7. The communication cards shown in Figure 16-7 *A* are on a chain worn around the neck of the person. The communication book shown in Figure 16-7 *B* and the board or display shown in Figure 16-7 *C* are based on letters/words/phrases or graphic symbols, respectively. The communication display in Figure 16-7 *D* is an example of an activity-specific communication display that is placed by the door to facilitate the choosing of a recess activity. Other low-tech approaches may include placing symbols on items around a room to develop labeling skills or using miniature objects as labels and formal systems like the Picture Exchange System (PECS) to teach requesting, as described earlier in this chapter.

There are several methods of selecting from low-tech systems. The most common is direct selection via pointing using a hand, arm, foot or a head pointer or eye gaze. It is also possible to apply the visual scene display approach (see next section) to low-tech AAC systems.[2] Partner-assisted scanning in which the partner points to the items sequentially and the AAC user responds when the correct item is indicated can be used with a low-tech system. The response can be a vocalization, an eye blink, head nod, the lifting of one finger or any other sign. Auditory scanning (see next section) can be used with low-tech systems.

High-Tech AAC Systems

The term *high-technology* AAC refers to devices that have electronic components. Figure 16-8 illustrates some examples of high-tech AAC devices. There are two broad categories that are discussed in Chapter 6: direct selection and scanning. Some devices with limited functions are called "lite technologies." The light pointer in Figure 16-8 *C* is an example of a direct selection light technology that has greater range and is easier to use than a mechanical head pointer. The lite technology devices in Figure 16-8 *B* and *D* use scanning to choose among a few items using a single switch. High-technology devices have many choices and typically provide speech output. They can use either direct selection (Figure 16-8 *E*) or scanning (Figure 16-8 *F*). Some AAC devices use mainstream technologies (computers, mobile phones, or tablets) with special software. These can use direct selection (Figure 16-8 *G*) or scanning (Figure 16-8 *H*).

The appeal of devices is important (Williams, Krezman, & McNaughton, 2008). Children want to have devices that look fun and do not set them off as different. Adults want

[2]For examples, see http://aac.unl.edu/intervention.html.

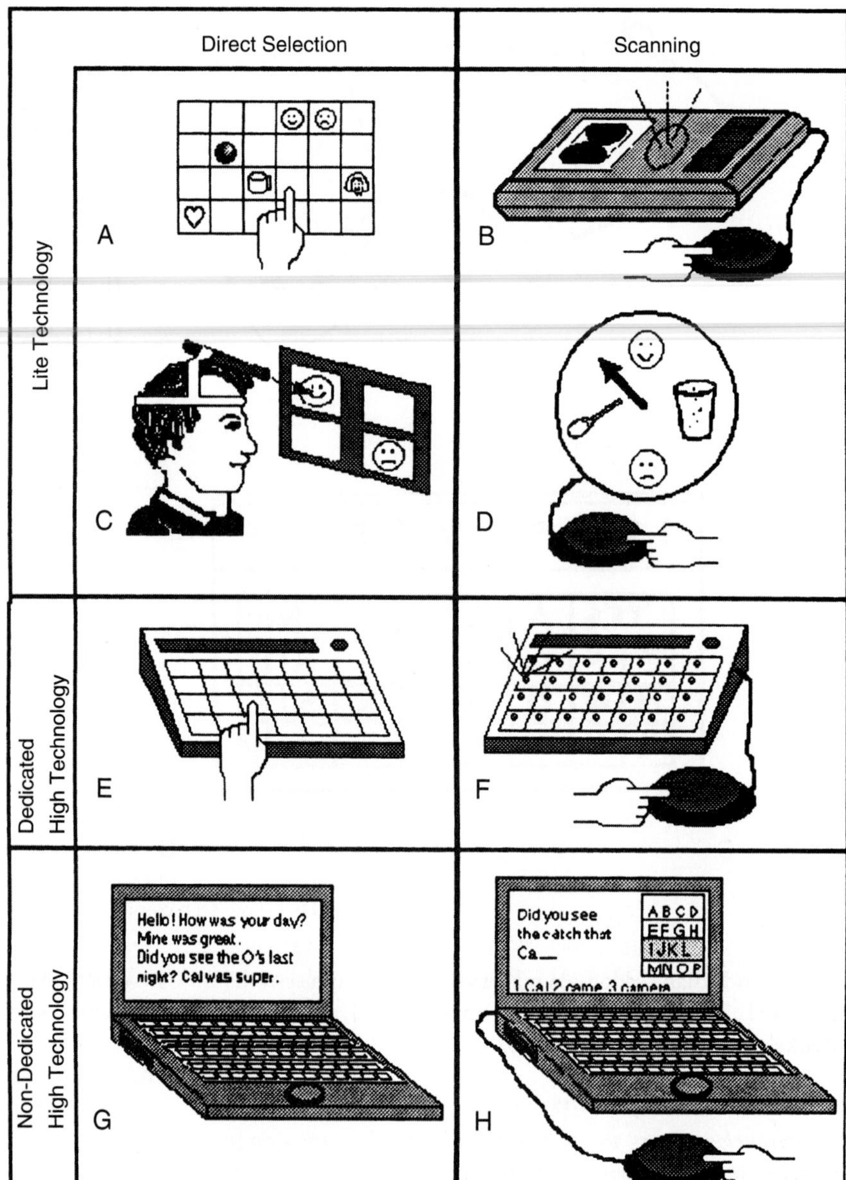

FIGURE 16-8 **A,** Manual communication display. **B,** Two choice voice output speech-generating device (SGD). **C,** Communication display accessed with a head-mounted light. **D,** Clockface communication device. **E,** Direct selection SGD. **F,** Scanning SGD. **G,** Direction-selection laptop computer-based SGD. **H,** Scanning laptop computer-based SGD. (From Glennen SL, DeCoste DC: *The handbook of augmentative and alternative communication,* 1997, San Diego, Singular Publishing.)

devices that are appropriate for academic, employment, and social activities. High-tech AAC systems typically use SGDs, some of which are specially designed for AAC and others of which are based on standard computers, mobile phones, or tablets. The salient general characteristics of these devices are described in this section.

Options for Making Selections in an AAC Device

There are many options for displaying the set of symbols so they can be selected. Static displays organized in a grid or matrix format are the most common. The displays or keyboards may contain all of the same alphanumeric characters as on a laptop computer. They may also contain words or nonalphabetic symbols or a small array of keys on a portable device. These may be physical keyboard-like panels or onscreen displays of the **selection set.** Low-tech AAC systems include printed static arrays.

Dynamic displays and visual scene displays are two other types of input devices that are well suited for AAC applications. All of these different ways of presenting vocabulary choices can be accessed by direct or indirect selection methods (see Chapter 6).

The person can make choices by directly selecting the item using a keyboard-like interface. Often the vocabulary items are displayed on a touch screen, and they are selected by directly touching the desired item. For indirect selection, choices are made by scanning using single or dual switches (see Chapter 6). Vocabulary choices can also be selected from a display using a pointing interface (mouse, trackball, or head pointer) to move a cursor around on the screen. There are many types of input devices or interfaces described in Chapter 7.

Most selection sets use visible symbols (e.g., letters, graphics, pictures) so individuals who have visual impairments

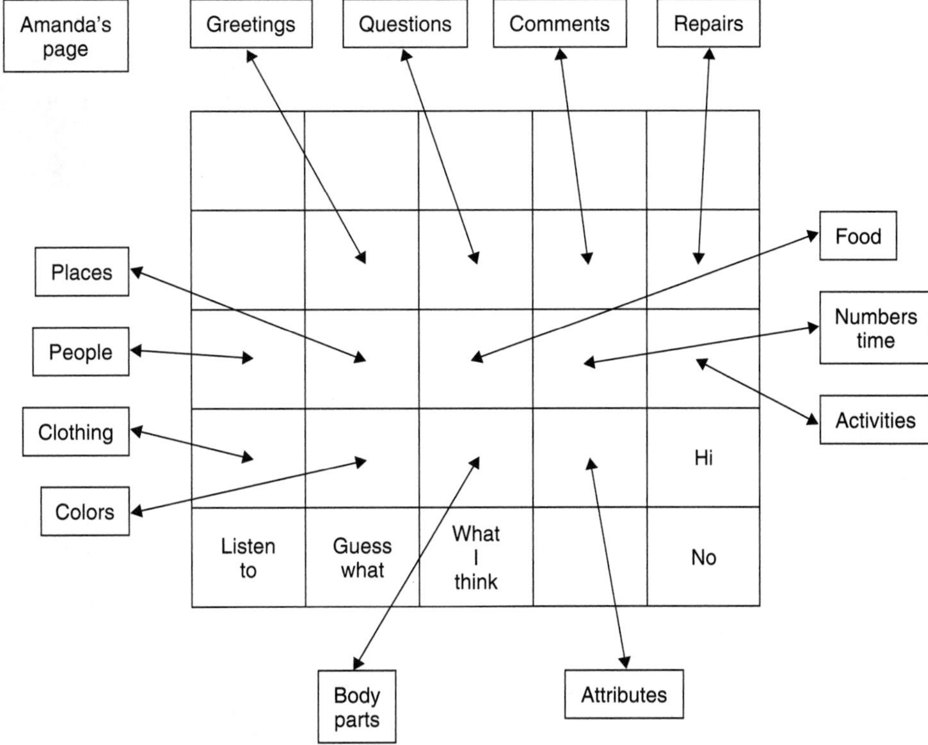

FIGURE 16-9 Dynamic display devices change the selection set presented to the user each time an entry is made.

and physical limitations requiring scanning may not be able to use visible arrays. For these individuals *auditory scanning* is used. Choices are presented in auditory form by a partner or an SGD and the user selects his or her choice from the auditory prompts. In some cases, both a prompting phrase and a selected auditory utterance are included and the user hears the prompting phrase through an earphone. In nonelectronic auditory scanning a list of vocabulary items is read aloud by the communication partner. The AAC user then chooses a vocabulary item by using a predetermined signal such as a vocalization to identify the desired vocabulary item. Kovach and Kenyon (1998) analyze a variety of approaches to auditory scanning, summarize current research in this area, and describe considerations to be included when developing an auditory scanning system for an AAC user.

Static Communication Displays

Communication displays that do not change with each entry are called *static displays*. The size of a static display can range from a few items (one to four or eight) up to 128 or more items. Considerations for selecting the most appropriate configurations for an individual are discussed in Chapter 7. Because static displays do not change, they are ideal for developing motor patterns that can dramatically increase the rate of selection and therefore the rate of communication. The key to motor patterns is that the individual items (symbols, letters, and icons) always remain in the same position. Thus a sequence of symbols always uses the same pattern of motor actions. Eventually this pattern becomes automatic. To get a sense of this, think about those cases in which you tried to remember a phone number, but you couldn't until you pretended to enter it on the telephone keypad. The number was still in memory, but it was stored as a motor pattern.

When the number of symbols or vocabulary is small, static display can work well. When the communication depends on the entry of sequences of symbols (e.g., iconic representations[3]) to generate large vocabularies, then static displays also work well. Static displays may also be indicated for cases in which the cognitive demands of dynamic displays are not present.

Dynamic Communication Displays

Dynamic communication displays change the selection set displayed when a choice is made. They are often used on smart phones, tablets, websites, and many other mainstream applications as well as many SGDs. When a choice is made the screen is reformatted to give a new set of options from which the user can select. For example, a general selection set may consist of categories such as work, home, food, clothing, greetings, or similar classifications. If one of these is chosen, either by touching the display surface directly or by scanning, then a new selection set is displayed. For example, a variety of food-related items and activities (eat, drink, ice cream, pasta, etc.) would follow the choice of "foods" from the general selection set. The symbols on the display can be varied, and this changes the targets for the user. Because each new selection set is displayed, the user does not have to remember what is on each level. This approach, illustrated in Figure 16-9, also

[3]Prentke Romich company, http://store.prentrom.com/.

TABLE 16-3 Comparison of Traditional Grid Displays and Visual Scene Displays

Variable	Typical AAC Grid	VSC
Type of representation	Symbols, traditional orthography, line drawings	Digital photos, line drawings
Personalization	Limited	High
Amount of context	Low	High
Layout	Grid	Full or partial screen, grid
Display management	Menu pages	Menu pages, navigation bars
Concept retrieval	Select grid space, pop-ups	Hotspots, speech key, select grid space

Traditional grid display

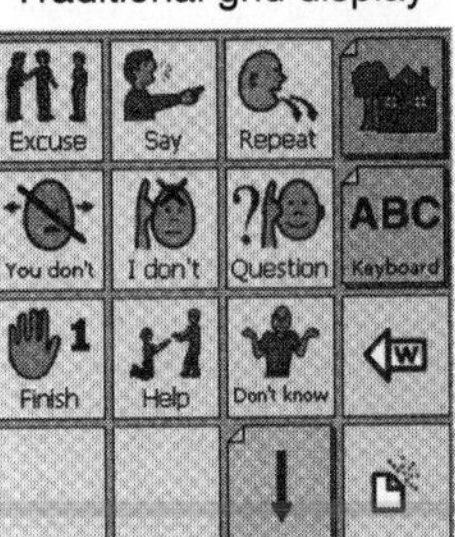

Visual scene display

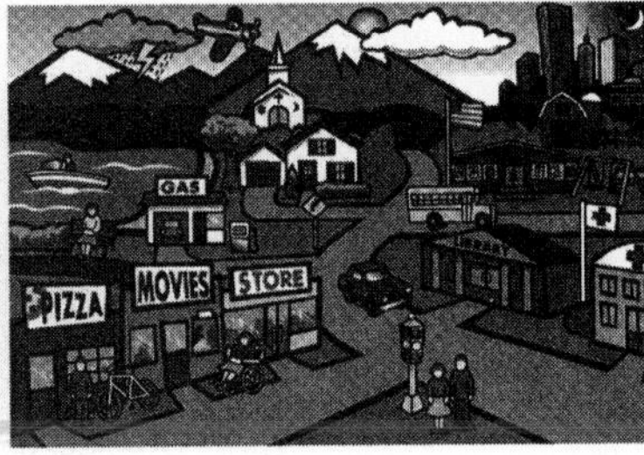

FIGURE 16-10 A comparison of a grid display (left) and a visual scene display (VSD) (right). (From Blackstone S: Visual scene displays, *Augment Commun News* 16(2):1-5, 2004.)

avoids having to squeeze several pictures into one square (of "x" dimensions) on a traditional grid display. A dynamic display also relies on recognition rather than recall memory for identification of the selection set elements, which can make it easier to use. Once an item is selected, the dynamic display automatically branches to the selected new page and displays it.

Blackstone (1994) describes a number of key features of dynamic displays. The nature of these devices allows the user to quickly change the screen and to configure the size, color, and arrangement of the symbols to match the topic. Dynamic displays reduce memory requirements because the user is prompted by the display after each choice. The constant vigilance to the screen requires a high level of visual attention and constant decision making. The user must also have mastered the concept of object permanence. These may be challenging for some individuals who have cognitive limitations.

Visual Scene Displays

Visual scene displays create displays that capture events in a person's life on the screen with "hotspots" that can be accessed to retrieve information (Blackstone, 2004). A hotspot is a region of a picture on the screen that the user can choose by pointing to it with a finger, a mouse, or a scanning cursor. VSDs may represent either a generic or personalized context. Generic context includes drawings of places (e.g., house, school room) whereas a personalized context is specific to one person (e.g., a picture of his or her house, a family outing). The images can be personal digital photographs of an event (e.g., a marriage or birthday party) or important people (e.g., family, friends, or teacher). The images can also be more generic photographs or other graphical representations that portray an area (e.g., child's room, kitchen) or event (e.g., going to the circus). Visual scene displays offer the user of AAC and his or her communication partner a greater degree of contextual information to support interaction. The richness of the display and the information content can also enable communication partners to participate more actively in a conversation. Table 16-3 describes the difference between a traditional AAC display (referred to as a grid) and a VSD (Blackstone, 2004).

The traditional grid supports communication of needs and wants and information exchange well. However, this type of display is usually restricted to symbols, text, or static drawings (although some animation is used with dynamic display items) and the vocabulary items are separated from any context to maximize their versatility. Personalization is also limited. Traditional grid displays present symbols out of context (i.e., language is presented in a box, isolated from the context in which it occurs) (Light & Drager, 2007). The grid display also does not preserve conceptual or visual relationships between elements in the grid display. In a traditional grid display, the line drawing of the apple used to represent *apple* may be as big as the head of the boy used to represent the concept *boy*, which in turn may be as big as the entire person used to represent the concept *run*.

Figure 16-10 illustrates the differences between a typical static grid display and a VSD (Blackstone, 2004). The VSD is developed for conversational support as a shared activity. Since it utilizes a range of information media, including video and family pictures in addition to text, symbols, and line drawings, it can be highly personalized, as shown in Figure 16-3 (Blackstone, 2004). In addition to communication of needs, wants, and information exchange, VSDs also support social closeness. Due to the dynamic nature of the VSD approach, it can also serve as a learning environment providing instruction, specific information, or prompts to help the user interact effectively. VSDs can be useful to individuals with cognitive (e.g., Down's syndrome) or language (e.g., aphasia, autism) limitations and young children.

Young (2.5 years old) typically developing children did significantly better at a birthday party communication task when using a schematic VSD layout (based on activities) than when using a grid layout (schematic or taxonomic) (Drager, 2003). One explanation is that the provision of a more meaningful context in the VSD reduced the language demand on the child. The VSD was organized around scenes of rooms: living room (arrival of children for party), kitchen (eating cake), family room (opening presents), and playroom (playing games); this reduces the demands on the child's working memory because the location of the item required fewer demands in the VSD. The grid was organized around the activities, which required more language processing by the child (e.g., categorizing, remembering the symbols).

For example, the topic of play could be illustrated by a digital photograph of the child's room including the toy box in the VSD and as a symbol for play on the grid. Clicking on the hot spot associated with the toy box in the VSD or on the grid element for play resulted in branching in both formats to more detailed information.

Light and Drager (2007) also studied the critical aspects of display layout and organization and the impact on children's learning to use AAC devices. The youngest of the children (age 2.5 years) were most accurate in locating vocabulary using the visual scene displays compared to the grid layouts, even though the displays were not personalized to the experiences of the children. By ages 4 and 5, the children located vocabulary with the visual scene displays and the grid layouts with similar levels of accuracy, but they had significant difficulty learning to use iconic encoding.

Children with developmental disabilities (ages 1 to 3) were able to use the visual scene displays to participate in social interactions, once their use had been modeled (Light & Drager, 2007). The children demonstrated significant increases in turn taking immediately upon introduction of the AAC technologies utilizing visual scenes. These gains in turn taking were sustained over the long term. All of the children also learned to use other types of displays over time, including traditional grid displays and hybrid displays

VSDs can stimulate conversations in which the communication partners play, share experiences, and tell stories. The dynamic nature of VSDs facilitates active participation of partners during these shared activities. For example, the topic of play could be illustrated by a digital photograph of the child's room including the toy box in the VSD and as a symbol for play on the grid. Clicking on the hot spot associated with the toy box in the VSD or on the grid element for play resulted in branching in both formats to more detailed information.

Vocabulary Storage and Retrieval Techniques

"Full participation in society requires access to, and the ability to use a full range of vocabulary at every step of an individual's life" (Williams, Krezman, & McNaughton, 2008). Speech allows communication at a rapid rate, 270 WPM during conversational speech and 160 to 180 WPM in oral reading (Shipley & McAfee, 2009). For an individual using an augmentative communication device to generate unlimited vocabulary, some form of letter or symbol selection is required; in many cases, persons who are unable to speak use a keyboard to type their messages, which are then spoken by an AAC device. This can result in significantly lower rates of communication than for speech. Many people who have disabilities must rely on single-finger typing for conversation. Using this mode, a person with a disability may only be able to type at a maximal rate of 10 to 12 words per minute. For individuals who use scanning (see Chapter 6), the maximal rates can be as low as three to five words per minute. Although there are several methods of increasing communication rate, the great disparity in rates of communication between a speaking person and an AAC system user often results in the speaking person's dominating a conversation with a nonspeaking person. Thus one of the goals in the design of augmentative communication devices is to reduce the magnitude of this disparity in communication rates. Many SGDs use approaches to increase input rate that are discussed in Chapter 6 (abbreviation expansion, word prediction, word completion). In addition, there are several methods for storing and retrieving vocabulary that are designed specifically for SGDs

Instant phrases are those used frequently for greetings, conversational repairs (e.g., "that's not what I meant") or similar actions. These are often included as single keystroke entries in an "activity row" or in a row of the scanning matrix, near the beginning of the scan. They can also serve as "floor holders" as in having the floor in a conversation (e.g., "please wait while I type my question/answer").

Coding of words, sentences, and phrases on the basis of their meanings is also known as semantic encoding or Minspeak® (Baker, 1982). This approach uses pictorial representations that can have multiple meanings as codes, making recall easier. For example, when a picture of an apple is used for "food" and a sun rising for "morning," then selection of "apple" and "sunrise" could be a code for "What's for breakfast." Icons can have multiple meanings. Thus the apple symbol can take on the meaning of "eat" or "red" or "fruit" rather than food. Several examples of Minspeak sequences are shown in Figure 16-11. Baker (1986) also developed an approach based on the use of syntactical labels coupled with icons. Figure 16-12 illustrates this concept. For example, the apple icon becomes "eat" when combined with the key labeled "verb" and becomes "food" when combined with the noun key.

With practice, these sequences of icons can be developed as motor patterns that can be generated at a more automatic, subconscious level. This has led to an approach that relies on motor planning and natural consequences for learning symbols. "Children learning to communicate with LAMP [Language Acquisition through Motor Planning] learn how to say the target words without initially learning the symbol or the associate of the symbol to the word" (Hallorn & Emerson, 2010, p. 13).

Unity is a family of Minspeak application programs included with Prentke Romich (Wooster, Ohio, www.prentrom.com) AAC devices. It includes 4, 8, 15, 32, 45, 84, and 128 location overlays that differ in the pointing resolution required by the user. Sequences of icons and their locations on the keyboard are kept as consistent as possible among the overlays to account for motor skill development while allowing growth in language usage. Versions of Unity vary from a few hundred words to more than 4000 words intended to address the core vocabulary that is responsible for the majority of conversational utterances.

When large numbers of sentences, words, and phrases are stored, the icon sequences can become difficult to remember. **Icon prediction** initially lights an indicator associated with each symbol that forms the beginning of an icon sequence. When one of these icons is selected, only those icons that are

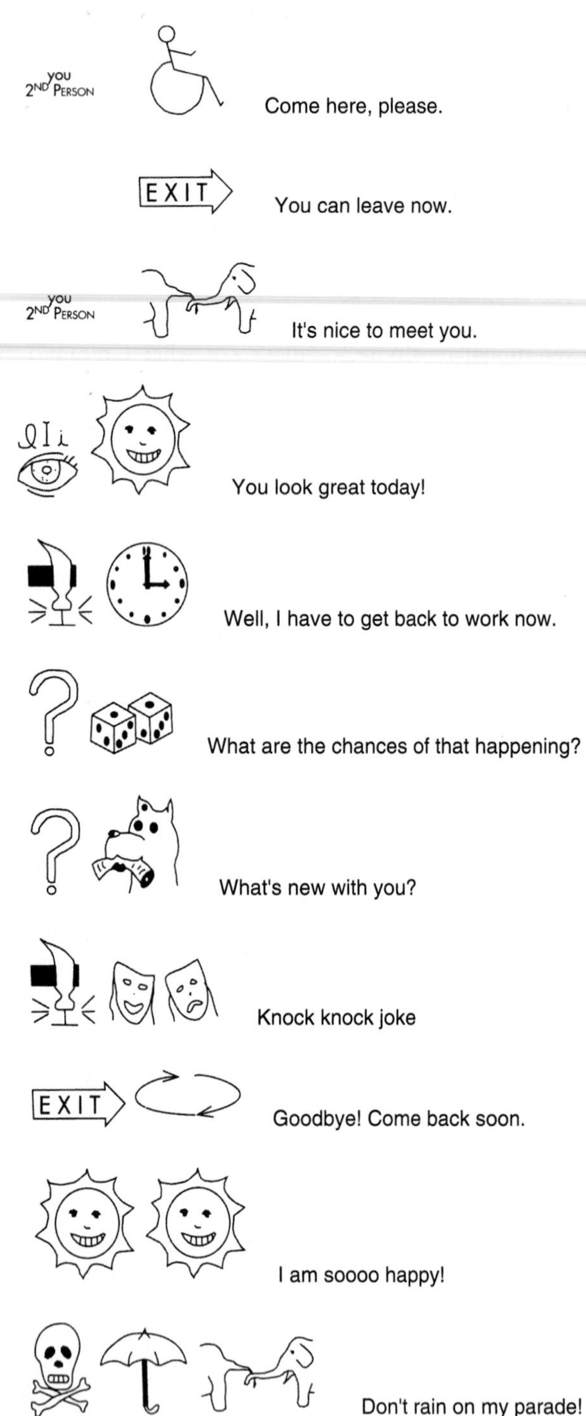
2ND PERSON YOU
Come here, please.
EXIT
You can leave now.
2ND PERSON YOU
It's nice to meet you.
You look great today!
Well, I have to get back to work now.
What are the chances of that happening?
What's new with you?
Knock knock joke
EXIT
Goodbye! Come back soon.
I am soooo happy!
Don't rain on my parade!

FIGURE 16-11 Examples of Minspeak symbol sequences. (From Romich B: *Liberator manual,* Wooster, OH: Prentke Romich.)

part of a sequence light up or flash, beginning with the first selected icon. This continues until a complete icon sequence has been selected. This feature can aid recall and increase speed of selection because the device limits the number of icons that must be visually scanned for each selection.

Williams (1991), an accomplished user of numerical abbreviation expansion and word-based Minspeak, describes several advantages of this approach. In comparison to sentence-based Minspeak, he states that he (and most of the rest of us) does not think in sentences but in words or short phrases. This makes a word-based device easier to use. Second, he indicates that of the three encoding approaches in which he has achieved skill (each after hundreds of hours of practice), the word-based Minspeak "offers powerful advantages over the rest" (p. 133). His major reasons for this are the ease with which words are recalled during use and the large vocabularies that are possible with the use of icons rather than arbitrary codes. Williams also points out that it requires a large amount of practice and effort to become proficient with this type of device, which must be built into training programs. Williams also addresses the initial reluctance that many cognitively able but physically limited adults with CCN have to using pictorial representations as codes.

Vocabulary Programs for Language Development

The *Gateway* (Dynavox Systems, Inc, Pittsburgh, PA, http://www.dynavoxtech.com/) series is an approach to vocabulary organizations that is based on language development in typically developing children. The levels of Gateway are designated by the number of elements in the selection set, from 12 through 75. These are intended for six distinct target user groups beginning with the 12- to 24-month language development level, progressing to two formats for mild/moderate cognitive disability for children or adults, arrays for children and adolescents/adults with typical cognitive/language development and physical limitations, and a high-end array for augmented communicators who have well-developed syntactical skills. Pop-up menus with frequently used items (word, phrases, or sentences) are available on the larger arrays.

WordPower (Inman Innovations, available on several commercial AAC systems) combines a core vocabulary of 100 words that represent about 50% of spoken communication. It includes approximately 100 single hit words, hundreds of two and three hit words, a core dictionary for word prediction of 30,000 words, automatic grammatical endings (-ed, -ing, -s), and a QWERTY keyboard for spelling. For literate users, this approach is intuitive and leads to efficient communication. There are both direct and indirect (scanning) versions available. Picture WordPower uses labeled symbols as word cues. The same basic core vocabulary is available.

Conversationally Based Vocabulary Storage and Retrieval

TALK (Todman, 2000) is based on the perspective of a typical conversation: person (me/you), queries (where, what, how, who, when, why), and tense (present, past, future). Figure 16-13 shows a typical TALK board with "where me/where/past" perspectives selected. This leads to the display of a particular set of phrases that can be chosen and spoken with one switch selection.

There are also a set of comments, repair phrases along the right side, and the conversation sections similar to CHAT along the top. The bottom of the screen has an area for letter-by-letter text entry. Using TALK and similar systems, the AAC user can obtain conversational rates of 30 to 60 wpm. One version of TALK is available with Speaking

Words Strategy Icon Sequences

+Noun	=family	+Noun	=dollar
+Prep.	=between	+Prep.	=by
+Adj.	=all	+Adj.	=real
+Conj.	=although	+Verb	=buy
+Adj.	=sick	+Verb	=wash
+Adj.+er	=sicker	+Verb+es	=washes
+Adj.+est	=sickest	+Verb+ing	=washing
		+Verb+ed	=washed

+A+Noun	=a wheelchair
+The+Noun	=the wheelchair
+The+Noun Pl.	=the wheelchairs

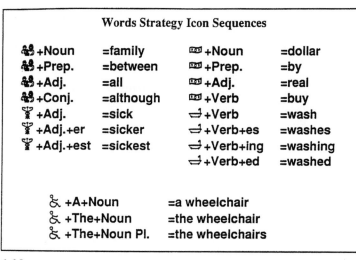

FIGURE 16-12 Symbols such as those used with Minspeak can be given syntactical meaning, as in this example from the Word Strategy application program. (From *Liberating the power of Minspeak*, Wooster, OH: Prentke Romich, 1991.)

Me
Greet | Stories | Storage | Switch | Finish
Ques | F'back
You
Sympa | Hedge
Saying | Sorry
Our first house was in Carnoustie | Most of my childhood we lived in Dundee | I was away at college in Motherwell for two years
Where
I don't remember it at all | We lived mainly in Charleston and Menziehill | It was really different living on the west coast
What
How
Uh huh | More
Agree | Disagree
Carnoustie is well known for its golf course | I really liked living there | I like the west coast of Scotland better than the east
When
Dunno | Thanks
Wait | Interupt
Good! | Bad!
Who
The first flat I had on my own was at Blackwood Court
Why
Yes | No
Oops! | Random
It was a real adventure living on my own for the first time
Past
Present
Future
Repeat | Quit
Edit Last
Edit Text | Go Edit
Speak

FIGURE 16-13 TALK board. (Courtesy Mayer-Johnson.)

Dynamically Pro.[4] When individuals who have limited experience with conversations are introduced to systems like TALK, significant training specifically oriented toward conversational flow is required (Todman, 2000).

Frame Talker (Higginbotham et al., 2005) is an AAC approach that allows the selection of natural language utterances by using a schematic format that represents the situational structure of communication events. The situational structure of communication events is represented by a communication frame. Frames can be used to semantically and functionally organize related conversational utterances. A communication frame consists of component frames, utterance constructions and lexical fields, a topic domain, and a frame hierarchy. The communication frame can be viewed as an utterance-based augmentative communication device designed to enable a person with CCN to communicate quickly and effectively. The internal structure of a communication frame consists of component frames and utterance constructions. Component frames uniquely identify typical subtopics or distinct situational portions within the larger communication frame (e.g., "severity" versus "cause" of pains) with utterance constructions located within them. A potentially large number of different utterances can be generated by each utterance construction in combination with its associated lexical field (i.e., group of semantically related terms). Topic domains are organized as clusters of individual communication frames that share similar generic topic interests.

[4]Mayer Johnson, Solana Beach, CA, www.mayer-johnson.com.

AAC System Outputs

SGDs or other AAC devices can produce a variety of *communication outputs*. Since AAC often involves conversation, electronic devices commonly produce speech as an output. Printed output is important for communication in written form. Often AAC devices also have outputs that control appliances or connect to other communication devices like computers, cell phones, or the Internet. Finally, AAC devices can be used to control power wheelchairs. These various outputs are discussed in this section.

Speech Output

The two major types of speech output use in SGDs are digitized and synthesized. These are both described in Chapter 6. Speech output allows use with partners who cannot read (e.g., small children or cognitively impaired persons). It is also the only type of output that can be used conveniently for speaking to groups (including use in classroom discussions) or speaking over the telephone (unless both the user of the device and the partner each have special TTY equipment; see Chapter 14).

In the end, the effectiveness of speech synthesis is how intelligible it is to human listeners. Although personal preference plays a part in this determination, there are objective ways in which to evaluate the intelligibility of various speech synthesizers. The environment in which speech is heard is also a factor in intelligibility. Most intelligibility studies are conducted under very controlled and noise-free conditions. When speech output communication devices are used, it is not in such highly controlled environments. One way to study the degrading of intelligibility in real settings is to add reverberation that simulates more natural conditions (Venkatagiri, 2004).

When reverberation is added to simulate a large room or a large lecture hall, the intelligibility of human speech degrades only slightly. Under the same conditions, synthetic speech intelligibility decreases by 28%. These tests were conducted without the benefit of linguistic and communicative context cues that would typically be available to the partners of an AAC user.

Drager, Reichle, and Pinkoski (2010) provided a scoping review of research on the intelligibility and listener comprehension of synthesized speech when young children are the listeners. If synthesized speech from SGDs used by children is intelligible to their peers then it may support more natural interactions. These interactions may lead to enhanced social relationships. There is also evidence that synthesized speech may help children learn to produce communication using AAC systems and symbols. Finally, if children use synthesized speech during naturalized language instruction, they may develop greater spoken language comprehension. Results of studies involving children showed a clear difference in synthesized word intelligibility compared to that for words produced via natural speech. There were also statistically significant differences in intelligibility scores between the 3-year-old children and the 4- and 5-year-old children but not between the 4-year-olds and the 5-year-olds in intelligibility of words and sentences with both synthesized and digitized speech. Intelligibility of synthesized speech signals was lower than natural speech. Intelligibility of synthesized speech was lower than for adults.

Written Output

Written output requires a printer. Most often people with complex communication needs use computer word processors and printers to generate written output. The AAC device may be connected to the computer (see Chapter 8) so that the stored vocabulary and other features such as indirect selection can be used by the person. Alternatively, the individual may use the computer directly with some of the built-in accessibility features (Table 8-2 in Chapter 8). Some SGDs allow connection of a printer via a USB port or Wi-Fi.

Outputs to Control Assistive Technologies

Specialized assistive technologies such as electronic aids to daily living (EADL) (e.g., remote controls for lights, television, other appliances, covered in Chapter 12), and powered wheelchairs (discussed in Chapter 10) are also often of use to individuals with CCN. Many SGDs either provide the functions of EADLs or interface with them through wireless remote connections. The real power in connecting people with CCN to the rest of the information society lies in granting them access to mainstream technologies. In addition to access to EADLs, SGDs allow connection to electronic games (e.g., Playstation, Wii) and other electronic devices. The most common types of wireless connection to external devices use infrared or Bluetooth signals. The infrared signals are often used for appliances or toys. Bluetooth control of appliances is increasing and this is the most common wireless connection to cell phones, computers, and other mainstream applications. Many SGDs have infrared outputs built in and an increasing number, especially those based on standard computers, also have Bluetooth signals available.

Access to Mainstream Technologies

"AAC access to today's mainstream technologies expands the focus from interpersonal communication to access of information and services over the expanding World Wide Web" (Shane et al., 2012, p. 3). The variety of communication functions and environments that have been enabled by access to mainstream technologies are listed in Table 16-4 (Shane et al., 2012). The focus has changed from technologies that enable face-to-face communication to a wide range of technologies that support worldwide communication options for people with CCN.

Features in mainstream technologies that were developed for people with disabilities (e.g., word completion/prediction, voice recognition, abbreviation expansion) are also being useful for the general public. This will further increase their availability to individuals with CCN. Digital photography built into cell phones also increases functionality for persons with CCN. In addition to the mainstream use (i.e., photography for recording family events, business, or school), the

TABLE 16-4 Communication Functions and Environments

Functions	Some examples
1. Interpersonal communication	Face to face–speech/text/symbol generating device Face to face-/text/symbol–non-electronic communication display Face to face–video chat Telephony–phone; cellphone; smartphone Social media–written (email, texting, twitter, instant messaging)
2. Information	Google/Ask/Yahoo News and weather websites
3. Online services	Online banking (money transfer, bill payment) Online shopping (countless consumer products) Tracking (e.g., orders)
4. Entertainment	Digital books, magazines, & newspapers Personal media library–video, music, games
5. Education	Online courses/distant education/eBooks Curriculum modifications
6. Employment	Telework Home, work site, mobile workstations
7. Health and safety	Telemedicine E-911 Patient provider communication accommodations
8. Tools	Telephone Address book Global positioning and maps Calculator Clock, timer, and reminders Dictionary
9. Public services & facilities	Online airport check-in Banking (ATM) Building keypads Public scanners requiring swiping (e.g., public transportation)

From Shane HC, Blackstone S, Vanderheiden G et al.: Using AAC technology to access the world, *Assist Technol* 24:3-13, 2012, Table 1, p. 5

camera features can be used as an additional AAC option for portraying vocabulary, reducing the descriptive information required to convey a message.

As we discussed in Chapter 15 for individuals with cognitive disabilities, the cloud can be utilized as a resource for people with CCN. Their user profiles as well as programs for text-to-speech conversion or vocabulary storage could be stored on cloud servers. Using simple technology such as Bluetooth-enabled keyboards or their own SGD, they could access these services and data with features matched to their skills and abilities. Alternatively, individuals could use an older computer or tablet as an interface to access the cloud resources as their main computer/AAC device to carry out functions like those in Table 16-4 (Shane et al., 2012). Computers available at school, community centers, libraries, or Internet cafes could be used by those with no personal computer.

Internet Access

The Internet is the name given to all data networks that are tied together and that use a common method for sharing information (IP or Internet Protocol). The Web refers to the collection of pages and services accessed using the Internet with a hypertext transfer protocol (HTTP) (Shane et al., 2012). The Internet and Web provide significant resources from the computer desktop. Quick, easy, and low-cost communication with individuals around the world is routine by use of email. Many people who have disabilities use email to communicate with friends, business associates, and organizations (Case Study 16-5). Many individuals with CCN access the Internet with their SGDs. Any stored vocabulary or special access methods are available for use while online. Some SGDs have AAC software on portable computers that can also function as Internet workstations.[5] The Internet also provides access to information through company, organization, and individual websites. By accessing this information, individuals who use AAC can learn about new technologies, conduct business independently, carry out research for academic pursuits, book airline reservations, and many other activities. Access to the Internet provides many opportunities for reading and writing, and this can have a positive impact on literacy skills for AAC users (Blackstone, 2003c). Temple University provides mentoring programs for individuals who rely on AAC.[6] The course consists of two weeks of intensive training on site and one year follow-up via the Internet. Program graduates mentor new students in the program.

CASE STUDY 16-5

Augmentative and Alternative Communication in Postsecondary Education

Heidi (Figure 16-14) is a doctoral student studying English at a major university. She has cerebral palsy, which limits her ability to speak and to use her hands for writing. She uses her computer to complete writing assignments and has written two plays (one for her master's degree thesis) and one book for teenagers who have cerebral palsy. She uses her notebook computer with a speech synthesizer for conversation and a word processor for writing. She also uses email to communicate with her PhD thesis advisor, colleagues, students, and friends. This technology allows her to keep in touch with people without the use of the telephone, which is difficult with her AAC device. Her computer system allows her several modes of communication, as well as providing the opportunity for her to work at home much of the time and avoid the hassles of special transportation arrangements. Her email contacts also prevent her from being isolated in her home environment.

Email allows composition at a slower speed because the recipient reads it at a later time (Blackstone, 2003c). Email also allows an AAC user to communicate with another person without someone else being present. Because the person's disability is not immediately visible, AAC users report that they enjoy establishing relationships with people who experience them first as a person and then learn of their disabilities.

[5]Medicare funding in the United States requires that these functions be locked and unavailable.

[6]http://disabilities.temple.edu/programs/aac/aces/.

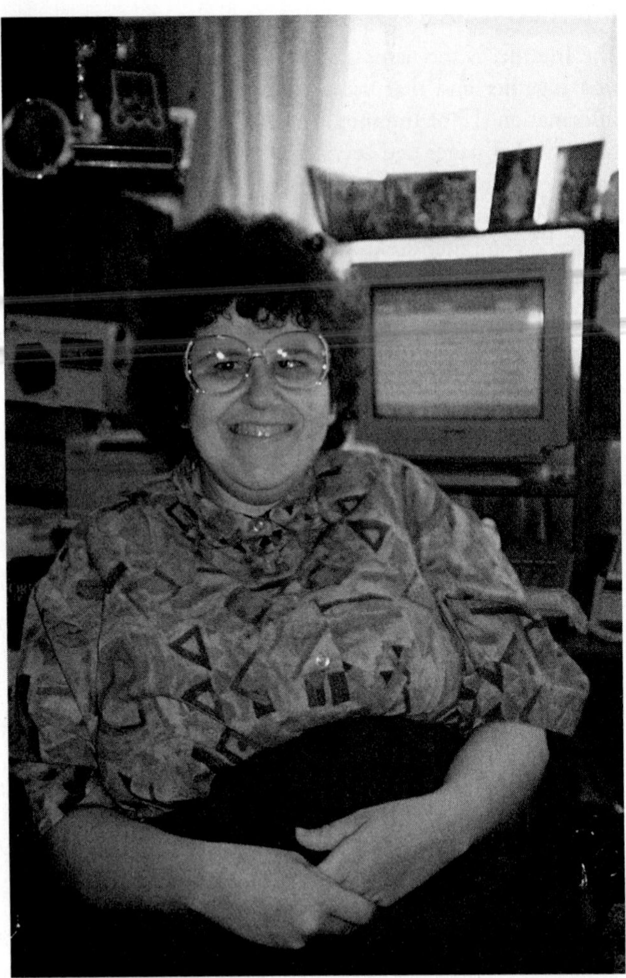

FIGURE 16-14 Access to the Internet provides Heidi with the tools necessary to pursue her PhD. She contacts her professors and students by email, conducts literature searches over the Internet, and participates in Web-based courses and discussion groups. This access is all obtained with the same laptop computer that she uses as an AAC device in face-to-face conversations.

Using social media (e.g., Facebook, Twitter) people not only obtain information from the Web, but they can also up-load and exchange information in real time and communicate with more people at once. For nondisabled people smart phones allow people to interact and get information much easier. However, Often smart phones are not easily accessible to people with CCN due to the small size of entry and display. Skype and other conferencing software can be useful in connecting people with disabilities to family and friends. Listserves, which consist of a group of individuals with common interests but are more like bulletin boards, also provide rich sources of information and friendly interaction. A popular AAC listserve is ACOLUG[7] hosted by Temple University.

Cell Phones

Physical, cognitive, and linguistic challenges facing people with CCN in accessing cell phones are very similar to those faced by individuals who have low vision or blindness (see Chapter 13). Four changes in cell phone technology described in Chapter 2 will increase access: (1) increased processing power, (2) ease of downloading into the phone, (3) wireless connection to a worldwide network, and (4) low cost and economic feasibility for persons with disabilities because these features will be built into standard cell phones (Fruchterman, 2003). The move away from proprietary software to an open source approach, much like personal computers of today, has led to greater diversity of software for tasks such as text-to-speech output, voice recognition, and downloadable user profiles that allow customization for a particular activity or task. For example, a specific stored vocabulary, word prediction/completion list, and key word index for text messaging could be resident on the Internet and downloaded as needed.

Features that were developed for people with disabilities (e.g., word completion/prediction, voice recognition, abbreviation expansion) are now built into cell phones and general-purpose computers (see Table 2-1), and these formerly specialized features are now available to individuals with CCN at low cost due to mass production of cell phones. In addition to the mainstream uses (e.g., photography for recording family events, business, or school), the camera features can be used to develop custom communication displays. For example, pictures can be integrated into visual scene displays and used as input devices. Pictures can also be used as vocabulary elements for nonliterate individuals or to enhance message generation for young children or others who have limited literacy skills, reducing the descriptive information required to convey a message.

Configurations of Commercial Speech-Generating Devices

In Chapter 2 (Figure 2-6) we described the multiple ways in which assistive technologies can be developed. AAC devices or SGDs can be based on mainstream technologies, based on software for standard computers, or developed as apps for mobile phones or tablets. We describe these three device realization approaches in this section.

Purpose-Built Speech-Generating Devices

To describe current SGDs, we have created seven categories of the major commercially available devices, shown in Table 16-5. The categories reflect different groupings of AAC device characteristics as well as the funding codes and categories for Medicare reimbursement of SGDs in the United States (Blackstone, 2001). Table 16-5 also includes accessories and mounting systems for AAC devices. We have opted for a few large categories on the basis of the most essential features, resulting in variability within each category. The format in Table 16-5 appropriately groups devices serving distinct populations. Within each category there is still significant opportunity for decision making that is based on a thorough assessment of skills and needs. Table 16-6 is a partial listing of manufacturers of AAC devices with web links that can provide up-to-date information.

[7]http://aac-rerc.psu.edu/index.php/projects/show/id/18.

TABLE 16-5 Feature Categories Commonly Combined in Commercial AAC Systems

Category	Speech Output**	Message Type**	Message Formulation Techniques**	Access Method**
Simple Scanners	None	Prestored	NA	1, 2, 4, or 5 switch scanning
Simple Speech Output (8 minutes or less) SCD, KO541**	Digitized	Prestored coverage vocabulary only	NA	Scan or direct selection, multiple methods
Simple Speech Output (greater than 8 minutes) SCD, KO542**	Digitized	Prestored coverage vocabulary only	Minimal rate enhancement or vocabulary expansion	Scan or direct selection, multiple methods
Direct Selection, Writing Only	No speech output	Message formulation	Spelling, rate enhancement	Direct selection
Spelling Only SGD, K0543**	Synthesized	Message formulation	Spelling	Direct selection
Multiple Selection Method with Rate Enhancement SGD, K0544**	Synthesized	Message formulation	Spelling and rate enhancement	Variety of selection methods and control interfaces
Software-based Multiple Selection Method with Rate Enhancement SGD, uses standard computer hardware as operating system, K0545**	Synthesized	Message formulation	Spelling and rate enhancement	Variety of selection methods and control interfaces
Mounts SGD, K0546**	NA	NA	NA	NA
Accessories, SGD K0547**	NA	NA	NA	NA

**Medicare Billing Codes

TABLE 16-6 Major Manufacturers of AAC Devices

Company	Website
AbleNet	www.ablenetinc.com/
Adaptivation, Inc.	www.adaptivation.com
Alexicom Tech	www.alexicomtech.com
Attainment Company	www.attainmentcompany.com
Augmentative Resources	www.augresources.com
CaDan Computers dba Technology for Education	www.tfeinc.com
DynaVox Mayer-Johnson	www.dynavoxsys.com
FRS Custom Solutions	www.frs-solutions.com
Jabbla	www.jabbla.com
LC Technologies	www.eyegaze.com
Possum, LTD	www.possum.co.uk
Prentke Romich Company	www.prentrom.com
Saltillo Corporation	www.saltillo.com
Sensory Software	www.sensorysoftware.com/
Therapy Box	www.tboxapps.com
Zygo Industries, Inc.	http://zygo-usa.com/

Simple scanners, the first category in Table 16-5, are generally operated by a single switch, although some can have dual-switch scanning and others allow four- or five-switch directed scanning. The devices in this category are distinguished by the use of a light to indicate the output selection, very limited vocabularies (32 items or less), no rate enhancement or built-in vocabulary, and the general absence of voice output as a standard feature.

The devices categorized as *simple speech output* are further delineated by length of recorded digital speech. They were all developed to provide a limited-vocabulary, easy-to-use output for very young children or individuals with limited language abilities. In general, they require direct selection, but some also allow scanning. Rate enhancement in this category varies from none, to levels, to simple codes or key sequences. Vocabulary storage varies from a low of a few seconds to several minutes.

The devices in the *direct selection, writing only* category are distinguished by their small size and focus on features that support writing. Some may have a built-in printer. Several devices in this category provide direct file transfer to a desktop computer, and several also have rate enhancement (generally abbreviation expansion, instant phrases, or word completion).

The devices in the *spelling only* SGD category are primarily distinguished by their dependence on spelling for message formulation. They also generally are a small size and use direct selection through a keyboard or touch screen.

The last two categories in Table 16-5 represent the highest level of sophistication in currently available devices. They incorporate all the rate enhancement approaches discussed in Chapter 6. Those in the *multiple selection method with rate enhancement* category are based on SGD hardware specifically designed for AAC. The devices in the last category are software applications that are designed to run on general-purpose computers such as laptops, tablets, or PDAs. Vocabulary storage capacity varies from a few hundred utterances to thousands of utterances. Interaction with other devices (e.g., computers, Chapter 8; power wheelchairs, Chapter 10; or EADLs, Chapter 12) and peripherals such as printers is possible for most of the devices in this group using

USB, Wi-Fi or Bluetooth connections. Within these two categories are devices that can meet the needs of a variety of consumers, from very young children who cannot spell to quantum physicists who make full use of sophisticated rate enhancement techniques. In some cases the same device can serve a wide range of needs because the software and vocabulary stored can be customized. In other cases the devices are relatively inflexible.

Devices in the last two categories provide great flexibility in control interfaces and selection methods. Several of the direct selection types allow both standard size and expanded or contracted keyboards as control interfaces. Several devices in these two categories allow scanning with single-switch or four- or five-switch directed scanning. Some also provide both one- and two-switch Morse code, and some provide direct selection by head pointing. For direct selection by head pointing, some devices use light pointers or sensors attached to the head, whereas others use reflective systems requiring the attachment of only a reflective dot. Some light pointers can also be held in the hand.

The flexibility provided by devices in these categories is particularly useful in dealing with degenerative diseases such as ALS. Initially a person may use direct selection with the hand. As this ability is lost, direct selection by head control is feasible. However, because the device has not changed, the stored vocabulary, rate enhancement strategies, and operational characteristics of the device remain the same. If direct selection by head control becomes impossible, scanning or Morse code can be used. Once again the device is not changed, and the vocabulary, rate enhancement, and operational features remain the same. This is a great advantage over having to learn a new device at each stage of the disease.

Mobile Technologies as Speech-Generating Devices

People with CCN can download applications (often called "apps") from the Internet as needed. Many of the available applications are for smart phones using the Android[8] operating system and the Apple iOS.[9] Many applications function like a full-featured SGD. The availability of these mainstream technologies will result in increasingly inexpensive hardware and software, availability of alternative access methods, and the opportunity to use standard software applications (Higginbotham & Jacobs, 2011; McNaughton & Light, 2013). Features include text-to-speech, voice personalization, a built-in default vocabulary of over 7000 items organized by category, and the availability of a variety of symbol systems. The cost is less that 10% of a purpose-built SGD. However, the individual must be able to access the smart phone or tablet both physically and visually. Mobile technologies utilize an array of highly coordinated fine motor movements for access (e.g., pinching, swiping left to right, touching) that require significant motor, cognitive, and sensory perceptual skills (McNaughton & Light, 2013). As with most SGD applications there is a set of individuals for whom this device is well suited and many for which other choices would be more successful. The number of AAC applications is growing rapidly, and there are many for people with disabilities.

Dolic, Pibernik, and Bota (2012) compared the technical characteristics and capabilities of purpose-built SGDs to mainstream tablet devices. As we have discussed, a major difference between most purpose-built SGDs and mainstream technologies is providing access to multiple communication functions (like those in Table 16-4) and electronic tools (e.g., accelerometers, GPS tracking, cameras) that could enhance access and functionality. Mainstream mobile technologies are frequently smaller than purpose-built SGDs. They also include a wide variety of mainstream smart phone applications such as texting, browsing the Internet, and GPS navigation (McNaughton & Light, 2013). For a child or adolescent user of AAC, having a purpose-built SGD carries a stigma that sends a message about being different and calling attention to a disability. On the other hand, using an iPad with an AAC app sends a message that says "I'm cool and I have the latest technology" (McNaughton & Light, 2013; Alliano et al., 2012).

Because purpose-built SGDs are often based on custom computer systems and software, the capability of the device cannot be expanded by installing additional applications made by the broader community as is the case with mainstream mobile technologies. Special-purpose SGDs are also often larger and heavier than the mainstream devices. They can be as much as 15 times more expensive than mainstream tablet devices, making them less accessible to users in countries where they are not subsidized by medical institutions. However, as pointed out by Hershberger, (2011), manufacturers repair devices that fail to operate properly, often providing service loaners while a device is being repaired. AAC device manufacturers assist clients during the assessment process by demonstrating equipment and assisting with obtaining funding for the SGD. The cost for the additional services that provide obvious benefits to clients is included in the price of the product, making traditional AAC devices significantly more expensive than comparable mainstream devices. The lack of support can be a major detriment, however, for those individuals who purchase a mainstream device and AAC app and then realize that there is little or no support for their use (Niemeijer et al., 2012).

Mainstream smart phone and tablet devices use operating systems developed and optimized for mobile devices whereas many purpose-built devices use customized PC operating systems. Mobile operating systems like iOS and Android are optimized for touch screen interfaces and consume low power. In contrast to purpose-built SGDs, mainstream mobile devices lack alternative input capabilities using switches, head control, or eye pointing. Bluetooth-enabled switch interfaces (see Chapter 8) can compensate for this in part. The Android operating system is open source, meaning that Google makes Android available to software developers (Higginbotham & Jacobs, 2011) Support for developers also means that many applications for people with CCN

[8]For Android examples, see http://www.appszoom.com/android_applications/augmentative%20communication.

[9]For iPhone, IPod Touch, and iPad apps, see http://store.apple.com/us.

can be developed at relatively low cost.[10] A negative result of Google's open-source approach is ensuring that developers produce quality apps. The lack of strong programming guidelines has resulted in a proliferation of user interfaces, with "inconsistent location and visual identity of application and system icons and control buttons" (Higginbotham & Jacobs, 2011, p. 54).

The new mobile technologies and apps have led to a consumer model for providing AAC solutions. Dave Moffatt, CEO of Prentke Romich Company, refers to this model as "Over-the-Counter AAC." Eliminating the funding process cuts time and expense, but also often eliminates the clinical component of selecting a device and creating a plan for clinical intervention (Hershberger, 2011, p. 30). In this model, the consumer buys the technology, typically a tablet, and downloads an AAC app. Because the operational requirements of AAC apps for the iPad resemble those used in other iPad apps, they may be more familiar to parents and clinicians (McNaughton & Light, 2013). The familiarity creates a level of comfort that might not exist for traditional SGDs. Consequently, many individuals show up at an assessment center with a tablet, PDA, or smart phone asking that it be made useful for their family member (Gosnell, Costello, & Shane, 2011a).

When AAC assessment and recommendation bypasses a speech-language pathologist, the results can be the purchase of AAC apps and technologies that do not match the needs and skills of the individual (Gosnell et al., 2011b; McBride, 2011). Increasingly, clinicians are asked to provide service to someone whose family has already obtained a tablet and an AAC app. Because most of the existing AAC apps are not based on research evidence, they may not meet the needs of individuals with CCN (McNaughton & Light, 2013). In contrast, developers of purpose-built SGDs collaborated with clinicians to discover better access methods, more robust vocabulary organization strategies, and more powerful customization options (Hershberger, 2011). Over the years this has resulted in products that meet many of the needs of individuals with CCN and are better matched to the user's skills and abilities.

The challenge is to maximize the potential hardware benefits and affordability of mobile technologies while also ensuring that the focus remains on enhancing communication and not on the technology (McNaughton & Light, 2013). It is also important that the support aspects of the traditional model not be lost (Hershberger, 2011). The need is to combine the consumer's access to the latest technology with the traditional SGD developers' focus on accessibility and functionality for individuals with CCN. It is possible that the clinical and consumer models for AAC will converge over the next few years, or they may remain separate. Either scenario will have profound effects on AAC service delivery.

[10]See http://www.appszoom.com/android_applications/augmentative%20communication.

A major question facing the AAC community is funding of devices and services. Funding agencies in some countries (e.g., Medicare in the United States) will not fund devices that have features that fall outside of the definition of SGDs (Hershberger, 2011). Functions such as computer or Internet access and phone (texting or voice) must be locked out if the funding agency is to pay. This limitation also applies to the service and support that is typically included with traditional solutions. Whether the funding process will evolve to allow individuals greater flexibility in acquiring products and services is a major question for the AAC community.

With so many AAC apps available, it can be overwhelming to sort through them to find the most appropriate one for an individual client. Gosnell, Costello, and Shane (2011a) provided a feature mapping tool for evaluating the suitability of AAC apps for individual users of AAC. This tool evaluates 11 clinical features: purpose of use, output, speech settings, representation, display, feedback features, rate enhancement, access, required motor competencies, support, and additional miscellaneous information. Alliano et al. (2012) applied this tool to describe the features of 21 AAC apps in three categories: symbols only, symbols and text-to-speech, and text-to-speech only. Of the 21 apps, 2 were available for free download and 19 required purchase.

Setting Up an AAC System for Use

Mounting SGDs to Wheelchairs

It is often necessary to attach the AAC device to a wheelchair and mount a switch or other control interface where the individual can easily access it. This is a critical step in the implementation process. For the SGD to be accessible by the user, it must be mounted so he or she can use it. If a switch or other interface is required to control the SGD, it must also be placed where it is accessible. Other changes need to be considered and their impact anticipated. For example, if the person is getting a new wheelchair and the assessment and recommendation were based on the old chair, things may not all fit together properly on the new chair.

The mounting of switches and other control interfaces for ease of use is discussed in Chapter 7. If the AAC user has a wheelchair, the SGD must be appropriately mounted to the wheelchair in a manner that is both sturdy and flexible. As shown in Table 16-5, mounting systems are considered accessories that are typically funded as part of the total AAC system. There are some companies that specialize in mounting systems,[11] and there are other systems that are available from manufacturers of SGDs. The complexity and need for flexibility in location varies by person.

There is a concept from prosthetics called "gadget tolerance" that refers to how much "stuff" people can stand to have around them in their personal space. Some people are happy to have many different gadgets available to them while others are overwhelmed by only one. This concept must be

[11]For example, Daedelus Technologies, Inc, http://www.daessy.com/; Blue Sky Designs, Inc, http://www.mountnmover.com/. Also see: http://www.abledata.com/abledata.cfm?pageid=19327&top=10857&trail=22,10825,10837.

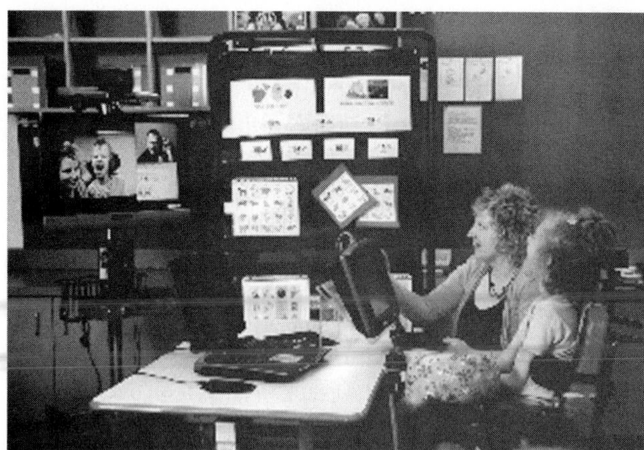

FIGURE 16-15 An AAC device can change the dynamics of interpersonal interaction (see text).

taken into account when mounting an SGD and associated switches to a wheelchair. The mounting for a switch may be a part of the seating and positioning system (e.g., switches attached to a head rest or to the lap tray).

Once the SGD is mounted, it may create a physical distance between the individual and communication partners (Figure 16-15). The location of the device when mounted on the chair needs to take this factor into consideration. The device must also be mounted with the option to move the device out of the way for transfers or times when it is not in use. Ease of removal from the wheelchair is also important for transportation on a bus or in a van (see Chapter 11). In Figure 16-15 there are a lot of factors at play. The mounting of the communication device is set so the child using it can see the display for scanning access, but this location for the display can block face-to-face interaction. Her mother is sitting next to her and this helps to see the display, but this location also limits face-to-face interaction and results in a close physical relationship between the person using AAC and their communication partner. This may not always be comfortable for one or both of the participants in the communication interaction.

Mounting systems that are specifically designed to mount SGDs to wheelchairs have several advantages. They are generally more stable because they are matched to the individual client's needs. These devices have a fixed orientation and position that do not change when they are moved out of the way for transfer or taken off of the wheelchair so they do not need to be re-adjusted. Most of these systems swing away so that the individuals can perform their activities of daily living or transfer out of the wheelchair without changing the position of the SGD on the mounting system. Commercial mounting systems generally have a main structure that provides support and a variety of mounting plates that are matched to the most common SGDs. They also provide mounting brackets for attaching the system to a wheelchair. Various types of wheelchair tubing are accommodated in these systems. For most mounting systems, the user is dependent on someone else to move the device out of the way and then move it

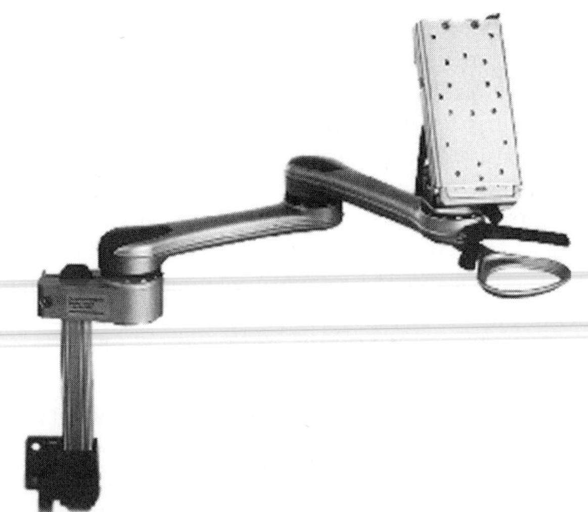

FIGURE 16-16 The user of this mounting system can move it out of the way by gripping and pressing on the silver ring. (Courtesy of Blue Sky Designs, Minneapolis, MN, http://www.mountnmover.com/.)

back for use. If the other person isn't paying attention, the user may have no access to a means of communication. The Mountnmover from Blue Sky Designs[12] (Figure 16-16) has provision for the user to move the SGD out of the way independently.

How to Choose Parts for a Mounting System[13]

Providing a stabilized and accessible custom mounting system involves many considerations. There are many different component parts and mechanisms available. The creation of a mounting system may include Velcro, glue, duct tape, carpet, pipe, rods, clamps, knobs, wood, fabric, paper clips, foam, corrugated cartons, or any other handy material as well as commercially available parts or complete systems. When designing a mounting system for an individual, it is often useful to obtain assistance from the SGD manufacturer or an assistive technology center or one of the companies specializing in mounting systems. This may require that digital photographs of the client be taken in a variety of locations where the SGD will be used (the easy chair in the living room, a bed, the wheelchair, at work, at school) together with the SGD to be mounted.

These digital photographs can then be emailed to share physical information and get help and suggestions on how to proceed. Box 16-3 contains a step-by-step approach to select an SGD mounting system for a wheelchair. Figure 16-17 shows an example of how a completed installation of an SGD will look. The clinician may be responsible for ensuring that all of the mounting components are adjusted for maximum efficiency and minimal effort by the person using AAC. Mounting systems also need to be checked frequently to be sure that the connections are tight and secure. Nuts and bolts can loosen from vibration during use.

[12] http://www.mountnmover.com/.

[13] Courtesy of Zygo Industries.

BOX 16-3 Suggestions for Developing a Mounting System for an SGD on a Wheelchair

Determine where in space the device needs to be when it's mounted:

- With a digital camera, take pictures of the user in the wheelchair from different vantage points. If possible, have someone hold the device in position for the photos. Otherwise, sketch on the pictures where the device should be.
- Determine where on the wheelchair the mount needs to attach and measure the diameter of the wheelchair tubing or note the cross-section configuration and dimensions (e.g., round, square, rectangular); look for mounting holes on the frame under the seat cushion sides.
- Decide how the mount and/or the device is to be removed from the wheelchair. Does the device need to swing out of the way for transfer or when getting close to tables? Does the device need to be placed flat on a table or desk when it's removed from the wheelchair? Does the device need to be moved from one mount to another?
- Determine the required strength of the mount: heavy duty mounts for heavy devices or for forceful users, medium strength or light weight for lighter, more protected units.
- Decide on the mounting components required.
- Select the wheelchair clamp from the wheelchair tubing diameter or frame configuration.
- Consider whether the vertical mount tubing can clear the parts of the wheelchair between the clamp and its supporting end.
- Is there a wheelchair lap tray to clear? Is there a joystick on the chair? If so, make sure that the mounting system will not interfere with these components.
- Select the style of the mount: fixed, right-angle tubing; straight tubing with a right-angle joint; folding, etc.
- Choose the device mounting tray or plate and tube clamp to secure it to the mounting tubing.

(Courtesy Zygo Industries, Portland, OR, zygo-usa.com)

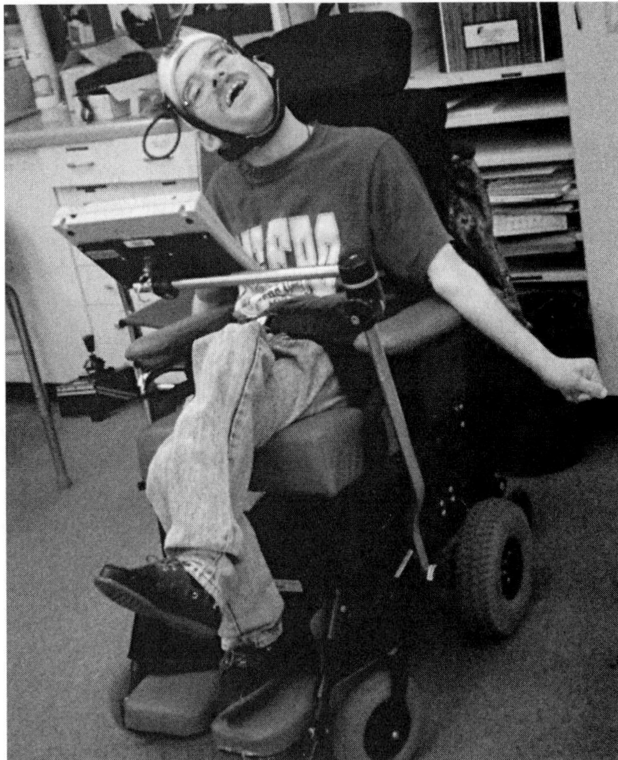

FIGURE 16-17 Implementation of an AAC system includes proper mounting of the AAC device and control interface to the wheelchair if necessary. Here is a completed installation ready for checkout.

BOX 16-4 Managing the AAC Implementation Process

Who will monitor the overall program of use of this system?
How much direct supervision does the individual require when using the system?
Who will provide supervision and assist in the day-to-day operation of the system?
Who should be called if the system does not work properly?

Implementation of Augmentative Communication Systems

As discussed in Chapter 5 in the total process of delivering assistive technologies, the recommendation of a communication device based on a formal assessment is only the beginning of the process. Once funding is obtained and the device(s) is/are procured, implementation begins. Other steps that may be required include customization to integrate components from different manufacturers (e.g., a communication device from one manufacturer and a control interface from another), programming of a device to include vocabulary specific to the individual consumer, fitting of the device to the consumer's wheelchair, and mounting a control interface in an accessible location. It is impossible in one chapter to cover all the issues related to AAC implementation. Beukelman and Mirenda (2013) is a source rich in practical information and case studies related to AAC implementation.

Once the AAC systems are obtained, the implementation of the AAC system begins. At this time, the clinician may be tasked with making the system work for the individual. A number of steps may be required to make the AAC device usable. Box 16-4 lists some important steps in managing the implementation process. Sometimes it is necessary to integrate components from different manufacturers (e.g., a communication device from one manufacturer and a switch or mounting system from others). Almost always it will be necessary to program (and plan on reprogramming) a device to add the specific vocabulary the individual user will need.

To gain more insight into this process, there are also frequent case studies presented in journals such as *Augmentative and Alternative Communication* and newsletters such as *Communication Matters*, *Augmentative Communication News*, and online with resources including YouTube and other video sites. These case studies vary from anecdotal reports written by individuals who use AAC devices or by those working with them. They include formal case studies and single-subject research designs. In this section, we discuss the most basic considerations related to training and follow-up. Things do not always progress smoothly when a new AAC system is being set up for an individual. Fields (1991) presents a case study indicating the steps that one family went through to implement an AAC system for their son (see Case Study 16-6). There is also a listserv for those who rely on AAC at http://listserv.temple.edu/archives/acolug.html. Many practical considerations related to the set-up and use of SGDs, strategies for using devices, and for augmented communication in general and related topics are discussed on this list.

Best practice suggests that the individual or family go through a trial period with the SGD as a means of obtaining valuable information. For example, the person's interest in using the SGD may increase when she sees how effective it is in meeting her needs. Or, conversely, their interest in using the SGD may decrease because she may not like how it sounds, how her friends react to it, or how difficult it is to use. A trial period can also help the multidisciplinary team to identify specific short- and long-term training goals for the person and her communication partners so she can develop communicative competencies that enable her to interact effectively and efficiently. If there are special features that require learning new skills (such as storing and retrieving information), these may be assessed during the trial. For individuals who prefer a longer trial period, many companies will lease a device for a 1- to 3-month period. The outcomes of an SGD assessment should include recommendations for the SGD, as well as any accessories or mounts and instructional strategies required to meet the person's unique needs and goals.

Vocabulary Selection

When a person needs an augmentative communication device, it is because he or she cannot rely exclusively on speech. In order for them to benefit from an augmentative communication device, it must have a stored vocabulary that they can access. Determining what that vocabulary should be can be very challenging.

The vocabulary is often not "built-in" or preprogrammed by the manufacturer (or if it is, it is so generic that it is useful only as a starting point), and once an AAC system is selected for an individual, it is necessary to create an initial vocabulary set that can be programmed into an electronic device or used with a nonelectronic system. Some dedicated SGDs and mobile device AAC apps may have many preprogrammed vocabulary sets provided from the manufacturer. The challenge is to determine a good fit between the individual using AAC and the vocabulary sets.

There are several categories of messages used by people who rely on AAC (Beukelman & Mirenda, 2013). The conversational categories shown in Table 16-7 provide a useful framework for initial vocabulary selections. Conversational messages begin with greetings and then often involve small talk as a transition between the greeting and information sharing. Small talk often utilizes scripts for initiating and maintaining conversations. In general, SGDs do not support small talk well because it is spontaneous and unpredictable. Small talk may be generic and usable in different conversations with different people. Specific small talk is more focused. Examples of both types of small talk are shown in Table 16-8.

TABLE 16-7 Categories to Be Included in Conversational AAC Systems

Category	Sample Vocabulary
Initiating and interaction	Hey, I've got something to say. Check this out. Come talk to me. May I help you?
Greetings	Hello, I'm pleased to meet you. I'm (name) and you are? Where have you been? I've been waiting forever. What's happening?
Response to greetings	I'm fine. Great, how are you? Not so hot, and you? I've had better days. Hanging in there.
Requests	I'd like a ___________. (object, event) I'd like to go to ________. (place, event)
Information exchange	What time is it? I have a question. The concert begins at 8:00 pm.
Commenting	I agree (disagree). What a great idea! Uh-huh. OK.
Wrap-up/farewell	Well, gotta go. See you later Bye, nice talking to you.
Conversational repair	Let's start over. That's not what I meant. You misunderstood me.

TABLE 16-8 Generic and Specific Small Talk

Generic	Specific
How is your family?	How is your wife?
What's happening?	What are you doing?
Isn't that beautiful!	That is a beautiful flower.
Good story!	Good story about your vacation.
She is great.	She is a great teacher.

A common form of conversational interaction for adults, particularly older adults, is story telling. Stories entertain, teach, and establish social closeness. An important role for those who support people using AAC systems is to help them remember and describe stories (often by interviewing family and friends as well as the AAC user or obtaining photographs, journals, or other records of past experiences). Once the stories are described, then the person will need assistance with programming the story into the device. The person can then retell/play back the story over and over for different audiences (individuals or groups). Devices typically allow playing back a stored message one sentence at a time by the individual pressing a key or hitting a switch to allow the pace of the story to be controlled.

BOX 16-5 Some Vocabulary Suggestions for a Zoo Outing

- Look at the poop!
- I want to see the ________
  - Monkeys
  - Giraffe
  - Lions
  - Birds
  - Etc.
- I'm hungry.
- Can we buy an ice cream?
- Let's ride the carousel.
- Look at the snake.

Vocabulary needs vary by the context (e.g., school, home, shopping mall), communication mode (SGD, communication board, gesture), and individual characteristics. Beukelman and Mirenda (2013) compiled a composite list of the 100 most frequently used words for a variety of categories, including age and gender. *Emerging communicators* are often preliterate (those who cannot read or spell) and they need to communicate essential messages. This is called a *coverage vocabulary*. Since generation of novel utterances by spelling isn't possible, the AAC team must ensure that as many messages as possible are stored in the device for easy retrieval. The specific vocabulary is highly dependent on the individual's needs. Most often the coverage vocabulary is organized by context with separate displays or pages for different activities. Preliterate individuals also need a developmental vocabulary that includes words and concepts that are not yet understood. These are selected on the basis of their educational value, not for functional purposes, and they encourage language and vocabulary growth. New words can be added around special events or activities, especially when an activity is to be experienced for the first time (e.g., going to the circus or to the zoo). The developmental vocabulary also encourages the use of different language structures reflecting semantic categories. A child's system could be programmed with things that he or she would want to do during the activity. Box 16-5 has suggestions for a zoo activity.

Required vocabulary resources for individuals who are literate include a core vocabulary that is used with a variety of situations and partners and occurs frequently. There are word lists based on successful general patterns, the needs of a specific individual, and the performance of natural speakers or writers in similar contexts (http://aac.unl.edu/). A list of 500 words covered 80% of total utterances for individuals who are operationally and socially competent with AAC systems (see training section of this chapter) (Beukelman & Mirenda, 2013). Words and messages that are unique to the individual are included in a *fringe vocabulary* that includes names of people, places, activities, and preferred expressions. This approach personalizes the AAC system by complementing the core vocabulary list. The fringe vocabulary content is often identified by family and friends as well as the individual. The initial items are those that are of high interest to the user and have potential for frequent use. It is important to include items that denote a range of semantic notions and pragmatic functions. To ease learning, the vocabulary should reflect the "here and now" and have potential for later multiword use. Ease of production by the individual and interpretation by the partner is also essential. It is also important to include conversational functions, such as those shown in Table 16-6.

In addition to word lists, there are a number of ways of determining what specific vocabulary is needed by an individual. One useful resource is the *Hearing Them Into Voice*[14] inventory that can be used by families and other informants to identify current language usage as well as identified communication needs. A nice feature of this form is that it poses questions in a functional way that makes it easy for families to respond. The Website also contains examples of filled-in forms to guide families in completing the form. While the format as presented on the Website is for children, it can easily be adapted for use with adults. Since it captures the specific things an individual needs to say as well as how the individual currently communicates, the *Hearing Them Into Voice* form is useful for group settings to ensure that a variety of communication partners communicate in a consistent way. The various partners can also identify a greater range of needs than any one respondent is likely to identify alone.

Environmental inventories document the individual's experiences by recording precipitating events and subsequent consequences (Beukelman & Mirenda, 2013). For example, if a resident of a group home hits another resident, it is important to note what caused the hitting (the precursor) and then to determine if vocabulary such as "I don't like what you did" might have provided an alternative for the person rather than hitting. The documentation includes words that might have been used by peers with and without disabilities. The identified pool of vocabulary items is reduced to a list of most critical words or concepts that the individual needs and can effectively use. *Communication diaries* and *checklists* are records of words and phrases needed by an individual for AAC that are kept by informants such as family members. There are some published lists that can also act as a shortcut to vocabulary selection (Beukelman & Mirenda, 2013).

Participants in adult programs (daycare and residential) who have intellectual disabilities have unique needs for vocabulary that differs from those of typical adults or children (with or without disabilities) (Graves, 2000). Using diaries compiled by staff working with adults who needed AAC, over 80% of the conversational topics were functional (e.g., physical needs and daily activities) for those with the most severe disabilities. For individuals with more moderate disabilities, the percentage of functional topics was twice that of physical needs. Emotional feelings (of anger, anxiety, fear, love) amounted to only 3.4% of all topics. Possible reasons for this low response may relate to the cognitive difficulties in expressing feelings and to cultural factors that limit the degree to which staff are able to provide emotional support

[14]Available from http://www.drsharonrogers.com/hearing-them-into-voice/.

to residents. These results differ from standard vocabulary lists in content and emphasis, and they reinforce the need for care in applying standardized vocabulary lists to AAC vocabulary selection.

Because most AAC devices are programmable, it is possible to continually add or change vocabulary as needs change for adults or children or as children's language skills develop. The choice of which additional vocabulary items to include is generally based on needs that occur frequently but are not part of the stored vocabulary. These needs may be identified by family, care providers, and other communication partners. Another reason for adding vocabulary is that new situations arise. For example, a grandchild may have been born recently and is being brought to his grandmother for the first time. Vocabulary about "proud parents," "he's adorable," "he has your grandfather's eyes," "is he a good eater?" would be added to allow her to talk about her grandchild during the visit and afterwards. In the majority of cases, vocabulary development (after the initial set is implemented) is relatively slow and occurs over a long period. Some devices (e.g., word completion or prediction systems) automatically add items to the stored vocabulary on the basis of the frequency of use.

Beukelman and his colleagues and students at the University of Nebraska at Lincoln have compiled a large number of resources relating to vocabulary selection and messaging in AAC. This information can be accessed through their Website (http://aac.unl.edu/vocabulary.html). Included in this resource are core vocabulary lists consisting of high-frequency words for preschool and school-age children, young adults, and older adults. They also include unabridged vocabulary lists (with use statistics) for nondisabled persons (20- to 30-year-old adults, older adults, and preschool children) and AAC users (four volumes). Vocabulary lists of small talk for children and adults, as well as context-specific messages suggested by AAC specialists, are also included. This site also provides vocabulary lists for school settings (preschool activities and classroom activities).

Finally, vocabulary lists for use as initial recommendations in AAC are reported, as well as references for AAC messaging and vocabulary selection. This site is a rich source of information for those charged with developing vocabulary for individuals who use AAC.

Physical Skill Development

AAC devices require physical skill, whether for direct selection or scanning, to operate them effectively. It takes practice to develop this skill, and it can be useful to separate the physical skills required for the use of an augmentative communication device from the communication skills required. This aspect of training is described in Chapter 6.

If the individual has insufficient motor skill to make reliable selections but is expected to develop the necessary motor control, it is important that this *physical competence* be developed separately from the *use* of the physical skill for communication. If the clinician attempts to teach motor skills by using the communication device, it is possible that errors in selection caused by lack of motor skill will be misinterpreted as lack of communicative skill; for example, the person may have intended to select the picture of the apple (signifying "eat") but missed the mark and selected the picture of the cup ("drink"). Conversely, errors caused by communication or language inability may be interpreted as motor selection difficulties. In the previous example, the person may have been capable of physically choosing apple but chose cup because he or she did not understand either the question or the communication task.

Training System Use: Developing Communicative Competence

When the installation is completed, the individual and those working with him or her (e.g., care providers, family, teachers, employers, therapists, and speech-language pathologists) can begin the process of learning to use the device. Depending on the complexity of the device and the sophistication of the features included, this process can take from a few hours to several months.

The development of communicative competence is most effective when a comprehensive program is used. One such approach is the System for Augmenting Language (SAL) (Sevick, Romski, & Adamson, 2004). SAL involves a multimodal approach to training of individuals who rely on AAC, their partners, and continuing follow-up. Sevick, Romski, and Adamson (2004) illustrate the application of SAL through a case study of a preschool child who used both a VOCA and a manual display consisting of PCS symbols. For young children with cognitive and language disabilities, the development of both expressive and receptive vocabulary can be developed by using a VOCA in an exercise to teach requesting (Brady, 2000). Children were taught to request objects using PCS symbols on a VOCA. After learning these symbols, the children's comprehension was evaluated. The use of the VOCA during the labeling instruction appeared to increase later comprehension of the symbols.

Scripts that are programmed into an AAC device can be used in a training paradigm. One formal approach is called "Script Builder."[15] The scripts are a way of training individuals to achieve greater social competence and more effective interactions. The scripts are coplanned and oriented toward the development of social closeness by encouraging social purposes and a sense of belonging. Typical topics of trivia, sports, gossip, hanging out, and "who's cute" allow the individual to display aspects of his or her personality through humor, teasing, whining, and joke telling. Scripts change perceptions of individuals who use AAC because greater social competence is evident. Some scripts focus on information content, others on conversation scripts (new information plus social closeness). Example scripts are shown in Box 16-6. There are three roles in the training: the individual who is developing AAC skills, his or her partner, and a "prompter" who prompts only when necessary in an unobtrusive way. The partner's role is communicating as naturally as possible, pausing when necessary, and not prompting at all. All social

[15]Linda J. Burkhart, Eldersberg, MD, www.Lburkhart.com.

BOX 16-6 Sample Scripts

The Prom—Getting Ready
Hey, come here.
Want to know a secret?
It's here in my bag.
It's one of my favorites.
I don't think you've seen this before.
Take a guess.
Want to see it now?
Naw, take another guess.
Oh, you've waited long enough.
Oops, can't get it out.
Oh all right—here it is.
Have you ever seen anything like this before?
I've got a ton of things in this bag.
Let's tell everyone but the teacher!
Hey, Mom!
Come here!
Oh no!
I've got to do my make-up for the prom!
It's getting late.
Hurry, Mom!
Remember, my dress is blue.
Let's do lipstick first.
Please . . . not purple!
Keep my lipstick on my lips.
Don't get it on my teeth.
I don't want to look like Bozo.
I have that red hair!
I want to look like Britney Spears.
She's beautiful.
Could I have a little more mascara, please?
Thanks!
I can't wait to get to the prom!
Mom, you did a great job.
I don't want to miss the dance.
Let's go!

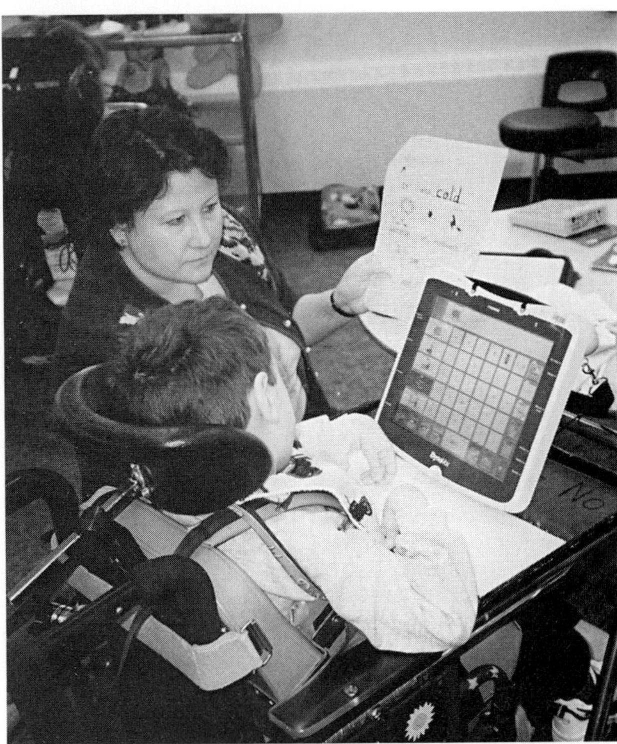

FIGURE 16-18 Development of operational competence with an AAC device requires a structured training program in which the device features are carefully explained and skill in their use is developed.

scripts start with a greeting and include a range of communicative functions such as positive and negative comments, teasing, and questioning. They provide for multiple turns and use topic maintainers like "tell me more." They need to be designed to ensure that the individual doesn't get "backed into a corner." The vocabulary chosen is appropriate to the individual's age, setting, and personality.

Communicative competence depends on many factors (Light, 1989). The context in the HAAT model affects competence in several ways. The partner and his or her skill in listening, the environment of use, and cultural factors all contribute to or detract from communicative competence. The degree of competence is also variable, and complete mastery of an AAC device is not necessary to have functional communication interactions. Light (1989) describes four areas of competence required for successful use of AAC devices: (1) operational, (2) linguistic, (3) social, and (4) strategic.

Operational competence requires the physical skills described earlier and an understanding of the technical operation of the AAC device. AAC devices must be made easier to learn. Current AAC devices (purpose-built and based on mainstream apps) require up to 2 years of organized study to become fluent in the operation of a device by older children, adolescents, and young adults (Williams, Krezman, & McNaughton, 2008). Once again, the degree of operational competence can be quite variable, from very basic operation to advanced features. An AAC device is like a musical instrument that can be played by an accomplished AAC communicator.

Operational competence includes the cognitive demands dictated by rate-enhancement techniques. Training operational competence requires a systematic introduction of technical features, coupled with ample opportunities for practice in their use, as shown in Figure 16-18.

The individual's facilitators must also be trained in certain operational features of the device (e.g., battery charging, connecting control interfaces), even though they will not develop the same level of competence as the individual.

The second phase, basic operation, includes how to connect the device to the control interface, how to charge batteries, how to attach it to a wheelchair, how to add vocabulary using rate-enhancement techniques (e.g., codes), and an introduction to troubleshooting in case the device fails to operate properly.

The last features to be introduced are those related to storage of new vocabulary, input acceleration techniques, and vocabulary manipulation features, such as text editing and reformatting the output. Often the first two phases are accomplished in one session. However, in some cases, they may require multiple training sessions, and the process is often a lengthy one that may be integrated with the other aspects of training in communicative competence.

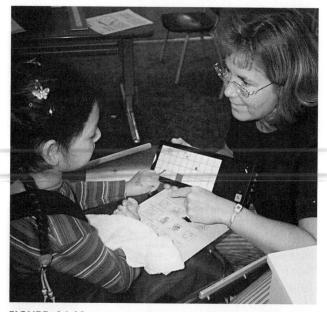

FIGURE 16-19 Development of linguistic competence is often taught in conjunction with other functional tasks, such as the one shown here.

Linguistic competence requires that the symbol system and rules of organization be understood by the individual using the AAC system. As Light (1989) points out, the individual often must be competent in two languages: the spoken language of the community and the language of the AAC device. It is likely that the individual also lacks models of proficient use in the language of the device. Development of competence in this area may require many hours of practice. Often this practice is built around a functional reading task, such as that shown in Figure 16-19.

In contrast to the typical "drill and practice" approach to developing vocabulary and AAC use, Mirenda and Santogrossi (1985) used a prompt-free strategy to teach a young child to use a picture-based communication board. The approach involved a four-step process, which began with a picture of a soft drink being available to the child during her regular therapy session. A drink was visible to her, as was the picture of the drink. The child was not told that touching the picture would result in her getting a drink, nor was she prompted in any way to touch the picture. If she touched the drink directly, she was told that she could have some later. If she accidentally or deliberately touched the picture, she was immediately given the drink with the explanation, "Yes, if you touch the picture, you may have the drink." Once the deliberate response had been established over several sessions, Mirenda and Santogrossi proceed to shape the pointing behavior by progressively moving the picture farther away, until it was out of sight and the child had to actively find it. As the child became proficient in this task, the number of pictures was increased to four and the process repeated for the other choices. Eventually the child was able to generalize to a language board of 120 pictures. The advantage of this approach is that the child learns the meaning and significance of the symbolic representation by discovery rather than by drill, which leads to greater generalization and more functional use of the AAC system.

Many people who use AAC devices have little or no experience in social discourse. Even individuals who have used natural language for communication and who have sustained a disease or injury are faced with a very different mode of interaction when an AAC device is used. Rules of conversation are altered, and the perception of the individual by his or her communication partners is different. To be socially competent, the individual must have knowledge, judgment, and skills in both sociolinguistic (e.g., turn taking, initiating a conversation, conversational repair) and sociorelational areas (Light, 1989). The latter term describes the understanding of interaction between individuals. The effective communication device user is described (Light, 1988) as having a positive self-image, interest in his or her partner, skill at drawing others into the conversation, ability to put a partner at ease, and active participation in the conversation. These are sociorelational skills, and the degree to which they are understood and used is one measure of social competence. These skills are best taught in the contexts in which they are to be used. One example of such training is shown in Figure 16-20, in which the child is being taught strategies for interacting with an adult partner.

Every person who uses an AAC system develops strategies to make that use more effective. Examples include letting the partner guess the next letter on a spelling board and using gestures (e.g., waving to indicate that a misunderstanding has occurred) in conjunction with an electronic device. Strategic competence describes the degree to which the person is able to develop adaptive strategies to make the most of the system. These may differ in different contexts. For example, a child's speech may be better understood at home than at school. He or she will rely on the electronic SGD more in school but will also develop strategies to make maximal use of both systems.

Just as the individual using the AAC system must develop several types of competencies, there are many ways of carrying out the training. One approach, shown in Figure 16-20, is to simulate a situation, model the types of interaction likely to occur, and have the user "practice" the strategies and skills necessary to make it a success. This step can be followed by an actual situation in which the clinician accompanies the user as he or she encounters the situation. The clinician can then prompt the user at appropriate times, add encouragement, and help to clarify when necessary. This combination of clinic-based practice and community-based skill development is often very effective.

For training to be effective, staff must have sufficient skill and experience to assist the AAC user, which requires training for those who are supporting AAC use. In a recent survey, close to 20% of the professionals and close to 30% of the family members and caregivers consider the professional supporting the AAC user only slightly knowledgeable on AAC (Niemeijer, Donnellan, & Robledo, 2012). To further complicate matters, in an inclusive educational environment, 16 teachers and educational personnel needed to learn how

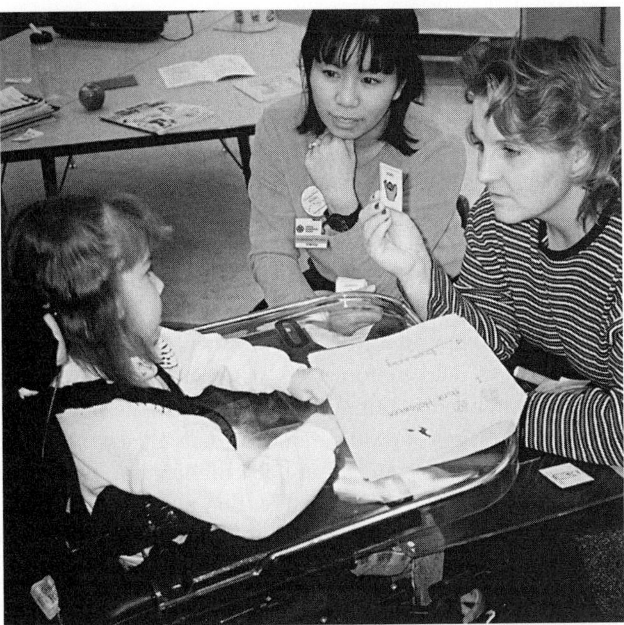

FIGURE 16-20 AAC users need to learn about conversational conventions and strategies. Training of these skills is often done in simulated situations. Here an aide is teaching the child how to use her AAC tools to interact with another adult partner.

to program and support the child's use of an AAC device over a 5-year period (Williams, Krezman, & McNaughton, 2008). Schepis and Reid (2003) identified seven basic steps in competence- and performance-based training for staff. These include specifying desired outcomes, roles for staff to support individuals in achieving these outcomes, providing both written and oral expectations and instructions to staff, demonstration of how to perform duties, and observation of staff performing the duties with corrective feedback as necessary.

Training of the individual who relies on AAC is only effective if communication partners are also trained. For children, the training of parents to recognize communication attempts and to understand the operational, linguistic, strategic, and social competencies is also important. Bruno and Dribbon (1998) evaluated a parent training program conducted as part of an AAC summer camp experience where parents attended the camp with their children. The camp featured structured therapy sessions, activities with nondisabled campers, and activities planned for families. The parent training had both device (conducted by manufacturers' representatives) and interaction training aspects. Parents reported making positive changes in both operational and interactional skills during the camp (Bruno & Dribbon, 1998). These changes were reflected in gains made by the children in skills related to the use of pragmatic functions (e.g., giving and requesting information, requesting assistance, responding, and protesting) over the course of the camp. The camp training significantly increased the degree to which parents gave their children access to the AAC system. In some cases, skills in these areas remained constant at the 6-month follow-up, and in some there was a decrease. The areas of social exchange and giving of information continued to increase at the 6-month follow-up evaluation.

AAC training can be both complicated and lengthy (Beukelman & Mirenda, 2013). Light and Binger (1998) have developed a seven-step process for developing AAC communication competence: (1) specify the goal, do baseline observations; (2) select vocabulary; (3) teach the facilitators how to support development of the target skill; (4) teach the skill to the target individual; (5) check for generalization; (6) evaluate outcomes; and (7) complete maintenance checks. Light and Binger provide data collection and assessment forms and strategies for implementing this program. ACETS (Augmentative Communication Employment Training and Supports)[16] has been developed specifically to assist those who rely on AAC in seeking employment. A formal training manual is available for this program that is based on three principles: (1) immersion in the workplace culture, (2) acquiring a broad base of employment-related skills and experience, and (3) support of individualized goals.

AUGMENTATIVE AND ALTERNATIVE COMMUNICATION EVALUATION AND ASSESSMENT

The goals of AAC intervention are: (1) to document communication needs, (2) to determine how many needs can be met through current communication methods, including speech, and (3) to reduce the number of unmet communication needs through systematic AAC intervention (Beukelman & Mirenda, 2013).

AAC assessment requires systematic consideration of many factors (Beukelman & Mirenda, 2013; Lloyd, Fuller, & Arvidson, 1997). These factors are described by the four components of the HAAT model. The most important step is to define the goals and needs of the person with CCN and his or her current and potential communication partners through a careful analysis of the desired activity or activities. The Social Networks tool is useful at this stage (Box 16-7). An evaluation of the various contexts in which communication will occur helps to further inform the assessment goals. The Participation Model (see below) helps to define opportunities and barriers in various contexts. Once the goals, needs (activity component of the HAAT model), and contexts (HAAT model) are clearly understood and agreed to by all team members (e.g., person with CCN, parent, spouse, teacher, employer, care provider, speech pathologist, OT, PT, and others), physical, sensory, cognitive, and language skills (the human component of the HAAT model) are assessed as they relate to augmentative communication. Finally, if a low- or high-tech AAC system component (e.g., SGD, computer) is indicated, the assistive technology characteristics can be matched to consumer skills and goals by systematically identifying the human/technology interface, the processing (e.g., SGD rate enhancement, vocabulary storage), and the activity output modes.

[16]Institute on Disabilities, Temple University, Philadelphia, PA, http://disabilities.temple.edu.

BOX 16-7 Social Networks

Social Networks is a formalized approach to the development of communication goals, the planning of AAC interventions, and measurement of progress. It is a tool that enables the perceptions of many AAC stakeholders to be considered when planning an intervention. It also provides a structure for gathering information on the basis of potential partners for communication. A pilot study of the *Social Networks Inventory* revealed some interesting features of AAC use related to the circle of partners shown in Figure 16-4. In the *First Circle*, people who use AAC tend to rely on speech, body language, and gesture. In the *Second Circle*, there is greater variety of AAC techniques that depend on both skill and access to systems and on vocabulary and trained partners. There is more reliance on high-tech devices and less on nonsymbolic modes in the *Third Circle*. Also, emergent and context-dependent AAC communicators often need lots of support when communicating with people in this circle. Many context-dependent communicators primarily use their AAC devices with service providers in the *Fourth Circle*. When communicating with unfamiliar partners (*Fifth Circle*), a range of conventional AAC approaches is required and significant partner support is needed when the individual does not use an SCD.

The Augmentative and Alternative Communication Team

AAC interventions require a collaborative team approach. Each member of the AAC team has important roles and responsibilities:

The client and family have the greatest knowledge of the daily communication needs of the person with CCN. Family members are often the individuals' primary communication partners and serve as advocates and facilitators. There is an ethical responsibility to involve individuals in decisions that affect them. "Individuals who use AAC also have a right to be present, receive clear information, and provide input regarding best practices in training for AAC professionals and the research and design of new systems" (Williams et al., 2008, p. 202).

The *speech-language pathologist* has the greatest general understanding of communication in general and can assess language and communication needs, abilities, and skills; select AAC materials and technologies; and teach the individual, family, and staff to use AAC system components effectively.

The *teacher* sets educational goals and oversees classroom implementation of each child's AAC system and has knowledge of literacy, social interaction, and education.

The *physical therapist (PT) or occupational therapist (OT)* carries out the motor evaluation, addresses seating and positioning, evaluates physical access to the AAC system, and has knowledge of how to support writing, drawing, and other activities of daily living.

The *teacher's aide/job coach* is also critical to the success of implementation. This individual supports the person in the school/work setting. Key team members are often referred to as "natural supports" because they have a continuing relationship with the individual (e.g., family, friends, coworkers, and employer). On occasion, physicians, psychologists, vision specialists, and other professionals also play an important role on AAC teams.

Assessment of Persons With Complex Communication Needs

Several types of AAC assessment may be conducted. A predictive assessment has a goal of understanding the client needs and status today, predicting future needs, and selecting a system to meet both of these. A serial assessment is a continuing evaluation to meet changing needs (e.g., as a child develops). A curriculum-based assessment is continuous in classrooms to help coordinate AAC interventions with the achievement of educational goals. In any case, the assessment process takes into consideration the individual's skills and abilities and current and future communication needs and preferences. From these, an intervention plan is developed.

The overall goals of AAC assessment are as follows: (1) to document communication needs, (2) to determine how many needs can be met through current communication methods, including speech, and (3) to reduce the number of unmet communication needs through systematic AAC intervention. Each member of the AAC team described earlier in this chapter has a specific role in the assessment process.

There are many tools available to the AAC team. However, assessment approaches designed for other populations often require adaptations of materials and procedures so that assessment results are valid and reliable, as described by Beukelman and Mirenda (2013). One tool is the Social Networks Inventory described later in this section. It enables the perceptions of many individuals to be considered when planning an intervention (Blackstone, 2003a) and it provides a structure for gathering of information. When used in combination, the HAAT model, Social Networks, and the Participation Model (Beukelman & Mirenda, 2013) provide a comprehensive framework for ensuring that all information needed for successful AAC implementation is obtained during the assessment process.

The Social Networks Inventory

The Social Networks Inventory,[17] described in Box 16-7, is based on a number of theoretical frameworks including the circle of friends (Falvey et al., 1994), the field of social networks, the Participation Model (Beukelman & Mirenda, 2013), and person-centered planning. This framework provides a systematic approach to identifying key communication partners, and the goals to be achieved and current communication methods for use with each group of partners (Blackstone, 2003a). It enables the perceptions of many individuals to be considered when planning an intervention and it provides a structure for the gathering of information. The Social Networks Inventory is administered by a speech-language pathologist or other person with expertise in AAC. The key informants are someone in the individual's first circle

[17]Social Networks: A Communication Inventory for Individuals with Complex Communication Needs and Their Communication Partners, www.augcominc.com/index.cfm/social_networks.htm.

and fourth circle and, if at all possible, the individual with CCN. The inventory is meant to be readministered over time to track progress. Sections on demographic and diagnostic information and the individual's skills and abilities in motor, sensory, language, speech, and cognitive areas are included.

For each circle, the inventory identifies key partners (e.g., favorite partner, partner who understands the person best, etc.), the primary communication modes a person uses in each circle (facial expressions/body language, gestures, vocalizations, manual signs, speech writing, nonelectronic communication display, and electronic communication devices), and all current use of AT. Information is also collected about the size of vocabulary the person can access and the effectiveness, efficiency, and intelligibility of the person's current means of communication.

Representational strategies (e.g., object, photograph, pictographic, manual sign language, auditory) and selection techniques (e.g., direct selection, scanning, coding using icons, alphanumeric coding) are also identified, as are topics the individual can (or would like to) talk about. The inventory also helps document which strategies communication partners rely on to support the individual's comprehension (e.g., aided language simulation, modeling AAC use, visual prompts, pictured sequences of tasks, social stories) and expression (e.g., gesture dictionaries, asking for repeat of utterance, suggesting slower speed, prompting for repair strategy use). Summary sheets are included for clinicians to use for intervention planning. This model is very useful for ensuring that all of the important current and future communication partners are considered.

Assessing Language Representation

There are a number of ways to determine if an individual understands the association between the symbol and its meaning (Beukelman & Mirenda, 2013). Visual matching—single stimulus to one item from a multiple symbol array or vice versa—presents an object and two symbols, one of which represents the object, or two different objects, one of which matches a single symbol presented. The individual is instructed to "Look at the different one" or "Look at the one that is the same" to match the symbol to the correct object or the correct object to the symbol. Confirmation of the choice can be via any controllable movement (e.g., eye gaze, head nod, pointing). The functional object approach asks the person to, "Show me what you do with this." Yes/no validation asks, "Is this a ______?" A question and answer approach asks, "Can you show me the ______ that does ______?" Finally, a requesting format presents 2 choices and asks, "I don't know what to do. Can you help me?" For this case, the symbol object could be a cup (drink), brush (brush hair), and or other object.

Clinicians may select from several assessment protocols (Beukelman & Mirenda, 2013). In one protocol (functional object use), the evaluator shows the person a symbol and says "Show me what you do with this." The response may be a gesture (e.g., hand to mouth for "eat it") or pointing at a picture or symbol (e.g., "drink" if prompt is a soft drink can). In another approach (visual matching) the evaluator asks the individual to find a single stimulus item from a multiple symbol array or vice versa.

Assessing Barriers to Participation

AAC must be effective in a variety of contexts, i.e., environments and social settings. The Participation Model provides a systematic method for understanding these *contexts* by defining communication opportunities and barriers (Beukelman & Mirenda, 2013). **Opportunity barriers** are those that involve *policies, practices, attitudes,* and *knowledge and skills* of those who support the person with CCN. As an illustration, consider the situation where a school district purchases an SGD for a child, but the child is required to leave it at school at all times for fear that it will be lost or damaged if taken off school property. This practice is a barrier to full societal participation and academic success of the child because the device is not available to him or her outside of school. Another example of an opportunity barrier is the employer who is resistant to a worker using an AAC device because the artificial-sounding voice output is distracting to other workers. Opportunity barriers are part of the social or institutional contexts of the HAAT model (Chapter 3). **Access barriers,** described by the human component of the HAAT model, are those that make it difficult for a person with CCN to communicate using an AAC device or technique. Access barriers include motor limitations (speech, fine and gross movement), hearing, and vision and cognitive ability (including language deficiencies).

Policies are formal rules put in place by an agency (e.g., the funder of rehabilitation services) or institution (e.g., a group home), or government agency or private company. These are hard to change and it may be necessary to work around them. *Practices* are less formal and are established within a facility to meet local demands. These may involve how time is allocated to various tasks such as supporting an individual who uses an SGD, and there may be insufficient time for training and programming due to constraints placed on staff. These barriers can be reduced or removed more easily than formal policies, but they may still require creativity and thoughtful consideration of local circumstances. *Attitudes* are also informal opinions, but they are generally specific to one individual or possibly a few people in the same facility. These might involve resistance to the use of technology or lack of willingness to devote the time necessary to support the user. For example, a teacher with 30 students in her class may not be willing or able to devote a large amount of time to one student who has CCN. Because attitudes are subjective, they can be changed through negotiation rather than a formal policy change process. Alternative approaches can be developed by the interdisciplinary team members and the family. *Knowledge* of AAC by the people who are supporting the person may be lacking due to lack of familiarity with the technologies or with AAC in general, leading to a fear of the technology due to its complexity. In-service education can help in this regard. Weakness in *skills* is usually the product of lack of direct experience that is most easily dealt with by on-the-job training by a more experienced person.

Assessment of access barriers is also included in the Participation Model. An "activity standards inventory" is developed in which desired communication-related activities of the person with CCN (termed "target person") are listed and then compared to the performance of a nondisabled peer doing the same activity (Beukelman & Mirenda, 2013). In a school, the peer would be a student in the same classroom. In a group home, it might be an adult without a disability. The level of participation of the target person is then rated as (1) independent, (2) independent with set-up (i.e., someone else needs to arrange the device so the person can use it), (3) requires verbal (e.g., prompting) or physical assistance cues (e.g., hand over hand) or (4) unable to participate. Any difference between the peer and the target person is determined to be either an opportunity or access barrier.

Once the type of barrier is determined, then a plan to reduce or remove that barrier is developed. The plan includes the possibility of: (1) increasing natural abilities (e.g., speech-language pathology to improve motor speech function), (2) making environmental adaptations (e.g., moving a child to the front of the class to encourage greater participation or adjusting dining room arrangements to allow greater participation by an AAC user in a **skilled nursing facility**), and (3) making use of AAC systems and/or devices to avoid or overcome barriers. If the third choice is included in the plan, then it is necessary to assess the skills and abilities of the target person in order to select appropriate AAC systems and devices. The Participation Model refers to this as a *capability assessment* that involves documenting the individual's speech, language, motor, sensory, cognitive, and social communication skills. When used in combination, the HAAT model (Chapter 1), the Social Networks Inventory, and the Participation Model provide a comprehensive approach for ensuring that all information needed for successful AAC implementation is obtained during the assessment process.

Beukelman and Mirenda (2013) present detailed information regarding the implementation of the Participation Model, including sample assessment forms and case examples. For example, opportunity barriers are those that involve policies, practices, attitudes and knowledge, and skills of those who support the person with CCN and that interfere with successful AAC interventions.

As an illustration, consider the situation where a school district purchases an SGD for a child, but the child is required to leave it at school at all times. This practice is a barrier to full societal participation and academic success. Keeping the device at school may be a policy of the district because uninformed administrators worry about the cost of the device and possible breakage or loss if it goes home. After all, schools allow students to take home band instruments, uniforms, books, and pencils. Another example of an opportunity barrier is the employer who is resistant to a worker using an AAC device. This may reflect the employer's attitudes about disability or a lack of knowledge about AAC or a lack of skill in supporting individuals with CCN.

BOX 16-8 Cognitive Skills Relevant to the Use of an AAC System

Alertness
Attention span
Categorization
Cause/effect
Vigilance (ability to visually and auditorily process information over time)
Express preference
Make choices
Matching
Sequencing
Sorting
Symbolic representation
Object or pictoral permanence

Another key element of the Participation Model is an "activity standards inventory" in which desired communication-related activities of the person with CCN (termed "target person") are listed. The standard of desired performance is that a nondisabled peer would carry out the same activity. The target person is then rated as to the level of participation (independent, independent with setup, verbal or physical assistance, or unable to participate), and the discrepancy between peer and target person (if any) are ascribed to "opportunity" or "access" barriers. These are evaluated in terms of potential needs: (1) to increase natural abilities, (2) to make environmental adaptations, and (3) to use AAC systems and/or devices. Finally, AAC potential is determined through an operational profile, a constraints profile, and a capability profile.

As described in Chapter 7, the human/technology interface evaluation is part of a capability profile. An important component of the capability assessment involves documenting the individual's speech, language, motor, sensory, cognitive, and social communication skills. Dowden (1997) describes assessment approaches for individuals with CCN who have some functional speech. There are many language tests for both children and adults. Cognitive assessments help to determine how the individual understands the world and how communication can be best facilitated within this understanding (Beukelman & Mirenda, 2013). There are no formal tests that accurately predict the ability of an individual to meet the cognitive requirements of various AAC techniques and technologies, and expressive language by use of AAC is itself required to accurately assess cognitive ability. Thus, the individual's cognitive ability is often estimated. Some cognitive skills that are important for AAC are shown in Box 16-8. Social communicative skills (e.g., degree of interaction, attention to task) are generally assessed by interviews with family, caregivers, teachers, and others and through observation during an assessment or during opportunities created specifically to encourage social interaction. One example of the information that may be required (and how it may be assessed) is delineated in the Medicare funding request for SGDs in the United States (shown in the first column of Table 16-5).

TABLE 16-9 Features Typically Included in an SGD

Input Features/Selection Techniques (also see Chapter 5)*	Message Characteristics*	Auditory Output Features*	Additional Features	Accessory Features*
Direct Selection Keyboards/display: Dynamic/static, size & # of keys/locations Activation type: Touch or pressure sensitive, adjustable *Indirect contact:* Head pointing, eye gaze	Types of symbols: Words, phrases, letters, tactile, pictures (color/B&W), pictographic Vocabulary size: # of words, phrases, etc. needed	Type: Digitized speech Synthesized speech Other sounds	Outputs: Electronic aids to daily living (also see Chapter 14) Infrared Bluetooth Computer access: USB Bluetooth (also see Chapter 8)	Mounts: Position of switches Position of device Portability Size, weight, transport/mount, case/carrier requirements
Scanning Display: # of elements, dynamic/static Mode: Visual/auditory Type of scan: Linear, row/column, group row/column, directed	Organization of messages: Message length, files of messages, # of different messages stored or formulated	Vocabulary expansion: Rate enhancement, prediction (word/icon), coding strategies, screens/levels	General computer-based: Laptop Tablet Palm PDA	Switches: pressure, feedback Pointing devices: Infrared, ultrasonic Feedback: Visual, tactile, auditory

Relating Goals and Skills to Augmentative and Alternative Communication System Characteristics

Chapter 5 describes the assessment and recommendation process in assistive technology as designing a total system for a specific person. This approach is particularly true in AAC because it is necessary to define a set of system characteristics that meets the needs of the person with CCN, is consistent with his or her skills, and will support communication across multiple partners and contexts. When an SGD is a part of the recommended AAC approach for the individual with CCN, it is important to determine a match between the needs and goals of the person and the characteristics of the SGD. Table 16-9 illustrates the relationship between assessment results and device characteristics. Input features, message characteristics, output features, and accessories are all specified on the basis of the assessment results. Blackstone (2001) includes several case studies that illustrate the application of this matching process for the selection of an AAC device and the preparation of a funding justification for submission to Medicare. This type of systematic approach to recommendations allows the characteristics and skills of the individual with CCN to be matched with available SGDs.

The individual or family may wish to use the SGD for a trial period, during which valuable information can be gained. For example, the person's interest in using the SGD may increase when he or she sees how effective it is in meeting needs or he or she may not like how it sounds or how friends react to it. A trial period can also help identify specific training goals for the person and his or her communication partners so that communicative competencies can be developed that enable the individual to interact effectively and efficiently. If there are special features that require learning new skills (such as storing and retrieving information), these may be assessed during the trial. For individuals who prefer a longer trial period, many companies will lease a device for a 1- to 3-month period. The outcomes of an SGD assessment should include recommendations for the SGD and any accessories or mounts and instructional strategies required to meet the person's unique needs and goals.

Matching assessment results to mainstream technologies (e.g., iPad, smart phone) should follow the same basic process as for any other AAC approach (McBride, 2011). As we have said, focusing on the needs of the communicator rather than the technology is critical. A survey of the ASHA Special Interest Group 12 (DAAC) and Quality Indicators in Assistive Technology (QIAT) email lists asked individuals who already had an iPod/iPad: "Was an evaluation conducted to determine if the iPod/iPad would be the most appropriate communication system?" Of concern, only 54.4% responded "Yes." We need to ensure that recommendations about the use of an AAC high-tech device truly come from the needs of the individual with CCN.

When the assessment involves mainstream technologies, there are a few additional steps that can be helpful to ensure that this goal is met (McBride, 2011). One resource that can be helpful when an AAC device has already been provided or requested by an individual, family, or team is *Asking and Answering the Right Questions*, a framework developed by AAC TechConnect.[18] Most of the questions parallel the process outlined above. One question that is useful in the case of a device already provided is whether the communicator is currently using the AAC device and how effective is he or she in using it to meet documented needs? Watching a child playing with his or her mother's iPod to find pictures or music can be informative in relation to physical and cognitive abilities and navigation. Ensuring that the procured

[18]http://www.aactechconnect.com/tools.cfm.

device (including any AAC app) is consistent with the communicator's language/linguistic ability including symbolic representation, amount and type of vocabulary, organization of vocabulary, message formulation, navigation, and device access (functions such as clear, on/off, speak, ability to use programming features) (McBride, 2011) is crucial.

OUTCOMES

The evaluation of communicative competence in the four domains (operational, linguistic, social, and strategic) will identify areas in which the AAC system is and is not adequately meeting the individual's needs. Periodic reevaluation of the individual's skills and needs may also result in changes in the training or the AAC system(s). The reevaluation may lead to new training goals in one or more of the four areas of communicative competence. In other cases, the caregivers, family, or other support staff may require additional training to facilitate the use of the AAC device.

The AAC device as it is configured may also be inadequate to meet the individual's needs. It may be possible to adjust some of the features (e.g., scanning rate, stored vocabulary), or it may be necessary to consider a completely new device. The magnitude of the changes in the device dictates the amount of additional operational training required. In some cases, the individual's skills may decrease (e.g., degenerative disease) or increase (e.g., a young child who develops greater language skills). In either case a reevaluation and adjustments in the AAC system (device plus training and support) will be required.

Murphy et al. (1996) identified obstacles to effective AAC system use in a study of 93 users of AAC systems and 186 partners (93 formal and 93 informal). The formal partners were speech-language pathologists (the majority), care providers in the day or living program, and teachers. Informal partners were family, friends, and others selected by the AAC users as those with whom they felt most comfortable using their AAC systems. In some cases one partner filled both the formal and informal roles. The majority of low- and high-tech AAC system use was in the day placement (90%), residential (70%), and leisure (60%) settings. Use was limited to organized therapy sessions in general.

AAC systems were available to only 48% of the users while shopping, 62% during outings such as day trips during their program, and 66% where they lived. SLPs were the most frequent (80%) formal partners, and residential or day care staff were the most common informal partners (62%). Friends and family were both reported as the primary informal partner in less than 10% of the cases. Only 57% of the low-tech and 59.4% of the high-tech AAC system users were able to independently access their systems (e.g., get a system out of a back pack on a wheelchair and set it up for use without a partner's help). Knowledge of the system sufficient to interact with the AAC user was reported in less than half of the formal partners and one third of the informal partners. Eighty-eight percent of the users received training from their formal partners. However, for the majority of the users, the training consisted of 60 minutes or less (or 40 hours per year on the basis of sessions conducted). This number is low compared with other types of therapy and training such as that for second language instruction (estimated by Murphy et al. to be more than 200 hours per year).

Murphy et al. found that basic vocabulary required for daily interactions (see Table 16-7) was not included in the AAC systems. Few users had greetings, wrap ups, or conversational flow vocabulary (e.g., comments, repair vocabulary). Thus, for these areas, the users most commonly used other modes of communication (e.g., eye gaze, gestures, facial expressions) rather than their AAC devices.

The preponderance of formal partners also reinforces the need for inclusion of both useful vocabulary and multiple modes of communication. The development of strategic competence is vital to increase the likelihood that an AAC user will be able to independently carry out conversations in a variety of settings and with a variety of partners. Availability and accessibility of AAC systems can be addressed by appropriate mounting of systems on wheelchairs and training to ensure that care providers understand the need to have the system available to the user at all times. The results reported by Murphy et al. also emphasize the importance of multiple modes of communication by AAC users.

Assessment of AAC outcomes can use the general measures (Family Impact of AT Scale (FIATS) PIADS, Quebec User Evaluation of Satisfaction with Assistive Technology (QUEST) described in Chapter 5. Because of the nature of communication, there are additional considerations. Because the major goal of AAC is the provision of expressive language capability, one of the most important considerations is the determination of communicative intent by the individual evaluating outcomes (typically SLP or special education teacher). Special education teachers tend to overassess intentionality (i.e., to assign intentionality more often than experienced researchers), whereas SLPs do so less often (Carter & Iacono, 2002). Individuals with different disorders are also assessed differently relative to intentionality, and observations are inconsistent across populations, sessions, and professional groups. These results are disturbing because intentionality is a key measure of communicative competence and effectiveness.

The Matching Person to Technology model (Chapter 5) has been adapted to AAC use as the *AAC Acceptance Model* (Lasker & Bedrosian, 2001). This model focuses on the prediction of acceptance of AAC by adults with acquired communication impairments. Although the technology may play a small role in acceptance or nonacceptance, other factors are more important. Among these other factors are the following: (1) the communication partners' acceptance of the technology, (2) the rate (sudden or gradual) of onset of the communication impairment, (3) affective, behavioral, and cognitive components of a user's attitude toward AAC technology, (4) perception of the user and other people toward the device, and (5) how other people view the person using the device. It is not clear whether this measure can be generalized to other populations (e.g., children with developmental disabilities).

There are a number of key reasons that provision of AAC systems may not achieve the goal of a "better life" for the AAC user (Beukelman & Mirenda, 2013): (1) payer resistance to or lack of acceptance of measures that reflect quality of life rather than more concrete functional outcomes, (2) increased costs of intervention necessary to achieve broader goals, (3) time limits set by payers on length of the intervention, (4) high demands on professionals to achieve and maintain skills, (5) family and user response to increases in their responsibilities in assuming a leadership role, (6) difficulty by families in envisioning the future for the AAC user, and (7) cultural differences between the user and professionals.

We can relate meaningful AAC outcomes to the three levels of the World Health Organization ICF classification system (see Chapter 1) (Beukelman & Mirenda, 2013). At the level of body structures and functions, the degree to which AAC intervention compensates for lost or absent speech or language function can be determined. Evaluations related to activity focus on the quality and quantity of communication interactions and the degree to which these meet the goals and needs of the individual. Evaluations related to participation focus on the socially defined role and tasks within a sociocultural and physical environment. Some "big picture" AAC outcomes are shown in Box 16-9 (Beukelman & Mirenda, 2013). There are several types of measures for AAC system outcome. Operational measures evaluate the user's ability to interact with the system itself (operational competence), whereas representational measures evaluate symbol and grammatical capability by the AAC user (Beukelman & Mirenda, 2013).

The most important result of the follow-up phase is to evaluate the outcomes of the AAC interventions to determine their effectiveness, including both the hard and soft technologies, and the appropriateness of the match between the originally specified needs and the resulting system. The principles of outcome measurement discussed in Chapter 5 apply to AAC system evaluation as well.

BOX 16-9 Big Picture Outcomes for AAC Intervention

Has the AAC system resulted in increased:
Self-determination for the user
Inclusion of the user in social groups
Independence, to the degree the AAC user wants it
Participation in the community
Gainful employment
Academic achievement
Social connectedness
Educational inclusion or decreased special class placement

Data from Beukelman DR, Mirenda P: *Augmentative and alternative communication: management of severe communication disorders in children and adults*, ed 3, Baltimore: Paul H Brookes, 2005.

SUMMARY

Augmentative and alternative communication systems serve needs for both writing and conversation for individuals who have difficulties in these areas. Low-technology AAC systems provide quick and easy help for meeting communication needs, whereas high-technology devices offer great sophistication in available vocabulary, speed of communication, and flexibility of access. The latter features allow persons who have very limited physical skills to use AAC systems. AAC systems also have great flexibility in required user cognitive skills, allowing for persons with a diversity of intellectual abilities to benefit from AAC. The rapid expansion in mainstream technologies such as tablets and smart phones and AAC applications that run on them has created opportunities for people with CCN. This explosion of technologies has also dramatically changed the AAC field with both opportunities and challenges growing dramatically. Thoughtful assessment, careful training, and thorough follow-through are essential to effective AAC intervention. "With the support of civil rights, disability rights, and human rights legislation worldwide, individuals who have access to AAC systems are finding education and meaningful employment to be increasingly achievable goals" (Williams et al., 2008, pp 203).

STUDY QUESTIONS

1. What are the two major communicative needs normally addressed by augmentative communication systems?
2. Distinguish between aided and unaided communication.
3. What are the five basic elements of language? Distinguish between speech and language.
4. What are the major goals for augmentative communication systems designed for conversational use?
5. What AAC needs do parents have for their nonspeaking children? Do mothers and fathers have the same needs for their children?
6. Describe differences in the conversational rules that apply between two speaking persons and those between one speaking person and one augmentative communication user.
7. Describe the relationship between the Social Networks model and the Participation Model. How does each of these relate to the HAAT model described in this text?
8. How do attitudes of the communication partners differ for the five circles of the Social Networks model?
9. What factors influence the attitudes of children toward their peers who use AAC?
10. What features distinguish competent augmentative communicators from those who are not successful?
11. Select three discourse functions from those listed in Table 16-7. Now pick an augmentative communication device (e.g., electronic, direct selection, with voice output; or a language board with letters and words) and develop a vocabulary and set of strategies for the implementation of each of the discourse functions that you choose.

12. What are the three types of graphical communication? List three ways in which they differ.
13. In what ways does the formal writing of adolescent AAC users differ from that of nondisabled adolescent writers?
14. Distinguish between formal writing and note taking in terms of the characteristics AAC devices must have to meet each need. What is the most important feature in each case?
15. Describe auditory scanning. Give an example of both a low-tech or no-tech approach and an electronic AAC approach. What are the essential features for the AAC auditory scanning device?
16. List three encoding methods used in AAC devices, and give one advantage and one disadvantage of each.
17. What are the major types of abbreviation approaches used in AAC devices, and what are the major advantages and disadvantages of each?
18. Pick three discourse functions and develop a logical coding scheme for each using (1) numerical codes, (2) abbreviation expansion, and (3) Minspeak codes.
19. Compare word completion and prediction with abbreviation expansion and Minspeak encoding.
20. What are the major approaches used to increase conversational rate when the individual is using scanning?
21. What are the seven steps to build communication competence through training?
22. What are dynamic displays, and what advantages do they provide?
23. What are visual scene displays and what unique features do they have?
24. What populations might benefit most from visual scene displays? Why?
25. Describe the major challenges and approaches for AAC intervention of individuals whose primary disorder is language- or cognitively based. How does this compare with individuals whose primary disorder is motor or physical?
26. List and discuss three advantages that the Internet provides for communication by AAC users.
27. What are the four types of competencies acquired in AAC training? Pick an AAC system for an individual and design the training. You must make assumptions regarding the person's skills and needs, and other people available to help facilitate the training.
28. For each of the categories of devices described in the section on current technologies, define a user profile (skills and needs) that would lead you to focus on that category in selecting a device for that person.
29. What are the primary advantages and risks associated with the use of mainstream technologies (smart phones and tablets) as SGDs?
30. How has the availability of mainstream AAC apps affected the AAC field clinically and from a manufacturer's perspective?

REFERENCES

Alliano A, Herriger K, Koutsoftas AD, et al.: A review of 21 iPad applications for augmentative and alternative communication purposes, *Perspect Augment Altern Commun* 21(2):60–71, 2012, DOI: 10.1044/aac 21.2.60.

Anderson NB, Shames GH: *Human communication disorders: An introduction*, Boston, 2006, Allyn and Bacon.

Angelo DH: Impact of augmentative and alternative communication devices on families, *Augment Altern Commun* 16:37–47, 2000.

Angelo DH, Kokoska SM, Jones SD: Family perspective on augmentative and alternative communication: families of adolescents and young adults, *Augment Altern Commun* 12:13–20, 1996.

Baker B, Minspeak: *Byte* 7:186–202, 1982.

Baker B: Using images to generate speech, *Byte* 11:160–168, 1986.

Ball LJ, Beukelman DR, Patee GL: Acceptance of augmentative and alternative communication technology by persons with amyotrophic lateral sclerosis, *Augment Altern Commun* 20:113–122, 2004.

Beck AR, Dennis M: Attitudes of children toward a similar-aged child who uses augmentative communication, *Augment Altern Commun* 12:78–87, 1996.

Beck AR, et al.: Influence of communicative competence and augmentative and alternative communication technique on children's attitudes toward a peer who uses AAC, *Augment Altern Commun* 18:217–227, 2002.

Beukelman DR, Ball LJ: Improving AAC use for persons with acquired neurogenic disorders: understanding human and engineering factors, *Assist Technol* 14:33–44, 2002.

Beukelman DR, Fager S, Ball L, et al.: AAC for adults with acquired neurological conditions: a review, *Augment Altern Commun* 23:230–242, 2007..

Beukelman DR, Mirenda P: *Augmentative and alternative communication: management of severe communication disorders in children and adults*, ed 4, Baltimore, 2013, Paul H Brookes.

Blackstone S: Dynamic displays, *Augment Commun News* 7:1–6, 1994.

Blackstone S: Amyotrophic lateral sclerosis, *Augment Commun News* 11:1–15, 1998.

Blackstone S: Assessment protocol for SGDs, *Augment Commun News* 13:1–16, 2001.

Blackstone S: Social networks, *Augment Commun News* 15:1–16, 2003a.

Blackstone S: Autism spectrum disorder, *Augment Commun News* 15:1–6, 2003b.

Blackstone S: The Internet and its offspring, *Augment Commun News* 15:1–3, 2003c.

Blackstone S: Visual scene displays, *Augment Commun News* 16:1–5, 2004.

Blackstone S: False beliefs, widely held, *Augment Commun News* 8:1–6, 2006.

Blackstone SW, Hunt Berg M: *Social networks: a communication inventory for individuals with complex communication needs and their communication partners—inventory booklet*, Monterey, CA, 2003, Augmentative Communication.

Blackstone SW, Williams MB, Joyce M: Future AAC technology needs: consumer perspectives, *Assist Technol* 14:3–16, 2002.

Blishcak DM, Lombardino LJ, Dyson AT: Use of speech-generating device: in support of natural speech, *Augment Altern Commun* 19:29–35, 2003.

Bondy A, Frost L: The picture exchange communication system, *Behav Modif* 25:725–744, 2001.

Brady NC: Improved comprehension of object names following voice output communication aid use: two case studies, *Augment Altern Commun* 16:197–204, 2000.

Bruno J, Dribbon M: Outcomes in AAC: evaluating the effectiveness of a parent training program, *Augment Altern Commun* 14:59–70, 1998.

Bryen DN, Cohen K, Carey A: Augmentative communication employment training and supports: some employment outcomes, *J Rehabil* 70:10–18, 2004.

Carlisle Ladtkow M, Culp D: Augmentative communication with traumatic brain injury. In Yorkston K, editor: *Augmentative communication in the medical setting*, Tucson, Arizona, 1992, Communication Skill Builders, pp 139–244.

Carter M, Iacono T: Professional judgments of the intentionality of communicative acts, *Augment Altern Commun* 18:177–191, 2002.

Clarke M, Kirton A: Patterns of interaction between children with physical disabilities using augmentative and alternative communication systems and their peers, *Child Lang Teach Ther* 19:135–151, 2003.

Colby KM, et al.: A word-finding computer program with a semantic lexical memory for patients with anomia using an intelligent speech prosthesis, *Brain Lang* 14:272–281, 1981.

Collier B: When I grow up… supporting youth who use augmentative communication for adulthood. In *Proceedings of the 2005 Alberta Rehabilitation and Assistive Technology Consortium Conference*, Edmonton, 2005, Canada. Accessed August 2007.

Crepeau EB, Cohn ES, Schell BAB: *Willard and Spackman's occupational therapy*, ed 11, Philadelphia, 2009, Lippincott Williams & Wilkins. 1154.

Dolic J, Pibernik J, Bota J: Evaluation of mainstream tablet devices for symbol based AAC communication. In Jezic G, Kusek M, Nguyen N-T, et al.: *Agent and multi-agent systems: technologies and applications*, Berlin, 2012, Springer, pp 251–260.

Dowden P, Cook AM: Choosing effective selection techniques for beginning communicators. In Reichle J, Beukelman DR, Light JC, editors: *Exemplary practices for beginning communicators*, Baltimore, MD, 2002, Paul H. Brookes, pp 395–432.

Dowden PA: Augmentative and alternative communication decision making for children with severely unintelligible speech, *Augment Altern Commun* 13:48–58, 1997.

Drager KDR: Light technologies with different system layouts and language organizations, *J Speech Hear Res* 46:289–312, 2003.

Drager KDR, Reichle J, Pinkoski C: Synthesized speech output and children: a scoping review, *Am J Speech-Lang Pathol* 19:259–2731, 2010.

Falvey M, et al.: *All my life's a circle: Using the tools of circles, MAPS and PATHS*, Toronto, 1994, Inclusion Press.

Fazzi E, Signorini SG, Piana R, et al.: Neuro-ophthalmological disorders in cerebral palsy: ophthalmological, oculomotor, and visual aspects. *Developmental medicine & child neurology* 54(8):730–736, 2012.

Fields C: Finding a voice for Daniel, *Team Rehabil Rep* 2(3):16–19, 1991.

Frager S, Hux K, Beukelman D: AAC acceptance and use by 25 adults with TBI, *CSUN Conference on Technology and People with Disabilities*, 2005. http:/aac.unl.edu. Accessed August 2007.

Fruchterman JR: In the palm of your hand: a vision of the future of technology for people with visual impairments, *J Vis Impair Blindness* 97:585–591, 2003.

Goldbart J, Marshall J: "Pushes and pulls" on the parents of children who use AAC, *Augment Altern Commun* 20:194–208, 2004.

Gosnell J, Costello J, Shane H: Using a clinical approach to answer "What communication apps should we use?" *Perspect Augment Altern Commun* 20(3):8796, 2011a, http://dx.doi .org/10.1044/aac20.3.87.

Gosnell J, Costello J, Shane H: There isn't always an app for that! *Perspect Augment Altern Commun* 20(1):7–8, 2011b, http://dx.doi.org/10.1044/aac20.1.7.

Graves J: Vocabulary needs in augmentative and alternative communication: a sample of conversational topics between staff providing services to adults with learning difficulties and their service users, *Br J Learning Disabil* 28:113–119, 2000.

Halloran J, Emerson M: *LAMP: Language Acquisiton through Motor Planning*, Wooster, OH, 2010, The Center for AAC and Autism.

Helsinger S: Teaching the Picture Exchange Communication System to adults with pervasive developmental disorder/autism, Presented at the Picture Exchange Communication System Exposition, Philadelphia, 2001.

Hershberger D: Mobile technology and AAC apps from an AAC developer's perspective, *Perspect Augment Altern Commun* 20(1):28–33, 2011, http://dx.doi.org/10.1044/aac20.1.28.

Higginbotham DJ et al.: The Frametalker project: building an utterance-based communication device, *Proceedings of the 2005 CSUN Conference on Technology For Persons With Disabilities*, 2005, Los Angeles, CA.

Higginbotham J, Jacobs S: The future of the Android Operating System for augmentative and alternative communication, *Perspect Augment Altern Commun* 20(2):52–56, 2011, DOI: 10.1044/aac20.2.52.

Hopkins HL, Smith HD, editors: *Willard and Spackman's occupational therapy*, ed 8, Philadelphia, 1993, JB Lippincott.

Jacobs B, et al.: Augmentative and alternative communication for adults with severe aphasia: where we stand and how we can go further, *Disabil Rehabil* 26:1231–1240, 2004.

Joseph D: The morning, *Commun Outlook* 8:8, 1986.

Kent-Walsh JE, Light JC: General education teachers' experiences with inclusion of students who use augmentative and alternative communication, *Augment Altern Commun* 19:102–124, 2003.

Kovach T, Kenyon P: Auditory scanning: development and implementation of AAC systems for individuals with physical and visual impairments, *ISAAC Bull* 53:1–7, 1998.

Kraat AW: Developing intervention goals. In Blackstone S, Bruskin D, editors: *Augmentative communication: an introduction*, Rockville, MD, 1986, American Speech-Language and Hearing Association.

Lasker J, Bedrosian J: Promoting acceptance of augmentative and alternative communication by adults with acquired communication disorders, *Augment Altern Commun* 17:141–153, 2001.

Light J: Interaction involving individuals using augmentative and alternative communication systems: state of the art and future directions, *Augment Altern Commun* 4:66–82, 1988.

Light J: Toward a definition of communicative competence for individuals using augmentative and alternative communication systems, *Augment Altern Commun* 5:137–144, 1989.

Light JC, Binger C: *Building communicative competence with individuals who use augmentative and alternative communication*, Baltimore, 1998, Paul H Brookes.

Light JC, Drager KDR: Improving the design of augmentative and alternative technologies for young children, *Assist Technol* 14:17–32, 2002.

Light J, Drager K: AAC technologies for young children with complex communication needs: State of the science and future research directions, *Augment Altern Commun* 23:204–216, 2007.

Lilienfeld M, Alant E: Attitudes toward an unfamiliar peer using an AAC device with and without voice output, *Augment Altern Commun* 18:91–101, 2002.

Lloyd LL, Fuller DR, Arvidson HH: *Augmentative and alternative communications: a handbook of principles and practices*, Boston, 1997, Allyn and Bacon.

Magiati I, Howlin P: A pilot evaluation study of the Picture Exchange Communication System (PECS) for children with autistic spectrum disorders, *Autism* 7:297–320, 2003.

McBride D: AAC evaluations and new mobile technologies: asking and answering the right questions, *Perspect Augment Altern Commun* 20(1):9–16, 2011.

McCarthy J, Light J: Attitudes toward individuals who use augmentative and alternative communication: research review, *Augment Altern Commun* 21:41–55, 2005.

McKelvey M, et al.: Performance of a person with chronic aphasia using a visual scene display prototype, *J Med Speech Lang Pathol* 15(3):305–317, 2007.

McNaughton D, Light J, Gulla S: Opening up a "whole new world": employer and co-worker perspectives on working with individuals who use augmentative and alternative communication, *Augment Altern Commun* 19:235–253, 2003.

McNaughton D, Light J: The iPad and mobile technology revolution: benefits and challenges for individuals who require augmentative and alternative communication, *Augment Alternat Commun* 29(2):107–116, 2013.

Mirenda P: Toward functional augmentative and alternative communication for students with autism: manual signs, graphic symbols and voice output communication aids, *Lang Speech Hearing Serv Schools* 34:203–216, 2003.

Mirenda P, Santogrossi J: A prompt-free strategy to teach pictorial communication system use, *Augment Altern Commun* 1:143–150, 1985.

Murphy J, et al.: AAC system use: obstacles to effective use, *Eur J Dis Commun* 31:31–44, 1996.

Niemeijer D, Donnellan A, Robledo J: *Taking the pulse of augmentative and alternative communication on iOS. Assistiveware.* Retrieved from http://www.assistiveware.com/taking-pulse augmentative-and-alternative-communication-ios, 2012.

Nolan C: *Dam-burst of dreams*, New York, 1981, St. Martin's Press.

Parette HP, Botherson MJ, Huer MB: Giving families a voice in augmentative and alternative communication decision-making, *Educ Train Ment Retard Dev Disabil* 35:177–190, 2000.

Rabins PV, Lyketsos C, Steele C: *Practical dementia care*, ed 2, Oxford UK Press, 2006.

Raghavendra P, Wood D, Newman L, et al.: Why aren't you on Facebook?: patterns and experiences of using the Internet among young people with physical disabilities, *Technol Disabil* 24:149–162, 2012.

Rush WL: *Journey out of silence*, Lincoln, NE, 1986, Media Productions and Marketing.

Schepis M, Reid D: Issues affecting staff enhancement of speech-generating device use among people with severe cognitive disabilities, *Augment Altern Commun* 19:59–65, 2003.

Scherer M: *Matching person and technology: a series of assessments for evaluating predispositions to and outcomes of technology use in rehabilitation, education, the workplace and other settings*, Webster, NY, 1998, The Institute for Matching Person & Technology.

Schlosser RW, Blischak DM: Is there a role for speech output in interventions for persons with autism? *Focus Autism Other Dev Disabil* 16:170178, 2001.

Schwartz IS: Beyond basic training: PECS use with peers and at home. Presented at the Picture Exchange Exposition, Philadelphia, 2001.

Sevick RA, Romski MA, Adamson LB: Research directions in augmentative and alternative communication for preschool children, *Disabil Child* 26:1323–1329, 2004.

Shane HC, Blackstone S, Vanderheiden G, et al.: Using AAC technology to access the world, *Assist Technol* 24:3–13, 2012.

Shipley K, McAfee J: *Assessment in speech and language pathology: a resource manual*, ed 4, New York, 2009, DELMAR Cengage Learning.

Simpson S: If only I could tell them, *Commun Outlook* 9:9–11, 1988.

Todman J: Rate and quality of conversations using a text-storage AAC system: single-case training study, *Augment Altern Commun* 16:164–179, 2000.

Venkatagiri HS: Segmental intelligibility of three text-to-speech synthesis methods in reverberant environments, *Augment Altern Commun* 20(3):150–163, 2004.

World Health Organization: *International classification of functioning, disability and health (ICF)*, Geneva, Switzerland, 2001, World Health Organization.

Williams MB: Message encoding: a comment on Light et al., *Augment Altern Commun* 7:133–134, 1991.

Williams MB, Krezman C, McNaughton D: "Reach for the stars": five principles for the next 25 years of AAC, *Augment Alternat Commun* 24:194–206, 2008.

Winter S: Cerebral palsy. In Jacobson J, Mulick J, Rojahn J, editors: *Handbook of intellectual and developmental disabilities*, New York, NY, 2007, Springer.

Resources for further information (courtesy of Gallaudet University)[1]

ABLEDATA
8630 Fenton Street, Suite #930
Silver Spring, MD 20910

V (800)227-0216 (800)227-0216 FREE
TTY: (301) 608-8912
Fax: (301) 608-8958
Email: ABLEDATA@verizon.net
Web page: http://www.abledata.com

1. **Alexander Graham Bell Association for the Deaf, Inc.**
3417 Volta Place NW
Washington, DC 20007

Voice/ TTY: (202) 337-5220
Fax: (202) 337-8314
Email: info@agbell.org
Web Page: http://www.agbell.org

2. **Described and Captioned Media Program National Association of the Deaf**
1447 E. Main Street
Spartanbrug, SC 29307
Local:

Voice: 864-585-1788 864-585-1788 FREE
TTY: 864-585-2617
Fax: 864-585-2611
Toll Free:

Voice: (800) 237-6213 (800) 237-6213 FREE
TTY: (800) 237-6819
Fax: (800) 538-5636
Email: info@cfv.dcmp.org
Web Page: http://www.dcmp.org

3. **National Association of the Deaf**
8630 Fenton Street, Suite # 820
Silver Spring, MD 20910-3819

Voice: (301) 587-1788 (301) 587-1788 FREE
TTY: (301) 587-1789
Fax: (301) 587-1791
Web Page: http://www.nad.org

4. **National Captioning Institute**
1900 Gallows Road, Suite #3000
Vienna, VA 22182

Voice/TTY: (703) 917-7600
Fax: (703) 917-9853

5. **Hearingloss Association of America**
7910 Woodmont Ave., Suite #1200
Bethesda, MD 20814

TTY/Voice: (301) 657-2249 (301) 657-2249 FREE
Fax: (301) 913-9413
Web Page: http://www.hearingloss.org

6. **Telecommunication for the Deaf, Inc.**
8630 Fenton Street, Suite #604
Silver Spring, MD 20910

Voice: (301) 589-3786 (301) 589-3786 FREE
TTY: (301) 589-3006
Fax: (301) 598-3797
Web Page: http://www.tdi-online.org/

7. ASHA provides public information about communication disorders, including deafness and the role of speech and hearing professionals in rehabilitation. Informational materials and Helpline is provided for inquires about speech, language or hearing problems.

8. **American Speech-Language Hearing Association**
2200 Research Blvd.
Rockville MD 20850-3289

HELPLINE: (800) 638-8255 (800) 638-8255 FREE (VOICE/TTY)
FAX: (301) 296-8580
Email: actioncenter@asha.org
Web Page: http://www.asha.org

Originally written by:
*Loraine DiPietro, M.A.; Pettyt Williams, Ph.D.; Hariet Kaplan, Ph.D.**

[1] (downloaded October 5, 2013; from: http://www.gallaudet.edu/clerc_center/information_and_resources/info_to_go/hearing_and_communication_technology/alerting_devices/alerting_and_comm_dev_for_deaf_and_hoh_ppl.html)

Glossary

Abbreviation expansion An augmentative and alternative communication or computer access technique in which a shortened form of a word or phrase (the abbreviation) stands for the entire word or phrase (the expansion); abbreviations are automatically expanded by the device

Acceleration The speed of change in velocity (increase or decrease)

Acceleration vocabularies Used by literate persons to increase the rate of communication through both selection of whole words and spelling

Acceptance time A method used for selection of an item in a scanning system that is based on the user's pausing for a preset period, after which the entry is made

Access Barriers Obstacles that make it difficult for a person with complex communication needs to communicate using an augmentative and alternative communication device or technique (e.g., motor limitations and hearing, vision, and cognitive abilities)

Accessibility software programs that enable accessibility to devices

Accessibility the capability of a device to allow use by individuals with disabilities

Accessibility options Software adaptations included in Windows that address common problems that persons with disabilities have in using a standard keyboard

Activation characteristics The method of activation, deactivation, effort, displacement, flexibility, and durability of a control interface

Activity The portion of the human activity–assistive technology model that defines what the individual needs or wants to do when using assistive technology

Activity analysis An occupational therapy process that involves deconstructing an activity followed by an analysis of the affective, cognitive, physical and sensory processes required for its completion and the environmental contexts that enable it

Activity output The action that is replaced or augmented by an assistive device, including communication, cognition, manipulation and mobility

Aesthetics The affective aspects related to how a device looks

Alerting devices Sensory devices that detect sounds (e.g., alarm clock, doorbell, telephone ring) and then cause a vibration or a flashing light signal, or both, to call attention to the sound for a person who is deaf

Alignment The degree to which the two structures are arranged in some systematic manner, e.g., the degree to which wheels on a wheelchair are parallel to each other

Alternative In assistive technologies, a different way of accomplishing the same task

Alternative input Technologies that offer the user different modalities for providing input commands or information to a device (e.g., voice recognition software)

Alternative mobility device An assistive device intended to assist a person who is blind in orientation and mobility

Alternative output Technologies that offer users a nontraditional means of acquiring feedback or information from a device (e.g., braille or auditory information substituted for visual displays)

Alternative sensory system The use of a different sensory channel to substitute for a nonfunctional one; common examples of this approach are the use of braille for reading by persons with visual impairment (tactile substitution for visual) and the use of manual sign language by persons who are deaf (visual substitution for auditory)

Ambient environment a network-based connectivity in which every electronic device used on a regular basis has both computing power and is linked to other devices through local networks (e.g., Wi-Fi) or the Internet

Amyotrophic lateral sclerosis (ALS) A rapidly progressing neuromuscular disease that affects speech in the majority of cases (see the following case study of Mr. Webster). There are two types of ALS: bulbar or brainstem ALS and spinal ALS

Android a smart phone operating system

Anti-tip devices Small wheels, attached to a rod and mounted at the back of the chair, that prevent the chair from tipping backwards

Aphasia Language disorder affecting both expression and reception of spoken and written language

Application program software that enables a particular function or supports an activity on a computer, smart phone or table

Attention deficit disorder A pattern of inattention, hyperactivity, and/or impulsivity that is more frequent or severe than for typical people of a given age

Apraxia An inability to plan motor movements, where the peripheral components necessary to execute the motion are generally intact

Assessment A process through which information about the consumer is gathered and analysed in a systematic manner with the purpose of identifying appropriate assistive technologies (hard and soft) and developing a plan for intervention

Assistive listening devices A class of assistive devices that are intended to be used in group settings such as in lecture halls, churches, business meetings, courtrooms, and broadcast television to amplify sounds and broadcast them to receivers worn by persons who are hard of hearing

Assistive technology A broad range of devices, services, strategies, and practices that are conceived and applied to ameliorate the problems faced by individuals who have disabilities

Assistive technology service Any service that directly assists an individual with a disability in the selection, acquisition, or use of an assistive technology device

Assistive technology system An assistive technology device, a human operator who has a disability, and a context in which the functional activity is to be carried out

Attention The mechanism for continued cognitive processing or the ability to focus on a particular stimulus

Attention deficit disorder (ADHD) A pattern of inattention, hyperactivity, and/or impulsivity that is more frequent or severe than typical behaviour of peers

Auditory function The degree to which the sensory and motor components of the human auditory system function

Augmentative Supplementation, by a device, of existing capabilities to support doing an activity in the manner in which it is typically done

Augmentative and alternative communication (AAC) Approaches and systems that are designed to ameliorate the problems faced by persons who have difficulty speaking or writing because of neuromuscular disease or injury

Augmentative manipulation Assistance in doing a manipulative task in the same manner as it is normally done

Autism spectrum disorder (ASD) A developmental disorder that is characterized by varying degrees of impairment in communication and social interaction skills, or the presence of restricted, repetitive, and stereotyped patterns of behaviour

Automatic scanning Items are presented continuously by the device at an adjustable rate, with selection of the choice made by activating the switch and stopping the scan; entry is by an additional switch press or acceptance time

Autonomy the right to self-determination and freedom from unnecessary constraints or interference without the loss of privacy.

Bariatrics A term that describes the practice of medicine concerning individuals who are significantly overweight; derived from the Greek baros meaning weight and iatrics meaning medical treatment

Bariatric chair A wheelchair that can accommodate individuals whose weight exceeds the maximum capacity of a standard wheelchair and whose mobility is limited by obesity and related chronic conditions

Beneficence An ethical principle ensuring that actions lead to good results that benefit

Bluetooth a wireless standard for short range communication between devices

Body structures and functions The components of the WHO International Classification of Functioning, Disability and Health that identify the physiological functions of body systems

Booster seat A seat designed to be used in a vehicle that positions the child so the vehicle seat belts fit properly. The vehicle seat belt provides restraint when a booster seat is used

Braille Raised dots that can be read by touch; a cell of either six or eight dots is used to portray letters and special computer symbols (e.g., cursor movement, uppercase and lowercase)

Camber The degree to which the wheel is mounted off vertical, usually 1 to 4 degrees. Camber tips the wheel so the top is closer to the user's body. When the wheels are set this way, the wheelchair becomes more stable and propulsion is more efficient

Capability theory A theory that proposes that includes essential capability that define what it means to be human and supports the right of the individual to choose to enact these capabilities. It suggests that the simple provision of human rights is insufficient if the human does not have the opportunity to enact those rights

Capacity Person's potential optimal performance of an activity given favourable and supportive circumstances

Captioning The process of generating a sentence or group of words that is written on or next to a picture to explain what is being shown

Cerebral vascular accident Incidence of irregular blood flow within the brain causing an interruption in brain function; also called *stroke*

Center of gravity The point in the body at which the acceleration caused by gravity is localized

Center of mass Point in the center of an object of any shape around which the gravitational forces acting on the body balance each other. The center of mass of an empty wheelchair is located under the seat, in front of the drive wheels

Center of pressure Center of gravitational forces when measured in posterior-anterior and lateral planes

Cerebral palsy a nonprogressive motor impairment due to a lesion or anomalies of the brain arising in the early stages of its development

Cerebral vascular accident/stroke Incidence of irregular blood flow within the brain causing an interruption in brain function, also called stroke

Child vehicle restraint system A car seat that provides occupant protection for children who are too small to be properly secured by the vehicle seat belt assembly

Circular scanning An approach in which the selection set is organized in a circular pattern

Client-centered practice Involvement of the client, the user of the assistive technology device and relevant others in the service delivery process to identify and pursue client goals; to recognize the client and her subjective experiences as central to the service delivery process

Clinical reasoning The thinking process that guides the health care professional's decision-making process. Four types of clinical reasoning have been identified: procedural, interactive, conditional and narrative

Closed captioning A process whereby the audio portion of a television program is converted into written words, which appear in a window on the screen

Closed circuit television (CCTV) A video camera and monitor used to enlarge text and other print material; also called video magnifiers

Cochlear implant An auditory prosthesis that provides some sound perception by directly applying electrical stimulation to the basilar membrane of the cochlea

Coded access A form of indirect selection in which the individual uses a distinct sequence of movements to input a code for each item in the selection set

Cognitive assistive technology (AT) An entire system of hardware, software, and personal assistance that is individualized to meet specific intellectual or mental processing needs

Cognitive skill Includes mental processes of orientation, attention, memory and executive function

Command domain The set of assistive device functions available to the user

Compact disk–read-only memory (CD-ROM) Optical storage of data and programs; uses lasers to read and write data to optical disks

Complex communication needs (CCN) Needs possessed by an individual who is not developing speech and language skills or has lost the ability to speak and/or understand spoken or written language

Compression Occurs when forces act toward each other (pushing together), such as the force of the vertebrae on the disks in the spinal column

Concept keyboard A keyboard in which the letters and numbers are replaced with pictures, symbols, or words that represent the concepts being used or taught

Context The portion of the human activity–assistive technology model that describes the influence of physical, social, cultural and institutional environments or contexts on the access to, service delivery and use of assistive technology

Context-Dependent Communicators A type of alternative and augmentative communication device that uses reliable symbolic communication; it is limited to specific contexts because it is either only intelligible to familiar partners, has insufficient vocabulary, or both.

Continuous control A type of control function used with electronic aids to daily living that results in successively greater or smaller degrees of output (e.g., closing the blinds, dimming the lights)

Contour Refers to seating devices that are moulded or shaped to conform to the human's body

Control enhancers Aids and strategies that enhance or extend the physical control (range or resolution) a person has available to use a control interface

Control interface The hardware (e.g., keyboard, joystick) by which the user operates an assistive technology system or controls a device

Control sites The body sites that can be used to control a device

Co-occupation An occupation in which two or more people are involved that cannot be done by a single person alone, e.g., teaching is a co-occupation that involves a learner and a teacher engaging with each other in the occupation of learning

Crashworthiness The process of determining the performance of a system under simulated vehicle crash conditions. Specifically, the performance of a wheelchair and seating system in a 21 g/48 km frontal impact crash simulation

Criteria for service The recognition of a need for assistive technology services that triggers a referral for services

Criterion-referenced measurement A measurement in which the person's own skill level when using an AT system is used as the performance standard

Cultural context The shared beliefs, practices, values and meanings that influence acceptance and use of technology

DAISY (Digital Audio-Based Information System) An international consortium of organizations that produce reading material for the blind; has developed standards for digital books

Dampening The ability of a material to soften on impact

Dementia A syndrome, or a pattern of clinical symptoms and signs, that can be defined by the following three points: (1) decline of cognitive capacity with some effect on day-to-day functioning, (2) impairment in multiple areas of cognition (global), and (3) normal level of consciousness

Deactivation characteristics The effort, displacement, flexibility, and durability required to release a control interface

Density The ratio of the weight of a material to its volume

Dependent mobility Mobility systems that are propelled by an attendant (e.g., strollers, geriatric wheelchairs, and transport chairs)

Desktop robots General-purpose manipulators that create full access to an area dedicated to the performance of a specific job or activity (a workstation)

Device A piece of hardware or software used by an individual to accomplish a task

Device characteristics General properties of the hard technology portions of an assistive technology system

Digital recording Human speech is stored in electronic memory circuits for later retrieval

Digital talking books (DTBs) Reading material for individuals who are blind; produced on digital media (usually CD-ROM) and that can be reproduced and read on a variety of hardware platforms and operating systems

Direct selection An approach in which the individual is able to use the control interface to randomly choose any of the items in the selection set

Directed scanning An approach in which the user activates the control interface to select the direction of the scan, vertically or horizontally, and then sends a signal to stop at the desired choice; entry is by an additional switch press or acceptance time

Discrete control A type of control function used with electronic aids to daily living in which each event requires a specific entry. Its selection produces a different result (e.g., on/off, open/closed)

Displacement Defines the position of a body in space; a change in displacement results in a new position

Distributed controls An approach used when multiple devices are controlled and each has its own control interface

Distributive justice Principles designed to guide the allocation of the benefits and burdens of economic activity

Driving evaluation Assessment by a trained evaluator of an individual's ability to drive a vehicle. A driving evaluation usually has two components: an off-road assessment that is paper or computer-based and an on-road component with a trained evaluator

Dynamic communication displays An input mode used in augmentative and alternative communication in which the selection set displayed to the user is changed as new choices are made; can be altered easily depending on previous choices and allows reliance on recognition rather than recall

Dysarthria A disorder of motor speech control resulting from central or peripheral nervous system damage; characterized by weakness, slowness, and incoordination of the muscles necessary for speech

Easy Access Software adaptations included in Apple Macintosh operating systems that address common problems that persons with disabilities have in using a standard keyboard

Ecological model Model comprised of different levels or components that form a system, which is viewed as an interactive and dynamic whole. Change in one component effects change in all others

Electrically powered page turners Devices that hold a book or other reading material and mechanically turn the pages when a switch or switches are pressed by the user

Electronic aid to daily living (EADL) Device that allows control of appliances (e.g., radio, television, CD player, telephone) through the use of one or more switches

Electronic travel aid (ETA) Sensory devices that supplement rather than replace the long cane or guide dog; designed to provide additional environmental information and to detect those obstacles typically missed by the long cane

Emergent Communicator Type of alternative and augmentative communication device that has no reliable method of symbolic expression and is restricted to communicating about here and now concepts

Enabler Someone or something that facilitates the performance of an occupation

Envelopment The degree to which the person sinks into a seating cushion and the degree to which the cushion surrounds the buttocks

Environmental interface The component of an assistive technology device that detects input from the environment, commonly sound and light, and converts it to some form that is usable by the consumer

Environmental sensor The portion of a sensory device that detects the data that the human cannot obtain through his or her own sensory system

Equilibrium The situation in which the force generated by one object is equal in magnitude and opposite in direction to the force generated by another object

Evaluation phase Involves activities in the service delivery process that identify needs; assess user knowledge, skills and performance; and trial device use

Evidence-informed Practice and service delivery that is informed by clinical and research evidence

Ethics A formal code of conduct that guides behaviour in different situations; includes professional codes of ethics

Expert Consumer who displays a high degree of competence when using an assistive technology device and who is able to use the device in novel ways or across novel situations

Feedback The modification or control of a process or system by its results or effects (e.g., visual, auditory or tactile); the output of the system that provides information to the user about the operation of the device

Fidelity the ethical principle that requires clinical practice in AT that is carried out with honesty, integrity, and trustworthy behavior

Fixed deformity A permanent change taking place in the bones, muscles, capsular ligaments, or tendons that restricts the normal range of motion of the particular joint and affects the skeletal alignment of the other joints

Flexible deformity Appearance of a deformity as a result of increased tone and muscle tightness causing the person to assume certain postures; externally applied resistance (passive stretch) in the opposite direction allows movement of the joint and reduction in the "deformity"

Follow-along The portion of the service delivery process in which a mechanism for regular contact with the consumer is established to see whether further assistive technology services are indicated

Follow-up The portion of the service delivery process that determines whether the system as a whole is functioning effectively; usually occurs after a set length of time from an initial or ongoing evaluation

Footplate Extension of the seat rails of a wheelchair on which the user places their feet

Force Anything that acts on a body to change its rate of acceleration or alter its momentum

Formal evaluation Consists of standardized outcome measurements and systematic data collection processes that evaluate general function and the specific outcomes of assistive technology use

Forward-facing child seat Child vehicle restraint system that is installed for long-term use in a vehicle and provides occupant protection for children over the age of 12 months who are between 20 and 40 pounds and up to 40 inches in height

Free and appropriate public education (FAPE) The right to an education of every child with a disability; established under the United States Individuals with Disabilities Education Act (IDEA)

Friction/Frictional forces Resulting forces from movement in opposite directions between two bodies in contact; may be static or dynamic

Front rigging Leg rests and footplates on a wheelchair that support the user's feet

Function allocation The allocation of functions in any human/device system in which some functions are allocated to the human, some to the device, and some to the personal assistant services

Funding Monetary resources that are available for certain types of assistive technology

Generalization the tendency to respond in the same way to different but similar stimuli.

General-purpose manipulation device Designed to accomplish a variety of manipulative tasks; examples are robotic systems and electronic aids to daily living

Graphical user interface (GUI) Characterized by three distinguishing features: (1) a mouse pointer, which is moved around the screen; (2) a graphical menu bar, which appears on the screen; and (3) one or more windows, which provide a menu of choices

Gravitational line The axis of the body along which the force of gravity acts

Gravity Acceleration of an object towards the center of the earth

Group-item scan An approach that is used to increase the rate of selection during scanning by grouping the selection set and allowing the user to first select a group and then the desired item in the group

Head pointers Devices with a pointer attached to a headband that are used for direct manipulation

Health-related quality of life The impact of health services on the overall quality of life of individuals; represents the functional effect of an illness and its consequent therapy

Hearing aids Sensory devices that provide amplification of sounds, including speech, for individuals who are hard of hearing

Hearing carry-over (HCO) For those who can hear but not speak, allows individuals to type their message and listen to the response using relay service

High technology Devices that are expensive, often complex, difficult to obtain and difficult to make

Human Component of the HAAT model that describes a person who uses assistive technology; includes the user's abilities in motor, sensory, cognitive and affective areas.

Human rights Fundamental opportunities or actions that belong to an individual and that cannot be denied by governmental or other organizations or persons

Human activity–assistive technology (HAAT) model A model guiding assistive technology research and development, service delivery and outcome evaluation. It consists of four parts: (1) activity, (2) human, (3) context, and (4) assistive technologies

Human/technology interface (HTI) The portion of the assistive technology system with which the user interacts

Icon prediction A feature of Minspeak-based devices that aids in recalling stored sequences

Immersion Describes the deformity that results when a load is applied to a material, including materials used to produce a seat cushion

Impairment Any loss or abnormality of psychological, physical, or anatomical structure or function

Implementation phase The portion of the service delivery process in which the recommended technology is ordered, modified, and fabricated as necessary; set up; delivered to the consumer; and initial training takes place

Independent manual mobility Systems in which the user has the ability to propel the device by body power only

Independent powered mobility Motorized wheelchairs that are controlled by the user

Indirect selection An approach in which there are intermediary steps involved in making a selection; includes scanning and coded access; typically the control interface used is a single switch or an array of switches

Individual Education Plan (IEP) Mandated by IDEA, the plan, written for each student, incorporates the student's specialized program. The IEP team must consider assistive technologies as a special factor when developing the learner's IEP

Informal evaluation a method of evaluating clients needs by observation or interview

Information Communication Technology (ICT) a communication device or application, including radio, television, cellular phones, computer and network hardware and software, satellite systems and the services and applications associated with them

Information processing the acquisition, recording, organization, retrieval, display, and dissemination of information

Informed consent includes two aspects: (1) not subjecting the individual to control by others without their explicit consent and (2) respectful interaction when presenting information, probing for understanding, and attempting to enable autonomous decision making

Infrared (IR) light transmission Devices that use invisible light to remotely control an electronic aid to daily living; consists of a transmitter unit, which is either hand held or mounted on a wheelchair, and a set of receivers, one for each appliance to be controlled

Input domain The number of independent inputs, or signals, generated by the control interface; may be either discrete or continuous

Integrated control An approach used when multiple devices are controlled with one control interface

International Classification of Functioning, Disability and Health (ICF) Classification system developed by the World Health Organization (WHO) for coding and classifying elements of the person, activity and environment to describe the interaction of these elements with a health condition and their collective influence on functioning

Intellectual or Developmental Disabilities A disability where one has a below-average score on an intelligence or mental ability test as well as a limitation in functional skills; skills include (but are not limited to) communication, self-care, and social interaction

Internet Worldwide computer network available by modem that connects users globally for electronic mail, file transfer, electronic commerce, and similar functions

Intrinsic enablers General underlying abilities that individuals use to perform activities and tasks

Inverse scanning An approach in which the scan is initiated by the individual's activating and holding a switch closed, with selection of the desired item indicated by releasing the switch; entry is by an additional switch press or acceptance time

iOS the operating system used by mobile devices manufactured by Apple, Inc.

Keyboard a control interface containing an array of switches, can be of varying sizes and shapes with the individual switches also varying in size and shape

Kinematics Aspect of mechanics that describe the motion of a mass, without consideration of forces involved in that motion

Kinetics Aspect of mechanics that describes the actions of forces to produce or change motion of a mass

Knowledge representation All the information and skills that have been learned (e.g., the alphabet, how to wash our hands, that gravity makes things fall, the colors of the rainbow)

Language a set of symbols and the rules for organizing their use

Language Skill The ability to successfully communicate using such tools as sequencing items, using symbol systems, combining language elements into complex thoughts, and using codes

Large accessible transit vehicles Public transit vehicles that provide transportation for multiple individuals with disabilities. Provision is made in these vehicles for wheelchair securement.

Latched control A control interface that is turned on by the first activation and off by the next activation

Learning disabilities Disorders in which one has near-normal mental abilities in general but a deficit in the comprehension or use of spoken or written language. These disabilities may be manifested as a significant difficulty with reading, writing, reasoning, or mathematical ability.

Least restrictive environment The degree of acceptable modification in a job or academic program

Leg rest A component of the front rigging of the wheelchair that supports the user's legs; may be fixed or removable

Leisure Activities done for recreation; often involving a significant element of choice

Lever arm The distance from the fulcrum to the point that a force is applied

Lifespan The time from birth to death; a lifespan approach considers both the commonalities and discrepancies that individuals experience at different ages and stages of life

Lightweight wheelchair A wheelchair that weighs less than the standard chair and has greater flexibility in choice of seat width and adjustment of back height

Lightweight high strength wheelchair A wheelchair that shares the same characteristics as a lightweight wheelchair but that is made from a high strength, more robust material

Line of application The particular direction along which forces are applied, either pushing or pulling

Linear The situation that occurs when all parts of a body move in the same direction, at the same time, and for the same distance

Linear scan An approach in which the selection set is organized in a linear (straight-line) format

Linguistic competence Process of developing and using sufficient vocabulary to enable the use of a device, for example, use of a wheelchair requires linguistic competence related to concepts of direction and space

Low-shear systems Systems in which the back hinges to the seat in a manner that reduces the movement of tissue across the seating surface during tilting or reclining of the seat

Low technology Devices that are simple to use, easy to produce and easy to obtain

Magnification aids Low vision aids for reading print material

Magnitude the amount or size of a measurement; when considering force, magnitude is measured in Newtons, pounds or kilograms

Mainstream smart phone a smart phone designed for use by the general public

Mainstream technology devices that are used by the general public rather than being designed specifically for people with disabilities. Examples include smart phones, tablets, and computers

Manual wheelchair Wheelchair that the user propels with his or her own muscle power

Marginalization Occurs when the needs of an individual or group, for participation in needed or desired occupations, are ignored or denied

Meaning Perceptions of a person, or shared meanings of a collective, of an experience or situation. It is influenced by everyday experiences, transactions and engagement with others (direct and indirect) and interaction with objects in the environment

Mechanisms mechanical components comprising the processor in the AT portion of the HAAT model

Media presentation The way in which information is presented on a computer screen, website, or other display. Careful attention to media presentation can avoid extraneous information that might be distracting.

Memory Often considered to have three components: (1) sensory memory, (2) short-term memory, and (3) long-term memory, each playing a role in assistive technology use

Mild cognitive disabilities Disabilities that have needs that are more subtle and harder to define than in the case of physical disabilities or more severe cognitive disabilities

Mobile assistive robots Devices that can move from one location to another to accomplish manipulative tasks under the control of a user who has a disability; two general classes: (1) wheelchair mounted and (2) mounted on a mobile base that is controllable by the user

Mobile technologies devices that are intended to be used in the community, typically battery powered, and lightweight

Mobility Allows movement that enables function in a seated or standing position

Momentary control An interface that controls a device or produces an action only for the length of time the switched is activated

Mouse a control interface used in conjunction with a Graphical user Interface to make selections

Mouthsticks Devices that are held in the teeth and are used for direct manipulation

Multitasking The capability of an operating system to pause while running one software program to run another program

Musical instrument digital interface (MIDI) A file used to store music as a series of notes with volume and duration attached; allows music to be played back through a sound card

Needs identification The portion of the assessment during which more detailed specification of the consumer's assistive technology needs is made

Nonmaleficence An ethical principle meaning do no harm

Nonproportional control Powered wheelchair control that operates the chair at a predetermined speed in a selected direction. The speed is not proportional to the displacement of the joystick.

Norm-referenced measurements The ranking of the performance of the individual or system according to a sample of scores others have achieved on the task

Novice User who has little to no experience in the use of an assistive technology device

Numerical codes A number is used to stand for a word, complete phrase, or sentence; when the user enters the number, the device converts it into the word, phrase, or sentence

Occupation Everything that people do to look after themselves and others, to contribute to their community and society, and to have fun and relax

Occupational alienation Experience of withdrawal or feeling of separation from one's community that results from limitation of resources or denial of opportunities to participate in daily and community activities

Occupational apartheid Segregation of individuals and groups with the intention of restricting or denying their access to resources and opportunities for participation in daily and community activities

Occupational balance The situation that exists when individuals are able to participate in a balance of different activities. This balance does not imply that all types of activities are performed equal amounts of time

Occupational competence The ability to meet the demands that are required for successful engagement in various life activities

Occupational deprivation Denial of the right and opportunity to participate in occupations due to circumstances beyond the control of an individual or community

Occupational engagement The degree of involvement of an individual in an occupation

Occupational imbalance Focus on one aspect of life to the detriment of others; for example, focus on work to the detriment of family or leisure occupations. Imbalance can result from personal choice or actions of others

Occupational injustice Political, social or economic barriers that limit opportunities or resources that support participation in daily and community activities

Occupational justice The creation of political, social or economic opportunities and resources that enable participation of individuals, communities and populations in daily and community occupations

Occupational marginalization The situation that occurs when the needs of individuals, communities and populations for engagement in occupation and community participation are unrecognized or ignored

Occupational Performance How a person does an occupation. Occupational performance may be observable as in the physical doing of an occupation or not as in the performance of mental operations

Occupational Satisfaction The affective component of occupational performance, describing the perception of the performance by the individual or group engaged in the occupation

On-screen keyboard Emulation method that uses a video image of the keyboard on the video screen, together with a cursor

Operational competence Skills required for the individual and his aides to use the basic features of the assistive technology device

Optical aids Devices that allow individuals with low vision to see print, do work requiring fine detail, or increase the range of their visual fields

Optical character recognition (OCR) A software program that runs on a standard PC; its primary function is to analyze the raw video data and assemble it into letters, spaces, and punctuation for synthetic speech or braille output

Opportunity barriers Barriers that involve policies, practices, attitudes, knowledge, and skills of those who support the person with complex communication needs

Orientation and mobility The process by which an individual who is blind is able to achieve independent movement in the environment

Original equipment manufacturer (OEM) The manufacturer that produces and markets products in their original format (e.g., an automobile company is considered to be the original equipment manufacturer of vehicles)

Outcome evaluation The process used to determine whether a given intervention has achieved the intended outcome. May be determined for both an individual and group

Outcome measures Used to evaluate the end result of the assistive technology intervention

Parallel port A computer output used to send bytes of data as a whole; requires a larger number of wires and is faster than a serial port; commonly used in printers and some speech synthesizers

Paralysis Significantly reduced (or absent) muscle strength preventing the use of certain effectors; muscle weakness caused by partial paralysis that makes it difficult to move but does not prevent movement is called paresis

Participation "involvement in a life situation" (WHO, 2001, p. 193)

Participation model A framework for the identification of potential barriers to educational access, especially those that can be addressed through the application of assistive technologies; two types of barriers are identified—opportunity and access

Peer training Instruction that introduces assistive technologies to the classmates of the learner who has a disability

Pelvic obliquity One side of the pelvis is higher than the other when viewed in the frontal plane

Pelvic rotation One side of the pelvis is forward of the other side with rotation in a lateral plane

Perception The interpretation and assignment of meaning to data received from biological sensors; involves an interaction between information derived from sensed data and information stored in memory on the basis of previous sensory experience

Performance Describes what a person actually does

Performance aid A document or device containing information that an individual uses to assist in the completion of an activity

Performance areas Activities of daily living, work and productive activities, and play and leisure

Phonology The sounds used in any particular language and the rules for their organization

Physical construction The properties of the assistive technology device that allow it to be mounted or positioned so that the client has reliable access to it; the portability of the device; its size and weight; and its aesthetics

Physical context Physical attributes of the environment that enable, hinder or affect performance of daily activities with or without assistive technology

Physical properties Characteristics of an assistive device; including but not limited to size and weight of the interface, its texture, hardness, size and brightness of the display, loudness of any auditory feedback, and the force required to use the interface

Physical skill The physical capacity and ability of an individual to perform and action; usually describes a motor behaviour

Planar Flat seating components that support the body only where it easily comes into contact with the supporting system

Powered wheelchair A wheeled mobility base with a power drive to the wheels, a control interface that the consumer uses to direct the movement of the wheelchair, an electronic controller, and powered accessories (e.g., recline, tilt)

Postural control Control provided by either internal (neuromusculoskeletal structures) or external positioning devices (e.g., seating components, tilt, recline) to enable a stable and functional position

Pragmatics The relationship between language and language users

Predictive selection A feature of scanning Minspeak-based augmentative and alternative communication systems in which only valid following icons in a sequence are scanned after the initial icon is selected

Pressure Force per unit area

Pressure mapping Data collection systems that involve quantification of pressure at an interface and translate these data into a visual map

Pressure redistribution Goal or outcome of seating technology that results in change in the distribution of pressure to relieve areas of high pressure, commonly under the ischial tuberosities or coccyx in sitting

Pressure ulcer A lesion that develops as a result of unrelieved pressure to an area and that results in damage to underlying tissue

Primary driving controls Adapted driving system components that are used to stop (brakes), go (accelerator), and steer

Privacy being free from being observed or disturbed by other people.

Problem solving A process for which the goal is to overcome obstacles obstructing a path to a solution.

Processor Component of an assistive technology device that translates information and forces received from the human into signals that are used to control the activity output

Productivity Commonly understand to be occupations involving work, volunteering or other contributions to the community

Professional ethics a code of values and norms that actually guide clinical practical decision making

Programmable controllers An electronic aid to daily living approach that is based on the storage of user-selected codes that are appropriate to a wide range of appliances; entering the correct code into the controller allows control of the appliance by the user

Prompting providing assistance for task completion via physical (e.g. "hand-over-hand"), verbal or visual (e.g., modeling) of the task

Propelling structure The portion of a manual wheelchair consisting of the wheels and an interface that the consumer uses to move the wheelchair; the portion of a power wheelchair consisting of a wheeled mobility base with a power drive to the wheels, a control interface that the consumer uses to direct the movement of the wheelchair, an electronic controller, and powered accessories (e.g., recline, ventilator)

Proportional control With 360 degree directionality, the wheelchair moves in whichever direction the joystick is displaced; the greater the displacement, the faster the chair moves

Prosodic features aspects of speech that give it a human quality, generated by changes in amplitude, pitch, and duration

Quality how good or bad something is

Qualitative assessment Assumes that each individual has a different experience and that it is important to provide the opportunity to capture that experience. There is no attempt to measure a particular construct. Rather, the purpose is to describe and understand the user's experience with the technology. Qualitative assessments may include observation, either directly or by videotape, or interview with the client and others.

Quality-of-life measures Assesses the effectiveness of assistive technology devices and services in the broader social context of the impact on the user's overall life

Quantitative measurement A measurement in which an indefinite amount or number is obtained (e.g., a numerical scale from 1 to 5 may be assigned to a given measurement, or the measurement may be in terms of a physical parameter such as weight)

Radiofrequency (RF) transmission Devices that use electromagnetic (radio) signals to remotely control an electronic aid to daily living; consists of a transmitter unit, which is either hand held or mounted on a wheelchair, and a set of receivers, one for each appliance to be controlled

Raising the floor An international coalition of individuals and organizations working to ensure that the Internet, and everything available through it, is accessible to people experiencing accessibility barriers due to disability, literacy, or age

Range of motion (ROM) The maximal extent of movement possible in a joint

Rate enhancement Augmentative and alternative communication and computer access approaches that result in the number of characters generated being greater than the number of selections the individual makes

Reacher A handle grip attached to a stem that is used to control the jaws of a device for grasping an object

Reading aid A sensory device designed to provide access to print materials for an individual who is blind

Rear-facing infant seat A child vehicle restraint system designed to provide occupant protection for children under the age of 12 months who weigh equal to or less than 20-22 pounds

Recline Systems that allow a change in the seat-to-back angle of the wheelchair that provides for greater hip flexion and a position of rest

Recovery The degree to which a seating cushion returns to a preloaded state when its load is removed

Referral and intake The portion of the assessment in which the consumer, or someone close to the consumer, has identified a need for which assistive technology intervention may be indicated and contacts an assistive technology practitioner; basic information is gathered and a determination of the match between the services provided and the identified needs of the consumer is made; funding is also identified and secured at this stage

Refreshable Braille display The use of mechanically raised pins to represent braille cells, organized in arrays of from 1 to 80 cells

Reliability An estimation of the consistency of a test when administered in different circumstances (e.g., over time, by different raters, or with different populations)

Remote control The absence of a physical attachment between the various components of an electronic aid to daily living

Resilience The ability of a material to recover its shape after a load is removed or to adjust to a load as it is applied

Resolution The smallest separation between two objects that the effector can reliably control

Resource specialist An individual associated with a local school who provides consultation regarding assistive technology applications

Restraint Any manual method or physical or mechanical device, material, or equipment attached or adjacent to a person's body that the individual cannot remove easily, which restricts freedom of movement or normal access to one's body

Rigid ultra lightweight wheelchair Has quick release rear wheels and a back that folds down to facilitate transfer and storage of the chair in a vehicle. The axle of the rear wheel of these chairs can be adjusted relative to the center of gravity of the user.

Rigid sport ultra lightweight wheelchair Category of wheelchair with quick-release rear wheels and back that folds down to facilitate transfer and storage of the chair in a vehicle. The axle of the rear wheel of these chairs can be adjusted to the centre of gravity of the user. Often designed for a specific type of sport

Robotic systems Electrically powered general-purpose manipulators that can carry out tasks under the control of a person who has a disability

Rotary scanning See circular scanning

Rotational Movements that occur around an axis (the *fulcrum*), involving the simultaneous change in direction, distance and time of motion

Row-column scanning A form of group-item scanning in which the items are arranged in a matrix and the row is first selected by a switch press, then the item is selected from that row by a second switch press; entry is by an additional switch press or acceptance time

Scanning The most common indirect selection method in which the selection set is presented by a display and is sequentially scanned by a cursor or light on the device, with the user selecting the desired choice by pressing a switch when it is indicated by the display; entry is by an additional switch press or acceptance time

Scoliosis Lateral or rotational curvature of the spine

Scooter A power wheelchair design featuring three or four wheels, a tiller steering system, and a bucket mounted to a single post coming up from the base; often used by marginal ambulators who need mobility assistance to conserve energy; often provided by grocery stores and shopping malls

Screen readers Systems that provide speech synthesis or Braille output for blind users

Scripts application software for assistive devices that is designed for specific types of programs, procedures or application (e.g., word processing, phone use)

Secondary driving controls Adapted driving system components that are needed for safe operation of a vehicle, including turn signals, parking brakes, lights, horn, turning on the ignition, temperature control (heat and air conditioning), and windshield wipers

Security the state of being protected or safe from harm

Selection methods An approach allowing the user to make choices from the selection set; includes scanning, directed scanning, and coded access

Selection set The items available from which user choices are made; in augmentative and alternative communication devices this is the component that presents the symbol system and possible vocabulary selections to the user

Self-care Commonly considered to be occupations that include activities of daily living such as dressing, eating and instrumental activities of daily living such as using transportation and banking

Self-efficacy The personal sense of how well one can perform an activity in an anticipated situation

Semantic encoding Coding of words, sentences, and phrases on the basis of their meanings

Semantics The relationship between words and their meaning

Sensory characteristics Auditory, somatosensory, and visual feedback produced during the activation of a control interface

Sensory function Performance of the human sensory systems, including hearing, vision, taste, tactile, somatosensory, olfaction and vestibular

Service delivery all facets of the process that starts with the identification of the client's needs for assistive technology and culminates with the ongoing outcome evaluation of the use of acquired technology

Set up The characteristics of an emulator that are customized for an individual application and user

Shearing (Shear) Occurs when forces are parallel (sliding across the surfaces), such as the movement that occurs as the head of the femur moves across the acetabulum during hip movement; when shear force is present, deep structures move in the direction of the applied force while superficial structures remain immobile

Shield an addition to a keyboard that blocks out certain keys

Short message service (SMS) the text communication protocol that enables text messaging using cell phones.

Sliding resistance A cushion property related to friction that describes the forces that influence movement of the user across the surface of a seat cushion

Skilled nursing facility (SNF) an institution or part of an institution that is regulated by government agencies for reimbursement

Smart home Denotes living environments in which automation is used to provide automatic functions including monitoring, communication, household functions (lights, air conditioning/heating, door locks), physiological measurements, or medication alerts

Smart wheelchair Either a standard power wheelchair to which a computer and a collection of sensors have been added or a mobile robot base to which a seat has been attached

Social competence Understanding the social implications and practices the influence the use of a device, for example, social competence is used when selecting vocabulary when using an alternative and augmentative communication device

Social context Individuals or groups in the environment who affect the performance of daily activities, either with or without assistive technology, directly or indirectly

Social justice Equitable access to rights and resources, initially from an economic perspective, but subsequently includes equal access to basic rights and freedom of choice

Somatosensory or tactile function The perception and interpretation of information through touch, either via actively touching something or passively receiving touch

Spatial characteristics The overall physical size (dimensions) and shape of the control interface, the number of targets available for activation, the size of each target, and the spacing between targets

Spatial display provides direct spatial information about the directions and distances to environmental locations in a navigation system

Special-purpose manipulation device A device designed to carry out only one manipulative task

Speech the oral representation of language

Speech-Generating Devices (SGDs) Electronic augmentative and alternative communication (AAC) systems that enable individuals with speech impairment to verbally communicate

Speech synthesis The generation of human-sounding speech by use of electronic circuits and computer software

Stability Postural control that allows an individual to maintain an upright seated position

Stability zone The balance limits for a person in either sitting or standing

Standard wheelchair base Generally useful for very short-term use such as rentals at an airport or shopping mall; do not accommodate any seating or positioning devices and cannot be modified to optimize position and function of the user

Standing frames Categorized as prone standers, supine standers, upright standers, and mobile standers. They support an individual in a standing position

Standing wheelchair Alters the position of the seat to support the user in a standing position. Many of these wheelchairs allow the user to move while in the standing position. The change to and from the standing position may be manually or electrically controlled

Step scanning An approach in which the user activates the switch once for each item to move through the choices in the selection set; entry is by an additional switch press or acceptance time

Stiffness How much a material gives under load

Stigma A mark of shame; an attribute that discredits the person who possesses it (Goffman, 1963)

Stimuli control Technologies that address attention or perception problems by limiting or manipulating the information presented to the user (e.g., noise reduction, uncluttered media presentation)

Strategic competence Skills in the use of strategies that maximize the effectiveness of the assistive technology system

Stress The resulting molecular change inside biological (e.g., soft tissue and bone) or nonbiological (e.g., metals, plastics, or foams) materials

Supporting structure Consists of the frame of a wheelchair and its attachments

Support surfaces Device designed to redistribute pressure or enable postural control; in seating technology, this term typically refers to a seat cushion or back

Surveillance in AT refers to monitoring an individual's actions, may occur in a living facility or in the broader community

Syntax The rules for organizing words into meaningful utterances

Technology abandonment A situation in which the consumer stops using a device even though the need for which the device has been obtained still exists

Telephone controllers Devices that allow a person with a disability to control a telephone using one or more switches; typically built around standard telephone electronics

Telerehabilitation The use of telecommunications technologies to capture and transmit visual and audio information, biomedical data (e.g., electroencephalograms, x-rays, ultrasound data), and consumer information

Tension Forces that act in the same line but away from each other (pulling apart), such as the force applied on the antagonist muscle during contraction of the agonist muscle

Text-to-speech programs Programs that analyze a word or sentence and translate it into the codes required by a speech synthesizer

Tilt Wheelchair systems in which all angles of the seating system (seat-to-back, seat-to-calf, calf-to-foot) are maintained for the wheelchair seat as it rotates around the axis formed by the seat to back angle

Touchscreen a control interface that allows selection by tapping, dragging, or other graphical movements (e.g., pinching or swiping)

Tracking and identification Of people or items; such devices often provide an extra degree of safety for users who might not have the cognitive skills required to work their way out of problematic situations

Traditional orthography The symbolic representation of language; based on letters and words

Trainable controllers Devices that provide functions of electronic aids to daily living by storing the control code for any specific appliance function

Traumatic brain injury (TBI) May occur when the head or brain is struck by an external force; one of these two criteria must be satisfied for the diagnosis: either the patient has amnesia from the traumatic event, or the patient has a documented loss of consciousness

Transparent access Two fundamental concepts that apply to all levels of computer adaptation: (1) 100% of the functions of the computer must be adapted if the user who has a disability is to have full access and (2) all application software that runs in the unmodified computer must also run in the adapted computer

Ultra lightweight wheelchair Retains the folding frame and is available with a lower seat-to-floor height for individuals who propel with their feet. The axle of the rear wheel is adjustable relative to the center of gravity of the user

Universal design The design of products and environments to be usable by all people, to the greatest extent possible, without the need for adaptation or specialized design

Universal docking interface geometry A wheelchair docking station for use in a large accessible transit vehicle that will secure a range of manufacturers' wheelchairs

Universal remote A remote control that is designed to operate multiple devices; may be trainable or programmable

Universal Serial Bus (USB) A serial bus standard to interface devices originally designed for computers but now commonplace on video game consoles, PDAs, portable DVD and media players, cell phones, televisions, home stereo equipment (e.g., mp3 players), car stereos, and portable memory devices

Usability Describes how well the person is able to access and use device functionality

USB switch connector An interface that allows switches to be connected to computers, phones an tablets through USB Port

User agent Software to access Web content; includes desktop graphical browsers, text and voice browsers, mobile phones, multimedia players, and software assistive technologies (e.g., screen readers, magnifiers, GIDEIs) used with browsers

User display The portion of a sensory device that portrays the sensory information for the human user

User satisfaction The consumer's perception of the degree to which the assistive technology system achieves desired goals

Validity Conclusions that are drawn from the interpretation of test results and the confidence that is derived from the interpretation that led to the conclusions

Vehicle seat belt assembly The seat belt system that is provided by the vehicle's original equipment manufacturer

Video magnifiers A video camera and monitor used to enlarge text and other print material; also called CCTVs

Vigilance Paying close and continuous attention over a prolonged period of time

Visual Scene Displays Create displays that capture events in a person's life on the screen. Regions of particular screen shots can be accessed to retrieve information.

Visual skill The ability to translate visual signals into meaningful information

Visual perception The ability to give meaning to visual information

Vocabulary expansion Methods by which the available vocabulary is increased through the use of codes or levels

Vocalization An oral utterance, may or may not be speech

Voice-carry-over (VCO) Allows communication by both voice and text. These individuals can use the relay service by speaking naturally and reading the responses on the screen.

Wheel locks The devices that prevent the wheels from moving during transfers and other stationary activities. They are available in a number of configurations, such as push or pull to lock, with lever extensions for individuals with limited reach, under the seat mounts, hill holders, and attendant controlled

Wheelchair tie-down system A strapping or docking system that secures a wheelchair and occupant in a vehicle. It does not provide protection for the occupant of the wheelchair

Wheelchair tie-down and occupant restraint systems (WTORS) A total system installed in a van, bus, or other vehicle that is designed to fasten the wheelchair and restrain the passenger to protect the passenger or driver who uses a wheelchair

Windows Generically, a portion of the computer screen that is devoted to a particular function; specifically, an operating system for computers developed by Microsoft Corp.

Windswept hip deformity When one hip is adducted and the other hip is abducted

Word completion A technique that displays stored words on the basis of the sequence of entered keys; the user selects the desired word, if any, by entering its code (e.g., a number listed next to the word) or continuing to enter letters if the desired word is not displayed

Word prediction A technique that displays stored words on the basis of previous words entered

Index

Page numbers followed by f indicate figures; t, tables; b, boxes.